PHARMACOLOGY IN NURSING

FIFTEENTH EDITION

ANNE BURGESS HAHN

R.N., B.S.N., M.A. (Nursing), M.A. (Biological Sciences)

Associate Professor and Science Coordinator of Nursing, University of Bridgeport,
Bridgeport, Connecticut; Consultant, Veterans Administration Medical Center,
West Haven, Connecticut; Adjunct Faculty of Respiratory Therapy Program,
University of Bridgeport, Bridgeport, Connecticut

ROBERT L. BARKIN

Pharm.B.S., M.B.A., R.Ph.

Faculty, Department of Pharmacology, Rush Medical College;
Faculty, College of Pharmacy, University of Illinois;
Assistant Director of Pharmacy, Rush Presbyterian
St. Luke's Medical Center, Chicago, Illinois

SANDY JEANNE KLARMAN OESTREICH

R.N.,C., B.S., M.S., Doctoral Candidate

Assistant Professor of Nursing, Adelphi University, Garden City, New York;
ANA-Certified Adult Health Nurse Practitioner, Community Health Program,
New Hyde Park, New York

with **95** illustrations

THE C. V. MOSBY COMPANY

ST. LOUIS • TORONTO • LONDON   1982

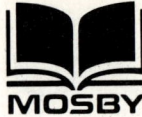

A TRADITION OF PUBLISHING EXCELLENCE

Editor: Thomas Allen Manning
Assistant editor: Nancy Mullins
Manuscript editor: Peggy Fagen
Design: Diane Beasley
Production: Debbie Wedemeier, Ginny Douglas

FIFTEENTH EDITION

Previous editions copyrighted 1936, 1940, 1942, 1945, 1948, 1951, 1955, 1960, 1963, 1966, 1969, 1973, 1976, 1979

Printed in the United States of America

International Standard Book Number 0-8016-0633-0

Library of Congress Catalog Card Number 66-10935

The C.V. Mosby Company
11830 Westline Industrial Drive, St. Louis, Missouri 63141

TS/VH/VH   9 8 7 6 5 4 3 2   03/C/307

CONTRIBUTORS

ANDRES GOTH, M.D.

Professor and Chairman,
Department of Pharmacology, Southwestern Medical School,
University of Texas Health Science Center at Dallas,
Dallas, Texas

RITA LENHART, R.N., B.S., M.A.

Nursing Instructor, Veterans Administration Medical Center,
West Haven, Connecticut

KAY SEE-LASLEY, M.S., R.Ph.

Clinical Pharmacist Oncologist, Lawrence, Kansas

MARY ANNE TOLL, R.Ph.

Clinical Instructor, Department of Pharmacy,
University of Kansas Medical Center, Lawrence, Kansas

SARA J. WHITE, M.S.

Associate Director of Pharmacy, Department of Pharmacy,
University of Kansas Medical Center, Lawrence, Kansas

JAMES S. WOODS, Ph.D.

Program Leader, Epidemiology and Environmental Health Research Program,
Health and Population Study Center, Battelle Human Affairs Research Centers,
Seattle, Washington

BRUCE WOOLLEY, Pharm.D.

Professor, Applied Pharmacology and Therapeutics, College of Nursing,
Brigham Young University, Provo, Utah

PREFACE

The reputation that *Pharmacology in Nursing* has gained over the years is a proud one. This textbook has served as an informative resource and guide to generations of nursing students learning the safe and therapeutic use of drugs in the care of patients. In order to keep pace with the constantly changing field of pharmacology, periodic revisions are required to introduce important new drugs and pharmacologic theories. This ensures a continually high level of contemporary information that provides a rational basis for intelligent application of modern drug therapy.

The fifteenth edition of *Pharmacology in Nursing* has undergone a significant revision. A major change includes the reorganization of the table of contents, whereby the chapters have been assembled into broad pharmacologic units. The units represent a more cohesive and consistent presentation of each major class of drugs. Accordingly, the chapters within a unit follow in a logical sequence so that the pharmacologic properties of a drug group are discussed in relation to their therapeutic effect on a specific organ system.

In addition, the reader will find that nearly every chapter has been extensively altered; most have been rewritten and a great deal of new material has been introduced. Current pharmacologic concepts and principles as well as descriptions of pharmacokinetic characteristics of the more important drugs have been incorporated. Two new chapters have been added—Chapter 5, "Assessment in Pharmacotherapeutics," and Chapter 6, "Plans, Implementation, and Evaluation." They deal with

the nursing process as an up-to-date tool for the safe and effective administration of drugs.

Also, this revision includes information on newly approved drugs and updates the new therapeutic uses of already established drugs. As an additional feature, we have inserted cross-references from one section of the book to another to direct the reader to the various properties and the multiple uses that may be associated with an individual agent.

Modern scientific advancements now presume knowledge of cell physiology as a basis for pharmacology. This involves the manner in which drugs alter the function of distinct cellular components in a disease process. For example, the response of specific receptors to various neurotransmitters and other chemicals, the role of Na^+-K^+ ATPase in the mechanism of action of digitalis glycosides, and the effect of antidysrhythmic agents on electrophysiologic properties of the cardiac cell are aspects of pharmacology that provide a deeper insight into *how* a specific drug alters a pathologic condition in a patient. Moreover, a focus on cellular function promotes progress toward an understanding of the mechanism of drug interactions. How drugs interact with each other has become a major clinical concern, and it is therefore essential that nurses become knowledgeable about this aspect of drug therapy.

At the end of each chapter, a summary of nursing considerations and questions for study and review have been added to reinforce content and stimulate critical thinking. The bibliographic references have been updated. Most of the books and periodicals cited in the list are generally available in the library so that the student will be encouraged to do additional reading.

Since nursing decisions are based on comprehension of pharmacologic concepts and principles, every effort has been made to provide this information. Throughout the book, emphasis has been placed on clinical application of drugs to ensure rational and optimal care of patients. Therefore, this edition will serve the clinical needs of both the student and the practitioner of nursing. However, we trust that the book also will be of value to students of other allied health sciences whose curriculum involves the study of pharmacology.

We wish to gratefully acknowledge the many people who were instrumental in the development of this revision. Particular thanks is extended to the editor who organized the vast amount of material into a consistent format, to the contributors who were willing to share their professional expertise, and to the staff of The C.V. Mosby Company. To Paul E. Carson, M.D.; Stephen Burgess, M.D.; Donald S. Ebersman, Ph.D.; Byong Moon, Ph.D.; Ronald D. Wise, M.D.; Gene W. Zdenek, M.D.; Patricia Flynn, R.N., M.S.; Jacqueline Rose Hott, R.N., Ph.D., F.A.A.N.; Joseph Greensher, M.D., F.A.A.P.; Howard C. Mofenson, M.D., F.A.A.P.; Rita Lenhart, R.N., M.Ed.; Justina Eisenhauer, R.N., M.Ed.; and illustrators Anne Kayser, B.F.A., and Cheryl Oestreich, special thanks is also extended. However it is the loyal support and help of our families for which we are most grateful, and to Diana, Stacy, Stephanie, Anne Marie, Eugene, Thomas, Charlie, Cheryl, and Lisa, we extend our love and appreciation.

Anne Burgess Hahn
Robert L. Barkin
Sandy Jeanne Klarman Oestreich

CONTENTS

NOTE TO THE READER

Great care has been used in compiling and checking the information in this book to ensure its accuracy. However, because of changing technology, recent discoveries, research, and individualization of prescriptions according to patient needs, the uses, effects, and dosages of drugs may vary from those given here. Neither the publisher nor the authors shall be responsible for such variations or other inaccuracies. We urge that before you administer any drug you check the manufacturer's dosage recommendations as given in the package insert provided with each product.

NOTE TO THE READER

The inclusion in *Pharmacology in Nursing* of a monograph on any drug in respect to which patent or trademark rights may exist shall not be deemed, and is not intended as, a grant of or authority to exercise any right or privilege protected by such patent or trademark. All such rights and privileges are vested in the patent or trademark owner, and no other person may exercise the same without express permission, authority, or license secured from such patent or trademark owner. The listing of selected brand name does not mean the publisher has any particular knowledge that the brand listed has properties different from other brands of the same drug, nor should it be interpreted as an endorsement by the publisher. Similarly, the fact that a particular drug has not been included does not indicate that the product has been judged to be unsatisfactory or unacceptable. Attention is called to the fact that *Pharmacology in Nursing* is fully copyrighted. Authors and others wishing to use portions of the text should request permission to do so from the publisher. No part of this book may be reproduced, stored in a retrieval system, or transmitted in any form by any means (electronic, mechanical, photocopying, recording, or otherwise) without written permission from The C.V. Mosby Company.

Great care has been used in compiling and checking the information in this book to ensure its accuracy. However, because of changing technology, recent discoveries, research, and individualization of prescriptions according to patient needs, the uses, effects, and dosages of drugs may vary from those given here. Neither the publisher nor the authors shall be responsible for such variations or other inaccuracies. We urge that before you administer any drug you check the manufacturer's dosage recommendations as given in the package insert provided with each product.

UNIT ONE

INTRODUCTORY ASPECTS OF PHARMACOLOGY

CHAPTER 1

Orientation to pharmacology

Historical origin and progress of pharmacology
Drug uses and mechanisms of action
Nursing scope and responsibilities
The nursing process as related to pharmacology
Goals of this text
Summary of nursing considerations

Medications are an essential part of patient care, and safe administration of drugs requires *sound* and *current* knowledge of their (1) mode of action, (2) side effects, (3) toxicity, (4) range of dosage, (5) rate and route of excretion, (6) individual differences in response, such as idiosyncratic or allergic reactions, and (7) interactions with other drugs. This knowledge can be obtained from textbooks and periodicals for health professionals, classroom lectures and discussions, and materials available in teaching laboratories. However, actual administration of drugs with careful observation of their effects in individuals and groups of patients will richly supplement and complement a student's knowledge of specific drugs.

There are several basic terms a nurse needs to know and understand to be properly oriented to pharmacology practice. The first is the word "pharmacology" itself.

Pharmacology is the study of the interaction between drugs and living systems. Branches of pharmacology include:

1 *Pharmacotherapeutics* (clinical pharmacology), which deals with the relative effects of drugs in the human system in specific applications
2 *Pharmacodynamics*, which deals with experimental science pertaining to theories of drug action
3 *Pharmacokinetics*, which is the study of a drug's alterations during its odyssey through the body as it is absorbed, distributed, bound to or localized in tissues, biotransformed, and excreted

4 *Pharmacogenetics*, which is the study of genetically induced drug responses that are often responsible for some "idiosyncratic" (unexplained) response

Chemotherapy is drug therapy to destroy or inhibit growth and reproduction of abnormal cells, such as cancer cells. This is the common use of the term, but it may also be applied to the treatment of infectious disease-causing organisms.

Drug is defined by the Food and Drug Administration (FDA) to be any substance for use in diagnosis, cure, mitigation (relief), treatment, or prevention of disease in humans or animals. This is the definition recognized by official standard-setters such as *The United States Pharmacopeia* and the *British Pharmacopoeia*. The terms "medication," "medicine," "medicament," and "medicinal" are used more or less synonymously with the term "drug."

Historical origin and progress of pharmacology

Historically the primitive person's belief that disease was caused by evil spirits inhabiting the body persisted throughout the Egyptian period of medicine until challenged by Hippocrates in 460 BC. This Greek priest-physician advanced the idea that disease resulted from natural causes and could only be understood

3

through study of natural laws. He believed in the body's recuperative powers and saw the physician's role in assisting the recuperative process. Called the Father of Medicine, Hippocrates influenced the sound principles that control the practice of medicine today. Building on the teachings and practice of Hippocrates, Galen (131 to 201 AD) established a system of medicine and pharmacy that made him the supreme authority for several hundred years.

The decline and fall of the Roman Empire marked the beginning of the medieval period (400 to 1580 AD). Germanic barbarians overran Western Europe and reverted to a medicine of folklore and tradition, similar to that of the Greeks before Hippocrates.

At the same time Christian religious orders developed whose members built monasteries that soon became repositories for all learning, including pharmacy and medicine. They aided the sick and needy with good food, rest, and medicinals from their monastery gardens.

The Arabs' interest in medicine, pharmacy, and chemistry was reflected in the hospitals and schools they built, the many new drugs they contributed and their formulation of the first set of drug standards.

Pharmacy came into its own during the sixteenth century. Valerius Cordus wrote the first pharmacopeia to be printed and authorized as an authoritative standard.

Paracelsus, professor of physics and surgery at Basel, denounced "humoral pathology" and substituted the idea that diseases were actual entities to be combated with specific remedies. He improved pharmacy and therapeutics for succeeding centures, introducing new remedies and compounds and reducing the overdosing so prevalent in that period.

In the seventeenth and eighteenth centuries great progress was made in pharmacy and chemistry. The first London pharmacopeia appeared in 1618. Many preparations were introduced that are still in use today, including tincture of opium, coca, and ipecac. In 1785, Englishman William Withering introduced infusion of digitalis for heart disease. Edward Jenner made his first public inoculation with smallpox vaccine in 1796.

During the nineteenth century, pharmaceutical chemistry emerged as an important subdivision of the highly specialized science of chemistry. Serturner's discovery of the alkaloid morphine in 1815 led to research on many vegetable drugs, resulting in discoveries of quinine, strychnine, atropine, codeine, and others. Ether and chloroform were first used as general anesthetics in the 1840s. The French *Codex* was the first of the important national pharmacopeias to be produced. Issued in 1818, it was followed by the United States' *Pharmacopeia* in 1820, that of Great Britain in 1864, and Germany's in 1872.

Accurate study of dosage became a reality in the nineteenth century, leading to the establishment of large-scale manufacturing plants for the production of drugs. Fewer drugs were prescribed, and knowledge of their expected action became more precise. Rational medicine had begun to replace empiricism.

Ehrlich's introduction in 1907 of salvarsan for syphilis and Banting's discovery of insulin for diabetes mellitus in 1922 constitute two early landmark events. The sulfonamides, penicillin, and other antibiotics revolutionized chemotherapy. The development of cortisone, first used in 1949, opened a new era in medical science. In 1955 and 1961, new poliomyelitis vaccines relieved humanity from another dread disease.

In the late 1950s, discovery that a chemical contraceptive taken by mouth could be a feasible approach to birth control had widespread effects on the per capita birth rate and sexual mores.

More recently, some of the most exciting research has turned up the existence of a whole new class of drugs that the body itself produces, such as interferon, enkephalins, endorphins, and endoxin (analogous to digoxin).

In the 1980s it is predicted that the most promising drug therapy research will be directed at drugs:

1 To reduce the nonfatal heart attack rate
2 That contain prostaglandins and prostacyclines for the treatment of diabetes, arthritis, coronary disease, ulcers, hypertension, and congenital heart malformations in infants
3 That will act to stimulate the immune system in immunosuppressed patients
4 That will be even broader spectrum antibiotics than those presently used

5 With greater antineoplastic action and less toxicity in the treatment of cancer

6 With antiviral activity for the treatment of herpes simplex, genital herpes, shingles, and hepatitis B

7 Like naturally occurring enkephalins and synthetic opiates that will not be addicting

8 To alleviate severe depression and many serious emotional disorders

9 To limit or reverse senility and failing memory

Two new general trends are emerging in health care related to pharmacology. First, people are becoming more concerned about the substances, including drugs, they ingest. The astute health care recipient now asks questions, and the person questioned is often a nurse. Second, the nurse is taking on greater responsibility in drug administration and drug therapy.

Drug uses and mechanisms of action

Drugs are typically used for the diagnosis, cure, relief, treatment, or prevention of disease. A drug cannot directly repair diseased tissues or organs, it can only facilitate normal cellular function. All drugs act by inducing one or more of the following mechanisms:

1 Stimulation or depression of targeted cell activity

2 Replacement of deficient subsystems

3 Killing or weakening foreign invading organisms

4 Irritation

These mechanisms may produce intended therapeutic responses in the patient, which are called the "intended" or "primary" effect or "therapeutic" effect, or they may affect other areas of the body and give rise to what is called "side" and "toxic" effects. Sometimes these are intended, but most of the time they are not. Side and toxic effects may run the gamut from merely annoying but acceptable side effects to unacceptable effects such as coma or death. Prime responsibility for observing intended and side and toxic drug effects in patients usually rests with nurses.

Nursing scope and responsibilities

Drugs have the power to help or to harm. Nurses, along with physicians and clinical pharmacists, are held legally responsible for safe and therapeutically effective drug administration. Nurses are liable for their actions and omissions and for those duties they delegate to others. They should know that they are personally responsible, legally, morally, and ethically, for every drug they administer or have administered, no matter who actually prescribed it. Nurses are not exonerated from responsibility when drugs are administered by medication technicians, pharmacy technicians, practical nurses, or even physicians. Indeed, all members of a health team may be held liable for a single injury to a patient. The continued increase in litigation against nurses and physicians indicates that society tolerates only a minimal margin of error in relation to human life. Claims have been brought against health professionals for drug errors that caused loss of life (*Norton v. Argonaut Insurance Co.*, the *Somera* case) and permanent injury (*Honeywell v. Rogers*).* When claims against health professionals are supported with evidence that the conduct of one or more health professionals helped to bring about the loss or injury, those parties are held liable. The law, a legal and social norm, requires health professionals to be safe and competent practitioners and permits compensation to those harmed or injured.

However, the law is a protective force for knowledgeable, competent, and skilled nurses. Nurses who are knowledgeable about the drugs patients are receiving, who use proper technique and precautions, who observe for and chart explicitly the drug effects, who keep up-to-date by referring to authoritative sources (pharmacist, pharmacologist, professional literature), who question a drug order that is unclear or that appears to contain an error, and who even refuse to administer a drug and intervene to prevent others from administering a drug if there is reason to believe harm may come to the patient are safeguarding and protecting patients from drug-induced harm. The law in turn will protect such nurses from unfair litigation.

Drugs deserve the respect of nurses, but that respect must be mingled with skepticism. Much remains to be learned about the actual mode of

---

*Murchison, I.A., and Nichols, T.S.: Legal foundations of nursing practice, New York, 1970, The Macmillan Co.

action as well as effects from prolonged use of many commonly prescribed drugs. Furthermore, there is increasing concern about drug-induced disease. Fortunately, drug therapy for most illnesses or for illness prevention is temporary. However, there are those diseases that require lifelong use of drugs to sustain life (such as insulin for diabetes mellitus) or prolonged use to maintain relatively normal physiologic or psychologic functioning.

Nurses are entrusted with potent and habit-forming drugs, and they must not abuse or misuse this trust. Used respectfully and intelligently, drugs are comforting and lifesaving. Used unwisely or with undue dependence, they can lead to irreparable tragedy. The nurse who combines diligent and intelligent observation with moral integrity and factual knowledge will be a safe and competent practitioner and a credit to the nursing profession.

Pharmacology is a challenging and interesting subject to study. It requires integrating knowledge from many different disciplines including anatomy and physiology, pathology, microbiology, organic chemistry and biochemistry, psychology, and sociology; thus, clinical drug therapy can be considered to be an applied science. The hundreds of drugs available would make the study of pharmacology formidable if they had to be studied as individual agents. Fortunately, drugs can be classified into a reasonable number of drug groups based on their chemical, pharmacologic, or therapeutic relatedness. Understanding the characteristic effects of a particular group of drugs at the subcellular, tissue, organ, or functional system level permits a student or practitioner to know a variety of facts about many drugs. An individual drug can then be studied according to those characteristics that differentiate it from other drugs within the same classification.

The doses of drugs and indications for use must not be regarded by the student as therapeutic dogma. New knowledge about drugs will be forthcoming from laboratory research and more scientific methods of clinical drug evaluation.

The constant advances in the field of drug therapy, the almost daily appearance of new drugs or new preparations of old drugs on the market and in the hospital, are a challenge to both the student and the graduate nurse to be students always. An examination passed and an R.N. acquired are no lasting guarantees of sufficient knowledge in the field of drugs to make a nurse helpful to the physician or even safe for the patient. Drugs change and will continue to change. Pharmacology books should become a permanent section of the nurse's and agency's library, and year by year as new editions or new books appear the library must be brought up-to-date. In addition, the official current literature on drugs must be followed carefully, since new drugs are slow in making their way into more permanent literature. For the nurse working in a hospital or health service, physicians, instructors, inservice educators, and pharmacists will be on hand to help. In a more isolated practice, greater personal effort will be required to keep abreast of current practices. In any case, a sustained interest in pharmacology will help to keep the nurse well informed about drugs.

Of primary importance is the understanding that learning is an active process and that learning does not take place without activity. Thus clinical experience with drugs is invaluable, for it enables the student to:

1 Note those drugs most commonly used to treat certain diseases or specific signs and symptoms
2 Note the frequency with which certain drugs are administered
3 Observe the degree of effectiveness between specific drugs for relieving particular signs and symptoms
4 Witness the individual differences in patients' reactions to a specific drug
5 Relate knowledge obtained from authoritative sources with real-life situations

Regardless of what subject matter is to be learned, reasoning and the ability to analyze and synthesize information and prerequisites to understanding. These cognitive skills, along with perceptual skills, permit an individual to see meaningful relationships, make comparisons, and determine significance, all of which are essential for sound decision making. The development of cognitive, perceptual, and manual skills is the foundation for professional competence.

The nursing process as related to pharmacology

There are many types of people and roles involved in teaching and planning with and for sick people. But only nurses "take care of" sick people.* True enough, basic human needs are the proper domain of nursing. The *nursing process* is a method for identifying patients' nursing needs and problems and for working toward alleviating them. It is a systematic guide through the maze of data about the patient. It points the way to rational nursing actions and evaluation of them. High-quality nursing care has always been characterized by this approach—only the name is new.

The nursing process has four steps: (1) assessment of data, (2) planning, (3) implementation, and (4) evaluation. In regard to drug therapy, nurses must *assess* the medication needs of the patient and their station to provide optimal therapy and an ample supply of drugs to be used when needed. Much of nurses' daily routines revolve around these varying activities. The *plan of action* includes ordering drugs from the pharmacy and goal-setting concerning a patient's medication administration and monitoring.

The *implementation* of the goals previously set involves the actual nursing care given to the patient and followthrough to make certain drugs are administered appropriately.

The final step, which is perhaps the most important, is the *evaluation* of the effectiveness previous activities to assure that the goals for the patient were met. Each time the evaluation process takes place, nurses' knowledge bases increase and, likewise, their professional value. The nursing process as it relates to pharmacology will be discussed in greater detail in Unit two: The Role of Pharmacology in the Nursing Process.

Goals of this text

The intent of this text is to provide a useful orientation to nursing pharmacology and therapeutics by presenting healthy attitudes and a practical approach to drug therapy in many settings.

The first part of the text gives basic information concerning general principles, theories, and facts about all drugs and how they are given. Practical information is presented on how the nursing process is integrated with pharmacology giving general principles of action to facilitate a student nurse's learning in both the academic and the clinical environments. The rest of the book provides drug information related to specific body systems and clinical indications giving specific nursing implications and considerations relative to each. Thus this book can be used as a text and as a reference in nursing pharmacology.

Summary of nursing considerations

Safe, therapeutically effective drug administration is a major responsibility of the nurses, dependent on sound, current knowledge of medications and careful monitoring of their effects on patients. Ongoing laboratory and clinical research modifies and enlarges available drug information, necessitating continued effort to keep one's knowledge up-to-date. The mode of action of many commonly prescribed drugs, effects of their prolonged use, and the possibility of drug-induced disease are yet to be completely understood. There are many sources of current drug information, but even the most diligent student of these sources requires clinical experience to develop competence in drug administration. Few, if any, areas of nursing demand more intelligence, integrity, and factual knowledge.

BIBLIOGRAPHY

Bordley, J., III, and Harvey, A.: Two centuries of American medicine, Philadelphia, 1976, W.B. Saunders Co.
Bowers, J.Z., and Purcell, E.F., editors: Advances in American medicine 1776-1976, Philadelphia, 1976, W.B. Saunders Co.
Clarke, F.H., editor: How modern medicines are discovered, Mount Kisco, N.Y., 1973, Futura Publishing Co., Inc.
Duffy, J.: The rise of the medical establishment, New York, 1976, McGraw-Hill Book Co.
Elliott, J.S.: Outline of Greek and Roman medicine, Boston, 1971, Milford House, Inc.

*Genrose Alfano, Director of Nursing, Loeb Center for Nursing, Bronx, N.Y.

Gerald, M.C.: Pharmacology, an introduction to drugs, Englewood Cliffs, N.J., 1974, Prentice-Hall, Inc.

Goodman, L.S., and Gilman, A., editors: The pharmacological basis of therapeutics, ed. 6, New York, 1980, Macmillan, Inc.

Gordon, M., and others: Nursing diagnosis: looking at its use in the clinical area, Am. J. Nurs. **80(4):**672, 1980.

Krantz, J.C.: Historical medical classics involving new drugs, Baltimore, 1974, The Williams & Wilkins Co.

Leake, C.P.: An historical account of archeology, Springfield, Ill., 1975, Charles C Thomas, Publisher.

Marriner, A.: The nursing process, a scientific approach to nursing care, ed. 2, St. Louis, 1979, The C.V. Mosby Co.

Poynter, N.: Medicine and man, London, 1971, C.A. Watts & Co. Ltd.

Price, M.R.: Nursing diagnosis: making a concept come alive, Am. J. Nurs. **80(4):**668, 1980.

Rogers, F.B.: A syllabus of medical history, Boston, 1972, Little, Brown & Co.

CHAPTER 2

NECESSARY KNOWLEDGE BASE I

Legal foundations of pharmacology practice

Drug standards

Drugs have been known to vary considerably in strength and activity. Drugs obtained from plants, such as opium and digitalis, have been known to vary in strength from plant to plant and from year to year, depending on where the plants are grown, the age at which they are harvested, and how they are preserved. Occasionally, one finds on the market drugs of low concentration or drugs that have been adulterated. Since accurate dosage and reliability of effect of a drug depend on uniformity of strength and purity, it has been necessary to find ways by which drugs can be standardized. The technique by which the strength or potency of a drug is measured is known as assay. The two general types of assay method used are chemical and biologic. Chemical assay really means chemical analysis to determine the ingredients present and their amount. A simple example would be the determination of the con-

centration of hydrochloric acid in a solution to be used medically. Thus the acid content of a solution might be measured by titration and then adjusted, for example, to a standardized tenth-normal solution.

Opium is known to contain certain alkaloids (*active principles* was the older term), and these may vary greatly in different preparations. The United States official standard demands that opium must contain not less than 9.5% and not more than 10.5% of anhydrous morphine. Opium of a higher morphine content may be reduced to the official standard by admixture with opium of a lower percentage or with certain other pharmacologically inactive diluents such as sucrose, lactose, glycyrrhiza, or magnesium carbonate.

In the case of some drugs either the active ingredients are not known or there are no available methods of analyzing and standardizing them. These drugs may be standardized by biologic methods—bioassay. Bioassay is performed by determining the amount of a preparation required to produce a definite effect on a suitable laboratory animal under certain standard conditions. For example, the potency of a certain sample of insulin is measured by its ability to lower the blood sugar of rabbits. The strength of a drug that is assayed biologically is usually expressed in units. For example, insulin injection possesses a potency of not less than 95% and not more than 105% of the potency stated on the label, expressed in U.S.P. insulin units. Both the unit and the method of assay are defined, so that national and sometimes international standards exist.

DRUG STANDARDS IN THE UNITED STATES

A book, *The Pharmacopeia of the United States of America* (abbreviated as *United States Pharmacopeia* or U.S.P.), sets standards for drugs used in the United States. Any drug included in it has met high standards for strength, quality, purity, packaging safety, labeling, and dosage form. Drugs meeting these criteria can be identified by the letters "U.S.P." following the official name. This U.S.P. compendium is revised every 5 years by a group of elected scientific experts from the fields of nursing, pharmaceutics, pharmaceutical chemistry, analytic chemistry, physical chemistry, radiochemistry, biochemistry, microbiology, and pharmacology. The 1980-1985 Committee of Revision added new members from the fields of nursing practice and consumer interest, among others. The 1980 revision of the U.S.P. combines material from *The National Formulary*, a volume that has in the past contained material that supplemented the U.S.P. A new and valuable supplement to the U.S.P. is the new publication, *U.S.P. Dispensing Information* (D.I.), which furnishes information of interest to the one who dispenses or administers the drug once it has been prescribed. It also contains a Patient Advice section. Chapter 7 describes the U.S.P. D.I. in more detail.

DRUG STANDARDS IN GREAT BRITAIN AND CANADA

British Pharmacopoeia (B.P.) is similar to the U.S.P. in its scope and purpose. Drugs listed in it are considered official and subject to legal control in the United Kingdom and those parts of the British Commonwealth in which the *British Pharmacopoeia* has statutory force. It is published by the British Pharmacopoeia Commission under the direction of the General Medical Council. Dosage is expressed in metric system, although in some cases dosage is indicated in both metric and imperial systems.

The United States Pharmacopeia is used a great deal in Canada, and some preparations used in Canada conform to the U.S.P. instead of the B.P. because many of the drugs used in Canada are obtained from the United States.

British Pharmaceutical Codex (B.P.C.) is published by the Pharmaceutical Society of Great Britain. In general, it resembles *The National Formulary*.

The Canadian Formulary contains formulas for preparations used extensively in Canada. It also contains standards for new drugs prescribed in Canada but not included in the *British Pharmacopoeia*. The publication has been given official status by the *Canadian Food and Drug Act*.

The Physician's Formulary contains formulas for preparations that are representative of the needs of medical practice in Canada. It is published by the Canadian Medical Association.

INTERNATIONAL STANDARDS

Various national pharmacopeias have been developed to meet the needs of different countries. *The United States Pharmacopeia* has been translated into Spanish for the Spanish-speaking parts of the Americas.

An international pharmacopeia, *Pharmacopoea Internationalis* (Ph.I.), was first published in 1951 by a committee of the World Health Organization. It represents an important contribution to the development of international standards in drugs and unification of national pharmacopeias. The work done on this publication has resulted in better working together and understanding of terms and in uniformity of strengths and composition of drugs throughout the world. The Ph.I. is published in English, Spanish, and French. The nomenclature is in Latin, and the system of measurement is metric. It is not intended to convey official status in any country unless it is adopted by the appropriate authority of that country.

Drug development and evaluation

In the United States, when a new drug is discovered the pharmaceutical company must obtain an *Investigational New Drug Exemption* (IND) from the Food and Drug Administration before any clinical tests can be conducted in humans. The pharmaceutical company must submit to the FDA all available information on the drug including a specific description of the drug, its active ingredients, and results of toxicity tests in animals. The drug must be tested in at least two different mammalian species using male and female animals. Routes of administration must be the same as those proposed for humans and magnitude of dose related to that intended for human use.

Drug development depends on the assumption that a high degree of correlation exists between the effects of drugs in animals and in humans. It is generally accepted that the principal physiologic and biochemical mechanisms in animals and humans are identical although variations exist in size, concentration, and activity in individual systems in different species. However, no amount of experimentation in animals will ensure absolute safety and complete predictablity in humans. Certain pathologic conditions in humans, such as psychiatric disorders, myocardial infarction, and bone marrow diseases, have no satisfactory equivalent in common laboratory animals. A major problem in correlation is that the pharmacodynamic data of healthy animals have to be adapted to the sick human. Attempts are now being made to reduce this source of error by "modeling" the disease in animals. Drug studies today are more intensive and extensive than was true in the past. For example, drug researchers are now trying to determine the following:

1 Toxicity reversibility (Is there recovery after a reaction to the drug?)
2 Tumorigenicity (Is the drug tumor or cancer producing?)
3 Reproductive toxicity (Is the drug teratogenic [causing malformed fetuses] or mutagenic [caus-

ing chromosomal changes]? Does it cause changes in fertility and general reproductive performance? Are there undesirable effects on fertility or reproduction or during the perinatal and postnatal periods? Observations are made for delayed or prolonged labor, abnormalities in lactation and maternal care, and the drug's direct toxic action on the offspring.)

Throughout the animal studies, detailed biochemical and hematologic measurements are made to determine drug absorption by different routes of administration, drug distribution throughout the body, and drug metabolism. These studies are often linked to pharmaceutical studies in which the drug's physical and physicochemical characteristics are altered to determine how this affects absorption of the drug. The animals' behavior is also closely observed during the study. To further assess the drug's effects on various body tissues, the animals are sacrificed and histopathologic examination of all body tissues is performed.

Clinical studies are divided into three phases by the FDA:

Phase I: Very limited investigations in humans to determine toxicity, metabolism, pharmacology, preferred route of administration, and safe dosage range
Phase II: Initial clinical trials on a limited number of patients for treatment or prevention of specific diseases
Phase III: Extensive clinical trials to establish the most effective therapeutic regimens for treating specific diseases and determining the therapeutic effect likely to be achieved, possible side effects, and safety of the drug

There should also be a follow-up phase after the drug is in general use, because the extent and severity of side effects often cannot be determined solely during the experimental stages.

Normal persons are usually used for phase I testing to permit assessment of the drug's effects in a person without disease. These can then be compared with those effects occurring in diseased persons to determine the extent to which disease modifies the drug's effects. In phase I testing all aspects of drug testing are fully known to both investigator and subject.

If the new drug appears to have a therapeutic effect the following questions need to be answered:

1 Does the drug have significant therapeutic effects when compared with placebo effects?
2 Is the new drug as good as, or superior to, the best drugs presently available for treatment?

There is little value in marketing an inferior product. Controlled studies in phases II and III are designed to answer these questions.

To minimize bias in drug evaluation various safeguards are used. These include:

1 Double-blind administration. Neither the subject nor the investigator is aware of which substance is administered: the new drug, a standard drug with which it is to be compared, or an inactive placebo. All are prepared in such a way that they appear identical.
2 Randomization of drug administration
  a Within-subject trials. All subjects receive each substance included in the study and their responses to each are compared.
  b Between-subjects trials. Subjects are divided into groups; each group receives only one of the substances in the study. Comparison is made between the responses of each group.
3 Exclusion of placebo reactors from within-subject trials.
4 Use of homogeneous subjects, such as all postoperative hysterectomy patients, and matching patients according to sex, age, weight, etc.
5 Formulation of criteria for measurement of effects and surveillance by trained observers for desired and undesired effects
6 Correlation of therapeutic and toxic effects with blood, tissue, or body fluid levels of drug
7 Comparison of the drug's effects to a standard drug such as morphine or aspirin
8 Proper statistical evaluation

The final FDA decision is based on whether the benefits of the drug outweigh the risks. How much risk is the public willing to take to obtain the benefits of a new drug when no drug is absolutely free of risk? For example, when a drug for the treatment of cancer is being judged, a somewhat higher degree of risk and adverse reactions may be deemed acceptable because the alternative may be death from the cancer itself. On the other hand, if the drug is a minor tranquilizer, a much lower degree of risk would be tolerable.

All participants in experimental drug studies should be true volunteers and not subjected to any coercion. Informed consent should be obtained from them only after they have been given careful explanation of the purpose of the study, procedures to be used, and risks involved. New drug studies in children and psychiatric patients require special consideration. The rights of human participants in medical research have come to be protected under the umbrella of the Nuremberg Code. This code was developed under the aegis of American physicians as a result of the post–World War II trials at Nuremberg of Nazi physicians who had conducted experiments on involuntary political prisoners. The Code states essentially that:

1 Truly voluntary consent of the human subject is critical
2 The experiment must be proved to be valid or made possible only through the use of human subjects
3 The results and risks are justified by the study
4 Unnecessary suffering, death, or disability will be avoided
5 The experiment will be conducted in a careful and professional manner by scientifically qualified persons
6 The subject or investigator may terminate the experiment at any point that it is felt unendurable or impossible.

Additionally, any experimental drug trials using humans that are supported by the U.S. Department of Health and Human Services must also meet federal guidelines for the protection of participants. Institutions supporting such investigational research have review boards that evaluate aspects of the research as it affects human subjects and that formally approve or disapprove research proposals accordingly.

Nurses involved in research projects concerning human subjects, whether tangentially or directly, must be knowledgeable about the Nuremberg Code and must protect patients by being ever alert to the possibility of subtle slipups in protocol or oversights in the adherence to the tenets of the Code. The most important elements of the Code relate to subjects' rights to informed consent and to participation that is without coercion and fully voluntary. Although this would seem to be naturally assumed, it has occasionally been abrogated in the past (for example, instances exist of forced sterilization of retarded persons and of uninformed inoculations of experimental drugs in military personnel).

Informed consent refers to the written consent to an experimental procedure by individuals after they have received full and adequate explanation of the procedure itself, their full role in it, the expected effects, and the risks. This particular consent is heir to the flaws of other patient consents: the information conveyed may be incomplete or not delivered in laymen's language, or perhaps it is presented at a time when the patient is sleepy or sedated and not fully cognizant of the ramifications of what is being signed. It is the nurse's obligation to assure that this does not happen and that it is the researcher or the physician, not the nurse, who gives the explanation and answers the pertinent questions.

Expanding roles in nursing often include nurses on the team researching experimental drug development. Indeed, more nurses than ever before are conducting research of their own, much of it clinical even if not directly related to investigational drugs, using human subjects. Because of a healthy professional commitment to patient well-being, nurses may find themselves caught in an ethical conflict. They likely may feel ambivalent about patients' right to know (vis-a-vis the Patients' Bill of Rights) and yet be uncomfortably aware that too much information may influence the person's behavior or condition unduly in some way and thereby adversely influence the variable under study. This is an area of ethics that awaits further study.

Nurses involved in clinical drug studies should be fully informed about the study and the drug under investigation. All information available to the physician, researcher, or pharmacist should also be available to the nurse. Ethical and legal responsibilities mandate that a nurse's actions be based on adequate knowledge and skill and that the patients be protected from foreseeable harm. This necessitates that the nurse know the recommended dosage range and route of administration, the desired therapeutic effect, and the undesired and toxic effects. Throughout the entire investigation the nurse must strictly adhere to the protocols of the study. Recordings of all observations should be as precise as possible for they will have a direct influence on the study outcome.

Drug legislation

Important though pharmacopeias, formularies, and other publications are to the maintenance of standards for drugs, unless provision is made to enforce the standards the public can be defrauded, drugs adulterated, and the market flooded with unreliable and unsafe preparations. Enforcement of standards is partly a responsibility of individual states, but federal legislation is needed to cover interstate commerce in drugs as well as in other items.

The twentieth century ushered in an era of rapidly expanding scientific knowledge. At the beginning of the century federal laws controlling drug distribution were nonexistent. Illness was treated primarily with well-known botanicals or time-honored products of nature, and many preparations of secret composition were sold to the public for all known diseases.

During the first decade of the twentieth century organic chemicals used in medicine increased in number, and it soon became evident that federal legislation was needed to protect the public in a complex area where individuals were unable to protect themselves. The result was enactment of the first federal drug law in 1906.

UNITED STATES DRUG LEGISLATION

Food, Drug, and Cosmetic Act. In 1906 the Food and Drug Act designated *The United States Pharmacopeia* and *The National Formulary* as official standards and empowered the federal government to enforce these standards. It was "an act for preventing the manufacture of adulterated or misbranded or poisonous or deleterious foods, drugs, medicines, and liquors, and for regulating traffic therein, and for other purposes." The federal drug law required that drugs comply with the standards of strength and purity professed for them, and it also required that labels on drugs and patent medicines containing morphine or other narcotic ingredients indicate the kind and amount of such substances.

In the second decade of the twentieth century the number of chemicals used in medicine continued to increase, and in 1912 Congress passed the Sherley Amendment prohibiting use of fraudulent therapeutic claims. Drug research continued to accelerate during the next two decades. Synthetic organic chemicals made their appearance, and the chemotherapeutic age began.

The Food and Drug Act of 1906 was updated by the federal Food, Drug, and Cosmetic Act of 1938. Impetus to revise the 1906 drug act was provided by more than 100 deaths in 1937 resulting from ingestion of a diethylene glycol solution of sulfanilamide. The sulfanilamide preparation had been marked as an "elixir of sulfanilamide" without benefit of investigation of the toxicity of the solvent. The only charge that could be made against the drug was that it was misbranded since it was labeled an "elixir" and the drug failed to meet the definition of an elixir as an alcoholic solution. The Food, Drug, and Cosmetic Act of 1938 contained a provision to prevent premature marketing of new drugs not properly tested for safety by requiring the manufacturer to submit an investigational new drug exemption to the government for review of safety studies before a product could be sold.

The Durham-Humphrey Amendment of 1952 further changed the 1938 drug act. This amendment restricts the dispensing of so-called legend drugs by the pharmacist to dispensing on prescription only. It also prohibits the refilling of such prescriptions without authorization of the physician. In addition, it provides for oral or telephone prescriptions of certain legend drugs. Finally, it provides for oral or telephone authorization of refills, subject to certain limitations. This provision modifies a previous provision that recognized only written prescriptions. Legend drugs are those that must bear the legend, "Caution: Federal law prohibits dispensing without prescription." These include all drugs given by injection as well as:

1 Hypnotic, narcotic, or habit-forming drugs or derivatives thereof as specified in the law.
2 Drugs that because of their toxicity or method of use are not safe unless they are administered under the supervision of a licensed practitioner (physician or dentist).
3 New drugs that are limited to investigational use or new drugs that are not considered safe for indiscriminate use by lay persons.

This amendment also recognized a second class of drugs, over-the-counter drugs (OTCs), for which prescriptions are not required.

In 1958, Senator Estes Kefauver of Tennessee began a senate investigation into the drug industry when it became known that the drug companies were making huge profits and that some drug promotion was false, misleading, and avalanche-like. This investigation received little support until given impetus by the thalidomide tragedy, although for the United States it was more a might-have-been catastrophe than a real one. Thalidomide, a hypnotic marketed in Europe, was found to be responsible for severe deformities in babies whose mothers had taken the drug during the early stage of pregnancy. These events led to passage of the Kefauver-Harris Amendment in 1962.

From 1938 to 1962 approval of a new drug application was based solely on proof of its safety for use in humans. Since passage of the Kefauver-Harris Amendment, proof of both safety and efficacy is required. To facilitate the enormous task of evaluating all drugs introduced between 1938 and 1962, the FDA signed a contract with the National Academy of Sciences and its research arm, the National Research Council (NAS-NRC) in 1966 to independently study all supporting data for all therapeutic claims. This program of study was called the Drug Efficacy Study Implementation (DESI). Early in the study it was agreed that each drug would be rated for effectiveness in each of its stated indications according to the following categories:

Effective: substantial evidence of effectiveness.
Probably effective: additional evidence required to rate the drug effective.
Possibly effective: effectiveness might be shown eventually, but at the present time there is little evidence of efficacy.
Ineffective: no substantial evidence of effectiveness.

Two other ratings were also formulated:

Ineffective as a fixed combination: even though one or more components might be effective if used alone, the product is not acceptable in fixed dosage combination for reasons of safety or because there is no evidence of contribution of each component to claimed effect.

Effective but: although effective there is an appropriate qualification or restriction imposed on the drug, which is still under consideration by the NASNRC and the FDA; the drug is effective for some recommended uses but not for all, requiring labeling changes.

Thousands of drugs and therapeutic claims have been evaluated and the "ineffective" drugs have been withdrawn from the market. Those rated as "possibly effective" or "probably effective" are being withdrawn or reformulated; however, the drug may remain on the market while claims are being modified and scientific data collected to substantiate the claims. Drugs in the "probably effective" and "possibly effective" categories must be upgraded to the "effective" category within time limits set by the FDA or the claims and drug withdrawn. The rating of a drug must be prominently displayed on the label.

Narcotic and drug abuse laws. The Harrison Narcotic Act passed in 1914 was the first federal law aimed at curbing drug addiction or dependence. This was the first narcotic act passed by any nation. It established the word "narcotic" as a legal term. This act regulated the importation, manufacture, sale, and use of opium and cocaine and all their compounds and derivatives. Marijuana and its derivatives were also subject to this act, as were many synthetic analgesic drugs that proved to produce or sustain either physical or psychologic dependence.

This act and other drug abuse amendments now have only historical import, since they have been superseded by the *Comprehensive Drug Abuse Prevention and Control Act of 1970,** also called the *Controlled Substances Act.* It became effective May 1, 1971. This law was designed to provide "increased research into, and prevention of, drug abuse and drug dependence; to provide for treatment and rehabilita-

*Current regulations can be obtained from the nearest Regional Director, Drug Enforcement Administration, or from the Drug Enforcement Administration, Department of Justice, Post Office Box 28083, Central Station, Washington, D.C. 20005.

tion of drug abusers and drug dependent persons; and to strengthen existing law enforcement authority in the field of drug abuse." This law is also designed to improve the administration and regulation of the manufacturing, distributing, and dispensing of controlled substances by legitimate handlers of these drugs to help reduce their widespread dispersion into illicit markets.

In July of 1973, the Drug Enforcement Administration (DEA) in the Department of Justice became the nation's sole legal drug enforcement agency; it replaced the Bureau of Narcotics and Dangerous Drugs.

Possession of narcotics. It is, of course, unlawful for any person to possess a controlled substance unless obtained by a valid prescription or order, or unless its possession is pursuant to actions in the course of professional practice. A nurse administering special controlled drugs, such as narcotics, from stock supplies must record the date, time of administration, patient's name, physician's name, and his or her own name. Stock supplies of narcotics must be accounted for, and nurses are responsible for maintaining accurate accounting of all narcotics dispensed to their hospital unit or clinic. Nurses need to know that it is a crime to transfer a drug listed in schedule II, III, or IV to any person other than the patient for whom the drug was ordered.

Food and Drug Administration. The Food and Drug Administration is charged with the enforcement of the federal Food, Drug, and Cosmetic Act. Seizure of offending goods and criminal prosecution of responsible persons or firms in federal courts are among the methods used to enforce the Act.

In addition, pharmaceutical firms must report at regular intervals to the FDA all adverse effects associated with their new drugs. The FDA also has an adverse-reaction reporting program with approximately 450 cooperating reporting sources. The purpose of this program is to detect reactions not revealed by previous clinical or pharmaceutical studies.

Public Health Service. The Public Health Service is an agency that is part of the U.S. Department of Health and Human Services. One of its many functions is the regulation of biologic products. This refers to "any virus, therapeutic serum, antitoxin, or analogous product applicable to the prevention, treatment, or cure of diseases or injuries of man." The control exercised by the Public Health Service over these products is done by inspecting and licensing the establishments that manufacture the products and by examining and licensing the products as well.

Product liability. In a majority of the states the rule of strict manufacturer's liability has been adopted. This doctrine holds manufacturers liable for injuries caused by defects in their products. Liability exists (1) if a product is defective or not fit for its reasonably foreseeable uses, (2) if the defect arose before the product left the control of the manufacturer, and (3) if the defect caused some person harm. If these three legal requirements are met, the manufacturer must pay money damages for the harm unless the liability can be shifted to some other party. Anyone harmed by a defective product has the right to sue the manufacturer for compensation.

Harm may be caused if the drug contains an ingredient whose danger is not commonly known, or if it contains an ingredient known to be harmful that one would not reasonably expect to find in such a product. Drugs containing potentially harmful ingredients must so state on the label warnings concerning its use; otherwise, the product will be considered defective and the manufacturer liable for resulting harm to unusually susceptible persons who unknowingly use it. Whether or not a product is defective depends on its compliance with current reasonable standards of safety. Manufacturers are legally responsible for knowing the effects of their products; if an unknown risk could have been discovered through a reasonable amount of research, the manufacturer will be held liable for any resulting harm.

The following are examples of drug liabilty awards:

A 43-year-old woman who sustained retinal damage as the result of taking Aralen, a prescription drug, was awarded $180,000 to be paid by the manufacturer. *Krug v. Sterling Drug, Inc.* (Mo S Ct 1967) ¶ 5789, 416 SW2d

The manufacturer of the drug Chloromycetin was

liable for the death of a 7-year-old girl of aplastic anemia. The parents were awarded $215,000. *Incollingo v. Ewing* (Pa Ct Com Pls 1969) ¶ 6388, 48 D&C. (Aff'd Pa S Ct 1971) ¶ 6941.

A 43-year-old male who developed cataracts as the result of taking MER/29, a prescription drug, was awarded $500,000 to be paid by the manufacturer *Toole v. Richardson-Merrel, Inc.* (Cal Ct App 1967) ¶ 5814, 60 Cal Rptr 398.

The parents of a 3-month-old infant who developed a permanent brain disorder as the result of injections of Quadrigen, a quadruple antigen, recovered $643,000 from the drug company. *Tinnerholm v. Parke-Davis & Co.* (Ca-2 NY 1969) 6178, 411 F2d 48.

Nurses should be alert to defects in the drugs they administer. Although detection of chemical defects is beyond the nurse's province, detection of observable physical defects is not. Nurses should be keenly aware of the proper physical characteristics of drugs they administer. Discoloration or improper consistency of tablets, pills, or liquids, or precipitates or foreign bodies in parenteral fluids, should be considered suspect. These should be referred to the pharmacist. It might mean that an entire stock supply or batch is defective. Recall of defective drugs may prevent unnecessary harm.

CANADIAN DRUG LEGISLATION

In Canada, the Health Protection Branch (HPB) of the Department of National Health and Welfare is responsible for administration and enforcement of the Food and Drugs Act, as well as the Proprietary or Patent Medicine Act and the Narcotics Control Act. These acts are designed to protect the consumer from health hazards and fraud or deception in the sale and use of foods, drugs, cosmetics, and medical devices. Canadian drug legislation began in 1875 when the Parliament of Canada passed an act to prevent the sale of adulterated food, drink, and drugs. Since that time there has been food and drug control on a national basis.

Canadian Food and Drugs Act. In 1953 the present Canadian Food and Drugs Act was passed by the Senate and House of Commons of Canada. Since that time the law has been amended yearly. The law states that no food, drug, cosmetic, or device is to be advertised or sold as a treatment, preventative, or cure for certain diseases listed in schedule A of the act. Among the diseases included in the list are alcoholism, arteriosclerosis, and cancer. When it is necessary to provide adequate directions for the safe use of a schedule G drug used to treat or prevent diseases mentioned in schedule A, that disease or disorder may be mentioned on the labels and inserts accompanying the drug. In addition, the act prohibits the sale of drugs that are contaminated, adulterated, or unsafe for use and those whose labels are false, misleading, or deceptive. According to the act, drugs must comply with prescribed standards as stated in recognized pharmacopeias and formularies listed in schedule B of the act, or according to the professed standards under which the drug is sold. This include the following:

Pharmacopoea Internationalis
The British Pharmacopoeia
The United States Pharmacopeia
Pharmacopée Française
The Canadian Formulary
The British Pharmaceutical Codex
The National Formulary

CSD means Canadian Standard Drug. This legend, or abbreviation, must appear on the inner and outer labels of a drug to signify that it meets the standards prescribed for it.

Sale of certain drugs is prohibited unless the premises where the drug was manufactured and the process and conditions of manufacture have been approved by the Minister of National Health and Welfare. These drugs are listed in schedules C and D and include injectable liver extracts, all insulin preparations, anterior pituitary extracts, radioactive isotopes, antibiotics for parenteral use, serums and drugs other than antibiotics prepared from microorganisms or viruses, and live vaccines. For some drugs the batch from which the drug was taken must meet safety approval, and these are listed in schedule E. Among the drugs listed are various arsphenamines and sensitivity disks and tablets. Distribution of samples of drugs is also prohibited, with the exception of distribution of samples of drugs to duly licensed individuals such as physicians, dentists, or pharmacists. Schedule F (Section 15) states that no person can sell any drug described in schedule F, Section 15. Thalidomide, a hypnotic known to be a teratogenic substance, is the only drug presently listed. However, thalidomide may be sold in powdered form to qualified investigators for experimental and investigational use in animals upon approval by the Minister of National Health and Welfare. Schedule F of the Act contains a list of drugs that can be sold only on prescription, and such prescriptions shall not be refilled unless the prescriber has so directed. Refills may be permitted at specified intervals but cannot exceed 6 months. Drugs listed in schedule F include the antibiotics, hormones, and tranquilizers. They must always be properly and clearly labeled and include directions for use. Labels on containers of schedule F drugs should be marked with the symbol $\boxed{\text{Pr}}$ (prescription required). These drugs cannot be advertised to the general public.

Controlled drugs are those listed in schedule G and include amphetamines, barbituric acid and its derivatives (barbiturates), methaqualone, pentazocine, and phenmetrazine. Controlled drugs must be marked with the symbol $\langle\!\langle C \rangle\!\rangle$ in a clear and conspicuous color and size on the upper left quarter of the label. The proper name of the drug must appear on the labels either immediately preceding or following the proprietary or trade name. Controlled drugs can be dispensed only on prescription.

When dispensed by prescription the labels of a controlled drug must carry the following:

1 Name and address of the pharmacy or pharmacist
2 Date and number of the prescription
3 Name of the person for whom the controlled drug is dispensed
4 Name of the practitioner
5 Directions for use
6 Any other information that the prescription requires be shown on the label

Prescriptions for controlled drugs cannot be refilled unless at the time the prescription was issued, the practitioner so directed in writing and specified the number of times it could be refilled and the dates for, or intervals between, refilling. All information on the labels must be clearly and prominently displayed and readily discernible. Controlled drugs cannot be advertised to the general public.

Designated drugs are the following controlled drugs: (1) amphetamines, (2) methamphetamines, (3) phenmetrazine, and (4) phendimetrazine. Physicians may prescribe a designated drug for the following conditions: (1) narcolepsy, (2) hyperkinetic disorders in children, (3) mental retardation (minimal brain dysfunction), (4) epilepsy, (5) parkinsonism, and (6) hypotensive states associated with anesthesia. Permission can be obtained to prescribe amphetamines for patients with diagnoses other than those listed.

Restricted drugs are those listed in schedule H and include the hallucinogenic drugs lysergic acid diethylamide (LSD), diethyltryptamine (DET), dimethyltryptamine (DMT), and dimethoxyamphetamine (STP; DOM). Sale of these drugs is prohibited. These drugs may be obtained for research by a qualified investigator if authorized by the Minister of National Health and Welfare. Precautions must be taken to ensure against loss or theft of a restricted drug.

The following are additional requirements to be found in the Food and Drugs Act:

1 Labels of drugs must show:
   a Proper name of the drug immediately preceding or following the proprietary or brand name.
   b Name and address of the manufacturer or distributor.
   c Lot number of the drug.
   d Adequate directions for use.
   e Quantitative list of medicinal ingredients and their proper or common names.
   f Net amount of drug.
   g Common or proper name and proportion of any preservatives used in parenteral drugs.
   h Expiration date if the drug does not maintain its potency, purity, and physical characteristics for at least 3 years from the date of manufacture.
   i Recommended single and daily adult dose; if the drug is for children the label must state: "Children: As directed by physician" or:

Age in years	Proportion of adult dose
10-14	One-half
5-9	One-fourth
2-4	One-sixth
Under 2	As directed by physician

   j A warning that the drug be kept out of the reach of children and any precautions to be taken (e.g., *"Caution:* May be injurious if taken in large doses for a long time. Do not exceed the recommended dose without consulting a physi-

cian." Warning is to be preceded by a symbol—octagonal in shape, red in color, and on a white background).
   k Contraindications and side effects of nonprescription drugs.
   l On and after July 1, 1974, the drug identification number assigned to the drug, preceded by the words "Drug Identification Number" or the abbreviation "D.I.N."; to be shown on the main labels of a drug sold in dosage form (i.e., one ready for use by the consumer).
2 Other specific regulations such as:
   a Manufacturers must be able to demonstrate that a drug in oral dosage form represented as releasing the drug at time intervals actually is released and available as represented.
   b Oral tablets must disintegrate within 60 minutes. Enteric-coated tablets must not disintegrate for 60 minutes when exposed to gastric juice but most disintegrate within an additional 60 minutes when exposed to intestinal juice.
   c Drugs containing boric acid or sodium borate as a medicinal ingredient must carry a statement that the drug should not be administered to infants or children under 3 years of age.
   d Safety factors such as sterility and absence of pyrogens must be assured in parenteral drugs.

The regulations allow the government to withdraw from the market drugs found to be unduly toxic. New drugs introduced to the market must have shown effectiveness and safety in human clinical studies to the satisfaction of the manufacturer and the government.

For more specific information, the nurse can obtain a copy of *Health Protection and Drug Laws* from Supply and Services Canada, Canadian Government Publishing Centre, Hull, Quebec K1A 059.

Canadian Narcotic Control Act. The regulations of the Canadian Narcotic Control Act govern the possession, sale, manufacture, production, and distribution of narcotics. The Canadian Narcotic Control Act was enacted in 1961. This act revoked the Canadian Opium and Narcotic Act of 1952. The 1961 act has been amended a number of times.

Only authorized persons can be in possession of a narcotic. Authorized persons include a licensed dealer, pharmacist, practitioner, person in charge of a hospital, or a person acting as an agent for a practitioner. A licensed dealer is one who has been given permission to manufacture, produce, import, export, or distribute a narcotic. Practitioners include persons registered under the laws of a province to practice the profession of medicine, dentistry, or veterinary medicine. However, persons other than these may be licensed by the Minister of National Health and Welfare to cultivate and produce opium poppy or marijuana or to purchase and possess a narcotic for scientific purposes. Members of the Royal Canadian Mounted Police and members of technical or scientific departments of the government of Canada or of a province or university may possess narcotics for the purpose of and in connection with their employment. A person who is undergoing treatment by a medical practitioner and who requires a narcotic may possess a narcotic obtained on prescription. This person may not knowingly obtain a narcotic from any other medical practitioner without notifying that practitioner that he is already undergoing treatment and obtaining a narcotic on prescription.

All persons authorized to be in possession of narcotics must keep a record of the name and quantity of all narcotics received, from whom narcotics were obtained, and to whom narcotics were supplied (including quantity, form, and dates of all transactions). In addition, they must ensure the safekeeping of all narcotics, keep full and complete records on all narcotics for at least 2 years, and report any loss or theft within 10 days of discovery.

The schedule of the act lists those drugs, their preparations, derivatives, alkaloids, and salts that are subject to the Canadian Narcotic Control Act. Included in the schedule are opium, coca, and marijuana. Before a pharmacist legally may dispense a drug included in the schedule or medication containing such a drug, he or she must receive a prescription from a physician. A signed and dated prescription issued by a duly authorized physician is essential in the case of all narcotic medication prescribed as such or any preparation containing a narcotic in a form intended for parenteral administration. Oral medication containing a narcotic may be dispensed by a pharmacist on the strength of a verbal prescription received from a physician who is known to the pharmacist or whose identity is established. Prescrip-

tions of any description calling for a narcotic may not be refilled.

There is one exception to the prescription requirement. Certain codeine compounds with a small codeine content may be sold to the public by a pharmacist without a prescription. In such instances the narcotic content cannot exceed 8 mg per tablet or 20 mg/28 ml. In products of this kind, codeine must be in combination with two or more nonnarcotic substances and in recognized therapeutic doses.

Additionally, items of this nature are required to be labeled in such a fashion as to show the true formula of the medicinal ingredients and a caution to the following effect: "This preparation contains codeine and should not be administered to children except on the advice of a physician." These preparations cannot be advertised or displayed in a pharmacy. It is also unlawful to publish any narcotic advertisement for the general public.

Labels of containers of narcotics must legibly and conspicuously bear the proprietary and proper or common name of the narcotic, name of the manufacturer and distributor, the symbol "N" in the upper left-hand quarter, and net contents of the container and of each tablet, capsule, or ampule.

Local or provincial laws modify to a certain extent regulations governing the sale and administration of narcotics.

Although the administration of the Canadian Narcotic Control Act is legally the responsibility of the Department of National Health and Welfare, the enforcement of the law has been made largely the responsibility of the Royal Canadian Mounted Police. Prosecution of offenses under the act is handled through the Department of National Health and Welfare by legal agents specially appointed by the Department of Justice.

The Narcotic Control Act defines a narcotic addict as "a person who through the use of narcotics, has developed a desire or need to continue to take a narcotic, or has developed a psychological or physical dependence upon the effect of a narcotic." A person brought into court for a narcotic offense may be placed in custody by the court for observation and examination. If the person is convicted of the offense and found to be a narcotic addict, the court can sentence him to custody for treatment for an indefinite period.

Amendments to this act place special restrictions on methadone. No practitioner can administer, prescribe, give, sell, or furnish methadone to any person unless the practitioner has been issued an authorization by the Minister of National Health and Welfare.

Application to nursing. A nurse may be in violation of the Canadian Narcotic Control Act if he or she is guilty of illegal possession of narcotics. Ignorance of the content of a drug in the nurse's possession is not considered a justifiable excuse. Proof of possession is sufficient to constitute an offense. Legal possession of narcotics by a nurse is limited to times when a drug is administered to a patient on the order of a physician, when the nurse is acting as the official custodian of narcotics in a department of the hospital or clinic, or when the nurse is a patient for whom a physician has prescribed narcotics. A nurse engaged in illegal distribution or transportation of narcotic drugs may be held liable, and heavy penalties are imposed in violation of the Canadian Narcotic Control Act.

INTERNATIONAL DRUG CONTROL

International control of drugs legally began in 1912 when the first "Opium Conference" was held at The Hague. International treaties were drawn up legally obligating governments to (1) limit to medical and scientific needs the manufacturing of and trade in medicinal opium, (2) control the production and distribution of raw opium, and (3) establish a system of governmental licensing to control the manufacture of and trade in drugs covered by the convention.

In 1961 government representatives formulated the "Single Convention on Narcotic Drugs," which became effective in 1964. This act consolidated all existing treaties into one document for the control of all narcotic substances by:

1 Outlawing their production, manufacturing, trade, and use for nonmedicinal purposes
2 Limiting possession of all narcotic substances to authorized persons for medical and scientific purposes

3 Providing for international control of all opium transactions by the national monopolies (countries designated to produce opium, such as Turkey) and authorizing production only by licensed farmers in areas and on plots designated by these monopolies
4 Requiring import certificates and export authorizations

An International Narcotics Control Board was established to enforce this law. Since this is an immense task it is impossible to prevent illicit trafficking of drugs. For example, during a 1 year period it was estimated that 1200 tons of opium were circulated in the illicit market when 800 tons were considered sufficient for world medical needs. Laws need to be frequently updated and strictly enforced.

Nursing legislation

Nursing practice is regulated not only by the previous drug standards and legislation but also by individual state nurse practice acts; joint policy statements among the state nursing associations, medical associations, and hospital associations; and institutional and agency policies. The last may set policies that interpret more specifically actions allowable under state nursing practice acts, but they may not modify, expand, or restrict the intent of such acts. Personal and professional ethical standards further govern actual nursing decisions and judgments in practice.

The nurse practice acts of individual states define conditions under which nurses may be licensed and practice professionally. One of its functions is to protect the public from unskilled, undereducated, and unlicensed nurses and to delineate clearly the scope of nursing as a health care profession. Another function is to protect nurses by defining clearly their responsibilities and freedoms. Every state nurse practice act includes laws and regulations on reciprocity and suspension or revocation of nurse licenses.

CHANGING NURSING ROLES AND NURSING LEGISLATION

Clearly, the traditional roles of the nurse are changing and expanding with newer techniques and approaches to drug therapy. These expanding roles often find the nurse in activities beyond accepted nursing practices, which challenge the judgment and accountability of the nurse legally. Two such areas are prescription writing and drug administration.

Prescribing of medications has been, in the past, a purely medical function, while medication administration has usually been delegated to nurses and occasionally to licensed pharmacists and other trained personnel. In reality, astute nurses have been indirectly prescribing for many years using diplomatic ploys with physicians to attend to changing patient needs: "Will you write an order for Dulcolax for Mrs. Rommel? She hasn't had a bowel movement for 5 days." Now certain expanding roles in nursing have necessitated changes to legalize the prescribing function. Two reports acknowledged this need, one from the American Medical Association in 1970 and the other from the Department of Health, Education and Welfare in 1971. Both clearly state that the prescribing of medications "may be the practice of medicine when carried out by a physician and the practice of nursing when carried out by the nurse." Several states as a result of this change have amended their nurse practice acts. These amendments have primarily given permission to the nurse to write prescriptions according to established protocols or under physician supervision.

As of 1980, Alaska, Idaho, Maine, New Hampshire, New Mexico, North Carolina, Oregon, Tennessee, Vermont, and Washington had revised their nurse practice acts to encompass prescribing as a nursing function.

In California, there is under review a study to broaden the scope of nurse prescribing. Three hundred nurse practitioners are participating in a 4-year program of education and supervision in prescription writing in order to assess the safety and cost-effectiveness of such activities.

Drug administration has been an accepted role of the nurse for some time. However, the function of giving medications directly into the vein has been reserved for the physician. In the past, nurses were given the freedom to administer large-volume continuous intravenous in-

fusions. More recently, nurses have begun administering medications by small-volume intermittent intravenous infusion (by "piggyback" or "rider"). Though not generally accepted as an appropriate nursing function, very small-volume, undiluted medications have been given by nurses either directly into a vein, by IV "push," or into IV tubing. Nurses who now perform this particular function are probably placing themselves in a tenuous legal position unless there exists written sanction by a jointly approved policy statement and they are qualified by virtue of adequate training, education, and experience.

Generally, changing roles and functions and the laws that govern them are not enacted simultaneously. There is usually a time lag between the adoption of a new function and official approval. Nurses who prepare and inject admixtures intravenously, whatever the delivery system, are breaking new legal ground. Since such procedures are potentially more risky than other medication procedures, policies should be drawn up jointly by the administration of the hospital or agency and nursing representatives. These policy statements must carefully delineate the roles of nurses and physicians and present guidelines for these procedures. They should include a list of drugs and routes to be used only by physicians and a listing of criteria for permitting nurses to give medications by an intravenous route or system.

Basically, at the level of implementation, three conditions must be met before a nurse may legally begin to administer a medication:

1 The medication order must be valid
2 The physician and nurse must be licensed
3 The nurse must know the purpose, actions, effects, and major side and toxic effects of the drug

A valid order is one that leaves no room for doubt as to the medication prescribed, its dose and route, and the prescriber's name/signature. More than that, the drug must also be deemed appropriate for that specific patient. Since nurses are legally, morally, and ethically responsible for their actions, even for each medication they administer to patients, they must assess the medication order for its preciseness, accuracy, and appropriateness.

The medication order must be written and worded in such a way that is correct, complete, legible, and clearly understandable. If it is not, clarification must be sought from the prescriber. Creating a healthy, open, questioning atmosphere in the prescriber-nurse relationship avoids the very real hazard lurking behind "guessing," "assuming," and not "bothering the doctor."

Although not every medication given in error results in actual patient harm, the potential always exists. It is always wise to avoid such prescribing situations as follows or to clarify them.

Verbal order. A physician's order is given verbally (often at a patient's bedside), such as "Just give her a little Mylanta." It is then appropriate to remind the prescriber that nurses cannot give medication unless the order is in writing. If the order is not written at that time, it is often forgotten. If the medication has already been given and it has not been "signed for," it is illegal until the order is written and signed. Managing this before the prescriber leaves the area is often not possible.

Telephone order. An order given over the telephone can easily be miscommunicated, misinterpreted, or not clearly heard, and such an order often remains too long unsigned by the prescriber. Many institutions have a specific policy that limits acceptance of verbal or telephone orders to emergency situations only. In any event, all orders should be signed by the prescriber as soon as possible. Nursing students should not follow or transcribe any unsigned telephone or verbal orders.

Incomplete order. Orders that are not fully complete in either the medication name, dose, route, time, or signature must be clarified and completed before administration. Medications by the intravenous route are the ones most often found incomplete; usually the rate of infusion is the part missing from the order.

Incorrect or inappropriate order. The order may be judged by the nurse to be incorrect or inappropriate for the patient (for example, a dose too high for the patient of low body weight or with renal function impairment as evidenced

by low creatinine clearance, or a medication ordered for a patient with a recent myocardial infarction that is noted to have secondary effects of tachycardia or arrhythmias). Here, the situation can be quite intimidating to the nurse who is now in position of challenging the judgment of the physician at the risk of incurring embarrassment, job threat, or both. Often physicians and some nurses (and many consumers) are under the mistaken impression that nurses who merely act by following a physician's order are absolved from any untoward results of that act. Actually, *no one can relieve a nurse of responsibility for actions;* to carry out an order that the nurse knows to be incorrect constitutes negligence. To change an order by modifying any part of it, if done without consultation with the prescriber, is similarly illegal.

If an order is believed to be in error, some suggested actions are as follows:

1 Validate the order by consulting an authoritative reference source (see Chapter 5 for suggested drug data references).
2 If the order is indeed apparently incorrect, objectively report the conflicting facts and discuss it with the prescriber in a factual, calm, nonblaming manner.
3 If the prescriber still wants the medication given as ordered after the nurse's objections have been raised, can the nurse give the medication if the prescriber takes full responsibility? Again, *no one can release nurses from full responsibility for every medication they give just because they are acting under a physician's order.* To do so is to court a suit for negligence. This fact must be made clear to the prescriber as the rationale for the nurse's refusal to medicate.

If the prescriber chooses to personally administer the medication after the nurse refuses to do so in the belief that it could be potentially harmful to the patient, the nurse should see that the facts of the situation are made known to the nurse's supervisors at least to the level of the Director of Nurses and possibly to the hospital administrator.

Invalid order. Orders signed by medical students, physicians' assistants, or nurse practitioners are not generally accepted as having been signed by a duly licensed physician (this is the wording of some nursing practice acts) and should not be implemented until actually signed by a physician. Validity of orders written and signed by a nonlicensed intern or resident may be equivocal, depending on local law or policy.

Order for unfamiliar drug. Orders for a medication that is unfamiliar to the administering nurse must stimulate a nearly reflex reaction to "look it up." Administration of an unfamiliar drug while remaining in ignorance of its actions and intended, side, and toxic effects (at the very minimum) is considered nursing negligence if it results in harm to the patient. For instance, a nurse was found liable when a 3-month-old infant died after being given an injectable form of digoxin instead of the pediatric elixir. In another instance, a nurse was found negligent when prolonged infiltration of a levarterenol (Levophed) infusion went unobserved, causing permanent injury.

• • •

Astute nurses are not only alert to the set limits of functioning but also to the quality of functioning within those limits. Although legal suits can be initiated when a nurse exceeds the limits of accepted practice, few have actually been instituted. However, more can be anticipated in the near future as the public becomes more aware of nurses' liability. Most suits, however, are brought against nurses by patients or their families who feel they have been subjected to behavior or to a procedure that was not of the quality of practice reasonably expected of someone having the nurse's professional education and experience and under the particular circumstances. This is identified legally as malpractice. Five major areas for potential malpractice through medication administration error can be safeguarded against by the nurse's observing the "Five Patient Rights." At the very least, the patient should be able to expect to be given:

1 The right medication (the one that was prescribed and one that is not contraindicated)
2 The medication meant for him as patient, not someone else's by mistake or one that looks similar
3 The correct dose as prescribed and appropriate (it may involve simple mathematical computations)
4 The medication's correct form, route, and appropriate technique as prescribed

5 The medication within an effective time interval (usually within half an hour of the time indicated and at beneficial intervals as ordered)

Samples of nursing actions that support and facilitate the meeting of these expectations of patients are:

1 Refusing to allow administration of a drug against good nursing judgment
2 Preparing medications in a quiet, undisturbed environment conducive to thoughtfulness and accuracy
3 Comparing the information on the medication ticket or Kardex with the prescriber's order and medication chart to prevent wrong dosage, double-dosing, or the like
4 Looking up information about all new or unfamiliar drugs before administering them
5 Reading medication labels and comparing them to the order
6 Carefully calculating dosage as necessary, especially when working with decimals
7 Administering only drugs that were self-prepared
8 Positively identifying the patient by comparing his armband and the name on the medication ticket or Kardex
9 Listening intently to patients when they question the administration of a particular drug, its color, size, dosage, or a possible allergy; patients frequently give nurses crucial data in this manner
10 Recording the administration of each dose as soon as possible
11 Observing carefully for side and toxic effects, reporting them, and documenting actions taken

Probably the most powerful fundamental force at work in the actual implementation of right and proper nursing practice is the nurse's own concept of ethical and moral correctness and responsibility. Both the American Nurses Association (1968)[1] and the International Council of Nurses (1973)[2] have each adopted similar codes of ethics for nurses, which can serve as a guide to standards of conduct, relationships, and practice. At the core of any such professional code is that its precepts spring from the reality that the patient is a person with rights and dignity not to be subsumed under the needs or rights of any other person or the machinations of the institution or society at large. For example, patients have every right to know necessary information about a drug they are receiving and to refuse to take it after having been given the courtesy of an explanation, no matter what the consequences.

For the nurse's part, accountability is a term that has gained increasing import, particularly as related to pharmacotherapeutics. Nurses are no longer considered to be merely "physicians' handmaidens" or to have the "umbrella protection from litigation" by the physician and the institution. Nurses are increasingly expected to take the responsibility for and be answerable for the service they provide or make available.

In summary, basic guides to clear, professional nursing practice, and medication administration in particular, include:

1 Know the limitations of nursing practice in the community through the hospital policies, joint medicine and nursing practice statements, nursing practice acts, and state and federal laws, then abide by them.
2 Know the limitations of one's own skills, expertise, knowledge, and experience and never exceed them.
3 Inform involved personnel of and document thoroughly and carefully all happenings related to patient care, especially those with legal implications.
4 Maintain a professional, caring, and collaborative relationship with patients and their families. Aside from this being a proper approach, it can act to divert potential dissatisfaction of patients with general health care delivery experiences, with the institution, or with its policies.

Summary of nursing considerations

Accurate dosage and reliability of effect of a drug depend on uniformity of strength and purity. Since drugs may vary considerably in strength and activity, it has been necessary to find ways by which they can be standardized. Two types of measurement are used: *chemical assay*—chemical analysis to determine ingredients and their amount—and *bioassay*—determining the amount of a preparation necessary to produce a given effect on a laboratory animal under certain standard conditions.

Official drugs in the United States are listed in *The United States Pharmacopeia* (U.S.P.) or *The National Formulary* (N.F.); drugs included are defined as to source, physical and chemical

properties, tests for purity and identity, assay, method of storage, category, and dosage. The U.S.P. is revised every 5 years by a committee of outstanding pharmacologists, physicians, and pharmacists. The N.F., which serves as a supplement to the U.S.P., is revised on a similar schedule and published in the same volume with the U.S.P. It contains information on single drugs, formulas for drug mixtures, and established standards for the agents and procedures used therein.

The British Pharmacopoeia (B.P.) is similar to the U.S.P. in scope and purpose. Both the U.S.P. and B.P. are used in Canada. *The British Pharmaceutical Codex* (B.P.C.) is the Canadian counterpart of N.F. *The Canadian Formulary* contains formulas for preparations used exclusively in Canada.

In 1951 a committee of the World Health Organization published the first *Pharmacopoea Internationalis*. Today it is published in English, Spanish, and French; nomenclature is Latin, and the system of measurement is metric.

Drug standards are established to ensure the safety and effectiveness of pharmaceutical preparations. In the United States, a pharmaceutical company must obtain an Investigational New Drug Exemption (IND) before any new drug can be clinically tested with humans. Drugs must be tested in two different mammalian species using both male and female animals to determine drug absorption, distribution, and metabolism as well as the following: (1) toxic reversibility, (2) tumorigenicity, and (3) reproductive toxicity. Following these animal studies, clinical studies in humans are divided into phase I (limited investigations in normal persons), phase II (initial clinical trials on a limited number of patients), and phase III (extensive clinical trials). The following safeguards are used to minimize bias:

1 Double-blind administration
2 Randomization of drug administration
3 Exclusion of placebo reactors
4 Use of homogeneous subjects
5 Formulation of criteria for measurement of effects
6 Correlation of therapeutic and toxic effects with blood, tissue, or body fluid levels of the drug
7 Comparison of drug's effects to a standard drug
8 Proper statistical evaluation

Nurses involved in clinical drug studies should have access to all information available to the physician, researcher, or pharmacist. The nurse's ethical and legal responsibilities demand that the patient's rights not be violated, in keeping with the principles of the Nuremburg Code.

Legislation facilitates enforcement of drug standards to protect the public against unreliable and unsafe drug products. See Table 2-1.

Careful records must be kept by nurses administering controlled drugs, since they are responsible for maintaining an accurate accounting of all narcotics dispensed to their hospital unit or clinic. Violation of this act is punishable by fine, imprisonment, and revocation of license.

The Food and Drug Administration enforces the federal Food, Drug, and Cosmetic Act. The

Public Health and Human Service, part of the U.S. Department of Health and Human Services, regulates biologic products such as serums and antitoxins.

Manufacturers are legally responsible for the quality and safety of their products; if a defective product causes any person harm, that person can sue the manufacturer for compensation. Nurses need to be alert to possible defects in drugs they administer. Any item of suspicion should be referred to the pharmacist.

Canadian drug legislation began on a national basis in 1875. Today the Health Protection Branch of the Department of National Health and Welfare administers and enforces the Food and Drugs Act, the Proprietary or Patent Medicine Act, and the Narcotics Control Act.

The abbreviation CSD (Canadian Standard Drug) must appear on inner and outer labels of

TABLE 2-1 Summary of important U.S. drug legislation

Legislation	Conditions of the law
Food, Drug and Cosmetic Act of 1938	This act which is implemented by the FDA, mandates that drug manufacturers must test all drugs for harmful effects and that labels and other literature enclosed be accurate and complete. It also requires that medical devices be safe and effective and that cosmetics be safe. The FDA has the power to prevent the marketing of any drug it has adjudged to be incompletely tested or dangerous.
Wheeler-Lea Act of 1938	This act defines the criteria for nonfraudulent advertising of drugs, food, or cosmetics: no false claims, full disclosure of chemical formulas including the amount of each ingredient. This act is implemented by the Federal Trade Commission.
Durkham-Humphrey Amendment of 1952	This amendment distinguishes more clearly between drugs that can be sold with or without prescription and those that should not be refilled without a new prescription and need to be so labeled. These latter are those drugs considered habit-forming, narcotic, hypnotic, or potentially harmful.
Drug Amendment of 1962 (Kefauver-Harris Act)	This act is a result of the thalidomide tragedy, wherein severely deformed babies were born to European mothers who had taken the hypnotic thalidomide. It was only through the staunch efforts of a woman investigator working for the FDA that this drug was not officially approved in the United States. This drug is now barred from the United States and its possessions. This act gave the FDA increased power to (1) tighten controls over drug safety and over statements about adverse reactions and contraindications, (2) evaluate the actual drug testing methods used by manufacturers, and (3) determine drug effectiveness (of both prescription and nonprescription drugs), not just their relative lack of toxicity. As a result, many drugs have now been determined to be "ineffective," "possibly effective," and so on (about 50% of all prescription drugs). These drugs must be so designated and must eventually be improved to "effective" status or be removed from the market.
Controlled Substances Act of 1970 (Title II of the Comprehensive Drug Abuse Prevention Act of 1970)	The FDA and Drug Enforcement Agency of the Justice Department have jurisdiction to regulate and control the flow of drug traffic. This act categorizes controlled substances (drugs such as narcotics, amphetamines, barbiturates, and tranquilizers and those that have potential for abuse) into five categories, called schedules, based on their relative potential for abuse and medical effectiveness. Drugs in schedule I offer the highest abuse potential. All controlled substances are limited in the number of times a prescription may be refilled.
Drug Regulation Reform Act of 1978	This act allows a shortened time period for new drug investigative efforts, thereby speeding new drug release to the public.

a drug to signify that it meets all standards prescribed for it.

The Canadian Narcotic Control Act, enacted in 1961, regulates the possession, sale, manufacture, production, and distribution of narcotics. Records comparable to those required by United States regulations must be kept on all transactions regarding narcotics.

The Proprietary or Patent Medicine Act was passed in 1908 to protect the Canadian public against unsafe or ineffective home medications. Proprietary or patent medicines (PPM) registered by the Health Protection Branch have been evaluated for dosage, efficiency, compatibility of ingredients, action, proper directions for use, and false or misleading claims.

International control of illicit drugs has been attempted since 1912. In 1964 the "Single Convention on Narcotic Drugs" became effective, and an International Narcotics Control Board was established to enforce it. However, the immensity of the task renders the board only partially effective.

Nursing practice is not only regulated by the previous drug standards and legislation but also by individual state nurse practice acts, by joint policy statements of the state nursing associations, medical associations, and hospital associations, as well as by institutional and agency policies.

Nurse practice acts define conditions under which a nurse may be licensed and practice professionally. Clearly, the traditional roles of nurses are causing nursing legislation to change, especially in the areas of prescription writing and drug administration. It is important that nurses know not only the limitations in their nursing abilities but also their legal limitations.

QUESTIONS

FOR STUDY AND REVIEW

1 State the purpose of the federal Food, Drug, and Cosmetic Act.
2 Explain the need for drug standards.
3 Explain the reason for testing new drugs in at least two different animal species.
4 Why are normal persons often used for phase I clinical testing of a new drug?

5 Discuss the various safeguards used to minimize bias in clinical drug studies.
6 Why would the effects of a new narcotic analysis be compared with those of a standard narcotic such as morphine or codeine?
7 What responsibilities does a nurse have when participating in new drug studies?
8 Formulate criteria for measuring the effectiveness of a new narcotic analgesic.
9 What is the purpose of using homogeneous subjects in clinical drug studies?
10 State the purpose of the Controlled Substances Act.
11 How does the Controlled Substances Act define a "drug-dependent person"? A "drug addict"?
12 Interview various hospital or clinic personnel to determine ways in which narcotics can be "pilfered" from hospital units or clinics.
13 Discuss the nurse's responsibility when a physician orders a narcotic for a patient by telephone.

OBJECTIVE QUESTIONS

Select the correct combination answer.

Controlled Substances Act (U.S.)

14 Schedule I drugs are those that:
a have high potential for abuse.
b do not have an acceptable medical use.
c include the hallucinogenics.
d lack accepted safety measures for use.
15 Schedule II drugs are those that:
a have an accepted medical use.
b have a high abuse potential.
c may cause severe dependence.
d include the barbiturates.
16 Schedule III drugs are those that:
a may cause moderate or low physical dependence.
b have low abuse potential
c may cause high psychologic dependence.
d include the barbiturates.
17 Schedule IV drugs:
a include major tranquilizers.
b may cause minimal dependence.
c include phenobarbital.
d have moderate potential for abuse.
18 Schedule V drugs:
a include over-the-counter drugs containing limited amounts of narcotics.
b lack potential for abuse.
c do not cause physical dependence.
d may cause psychologic dependence.

Canadian Food and Drugs Act

19 Match the following:
a _____ Designated   1. Sale of these drugs
     drugs   is prohibited

b —— Restricted drugs

c —— Controlled drugs

2. Prescription drugs
3. These drugs to be prescribed only for specific listed conditions

20 Which of the following statements are correct?
  a Hallucinogenics are restricted drugs.
  b Obesity is one of the listed conditions for which amphetamines may be prescribed.
  c The legend "CSD" on a drug label indicates that the drug meets the standards prescribed for it.
  d Amphetamines and barbiturates cannot be advertised to the general public.

21 What law establishes the criteria for nurse licensure?

22 What groups would draw up policies and procedures for the administration of intravenous medications?

REFERENCES

1 Code for nurses with interpretive statement, New York, 1968, American Nurses' Association.
2 International Council of Nurses Code for Nurses, Am. J. Nurs. **73:**1350, 1973.

BIBLIOGRAPHY

A.M.A. Committee on Nursing: Medicine and nursing in the 1970's, a position statement, Chicago, June 1970, The Association.

Black, J.B., editor: Safeguarding the public—historical aspects of medical drug control, Baltimore, 1970. The Johns Hopkins Press.

Blackwell, B.: For the first time in man, Clin. Pharmacol. Ther. **13:**812, 1971.

Blissett, C.W., Webb, O.L., and Stanaszek, W.F.: Clinical pharmacy practice, Philadelphia, 1972, Lea & Febiger.

Bomar, D.P., and others: Intravenous medications, Philadelphia, 1980, J.B. Lippincott Co.

Burke, J.: The rural health clinic services act—impetus for state legislation, Nurs. Prac. **3**(2):9, 1978.

California nurse practitioners begin prescription test project, Am. J. Nurs. April 1979.

Creighton, H.: The nurse's right to question a physician's order, Supervisor Nurse **2:**12, 1971.

Creighton, H.: Nurse's adding of drugs to I.V.'s, Supervisor Nurse **4:**62, 1973.

Creighton, H.: Law every nurse should know, ed. 3, Philadelphia, 1975, W.B. Saunders Co.

Dexter, P.: How to solve a math problem, J. Nurs. Ed. **19** (2):49, 1980.

DiPalma, J.R.: Drill's pharmacology in medicine, ed. 4, New York, 1971, McGraw-Hill Book Co.

Gerald, M.C.: Pharmacology, an introduction to drugs, Englewood Cliffs, N.J., 1981, Prentice-Hall, Inc.

Leitch, C., and others: A state-by-state report: the legal accommodation of nurses practicing expanded roles, Nurs. Prac. **2**(8):19, 1977.

Michigan Nurses' Association: Position on nursing practice, East Lansing, 1971, The Association.

Nichols, T.S.: Human experimentation in clinical nursing research. In Anderson, E.H., and others, editors: Current concepts in clinical nursing, vol. 4, St. Louis, 1973, The C.V. Mosby Co.

Palmer, R.F.: Products liability—minimizing the hazard, New York, 1971, Commerce Clearing House, Inc.

Palmer, R.F.: Controversies in clinical pharmacology and drug development, Mount Kisco, N.Y., 1972, Futura Publishing Co., Inc.

Passos, J.: Accountability: myth or mandate, J. Nurs. Admin. **3:**16, 1973.

Perlstein, P.H., and others: Errors in drug computations during newborn intensive care, Am. J. Dis. Child. **133:**376, 1979.

Regan, W. A.: Levophed infiltration due to R.N. negligence, Regan Rep. Nurs. Law **11**(2):1, 1970.

Silverman, A., and Lee, P.R.: Pills, profits and politics, Los Angeles, 1974, University of California Press.

Tennessee nurse practitioners fight ban on prescribing, Am. J. Nurs. Nov. 1979.

Turner, P., and Richens, A.: Clinical pharmacology, London, 1973, Churchill Livingstone.

Uehleke, H.: Animal data in perspective, Int. J. Clin. Pharmacol. **8:**239, 1973.

Wolfe, S., and others: Pills that don't work, Public Citizen Health Research Group, Washington, D.C., 1980; reprinted in Sci. Nurs., Feb. 7, 1981, p. 92.

OFFICIAL PUBLICATIONS

Code of Federal Regulations, No. 21, Food and Drugs, Washington, D.C., 1973, U.S. Government Printing Office.

Department of Health, Education, and Welfare: A primer on new drug development, FDA Consumer, HEW Pub. No. (FDA) 74-3021, Rockville, Md., 1974.

Department of Health, Education, and Welfare: Extending the scope of nursing practice, Washington, D.C., 1971, U.S. Government Printing Office.

Department of Health, Education, and Welfare: We want you to know about today's FDA, HEW Pub. No. (FDA) 77-1021, Rockville, Md., 1977.

Food and Drugs Act and Regulations, 1972, with Amendments to December, 1977, Roger Duhamel, F.R.S.C. Ottawa, Ontario, Queen's Printer and Controller of Stationery.

Health Protection and Drug Laws, 2/80, Minister of National Health and Welfare, Educational Services, Health Protection Branch, Department of National Health and Welfare, Canada.

Narcotic Control Act and the Narcotic Control Regulations, Roger Duhamel, F.R.S.C. Ottawa, Ontario, Queen's Printer and Controller of Stationery.

Patent Medicines, No. 14, Educational Services, 1971, Food and Drug Directorate, Ottawa, Ontario, Department of National Health and Welfare.

United States Pharmacopeia, ed. 20, and The National Formulary, ed. 15, Rockville, Md., 1980, The United States Pharmacopeial Convention, Inc.

Public Law 91-513, 91st Congress, H.R. 18583, Washington, D.C., 1972, U.S. Government Printing Office.

United States Pharmacopeia Dispensing Information, Easton, Pa., 1980, Mack Publishing Co.

CHAPTER 3

NECESSARY KNOWLEDGE BASE II
Drug characterization

Names of drugs

Sources of drugs

    Active constituents of plant drugs

Drug classification

Pharmaceutical preparations

    Solutions and suspensions
    Dosage forms
    Additional formulations
    Miscellaneous drug delivery systems
    Pharmaceutical accessories

Drug stability and storage

Summary of nursing considerations

Names of drugs

As a drug passes through the investigational stage and the stages when it becomes accepted and marketed, it collects and keeps as many as three different types of names: the chemical name, the generic or nonproprietary name, and the trade name.

The *chemical name* is a very precise description of the drug's chemical composition and molecular structure. As such it is meaningful primarily to the chemist. For example, the chemical name of one of the common antibiotics is 4-dimethylamino-1,4,4a,5,5a,6,11,12a-octahydro-3,6,10,12,12a-pentahydroxy-6-methyl-1,11-dioxo-2-napthacenecarboxamide. Its generic name is tetracycline and it is also sold under a number of trade names—Achromycin, Mysteclin, and Panmycin, among others.

The *generic* or *nonproprietary name* is often assigned by the manufacturer to denote pharmacologically related drugs. The generic name is simpler and often derived from the chemical name, but it may not be as easy to pronounce or

as catchy as its trade names. It is not as easily remembered, and as a result it is not as frequently prescribed by the physician. Some would argue that the trade name drug is likely to be more reliable than a generic drug with regard to the properties of consistency, dissolution, potency, and bioavailability, but this has not been proved. It *has* been shown that there is variability among different preparations of the same drug. A few of the drugs that can have different bioavailabilities when they come from different sources, yet supposedly be the same preparation, are as follows*:

Chloramphenicol	Phenytoin
Digoxin	Prednisone
Griseofulvin	Sulfadiazine
Hydrochlorothiazide	Tetracycline
Nitrofurantoin	Thyroid extract
Oxytetracycline	Tolbutamide
Phenacetin	Triamterene
Phenylbutazone	

*Data from Bowman, W.C., and Rand, M.J., editors: Textbook of pharmacology, ed. 2, Oxford, 1980, Blackwell Scientific Publications, p. 40.10.

A nurse should advise a patient to keep the same brand name drug or source of the generic medication in order to maintain the same therapeutic response. This is especially important in the treatment of epileptic individuals with phenytoin (Dilantin).

The *trade name, brand name,* or *proprietary name* is selected by the drug company selling it and is copyrighted; it is a proper noun and the first letter is capitalized. The trade names of drugs discussed in this book will be found enclosed in parentheses following the generic name.

Skilled marketing specialists work on giving their drugs an easily spelled, short trade name that in some way infers by association its major action or ingredient. When a prescription is written using the trade name, it limits the consumer's purchase to that specific formulation of the drug as produced by a specific drug company and usually increases its cost above that of its generic analog.

In order to promote sales under the trade name, extensive advertising is usually necessary. This involves considerable expense, which is borne mainly by the consumer. On the other hand, much of the research in new drugs is done in laboratories of reputable drug firms, and in order to realize a legitimate return for the cost of research, they need to patent their product and have exclusive rights to its manufacture and sale.

Health care–related organizations have recognized the growing confusion among the public and among health care providers and prescribers that has resulted from the current proliferation of "new" drugs and the problem of triple names for each. Most of these "new" drugs are just reformulations of established drugs, some whose patents may have expired after 17 years, in order to capitalize on an existing market. The United States Adopted Name (USAN) Council of the U.S. Pharmacopeia Committee and the World Health Organization are working to facilitate world-wide standardization of drug names, and the AMA-USP Nomenclature Committee and the American Pharmaceutical Association are working to create simpler, more useful generic names through the use of more logical syllables. It is anticipated that these approved names will eventually be adopted as the official drug nomenclature.

Sources of drugs

Drugs are derived from four main sources: (1) plants, examples of which are digitalis, vincristine, and colchicine; (2) animals, from which drugs such as epinephrine, insulin, and ACTH are obtained; (3) minerals or mineral products, such as iron, iodine, and Epsom salts; and (4) chemical substances made in the laboratory. The drugs made of chemical substances are pure drugs, and some of them are simple substances, such as sodium bicarbonate and magnesium hydroxide, whereas others are products of complex synthesis, such as the sulfonamides and the adrenocorticosteroids.

ACTIVE CONSTITUENTS OF PLANT DRUGS

The leaves, roots, seeds, and other parts of plants may be dried or otherwise processed for use as medicine and, as such, are known as crude drugs. Their therapeutic effect is caused by chemical substances contained in the crude preparation. When the pharmacologically active constituents are separated from the crude preparation, the resulting substances are more potent and usually produce effects more reliable than those of the crude drug. As might be expected, these active principles are also more poisonous, and the dosage must be smaller. Some of the types of pharmacologically active compounds found in plants, grouped according to their physical and chemical properties, are alkaloids, glycosides, gums, resins and balsams, and oils.

Alkaloids. Alkaloids (alkali-like) are compounds composed of carbon, hydrogen, nitrogen, and oxygen. Alkaloids have a bitter taste; they are often poisonous and hence preparations of them are administered in small doses. They are, for the most part, white crystalline solids. The name of an alkaloid ends in "ine," for example, caffeine, atropine, and morphine. Alkaloids will combine with an acid to form a salt. The salts of alkaloids are used in medicine in preference to pure alkaloids because they are more soluble; for example, morphine sulfate is preferred to morphine since it is much more soluble in water. Increased solubility may make possible administration by injection. A number of alkaloids have been chemically synthesized in the laboratory.

Both alkaloids and their salts are precipitated by tannic acid and oxidized by potassium permanganate. Hence these substances can be used under certain circumstances as antidotes for poisoning from alkaloids.

Glycosides. Glycosides are active principles that upon hydrolysis yield a carbohydrate (a sugar) and some other chemical grouping such as an aldehyde, acid, or alcohol. The carbohydrate may be glucose, in which case the compound may be called a glucoside, but carbohydrates other than glucose may occur in the molecule, hence the use of the more general term *glycoside*. The carbohydrate molecule is usually not necessary for the action of the glycosides, and in the body it may be removed to liberate the active aglycone or genin. The presence of a sugar in the molecule of the glycoside is thought to modify activity by increasing solubility, absorption, permeability, and cellular distribution. An important glycoside used in medicine is digitoxin.

Gums. Gums are exudates from plants. They are polysaccharides that vary in the degree of their solubility in water. On the addition of water some of them will swell and form gelatinous or mucilaginous masses. Some remain unchanged in the gastrointestinal tract, where they act as hydrophilic (water-loving) colloids; that is, they absorb water, form watery bulk, and exert a laxative effect. Agar and psyllium seeds are examples of natural laxative gums. Synthetic hydrophilic colloids such as methylcellulose and sodium carboxymethyl cellulose may eventually replace the natural gums as laxatives. Gums are also used to soothe irritated skin and mucous membranes. On the addition of water, tragacanth gum forms an emulsion used as a base for a greaseless catheter lubricant or for chapped skin. Acacia (gum arabic) is used as a suspending agent in making emulsions and mixtures.

Resins. Resins are crude drugs or an extraction from a crude drug. The rosin used by violinists is an example of solid resin. A few resins are devoid of color, and some give off an aromatic fragrance as a result of admixture of a volatile oil. Resins form the sap of certain trees. They are insoluble in water but soluble in alcohol, ether, and various oils. Resins are local irritants and some have been used in medicine as cathartics. Podophyllum resin is a constituent of aloin, belladonna, cascara, and podophyllum pills (Hinkle's Pills) and is a rather irritating cathartic.

Balsams also contain resins in addition to benzoic or cinnamic acids. Benzoin, Peruvian balsam, and tolu balsam, are examples.

Oils. The term "oil" is applied to a large number of liquids characterized by being insoluble in water and highly viscous. Their greasy feel is the result of these properties. Oils are of two kinds, volatile and fixed.

Volatile oils are liquids that impart an aroma to a plant. They evaporate easily and leave no greasy stain. Because of their pleasant odor and taste they are frequently used as flavoring agents. Because of their volatility and consequent power of penetration they may be irritating, mildly stimulating, and antiseptic in effect. Peppermint oil and clove oil are listed in the U.S.P. and the B.P. and are occasionally used in medicine.

Fixed oils are those that feel greasy and do not evaporate readily. They hydrolyze to form fatty acids and glycerin. Some fixed oils are used as food, for example, olive oil. Others are used in medicine, such as castor oil, and some as vehicles in which to dissolve other drugs, such as sesame oil.

Drug classification

Drug classification can be approached from two perspectives, by clinical indication or by body system. This book uses both approaches where appropriate. Examples of drugs classified by clinical indication include:

Chapter 9—Anesthetic agents
Chapter 11—Psychotherapeutic drugs used in treatment of emotional disorders
Chapter 23—Antimicrobial agents

Examples of drugs classified by body system are:

Chapter 8—Central nervous system drugs

Chapter 14—Respiratory system drugs
Chapter 30—Dermatologic agents

These drug groupings can assist the nurse to understand and memorize the vast number of individual agents available for drug therapy. Learning pharmacology becomes easier when one understands the common characteristics of each drug classification and when each prototype drug within the group is studied thoroughly. When a new drug becomes available, the nurse will be able to immediately associate it with its drug classification and know many of its basic qualities before reading anything about its therapeutic indications. Learning which of its qualities are different from the prototype drug and its dosage will be most important.

Nurses need not be overwhelmed by long, involved drug names. Certain syllables can suggest information, such as the suffix "-caine" and its association with anesthetics; the syllable in cortisone derivatives "-cort-"; "ceph-", relating to cephalosporin-type antibiotics; and so on. Basic information that should be learned about each major drug includes its generic name and one trade name, the category to which it belongs, its clinical uses, its mechanism of action, side effects and toxic effects, and other specifics associated with the nurse's role in administration of that drug. "Looking it up" should become second nature to the nursing student and to the practicing nurse, who should also encourage or initiate the development of a nurses' library shelf and a file of informative inserts about drugs frequently used in the clinical area. For those who question, "Do nurses really need to know 'all that'?" it must be remembered that nurses are professionally, morally, legally, and personally responsible for every dose of medication they give! The nurse who does not stay up-to-date courts a lawsuit.

Pharmaceutical preparations

Pharmaceutical preparations are the preparations that make a drug suited to various methods of administration. They may be made by the pharmacist or by the pharmaceutical company from which they are purchased. The nurse who has some knowledge of these preparations is likely to bring more understanding to the task of administering drugs.

SOLUTIONS AND SUSPENSIONS

Aqueous solutions. Aqueous solutions have one or more substances dissolved in water. *Waters* are saturated (unless otherwise stated) solutions of volatile oils or other aromatic substances in distilled water. Peppermint water and concentrated peppermint water are examples. Other aqueous solutions, sometimes referred to as *true solutions,* are made by dissolving a nonvolatile substance in water. Examples are strong iodine solution (Lugol's Solution), epinephrine nasal solution, and aluminum acetate solution.

Syrups are sometimes used for their demulcent (soothing) effect on irritated membranes of the throat. Syrup as listed in the U.S.P. is an aqueous solution of sucrose (85%). Syrups may be flavored and used as a vehicle in which to disguise unpleasant-tasting medicines and also as a preservative. Examples listed in the *National Formulary* are orange and cherry syrups. Promethazine hydrochloride syrup, an antihistaminic, is an example of a syrup that reflects medicinal content.

Aqueous suspensions Aqueous suspensions are defined in U.S.P. XIX as preparations of finely divided drugs either intended for suspension or already in suspension in some suitable liquid vehicle. Sterile suspensions are prepared by adding sterile, distilled water for injection to the preparation, for example, sterile chloramphenicol for suspension. A sterile suspension ready for use is sterile penicillin procaine G suspension. Sterile suspensions are intended for intramuscular or subcutaneous injection, but they cannot be given intravenously or intrathecally. Oral suspensions may be prepared in much the same way, but they are not sterile and must not be injected. Suspensions for ophthalmic use are sterile and contain a bacteriostatic agent. Hydrocortisone acetate ophthalmic suspension is a good example. Suspensions tend to settle slowly and should be shaken well before use to provide uniform distribution of the drug in the aqueous medium.

Mixtures. Mixtures are any solid material suspended in a liquid. No mixtures are listed in the U.S.P. The B.P. records a mixture of magnesium hydroxide. The term "mixture" is also used to mean any preparation of several drugs, such as a cough mixture. However, the term is usually restricted to mean only preparations for internal use.

Emulsions. Emulsions are suspensions of fats or oils in water with the aid of an emulsifying agent, which lowers the interfacial tension between the two substances, masking its oily feel. These oils are more easily digested than undispersed oils. Emulsions are stabilized by agents such as acacia and gelatin, which coat the tiny droplets of oil and prevent them from coming in direct contact with water. An example is cod liver oil emulsion.

Magmas. Magmas are sometimes called milks because they are white and resemble milk. They are bulky suspensions of insoluble preparations in water. Milk of magnesia or magnesium hydroxide mixture is an example. Magmas tend to settle or separate on standing and should be shaken well before they are poured.

Gels. Gels are aqueous suspensions of insoluble drugs in hydrated form. The particles suspended are approximately the size seen in colloidal dispersions. Magmas and gels are similar except that the particles suspended in a magma are larger; aluminum hydroxide gel is an example.

Spirits. Spirits are concentrated alcoholic solutions of volatile substances. They are also known as essences. The dissolved substance may be solid, liquid, or gaseous. Most spirits contain from 5% to 20% of the active drug. The alcohol serves as a preservative as well as a solvent. Peppermint spirit is sometimes used as a carminative and also as a flavoring agent.

Elixirs. Elixirs are aromatic, sweetened, alcoholic preparations, frequently used as flavored vehicles, such as aromatic elixir, or as active medicinal agents if they are medicated elixirs, such as phenobarbital elixir, or cascara elixir.

Tinctures. Tinctures are alcoholic or hydroalcoholic solutions usually prepared from plant drugs or from chemical substances. Tinctures of potent drugs contain 10 g of drug in 100 ml of tincture. Most other tinctures contain 20 g of drug in 100 ml of tincture. Tinctures are prepared by extracting the drug from its crude source or by making an alcoholic solution of the drug. Iodine tincture is made by dissolving iodine in an alcoholic solution of sodium iodide. The alcoholic content of tinctures improves their stability and facilitates solution of drugs that are poorly soluble in water. Tinctures listed in the B.P. are preparations extracted from crude drugs, not simple solutions. The usual dose of a potent tincture is about 1 ml (0.3 to 1 ml) or 5 to 15 minims.

Fluidextracts. Fluidextracts are alcoholic liquid extracts of vegetable drugs made so that 1 ml of the fluidextract contains 1 g of the drug. They are the most concentrated of any of the fluid preparations, being of 100% strength and 10 times stronger then potent tinctures. Since many of them precipitate in light, they should be kept in dark bottles and not used if a precipitate has formed. Glycyrrhiza fluidextract is used as a flavoring agent, whereas aromatic cascara sagrada fluidextract and cascara liquid extract are used as cathartics.

NOTE: Spirits, medicated elixirs, tinctures, and fluidextracts are preparations that tend to be potent and therefore the dosage is likely to be small. A nurse would never expect to administer as much as 30 ml (a fluidounce) of any of them. A fraction of a milliliter (a few minims) up to as much as 2 to 4 ml (1 to 2 fluidrams) is likely to be the range of dosage. Furthermore, these preparations are never injected, one reason being that they all contain alcohol. Most tinctures contain resins that make them incompatible with water.

Extracts. Extracts are concentrated preparations of vegetable or animal drugs obtained by removing the active ingredients of the drugs with suitable solvents and then evaporating all or part of the solvents. Extracts are made in three forms: semiliquids or liquids of syrupy consistency, plastic masses or pillular extracts, and dry powders known as powdered extracts. Extracts are intended to preserve the useful constituents of a drug in a form suitable for medication or for the making of other dosage forms such as tablets or pills. Liver extract is a dry extract. Cascara dry extract is used to make cascara tablets.

DOSAGE FORMS

Capsules, sustained-release capsules, tablets, pills, and troches are used to divide a drug or mixture of drugs into definite doses and avoid the inconvenience of preparing the dose from dry powders. They are therefore referred to as dosage forms. Capsules and coated tablets are a convenient way of giving drugs that have an unpleasant taste. It has been true in the past and to some extent continues to be true that some patients are more impressed with a vile-tasting medicine than a pleasant-tasting or tasteless preparation. However, most patients appreciate preparations that are not unpleasant to take.

Capsules. Capsules are one of the most popular dosage forms for the oral administration of powders, oils, and liquids. They dissolve readily in the stomach and make the contents available for absorption only slightly less quickly than a liquid medicament. New drugs for oral use are often introduced in capsules in order to avoid problems of disintegration, stability, or taste. When these problems have been solved, tablet forms of the drug are generally used because they are less costly to produce. Capsules are usually made of gelatin and may be hard or soft, depending on the amount of glycerin in the gelatin. Gelatin capsules may be coated with a substance that resists the action of gastric juice and so will not disintegrate until they reach the alkaline secretions of the intestine. Such capsules are said to be *enteric coated*. Sizes of capsules range from 5 to 000 (Fig. 3-1).

Capsules are often of a distinctive color or shape to identify the manufacturer.

Dosage forms providing for gradual but continued release of drug are sold under a number of different names, such as Spansules, Gradumets, and Timespans. Sustained-release dosage forms contain small particles of the drug coated with materials that require a varying amount of time to dissolve. This provides for a long continuous period of absorption and effect. Some particles dissolve and are absorbed almost immediately, others require 2 or 3 hours, and some do not dissolve for 10 or 12 hours. An increasing number of drugs are available in sustained release form; prochlorperazine edisylate (Compazine Edisylate), is available in this dosage form.

Tablets. Tablets are preparations of powdered drug that are compressed or molded into small disks. They may be made with or without a diluent (dextrose, lactose, starch), and they may differ greatly in size, weight, and shape. *Compressed tablets* are made with heavy machinery. The granulated form of the preparation is formed, under great mechanical pressure, into tablets. Compressed tablets usually contain in addition to the drug a diluent, a binder, a disintegrator, and a lubricant. Binders are substances that give adhesiveness to the powdered drug. Diluents are used when the amount of active igredient is small, and lubricants keep the tablet from sticking to the machines. A disintegrator, such as starch, helps the tablet to dissolve readily when it is placed in water, because the starch expands when it gets wet. Tablets are sometimes scored (marked with an indented line across the surface) so that

FIG. 3-1. Various sizes and numbers of gelatin capsules, actual size.

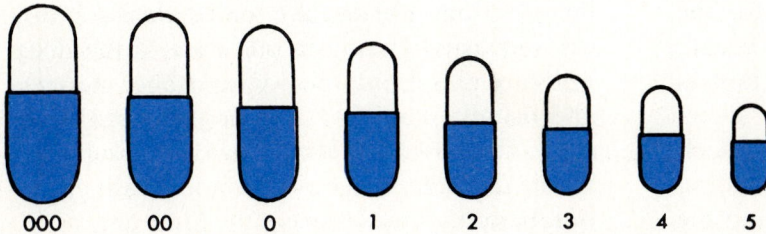

000   00   0   1   2   3   4   5

they can be broken easily if half a tablet is the dose required. Tablets may be coated with sugar or chocolate to enhance their palatability. They may be covered with a colored coating to make them more attractive to patients, easier to swallow, or identifiable by the use of distinctive colors and legible imprinting. Both tablets and capsules may be enteric coated, either to protect the drug from the effect of the gastric secretions or to prevent drug irritation of the gastric mucosa.

Enteric coatings should never render the drug ingredient less available, but this problem may occur. When enteric-coated medication seems to fail or proves less effective than expected, the patient may be excreting the tablets intact.

The absorption of drugs from tablets and capsules is receiving much attention these days. It was discovered that the absorption may vary greatly depending on the manufacturing practices of different firms. For this reason the Food and Drug Administration is paying more and more attention to "bioavailability" in the approval of different medical preparations. This concept takes into consideration not only the amount of active drug in a preparation but also the percentage of its absorption. A tablet may be so poorly made that its dissolution and absorption are defective. It has been shown, for example, that digoxin tablets made by different manufacturers may produce quite different blood levels although the amount of the active drug in the tablets is the same. There is every reason to believe that eventually bioavailability data will be available on virtually all drugs.

Compressed tablets are usually administered orally. *Molded tablets* or *tablet triturates* are made by mixing the moistened powdered drug with dextrose or lactose and powdered sucrose, so as to make a plastic mass suited for manual pressure into small molds. Later the tablets are ejected and dried. They disintegrate readily when placed in water. Molded tablets are administered orally, sublingually, or sometimes by inserting them in the buccal pouch (between the cheek and the teeth), depending on the type of medication they contain and the purpose for which they are given. Hypodermic

tablets are compressed or molded tablets that dissolve completely in water, making a solution suitable for injection. They must be prepared under aseptic conditions and dissolved suitably before administration.

Tablets may "case harden" on storage, which would interfere with absorption, or deteriorate when exposed for long periods of time to high humidity, thereby reducing the availability of the drug. Tablets so affected should be discarded.

Numerous sustained-release products are also available as tablets that may (1) disintegrate into discrete articles in the gastrointestinal tract, (2) gradually erode but retain their original shape while getting smaller, and (3) retain their original shape but give up active drug by leaching.

Troches. Troches or lozenges are flat, round, or rectangular preparations that are held in the mouth until they dissolve, liberating the drug or drugs involved. They usually contain water, sugar, and a mucilage in addition to the drug and are dried in hot air. They temporarily produce a high concentration of the drug in the oral cavity. They are held in the mouth until entirely dissolved. That which is swallowed may produce systemic effects.

Pills. Pills are mixtures of a drug or drugs with some cohesive material. The mass is molded into globular, oval, or flattened bodies convenient for swallowing. Pills are not suitable for injection. They have been replaced to a great extent by capsules and tablets. Although "pill" is a popular, general term for tablets or capsules, this is a misuse of the term. In fact, very few true pills are on the market today.

Powders. Powders are finely divided solid drugs or mixtures of drugs for internal or external use.

Ampules and vials. Ampules and vials contain powdered or liquid drugs usually intended for injection. *Ampules* are sealed glass containers and usually contain one dose of the drug. *Vials* are glass containers with rubber stoppers and usually contain a number of doses of the drug. The powdered drug must be dissolved in sterile distilled water or in isotonic saline solution before administration.

Disposable syringes. Disposable syringes

FIG. 3-2
How to use Tubex-sterile needle units. *(Courtesy Wyeth Laboratories, Philadelphia, Pa.)*

**How to use
Tubex®-sterile needle units**

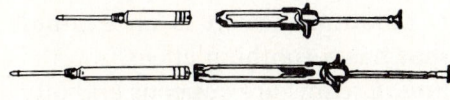

To load the syringe

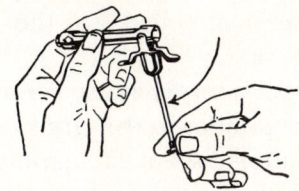

1
Grasp barrel of syringe with one hand. With the other hand, pull back firmly on the plunger and swing the entire handle section downward so that it locks at right angle to the barrel.

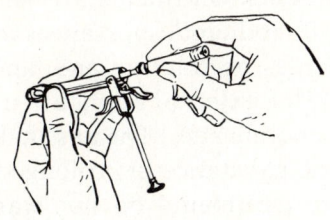

2
Insert Tubex-sterile needle unit, needle end first, into the barrel. Engage needle ferrule by rotating it clockwise in the threads at front end of syringe.

To administer
Method of administration is the same as with conventional syringe. Remove rubber sheath, introduce needle into patient, aspirate, and inject.

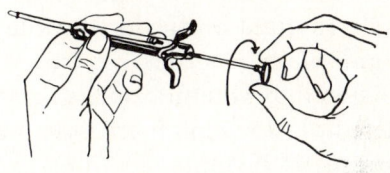

3
Swing plunger back into place and attach end to the threaded shaft of the piston. Hold the syringe barrel with one hand and rotate plunger until both ends of Tubex are fully but lightly engaged. To maintain sterility, leave the rubber sheath in place until just before use. To aspirate before injecting, pull back slightly on the plunger.

To remove the empty Tubex

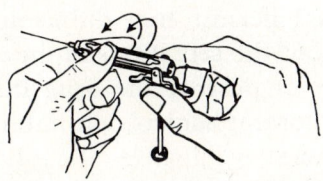

4
Disengage plunger from piston by rotating counterclockwise and open syringe as in step 1. Do not pull plunger back before disengaging or syringe will jam. Rotate Tubex-sterile needle unit counterclockwise to disengage at front end of syringe, remove from syringe, and discard.

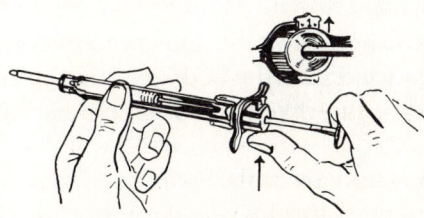

**TO ADAPT 2 CC SYRINGE
TO 1 CC TUBEX**

The 2 cc syringe can be used for a 1 cc. Tubex. Engage both ends of Tubex and push the slide through so the number "1" appears. After use, the syringe automatically resets itself for 2 cc Tubex.

containing doses of drug preparations are widely used. Various antibiotic preparations are commonly given this way. Another dosage form employs the cartridge type of container, which is fitted into a metal framework and a needle attached, such as Tubex. The cartridge contains the drug that is given by injection and the whole resembles a hypodermic (Fig. 3-2).

Large-volume intravenous solutions. Large-volume intravenous infusion solutions are available in glass, flexible plastic, or semirigid plastic, usually in volumes of 250, 500, or 1000 ml. Medications are added to them by needle and syringe, by pump-action vials, or by special double-needles attached to the medication vial.

Intermittent intravenous solutions. These solutions are similar to the large-volume intravenous solutions except they come in smaller volumes. These are used when the medication is to be diluted in a small amount of fluid. They are run intermittently at scheduled times according to the dosage ordered. After the drug is administered, the continuous large volume intravenous solution is reinstated. They are available in glass bottles or flexible plastic or semirigid plastic bottles or bags. Some are administered by volume-control sets, which are calibrated plastic containers hung beneath the primary set of IV tubing.

Direct intravenous injection. Direct intravenous injection is accomplished by the fairly rapid injection of a small amount of medication directly into a vein, into the tubing, or into a vein via heparin lock without continuous infusion or solution between doses.

ADDITIONAL FORMULATIONS

Drops. Drops are aqueous solutions that anesthetize, soothe, or medicate eyes, ears, or nose.

Instillations. Instillations are aqueous solutions instilled into the body cavities or wounds and allowed to dwell there in contact with tissue.

Foams and aerosols. Foams and aerosols are powders or solutions for spraying on skin as topical anesthetics, to soothe or protect, or for inhalation for the purposes of anesthesia or bronchodilation.

Liniments. Liniments are liquid suspensions or dispersions intended for external application. They are applied to the skin by rubbing. In addition to one or more active ingredients they may contain oil, soap, water, or alcohol. The oil and the soap of liniments adhere to the skin and serve as lubricants while the preparation is being rubbed on. Liniments usually contain an anodyne (to relieve pain) or a rubefacient (to redden the skin). Liniments may tem-

porarily relieve pain and swelling by counterirritation and by improving circulation of blood to the part.

Lotions. Lotions are liquid suspensions or dispersions intended for external application. Lotions usually should be patted on the skin and not applied by rubbing. This is particularly true if the skin is irritated or inflamed. Lotions can be protective, emollient, cooling, cleansing, astringent, or antipruritic, depending on their content. Calamine lotion is an example of a lotion that has a soothing effect.

Creams. Creams are aqueous and oily emulsions to soothe skin or to act as moisturizers.

Ointments. Ointments are semisolid preparations of medicinal substances in some type of base such as petrolatum and lanolin. They are intended for external application to the skin or mucous membranes. The base helps to keep the medicinal substance in prolonged contact with the skin. Ointments do not wash off readily unless surfactants have been added. A number of other bases can be used in ointments, some of which are miscible with water. Ointments are used for their soothing, astringent, or bacteriostatic effects, depending on the drug or drugs contained in the preparation. Sulfur ointment, rose water ointment, and zinc oxide ointment are examples.

Ophthalmic ointments are sterile, specially prepared ointments for use in the eye. The ointment base selected must be nonirritating to the eye, must permit free diffusion of the drug throughout the secretions of the eye, and must not alter or destroy the drug that it incorporates. Chloramphenicol ophthalmic ointment is an example.

Pastes. Pastes are ointment-like preparations suited only for external application. Many of them consist of thick stiff ointments that do not melt at body temperature. They tend to absorb secretions and they soften and penetrate the skin to a lesser extent than do ointments. Zinc oxide paste and compound zinc paste are examples.

Plasters. Plasters are solid preparations that serve as either simple adhesives or counterirritants. When applied to the body the heart softens them and makes them adhere. The base is usually a rubber mixture called rubber plaster.

Adhesive tape and salicylic acid plaster are two examples.

Suppositories. Suppositories are mixtures of drugs with a firm base that can be molded into shapes suitable for insertion into a body cavity or orifice. The base may be glycerinated gelatin, a hard soap, cacao butter (cocao butter), or Carbowax, (a polymer of ethylene glycol). These substances melt at body temperature and dissolve in the secretions of mucous membranes to produce local or systemic effects. The shapes and sizes are suitable for insertion into the rectum, vagina, or urethra. Urethral suppositories are called *bougies*. Aminophylline suppositories and aspirin suppositories are listed in the U.S.P.

Poultices. Poultices are soft moist preparations, the purpose of which is to supply moist heat to a skin area. If applied too long they cause maceration of the skin. They tend to be regarded as home remedies. There are no poultices listed in the U.S.P.

MISCELLANEOUS DRUG DELIVERY SYSTEMS

The drug delivery system has become even more sophisticated with *implanted drug deposits*, *membrane drug delivery systems*, and *needle-syringe pump assemblies* used to administer a steady, continuous dose of a drug when required.

PHARMACEUTICAL ACCESSORIES

Coloring substances. Coloring substances may be added to medicines to make them more acceptable to patients. Red and green colors seem to be favorites. The coloring agent must be either an official agent or one that has been certified under the Food, Drug, and Cosmetic Act. Amaranth solution imparts a vivid red color to a preparation such as phenobarbital elixir. Compound amaranth solution is listed in the N.F.

Other additives. Common additives to drug forms are preservatives, PH stabilizers, bacteriostatic agents, diluents, binding agents, lubricants, disintegrators, coatings, flavorings, and colorings. The active ingredients in an administered drug may actually constitute only a small portion of the drug form.

Table 3-1 summarizes and expands the pharmaceutical preparations available to clinical medicine, with more examples of how they are used in the practice of medicine.

Drug stability and storage

Deterioration, decomposition, or alteration of any drug or chemical compound begins and proceeds gradually as soon as it has been produced. Eventually this may result in altered effectiveness or toxicity of the drug. This fact guides nurses in ordering, storage, and administration of drugs.

Most drugs can be stored right on the stock supply shelves or in the patient's own supply box, but some must be stored according to specific manufacturer's directions (on the label or package insert) in order to retard deterioration (for example, live vaccines, most reconstituted drugs, and most suppositories). Many drugs change composition or potency when exposed to light, heat, moisture, or gases in the environment. The *United States Pharmacopeia* has defined the nomenclature used in instructions for prevention of changes due to heat*:

Freeze—store below 0° C (32° F)
Store in a cold place—temperature no higher than 15° C (59° F)
Refrigerate—2° to 15° C (36° to 59° F)
Avoid excessive heat—temperature no higher than 49° C (120° F)

Medication refrigerators in agencies should be used solely for the storage of drugs and related necessities and should be cleaned out regularly and expired drugs discarded. There should be at least one thermometer inside to monitor temperature maintenance (either on the top shelf or the door). The recent incident of several "immunized" children contracting measles was traced to a single physician's office where live measles vaccine was routinely stored on the refrigerator door shelf. Such storage has occasionally been shown to allow the temperature of the medications there to fluctuate unduly and to cause them to become inactivated, lose potency, or increase the rate of deterioration, since the area is flooded with warm

*Modified.

T A B L E 3 - 1   Various forms of drug preparations

Form	Examples/remarks
Preparations for oral use	
Liquid	
Aqueous solutions	Substances dissolved in water: waters (volatile substances in water) and syrups
Aqueous suspensions (shake well before administering)	Mixtures (solid particles suspended in liquid), emulsions (fats or oils suspended in a liquid with an emulsifier), magmas (milky suspensions), gels (suspension of an insoluble substance)
Spirits (alcohol solutions)	
Elixirs (aromatic, sweetened solutions containing a dissolved substance or medication)	Potent; prescribed in small doses
Tinctures (extracts with or without alcohol)	
Fluidextracts (concentrated alcoholic liquid extracts of vegetables)	
Extracts (syrup or dried extract of the active drug ingredients)	
Solid	
Capsules (gelatin-covered dry drug, used to avoid the problems of disintegration, instability, or taste; or in tiny beads for continuous release); do not open capsules before administering	Tetracycline (Achromycin)
Tablets (powdered drug that is compressed and molded into small disks); may be scored to allow for half doses; may be coated for palatability, for ease in swallowing, to make identifiable or layered for sustained release or enteric coated (to protect drug from gastric secretions or to protect gastric mucosa from effects of the drug)	Aspirin (acetylsalicylic acid) — Enteric tablets/capsules have been found undigested in patients' stool and may cause local mucosal irritation; both capsules and tablets may "case harden" or deteriorate with age
Troches (lozenges that dissolve in the mouth)	Cēpacol throat lozenges
Powders and granules (loose or molded); for use with or without mixing in liquid	Potassium chloride for oral solution (K-Lor); psyllium hydrophilic mucilloid (Metamucil)
Preparations for parenteral use	
Ampules (small sealed all-glass containers for liquid injectable medication; must be broken open for use)	Diazepam (Valium)
Vials (glass containers with rubber stoppers for liquid or powdered medication—diluent must be added); before medication is withdrawn, air equivalent to the dosage volume must be added	Mix-O-Vial
Cartridges (usually a single-dose unit of parenteral medication that comes with or without needle attached to the glass cylinder); to be used with a specific injecting assembly mechanism	Tubex sterile needle units
Large-volume intravenous infusions	D₅W, normal saline
Glass bottles, various sizes containing from 150 to 1000 ml for continuous infusion of fluid replacement with or without medications added via medication port; rubber stoppers with an air vent, either a long plastic tube through the solution and opening into air at top of inverted bottle (without air filter) *or* air inlet on administration set at juncture with bottle (with air filter); rigid, easy to handle, and biologically inert glass, but heavy and breakable	Large-volume infusions are used for drugs that must be highly diluted (KCl) or that require steady blood levels (e.g., nitroprusside, oxytocin), or for total parenteral nutrition
Flexible, collapsible plastic bags of polyvinyl chloride containing 150 to 1000 ml for continuous infusion of fluid replacement with or without medications added via small auxiliary tube port; needs no air vent; unbreakable, lightweight, but not biologically inert (may adsorb some medication to inside of container and some constituents of the plastic [plasticizers] may leach out into solution; this creates no currently known hazard to patient)	

TABLE 3-1 Various forms of drug preparations—cont'd

Form	Examples/remarks
Semirigid plastic container made of polyolefin in a (currently) limited variety of volume sizes for continuous fluid replacement with or without added medication via port; needs no air vent; biologically inert, impermeable to moisture, lightweight, unbreakable	
Ampules and vials as discussed previously	
Pump-action vials with a plastic spike on top for inverting and injecting into a large-volume infusion	
Special double needles inserted into both the medication vial and the bottle for mixing and injecting into the large volume-intravenous infusion	
Intermittent intravenous infusions	
Small plastic or glass bottles (volume: 50 to 250 ml solution) to which medication is added; to run as "piggyback," hung separately from primary (main) IV infusion, and run via a secondary administration tubing set for a period of 20 minutes to 2 hours; primary IV solution is run during the time between medication doses; volume-control sets are small-volume (100 to 250 ml solutions), semirigid, calibrated plastic chambers or flexible plastic bags to which medication is added; the volume-control set is hung below an IV solution, which acts as diluent-reservoir for intermittent medication administration or as the primary infusion between doses of medication	Medication: antibiotics Soluset (Abbott Laboratories) Volu-Trole-A (Cutter Laboratories) Pedatrol (Travenol Laboratories)
Direct intravenous rapid injection	
Intermittent infusion device consisting of a winged infusion needle with a short length of narrow tubing for intermittent injection of small doses of medication by needle and syringe; device stays in place between doses without any solution infusing; needle and syringe injection of very small volume of a drug directly into IV tubing via a port or the rubber bulb or directly injected into a vein itself; injection completed over a 1 to 2 minute period, or occasionally more rapidly; no solution infuses between doses	Heparin lock Emergency drugs Cancer chemotherapy
Preparations for topical use	
Liniments (liquid suspension for lubrication; apply by rubbing)	
Lotions (liquid suspensions; apply by patting on); can be protective, emollient, cooling, astringent, antipruritic, cleansing, etc.	
Ointment (semisolid medicine in a greasy base) for protective, soothing, astringent, bacteriostatic effects	
Pastes (thick ointments) primarily for skin protection	
Plasters (solid preparations that are adhesive, protective, or soothing)	
Creams (emulsions containing an aqueous and an oily base)	
Aerosols (fine powders or solutions in volatile liquids with a propellant)	
Preparations for use on mucous membranes	
Drops (aqueous saline solutions with or without gelling agent to increase retention time in the eye); dropper tip should not touch anything except the solution itself to retain sterility	For eyes, ear, or nose
Instillation (aqueous solution of medications for topical action or occasionally for systemic action)	Enemas, douches, mouthwashes, throat sprays, gargles
Aerosol sprays, nebulizers, inhalers (aqueous solutions of medication delivered by container designed to make droplets of a size appropriate to the location of the target membrane; i.e., the smaller the droplet, the farther it will travel down the bronchial tree); with or without a propellant, for bronchodilation or topical anesthesia	Bronchodilators: metaproterenol sulfate (Alupent); teach patients to exhale fully before inhaling medication and to hold breath momentarily after deep inhalation; tolerance may build—do not overuse
Foams (powders or solutions of medication in volatile liquids with a propellant)	Vaginal foams: for contraception
Powders, tablets, creams	Vaginally, for contraception or vaginitis, etc.
Suppositories (medicinal substances mixed with a firm but malleable base, e.g., glycol, to facilitate insertion into a body cavity); should be refrigerated	Laxatives, etc.

Continued.

TABLE 3-1 Various forms of drug preparations—cont'd

Form	Examples/remarks
Miscellaneous drug delivery systems (examples)	
Intradermal implants	
Pellets containing a small deposit of medication inserted in a dermal pocket; designed to allow medication to leach slowly into tissue	Testosterone Estradiol
Micropump system	
Small external pump attached by belt that delivers medication by needle (e.g., insulin) in a continuous steady dose	
Membrane delivery systems	
Drug-laden polymer membrane installed in the conjunctival fornix of the eye to deliver a steady flow of medication (e.g., pilocarpine, corticosteroids, or other)	
Pessaries and IUDs	
Drug enveloped or impregnated within the device for slow release of medication (e.g., hormones, copper, or other substance) to prevent contraception, etc.	
Common additives to drug preparations (inactive ingredients; excipients)	
Preservatives (none in some medications because they inactivate the drug)	Chloroform, benzoic acid
pH stabilizers	
Bacteriostatic agents	
Diluents as "fillers" where the drug dose is too small to work with	Sterile water, normal saline, bacteriostatic water, dextrose, lactose, starch, bentonite, kaolin, Fuller's Earth
Binding agents provide adhesion to a powdered drug	Acacia gum, methylcellulose
Lubricants prevent the drug product from sticking to the machinery in formulation of tablets, etc.	Starch, lactose
Disintegrators to facilitate dissolution of product when appropriate	Starch (expands when exposed to water), sodium bicarbonate
Coatings	Gels, gums, waxes
Flavoring	Sugar or chocolate
Coloring	Dyes

air and light each time the door is opened. The need to maintain a cool temperature of these specific drugs does not end when they are to be administered; for example, if given by too slow an intravenous infusion, their effectiveness is similarly undermined.

Even room temperature may be subject to radical changes that may go unobserved. Storage of medications on a window sill may subject them to late afternoon sun. This same storage spot may seem safe in the summer but actually subject the medication to high radiator heat in the winter.

Amber colored containers are necessary to protect some medications against deterioration by light (such as furosemide and nitroglycerin). This fact and its significance should be pointed out to patients who are self-medicating and who might otherwise transfer medications to a different container (to take to work, on vaca-

tion, and the like). Storage in a closed cabinet or other dark place should also be advised. If feasible, patients should be given information about how to tell if their medication has deteriorated (nitroglycerin no longer tingles under the tongue), and they should be told that the medication may need replacement if storage requirements have been abridged or if the medication's appearance or effects have changed.

Tight lids can prevent degradation or change of the drug form or its active constituents by preventing exchange of moisture or gases within the container.

Patients who store drugs at home should be reminded that they *must* be stored out of reach of children. The child under 5 is an insatiably curious little being who may mimic adults' drug-taking behavior. The drug's childproof cap may only serve to slow the child down.

The expiration dates as printed on drug

labels mean simply that the drug contained is probably at its peak effectiveness until some point in time around that date. Since quality controls in drug production are subject to error rates similar to all other control programs, pharmaceutical companies tend to estimate these expiration dates somewhat conservatively. This does not mean that the drug is instantly rendered useless or harmful by that date. It does mean that effectiveness of the therapy may be gradually diminished and give inadequate or occasionally toxic results some time after the printed date. The nurse should not administer doses from that lot of drug or container; a fresh supply must be obtained.

When ordering drugs for the day, the nurse should keep in mind those medications with limited stability times and special storage requirements. The nurse needs to anticipate those medications that have expired so that a fresh supply of the drug is available when needed. There is usually a lag time between the recognition of a low stock of drugs, reordering, and delivery, and these time factors must be kept in mind.

When the drugs are received, they should be checked against the order and for broken or defective containers, cloudy solutions, unusual color or odor, and sediment. Expiration dates should also be checked.

Summary of nursing considerations

The same drug may be known by a variety of names: the *chemical* name, which describes the precise chemical constitution of the drug; the *generic* or *nonproprietary* name, usually simpler than but similar to the *chemical* name; and the *trade, brand,* or *proprietary* name(s) registered by the manufacturers.

Drugs are derived from four principal sources: (1) plants, (2) animals, (3) minerals or mineral products, and (4) chemical substances made in the laboratory. Pharmaceutically active compounds found in plants include alkaloids, glycosides, gums, resins and balsams, and volatile and fixed oils.

Knowledge of the kinds of pharmaceutical preparations available is essential to competent drug administration. *Aqueous solutions* contain one or more substances dissolved in water and include waters, true solutions, and syrups. *Aqueous suspensions* are finely divided drugs in suspension in a suitable liquid vehicle. Among these are mixtures, emulsions, magmas, and gels.

Spirits are concentrated alcoholic solutions of volatile substances, also known as essences. *Elixirs* are aromatic, sweetened alcoholic preparations. *Tinctures* are alcoholic or hydroalcoholic solutions usually prepared from plant drugs or from chemical substances. *Fluidextracts* are alcoholic liquid extracts of vegetable drugs in which 1 ml of the fluidextract contains 1 g of the drug. *Extracts* are concentrated preparations of vegetable or animal drugs obtained by removing the active ingredients of the drugs with suitable solvents and then evaporating all or part of the solvents.

Drugs and mixtures of drugs are available in various dosage forms. *Capsules* are usually of gelatin and range in size from 5 to 000. *Sustained-release capsules* contain small particles of a drug coated with materials that require varying amounts of time to dissolve. *Tablets* are preparations of powdered drug compressed or molded into small disks. *Troches* or *lozenges* are flat, round, or rectangular preparations held in the mouth until they dissolve. *Pills* are mixtures of a drug or drugs with some cohesive material, molded into globular, oval, or flattened bodies convenient for swallowing. *Powders* are finely divided solid drugs or mixtures of drugs. *Ampules* are sealed glass containers, usually holding only one dose of a drug intended for injection. *Vials* are glass containers holding a number of doses of an injectable drug. Prefilled, *disposable syringes* have become the most popular form for injectable drugs. *Large-volume intravenous solutions, intermittent intravenous solutions,* and *direct intravenous injections* have become major modes of drug therapy in the institutional setting.

Drops are aqueous solutions used for eye, ear, and nose preparations. *Aerosols* and *foams* have been useful in drug delivery for bronchial and vaginal disorders.

Liniments are liquid suspensions or dispersions intended for external application by rubbing on the skin to relieve pain and swelling. *Lotions* are also liquid suspensions or dispersions for external application but should be *patted* on the skin and can be protective, emollient, cooling, cleansing, astringent, or antipruritic. *Creams* are emulsions used to soothe or moisturize skin.

Ointments are semisolid preparations of medicinal substances in a base such as petrolatum and lanolin, intended for external application to the skin or mucous membranes for soothing, astringent, or bacteriostatic effects.

Pastes are ointment-like preparations that do not melt at body temperature. *Plasters* are solid preparations that serve as simple adhesives or counterirritants.

Suppositories are mixtures of drugs with a firm base, molded into shapes suitable for insertion into body cavities—rectal, vaginal, or urethral. *Poultices* are soft, moist preparations designed to supply moist heat to a skin area.

Newer drug delivery systems have also been developed. Other accessories to pharmaceutical formulations are colorings, preservatives, pH stabilizers, "fillers," flavorings, and others.

Drug stability and storage are important factors to monitor in the nursing process. Nursing responsibilities include proper storage, ordering to ensure availability, and proper and safe drug administration.

QUESTIONS

FOR STUDY AND REVIEW

1 What is meant by the generic name of a drug? How does it differ from a trade name?
2 What is the advantage of labeling drugs with both their generic and trade names?
3 Through library research determine which commonly used drugs must still be obtained from plant sources; from animals. Explain why.
4 Describe an important characteristic of suspensions.
5 Differentiate between the various medicinal preparations that contain alcohol.
6 What advantages, if any, do capsules have over tablets?
7 What is meant by an enteric-coated tablet? What is the purpose of the enteric coating?
8 What purpose is served by sustained-release dosage forms of drugs?
9 What is the difference between an ampule and a vial?

BIBLIOGRAPHY

Bowman, W.C., and Rand, M.J.: Textbook of pharmacology, Oxford, England, 1980, Blackwell Scientific Publications.

DiPalma, J.R., editor: Drill's pharmacology in medicine, ed. 4, New York, 1980, McGraw-Hill Book Co.

Goodman, L.S., and Gillman, A., editors: The pharmacological basis of therapeutics, New York, 1980, MacMillan, Inc.

Hallister, L.E.: Studies of delayed action medication, N. Engl. J. Med. **266**:281, 1962.

Nursing '80 Skillbook: Managing I.V. Therapy, Horsham, Pa., 1980, Intermed. Communications.

Osol, A., and others, editors: Remington's pharmaceutical sciences, ed. 15, Easton, Pa., 1975, Mack Printing Co.

Sager, D.P., and Bomar, S.K.: Intravenous medications, Philadelphia, 1980, J.B. Lippincott, Inc.

Sprowis, J.B., editor: American pharmacy; an introduction to pharmaceutical techniques and dosage forms, ed. 7, Philadelphia, 1974, J.B. Lippincott Co.

OFFICIAL DRUG COMPENDIA

British Pharmacopoea, ed. 10, London, 1980, The Pharmaceutical Press.

The United States Pharmacopeia and the National Formulary, XX, ed. 15, Rockville, Md., 1980, The United States Pharmacopeial Convention, Inc.

CHAPTER 4

General principles of drug action

Mechanisms of drug action
    Pharmaceutical phase
    Pharmacokinetic phase
    Pharmacodynamic phase
Adverse responses to drugs
Summary of nursing considerations

Because of the constantly increasing number of drugs utilized in medical therapeutics and the nurse's expanded responsibility in this area, it is essential that the nurse have a coherent, rational, and scientifically accurate understanding of the principles underlying pharmacology. The time is long past when anyone can expect to acquire complete knowledge about all drugs. Thousands of drugs exist, requiring that health professionals have some fundamental theoretical framework through which to approach their study and understanding of drug therapy.

Historically, the administration of drugs has been a prominent nursing task. This task, however is changing in nature and prominence. A shift in responsibility is occurring away from the actual administration of drugs to greater responsibility in relation to other aspects of drug therapy. The nurse's expanded role currently includes a variety of functions, all of which are predicated on a sound understanding of drug action. In many health care delivery settings, for example, the nurse is no longer the primary administrator and dispenser of drugs. In such settings, the nurse's responsibility has shifted to assuring safe administration of drugs by a variety of specially educated health workers and to observing and interpreting the patient's response to drug therapy. However, the moral, ethical, and legal responsibility of drug administration remains the nurse's. In

addition, other nursing roles in relation to drug therapy have been developed and expanded. Today, more than before, nurses have the responsibility of *teaching* patients about the drugs they are receiving. They have a *data-gathering role* in relation to the patient's previous drug therapy and present and past responses to drug therapy, as exemplified in the function of obtaining a drug history from the patient. They are *decision-makers* regarding p.r.n. medications. By virtue of their interpersonal skills, they may also function as *potentiators* of drug effects. Nurses are *communicators* of knowledge and observations to other health care professionals, notably to the physician who prescribes drug therapy. There is also a change in nurses' roles in relation to drug prescriptions. In some states nurse practice acts have been changed to give nurse practitioners limited authority in the prescribing of drugs.

These responsibilities require more than memorization of specific drugs, their actions, and their dosages. Rather, their effective implementation depends on a sound comprehension of the theories of drug action, knowledge the nurse can transfer to the individual patient with a specific diagnosis and definable, individualistic needs. Such a background necessitates knowledge of theories of drug action, physiologic processes mediating drug action, variables affecting drug action, and unusual and adverse responses to drug therapy.

Mechanisms of drug action

In order to produce its optimal desired or therapeutic effects, a drug must reach appropriate concentrations at its sites of action. This means that the molecules of the chemical compound must proceed from their point of entry into the body to the vicinity of the tissues with which they react. The concentration that the drug attains at its site of action is influenced by various processes, which may be divided into three phases of drug activity: (1) pharmaceutical phase, (2) pharmacokinetic phase, and (3) pharmacodynamic phase. The sequential order of these phases occur as shown in Fig. 4-1.

PHARMACEUTICAL PHASE

Disintegration and solubility. In order to be absorbed, a drug must be in solution. Oral drugs given in liquid form, being already in solution, are generally more rapidly available for absorption than those given in solid form (capsule or tablet). After ingestion, a solid drug must first disintegrate and then be readily soluble in the gastrointestinal fluids. Thus the drug form is important, for the more rapid the rate of dissolution of a drug, the greater will be the rate of absorption. (See Fig. 4-2.)

PHARMACOKINETIC PHASE

Pharmacokinetics is the study of the movement of drug molecules in the body in relation to its absorption, distribution, metabolism, and excretion. The concentration the drug attains at its site of action is influenced by four primary factors: (1) the rate and extent to which the drug is *absorbed* into body fluids; (2) the rate and extent to which the drug is transported or *distributed* to sites of action or storage in the body; (3) the rate and extent to which the drug is *biologically transformed* or *metabolized* in the

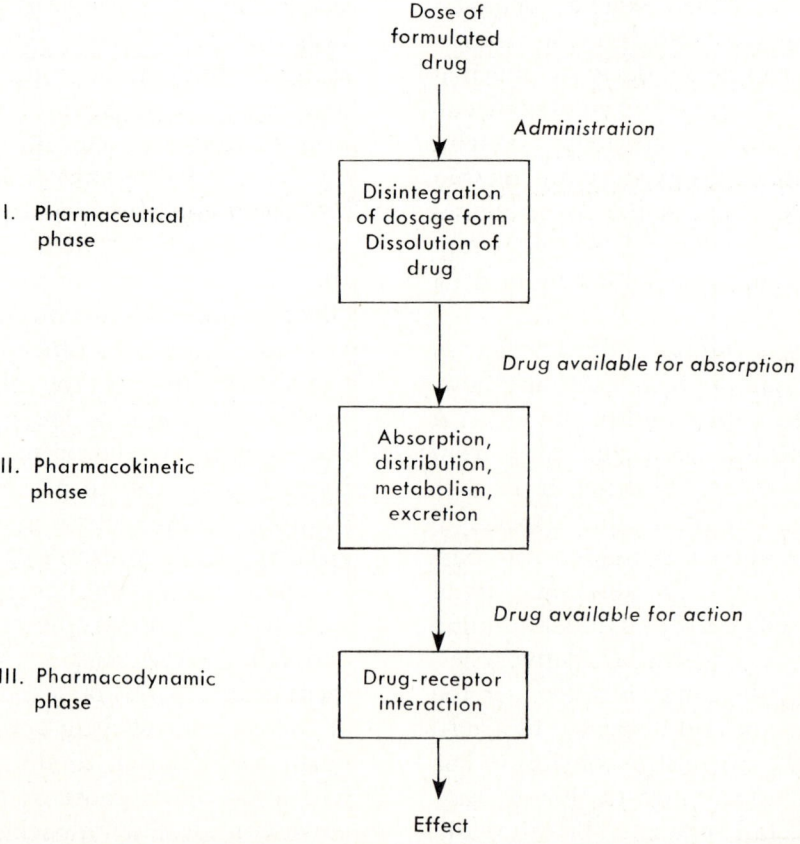

FIG. 4-1. Three phases of drug activity. (Modified from Ariens, E.J., and Simonis, A.M.: Molecular pharmacology. New York, 1964, Academic Press, Inc.; from Bowman, W.C., and Rand, M.J.: Textbook of pharmacology, ed. 2, London, 1980, Blackwell Scientific Publications.)

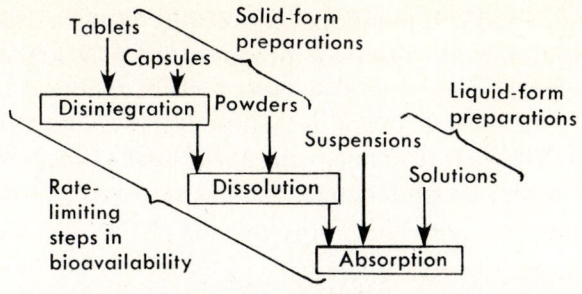

FIG. 4-2. Preparations for oral administration. (From Bowman, W.C., and Rand, M.J.: Textbook of pharmacology, ed. 2, London, 1980, Blackwell Scientific Publications.)

body to breakdown products; and (4) the rate and extent to which the drug is *excreted* from the body by various routes.

Drug molecules free to move to sites of action are transported from one body compartment to another by way of the plasma. However, free movement may be somewhat limited because these various sites are enclosed by membranes. Barriers to drug transport may be a single layer of cells, as in intestinal epithelium, or several layers of cells, such as that of the skin. Nevertheless, in order for the drug to gain access to the interior of a cell or a body compartment, it has to penetrate cell membranes. Despite structural differences, the drugs do manage to cross these boundaries by one of two mechanisms: passive transport or active transport.

Passive transport. Drugs may act at the outer membrane surface or inside the cell. Cell membrane, which consists of lipids and proteins, is penetrated at intervals by aqueous channels or pores through which small water-soluble molecules (dimensions smaller than those of the pores) and ions (such as K^+ and Cl^-) pass; this process is called *filtration*. Lipid-soluble molecules, like those in anesthetic gases, diffuse readily through cell membranes, a process called *simple diffusion*. The higher the lipid/water coefficient, the greater its lipid solubility and the greater the ease with which the drug moves from the fluids outside the cells into the lipid material in the cell membrane. *Facilitated diffusion* is a carrier-mediated transport in which a compound is not moving against a concentration gradient, and energy

source is not required. Glucose, for example, is transported into most cells by this process. Transport is facilitated by attachment to a carrier in the membrane, and the release of the molecule into the cell makes the carrier available for transport of other molecules. Thus all these various forms of diffusion represent passive transport of drugs.

Active transport. Moderate sized water-soluble molecules as well as moderate sized ions, including the ionic form of most drugs, do not readily enter cells but require some means of transport. *Active transport* is believed to be conducted by "carriers" that form complexes with drug molecules on one surface of the membrane, carry them through the membrane, and then dissociate from them. Active transport requires an energy source and involves the movement of drug molecules against the concentration gradient (from areas of low concentration to areas of high concentration) or, in the case of ions, against the electrochemical potential gradient such as occurs with the "sodium pump." Active transport is usually more rapid than passive diffusion.

All of the physiologic processes mediating drug action—absorption, distribution, metabolism, and excretion—are predicated on these two transport processes.

Absorption

Absorption refers to the process by which a drug is transferred from its site of entry into the body to the circulating fluids of the body, the bloodstream and the lymphatic system. With the exception of locally acting drugs, all drugs must reach the bloodstream in order to be carried to their sites of action. Absorption of the drug from its site of administration is largely influenced by the following factors.

Routes of drug administration. A drug may enter the circulatory system either by being injected there directly—for example, intravenously—or by absorption from depots in which it has been placed. The routes of drug entry into the body can be classified into three categories: the enteral (drugs administered via any portion of the gastrointestinal tract), the parenteral (drugs administered by routes that bypass the gastrointestinal tract and that are generally given by injection, thereby avoiding the necessity for absorption across a mucosal barrier), and the percutaneous (drugs absorbed from mucous membranes, either through sublingual administration or by inhalation).

Generally, the oral route of drug administration is the safest, most convenient, and most economical method of drug administration. However, the frequent changes of the gastrointestinal environment produced by food, emotion, and physical activity make it the most unreliable and slowest of the commonly used routes in terms of both the amount and the rate of drug absorption. Generally, slowing the gastric emptying rate will decrease drug absorption and vice versa. This is why so many drugs are administered on an empty stomach with sufficient water to ensure their rapid passage into the small intestine, where drug absorption is usually increased because of the larger surface area available to the dissolving drug. An additional limitation of the oral route of administration is that this route cannot be used for drugs that are susceptible to alteration by the biochemical processes involved in digestion. Insulin, for example, is destroyed by the digestive enzymes and must be administered by parenteral routes if it is to be absorbed. Drugs administered sublingually or rectally are not changed by the digestive processes, but sublingual drugs must be readily soluble and depend on the patient's ability to cooperate, while drug retention is frequently unpredictable with rectal administration. Parenteral administration affords relatively rapid drug absorption since the drugs bypass the epithelial barrier. Absorption from these sites is more reliable than from enteral routes. The intravenous route of administration completely bypasses the process of absorption, and this route represents the most rapid means of introducing drugs into the bloodstream. Inhalation drugs, such as gaseous drugs or aerosol drugs, are also rapidly absorbed from the respiratory tract or alveolar surfaces.

Drug solubility. As already discussed, in order to be absorbed, a drug must be in solution. The more soluble the drug the more rapidly it will be absorbed. Moreover, because cell membranes contain a fatty acid layer, lipid solubility is a valuable attribute of a drug that is to be absorbed from the alimentary tract; this attribute is also necessary for drugs to cross the placental barrier. Because the skin has a lipid barrier, topically applied drugs are poorly absorbed, if at all. However, if this lipid barrier of the skin is altered—for example, by cuts, abrasions, or burns—toxic drug dosage may result. Chemicals and minerals that form insoluble precipitates in the gastrointestinal tract, such as barium salts, or drugs that are not soluble in water or lipids cannot be absorbed. Parenterally administered drugs prepared in oily vehicles, such as streptomycin, will be absorbed more slowly than drugs dissolved in water or isotonic sodium chloride.

Influence of pH. When in solution, drugs are a mixture of ionized and nonionized forms. Nonionized drug is lipid soluble and diffusible (referred to as *nonionic diffusion*); ionized drug is lipid insoluble and nondiffusible. The proportion of drug in the nonionized form depends on the dissociation constant of the drug (pK_a) and on the pH of the medium in which it is dissolved. Most drugs are weak acids or bases. In aqueous solutions drugs that are acid produce hydrogen ions (H^+); drugs that are bases produce hydroxyl ions (OH^-). A drug that is acidic tends to dissociate less in an acid medium while a drug that is a base will dissociate to a greater extent in an acid medium. The reverse occurs when the drugs are in an alkaline medium.

In the stomach the pH is low (about 1.4), and drugs such as the barbiturates, which are slightly acidic, tend to remain in a nonionized state and thus are readily absorbed from this area. Morphine and quinine are slightly basic; they tend to ionize in the stomach and thus are poorly absorbed from this area. The neutralization of the stomach contents by giving sodium bicarbonate may facilitate the absorption of basic drugs in the stomach.

In the intestines the pH is higher (6 to 8). Nonionized basic drugs will tend to remain nonionized and be readily absorbed in this area while the reverse is true for acidic drugs. Plasma pH is about 7.4, and only drugs that are substantially nonionized in this pH will be widely distributed.

Urinary pH varies between 4.6 and 8.2 and affects the amount of drug reabsorbed in the renal tubule by passive diffusion. Weak acids are excreted more readily in alkaline urine and more slowly in acidic urine; the reverse is true for weak bases. In cases of poisoning by aspirin or phenobarbital, alkalinizing the urine can result in increased urinary drug excretion. However, acidifying or alkalinizing urine to promote drug excretion is seldom of great importance.

Local conditions at the site of administration. These local conditions include circulation to the site and the area of the absorbing surface. Generally, the more extensive the absorbing surface, the greater the absorption of the drug and the more rapid its effects. For example, anesthetics are very rapidly absorbed from the pulmonary epithelium because of its vast surface area and its vascularity. Circulation to the site of administration is also a significant factor in the absorption of parenteral drugs. A patient in shock, for example, may not respond to intramuscularly administered drugs because of poor peripheral circulation. Drugs injected intravenously, on the other hand, are placed directly into the circulatory system and are totally absorbed. This route of administration is desirable when speedy drug effects are necessary, but it carries the potential danger of achieving temporarily toxic effects in vital organs such as the heart or the brain.

Circulation to the site of administration can also be externally manipulated in order to hasten or retard the rate of drug absorption. Local cooling of the site will hinder absorption, as will the application of a tourniquet proximally to the injection site. On the other hand, applying heat or friction to the site of administration will hasten absorption.

Drug concentration or dosage. Drugs administered in high concentrations or dosages are more rapidly absorbed than drugs administered in low concentrations. In certain situations, a drug may be initially administered in large doses that temporarily exceed the body's

capacity for excretion of the drug. In this way, active drug levels are rapidly reached at the receptor site. Once an active drug level is established by such cumulation of effects, smaller daily doses of the drug can be administered to replace only the amount of the drug excreted since the previous dose. The initial and temporary overloading doses of the drug are *priming doses*, while the smaller daily doses are *maintenance doses*. Such manipulation of drug dosage is frequently used, for example, with digitalis and steroid preparations in acute situations.

Bioavailability. Bioavailability refers to the proportion of active principles in a drug that is absorbed and available to exert a systemic effect. Different brands of the same drug can vary, and even different lots of preparations from a single manufacturer may show discrepancy in its effectivenss. Thus the Food and Drug Administration is paying more attention to this aspect of drug preparation. The goal is to ensure that the bioavailability of a drug conforms to uniform standards. Both the proportion of active drug in the preparation and the percentage of its absorption are essential for attaining therapeutic equivalence of all chemically similar drugs.

Another way in which drug concentration can be manipulated is by pharmaceutical processing. It is possible to combine an active drug with a resin or another substance from which it is only slowly released or to prepare a drug in a vehicle that offers relative resistance to the digestive action of stomach contents (enteric coating). Enteric coatings on drugs are used for the following reasons: (1) to prevent decomposition of chemically sensitive drugs, (2) to prevent dilution of the drug before it reaches the intestine, (3) to prevent nausea and vomiting, and (4) to provide delayed action of the drug. Capsule forms of drugs are absorbed more rapidly than tablets because the powder inside capsules affords a larger surface area than the compressed tablet. Repository dosage forms are produced by suspension of a drug in a substance from which it is slowly released, producing uniform drug absorption for at least 8 hours or longer. For example, protamine zinc insulin is suspended in protamine for slow, sustained release so that its duration of action is 24 to 36 hours. Drug "Spansules" are gelatin capsules containing drug pellets having different coatings designed for timed release of the drug contained within. Advantages of this dosage form include decreased frequency of administration and prolonged maintenance of therapeutic effects. Disadvantages are related to possible failure of the sustained release mechanism, which could result in release of unexpectedly high and toxic levels of the drug or in therapeutically inadequate levels.

Distribution

After a drug is absorbed or injected into the bloodstream, it is distributed throughout the body by means of the circulation. Drug distribution is the transport of a drug across cell membranes, resulting in accumulations of the drug in certain tissues. The rate of entry of a drug into the various tissues of the body depends on the relative rate of perfusion and the permeability of the capillaries for the particular drug molecules. The distribution may be general or restricted. Some drugs cannot pass particular cell membranes and are restricted in their distribution, while other drugs, such as ethyl alcohol, can eventually be found in solution in all body fluids.

Plasma binding. Differential distribution of drugs may result from the binding of a drug to plasma proteins and from the unequal passage of a drug across biologic membranes, most notably into the central nervous system and the placenta. The same kinds of bonds that are formed when a drug interacts with its receptor can be formed between drug molecules and other macromolecular tissue components. The difference in these bonds is that the drug-receptor combination leads to drug action, while binding with a nonreceptor substance does not. Binding of drugs can occur at sites of absorption, in plasma, or at extravascular sites, but *the proteins of plasma appear to be the most common site of drug binding. Albumin is the protein with which the greatest variety of drugs combine.* The binding of drugs decreases the concentration of free drug in circulation and prevents the drug from reaching its site of action in full concentrations. As the free drug is eliminated from

the body more drug can be dissociated from the protein to replace what is lost.

Hypoalbuminemia. Hypoalbuminemia occurs in patients who have a low level of plasma protein caused by hepatic damage or some type of body cavity drainage. Patients who require drugs that are dependent on protein binding for distribution generally receive albumin replacement. The drug dosage in the meantime is adjusted until the normal level of the plasma protein (the vehicle for drug distribution) is restored.

Storage reservoirs. Other tissues of the body can also act as reservoirs, or depots, for drugs. Some drugs have preferential sites of accumulation in certain tissues. For example, body fat has a high affinity for some drugs, such as thiopentone. Another common site of drug accumulation is muscle, which may be considered as a storage depot for a drug. The stored drug is in equilibrium with the amount of drug contained in plasma and is released as plasma levels are reduced. Consequently, plasma levels of the drug are maintained for longer periods and, therefore, pharmacologic effects are predicated on the administration of initially adequate priming doses in order to saturate the storage depots or binding sites.

Distribution barriers. In relation to the passage of drugs into the central nervous system, it has long been noted that many drugs fail to penetrate into those tissues as readily as into other tissues. This phenomenon has led to the conceptualization of a *blood-brain barrier.* Currently, this concept is undergoing scrutiny, and recent research indicates that what has been termed the "blood-brain barrier" is not an absolute barrier. It has been postulated that it is a quantitative rather than a qualitative difference in capillary permeability as compared with other tissues. Still, the fact remains that the distribution of some drugs will be more readily achieved into other parts of the body than into the central nervous system. There is a very slow rate of entry of water-soluble and ionized drugs, such as penicillin, into the brain and spinal cord. Lipid-soluble compounds, on the other hand, enter the brain easily and rapidly. Moreover, some drugs that have no effects on the central nervous system when administered systemically have striking effects when injected directly into the cerebrospinal fluid.

Passage of drugs across the *placenta to the fetus* is a well-established fact. Again, lipid-soluble substances diffuse across the placenta readily and other substances are assisted by energy-coupled specific transport systems. Some drugs that are easily transported across the placenta include steroids, narcotics, anesthetics, various teratogenic agents, and some antibiotics. The rate of maternal blood flow to the placenta limits the availability of the drug to the fetus. This explains why an alert infant can be delivered to an anesthetized mother, provided that delivery occurs within 10 to 15 minutes after the drug is administered to the mother. Long-term administration of drugs to the mother, however, may produce adverse effects on the fetus. For example, infants born to mothers dependent on narcotics will manifest withdrawal symptoms when the infants are no longer supplied with these drugs after delivery. *Teratogenic effect* of drugs pertains to exposure of the pregnant woman to certain toxic agents that cause physical defects in the embryo, especially during early stages of fetal development. Many drugs can be found in breast milk and may be potentially harmful to infants.

Metabolism (biotransformation)

The liver is the primary site of metabolism of drugs, but other tissues may also be involved in this process.

Hepatic first-pass elimination. Drugs absorbed from the gastrointestinal tract into the bloodstream will travel first to the portal system and the liver before reaching the systemic circulation. As a result, a drug may be taken up by the liver cells and metabolized. Loss of drug on passage through the liver from the bloodstream is called *hepatic first-pass effect*. Because drugs such as lidocaine and morphine have such extensive first-pass metabolism, these agents cannot be given orally. In some cases, the first-pass effect may result in complete elimination of the drug. Parenteral administration is used to prevent this occurrence.

Hepatic metabolism. Most drugs, once absorbed, are distributed to their sites of action and then undergo metabolic changes or biotransformation. This process, which usually takes place in the liver, converts the drug into products that are generally less active and more water soluble. Hence these compounds are more easily excreted than the original form. For example, most drugs are fat soluble, but the kidney excretes water-soluble compounds; therefore, one function of metabolism is to convert lipid-soluble drugs to water-soluble products.

Detoxication has often been used to describe the metabolism of drugs, but it is not an optimally accurate conceptualization of the process. The term implies that all drugs are toxic to the body and that all are metabolized to less toxic products, which is not always the case. Although most types of biotransformation result in inactivation of a drug, occasionally the result of this metabolic process is a more active compound that requires further biotransformation before being excreted. For example, the active ingredient of chloral hydrate is its metabolite, which must then undergo a second reaction to facilitate its excretion. In addition, drugs may be changed to other chemical forms or inactivated before excretion. In other instances, drugs may be excreted from the body unchanged, as is the case with ether, for example.

The chemical alterations of biotransformation are produced by enzyme systems in the blood and in all body cells, but particularly those of the liver. The hepatic enzyme systems responsible for the biotransformation of many drugs seem to be located in the hepatic endoplasmic reticulum and are generally called microsomes, because they are located in the microsomal fraction of the liver. These hepatic microsomal enzymes effect the process of biotransformation through two general classes of chemical reactions: the synthetic and the nonsynthetic. The synthetic chemical reactions, also called *coupling* or *conjugation*, involve the union of the drug (or its metabolite) with another substance. This chemical reaction produces a soluble, inactive product that is readily excreted. Nonsynthetic chemical reactions of drug metabolism include oxidation, hydrolysis, or reduction, which can result in activation, a change in activity, or inactivation of a drug.

Research indicates that drug metabolism can be depressed or stimulated. Depression of the microsomal drug-metabolizing system can be produced by conditions that have a deleterious effect on hepatic function, such as starvation and obstructive jaundice. Individuals with any type of hepatic disease, severe cardiovascular disease, or renal disease may be expected to have prolonged drug metabolism. Immaturity of drug-metabolizing enzymes in infants and degeneration of these enzymes in the aged also produce depression of biotransformation. In addition, some drugs are known to inhibit the metabolism of other drugs when they are administered simultaneously. If metabolism of drugs is delayed, cumulative drug effects may be expected and may be manifested as excessive or prolonged responses to ordinary doses of drugs. Stimulation of drug metabolism, on the other hand, may produce a state of apparent drug tolerance. A number of substances are also known to cause an increase in the activity of hepatic microsomal drug-metabolizing enzymes. These include CNS depressants, xanthines, pesticides, food preservatives, and dyes. It is possible that repeated administration of some drugs stimulates the formation of new microsomal enzymes. This is thought to be the case with some hypnotic drugs, whose effect diminishes with prolonged administration.

Biotransformation of drugs does not occur exclusively in the liver. The plasma, the kidneys, the lungs, and the intestinal mucosa also contain enzymes and function to metabolize drugs, although to a lesser degree.

Excretion

A drug continues to act in the body until it is changed or excreted. Drug molecules, intact, changed, or inactivated, ultimately must be removed from their sites of action by the physiologic channels and mechanisms of excretion. The lungs are the major organs of excretion for gaseous substances such as some alcohols and anesthetics. The most important route of excretion for nonvolatile substances, however, is the kidney. Some drug metabolites are also excreted through the intestines via the feces, but the liver, through its secretion of bile into the small intestine, contributes to the major portion of material excreted in this manner. Many of these drug metabolites are also reabsorbed into the blood and excreted in the urine.

Some drugs are excreted almost unchanged in the urine, while other drugs are so extensively metabolized that only a small fraction of the original chemical substance is excreted in intact form. Other routes of drug elimination include the nursing mother's milk, perspiration, tears, and saliva, although the last three constitute relatively unimportant routes.

Drugs may also be eliminated through the use of extracorporeal dialysis, which was originally designed to substitute for renal function in cases of severe but temporary renal shutdown. Overdosage of drugs may lead to just such a situation. By an artificial process resembling glomerular filtration, dialysis can achieve rapid reduction of high plasma levels of the drug. As a general rule, substances that are completely or almost completely excreted by the normal kidney can be removed by hemodialysis. Such substances include some CNS stimulants and depressants, some nonnarcotic analgesics, and some metals.

Excretion via the kidneys remains by far the most important route of drug elimination. This process is accomplished through passive glomerular filtration, active tubular secretion, and partial reabsorption. The availability of a drug for glomerular filtration depends on its concentration in unbound form in plasma. Some drugs are cleared by tubular secretion and all of the drug, bound and free, becomes available for active secretion. The renal excretory mechanisms, then, have the net effect of removing the amount of free drug that is brought to the kidneys by the renal arterial blood.

There are several factors that influence the rate of drug excretion. Prerequisite to successful excretion is the maintenance of effective physiologic mechanisms of distribution (the circulatory system) and excretion (kidney and bowel function, respiratory function, and sweating). Immaturity or deterioration of the renal system, for example, will influence the rate of drug excretion. In newborn infants, whose renal tubular secretory mechanisms are incompletely developed, and in individuals with renal dysfunction, drug elimination is severely hampered and drug toxicity may result. The rate at which the drug is presented to the kidney and the rate of glomerular filtration also influence the rate of excretion.

Biologic half-life. Excretion and metabolism determine the biologic half-life of a drug. (The half-life of a drug is the amount of time required for the plasma level concentration of the drug to decrease to 50% of the original concentration.) This half-life will not change with the drug dose; it will always take the same amount of time to eliminate one half of the drug present in the body. If, for example, 10,000 units of a drug is administered and that drug has a half-life of 4 hours, then 5000 units of the drug will be excreted in 4 hours. In the next 4 hours, 2500 units will be excreted, with 1250 units more excreted in the third 4-hour period.

PHARMACODYNAMIC PHASE

Pharmacodynamics is the study of biochemical and physiologic effects of drugs and their mechanisms of action on living tissue. As such, it is concerned with the response of tissues to specific chemical agents at various sites in the body.

The effects of drugs can be recognized only by alterations of a known physiologic function or process. That is, drugs *modify* physiologic activity but *cannot confer any new function* on a tissue or organ in the body. Alteration in function is achieved by drugs that can *replace, interrupt,* or *potentiate* a physiologic process in specialized tissues. For example, drugs used to treat anemia can *replace* iron deficiency and restore the adequate production of red blood cells. On the other hand, atropine can *interrupt* the rate of salivation in preoperative patients, which is an essentially abnormal state but a necessary one to decrease the surgical risk of aspiration. Finally, the administration of a cathartic can *potentiate* the rate of evacuation of the large intestine.

When a drug enters a living system, one can think of its molecules immediately beginning to react with the molecules of the cells and tissues with which it comes in contact. The effects a drug produces must be regarded as ultimate consequences of complex physical and chemical interactions between the drug and molecules in the living organism. The goal of all drug therapy is to attain a therapeutic effect in a patient, but in some instances adverse reactions to the compound are manifested.

Theories of drug action

The means by which drugs produce an alteration in function at its site of action is known as their *mechanism of action.* The mechanism of action of most compounds is believed to involve a chemical interaction between the drug and a functionally important component of the living system. Most drugs produce their effects by one of the following ways:

1 Selectively combining with specific cellular sites called *receptors*
2 Interacting with *enzyme systems*
3 Effecting a change caused by *physicochemical properties*

Receptor theory. Structural specificity is an essential postulate of the receptor theory of drug action. Receptor theory hypothesizes that drugs are selectively active substances that have a special affinity for certain chemical groups or parts of cells and not for others. That is, drugs act at some sites to produce their characteristic biologic effects, whereas their presence at other cells, tissues, or organs leads to no measurable biologic response. Therefore, receptor theory states that drugs exert their action by becoming attached to specialized regions of a cell. The cellular components with which drugs interact to produce their characteristic biologic effects are called *receptors.* The relationship of a drug to its receptor has often been likened to the fit of a key into a lock. That is, some sort of reciprocal, or *complementary,* relationship exists between the chemical structure of the drug molecule and the drug receptor. The drug must interact by combining or binding with the macromolecular tissue element at the site of action in order to produce its characteristic biologic effects. Therefore, there must be some forces that not only attract the drug to its receptors but also hold it in combination with the receptor long enough to initiate the chain of biochemical reactions leading to the drug effect. It is believed that drug receptor binding may result from the formation of hydrogen, covalent, or ionic bonds or from weak binding forces that operate when any atoms are brought together.

Affinity is used to describe the propensity of a drug to be found at a given receptor site, and *efficacy* is used to describe the drug's ability to initiate biologic activity as a result of such binding. A drug that combines with receptors and initiates a sequence of biochemical and physiologic changes is said to possess both properties and is termed an *agonist*. However, many drugs are *antagonists,* designed to inhibit or counteract effects caused by other drugs or undesired effects caused by cellular components during illness. A *competitive antagonist* has an affinity for the same receptor site as an agonist; the competition with the agonist for the site inhibits the action of the agonist; increasing the concentration of the agonist tends to overcome the inhibition. Competitive inhibition responses are usually reversible. A *noncompetitive antagonist* combines with different parts of the receptor mechanism and inactivates the receptor so that the agonist cannot be effective regardless of its concentration. Noncompetitive antagonist effects are considered to be irreversible or nearly so. *Partial agonists* have affinity and some efficacy but may antagonize the action of other drugs that have greater efficacy. Not infrequently, antagonists share some structural similarities with their agonists.

Drug enzyme interaction theory. Because of some basic similarities between the receptor theory and theories of enzymatic action, many drugs are thought to produce their effects by combining with enzymes. Those drugs that are believed to combine with enzymes are thought to do so by virtue of their structural resemblance to an enzyme's substrate molecule (the substance acted upon by an enzyme). A drug may resemble an enzyme's substrate so closely that it may combine with the enzyme instead of with the normal substrate. Drugs resembling enzyme substrates are termed *antimetabolites* and can either block normal enzymatic action or result in the production of other substances with unique biochemical properties. The enzyme, then, becomes the receptor for the drug. However, while enzymes may be receptors, not all receptors are enzymes.

Rate theory of drug action. The rate theory assumes that the most important factor determining drug action is the rate at which drug-receptor combinations take place. It postulates that if a drug-receptor complex dissociates rapidly, it has high efficacy. Conversely, if there is slow dissociation, there is firm binding, prolonged occupancy, and low efficacy. Therefore drug antagonism is associated with slow kinetics and drug agonism with fast kinetics.

The validity of rate theory is controversial at this time, although it does explain drug phenomena in quantitative as well as qualitative terms.

Physicochemical theory. Some drugs demonstrate no structural specificity and presumably act by more general effects on cell membranes and cellular processes. These drugs may penetrate into cells or accumulate in cellular membranes where they interfere, by physical or chemical means, with some cell function or some fundamental metabolic processes.

Cell membranes are complex lipoprotein structures that regulate the flow of ions and metabolites in a highly selective manner, thereby maintaining an electrochemical gradient between the interior and exterior surfaces of the cell. Structurally nonspecific drugs are exemplified by the general anesthetics, which are lipid-soluble compounds of unrelated chemical structure but having similar properties. It is believed that general anesthetics alter the properties of lipids in cell membranes of nerves rather than acting on specific receptors.

Other structurally nonspecific drugs may act by biophysical means that do not affect cellular or enzymatic functions. Drugs acting as a result of their obvious physical properties include the ointments and emollients. Hydrophilic indigestible substances exert a cathartic action because of their physical action on the bowel. The interaction of a molecule like lead with an antidotal drug is a true chemical reaction that produces biologic effects. The neutralization of hydrochloric acid present in gastric juice by antacid drugs is a true chemical reaction that also produces a biologic effect. It is not considered a receptor interaction because there are no macromolecular tissue elements involved. Detergents, alcohol, oxidizing agents such as hydrogen peroxide, and phenol derivatives such as Lysol are also structurally nonspecific and act by irreversibly destroying the functional integrity of the living cell.

Dosage concentration curve

The dosage concentration curve is the curve of intensity of the pharmacologic action of a drug. To attain a therapeutic effect, the concentration of a drug must be high enough to produce the intended pharmacodynamic response. After administration of a single dose, the time course of the amount of drug in the body depends on the rates of administration and elimination. By monitoring the plasma level of a compound, the efficacy and safety of drug therapy can be more closely controlled.

Following a single oral dose, there is a delay in concentration time until the drug is absorbed and the minimum effect of plasma level is reached. (See Fig. 4-3 for time concentration curve.) This indicates the first sign of a drug effect or the *onset of drug action* and signifies the *minimum effective concentration* of the drug. The plasma level than gradually rises until it reaches the *peak level* or the maximum

therapeutic concentration of drug in the plasma. Continued entry of the compound into the body represents the *duration of action*. Thus with a slower rate of absorption, the duration of action will become longer. As the drug disappears from the body, the rate of decline of the plasma level can be seen on the curve. The *rate of elimination* of the drug corresponds to its half-life. In hepatic dysfunction, which interferes with drug metabolism, or in renal disorders, where elimination may be prolonged, the half-life of the drug is lengthened. This usually necessitates an adjustment of drug dosage to a smaller amount. *Cumulation* occurs when drugs are excreted more slowly than absorbed and this condition increases the potential for toxic drug reactions. In this situation, the plasma level may rise until adequate time is given to remove the drug from the body.

The repetitive administration of a drug can produce a rise in plasma concentration until a *steady state* or *plateau* plasma level is reached. A continuous intravenous infusion maintains this type of curve as long as absorption equals drug elimination. An advantage of maintaining a plateau of drug concentration is that the thera-

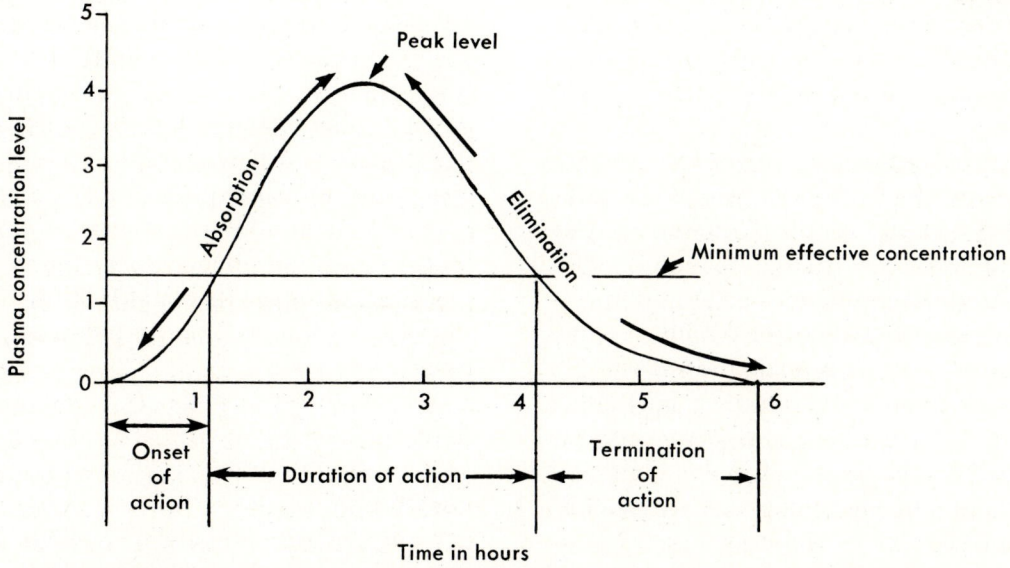

FIG. 4-3. The time-concentration curve correlates the plasma drug level with the therapeutic effectiveness of a drug in time. *Onset of action*—following oral administration, it takes 1 hour until the drug is absorbed and the minimum effective concentration level in the plasma is reached. *Duration of action*—this begins from the time of onset of perceptible effects with continued absorption until the peak level of the drug is reached. This period lasts 3 hours, ending with the decline of the curve, which indicates the elimination of the drug. *Termination of action*—when the plasma level falls below the minimum effective concentration, the drug action is terminated. Time of complete absorption and elimination of drug varies with each compound.

peutic level can be prolonged for a period of time until the infusion is discontinued.

Predictable variables influencing drug action

There are some factors that will alter an individual's response to drug therapy. Deviant drug reactions can frequently be traced to the predictable influence of such variables. It is important for the nurse to be cognizant of factors that modify cell conditions and, therefore, modify the activity of a drug. Some of these factors include the following.

Age. It is generally recognized that children and elderly persons are highly responsive to drugs. Infants often have immature hepatic and renal systems and, therefore, incomplete excretory and metabolic mechanisms. Aged individuals may demonstrate different responses to drug therapy because of deterioration of hepatic and renal function, which is often accompanied by concurrent disease processes, such as cardiovascular disease. Modifications of dosage for children may be calculated as a fraction of the adult dose on the basis of body weight or surface area.

Body mass. The relationship between body mass and amount of drug administered influences the distribution and concentration of a drug. In order to maintain a desired drug concentration in individuals of various sizes, drug dosage must be adjusted in proportion to body mass. For a given dose of drug, the greater the volume of distribution, the lower the concentration of drug reached in various body compartments. Since the volume of interstitial and intracellular water is related to body mass, weight has a marked influence on the quantitative effects produced by drugs. The average adult drug dose is calculated on the basis of the drug quantity that will produce a particular effect in 50% of the population who are between the ages of 18 and 65 and weigh about 150 pounds (70 kg). Therefore, particularly for children and for very lean and for very obese individuals, drug dosage is frequently determined on the basis of amount of drug per kilogram of body weight or body surface area.

Sex. Differential drug effects related to the variable of sex result, in part, from size differences between men and women. Women are usually smaller than men, which will lead to high drug concentrations if dosage is prescribed indifferently. There are also demonstrable differences in relative proportions of fat and water in the bodies of men and women, and some drugs may be more soluble in one or the other. Some authorities also indicate that subjective factors regarding drug effects may vary with sexual differences, stating that women are more suggestible to drug effects than men. This, however, is a controversial hypothesis. Differential drug reactivity by sex is most pronounced during pregnancy, since drugs taken by the pregnant woman might affect the uterus and/or the fetus as a result of placental transfer. As a precaution, the use of drugs is best avoided during pregnancy unless an absolute necessity exists.

Environmental milieu. Drugs affecting mood and behavior are particularly susceptible to the influence of the patient's environment. With such drugs one has to consider effects in light of four factors: (1) the drug itself, (2) the personality of the user, (3) the environment of the user, and (4) the interaction of these three components. Sensory deprivation and sensory overload may also affect responses to drugs. Physical environment may also modify drug effects. For example, temperature affects drug activity: heat relaxes peripheral vessels and so intensifies the actions of vasodilators, while cold has the opposite effect. The relative oxygen deprivation at high altitudes may also increase sensitivity to some drugs.

Time of administration. It is well known that drugs are absorbed more rapidly if the gastrointestinal tract is free of food, while irritating drugs are more readily tolerated if there is food in the stomach.

Although admittedly highly speculative, if findings from drug research on animals are applicable to humans, the time of drug administration in relation to human biologic rhythms can significantly affect the response to various drugs. It seems quite plausible that in humans the sleep-wake rhythm, deep sleep and dreaming sleep cycle, drug-metabolizing enzyme rhythms, corticosteroid secretion rhythm, blood pressure rhythms, as well as circadian (24-hour) variation in absorption and urinary excretion contribute to the effective, ineffective, adverse, or toxic response to particular drugs. There may also be a circadian rhythm in drug receptor susceptibility. Chronopharmacology and chronotoxicology are new areas of interest, and the frequency with which drug rhythm reports are appearing in the literature is increasing. Nurses should make every effort to understand their patient's normal and abnormal rhythms and seek to determine possible relationships between the patient's reactions to drug therapy and his biologic rhythms.

Pathologic state. The presence of a pathologic condition and the severity of symptoms may call for careful consideration of the type of drug administered and for adjustment in dosage. For example, the presence of severe pain tends to increase a patient's requirement for opiates, and an extremely anxious patient can prove resistant to very large doses of tranquilizing and sedating drugs. When aspirin is administered to a patient with a fever, he will respond with a decrease in temperature, whereas a patient taking the drug for its analgesic effects will show no temperature change at all. Larger doses of insulin may be required for the diabetic patient whose condition is complicated by fever or infection. In addition, it bears repeating that the presence of circulatory, hepatic, and/or renal dysfunctions will interfere with the physiologic processes of drug action.

Genetic factors. Genetic differences may alter greatly the response of individuals to a number of drugs. Such differences may arise from genetically conditioned deficiencies in drug metabolism or in receptor sensitivity. These pharmacogenetic abnormalities often manifest themselves as "idiosyncrasies" and may be mistakenly diagnosed as drug allergies. For example, an individual may lack pseudocholinesterase activity in his plasma. If he receives an injection of succinylcholine, which is normally hydrolyzed by plasma cholinesterase, he may remain paralyzed for a long time. The field of pharmacogenetics is of great interest since it may provide a rational explanation for many so-called drug idiosyncrasies.

Psychologic factors. The patient's symbolic investment in drugs and his faith in their effects strongly influence and usually potentiate drug

effects. The placebo effect is an outstanding example of how strong motivation can influence the emergence of desired drug effects. Conversely, hostility and mistrust of medicine and health personnel can diminish drug effects. It is important for nurses to realize that their attitudes and the impressions created at the time of drug administration may influence the therapeutic result.

Adverse responses to drugs

There are many ways in which drugs may react in the body to produce unpredictable, harmful, and somtimes unexplainable responses. No drug is totally safe and absolutely free of toxic effects. Sometimes these effects are immediately apparent. At other times, they may take weeks or months to develop. Some drugs result in aberrant pharmacologic actions when administered individually; other aberrant actions are precipitated by the concurrent administration of certain chemicals. Some adverse reactions to drugs are relatively mild; others can be fatal. With the increasing numbers of drugs being utilized, the incidence of adverse reactions has increased and is presently a significant problem in medical therapeutics.

Untoward effects of drugs can be classified as iatrogenic diseases or as adverse reactions. Generally, iatrogenic diseases refer to groups of adverse effects produced unintentionally by the physician in treating the patient. Iatrogenic diseases induced by drugs manifest themselves in five major syndromes; (1) blood dyscrasias, such as agranulocytosis, thrombocytopenia, aplastic anemia, and bone marrow depression; (2) hepatic toxicity, which is common and may take the form of biliary obstruction, hepatitis-like syndromes, and hepatic necrosis; (3) renal damage, particularly glomerular damage, which is a significant toxic effect of a number of drugs, including some antibiotics; (4) teratogenic effects, or drug effects causing malformations in the fetus as a result of placental transfer of drugs taken by a pregnant woman; and (5) dermatologic effects, such as acne, psoriasis, eczema, maculopapular rashes, and, rarely, erythema multiforme.

In addition to these common and well-known drug-induced diseases, there are numerous other iatrogenic syndromes specific to certain drugs. Ulceration of the gastrointestinal tract, for example, is a common result of long-term therapy with drugs such as aspirin, steroids, and potassium chloride. The relationship being investigated between oral contraceptive agents and thromboembolic phenomena is another untoward effect that may eventually be defined as an iatrogenic disease.

Adverse drug reactions, on the other hand, refer to one way of characterizing unpredictable and sometimes unexplainable drug responses that have not been optimally, clearly, and distinctly defined. Among the most common and best defined adverse drug reactions are the following.

Drug allergy is an altered state of reaction to a drug resulting from previous sensitizing exposure and the development of an immunologic mechanism. Substances foreign to the body act as antigens to stimulate the production of antibodies or immunoglobulins. Later, when a previously sensitized individual is again exposed to the foreign substance, the antigen reacts with the antibodies in ways that are damaging to body tissues. The antigen-antibody complex is not directly responsible for the manifestations of allergy. Rather, the complex reacts with various tissues and cells of the body by processes not clearly understood and causes them to release certain sustances (for example, histamine), which then provoke the symptoms of allergy.

Allergic reactions may manifest themselves in a variety of symptoms ranging from minor skin rashes to fatal hypotension. Reactions may be localized or widespread, and the symptoms may appear immediately or within hours to days following drug administration.

Immediate reactions occur within minutes of exposure to the chemical to which the person has been previously sensitized. Immediate and severe reactions are called anaphylactic reactions and are frequently fatal if not recognized and treated quickly. Signs and symptoms are severe, occur suddenly, and produce shock. The most dramatic form of anaphylaxis is sudden, severe bronchospasm, vasospasm, severe hypotension, and rapid death. Signs are largely caused by contraction of smooth muscles and may begin with irritability, extreme weakness, nausea, and vomiting and may proceed to dyspnea, cyanosis, convulsions, and cardiac arrest. Antihistamine drugs, epinephrine, and bronchodilators are indispensable in the treatment of anaphylactic shock.

Mild allergic reactions may be characterized by the development of a rash, angioedema, rhinitis, fever, asthma, and pruritus. Some allergic reactions are delayed and may appear anywhere from 7 to 14 days after initial administration of the drug. Delayed reactions are frequently analogous to "serum sickness" and are characterized by angioedema, arthralgia, fever, lymphadenopathy, and splenomegaly. Contact dermatitis, which results from direct skin contact with the eliciting drug, is also a delayed allergic response.

An individual who has had a mild allergic response to a particular drug should avoid reexposure to that drug and, optimally, should have skin tests performed in order to more definitely diagnose his response. Reinstitution of therapy with the same drug to patients who manifest allergic reactions is always dangerous, since an anaphylactoid reaction may occur.

The term "hypersensitivity" is frequently used synonymously with allergy, but it is inappropriate because it is frequently confused with other kinds of adverse drug reactions. Since there is a lack of precision to defining hypersensitivity, it may be wisest to avoid use of the term.

Idiosyncrasy is any abnormal or peculiar response to a drug that may manifest itself by (1) overresponse or abnormal susceptibility to a drug; (2) underresponse, demonstrating abnormal tolerance; (3) a qualitatively different effect from the one expected, such as excitation after the administration of a sedative; or (4) unpredictable and unexplainable symptoms. Idiosyncratic reactions are generally thought to result from genetic enzymatic deficiencies that lead to abnormal mechanism of metabolizing drugs. This term has been used rather vaguely to describe drug reactions that are qualitatively different from the usual effects obtained in the majority of patients and that cannot be attributed to drug allergy.

Tolerance is said to exist when there is a decreased physiologic response to the repeated administration of a drug or a chemically related substance. It is a reaction that necessitates an excessive increase in dosage to maintain a given therapeutic effect. Drugs well known for their propensity to produce tolerance are tobacco, opium alkaloids, nitrites, barbiturates, and ethyl alcohol. The actual mechanism of tolerance is unknown. In some instances, prolonged administration of some drugs somehow induces the synthesis of extra drug-metabolizing enzymes in the liver, which may account for the patient's increased ability to tolerate drug doses that previously affected him. Cross tolerance between related chemicals (such as between alcohol and some anesthetics) is a well-documented phenomenon. It is quite clear, however, that not all cases of tolerance are attributable to a drug's increased rate of metabolism. For example, the remarkable tolerance to morphine cannot be caused by its more rapid metabolic degradation.

Cumulation occurs when the body cannot metabolize one dose of a drug before another dose is administered. In other words, when drugs are excreted more slowly than they are absorbed, each new dose adds more to the total quantity in the blood and organs than is lost in the same amount of time by excretion. Unless drug administration is adjusted, sufficiently high concentrations can be reached to produce toxic effects. Cumulative toxicity can occur rapidly, as dramatically ilustrated in ethyl alcohol intoxication, or it can occur insidiously, as is the case in poisoning with heavy metals, such as lead. The latter is stored in many body tissues and deposited in bones, therefore having prolonged effects on the body while accumulation continues.

Tachyphylaxis refers to a quickly developing tolerance to the rapid, repeated administration of a drug. It is quick in onset and the patient's initial response to the drug cannot be reproduced with even larger doses of the drug.

Drug dependence is the term preferred over the previous terminology of "habituation" and "addiction." The World Health Organization has suggested the use of *dependence* in conjunction with the drug being described (for example, barbiturate dependence or opiate dependence). Dependence can be physical or phychic. Physical dependence refers to an adaptive physiologic state to a drug that manifests itself by intense physical disturbance when the drug is withdrawn. Psychic dependence is a state of emotional reliance on a drug in order to maintain a state of well-being. Its manifestations may range from a mild desire for a drug, to craving, to compulsive use of the drug. Drug dependence will be explored in greater breadth and depth in Chapter 12.

Summation, *additive effect*, and *synergism* refer to different situations in which the combined effect of two or more drugs acting simultaneously is either equal to or greater than the effect of each agent given alone.

Drug antagonism occurs when the conjoint effect of two drugs is less than the sum of the drugs acting separately.

Drug interaction results from the concurrent administration of two or more drugs and may be based on several mechanisms. (See also Chapter 5.)

Summary of nursing considerations

The optimal therapeutic effect of pharmacologic agents depends on their concentration at the sites of action. The time course of this concentration involves complex processes that may be divided into the following phases: (1) pharmaceutical phase, (2) pharmacokinetic phase, and (3) pharmacodynamic phase.

The principal method of giving drugs is by mouth. Therefore, most agents are absorbed from the intestine. The *pharmaceutical phase* refers to the drug or dosage form (liquid, tablet, or capsule), all of which must be in solution for absorption to occur. The solid form (tablet or capsule) must undergo disintegration and dissolution in the gastrointestinal fluids, whereas the liquid form is already in solution. This means that the drug form is important, for the more rapid the rate of dissolution, the greater will be the rate of absorption. The concentration the drug attains at its site of action is determined by the *pharmacokinetic phase*. This process primarily is influenced by (1) the rate and extent to which the drug is *absorbed* into body fluids; (2) the rate and extent to which the drug is transported or *distributed to* sites of action or storage in the body; (3) the rate and extent to which the drug is *biologically transformed* or *metabolized* in the body to breakdown products; and (4) the rate and extent to which the drug is *excreted* from the body via various routes.

To reach their site of effectiveness, drug molecules must cross cell membranes that in some instances may act as barriers to transport. Despite structural differences, the drugs cross these boundaries by one of two mechanisms: passive transport and active transport. The drug then enters the *pharmacodynamic phase*, which deals with the biochemical and physiologic effects of drugs and their mechanisms of action. It is concerned with the response of tissues to specific chemical agents. Drugs may increase or diminish the normal functions of tissues or organs, but they cannot confer any new functions on them. During this phase of action, pharmacologically active compounds can be divided into three groups: (1) drugs that selectively combine with specific cellular sites called receptors, (2) drugs that interact with enzyme systems, and (3) drugs that effect a change because of physicochemical properties.

The nurse must be cognizant of factors that modify cell conditions and thus the activity of a drug. Some of these factors include age, body mass, sex, environmental milieu, time of administration, pathologic state, genetic factors, and psychologic factors.

Unfavorable effects of drugs can be classifed as iatrogenic diseases or as adverse reactions. Iatrogenic diseases refer to groups of adverse effects produced unintentionally by the physician in treating the patient. Five major syndromes of iatrogenic diseases are blood dyscrasias, hepatic toxicity, renal damage, teratogenic effects, and dermatologic effects. On the other hand, adverse drug reactions include unpredictable responses such as drug allergy, hyper-

sensitivity, idiosyncrasy, tolerance, cumulation, tachyphylaxis, dependence, summation, additive effect, synergism, antagonism, and drug interaction.

QUESTIONS

FOR STUDY AND REVIEW

1. Define and describe the three phases of drug action that occur between administration of a drug and the production of its effects.
2. Briefly explain the receptor theory of drug action.
3. Define *affinity* and *efficacy* as they relate to drug action. What is bioavailability?
4. Describe how the following factors may influence drug absorption: route of drug administration, drug solubility, pH, local conditions at site of administration, and drug concentration.
5. Define and explain the rationale underlying the administration of drugs in "priming" and "maintenance" doses.
6. Define *active transport*.
7. Explain the meaning of *agonist* and *antagonist*.
8. Identify the system primarily responsible for the biotransformation of drugs.
9. Explain how drug metabolism can be depressed or stimulated.
10. Describe how the following variables influence drug action: age, body mass, sex, environmental milieu, time of drug administration, and pathologic state.
11. Define *iatrogenic disease* and identify the five major syndromes by which drug-induced iatrogenic disease may be manifested.
12. Define *adverse drug reactions* and list some of these reactions.
13. Explain why drug interaction has become a vital issue in contemporary medical therapeutics.

BIBLIOGRAPHY

Anders, M.W.: Enhancement and inhibition of drug metabolism. Annu. Rev. Pharmacol. **11**:37, 1971.

Avery, G.S., editor: Drug treatment, ed. 2, Acton, Mass., 1980, Publishing Sciences Group, Inc.

Benet, L.Z., editor: The effects of disease states on drug pharmacokinetics, Washington, D.C., 1976, American Pharmaceutical Association.

Bowman, W.C., and Rand, M.J.: Textbook of pharmacology, ed. 2, London, 1980, Blackwell Scientific Publications.

DiPalma, J.R., editor.: Basic pharmacology in medicine, New York, 1976, McGraw-Hill Book Co.

Dittert, L.W., and DiSanto, A.R.: A background chapter for the practitioner—the bioavailability of drug products, J. Am. Pharm. Assoc. **13**:421, 1973.

Drayer, D.E.: Pathways of drug metabolism in man, Med. Clin. North Am. **58**:927, 1974.

Feldman, S.: Drug distribution, Med. Clin. North Am. **58**:917, 1974.

Glauser, S.C.: Drug metabolism: conjugations and multiple pathways. Med. Clin. North Am. **58:**945, 1974.

Goldstein, A., Aronow, L., and Kalman, S.: Principles of drug action: the basis of pharmacology, ed. 2, New York, 1974, John Wiley & Sons, Inc.

Goodman, L.S., and Gilman, A.: editors: The pharmacological basis of therapeutics, ed. 6, New York, 1980, Macmillan, Inc.

Goth, A.: Medical pharmacology, ed. 10, St. Louis, 1981, The C.V. Mosby Co.

Greenblatt, D.J., and Koch-Weser, J.: Drug therapy: clinical pharmacokinetics, N. Engl. J. Med. **293:**702, 964, 1975.

Gringauz, A.: Drugs: how they act and why, St. Louis, 1978, The C.V. Mosby Co.

Herd, A.K., and Haleblian, C.A.: Pharmaceutical sciences—1973: literature review of pharmaceutics, J. Pharm. Sci. **63:**995, 1974.

Hussar, D.: Drug interactions: good and bad, Nursing '76 **6:**(9):61, 1976.

Julien, R.M.: A primer of drug action, ed. 2, San Francisco, 1978, W.H. Freeman and Co., Publishers.

Kappas, A., and Alvares, A.: How the liver metabolizes foreign substances, Sci. Am. **232:**22, 1975.

Koch-Weser, J., and Sellers, E.M.: Drug therapy: binding of drugs to serum albumin, N. Engl. J. Med. **294:**311, 1976.

Koch-Weser, J., and Sellers, E.M.: Drug therapy: binding of drugs to serum albumin, N. Engl. J. Med. **294:**526, 1976.

Leff, D.: Receptors, Med. World News, pp. 70-81, July 10, 1978.

Levine, R.R.: Pharmacology: drug actions and reactions, ed. 2, Boston, 1978, Little, Brown & Co.

Lowenthal, W.: Factors affecting drug absorption—a programmed unit, Am. J. Nurs. **73:**1391, 1973.

Meyers, F., Jawetz, E., and Goldfein, A.: Review of medical pharmacology, ed. 7, Los Altos, Calif., 1980, Lange Medical Publications.

Parker, C.W.: Drug allergy, Parts I to III, N. Engl. J. Med. **292:**511; 732; 957, 1975.

Rowland, M.: Hemodynamic factors in pharmacokinetics, Triangle, Sandoz J. Med. **14:**3, 1975.

Wagner, J.: Drug bioavailability studies, Hosp. Pract. **12:**119, 1977.

Wilkinson, G.R.: Pharmacokinetics of drug disposition: hemodynamic considerations, Annu. Rev. Pharmacol. **15:**11, 1975.

UNIT TWO

THE ROLE OF PHARMACOLOGY IN THE NURSING PROCESS

CHAPTER 5

Assessment in pharmacotherapeutics

The nursing process

Assessment of data

    Taking a drug history
    Patient and environmental data
    Drug data
    Primary, side, and toxic drug effects
    Drug interactions
    Exploring drug data

Nursing problems/nursing diagnostic statements

Summary of nursing considerations

The nursing process

As briefly described in Chapter 1, the nursing process is a systematic method of identifying nursing problems by using an organized approach to handling the data about patients and their drugs. It facilitates clear thinking, resulting in rational nursing action to provide optimal patient care. It involves four phases: (1) assessment, (2) planning, (3) implementation, and (4) evaluation. Fig. 5-1 schematically presents these four phases.

The nursing process is the foundation of clinical practice, and it is no more effectively used than when applied to nursing care procedures related to pharmacology. The nursing process and the various areas from which pharmacology data are drawn are described here.

Assessment of data

The assessment phase of the nursing process is not only the first phase but also a continuous phase that ends only on discharge of the patient. During assessment of data, all the facts relating to the patient and his/her drug therapy, to relationships with others, to the health history, and to the environment are collected and organized so that the nurse can begin to determine any problems related to drug therapy.

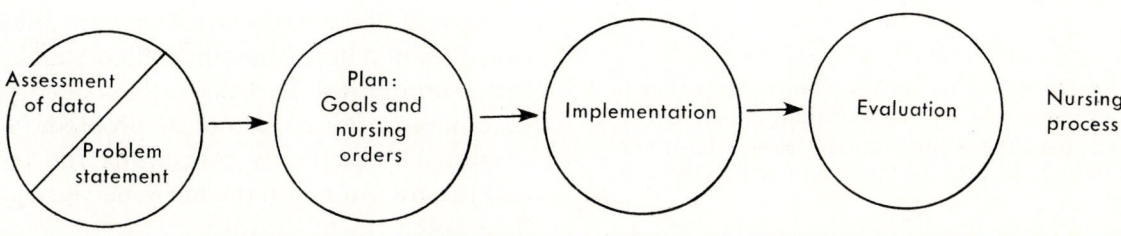

FIG. 5-1. Nursing process.

The patient's status and the assessment data derived from the sources mentioned are constantly changing. Nursing problems or diagnostic statements will change as well, which may result in drug deletions or additions or dosage changes in a patient's regimen.

Nurses must have a sound knowledge base of a patient's disorder and of drugs being administered, as well as the ability to use references to answer questions that arise. The ability to ask questions and seek answers about the data collected will form a solid foundation for the planning, implementation, and evaluation phases of the nursing process and will provide for optimal care of the patient.

TAKING A DRUG HISTORY

Taking a drug history can be extremely useful for gathering data about an individual's experience with medications. Pharmacists have been the prime movers in pushing for the ongoing assessment of this information in clinical settings and in pharmacies (where it is called a drug profile). Nurses are well suited to gather this information since they can combine their interviewing skills with a little detective work. Practical usefulness of this information will be demonstrated time after time. A drug history can:

1 Explain a mysterious new symptom reported by the patient
2 Provide clues about unreported chronic disorders
3 Reveal learning needs or problems in compliance
4 Provide information crucial to prevent drug interactions, allergies, or side or toxic effects
5 Help interpret laboratory tests reliably

Probably the best drug history form is the simple one: not so detailed that it will not be filled out or read by busy practitioners. Basically the medication history should include at least:

1 Current prescription medications—those taken regularly and those p.r.n. and their effectiveness
2 Current over-the-counter medication—those taken regularly and those p.r.n. and their effectiveness
3 Prescription medications discontinued within the last 6 months

4 Secondary reactions specifically described (do not accept "allergic reaction" without pursuing an accurate description of the reaction to rule out a quite different reaction)
5 Other pertinent comments

When taking a drug history it is best to avoid medical jargon and to accept and be familiar with local terms such as "high blood" for hypertension, "water pills" for diuretics, "low blood" for anemia, "bad blood" for syphilis, "nerve pills" for tranquilizers, and the like. When asking about over-the-counter drug categories, the nurse should use common brand names such as Anacin, Bufferin (may not be recognized as containing aspirin), or Rolaids (not "antacids"). The nurse should ask specifically whether the individual takes birth control pills, vitamins, cold tablets, nerve pills, or laxatives; these are not always viewed as drugs by the patient. Caffeine, tobacco, and alcohol are not usually considered by patients to be drugs, so the nurse must specifically ask about their use. These are substances often implicated in common drug interactions.

PATIENT AND ENVIRONMENTAL DATA

Patient and environmental data are collected from patients, their friends, or their relatives by subjective and objective observations of patients and their environment, including their interactions with others, and from patients' chart in the history and physical examination section. At the initial interview the practitioner notes a patient's past health history and does a physical examination to assess the current status of the patient. Often the resulting diagnosis is a prioritized problem list that reveals quickly the emphasis of therapy and the approach toward the patient.

Before compiling the nursing data base, the nurse must establish friendly rapport to begin the interview.

Second, the nurse must review the information obtained in the patient's history and physical examination. In order to have a complete data base to use to formulate problem lists or diagnostic statements concerning the patient and the environment, the nurse needs to gather data about the following:

Diagnosis. What are the patient's medical

Nursing process applied to pharmacology

STEP 1a: Assessment of data

A. Patient data
   1. Patient interviews; drug history
   2. Relatives and others
   3. Chart (patient history and physical examination)
B. Environmental data
   1. Patient/other relationships
   2. Patient/health professional relationships
   3. Adequate equipment
   4. Sufficient supplies
   5. Room atmosphere and surroundings conducive to optimal therapy
   6. Patient compliance with therapy
C. Drug data
   1. Physicians' orders or prescriptions
   2. Patient observations and evaluations (primary, side, toxic drug effects)
   3. Chart (laboratory values)
D. Exploring drug data
   1. Drug information references
   2. Other drug information sources

STEP 1b: Nursing problems/nursing diagnostic statements

STEP 2: Planning (goal-setting and specific planning)

A. Outline goals for patient care pertaining to drug therapy.
B. Write nursing orders to provide adequate drugs and equipment to meet patient's needs from pharmacy and central supply.
C. Try to resolve suboptimal relationships or room surroundings.
D. Establish specific drug dosage times and routes for administration; note in Kardex.

E. Anticipate laboratory data returns and orders to monitor drug therapy.
F. Plan patient learning and discharge information concerning medications or disorder (i.e., diabetes).

STEP 3: Implementation

A. Replace ward stock, narcotic, or emergency drug supplies.
B. Administer medications.
   1. Calculate drug.
   2. Prepare drug.
   3. Administer drug.
   4. Record drug administration.
C. Consult with prescriber concerning patient needs and orders.
D. Give patient discharge consultations.

STEP 4: Evaluation

A. If goals were successfully accomplished, continue the process with ongoing refinements.
B. If goals were not met, reappraisal of steps is necessary:
   1. Is there an adequate data base? Are there new data about primary effects or side and toxic effects?
   2. Are problems or nursing diagnoses stated effectively and accurately?
   3. Are problems appropriately prioritized?
   4. Are patient outcomes (goals) realistic?
   5. What other approaches to implementation could be attempted?
   6. Revise process accordingly.
C. Document the nursing process succinctly in acceptable manner.

diagnosis and social problems? Are the drugs ordered in the practitioner's plan of action clinically indicated and based on medical-nursing judgment according to the literature? Rarely, an ordered drug may be inappropriate for the therapeutic need. Though this is rare, the administering nurse is held legally accountable.

Age. Has the drug therapy taken into consideration the age of the patient and past drug reactions? Both the very young and the elderly are subject to a wider range and greater intensity of side and toxic effects than the average patient, mostly because of the less-than-optimal functioning of their various body systems for the absorption, transport, metabolism, and excretion of drugs. The first three can result in

apparent drug ineffectiveness, and the last can prolong drug effects and accentuate them beyond desirable limits.

In the very young patient there is a high potential for side and toxic effects because systems may be immature or because the proportion of body mass to body fluid is so different from the adult and is constantly changing. Liver immaturity may interfere with the ability to metabolize or degrade certain drugs, allowing them to remain in the body to act longer because crucial enzymes may only be produced at low levels.

Depending on individual health and age status, the elderly can be expected to exhibit the same decrement in one or more body systems with similar exaggeration of side effects. Gastrointestinal absorptive powers may be slowed, circulation may be diminished, and distribution may be uneven due partly to altered protein binding capacity. Additionally, there may be impairments of biotransformation activities as a result of liver enzyme deficiencies and of kidney dysfunction resulting in reduced renal clearance, all caused by the aging of cells critical to the body's processing of drug chemicals. Other contributing factors can include a possibly disordered response of drug receptor sites in the aging, overall decreased height-weight–blood volume ratio, and increased permeability of the blood-brain barrier. The cumulative effects are circulation of large amounts of the free unbound drug and prolongation of the drug half-life, giving rise to enhanced drug effects and a concomitant potential for toxicity in many elderly patients.

Body mass. Was the patient's body mass taken into consideration in drug dosage calculations? Dosages should be assessed in relation to such patient factors as total body weight, body surface area (patient's weight-to-height ratio), and lean body mass. For prescribing purposes, the person 12 years old or younger is usually considered to be a child and accordingly is administered the pediatric dosage, often half the average adult dosage. Average weight of a 12-year-old child is around 90 pounds. An adult at or near that weight who receives the "average adult dose" (with the "average" adult weighing approximately 150 pounds) may exhibit signs of overdosage and develop side effects or toxic effects.

Inherited factors. Does the drug therapy need to be altered because of genetic factors? Genetic differences (pharmacogenetic variations) in enzyme production, destruction, or absence or presence will cause apparent therapeutic failure or side or toxic effects when a drug is too rapidly metabolized to be effective or when the medication is too slowly or incompletely metabolized. Other aberrant reactions, occasionally termed "idiosyncrasy," are often actually caused by genetic abnormalities. An example is the lack of the enzyme glucose-6-phosphate dehydrogenase, found in a small percentage of people of Mediterranean descent and some black Americans. Quite a few common drugs (such as aspirin and sulfonamides), if tak-

en by susceptible individuals, will cause hemolytic anemia. Also, hypersensitivity (allergy) to specific medications often correlates with a tendency to other common allergies such as hypersensitivity to certain foods, grasses, trees, molds, or animal dander, thereby alerting the nurse during data gathering.

Coexisting conditions. Are there any disorders that affect any of the major body systems, especially those of the gastrointestinal tract or circulatory, hepatic, or renal systems, that will interfere with the normal body processes of digestion, absorption, transport, metabolism, degradation, and detoxification or excretion of the drugs prescribed? Impaired capacity for biotransformation will alter drug action and increase the possibility of toxic effects or therapeutic failure. It is important to note that pregnancy or breast-feeding preclude administration of all but essential medications.

Patient concurrence with therapy. There are factors that influence whether the patient will actually adopt a positive attitude toward and go along with the treatment suggested, will accept and follow the therapeutic plan, and will participate in self-care management (termed "compliance" by many). Are there any factors affecting patient concurrence with therapy? Of all the classes of data that should be gathered to assess nursing pharmacotherapeutics, this is the most likely to be ignored, yet the effects of these factors may be at least as significant to therapeutic outcomes as the others.

Attitudes and behavior conducive to positive health have several bases. These are traits from the psychosocial, cultural, economic, cognitive, and physical spheres. Whether an individual actually "takes the pills" or achieves the desired therapeutic effect may also depend on how he/she views and values health and illness; understands or accepts illness; knows about the drug in question; relates to the health care surroundings, system, and practitioners; assigns control and decision-making; thinks logically; has been educated; and has an ability with manipulative skills, among others. Studies also show that having faith in a therapy has a decidedly favorable effect on its outcome. All of these subjective beliefs and attitudes demand a subtler approach than other areas of a health history.

DRUG DATA

Drug data are comprised of the information derived from the prescriber's orders or prescription and that gained from assessment of the drugs' primary or side effects on the patient using observation, vital signs, and laboratory reports. The characteristics of the drugs administered and the way they are ordered by the prescriber have an impact on the nursing care of the patient.

Prescribers' orders

"Medicating" a patient begins when the medication is suggested and authorized by a legally sanctioned prescriber, usually a licensed physician or dentist. These two professionals are currently the only ones legally allowed to initiate medication plans in all states. In several states, nurse practitioners or physicians' assistants have also been given that function legally; in other states this is under current consideration. The practicing nurse should be aware of and follow the limitations outlined in the state nurse practice act.

The prescriber's orders are meant for the one who dispenses the medication. There are two different formats, the prescription blank and the order sheet. The prescription blank is carried by the client to be filled by a community pharmacist; it may look similar to Fig. 5-2. For patients in a clinical setting, the order is written on an order sheet found in the patient's chart (Fig. 5-3). It is filled by the pharmacy within the institution and sent to the medication room on the patient's floor for access by the patient's medicating nurse.

A prescription blank has two available places for the prescriber's signature. Where the prescriber chooses to sign can be a key factor in the cost to the consumer. Though the medication itself may be prescribed by either its trade name or its generic name on the blank, in 45 states the law allows pharmacists to select which product of the prescribed category to dispense unless the prescriber insists on a specific brand name by signing the blank above the words "Dispense As Written." When drugs are marketed by more than one company, significant cost differences usually exist; a generic product may save the consumer even more. The *Guide to Prescription Drug Costs,* published by the U.S. Department of Health and Human Services, compares the costs of common drugs to community pharmacies, thereby giving a basis for comparison to promote cost consciousness among prescribers and pharmacists without compromising the quality of health care.

The prescriber's order has seven elements that should be present and identifiable:

1 Patient's name and other identifying data
2 Date that the order was written

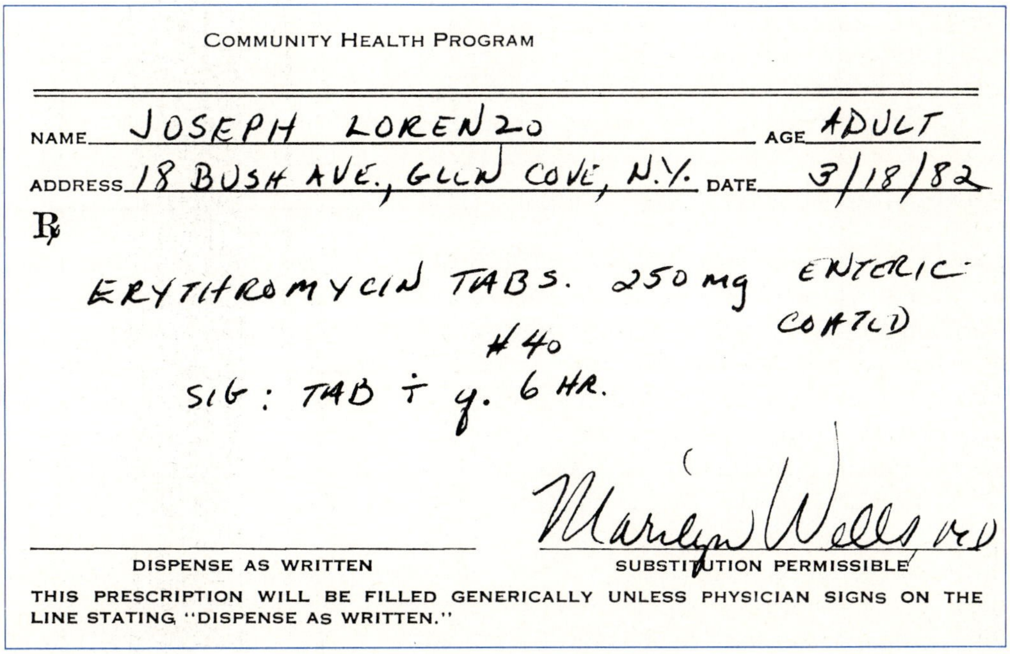
COMMUNITY HEALTH PROGRAM

NAME JOSEPH LORENZO AGE ADULT

ADDRESS 18 BUSH AVE., GLEN COVE, N.Y. DATE 3/18/82

℞

ERYTHROMYCIN TABS. 250 mg ENTERIC-COATED

#40

SIG: TAB i q. 6 HR.

Marilyn Wells, MD

DISPENSE AS WRITTEN — SUBSTITUTION PERMISSIBLE

THIS PRESCRIPTION WILL BE FILLED GENERICALLY UNLESS PHYSICIAN SIGNS ON THE LINE STATING "DISPENSE AS WRITTEN."

FIG. 5-2.
Prescription blank.

FIG. 5-3. Order sheet.

DATE	TIME	PROB. NO.	ORDERS	DOCTOR	NOTED BY	TIME	CODE NO.
3/18/82	3 PM	6	ERYTHROMYCIN 250 mg p.o. q.6hr.	M. Wells	Io		

DOCTORS ORDER SHEET

5 25345-0

3 Medication name
4 Dosage to be administered each time
5 Route of administration
6 Frequency of administration and any special instructions (for example, "Give with orange juice" if the medication taste is strong or unpleasant and would not interact with the acidic solution)
7 Prescriber's signature

The "five rights" of medication administration referred to in many nursing skills books are derived from these seven elements (omitting numbers 2 and 7). All parts of the order as listed should be clearly legible, with no room for doubt as to the intent or meaning. If there is any doubt the prescriber must be contacted to validate or clarify. Obviously, to administer a drug under questionable instructions is to risk harm to the patient in an area with a high potential for error (see Chapter 6).

Safe nursing practice is to follow procedures as accepted in the particular work environment and to administer only such drugs as are ordered in writing. Nursing *students* in particular should be advised to follow only written orders. However, there are times when following a verbal or telephoned order from a physician, often in response to the nurse's telephoned request, is unavoidable. When it is necessary to receive a verbal order, it is best to copy the order as it is being given, then verify it by repeating it back to the sender. This is only rarely acceptable behavior, and then only under circumstances of some urgency, *not* merely to suit someone's convenience. The order must be clearly communicated and noted on the patient's chart by the nurse. It must be countersigned by the physician, usually within 24 hours, in most institutions, *to be legal*. It is careless and negligent to allow it to remain unsigned because it violates the law and institution policy. This allows a precarious period of vulnerability to malpractice charges. (See Chapter 2.)

TYPES OF MEDICATION ORDERS

Some medication orders leave nurses to their own discretion and judgment. A p.r.n. order (one that is to be implemented "as necessary") allows the decision of whether or not to administer medication up to the nurse based on certain criteria included in the order (such as the time interval).

Other types of orders dictate the conditions under which the medication should be administered, leaving varying degrees of freedom for nursing judgment. These include:

Routine order. This is the most common type and is meant to be administered until a discontinuation order is written or until the termination date is reached. Termination dates may be included in the order or may be explicit in agency policy, as, for example, narcotic or barbiturate orders, which are frequently meant to be discontinued automatically after 48 hours.

Single order. A single order is to be administered only once, at the time indicated. An example is a preoperative medication.

Stat order. This is a single order that is to be administered immediately.

Protocol. A protocol is a set of criteria that serves as a directive under which medication may be given. Protocols may typically be one of two types: *standing orders* or *flow diagram protocols*. Standing orders are officially accepted sets of orders (not only for medications) to be applied routinely by nurses to the care of patients with certain conditions or under certain circumstances (for example, as part of admission orders in some critical care units). Flow diagram protocols are criteria that give nurse practitioners guidelines for administration of certain treatments and medications based on patient variables. These protocols provide the widest scope for application of nursing judgment and decision making of all the types of orders. Criteria and direction may either be very specific, for those with limited expertise or responsibility, or less specific and allow for greater latitude, self-reliance, and sophistication in decision making for others.

ASSESSMENT OF MEDICATION ORDERS

Patient. Every possible effort should be made to ensure that the right patient gets the medication intended for him/her and in the manner intended by the prescriber. Toward this end, patients with similar names should be widely separated in the health care setting, and all their paperwork must be clearly distinguished from one another. An identifying armband must be kept on every patient and compared to identifying information that accompanies each dose of medication.

Date. The date that a medication order was written becomes important so that it can be checked against other information for accuracy or to check when medication must be discontinued or when the last dose is to be given. For example, a drug may be ordered for just 3 days, or there may be a policy that narcotics may be given based on the original order for just 48 hours, or an antibiotic must be terminated routinely in 72 hours unless a renewing order has been written.

Medication. The medication's name may be written either in generic or trade name form. The patient should know the name of the medication if it is agency policy. If it is not, then the nurses in the agency should be actively working with administrative leaders to reverse the policy. It is illogical to keep patients uninformed about the names of their drugs while hospitalized only to expect that on discharge they will be able to self-administer their drugs successfully at home! It is also dangerous to keep patients ignorant of their medication. Nurses who have worked in emergency situations have seen all too many patients interviewed who can only describe their "white heart pill" or their "water pill." Yet the exact name and dosage are crucial information for attending physicians to know before emergency treatment can be begun.

Dosage and frequency. Drug dosages should be given as prescribed in the medication order unless nursing judgment detects, for example, that the size of the dose ordered falls outside the range of normal or usual limits or that there are intervening factors in the patient-dosage relationship that warrant reevaluation of the dosage, its frequency, or the route of administration. The drug would then not be administered or would be held until the nurse and prescriber consult on the question.

During the development of a drug there is a determination made of the range of dosage, frequency, and effective route for administration. These are based on the known pharmacokinetics of the drug. For example, one drug that routinely undergoes biotransformation slowly may dwell in the body system longer and produce more prolonged effects than another. Therefore, it may effectively be given on a once-a-day basis, but a drug that is excreted rapidly may need to be given every 4 hours around the clock if effective tissue levels of the drug are to be maintained. Nursing judgments must be made to align an individual patient's medication schedule with agency policy at appropriate intervals or to keep to a single schedule to meet a specific need of the patient. Some reasons to individualize administration time include avoiding disturbing the patient's rest, sleep, meals, visiting hours, other activities, or treatments or patient convenience. Rationale for other modifications in the medical plan should be discussed with prescriber.

Route. Every medication order should include a specified route for administration. Making assumptions in this area is negligent. However, choice of the actual *site* of administration of injectables may be a nursing or nurse-patient decision. For example, subcutaneous, intramuscular, and intravenous sites to avoid would include any areas of obvious injury, disease, or lesions, even if minor. Such areas would include any that are noticeably erythematous (reddened), vesicular (blistered), open and weeping or pustular, ecchymotic (bruised), scarred, or previously overused for injection. The rationale is that such areas may have impaired circulation or that they may be adversely affected by the injection itself or by the material injected.

The ordered route of administration should routinely be assessed as to its efficacy, feasibility, or practicality. The oral route would naturally be precluded for the patient who is nauseated or vomiting. Prior consultation with the prescriber must be made before administering the drug by a different route, because dosage or other factors may have to be readjusted if bioavailability is affected by such changes.

PRIMARY, SIDE, AND TOXIC DRUG EFFECTS

The ultimate effects of drugs on the body can be divided into two types. The main purpose of administering a medication to a patient is to utilize its primary therapeutic effect. All other consequences can be thought of as side and toxic effects, largely unintended and often nontherapeutic.

Although drugs are developed and formulated to promote specific effects, the appearance of side or toxic effects demonstrates a continuing challenge to drug manufacturers. The crux of this problem is that most drugs cannot be made selective enough to be targeted at only one body system, organ, tissue, or cell. There is enough random direction that the drug is circulated or distributed to other areas as well. These areas respond with reactions that may range in severity from merely inconvenient or annoying side effects to very serious toxic effects. On the other hand, occasionally a side effect may actually be the sought-after primary effect under certain circumstances or may exploited by the prescriber as a therapeutic effect along with the primary effects. For example, the fact that morphine sulfate happens to produce some respiratory depression with a resultant salutary effect on cardiac work load as well as producing analgesia in myocardial infarction (its primary effect) makes it most useful in this condition. Such primary and side effects are often dose-related, that is, directly related to increases in dosage, or they may be related to the duration of that specific therapy.

It is essential that the medicating process be assessed with regard to each medication's clinical indications and potential efficacy and any contraindications, especially any hypersensitivity (allergy) to the drug or any pathologic condition, etc., that would preclude its administration.

An allergic history of any sort, even if unrelated to the medication, must be explored to rule out and prevent any possible allergic reaction to it. The occurrence of drug hypersensitivity reactions is extremely individualized, unpredictable except for history, and not usually closely dose-related. The reaction may result in a very serious and life-threatening situation. Consequently the drug must not be given. Responses may vary from mild rash to severe exfoliative dermatitis, or asthma to anaphylactic shock, and may include urticaria, angioneurotic edema, and fever.

Some medications that cause frequent allergic reactions include sulfa drugs and the penicillins. It is essential to check the chart or Kardex before giving any medications, especially these, for any alerting stickers or notations as to an allergic history. Records may denote "no known allergy" (NKA), but usually this refers to drugs. Since there is often a correlation between one allergic response and the development of another, the patient's description of *any* past allergic manifestations—to drugs, inhalants, contactants, foods (typically: eggs, orange juice, chocolate, shellfish, strawberries), or whatever—must be clarified and evaluated. Often the patient erroneously defines any unexpected response as an allergic one. For example, the nausea following a meperidine (Demerol) injection may be labeled an allergic reaction by the patient, when in actuality it is likely to be only a normal, if exaggerated, side effect.

When a true allergy exists, administration of the drug is positively contraindicated. Withholding the drug is the best approach if allergy is suspected. Treatment depends on the type of hypersensitivity reaction that occurs. Drugs often used to treat severe reactions include antihistamines, such as diphenhydramine (Benadryl) and epinephrine.

Another contraindication to drug therapy may be the existence of a pathologic condition in an organ system essential to the drug's biotransformation in some way. Assessing for the presence of contraindications is essential in this first phase of the nursing process in pharmacotherapeutics. The wider spectrum of possible unintended effects aside from contraindications is discussed appropriately in Chapter 6.

DRUG INTERACTIONS

The complexity of modern pharmacotherapy is nowhere more obvious than in the ever-growing list of drugs that interact nontherapeutically with one another, with foods, and with fluids and that distort laboratory test results. That these chemical substances will interact with or potentiate one another is not surprising; this fact should always be kept in mind when medications appear either ineffective or harmful or when the accuracy of laboratory tests is crucial.

Variables influencing drug interaction include the following: (1) intestinal absorption,

(2) competition for plasma binding, (3) drug metabolism or biotransformation, (4) action at the receptor site, (5) renal excretion, and (6) alteration of electrolyte balance. The following are examples of these variables' effects.

1 Intestinal absorption: antacids that contain calcium, magnesium, or aluminum interfere with the absorption of tetracycline.
2 Competition for plasma protein binding: tolbutamide can be displaced from its binding on plasma proteins by bishydroxycoumarin, resulting in severe hypoglycemia. Many drugs are weak acids that are bound largely to plasma proteins. These weak acids may compete for binding sites on plasma proteins, thus increasing the free, active drug that may have potent effects.
3 Drug metabolism or biotransformation: the monoamine oxidase inhibitors prevent the biotransformation of tyramine, which is present in cheese and other fermented foods. As a consequence, patients taking monoamine oxidase inhibitors as antidepressants have developed hypertensive crises caused by the release of large amounts of stored norepinephrine after ingesting tyramine-containing foods and drinks.
4 Action at the receptor site: there are numerous examples of one drug intensifying or antagonizing the action of another drug at the receptor site. For example, the antihistaminics decrease many effects of histamine, while cocaine increases the actions of epinephrine.
5 Renal excretion: probenecid inhibits the renal clearance of penicillin.
6 Alteration of electrolyte balance: the thiazide diuretics may cause hypokalemia, which predisposes to digitalis toxicity.

It should be remembered that not all drug interactions are dangerous; some are insignificant or even beneficial. Tables listing all known drug interactions should be posted and available to the nurse when dangerous drug interaction is suspected.

Drug-drug interactions

Some drugs commonly found in clinically significant drug-drug interactions include coumadin, tricyclic antidepressants, aminoglycosides, amphetamines, corticosteroids, digitalis glycosides, diuretics, sulfonamides, alcohol, and theophylline. Before any such medication is given, an appropriate source should be consulted to assess the interactive drug, its mechanism, and any other medications given concurrently to determine the probability of difficul-

ties developing. This text gives this information in the context of specific drug data.*

Other drug interactions

Pharmacologically active substances in foods can be categorized in four groups: foods of plant and animal origin (oxalates, metals, hydroxytryptamine, dihydroxylphenylalanine); foods of marine origin (neurotoxins, pesticides, and heavy metal residues); food additives and contaminants (preservatives, antioxidants, surface-active agents, stabilizers, thickeners, bleaching and maturing agents, buffers, acidulents, food colors, dietary sweeteners, flavors, mycotoxins, antibiotics, etc.); and water, soft drinks, and alcoholic beverages (may contain various metals, xanthines, and histamines).

Although not as common, certain drugs in combination with these foods or fluids can cause interaction problems.

Drug-induced malabsorption of foods and nutrients. Drugs that change gastric or intestinal motility can alter the digestion or absorption of certain nutrients. Important drugs that effect these changes are stimulant cathartics and mineral oil and, at the other extreme, anticholinergics and narcotics. Long-term use of diuretics to treat such conditions as congestive heart failure can lead to serious potassium depletion. If the potassium loss is not corrected in patients taking digitalis, the heart may overrespond to the usual dose of digitalis. Some oral contraceptives impair folic acid absorption in undernourished patients.

Food-induced malabsorption of drugs. Food in the gastrointestinal tract can slow the amount and/or rate of drug absorption (see Chapter 4). Fatty foods or foods low in fiber will delay stomach emptying by up to 2 hours. Many tetracyclines can form insoluble complexes in the gastrointestinal tract if given at the same time as foods or drugs containing ions of calcium, aluminum, magnesium, or iron. Thus administering tetracycline medication along with milk-based tube feedings or common antacids should be avoided. Ascorbic acid from cit-

---

*An extensive listing of the clinically more important drug interactions may be found in Avery, G. S., editor: Drug treatment, principles and practice of clinical pharmacology and therapeutics, ed. 2, New York, 1980, Adis Press.

rus fruits or juices enhances absorption of iron, but carbonated soft drinks or acid juices (fruit or vegetable) can cause drugs to dissolve more quickly in the stomach than in the intestine or can neutralize them, thereby changing the intended rate or completeness of absorption.

Alteration of enzymes. Enzyme alterations, either induction or inhibition, may affect the metabolism of the food or drug. The natural extract of licorice is chemically similar to steroids and therefore if taken in excess can cause hypokalemia, retention of sodium and water with resultant hypertension, and alkalosis. Ingestion of large amounts would be contraindicated for patients concurrently taking potassium-losing diuretics or with cardiovascular disease.

Likewise, foods high in vitamin K (such as liver and green leafy vegetables) may hinder the effectiveness of oral anticoagulants. Brussels sprouts and cabbage ingestion will reduce the rate of metabolism of antipyrine and phenacetin; charcoal-broiled beef ingestion will reduce the effects of theophylline, antipyrine, and phenacetin.

Monoamine oxidase inhibitors (antidepressants) act by inhibiting the breakdown of norepinephrine, a vasopressor substance. This excess norepinephrine is then stored in the neurons. The ingestion of certain tyramine-containing foods (aged cheeses, beef and chicken liver, pickled herring, broad beans, canned figs, bananas, avocados, soy sauce, active yeast preparations, beer, sherry in large quantities, Chianti wine, chocolate, and many fermented foods) elevates the quantity of norepinephrine to toxic levels, thereby precipitating hypertensive crises. Over-the-counter cold remedies containing ephedrine, phenylephrine, and phenylpropanolamine and amphetamines in general can act similarly, releasing stored quantities of norepinephrine. The net effect can be a headache, sudden climb in blood pressure to dangerous levels, cardiac arrhythmias, or intracranial bleeding.

Alcohol consumption. Of the more than 100 most frequently prescribed drugs, more than half contain at least one ingredient known to interact adversely with imbibed alcohol. An interaction is probable if the drug is known to

---

Relationship of drug administration to meals (partial listing of some commonly prescribed drugs)

Take on an empty stomach (2 hours after meals or 1 hour before meals):

Erythromycin
Penicillins (especially penicillin G)
Tetracyclines (except doxycycline [Vibramycin])

Take ½ hour before meals:

Librax
Donnatal
Propantheline bromide (Pro-Banthine)

Take with meals or food:

Aminophylline
Antidiabetic drugs (tolbutamide [Orinase])
Chlorothiazide (Diuril, Hydro-DIURIL)
Mefenamic acid (Ponstel)
Metronidazole (Flagyl)
Nitrofurantoin (Furadantin, Macrodantin)
Phenytoin (Dilantin)
Prednisone
Reserpine (Serpasil)
Theophylline, aqueous (Theolair)
Triamterene (Dyrenium)

Do not take with milk:

Bisacodyl (Dulcolax)
Potassium chloride
Potassium iodide
Tetracyclines except doxycycline (Vibramycin)

Do not take with fruit juices:

Ampicillin
Cloxacillin (Tegopen)
Erythromycin
Penicillin G

Do not drink alcohol while taking:

Acetohexamide (Dymelor)
Antihistamines (diphenhydramine [Benadryl], chlorpheniramine [Chlor-trimeton], etc.)
Chloral hydrate
Chlordiazepoxide (Librium)
Chlorpropamide (Diabinese)
Diazepam (Valium)
Diphenoxylate (Lomotil)
Flurazepam (Dalmane)
Meclizine (Antivert)
Methaqualone (Quaalude)
Metronidazole (Flagyl)
Monoamine oxidase inhibitors
Narcotics (Percodan, Tylox, codeine)
Tolbutamide (Orinase)

Modified from Lambert, M. L., Jr.: Drug and food interactions, Am. J. Nurs. **75**(3): 402-406, 1975.

affect the central nervous system or is metabolized by the liver. The effects are dose-related, and whether quantities of alcohol are used habitually, chronically, or only occasionally often makes a distinct difference in the direction of interactive effects. Patterns of alcohol consumption will likely have a bearing on the patient's concurrence with drug treatment and follow-through as well. Thus it is obvious that patterns of alcohol consumption are significant when taking a history. Some of the drugs whose effects are known to be either potentiated or diminished by alcohol ingestion are listed in Table 5-1.

The fact that many elixirs and tinctures are liquid formulations of drugs dissolved in alcohol is significant, especially in the assessment of pharmacotherapy of children. These preparations must be reassessed and cannot be assumed to have the same rate and degree of absorption as the same drug in aqueous solution since bioavailability may be altered.

Cigarette smoking. The main pharmacokinetic effect of heavy cigarette smoking is the lowering of drug plasma levels by nicotine and other tobacco constituents by inducing microsomal enzyme systems responsible for increased drug metabolism or excretion. The rate of theophylline breakdown is increased, necessitating an increase in dosage of from 1½ to 2 times the average dose. The usual doses of other drugs are found to be diminished in effectiveness in the heavy smoker: the antidepressant imipramine; analgesics such as pentazocine, antipyrene, phenacetin and propoxyphene; vitamins C, B$_{12}$, and B$_6$; and the influenza vaccine, for example. Smoking also interacts with glutethimide, furosemide, and propranolol. CNS depression is less frequent with diazepam (Valium) and drowsiness is reduced with chlorpromazine (Thorazine). When smoking is combined with use of estrogens, the risk of heart attack, stroke, and other circulatory disorders goes up. Laboratory test results may also be somewhat outside the range of normal, especially with regard to duration of smoking history and inhalation practices: the white cell count is increased (in the absence of clinical infection), hemoglobin concentration, hematocrit, and red blood cell size are increased, and

TABLE 5-1 Drugs that commonly interact with alcohol

Drug(s)	Effects
Antianginals (some)	Potentiated
Antibiotics (some)	Nausea, vomiting, headache, possible convulsions
Antidepressants (some)	Potentiated
Antihistamines	CNS effects potentiated
Antihypertensives (some)	Potentiated
ASA	Bleeding of gastrointestinal tract potentiated
Barbiturates	Lethal dose 50% lower; effects potentiated
Chloral hydrate	Potentiated
Hypoglycemics, oral (many)	Potentiated; disulfiram-like effects: nausea, vomiting, stomach pain
Isoniazid	Diminished
Major tranquilizers	Possibly fatal; respiratory depression
Metronidazole	Disulfiram-like effects: nausea, vomiting, stomach pain
Minor tranquilizers	Potentiated
Narcotics	Effects potentiated, except codeine
Phenytoin (Dilantin)	Diminished
Warfarin	Potentiated

clotting time reduced. Some investigators of cigarette smoking have found an abnormal increase in cholesterol and others have found carcinoembryonic antigen levels as high as for persons with colon cancer, yet without other evidence of it. Therefore smokers can be expected sometimes to exhibit more numerous drug therapy "failures" or adverse effects, or even to have fewer or different reactions to drugs, than nonsmoking patients. Certain laboratory test results must be interpreted in light of cigarette smoking history.

Food-initiated alteration of drug excretion. Changes in the pH of urine caused by food (making the urine overly acidic or alkaline) can have a significant effect on the excretion rates of some drugs, since pH influences the ionization of weak acids and bases. A drug will diffuse more easily from the urine back into the blood in its nondissociated state, thereby prolonging drug action. The action of acidic drugs is prolonged, for example, when urine is acid. Though it is quite difficult to override the kid-

TABLE 5-2 Miscibility (compatibility) of intramuscular injectables

General rules:

1. All mixtures should be inspected for clarity before injection.
2. Injections should be administered within 15 minutes of mixing.
3. If a combination is ordered that does not occur in this list, contact pharmacy for evaluation before mixing.
4. When reconstituting always use the recommended diluent.

Please note:

This chart has been prepared as a convenient reference guide for some combinations which do or do not show visual incompatibility within 15 minutes.

Drug	Compatible? No	Compatible? Yes	Drug	Compatible? No	Compatible? Yes
Atropine	Librium Luminal Seconal Valium	Benadryl Benadryl+Demerol Compazine Demerol Demerol+Phenergan Inapsine Innovar Morphine Nembutal Phenergan+Demerol Sparine Sublimaze Talwin Thorazine Vistaril	Innovar (fentanyl and droperidol)	Librium Luminal Seconal Valium	Atropine Scopolamine
			Librium (chlordiaze- poxide)	No mixing	
Benadryl (diphenhy- dramine)	Librium Luminal Nembutal Valium	Atropine Demerol Morphine Phenergan	Luminal (pheno- barbital)	No mixing	
Compazine (prochlor- perazine)	Librium Luminal Nembutal Phenergan Seconal Talwin Valium Vistaril	Atropine Demerol Morphine Scopolamine Thorazine	Morphine	Librium Luminal Nembutal Seconal Talwin Valium	Atropine Benadryl Compazine Phenergan Pro-Banthine Scopolamine Sparine Thorazine Vistaril
Demerol (meperidine)	Librium Luminal Nembutal Seconal Talwin Valium	Atropine Benadryl+Atropine Compazine Dramamine Phenergan+Atropine Pro-Banthine Scopolamine+Phenergan* Sparine Thorazine Vistaril	Nembutal (pento- barbital)	Benadryl Compazine Demerol Morphine Phenergan Scopol- amine Sparine Talwin Thorazine Vistaril	Atropine
Dramamine (dimenhy- drinate)	Librium Luminal Seconal Valium	Demerol	Phenergan (prometh- azine)	Compazine Librium Luminal Nembutal Seconal Valium	Atropine Atropine+Demerol Benadryl Codeine Demerol Epinephrine Morphine Nisentil Nisentil+Atropine Scopolamine Sparine Talwin Vistaril
Inapsine (droperidol)	Librium Luminal Seconal Valium	Atropine Scopolamine			

Reprinted by permission from Pharm Alert, June 1974, Bess Kaiser Hospital, Portland, Oregon.
*Mix Phenergan and Scopolamine together first, then draw this mixture into the Demerol. Use immediately.

Continued.

T A B L E 5 - 2 Miscibility (compatibility) of intramuscular injectables—cont'd

Drug	Compatible? No	Compatible? Yes	Drug	Compatible? No	Compatible? Yes
Pro-Banthine (propantheline)	Librium Luminal Seconal Valium	Demerol Morphine Sparine	Sublimaze (fentanyl)	Librium Luminal Seconal Valium	Atropine Scopolamine
Seconal (secobarbital)	No mixing		Talwin (pentazocine)	Compazine Demerol Librium Luminal Morphine Nembutal Seconal Valium	Atropine Phenergan Scopolamine Thorazine Vistaril
Scopolamine	Librium Nembutal Seconal Valium	Compazine Demerol+Phenergan* Inapsine Innovar Morphine Phenergan+Demerol* Sublimaze Talwin Thorazine Vistaril	Thorazine (chlorpromazine)	Librium Luminal Nembutal Seconal Valium	Atropine Compazine Demerol Morphine Scopolamine Talwin
			Valium (diazepam)	No mixing	
Sparine (promazine)	Librium Luminal Nembutal Seconal Valium	Atropine Codeine Demerol Demerol+Atropine Morphine Nisentil Nisentil+Scopolamine Phenergan Pro-Banthine Scopolamine	Vistaril (hydroxyzine) same as Atarax	Compazine Librium Luminal Nembutal Seconal Valium	Atropine Demerol Morphine Phenergan Scopolamine Talwin

neys' ability to regulate urine pH, an alkaline ash or acid ash diet, whether by purpose or not, can drive urinary pH above 8 or below 5, creating a medium for potential drug reactions. Continued taking of many antacid tablets each day in concert with quinidine administration was seen in one instance to create quinidine intoxication by shifting urinary pH toward the base and causing a serious arrhythmia necessitating hospitalization.

Drug incompatibilities

Interactions occurring when drugs are mixed before administration, as in a single syringe or in intravenous fluids, are termed incompatibilities. Such mixtures may precipitate or be neutralized in such solutions. Lists of incompatible drugs are usually posted in areas where nurses prepare medications for administration. Agency pharmacists can also provide helpful consultation. Some of the most common drugs involved in incompatibilities are listed in Table 5-2.

EXPLORING DRUG DATA

Any nursing process will only be as effective as the analytic thought that goes into it. Logic and judgment improve as the nurse's information base is perfected, partly as experience is tested against knowledge. Nowhere is ongoing self-learning more essential than in nursing pharmacotherapeutics. The "need to know" escalates, for example, when nurses who are responsible for administering medications are confronted with an order for an unfamiliar drug or by an unexpected patient symptom not usually associated with the diagnosis.

Realistically, it is not possible to know everything about all medications on the market, even the ones nurses use frequently. It *is* important to know where to get essential information as it becomes required. Various reference sources exist, each with its own emphasis, yet most are inadequate to meet the specialized needs of nursing pharmacotherapeutics.

Drug information references

The following are references frequently used as drug information sources by nurses.

Physicians' Desk Reference (P.D.R.) (Oradell, N.J.: Medical Economics, Inc.) is the most commonly consulted reference in clinical settings. It is a concise compilation of specific information similar to that found enclosed with medication as it comes from the pharmaceutical distributor (package inserts). As such, it is of limited value for the nursing process since it is written in "medicalese," lacks any nursing methodology, and lists long strings of secondary effects without regard to relative frequency or severity. It is probably best used as a quick reference with another source handy to fill in the information gaps left. However, both the P.D.R. and package inserts can be considered to give an FDA-approved and reliable discourse on drugs' clinical indications and safe ranges of dosages.

Users of this information for the purpose of prescribing should be aware that individual cases may allow for variation in use and dosage of a drug, even to exceed suggested dosage range, but that such individual variation should have a valid rationale. When using this source, it should be borne in mind that the material it contains is submitted by the pharmaceutical company producing the drug.

American Hospital Formulary Service (Bethesda, Md.: American Society of Hospital Pharmacists) is a fairly objective overview in monograph form of every available drug in the United States.

A.M.A. Drug Evaluations (Chicago: American Medical Association) is a source of information about specific drugs, even those that are being used for valid clinical applications different from those that have been approved thus far.

Nursing journals such as *American Journal of Nursing, Nursing '82 ('83,* etc.), and *R.N.* will offer both general and specific drug informa-

tion in nursing terminology, giving it a nursing emphasis.

Many *nursing pharmacology texts* such as this one follow the same approach as the nursing journals but also include a greater depth of information about physiology and pathology of specific medication uses. Some offer the specifics only, as quick reference.

FDA Drug Bulletin (Rockville, Md.: Department of Health and Human Services, Public Health Services) is a free six-page newsletter published several times a year to inform health professionals about the results of recent FDA reviews of various drugs (usually common ones) and their new clinical findings. Each issue also includes a form for reporting unusual clinical experiences with drugs.

Nurses' Drug Alert (New York) is a monthly newsletter that discusses recent findings as to the more serious side effects of various commonly administered drugs. It includes a paragraph under each drug that discusses nursing implications. The staff includes registered nurses as well as pharmacists.

Physicians' Desk Reference for Nonprescription Drugs (Oradell, N.J.: Medical Economics, Inc.) was first published in 1980 in recognition of the many laypersons with growing health awareness who are eager to participate in self-care management and the massive proliferation of over-the-counter drugs. The format is similar to that of the *P.D.R.*, with identifying photographs of the drugs, pharmaceutical company addresses, and descriptions of individual drugs and compounds. It also includes a section on the self-care of minor health problems.

Handbook of Nonprescription Drugs (Washington, D.C.: American Pharmaceutical Association) deals with over-the-counter drug information in general categories. Each chapter presents the relevant physiologic background first, and concludes with a table comparing specific drugs.

United States Pharmacopeia (Rockville, Md.: U.S. Pharmacopeial Convention, Inc.) includes source, formula, property, tests, assays, methods of storing, and dosages of drugs. To be included in the U.S.P., drugs must be demonstrated by their developer to be of therapeutic value and low in toxicity.

The *National Formulary* (Rockville, Md.: U.S. Pharmacopeial Convention, Inc.) enlarges upon the U.S.P. and contains formulas and preparations of drugs. It is now published in the same volume as the U.S.P.

United States Pharmacopeia Dispensing Information (Easton, Pa.: U.S. Pharmacopeial Convention, Inc.) is a reference first published in 1980 to meet the needs of those involved in the dispensing and administration phases of medicating themselves or others *after* the prescription has been written and filled. It includes information on each drug including its category, precautions to consider, side effects, what to tell the patient or client, dosage forms, and labeling. A section entitled "Advice for the Patient" gives the reader in nontechnical language pertinent essentials about the drug, describes its ramifications, and tells how to tailor its administration to life-style. As such, it seems to be a highly relevant source for nurses.

The Pharmacological Basis of Therapeutics (A. G. Gilman, L. S. Goodman, and A. Gilman, editors; New York: Macmillan, Inc.) is a thorough and respected textual reference that is considered an authoritative source for those learning or working with pharmacology. It is not geared especially for nurses nor does it contain specifics related to nursing pharmacotherapeutics, but it is an excellent reference text.

Drugs of Choice (W. Modell, editor; St. Louis: The C.V. Mosby Co.) is a handy reference for understanding the clinical applications of drugs under varying circumstances.

Other drug information sources

Drug information centers are located in many areas of the United States for the express purposes of enlightening professionals who contact them and disseminating information about the clinical uses of drugs and related equipment. A wide variety of either general or specific information can be obtained with advice based on scientific literature. The contact is usually a team of specially trained pharmacists, often located within a large, medical center setting. Many difficult pharmacologic questions related to patient care can be dealt with quickly by contacting the nearest Drug Information Center.

Pharmacists located in hospitals, skilled care facilities, and other agencies can also be a source of similar information or provide access to it as needed.

Agencies often can supply a wealth of similar sources of information. The area or floor where a nurse works often has a card file of package inserts at the very least, and ideally has its own nursing library shelf which might contain pharmacology information and other material of interest. Any nurse could initiate the development of such material and request funds or supplies to do so. The agency nursing inservice or education department has the goal of promoting ongoing and updated learning and, as such, could be the facilitator via audiovisual aids, references, or seminars.

Building one's own library and maintaining its currency are important professional activities.

None of the previously discussed texts is a complete source of all pharmacology information necessary for nursing practice. The nurse must choose from among these and other materials to gather reliable resources that meet the clinical needs of the particular specialty area.

Nursing problems/nursing diagnostic statements

Nursing, in its striving for independence from the medical model, is struggling toward a standard nomenclature to facilitate communication among its practitioners. it is hoped that by identifying groups of nursing diagnoses in classes and subclasses, patterns and relationships will evolve. Campbell,[1] in her voluminous work, has done a most extensive survey of the situation.

The first National Conference on Classification of Nursing Diagnosis was held in St. Louis in 1973. Two subsequent conferences have been called. There is little consensus reached that is acceptable to the majority of practitioners.

Price[3] rationalizes this nonacceptance as deficiencies in the skill of the practitioners themselves, while Henderson[2] offers more hope: "Nursing and medicine will develop a thoroughly collaborative role in which the patient will benefit from the medical emphasis on specific pathology and the nurse's sensitivity to the psychosocial needs of the patient."

Assessment for the purpose of identifying nursing problems and developing the diagnoses related to medication administration is similar. First, data pertaining to a particular subject are compared to the knowledge base for significance and relevance. They are collected and analyzed for accuracy, adequacy (of kind as well as amount), and similarities. Synthesizing and analyzing of data in light of the knowledge base plus experience result in the identification of a nursing problem or problems. When a phrase is added to this simple problem statement about its etiology or cause and the signs and symptoms resulting, it becomes a nursing diagnosis. This is the PES format—problem, etiology, sign and symptoms. The PES format is one current conceptual interpretation of nursing diagnosis.

The development of a nursing diagnosis follows; note that there could be countless ways to say the same idea, all equally correct.

Problem statement: Patient has a potential for an allergic drug reaction.

Then, to create a nursing diagnosis, the etiology of the problem and the signs and symptoms are added:

Nursing diagnosis: Patient has a potential for an allergic drug reaction to Gantrisin due to a past history of allergy to other medications and the presence of a slight rash on his back.

Of course, even this could be elaborated to describe more thoroughly parts of the diagnostic statement; for example, the rash could be described more specifically as to its exact anatomic location, size of patch, type of lesions, and the like. More about specific allergies could also be detailed. Following this, the phases of planning, implementation, and evaluation would proceed, including the action of with-

holding the suspect medication after collaboratim with the prescribing health care provider.

Another example is as follows:

Problem statement: Potential for side and toxic effects of medication.

Nursing diagnosis: Potential for hemorrhage due to the administration of both coumadin and acetylsalicylic acid.

Assessment in nursing pharmacotherapeutics is the ongoing collection and analysis of data when inferences have been made that a patient (1) needs or could benefit from a medication not yet ordered or (2) no longer needs or no longer is benefitting from a medication because either the disorder has resolved or the side and toxic effects outweigh possible gains from the primary effects of the medication.

Summary of nursing considerations

The nursing process is the problem-solving system used in professional nursing today to organize and facilitate patient care. It is divided into four steps: assessment, planning, implementation, and evaluation. This chapter explores the assessment phase and the way in which it is used in clinical nursing to organize the giving of medications to patients.

Assessment is the phase in which data are gathered on which to base nursing decisions. Data include patient, environmental, and drug information. Common problems inherent in these areas are explored and suggestions are made to avert them.

Accountability and the seriousness of the nurse's responsibility in proper drug administration are underscored. Official and proprietary sources of drug information are listed for the convenience of the reader.

Nursing diagnosis, as the final step of the assessment phase, is described and given a historical overview.

QUESTIONS

FOR STUDY AND REVIEW

1 The nursing process consists of four phases, the first of which is _____.

2 A medication order must be signed by the prescriber to be _____.

3 A nurse may not legally change the route of administration of a medication because _____.

4 The United States Pharmacopeia now incorporates _____.

5 The first phase of the nursing process culminates with the determination of a _____.

REFERENCES

1. Campbell, C.: Nursing diagnosis and intervention in Nursing practice, New York, 1978, John Wiley & Sons, Inc.

2. Henderson, V., and Nite, G.: Principles and practice of Nursing, ed. 6, New York, 1978, Macmillan, Inc., p. 430.

3. Price, M.R. Nursing diagnosis: making a concept come alive, Am. J. Nurs. 80(4):668-671, 1980.

BIBLIOGRAPHY

Alcohol-drug interactions, F.D.A. Drug Bull. **9(2)**:10-12, 1979.

Alvares, A.P.: Interactions between environmental chemicals and drug biotransformation in man, Clin. Pharmacokinetics **3**:462, 1978.

Bell, S.K.: Guidelines for taking a complete drug history, Nursing '80 **10**:10, 1980.

Clinical implications of the Surgeon General's Report on Smoking and Health, FDA Drug Bull. **9(1)**:4, Feb.-Mar. 1979.

Conney, A.H., and others: Enhanced phenacetin metabolism in humans fed charcoal broiled beef, Clin. Pharmacol. Ther. **20**:633, 1976.

Drug effects can go up in smoke, The Consumer, H.E.W. Pub. No. (FDA)79-3086, Washington, D.C., 1979, U.S. Government Printing Office.

Food and drug interactions, FDA Consumer, H.E.W. Pub. No. (FDA)78-3070, Washington, D.C., 1978, U.S. Government Printing Office.

Franke, D.E., and Whitney, H.A.K., editors: Perspectives in clinical pharmacy, Hamilton, Ill., 1972, Drug Intelligence Publications.

Gebbie, K., and Lavin, M.A.: Classifying nursing diagnosis, Am. J. Nurs. **74**:250, 1974.

Gordon, M., and others: Nursing diagnosis: looking at its use in the clinical area, Am. J. Nurs. **80**:672, 1980.

Greenblatt, D., and Koch-Weser, J.: Intramuscular injection of drugs, N. Engl. J. Med. **295**:542, 1976.

Guide to prescription costs, Department of Health and Human Services, Health Care Financing Administration Pub No. HCFA-02104-A, Washington, D.C., June 1980, U.S. Government Printing Office.

Handbook of nonprescription drugs, ed. 6, Washington, D.C. 1979, American Pharmaceutical Association.

Hansten, P.D.: Drug interactions, Philadelphia, 1979, Lee & Febiger.

Hayes, S.L., and others: Effect of ethanol on drug absorption, N. Engl. J. Med. **296**:186, 1977.

Itasalo, E., and Ruikka, I.: Serum levels of antibiotics and renal excretion of digoxin in the elderly, Acta Med. Scand. **196**:59, 1974.

Jeffery, W.H., and others: Loss of warfarin effect after occupational insecticide exposure, J.A.M.A. **236**:2881, 1976.

Lambert, M.L., Jr.: Drug and food interactions, Am. J. Nurs. **75(3)**:403, 1975.

Newton, D.W., and Newton, M.: Route, site and technique, Nursing '79 **9**:18, 1979.

Ochs, H.R., and others: Reduced quinidine clearance in elderly persons, Am. J. Cardiol. **42**:481, 1978.

Oglivie, R.I.: Clinical pharmacokinetics of theophylline, Clin. Pharmacokinetics **3**:267, 1978.

Shader, R.I., and others: Absorption and disposition of chlordiazepoxide in young and elderly male volunteers, J. Clin. Pharmacol. **17**:709, 1977.

Smith, D.: A clinical nursing tool, Am. J. Nurs. **68**:2384, 1968.

United States Pharmacopeial Convention: The United States Pharmacopeia, rev. XX, and The National Formulary, rev. XV, Rockville, Md., 1980, United States Pharmacopeial Convention, Inc.

Yaffee, S.J.: Comment, Pediatric Alert **2(3)**:3, 1977.

CHAPTER 6

Plans, implementation, and evaluation

Goal setting and specific planning
Implementation
Administering medications
Recording drug administration
Preventing and reporting errors
Patient teaching
Evaluation
Summary of nursing considerations

In the nursing process, once an assessment of a problem has been made and the specific problems have been stated and given priorities, the first definitive step has been taken. This chapter deals with the remaining phases of the nursing process as they relate to the medication needs of patients: the planning, implementation, and evaluation phases. The planning phase has two parts: goal setting and specific planning for implementation. The implementation phase comprises all those nursing interventions necessary for actually carrying out the plans that have been projected. Evaluation consists of a review of the patient's condition or behavior after the plans have been carried out to determine whether the stated goals have been met. If no goals were met, a reassessment is made, and the cyclic process is repeated. Once again, we are reminded that the nursing process is a systematic process for problem solving in nursing that facilitates the efficiency of providing optimal drug therapy to the patient in the clinical environment. Our written communication tool, the nursing care plan, is the medium for exchange of information about our patient.

Goal setting and specific planning

The planning to meet the pharmacotherapeutic nursing needs of patients should be characterized by the following: (1) patient orientation, (2) environmental orientation, and (3) future orientation. These in turn should be characterized by a balance between the real and the ideal.

Goals associated with medication needs of patients may be stated in many ways to encompass these three directions. They must actually be stated (for example, in the nursing care plan) to provide communication with the rest of the staff and to give clear direction for the subsequent implementation and evaluation phases. Otherwise implementation and evaluation of the nursing care will be based on vague events and partially remembered and incomplete actions.

Goals are objectives to be met sometime in the future. Therefore, the use of the words "will be" in the goal statement is appropriate. An approximation of time limits for the goal to be accomplished should be included in the statement as a measurement of progress toward the goal, whether short term, intermediate, or long term. Completion of the plan of care should be stated in the goal: "by date of discharge," "in 3 days," "by 2 PM today." The time limit should be the best estimate, not an edict carved in stone. The goal should be patient oriented in that it *should describe what the patient's condition or behavior will be at the* **outcome** *of nursing care*, not what the nurse intends to do for the patient. For example, a goal is best stated as "Patient will demonstrate understanding of drug regimen before discharge from the hospital," rather than "To promote understanding of the drug regimen by the time of discharge from the hospital." If the terms describe only what nurses do, they could work diligently to promote patients' understanding of a drug regimen, and success would merely be measured in the evaluation of what procedures were performed; yet the patient may never be able to demonstrate learning, which is the actual goal desired.

The nurse can prevent the blurring of goals and intervention—two entirely different phases of the nursing process—by stating goals in terms of behavioral objectives for the patient. If goals are stated in words that depict nursing interventions or actions, such as "prevent," "provide," or "promote," then evaluation of care becomes more an appraisal of what the nurse did by intervening than of the patient's condition.

Finally, goals related to each nursing problem or diagnosis identified earlier can be ranked in priority to meet the patient's needs.

The rest of the planning phase lays the groundwork for carrying out specific actions in the implementation phase. Such plans for nursing actions should be supportable by applicable principles from the arts, sciences, and humanities, which are the foundations of nursing.

Development of a positive, assertive attitude through goal setting and specific planning for each nursing action strengthens what nurses do for patients and why. Goal setting and specific planning provide documentation for peers and preclude legal challenge, while first and foremost guiding the selection of appropriate caring actions. The completed abbreviated nursing care plan, as a blueprint for action, can be entered in writing in the Kardex or in the patient's chart and makes up the plan for nursing management.

Implementation

Implementation is the actual giving of care as prescribed by the nursing care plan or nursing orders. Guided by the nursing care plan as outlined, with goals clearly in focus, proposed actions can be initiated. They should be reviewed with the patient continually as they change. Any action not viewed by patients as congruent with their goals will not likely be fully successful.

The implementation phase in the nursing process of pharmacotherapeutics relates predominantly to any phase of actually administering medications. It encompasses the act of medicating patients according to prescribers' orders (depending on patient response), offering to the prescriber suggestions about the need to add a new medication to the patient's therapy or to change an existing one, to change a dosage order, to alter the route, site, or frequency of dosage; and temporarily withholding or discontinuing the drug and consulting with the prescriber about a dose of medication carefully judged by the nurse to be inappropriate. In order to perform these complex nursing functions, the nurse needs to be able to rely on interpersonal, cognitive, and psychomotor skills. These actions are the culmination of effort from foundation course work in the biologic as well as the psychosocial sciences.

ADMINISTERING MEDICATIONS

The most visible function of nurses, one most closely identified by the public with nursing and one with the most legal vulnerability, is that of administering medications. It requires much preparation, a solid knowledge base, and skilled decision-making abilities.

Technically, written medical orders are the only legal means for the administration of medications by nurses. Written orders constitute permanent legal records of the prescriber's plans and can be submitted as evidence in case of litigation. As such, nurses must routinely ensure that (1) each order is appropriate, accu-

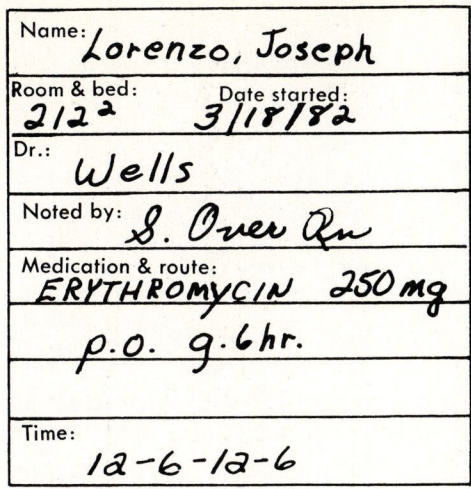

Name: *Lorenzo, Joseph*

Room & bed: *212²* Date started: *3/18/82*

Dr.: *Wells*

Noted by: *S. Over Rn*

Medication & route: *ERYTHROMYCIN 250 mg*

p.o. q·6 hr.

Time: *12-6-12-6*

FIG. 6-1. Transcription of a medication order onto the Kardex or a medication card or ticket.

rate, and complete, and (2) the order is followed unerringly to completion, for they are held legally accountable for every dose of medication that they administer. Free flow of communication between prescriber and nurse is crucial to fulfillment of this responsibility. Nurses must be ready to consult with the prescriber as necessary to clarify, understand, or suggest medication therapy as needed. Assertiveness is a quality that must be developed in the character of professional nurses if they are to deal from an appropriate position of strength within the health care system to promote their patients' best interests while achieving equity for their own contributions.

What is the process by which a prescriber's order is translated into the administration of a medication? It is first transcribed by a ward clerk, head nurse (or nursing care coordinator), or primary nurse from an order sheet onto the Kardex or onto a medication ticket or card (Fig. 6-1). The drug is then requested in a small supply from the institution's pharmacy department. When the supply arrives, it is stored in the medication room either as stock supply to meet general needs of patients on the floor or in an individual patient's own medication box or drawer of a medication cart.

The nurse administers a drug by following the order as written on the medication card, ticket, or Kardex. Because of space limitation, physicians, pharmacists, and nurses rely on

pharmacologic symbols for communication. These are usually from the Latin and are universally used. Table 6-1 includes the most commonly used of these Latin abbreviations, along with some symbols that are common to clinical practice.

The physician's order when transcribed must contain all the elements described in Chapter 5. It must contain the *full name* of the patient; the *date* the order was written; the *medication name, dosage, route,* and *frequency;* and, according to agency policy, the *name* or *initial* of the nurse responsible for the transcription. In addition, the exact *location* of the patient's bed should be noted (for example: Room 202 Bed 2). The physician should later sign the order.

Drug delivery systems and storage

There are several pharmacy-nursing approaches to distributing and dispensing drugs to patients in an institutional setting: the floor stock system, individual patient prescription orders, unit dose drug distribution, and a combination of these. In a complete floor stock system, all medications except infrequently used ones are stored on the nursing unit in the medication room. The disadvantages of this system are the increased potential for medication errors because of the large array of stock medications to choose from, the economic loss caused by misplaced or forgotten charges and increased amounts of expired drugs to be discarded, the need for frequent total drug inventorying, and storage problems. The individual order method of dispensing each medication to individual patients is an improvement but is rather unwieldy and time consuming. A combination of floor stock and individual orders is superior but has the disadvantages of both systems.

Unit dose drug distribution uses single unit packages of drugs that are dispensed to fill each dosage requirement as it comes up. It is the safest and most economical method of drug distribution in institutions. The disadvantages of using the unit dose system are primarily those of space for storage. Small and inexpensive single unit package machines are available for purchase that permit hospital pharmacists to make up unit dose packages from their own

T A B L E 6 - 1 Common abbreviations and symbols

Abbreviation	Unabbreviated form	Meaning	Abbreviation	Unabbreviated form	Meaning
a.c.	ante cibum	before meals	p.r.n.	pro re nata	according to necessity
ad lib.	ad libitum	freely			
a.m.	morning	morning	pt	patient	patient
b.i.d.	bis in die	twice each day	q.	quaque	every
$\bar{c}$	cum	with	q.d.	quaque die	every day
cap	capsule	capsule	q.h.	quaque hora	every hour
cc, cm³	cubic centimeter	cubic centimeter	q.4h., q4°	every 4 hours	every 4 hours around the clock
clt	client	client			
dc	discontinue	terminate	q.i.d.	quater in die	four times each day
dl, dL	deciliter	one tenth of a liter			
D_5W	dextrose 5% in water	dextrose IV solution	q.o.d.	quaque aliem die	every other day
			q.s.	quantum satis	sufficient quantity
elix	elixir	elixir	R	right	right
g	gram	1000 milligrams	R_x	receipt	take
gr	grain	60 milligrams	$\bar{s}$	sine	without
gtt	gutta	drop	S.O.S.	si opus sit	if necessary
h.s.	hora somni	at bedtime	ss.	semis	a half
IM	intramuscular	into a muscle	stat.	statim	at once
IV	intravenous	into a vein	subcu, SQ, SC	subcutaneous	into subcutaneous tissue
IVPB	IV piggyback	secondary IV line			
kg	kilogram	2.2 lb	tbsp	tablespoon	tablespoon
KVO	keep vein open	very slow infusion rate	T.O.	telephone order	order received over the telephone
L	left, liter	left, liter			
mcg, μg	microgram	one millionth of a gram	tsp	teaspoon	teaspoon
mg	milligram	one thousandth of a gram	V.O.	verbal order	order received verbally
mEq	milliequivalent	milliequivalent	ī, ī̄ī	one, two	one (as in gr ī), two
min. or ℥	minimum	minim	ʒ	dram	0.0625 ounce
ml, mL	milliliter	milliliter	℥	ounce or fluid-ounce	ounce (30 milliliters)
NS	normal saline	0.9% sodium chloride IV solution	×	times	as in two times a week
$\bar{o}$	no or none	no or none	>	greater than	greater than
o.d.	oculus dexter	right eye	<	less than	less than
o.s.	oculus sinister	left eye	=	equal to	equal to
os	os	mouth	↑, ↗	increase or increasing	increase or increasing
OTC	over-the-counter	nonprescription drug	↓, ↙	decrease or decreasing	decrease or decreasing
o.u.	oculus uterque	each eye			
p.c.	post cibum	after meals			
P.O.	per os	by mouth, orally			

stock supplies for medications ordered for patients in their hospital. The hazard is that the nurse is responsible for the administration of a medication whose accuracy is determined by someone else.

The advantages of using unit dose packages far outweigh their disadvantages. The most important advantage is medication safety and a decrease in error, since drug computations are eliminated. The drug is already properly labeled and does not have to be prepared. All the nurse needs to do is deliver the package to the patient, where it is opened at the bedside and administered. This may permit patients to check on their own drugs and be assured of proper medication and dosage. Unit dose packaging also decreases chances of deterioration and permits giving financial credit to the patient for drugs not used. Otherwise, because of fear of contamination, bottles of unused drugs may often be discarded and not relabeled for any other patient. Because of this the patient for whom the drug was originally ordered does not get financial credit for drugs he did not receive.

Strip packages permit ease of narcotic

counting, since all packages in the strip are numbered and only the number needs to be checked. This also prevents contamination caused by pouring narcotic tablets into the hands for counting, which is a grossly improper technique. Prefilled disposable syringes for medications to be given subcutaneously, intramuscularly, and even intravenously are available through the unit dose system. Their advantages are:

1 Accuracy of dosage
2 Sterile product
3 Sharp needle
4 Elimination of suspected source of serum hepatitis
5 Less danger of allergic sensitization of personnel handling the drugs
6 Immediate availability of drug for use
7 Charge only for medicine used
8 Reduced likelihood of pilferage of narcotics
9 Less waste by breakage or incomplete use
10 Safer use of nonprofessionals permitted to administer subcutaneous or intramuscular drugs

Unit dose dispensing systems in hospitals may be centralized, decentralized, or a combination of both. In the centralized system the pharmacist and pharmacy are located in a central area from which doses for all patients are prepared and distributed to patient care areas. In the decentralized system, clinical pharmacists and satellite pharmacies are located in patient care areas and doses are prepared and distributed to patients in those particular areas. In the combined system, patient medications are prepared in a central area with clinical pharmacists assigned to various patient care areas to oversee drug therapy, thus providing safer and more controlled drug ordering and drug distribution.

Medication carts are used in some hospitals for distributing unit doses to the nursing unit and to the patient's bedside. Each patient has a drawer or tray for his medications, which are stocked by the pharmacy staff.

Clinical pharmacists. The present trend is toward more extensive use of clinical pharmacists who are stationed in nursing areas to work closely with physicians, nurses, and dietitians.

Since pharmacists are well educated in the compounding, dispensing, and control of drugs,

it is only natural that they become more involved in drug therapy for the hospitalized patient. They should not be isolated from the clinical areas where much of the actual compounding and dispensing of drugs in the hospital really takes place.

There are also hospital pharmacies with special "clean rooms" and specially filtered air for compounding various parenteral solutions. The pharmacist may be responsible for putting all additives into intravenous solutions and checking all such solutions for compatibility reactions.

Role of the nurse. Regardless of the changes that may come about in the ordering, distribution, or administration of drugs, nurses are still responsible for their patients and their care 24 hours a day. Automation, clinical pharmacists, and unit package doses do not simplify the task of the nurse but serve to increase the complexity of patient care and responsibility of the nurse. As a result of these changes nurses need to be better informed about drugs and their actions. Nurses still need to make their observations of patients, determine whether p.r.n. orders are to be given, and consult with prescribers about withholding, discontinuing, or changing the drug dosage. They will continue to teach patients about drugs and their effects, to help patients plan their drug therapy upon returning home, and take drug histories.

Drug storage. Certain precepts should guide the way patients' drugs should be stored, distributed, and accounted for. Health care agencies have developed policies that, with variation, support these precepts as rules for patient protection and save nurses from making errors. They are not to be followed so blindly that rational nursing judgments do not enter into the process of decision making. Sometimes departure from these rules is a wise and necessary decision, but it should never be undertaken lightly. It should be a practice to consult other experienced personnel or authorities.

The following guidelines are not necessarily listed in order of importance.

1 All medicines should be kept in a special place, which may be a cupboard, closet, or room. It should not be freely accessible to the public.
2 Narcotic drugs and those dispensed under special legal regulations must be kept in a locked box or

compartment and accounted for at the end of each shift. Any dose that is wasted or discarded must be attested to by another nurse by initialing such a notation.

3 In some hospitals each patient's medicines are kept in a designated place on a shelf or compartment of the medicine cupboard or room or in a drawer of the medication cart. Such an arrangement means that the nurse must be careful to keep the patient's medicines in the right area and to make certain that, when the patient leaves the hospital, the medicines are returned to the pharmacy or are taken home by the patient.

4 If stock supplies are maintained, they should be arranged in an orderly manner. Preparations for internal use should be kept separate from those used externally.

5 Some preparations, such as serums, vaccines, certain suppositories, certain antibiotics, and insulin, need to be kept on a refrigerator shelf, not on the door.

6 Labels of all medicines should be clean and legible. If they are not, they should be sent to the pharmacist for relabeling. *Nurses should not label or relabel medicines.*

7 Bottles of medicines should always be stoppered and protected from light, heat, and high humidity as necessary.

Preparing to administer medications

Dosage and scheduling. Medical rationale for selection of a particular dosage for a patient and the frequency of administration requires that the nurse have some basic understanding of the drug in question. The most influential factors are pharmacokinetic variations in a patient's system or malfunctioning of particular organ systems of the patient. These factors account for many of the observable variations in response to specific drug therapy.

In general, increasing the dose of a drug or the frequency with which it is given increases its pharmacologic effects but can also increase the risk of side and toxic effects. Studies to determine optimal dosages of individual drugs involve *dose-response* relationships; studies to determine optimal frequency or intervals of dosages involve *time-response* relationships. Dose-response relationships involve interaction of the following three variables: *drug potency* (absolute amount of drug required to produce a desired effect); *therapeutic index*, or relative margin of safety (ratio of lethal dose to effective dose); and *maximum effect* (the greatest response possible regardless of dosage given).

In general, to avoid wide fluctuations in serum concentration of a drug, the intervals between doses are chosen so that as close to a steady state as possible is maintained without accumulation of the drug above the plateau level. If the dosage interval is too short, accumulation with potential for toxicity will occur. If it is too long, serum concentration will drop because of increased relative excretion of the drug. Accumulation of drugs with very short half-lives will not occur if they are given orally and frequently, since very frequent doses are needed for accumulation. With a drug that has a very long half-life, once-daily dosing may be sufficient.

Time-response relationships involve the association of the following variables: *latency* (time necessary for onset of response), *maximum effect* (time after administration for the drug's effect to peak), and *duration of action* after a single dose, all of which are affected by the route used and pharmacokinetics involved. These factors also influence the drug's response variability in patients.

In studies of drugs, results are interpreted on the basis of a normal curve, and dosages and dosage intervals are derived for treating the ideal "average" person in a population. This explains why certain medications with relatively long half-lives can be given on a once-a-day basis for most people. Likewise, it explains why a drug scheduled to be given every 6 hours should not be expected to be as effective for most people if given arbitrarily instead by the nurse four times a day during daylight hours; it is less likely that optimal serum levels or tissue levels will be maintained by the latter schedule. It also explains why, although dosage and dosage intervals have been studied statistically, the need for individualization of drug therapy regimens must continually be reassessed. Because of the many variables inherent in the population, some people will fall outside the average range with regard to a drug's response. In addition, dosage intervals should be modified by consideration of patient convenience and its effect on compliance.

Within the limitations of a drug's pharmacokinetics and patient characteristics, the exact schedule for administering the drug may be determined by policy of the agency's nursing department. For example, times for q.i.d. administration of drugs may be routinely set at 10 AM, 2 PM, 6 PM, and 10 PM, or at 9 AM, 1 PM, 5 PM, and 9 PM, or at other sequences based on patient convenience and the need to avoid mealtimes or other activities that might interfere with either drug administration or its pharmacokinetics.* Drugs administered only once a day, for example, can usually be given with some flexibility in scheduling, just before or after a treatment that would interfere with a dosage time, such as a patient's trip off the floor to the physical therapy department or x-ray department. Drugs should be administered to patients as close to the time indicated as possible, but obviously a nurse cannot medicate each of a group of assigned patients all at the same time. Agency policies may vary, but usually they stipulate that individual drugs should be administered within ½ hour before or after the indicated time. Thus a drug scheduled to be given at 10 AM could be given any time from 9:30 to 10:30 AM. Exempt from this flexibility in policy are stat or one-time-only drug orders, such as those given before diagnostic procedures or surgery.

Drug effects are monitored by the prescriber in either *direct ways* (observation for clinical responses) or *indirect ways* (laboratory values or serum concentrations of the drug). Nurses, because of their unique function and expertise, are most capable in assisting the prescriber in the drug assessment process by giving their observations and suggestions concerning the efficacy of response to a drug, its schedule, or the need to add or remove a drug from a particular medication plan.

Dosage measurement. When the correct amount of a drug is not prepackaged in single-unit doses, the nurse must be able to choose by label from among numerous drugs for the patient the right drug and the right dose. If the drug is formulated in units that are multiples of the dosage ordered, whether tablet or liquid, the computation to determine the correct dose is simple. If, however, the drug does not come in units that are multiples of the dose prescribed, if the drug must be dissolved in water, or if the

order is written in the apothecary system and the drug is available only in metric units, some nurses may have difficulty in dosage calculations. This may present drug administration as a forbidding task and lend tension to the atmosphere of drug preparation, making it conducive to error. But the clinician, as a responsible professional, will correct any shortcomings and improve skills.

Flow rate calculations are necessary for certain therapies in order to set the proper amount for the desired dose effect. Intravenous (IV) infusions (some deliver no more than 170 to 200 calories/1000 ml and even those are derived solely from carbohydrates), hyperalimentation or total parenteral nutrition (often capable of delivering the patient's total nutritional needs), and oxygen therapies necessitate careful flow rate calculation. These therapies should be ordered by the prescriber in definitive amounts and rates.

The rate of replacement fluids with or without other additives by IV infusion may be regulated in one of two basic ways. One is by a simple *roller clamp* on the tubing, which can be manually adjusted to deliver the number of drops per minute that will provide the prescribed total amount in a given time. Given the total volume of solution to be infused, the total number of minutes the solution is to be infused, and the drop factor (number of drops per milliliter that the tubing delivers—a number that varies among tubing maufacturers), the prescribed drops per minute can be calculated and the set regulated by counting drops in the drip chamber of the tubing. A simple formula for IV flow rate calculation can be found among the Exercises, in later material.

Another way that infusions can be made to run more precisely is by the use of instrumentation such as IV controllers and pumps.* These can be used in situations that warrant more accurate titration of infusion fluids or nutrients than provided by hand-adjusted roller clamps, which can allow up to a 5% error in flow rate within the first 15 minutes of flow. One study in a Boston hospital revealed that 37% of their hospitalized patients who died

*Special units, such as pediatrics, have medication hours set to coincide with the special needs of their patients.

*Our appreciation is extended to Mr. R. Pentell of IVAC Corporation for his review of the material on IV controllers and pumps.

from drug-related causes did so from fluid overload or potassium excess (potassium is a frequent additive to intravenous infusions). A rise in use of instrumentation for regulating IV flow rate can be predicted in the future.

Most of the instrumentation to regulate infusions consists of various applications of either infusion controllers or infusion pumps (at least two types). They are small boxlike devices attached to special IV poles and through which the infusion tubing is strung for regulation of rate to assure automatic delivery of solutions at preselected rates or volumes.

Infusion controllers (Fig. 6-2) work simply by utilizing the force of gravity; they are not capable of delivering the accuracy of *infusion pumps*, which may be more useful in special situations where there will be rises in back pressure that are transmitted to the fluid in the tubing. Such is the situation when the patient is a screaming child or a woman in labor or in arterial infusions. However, unlike the infusion pumps, *IV controllers* will not pump fluid into interstitial tissue if the infusion needle infiltrates. *Controllers* are useful in 80% to 85% of cases calling for intravenous therapy.

Infusion pumps are of at least two kinds, both delivering infusion fluids under positive pressure: (1) nonvolumetric ("infusion pumps"; Fig. 6-3), which measure fluid volume delivery by drop rate (not as accurate since drop volume may vary), and (2) volumetric ("volume pumps"; Fig. 6-4), which can measure very precisely even smaller volumes of infusion solution by ml/hour. This latter pump is especially useful for small children, total parenteral nutrition, etc.; alarm readout messages (for example, "Fix Me") may be displayed on the front panel of the instrument.

Similar instrumentation is made by several different manufacturers and utilizes various physical principles to sense pressures and pump fluid and read out the flow-rate settings and the like. Their capabilities include greater accuracy than other modes of infusion delivery systems and alarms to warn of blocked tubing, air in the tubing, or empty solution containers. All this capability sounds ideal, but like all mechanical devices, infusion pumps are subject to malfunction and therefore require continued watchfulness by nurses to assure reliability and

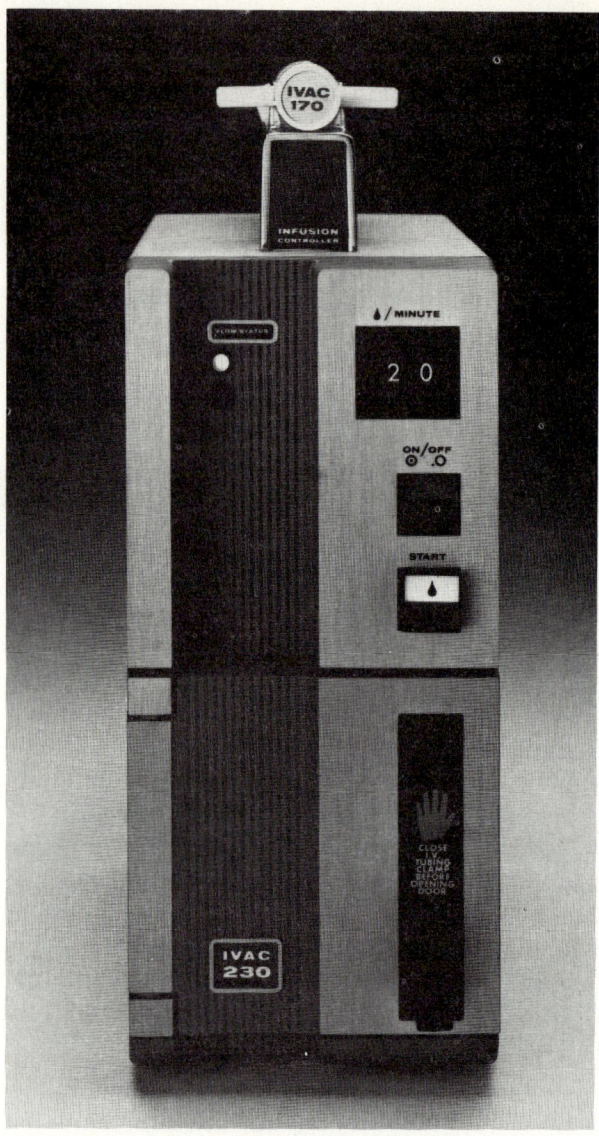

FIG. 6-2. Infusion controller, which is used when gravity alone can provide sufficient force to control accuracy of preset drop rate. It is the most commonly used type of infusion instrumentation. (Courtesy IVAC Corp.)

to maintain personal contact with the purpose of it all—the patient. There is currently a growing fund of literature on this type of equipment. Its intricacy presents nurses with still another challenge. It is not an insurmountable one. The reader is referred to the excellent references at the end of the chapter to learn more.

Oxygen therapy is also ordered in units of flow rate. Oxygen is a medication that should be administered with care, expecially to a patient with a chronic pulmonary disorder or one who requires longer-than-usual continuous oxygen supportive therapy. Regardless of the

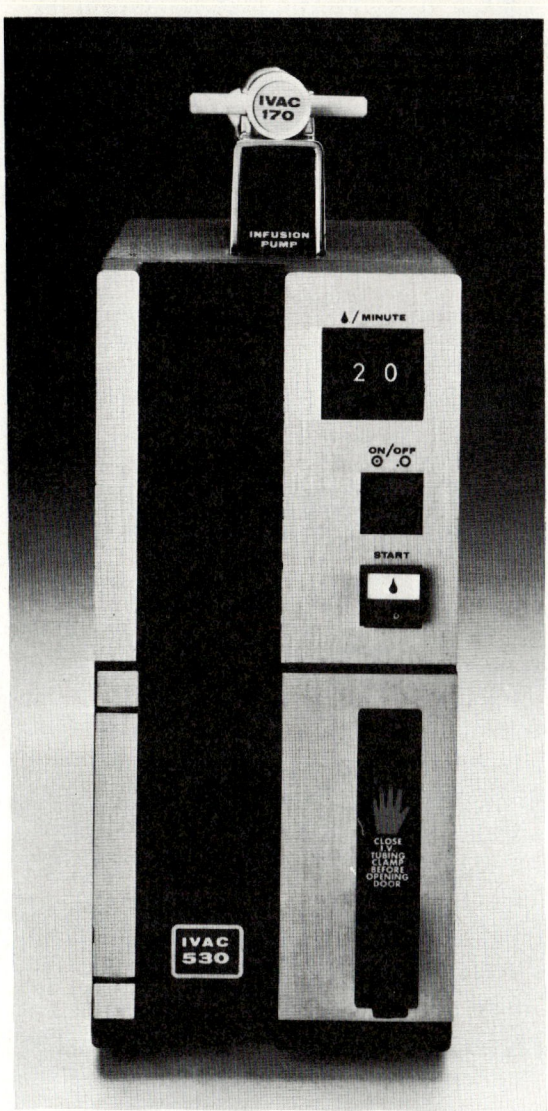

FIG. 6-3. Typical infusion pump used when positive pressure provided by peristaltic action on the tubing produces the preset drop rate. (Courtesy IVAC Corp.)

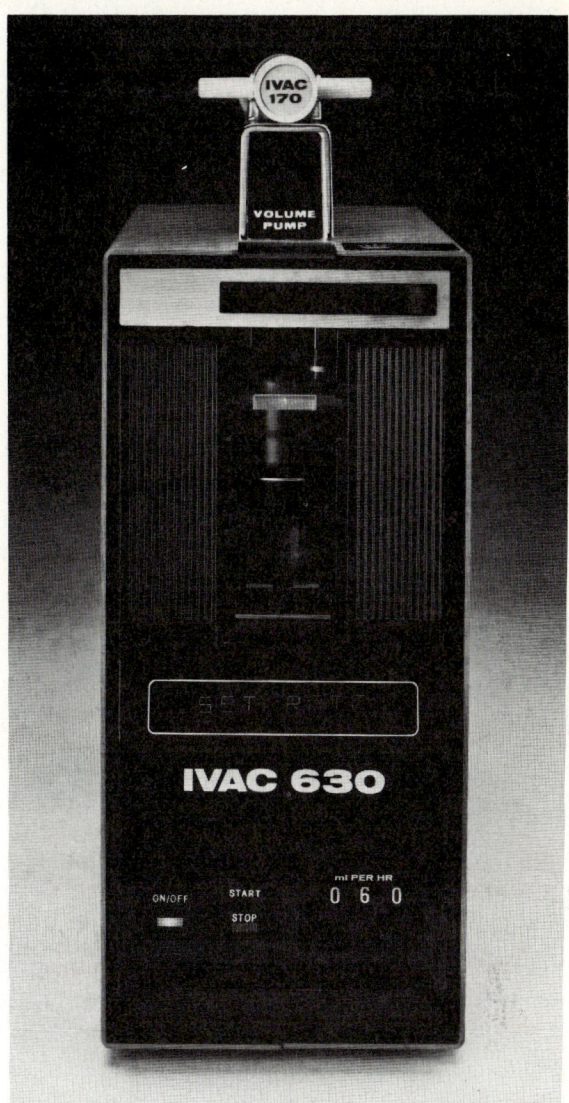

FIG. 6-4. A positive pressure volumetric infusion pump, which assures close accuracy of the infusion in volumes of milliliters per hour rather than the slightly less accurate drops per minute of other types of pumps. (Courtesy IVAC Corp.)

delivery equipment (cannula or "prongs," catheter, mask, or tent), the oxygen order should specifically state the desired flow, usually in liters per minute (often 2 to 4 liters/minute) and, if necessary, by concentration desired. Regulation is usually by a flow meter calibrated in liters per minute, which is attached to a jar of oxygen-humidifying sterile distilled water to alleviate the drying effect of oxygen on respiratory mucosa.

Frequently oxygen is ordered to be given at a certain rate, "p.r.n.," or "on standby" for the patient who can be anticipated to have occa-

sional bouts of dyspnea or chest pain caused by coronary insufficiency. Full, continuous oxygen therapy for more than 24 hours can have serious consequences, since oxygen works to fuel oxidative body processes; certain tissues (especially lung and retinal tissues in the newborn) may literally burn themselves out. Patients with a history of chronic obstructive pulmonary disorders may also be at risk if the rate of flow routinely exceeds about 2 liters/minute. The bodily oxygen sensors in these patients have become accustomed to lower than normal blood oxygen levels accompanied by higher carbon dioxide levels. Their sensors have adapted to regulating respiratory excursions via higher than normal carbon dioxide levels. If these sensors are suddenly flooded with normal or high oxygen levels and correspondingly reduced carbon dioxide levels, the drive to initiate respirations is reduced or eliminated. Thus patients with chronic obstructive pulmonary disease may stop breathing if oxygen is delivered at a normal or high flow rate.

A dosage problem may be as simple as giving 10 grains of acetylsalicylic acid from a container of 5-grain tablets. It is almost as easy to figure out how many milliliters of morphine sulfate one must give if the container is labeled "15 mg = 1 ml" and the order reads "10 mg morphine sulfate s.c." Problems arise when the units of measurement in the medication order must be converted to the type of unit in which the drug is available.

Currently three systems of measurement are in use for administering medications: the metric system (the most widely adopted and the most convenient); the apothecary system (rapidly being phased out except for a few drugs); and the household system (the least accurate and not widely used except in home settings).

Metric system. The metric system of weights and measures was invented by the French at the end of the eighteenth century, and toward the end of the nineteenth century the Bureau of Weights and Measures was formed and given the challenge to develop metric standards for international use. The United States finally joined the worldwide trend toward adoption of the metric system with the enactment of the Metric Conversion Act of 1975, calling for the country's conversion over a 10-year period.

The basic metric units of measurement are the meter, the liter, and the gram. The *meter* is the unit for linear measurement, the *liter* for capacity or volume, and the *gram* for weight. A meter is a little longer than a yard; a liter is a little more than a quart; and a gram is a little more than the weight of a paper clip.

The metric system is a decimal system; the basic unit can be divided into 10, 100, or 1000 parts; or the basic unit can be multiplied by 10, 100, or 1000 to form secondary units that differ

TABLE 6-2 Metric prefixes, meanings, and relationships

Prefix	Meaning
Giga*	Billions
Kilo†	Thousands
Hecto	Hundreds
Deka	Tens
Base units of meter, liter, gram	One unit
Deci	Tenths
Centi†	Hundredths
Milli†	Thousandths
Micro	Millionths
Nano	Billionths

Data from The International System of Units, National Bureau of Standards Publications No. 330, August 1977, U.S. Department of Commerce.
*Abbreviated G, as opposed to g for gram.
†Prefixes most commonly encountered in nursing.

from each other by 10 or some multiple of 10. The names of the secondary units are formed by joining Greek and Latin prefixes to the names of the primary unit (Table 6-2). Subdivisions of the basic unit are made by moving the decimal point to the left, and multiples of the basic unit are indicated by moving the decimal point to the right.

The *meter* is the unit from which the other metric units were derived. Centimeters and millimeters are the chief linear measures used in hospital work. Measurement of the size of body organs is made in centimeters and millimeters, and students will recall that the sphygmomanometer used in measuring blood pressure is calibrated in millimeters. There are approximately 2.5 cm (25 mm) in 1 inch.

The *liter* is the unit of capacity or volume and is equal to approximately 1000 cc and to 1000 ml. The weight of a liter of water at 4° C is 1 kg. The contents of a cube whose sides measure 1 decimeter (10 cm) constitute the unit of capacity. It was originally intended that the liter and the cubic decimeter should be exactly the same. Because of the difficulty of measurement, however, the liter is slightly larger than 1 cubic decimeter.

The liter, therefore, is 28 parts per 1,000,000 larger than intended. However, since the liter in common use is acutally 1000.028 cc, the cubic centimeter is less than the milliliter by 0.000028 cc. *In practice the cubic centimeter and*

T A B L E 6 - 3 **Approximate equivalents of weights and measures**

Metric	Apothecary	Household
Weight		
1 kg*	2.2 pounds	
1000 mg = 1 gram*	gr xv	
60 mg* (occasionally seen as 65 mg)	gr i̇	
30 mg	gr ss (one half)	
1 μg (mcg) = 0.001 mg		
Volume		
	4 quarts	1 gallon
1000 ml* = 1 liter or approx 1000 cc (cm³)	Approx 1 qt	
500 ml	Approx 1 pint (½ qt)	16 ounces
240 ml	ʒ viii (8 fluidounces)† = approx ½ pint	1 cup or 1 glass
30 ml* = approx 30 cc (or cm³)	ʒ i̇ (1 fluidounce)	2 tbsp
Approx 16 ml = approx 16 cc (cm³)	ʒ iv (4 fluidrams)	1 tbsp
8 ml	ʒ ïi (2 fluidrams)	2 tsp
4 to 5 ml	ʒ i̇ (1 fluidram)	1 tsp
1 ml* = approx 1 cc (cm³)	Minims xv or xvi	Minims cannot be compared with drops

*These equivalents may be committed to memory for ready application to dosage problems.
†Note the small difference in the symbols for fluidounce and fluidram.

the milliliter are considered equal. The difference is so small that it is of no importance except in determinations of great precision.

Fractional parts of a liter are usually expressed in milliliters or cubic centimeters. For example, 0.6 liter would be expressed as 600 ml or 600 cc.* Multiples of a liter are similarly expressed: 2.4 liters would be 2400 ml or cc.

The *gram* is the metric unit of weight that is used in weighing drugs and various pharmaceutical preparations. Originally, the unit of measurement of weight was the kilogram, but this proved too large to meet the practical needs of the pharmacist. The gram is the weight of 1 ml of distilled water at 4° C.

The approved abbreviation for gram is g; G as the abbreviation for gram is no longer approved, as it conflicts with the abbreviation for the prefix giga. Gm is also not approved by the National Bureau of Standards.

As a review of Table 6-2 indicates, 1 decigram is 10 times greater than a centigram and 100 times greater than a milligram. To change decigrams to centigrams one would therefore multiply by 10; to change decigrams to milligrams one would multiply by 100. To change milligrams to centigrams one would divide by 10; to change milligrams to decigrams one would divide by 100; to change milligrams to grams one would divide by 100; and so forth.

The International System of Units (referred to as SI) has a standard style of notation that everyone should follow except when it is in conflict with proper English language norms:

Units are not capitalized (gram not Gram).
No period should be used with abbreviations of units (ml not m.l. or ml.).
A single space should be left between the quantity and the symbol (25 kg not 25kg).
Large numbers may be separated into groups of three numbers, without comma (25 000 not 25,000).
Only decimal notation should be used, not fractions (0.25 kg not ¼ kg).
Numerical quantities less than 1 should have a zero placed to the left of the decimal point (0.75 mg not .75 mg).
Abbreviations should not be pluralized (kg not kgs).

Nurses need the foregoing as part of their knowledge base not only for use in preparing medications but also for interpreting laboratory data (some are reported in milliliters, others in deciliters or nanograms, and so forth), for weighing patients (kilograms instead of pounds), and figuring flow rates of IV infusions.

Until the metric system is fully accepted and used in clinical practice, nurses will need to

* The abbreviation cc is in the process of being dropped and is considered obsolete; ml or mL or cm³ is to be used (Source: National Bureau of Standards).

deal with all three systems of measurement; metric, apothecary, and household. The most practical approach may be to gain a basic understanding of the logic of each system and then review the interrelationships between the systems (Table 6-3). Then a few crucial relationships can be extracted and memorized. These data can then be readily inserted where applicable as part of a formula or as half of a ratio-and-proportion equation so often used for dosage calculation. A suggested practical list of equivalents that nurses should know is presented in Table 6-3.

Apothecary system. Only a few medications are now ordered or available in units of the apothecary system. It is less convenient and less precise than the metric system. The basic unit of weight is the *grain,* which is derived from the age-old standard of the weight of a single grain of wheat, a weight now variously accepted as approximately equivalent to 60 or 65 mg (60 mg is the more widely accepted of the two). Other units of weight commonly used in the apothecary system are the dram, the ounce, and the pound.

The basic unit of fluid volume is the *minim,* approximately equal to the volume of water that would weigh a grain, a very small amount equal to about 0.005 or 0.006 ml. Other volume measures, which may also be considered household measures, are the pint and quart.

The placement of abbreviations and the type of numerals used in the apothecary system are a more complex arrangement than in the metric system. Usually the abbreviation is placed before the numeral. Whole numerical quantities usually are expressed in roman numerals (for example, gr x for 10 grains). Fractional quantities are usually expressed by arabic numerals rather than by decimals (for example, gr ¼, not gr 0.25, for one-quarter grain). When comparing fractional amounts, remember that the larger the bottom number (the denominator), the smaller the quantity involved, given the same numerator. In other words, gr $\frac{1}{200}$ is a smaller quantity than gr $\frac{1}{150}$.

Household measures. With the increase of nursing care in the home, household measures may be used for medication administration,

though it is to be discouraged because of the wide variation among measuring instruments found in the home. Measures include the glass, cup, tablespoon, teaspoon, and drops; pints and quarts are often included here as well as in the apothecary system. Because standardized measurements of household equipment usually do not exist, the community health nurse may not have access in the home to an accurately calibrated measuring device. For example, the average teacup or coffee cup can hold anywhere from 5 to 9 oz or more, not the accepted 8 oz or half pint; the average household teaspoon can hold 4 or 5 ml or more of liquid medication, rather than the standard 5 ml. A drop and a minim *cannot* be considered equivalents, since drop size will vary with viscosity of the medication and other variables even when measured by an approved dropper. Therefore, any listing of household measurements on a table of equivalent measures must be considered only approximate measures. Depending on the situation and the need for precise dosage, such measures may or may not be acceptable.

Dosage calculation. Serious challenges to the computational skills of nurses occur infrequently in the administration of medications. Most calculations can be done with confidence by the average nurse or nursing student based on high school experience with ratio-and-proportion logic or any other competent mechanism to which one has become accustomed. An equation can be set up in a way that applies what the nurse has learned about a few crucial equivalents and how that relates to what needs to be solved—all in a logical sequence or relationship. Calculators are not acceptable in the nursing unit, for they tend to be too bulky, to have exasperating battery failures, or to disappear from busy hospital units. It is best to develop and maintain one's competence in mathematical calculations. If distractions impede concentration, the nurse should work dosage problems out on paper. Seeing the problem and thinking it through help avoid error.

Following are some typical exercises to do, accompanied by explanations and answers. These exercises assume a working knowledge of decimals, fractions, and a ratio-and-proportion approach to problem solving. Again, if you are used to working with another method that works as well, use it instead—just check your answers and rationale with the following.

EXERCISES

1. If a drug is ordered in metric units different from the units on hand, the order must be mathematically translated into the units available. Thus if the medication order is written in terms of milligrams, yet the patient's drug is supplied in grams, for example, you must translate the needed dose into grams.

   Example: A drug is ordered to be given in the amount of 1500 mg. How many grams would you give?

   Answer: Knowing that there are 1000 mg in a gram, set up the ratio in logical sequence. The logic of the relationships ("this is to this as that is to that") remains constant in a ratio-and-proportion approach, but which of the relationships is set down first in the equation does not matter. Some people set down first, on the left side of the equation, the relationship between what has been ordered or what information is wanted in the problem and the unknown quantity, or x. Then on the right side of the equation they set down the known quantities, or the "givens." Once set up, the equation is solved by multiplying the means (middle adjacent numbers) by the extremes (numbers on each end):

   $$1500 \text{ mg}: x = 1000 \text{ mg}: 1 \text{ g}$$
   $$1000x = 1500$$
   $$x = 1.5 \text{ g}$$

2. *Example:* A dosage of 30 ml of cough syrup is ordered to be given q.i.d. The label on the bottle of medication states that it contains a total of 240 cc. How many cubic centimeters would you give?

   Answer: You need to know that 30 ml is roughly equivalent to 30 cc.

3. *Example:* Ten mEq of potassium chloride (KCl) is to be added to an IV infusion solution. KCl is available for this application in vials of 40 mEq/20 ml. How many milliliters would you give?

   Answer: Again, set up the equation in logical sequence, possibly starting with the desired ingredient and ending with the unknown quantity:

   $$10 \text{ mEq}: x = 40 \text{ mEq}: 20 \text{ ml}$$
   $$40 x = 200$$
   $$x = \frac{200}{40} = 5 \text{ ml.}$$

4. Sometimes medication for injection comes in powdered or concentrated liquid form and must

be dissolved (reconstituted) or diluted before it can be injected. Most often directions as to how much diluent (dissolving or diluting solution) and what kind should be added by needle and syringe to the powder or liquid are on the label of the container of the drug. All that the nurse needs to know to figure out the amount to give is on the label.

   Example: A certain antibiotic has been ordered "750 mg IM." The drug comes in a 10-g multiple-dose vial (there is more than enough of the drug in the vial for one dose) in powdered form. The label reads, "Add 7.2 ml sterile water or sodium chloride solution for injection to yield 10 ml of reconstituted drug." After the diluent has been added, how many milliliters would you give?

   Answer: Ten ml now contains 10 g; thus 1 ml equals 1 g. You should already know or be able to refer to a listing of standard equivalents to find out that 1 g equals 1000 mg. You may then start the equation by setting down the relationship between what you want to give and the volume that contains it. Then follow the same sequence of relationship on the other side of the equation that denotes what is available in what volume:

   $$750 \text{ mg}: x = 1000 \text{ mg}: 1 \text{ ml}$$
   $$1000x = 750$$
   $$x = \frac{750}{1000} = 0.75 \text{ ml}$$

   Whenever a drug appears in concentrated form (powder or liquid), after the appropriate diluent has been added and well dispersed or dissolved, the same mathematical approach can be used, no matter what the size of the finished solution.

5. *Example:* The quantity of a certain medication is ordered as "gr xv," and the tablets on hand are in gr v dosage. How many tablets should be given?

   Answer:

   $$\text{gr } 15: x = \text{gr } 5: 1 \text{ tablet}$$
   $$5x = 15$$
   $$x = \frac{15}{3} = 3 \text{ tablets}$$

6. *Example:* One quart bottle of potassium permanganate has been sent up from the pharmacy for a patient's use. The patient's order reads that 1 pint of potassium permanganate is to be used in each treatment of the patient's skin condition. How much solution will be left after the first treatment?

   Answer: One pint. You should know that 2 pints make 1 quart.

7. *Example:* How many pints should be requested from the pharmacy if a medication is to be given in 4-oz doses three times a day for 2 days?

Answer: You need to know that 16 oz are in 1 pint. Total number of ounces for the course of therapy = 4 × 3 × 2 = 24 oz, or 1½ pints.

8. *Example:* A patient's medication has been ordered for him based on body weight. If he weighs 150 pounds, how many kilograms is that?

Answer: You need to know that 1 kg is equal to 2.2 pounds.

$$150 \text{ lb} : x = 2.2 \text{ lb} : 1 \text{ kg}$$
$$x = 68.2 \text{ kg}$$

9. *Example:* A patient's order calls for ½ ml of a medication. If available syringes are calibrated only in minims, how many minims will you give?

Answer: You need to know that there are between 15 and 16 minims in 1 ml. Choose either figure to use.

$$0.5 \text{ ml} : x = 1 \text{ ml} : 16 \text{ minims}$$
$$x = 0.5 \times 16$$
$$x = 8 \text{ minims}$$

10. *Example:* Morphine sulfate gr $\frac{1}{150}$ is ordered. How many tablets would you give if the available supply is in tablets of 0.2 mg?

Answer: First you need to know that 1 grain is equivalent to 60 mg; then you can find how many milligrams are equivalent to gr $\frac{1}{150}$. Second, you need to find out how many tablets will provide the milligram equivalent of gr $\frac{1}{150}$.

$$\text{gr } \tfrac{1}{150} : x \text{ (mg)} = \text{gr } 1 : 60 \text{ mg}$$
$$x = 60 \left(\frac{1}{150}\right)$$
$$x = \frac{60}{150} = 0.4 \text{ mg}$$

The second step may certainly be done without pencil and paper, but it is more likely to be accurate if not calculated in the head.

$$0.4 \text{ mg} : x = 0.2 \text{ mg} : 1$$
$$0.2\, x = 0.4$$
$$x = \frac{0.4}{0.2} = 2 \text{ tablets}$$

11. *Example:* You may also be confronted with the reverse of the preceding question. How many grains would you give if 0.6 mg morphine sulfate has been ordered?

Answer:

$$0.6 \text{ mg} : x \text{ (gr)} = 60 \text{ mg} : \text{gr } 1$$
$$60\, x = 0.6$$
$$x = \frac{0.6}{60}$$
$$x = \text{gr } 0.01 = \text{gr } \tfrac{1}{100}$$

12. *Example:* Codeine gr ss is ordered; how many milligrams would you give?

Answer: You need to know that the symbol "ss" indicates the quantity one half.

$$\text{gr } \tfrac{1}{2} : x = \text{gr } 1 : 60 \text{ mg}$$
$$x = 60 \left(\frac{1}{2}\right)$$
$$x = \frac{60}{2}\ 30 \text{ mg}$$

13. *Example:* The patient is to take 6 oz of magnesium sulfate solution, and the calibrations on the available measuring device are in milliliters. How many milliliters would you give?

Answer: You need to know that 1 oz is equivalent to 30 ml.

$$6 \text{ oz} : x \text{ (ml)} = 1 \text{ oz} : 30 \text{ ml}$$
$$x = 6 \times 30$$
$$x = 180 \text{ ml}$$

14. Although some practitioners may not technically consider IV infusions to be medications, we will practice figuring IV infusion rates here.

The amount of IV solution to be infused during a given length of time is the IV flow rate. It is dictated by the prescriber's order, which should give the total amount of fluid and the number of milliliters that should be infused over each 1-hour period or less *or* the number of drops per minute that should be infused. Some IV orders are still being written giving only the total volume of solution to be infused (for example, 1000 ml) over a longer period (for example, 8 hours). Technically, anything less than such specific information is an inadequate order and should be clarified.

If the order does not spell out the rate of flow in drops per minute, the following formula may be used to figure this out:

$$\frac{\text{Total number of milliliters to be infused}}{\text{Total number of minutes infusion is to run}} \times$$

$$\text{Drop factor} = \text{Rate in drops per minute}$$

Example: If an order is given for 1000 ml D_5W to run for 8 hours and the drop factor is 10 drops/minute for the particular tubing used (other types deliver 15 drops or 60 drops—often used to infuse children), how fast should the IV infusion be set to run?

$$\frac{1000 \text{ ml}}{480 \text{ minutes}} \times 10 = x$$

$$\frac{100}{48} \times 10 = 20.8 \text{ drops (gtt)/minute} = 21 \text{ gtt/minute}$$

15. A bit more challenging are some of the mathematics involved with IV rates via infusion pumps. These pumps are often used for giving drugs that must be calculated more closely.

Example: Dopamine 400 mg is ordered to be added to 250 cc D_5W to be infused at a rate of 350 μg/minute. It is to be regulated by a volumetric infusion pump that is calibrated to deliver the fluid in units of cubic centimeters per hour. At how many cubic centimeters per hour should the pump be set?

Answer: Here you are asked to convert the "language" of one flow rate to the language of another. First you need to know that 1 μg is equal to 0.001 mg, so:

$$350 \ \mu g : x \ (mg) = 1 \ \mu g : 0.001 \ mg$$
$$x = 0.350 \ mg \ or \ 0.35 \ mg$$

Thus 0.350 mg is being infused every minute. Now you need to go on and figure out the rate per hour. That is, if 0.35 mg is infused every minute, how many will be infused per hour?

$$x : 60 \ minutes = 0.35 \ mg: 1 \ minute$$
$$x = 60 \times 0.35$$
$$x = 21 \ mg$$

Now convert to cubic centimeters per hour:

$$21 \ mg: x \ (cc) = 400 \ mg : 250 \ cc$$
$$400x = 21 \times 250 = 5250$$
$$x = 13.125 \ or \ 13 \ cc/hour$$

Some rules of thumb will become more important as the metric system predominates. It can help to:

Place a zero to the left of the decimal point when there is no integer in the decimal.

Carry out problems to the hundredths place and then round off only in the final answer.

Use judgment in rounding off numbers. The smaller the answer (the lower the number), the more significant the change in the answer made by rounding off.

Many excellent nursing texts are available that one can use to develop and practice arithmetic skills necessary in the administration of medications. (See the references at the end of this chapter.) Much more practice is necessary than is presented here for introductory purposes.

Procedures and techniques of medication administration

Accurate and full identification of the patient before each dose of medication is given ensures that the right patient gets the right medication. Using the patient's full name on all paperwork and in reference to her or him helps prevent mixups, as does being alert to similarities in names and geographically separating

people with similar names. Nurses should not rely on memory to identify patients. *Checking the patient's name on the armband* against the name on the accompanying medication ticket is the *most reliable* mode of identification. Asking the patient her or his name and comparing it with the name on the medication order is not foolproof. For example, a patient may give his name, "William" (first name), and then be given medication intended for "Mr. Williams" (last name). Checking the patient's name by calling it out and waiting for a corroborating answer is particularly risky; in a sleepy state, patients have been known to answer to almost any name. Reliance on names on bed tags or labels is dangerous because patients are often away from their beds and their beds can be inadvertently occupied by another patient who is in a groggy state after returning, for example, from a laboratory test. Again, the *surest* way to properly identify a patient before giving medication is to *check the armband*.

Before administering medications, the nurse must also make sure that the drug order has not been changed in any way (such as discontinued or dosage changed) from what appears on the medication ticket or Kardex. It is also wise to check that the dose about to be given has not already been given by someone else caring for the patient (private duty nurse, nursing student, and so forth). Individual agency policies spell out the checking procedure to be used; these policies should be followed routinely to avoid error.

The following are recommended guidelines to follow when distributing or administering drugs to patients.

1 When preparing or giving medicines, concentrate your whole attention on what you are doing. Do not permit yourself to be distracted while working with medicines.

2 Make certain that you have a written order for every medication for which you assume the responsibility of administration. (Verbal and telephone orders should be written out and signed by the prescriber as soon as possible.)

3 Make a habit of reading the label of the medicine carefully before removing the dose from the container.

4 Make certain that the data on the medicine card (or whatever is used) corresponds exactly with the doctor's written order and with the label on

the patient's medicine. If the card system is used, a card should accompany each dose. Sometimes skipping a dose of medicine may be as dangerous as an overdose.

5 Never give a medicine from an unlabeled container or from one on which the label is not legible.

6 If you must in some way calculate the dosage for a patient from the preparation on hand and you are uncertain of your calculation, verify your work on paper by having some responsible person—an instructor, nurse in charge, or pharmacist—check it.

7 Measure quantities as ordered, using the proper equipment: graduated containers for milliliters, fluidounces, or fluidrams, minim glasses or calibrated pipets for minims, and droppers for drops. When measuring liquids, hold the container so that the line indicating the desired quantity is on a level with the eye. The quantity is read when the lowest part of the concave surface of the fluid (meniscus) is on this line.

8 Dosage forms such as tablets, capsules, and pills should be handled in such a way that the fingers will not come in contact with the medicine. Use the cap of the container or a clean medicine card to guide or lift the medicine into the medicine glass or container you will be taking to the bedside of the patient.

9 Avoid waste of medicines. Medicines tend to be expensive; in some instances a single capsule may cost the patient several dollars. Dropping medicine on the floor is one way of wasting it.

10 When pouring liquid medicines, hold the bottle so that the liquid does not run over the side and obscure the label. Wipe the rim of the bottle with a clean piece of paper tissue before replacing the stopper or cover.

11 Never administer medication prepared by another person. In doing so, you accept the responsibility for accuracy, dose, correct medication, and so forth. If the person who prepared the medication has made an error, you are accountable for any harm done to the patient.

12 If a patient expresses doubt or concern about a medication or the doage of a medication, do everything possible to make certain that no mistake has occurred. Occasionally, the patient is right. Reassure the patient as well as yourself by rechecking to make certain that there is no error. You may need to recheck the order, the label on the medicine container, or the patient's chart. The astute and caring nurse also recognizes that, when a patient refuses medication, he has the right to do so and that his behavior is giving a message about unexpressed feelings. The understanding nurse is not content to simply chart that the patient refused 10:00 AM medication. You may encourage the patient to talk about things

that are deeply upsetting and thus help the patient feel that his reaction, whatever it may be, is accepted. You thus provide the patient opportunities to exercise some control over his environment.

13 Assist weak or helpless patients in taking their medications.

14 Most liquid medicines should be diluted with water or other liquid. This is especially desirable when medicines have a bad taste. Exceptions to this rule include oils and cough medicines that are given for a local effect in the throat. The patient should be supplied with an ample amount of fresh water after swallowing solid forms such as tablets or capsules, unless for some reason the patient is allowed only limited amounts of fluid.

15 Remain with the patient until the medicine has been taken. Most patients are very cooperative about taking medicines at the time that the nurse brings them. However, sometimes patients are more ill than they appear and have been known to hoard medicines until they have accumulated a lethal amount and then have taken the entire amount, with fatal results. In some instances patients may be permitted to keep medicines at their bedside and take them as necessary, such as nitroglycerin and antacids.

16 Do not leave a tray of medicines unattended. If you are in a patient's room and must leave, take the tray of medicines with you (Fig. 6-5).

17 Never chart a medicine as having been given until it has been administered. It is often necessary to check the order in the chart before giving the medication. All medications are recorded, but the manner of recording may vary from hospital to hospital. The name of the drug, the dosage, the time of administration, and the route of administration should be noted on the medication record in the chart. The patient's response to the medication should be recorded in the progress notes or nursing notes.

The medicine containers from which the patient is served his medicine should be scrupulously clean, and water supplied immediately after the medicine should be fresh. Carelessly prepared medicines and lack of consideration in the way a medicine is handed to a patient can convey a demeaning or insulting message, whether intended or not.

When a medicine with an unpleasant taste is given, it is better to admit that it is unpleasant and thereby agree with the patient than to make him feel that his reaction is grossly exaggerated or silly. The nurse can attempt to improve the taste by diluting the medicine (if

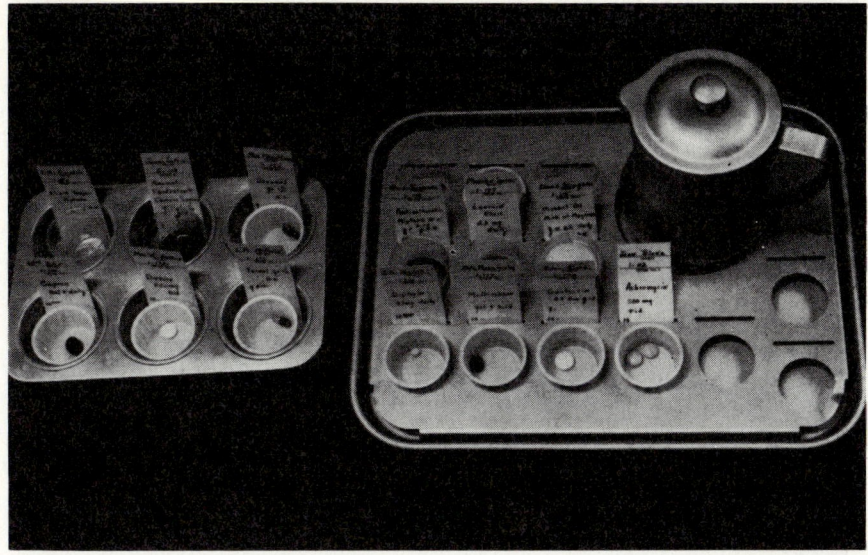

FIG. 6-5. Two medicine trays with cards. The small tray at the left may be used for a number of patients, as in a double room or a small ward. Souffle cups instead of medicine glasses may be used for capsules or tablets. The large tray is arranged for the administration of medications to a group of patients.

possible) or by offering chewing gum or a Life Saver immediately after the medicine.

If an injection is likely to sting or hurt, it is more honest to tell the patient beforehand. The patient is also more likely to deal with it better than if he were not told. It is better to tell a child just before the injection rather than much beforehand so that there is little time for the child to anticipate and grow anxious, thereby actually increasing the pain.

The route of administration of a drug is determined by its physical and chemical properties, the condition or status of the patient, the desired action of the drug, its speed of absorption, and the rapidity of response desired. As a rule, drugs are administered for one of two effects: *local*, in which the effects are confined to the site of application, or *systemic*, in which the results are realized after the drug is absorbed into the blood and diffuses into one or more tissues of the body. Some drugs given locally may produce both local and systemic effects if they are partly or entirely absorbed. Yet a drug may be injected into a joint cavity and have little or no effect beyond the tissues of that structure. Some drugs, such as nitroglycerin ointment, may be topically administered for a distant effect.

FOR LOCAL EFFECTS

Application to skin. Medications are applied to the skin primarily for the following effects:

1 *astringent:* resulting in vasoconstriction, tissue contraction, and decreased secretions and sensitivity, thereby counteracting inflammatory effects
2 *antiseptic* or *bacteriostatic:* to inhibit growth and development of microorganisms
3 *emollient:* for a soothing and softening effect to overcome dryness and hardness
4 *cleansing:* for the removal of dirt, debris, secretions, or crusts

These medications may be applied in the form of a lotion, tincture, ointment or cream, wet dressing, baths, or soaks. Effectiveness of medicinals applied to the skin is limited by the fact that highly specialized layers of skin resist penetration of foreign substances to protect the internal body environment. However, absorption is increased when the skin is thin or macerated, when there is increased drug concentration, or when there is prolonged contact of the drug with the skin.

Application to mucous membranes. Drugs are well absorbed across mucosal surfaces, and therapeutic effects are easily obtained. However, mucous membranes are highly selective in their absorptive action and differ in sensitivity. A drug applied to oral (buccal or sublingual) mucosa may be twice as concentrated as that applied to nasal mucosa, while its concentration may be reduced one fourth to one half for delicate membranes of the eye or urethra. Aqueous solutions are quickly absorbed from mucous membranes, whereas oily liquids are not. Oily preparations should not be applied to nasal or respiratory mucosa by sprays or nebulae, since the droplets of oil may be carried to terminal portions of the respiratory tract and retained there, causing lipoid pneumonia.

Respiratory mucosa may be medicated by means of inhalation or insufflation. The *inhalation* method utilizes sprays or nebulae, whereby the drug is sprayed into the throat by a nebulizer, or aerosols, whereby a flow of air or oxygen under pressure disperses the drug throughout the respiratory tract. In the *insufflation* method a fine powder is blown or sprayed onto nasal mucosa. Drugs so administered tend to have both a local respiratory and a systemic effect. The respiratory mucosa offers an enormous surface of absorbing epithelium. If the drug is volatile and capable of being absorbed and if there is more in the inspired air than in the blood, the drug is instantaneously absorbed. This fact is of significance in emergencies. Amyl nitrite, ether, oxygen, and carbon dioxide are examples of volatile and gaseous agents that are given by inhalation.

Drugs in suppository form can be used for their local effects on the mucous membranes of the vagina, urethra, or rectum. Packs and tampons may be impregnated with a drug and placed in a body cavity; these are used particularly in the nose, ears, and vagina. Drugs may also be painted or swabbed on a mucosal surface, instilled, or administered via a douche, irrigation, or injection (such as intralesional for psoriasis or intraarterial for cancer).

FOR SYSTEMIC EFFECTS

Drugs that produce a systemic effect must be absorbed and carried to the cells or tissues capable of responding to them. The route of administration used depends on the nature and amount of drug to be given, the desired rapidity of effect, and the general condition of the patient. Routes selected for systemic effect include the following: skin,* oral, sublingual, rectal, and parenteral (injection). Types of parenteral administration include intradermal (or intracutaneous), subcutaneous, intramuscular, intravenous, intraspinal (or intrathecal), and sometimes intracardiac, intrapericardial, intraosseous, and intraperitoneal injection.

Oral administration. Oral administration is the safest, most economical, and most convenient way of giving medicines. Therefore, medications should be given orally unless some distinct advantage is to be gained by giving them another way. Most drugs are absorbed from the small intestine; a few are absorbed from the stomach and colon. This explains the ineffectiveness of cathartics and enemas in the attempt to remove most toxins and overdoses in cases of poisoning.

Following oral administration, drug action has a slower onset and *more prolonged* but *less potent effect* than when drugs are given parenterally. This may result from: (1) variation in absorption as a result of drug composition, gastric or intestinal pH and motility, food content, and a pathologic condition within the gastrointestinal tract; or (2) alteration of the drug resulting from its retention, inactivation, or partial destruction by the liver if the drug traverses the hepatic circulation before entering the general circulation. Some drugs meant for intramuscular administration, such as those containing propylene glycol or alcohol, may actually be absorbed slower than if administered orally.

Disadvantages of oral administration of certain drugs are: (1) they may have an objectionable odor or taste; (2) they may harm or discolor the teeth; (3) they may irritate the gastric mucosa, causing nausea and vomiting; (4) they may be aspirated by a seriously ill or uncooperative patient; (5) they may be destroyed by digestive enzymes; and (6) they may be inappropriate for some patients, such as those who must be given nothing by mouth.

Sublingual administration. Drugs given sublingually are placed under the patient's

---

*Nitroglycerin ointment is applied to the skin in small amounts for absorption and dissemination to the heart.

tongue, where they must be retained until dissolved and absorbed. The thin epithelium and rich network of capillaries on the underside of the tongue permit both rapid absorption and rapid drug action. In addition, there is greater potency, since the drug gains access to the general circulation without traversing the liver or being affected by gastric and intestinal enzymes.

The number of drugs that can be given sublingually is limited (for example, nitroglycerin tablets). The drug must dissolve readily, and the patient must be able to cooperate; the patient must understand that the drug is not to be swallowed and that he must not take a drink until the drug has been absorbed.

A drug may be applied against the mucosa of the cheek for *buccal absorption*.

Rectal administration. Rectal administration can be used advantageously when the stomach is nonretentive or traumatized, when the medicine has an objectionable taste or odor, or when it can be changed by digestive enzymes. It is also a reasonably convenient and safe method of giving drugs when the oral method is unsuitable, as when the patient is unconscious.

Use of the rectal route avoids irritation of the upper gastrointestinal tract and may promote higher bloodstream drug titers because venous blood from the lower part of the rectum does not traverse the liver. The suppository vehicle is far superior to the retention enema because the drug is released at a slow but steady rate to ensure a protracted effect. One disadvantage of the retention enema is unpredictable retention of the drug; another is that much of the fluid passes above the lower rectum and then is absorbed into the portal circulation. An evacuant enema before administra-

TABLE 6-4 Suggested injection guides

Route	Common areas	Region	Needle sizes	Volume injected (milliliters) Average	Range	Examples of medications by this route
Intradermal (intracutaneous)	Skin (corium)	Inner aspect of midforearm and scapula	26 or 27 gauge × ⅜ in.	0.1	0.01 to 1.0	Tuberculin, allergens, local anesthetics
Subcutaneous	Beneath the skin	Lateral upper arms, thighs; abdominal fat pads below and lateral to navel; upper back; upper hips	25 to 27 gauge × ½ to ⅝ in.	0.5	0.5 to 1.5	Epinephrine (non-oily), insulin, some narcotics, tetanus toxoid, vaccines, vitamin B_{12}, heparin
Intramuscular	Gluteus medius	Dorsogluteal	20 to 23 gauge × 1½ to 3 in.	2 to 4	1 to 5	Most intramuscular and Z-track injections
	Gluteus minimus	Ventrogluteal	20 to 23 gauge × 1½ to 3 in.	1 to 4	1 to 5	All intramuscular medications
	Vastus lateralis	Anterolateral midthigh	22 to 25 gauge × ⅝ to 1 in.	1 to 4	1 to 5	Almost all intramuscular medications
	Deltoid	Upper arm below shoulder	23 to 25 gauge × ⅝ to 1 in.	0.5	0.5 to 2	Vaccines, absorbed tetanus toxoid, most narcotics, epinephrine, sedatives, vitamin B_{12}, lidocaine
Intravenous	Cephalic and basilic veins	Dorsum of hand and forearm; antecubital fossa	19 to 23 gauge × 1 to 1½ in.	1 to 10	0.5 to 50	Antibiotics, vitamins, fluids and electrolytes, antineoplastics, vasopressors, corticosteroids, aminophylline, blood products

Modified from Newton, M., and Newton, D.W.: Guidelines for handling drug errors, Nursing '79 **9**(7):18, 1979.

tion of rectal medication is usually advisable. The amount of solution that can be given rectally is usually small.

Parenteral administration. Strictly speaking, parenteral administration means administration by any route other than oral; thus technically it could be defined to include topical or inhalation administration. In practical use, however, parenteral usually means administration by the use of a needle (see Table 6-4).

Parenteral administration of drugs includes all forms of drug injection into body tissues or fluids using a syringe and needle or catheter and container (Figs. 6-6 and 6-7). Drugs given parenterally must be sterile, readily soluble and absorbable, and nonirritating. Since parenteral administration of drugs can be hazardous, precautions are required: (1) aseptic technique must be used to avoid infection, and (2) accurate drug dosage, proper rate of injection, and proper site of injection are essential to avoid harm such as abscesses, necrosis, skin slough, nerve injuries, prolonged pain, or periostitis. *An injected drug is irretrievable,* and an error in dosage or method or site of injection is not easily corrected.

With drugs given parenterally rather than orally (1) the onset of drug action is more rapid (except as noted previously) but of shorter duration; (2) the dosage is often smaller, since drug potency tends not to be altered; and (3) the cost of drug therapy may be greater. Parenteral administration of drugs requires specialized knowledge and manual skill to ensure safety and therapeutic effectiveness. Various methods of parenteral administration may be performed by the nurse, but some are done only by a physician. The nurse should know and adhere to agency policy.

Intradermal. Intradermal or intracutaneous injection means that the injection is made into the upper layers of the skin (Fig. 6-8). The amount of drug given is small and absorption is slow. This method is used to advantage when testing for allergic reactions of the patient and for giving small amounts of a local anesthetic. In a test for allergic reactions minute amounts of the solution to be tested are injected just under the outer layers of the skin. The medial surface of the forearm and the skin of the back are the sites frequently used. These injections are best made with a fine, short needle (26 or 27 gauge) and a small-barrel syringe (such as a tuberculin syringe) (Fig. 6-9).

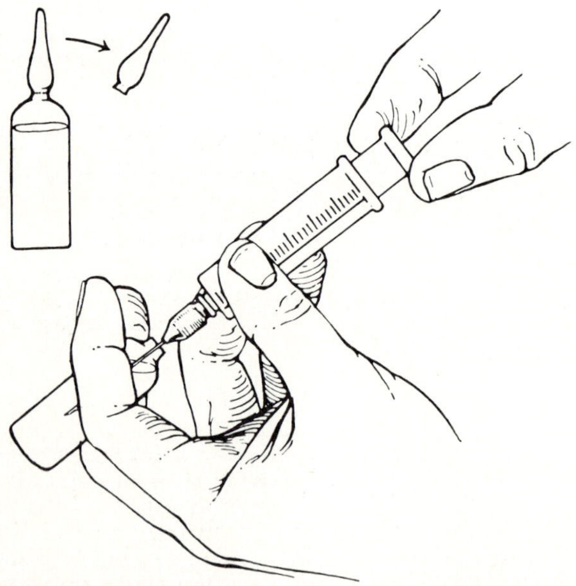

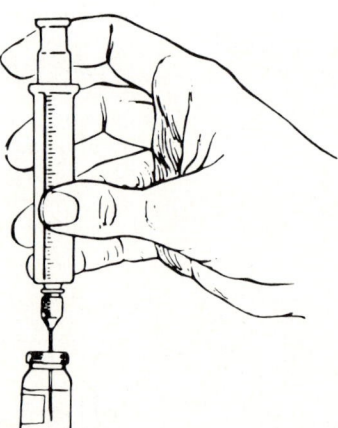

FIG. 6-6. Withdrawing medication from an ampule. The ampule on the left will break easily when pressure is exerted at the constricted portion. An ampule may be made so that a metal file must be used at the neck to secure a clean break.

FIG. 6-7. Inserting needle into a stoppered vial. When a needle is inserted into a vial of this type, it is important that air be injected into the vial first to facilitate withdrawal of the liquid medication. The desired amount is then drawn into the syringe, aided by the increase of air pressure in the vial. Current literature also supports the procedure of drawing up an additional 0.1 to 0.3 ml of air into the syringe after the proper amount of medication has been drawn into it. This bubble should rise to the top of the medication in the syringe and form an absorbable plug so that medication cannot back up the track made by the needle.

Subcutaneous. Small amounts of drug in solution are given subcutaneously usually by means of a 25-gauge (or thinner) needle and syringe. The needle is inserted through the skin with a quick movement, but the injection is made slowly and steadily. The nurse should slightly withdraw the piston of the syringe before injecting the drug to make sure that a blood vessel has not been entered. The angle of insertion should usually be 45 to 60 degrees (but can be any angle from 30 to 90 degrees, depending on needle length and depth of fat pads) and should be made on the fat pads of the abdomen, the outer surface of the upper arm, or the anterior surface of the thigh, and occasionally the lower abdominal surface (heparin). In these locations there are fewer large blood vessels, and sensation is less keen than on the medial surfaces of the extremities. Massage of the part after injection tends to increase the rate of absorption but should be avoided after injection of some drugs, such as heparin, to

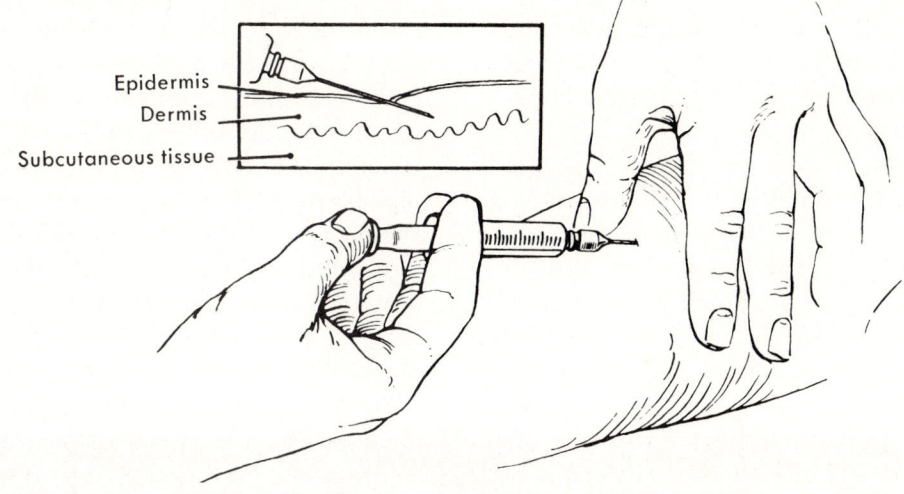

Epidermis
Dermis
Subcutaneous tissue

FIG. 6-8. Intradermal injection. Needle penetrates epidermis and goes into dermis.

FIG. 6-9. These syringes are used to accurately measure varying amounts of liquids and liquid medications. The uppermost syringe is known as a tuberculin syringe and is graduated in 0.01 cc (ml). It is a syringe of choice for administration of very small amounts. The 2-cc syringe is the one commonly used to give a drug subcutaneously. It is graduated in 0.1 cc. The larger syringes are used when a larger volume of drug is to be administered.

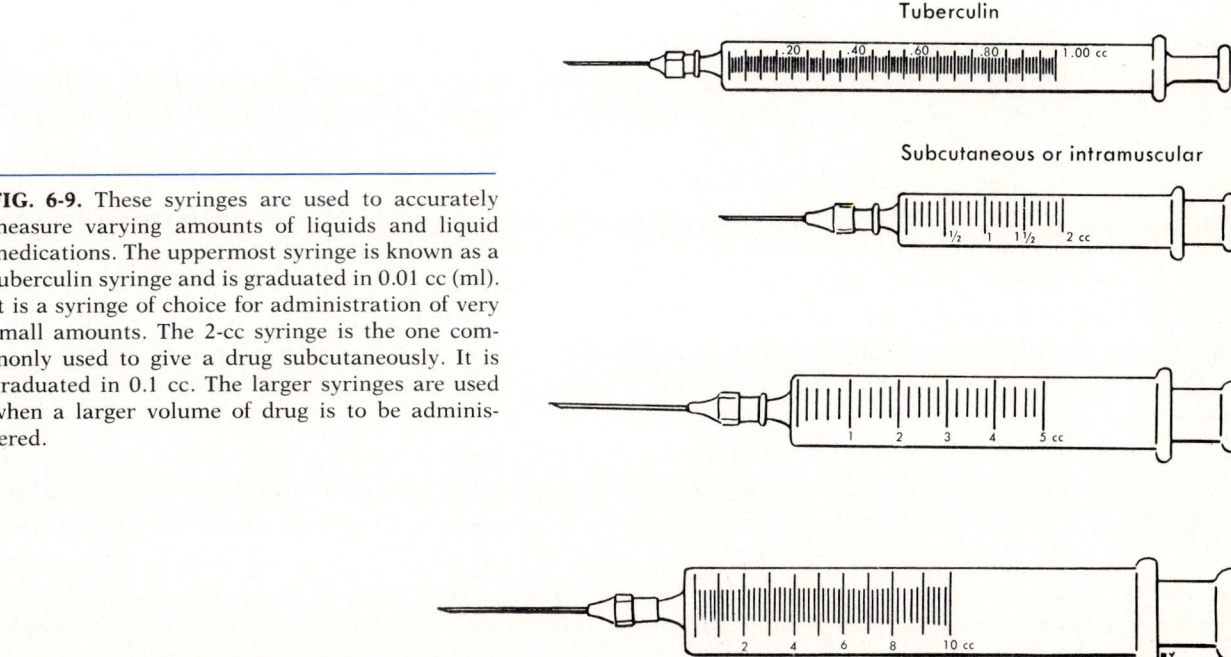

Syringes:

Tuberculin

Subcutaneous or intramuscular

minimize bruising as the drug spreads through the tissues. Disposable syringes and needles contribute to safety of the procedure but also to cost and problems of storage and disposal. Subcutaneously injected medicines are limited to the administration of drugs that are highly soluble and nonirritating and to solutions of limited volume (ideally no more than 1 ml).

Irritating drugs given subcutaneously can result in the formation of sterile abscesses and necrotic tissue. Infection can also occur more easily after subcutaneous administration than when drugs are given intravenously. Care should be exercised to avoid contamination and to rotate sites. Subcutaneous injections are not satisfactory in individuals with sluggish peripheral circulation.

The introduction of large amounts of solution (500 to 1000 ml in adults) into subcutaneous tissues is known as *hypodermoclysis.* Isotonic solutions of sodium chloride or glucose are administered this way. The needle is longer than that used for a hypodermic injection, and it is inserted into areas of loose connective tissue such as that under the breasts, in the upper surfaces, of the thighs, and into the subscapular region of the back. Fluids must be given slowly to avoid overdistention of the tissues. Hyaluronidase is sometimes added to the solution to facilitate the spread and absorption of fluid by decreasing the viscosity of the ground substance in connective tissues. Some physicians prefer IV infusion of fluids to hypodermoclysis because the amount of absorption is more readily determined.

Intramuscular. Injections are made through the skin and subcutaneous tissue into muscular tissue when prompt absorption is desirable or when the drug is too irritating to be given subcutaneously. Intramuscular absorption is delayed in circulatory collapse; the IV route is then chosen. Irritation may not be obvious following intramuscular injection. Larger doses can be given intramuscularly than can be given subcutaneously (up to 4 to 5 ml in divided doses, twice daily).

A drug may be given intramuscularly in an aqueous solution, an aqueous suspension, or a solution or suspension of oil. Suspensions form a depot of drug in the tissue, and slow, gradual absorption usually results. Two disadvantages are sometimes encountered when preparations in oil are used: the patient may be sensitive to the oil, or the oil may not be absorbed. In the latter case, incision and drainage of the oil may be necessary.

Criteria for selection of a safe intramuscular injection site include distance from large, vulnerable nerves and blood vessels and from bruised, scarred, previous injection or infusion sites. The type of needle used for intramuscular injection depends on the site of the injection, the condition of the tissues, and the nature of the drug to be injected. Needles from 1 to 1½ inches in length may be used. The usual gauge is 20 to 25 (the larger the number, the finer the needle). Fine needles can be used for thin solutions and heavier needles for suspensions and oils. Needles for injection into the deltoid area should be ⅝ to 1 inch in length, the gauge again depending on the material to be injected. The deltoid can readily absorb up to 2 ml of drug. For many intramuscular injections the preferable site of injection is the buttock because of fewer nerve endings at this site. The needle must be long enough to avoid depositing the solution of drug into the subcutaneous or fatty tissue. The depth of insertion depends on the amount of subcutaneous tissue and will vary with the weight of the patient.

It is essential to locate the appropriate landmarks to delimit the areas safe for injections (Table 6-4). Intramuscular injections may be given into such clearly defined areas of muscularity as the gluteal region of the lower back (provides slowest absorption), deltoid area, and anterolateral thigh. At first to most nursing students it seems that the fleshy part of the buttock is a logical intramuscular site. It is not, since underneath, centrally, and running diagonally is the sciatic nerve, which if damaged can result in permanent leg paralysis. Every attempt must be made to avoid this area.

There are now two acceptable ways to map appropriate intramuscular sites in the gluteal region. The formerly used method of dividing the gluteus medius into imaginary quadrants and injecting into the upper outer quadrant is out of favor because it does not necessarily prevent an injection into the sciatic nerve, espe-

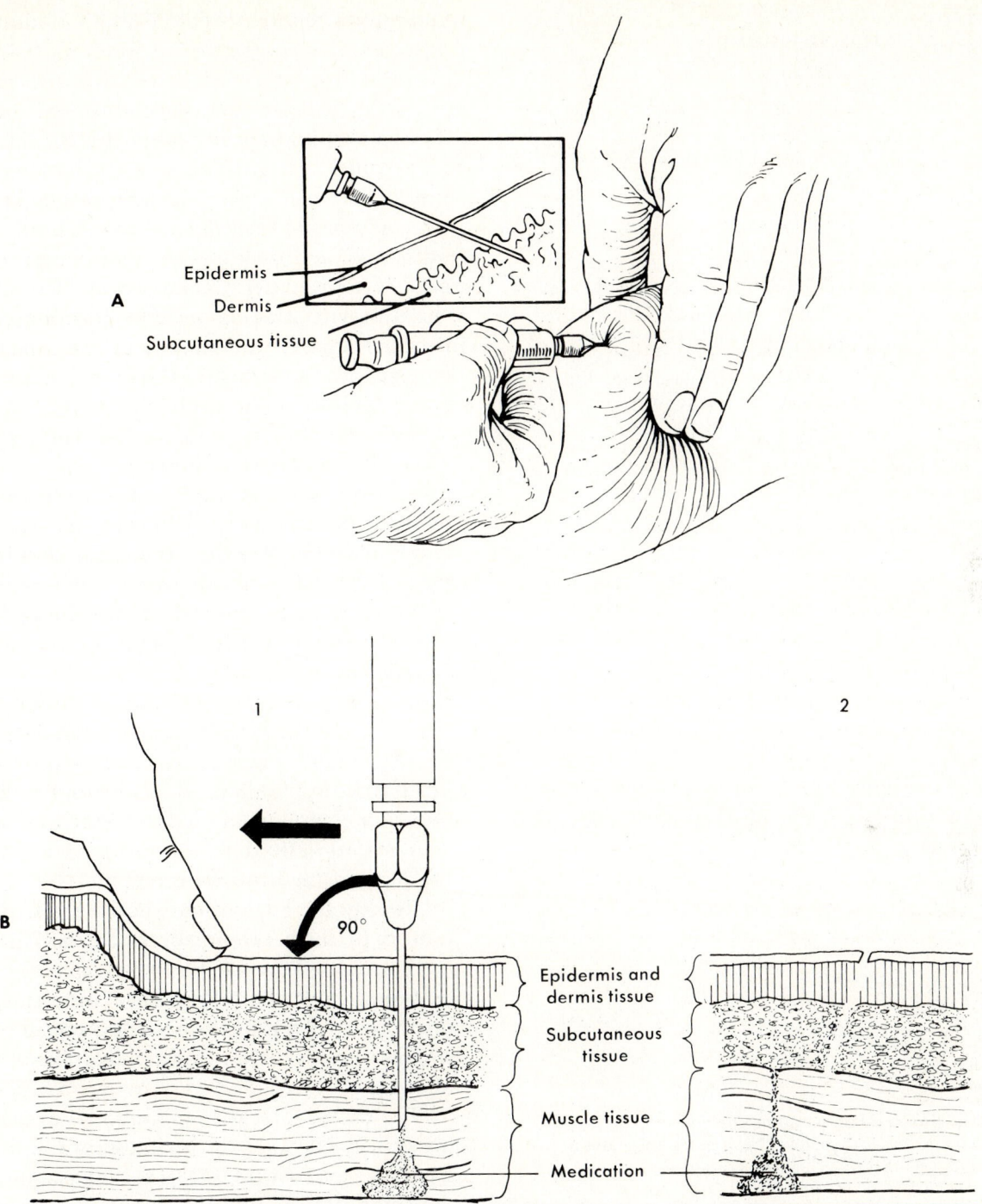

FIG. 6-10. A, Subcutaneous injection. The skin surface has been cleansed, and the syringe is held at the angle at which the needle will penetrate the tissue. The left hand is used to pinch the arm gently but firmly. When the needle has been inserted into the subcutaneous tissue, the tissue of the arm is released and the solution is steadily injected. Based on the patient's condition or the medication to be injected, nursing judgment may dictate a different angle or an approach different from pinching up the skin. **B,** Z-track intramuscular injection method, which is useful for administration of medication known to cause pain or permanent staining of superficial tissues. *1,* The skin is stretched to one side and medication injected as usual. *2,* Needle is then removed and the skin allowed to return to resting position, sealing off the deposited medication from the track made by the needle. The site is not massaged in this method. (**B** modified from Kozier, B., and Erb, G.: Fundamentals of nursing, Menlo Park, Calif., 1979, Addison-Wesley Publishing Co.)

FIG. 6-11
Intramuscular injection.

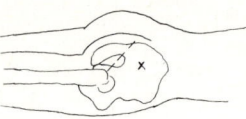

A

Posterior gluteal site, located above the diagonal line from the trochanter to the posterior iliac spine. An injection near the middle of the buttocks may result in an injury to the sciatic nerve. It is, of course, important to vary the sites of injection, preferably using alternate buttocks. The needle is inserted in with a quick firm movement, entering perpendicular to the skin. After aspiration to make certain the needle is not in a blood vessel, the solution is injected slowly and steadily.

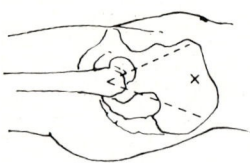

B

Ventrogluteal intramuscular injection site. The V fans out from the greater trochanter. The injection site (X) is centered at the base of the triangle.

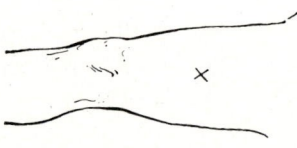

C

Midlateral thigh intramuscular injection site— a handsbreadth below the greater trochanter and a handsbreadth above the knee.

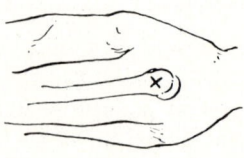

D

Mid-deltoid intramuscular injection site— below the acromion and lateral to the axilla.

cially if its course runs abnormally in that individual.

The nurse can best locate the dorsogluteal site (the muscle underneath is the gluteus medius) by asking the patient to lie face down and exposing the entire area so that the landmarks and injection site can be clearly located. The proper site for this injection is outlined by an imaginary diagonal line drawn from the area of the greater trochanter of the femur to the posterior iliac spine. The injection should be given at any point between that imaginary straight line and below the curve of the iliac crest (hipbone) (Fig. 6-11, *A*).

The ventrogluteal site can be made accessible with the patient in a supine, prone, or side-lying position. This site is used for intramuscular injections in either children or adults. To locate it on the left side, the nurse should palpate for the left greater trochanter with the right palm, place the right index finger on the anterior superior iliac spine, and extend the middle finger to the iliac crest. The injection should be made into the center of the V formed between the index and middle fingers (Fig. 6-11, *B*). The left hand is likewise used to detect landmarks in the right hip. Either of the gluteal two sites is preferred for the Z track method.

The mid-deltoid area is the muscular area in the arm formed by the rectangle bounded on the top by the edge of the shoulder and on the bottom by the beginning of the axilla (Fig. 6-11, *D*). The deltoid muscle has a considerably higher blood flow than the other intramuscular injection sites and is the area of choice for most small-volume (2 ml or less) medications for rapid onset.

The vastus lateralis is a muscular area in the upper leg. The area for injection is a long rectangular area just lateral to the frontal plane of the thigh. Its top boundary is found about one handsbreadth below the greater trochanter and about one handsbreadth above the knee (Fig. 6-11, *C*). This area can accommodate volumes of medication the same size as the gluteus medius and is distant from any major blood vessels or nerves but injection here may be more painful than in the gluteals.

If the needle is inserted all the way to the hub, it should be withdrawn just enough to have something to grasp if the needle breaks.

After the needle is inserted, the plunger should be slightly withdrawn to make certain that the needle is not in a blood vessel. Although this problem seldom occurs when the injection is made in the sites mentioned, it is not justifiable to take a chance of injecting a drug into a blood vessel when this is not the route of administration selected for the drug. In certain instances injection of oily or particulate medicines or killed bacteria by inadvertent IV administration could result in a serious emergency.

When an intramuscular injection is given, it is usually preferable to have the patient in a prone position, with the head turned to one side and with a pillow under the legs just below the knees. The patient should be instructed to toe inward; this will help promote relaxation of the gluteal muscles. If this is not a convenient position for the patient to take he/she may be placed on the side with the leg flexed at the knee.

To prevent excessive scar formation or tissue irritation, no two injections should be made in the same spot during a course of treatment. When injection is made into the buttocks, it should be given first on one side and then on the other. The technique in which the tissue is pinched between the fingers, rather than spread, may be desirable for patients with very little subcutaneous tissue but is contraindicated for patients who are bruised as a result of repeated injections.

Contrary to popular belief, needle puncture of the skin may not always be the source of most pain associated with injections, although a dull needle (such as one that was inserted through a rubber stopper) will certainly contribute to pain. Also, it is not the length of the needle that causes pain, but the diameter; a 3-inch needle will hurt no more than a ⅝ inch one if the diameter is the same. Except for the psychologic aspect of anxiety about needles, most injection pain is thought to result from stretching of tissue as it accommodates the volume of the drug, from the irritation of the drug itself, or from contact with antiseptics remaining on the needle if the skin antiseptic was not allowed to dry before the skin was punctured.

Intravenous. When an immediate effect is desired, or when for any reason the drug cannot be injected into other tissues, or when absorption may be inhibited by poor circulation, it may be given directly into a vein as an *injection* or *infusion*. The technique of this method requires skill and asepsis, and the drug must be highly soluble and capable of withstanding sterilization. This method is of great value in emergencies. The dose and amount of absorption can be determined with accuracy, although the rapidity of absorption and the fact that there is no recall once the drug has been given constitute dangers worthy of consideration. From this standpoint it is one of the least safe methods of administration. Precautions must be taken to prevent extravasation of drug or fluids into surrounding tissue.

In IV *injection* (IV push) a comparatively small amount of solution (also referred to as a bolus) is given by means of a syringe into IV tubing, into a heparin lock, or directly into a vein over a 1- to 7-minute period. The drug is dissolved in a suitable amount of normal (physiologic) saline solution or some other isotonic solution. The injection is usually made into the median basilic or median cephalic vein at the bend of the elbow (Fig. 6-12). However, any accessible vein may be used. Factors that determine the choice of a vein are related to the thickness of the skin over the vein, the closeness of the vein to the surface, and the presence of a firm support (bone) under the vein. The veins in the antecubital fossa are readily accessible, although the veins of the hands are also sometimes used.

A vein that is normally distended with blood is much easier to enter than a partially collapsed vein. If a vein of the arm has been chosen, a tourniquet is drawn tightly around the middle of the arm to distend the vein, the air is expelled from the syringe, and the needle should be introduced quickly and forcefully pointing proximally. A few drops of blood aspirated into the syringe indicates that the needle is in the vein; the tourniquet is then removed, and the solution is injected very slowly. The needle, syringe, and solution must be sterile, and the hands of the doctor and nurse and the skin of the patient at the point of insertion of the needle must be clean.

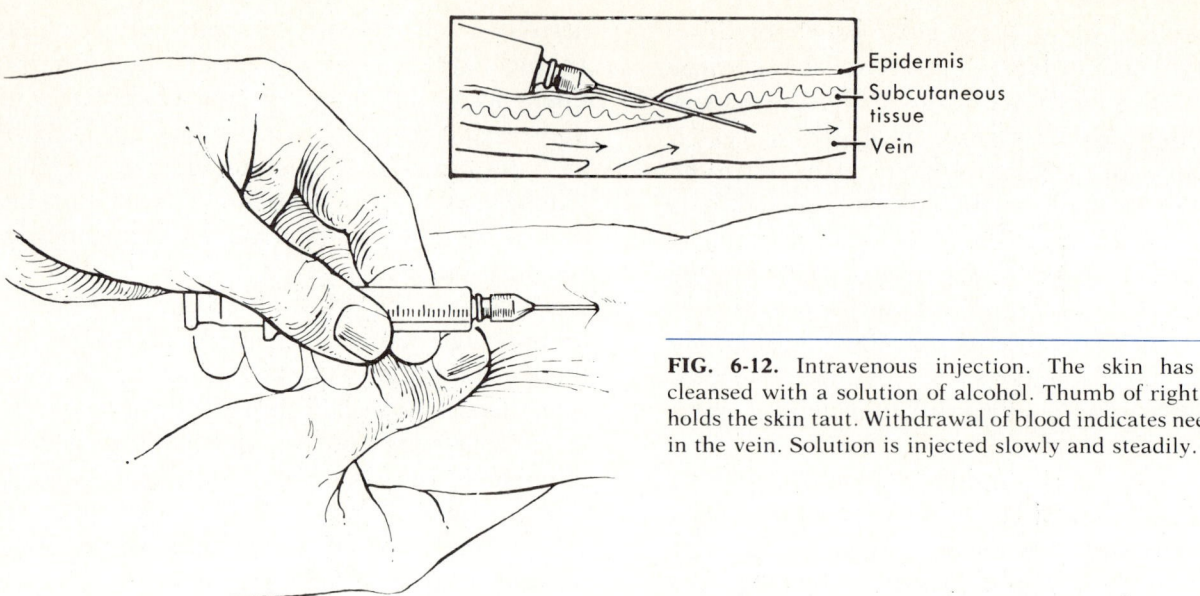

FIG. 6-12. Intravenous injection. The skin has been cleansed with a solution of alcohol. Thumb of right hand holds the skin taut. Withdrawal of blood indicates needle is in the vein. Solution is injected slowly and steadily.

In IV *infusion* a larger amount of fluid is usually given, varying from 1 to 5 pints. The solution flows by gravity from a graduated glass bottle or plastic bag through tubing, connecting tip, and needle or catheter into a vein.

Infusions are most commonly given to relieve tissue dehydration, to restore depleted blood volume, to dilute toxic substances in the blood and tissue fluids, to supply electrolytes and drugs, and to run very slowly to provide an IV line if an emergency is anticipated.

The fluid is usually given slowly to prevent reaction or fluid overload, which may impair cardiac and pulmonary function, especially in elderly patients or patients with cardiac disease. Ordinarily 8 hours are required for every 1000 ml of fluid, depending on the condition of the patient, the nature of the solution, and the reasons for giving it. For children the rate will be slower and is determined by age, weight, and urinary output.

Sodium chloride (0.9%) solution, commonly known as physiologic or isotonic salt solution (normal saline, NS), is the fluid of choice for IV infusion to relieve dehydration not complicated by acidosis.

Five percent dextrose (D_5W) solution is frequently administered and is of value because it provides a means of administering water and a sugar, but it is a small source of energy (1000 ml D_5W contributes only 200 calories). (Basically, there is *no* IV solution that contains all essential nutrients to keep patients from starving. Patients should be progressed to a regular diet as soon as possible.) A concentration of 5.5% is approximately isotonic with normal body fluids. Dextrose in physiologic saline (D/NS) solution is sometimes given.

A dextran solution may be given intravenously as an infusion colloid to support blood volume in the management of various types of shock.

A number of commercial solutions are used in IV replacement therapy. Some solutions contain not only salts of sodium and potassium but also salts of calcium and magnesium. Vitamins are also added to IV fluids when necessary.

Total parenteral nutrition (TPN) or hyperalimentation is the infusion of an individual's total basic nutritional needs via an infusion catheter to a large central vein and/or to a peripheral one. The choice of site depends partly on the phlebitis-causing potential of the medium.

Whole blood and blood plasma are likewise given intravenously to restore depleted blood volume as well as constituents of the blood. Blood products should be introduced through

TABLE 6-5 Common intravenous needle site complications

Data	Infiltration	Clot over needle opening or obstruction	Phlebitis	Infection at site of needle insertion
Color	Pale	No change	Red	Red at site
Temperature	Cool to cold	No change	Warm to hot	Warm at site
Swelling	Rounded	None	Cordlike vein path	Small amount at site
Pain	Yes, usually	None	Yes	None usually
Flow	Slowed or stopped	Slowed or stopped	No change or may be slowed	No change
Nursing actions	Tourniquet; lower bottle Discontinue IV Call IV team Get order for warm compresses and elevate part	Lower bottle Reposition arm Pinch tube and squeeze ball Aspirate clot into needle	Discontinue IV *usually* Call IV team Note irritating solution (Valium, Keflin, KCl running too fast) Warm compresses; elevate and immobilize part	Do not discontinue IV until advice has been sought or physician has been notified (it may be the only vein available for essential infusion)

IV tubing that has been primed with a normal saline infusion solution rather than dextrose solution, which would cause "stickiness" of red blood cells, causing them to clump artificially, possibly clogging the needle and/or hemolyzing. Insertion of a rather large-gauge needle when blood products are expected to be infused will help minimize trauma to cells. Tubing should also be of the sort that incorporates a filter to trap cell particles and clumped cells to prevent them from circulating or clogging the needle.

Some drugs, such as antibiotics, are administered by intermittent infusion (known as "IV piggyback" [IVPB] or "IV rider" in some parts of the country). They are given via a setup that is secondary to the primary IV infusion and that is hung in tandem and connected to the primary setup. The secondary setup may consist of a drug infusing from a small volume of fluid in either a small bag or bottle (up to 250 ml) or from a volume-control set made up of a calibrated chamber hung under the primary IV solution container that can provide the necessary 50 to 250 ml of diluent per dose of the drug. Most intermittent diluted drug infusions are meant to have a total infusion time of 20 or 30 minutes to 1 hour, depending on factors such as package insert instructions related to the amount of diluent required or the potential for vein wall irritation by the drug. Again, references for more detailed information can be found at the end of this chapter.

Particulate matter found in IV infusion solutions is disturbingly common. It can be introduced during manufacture, during hanging of the solution, or during administration of a medication. It consists of tiny chunks of rubber stoppers or glass slivers from ampules. One study showed that all twelve antibiotic injectables tested contained extraneous particles. The resulting potential for phlebitis is high. It is recommended that in-line filtering devices be used for all IV therapy. Optimal filtration is provided by 0.22 μm filters; most organisms, except certain strains of *Pseudomonas* and the viruses, are filtered out by 0.45 μm in-line filters. To prevent injection of larger particles, disposable needles with 5-μm filters can be used to draw medication up.

Stainless steel scalp-vein needles ("butterfly needles") produce lower rates of infection and phlebitis, but plastic catheters or cannulae tend to decrease the incidence of infiltration and work best when an infusion needle will be in place for a long period. Advantages and disadvantages must be weighed at the time of insertion.

Although it was traditionally the duty of physicians, many nurses today are being trained to start infusions and draw blood, especially in critical care areas. Probably one of the most effective approaches is the training of IV teams whose sole job is to maintain, remove, and replace IV needles, catheters, and so forth. However, such teams may prove to be a mixed blessing insofar that, although they become very proficient at their job, they also may serve to further fragment a patient's care.

Table 6-5 lists data to assess for IV needle site complications and suggests concomitant nursing interventions.

Intraspinal. Intraspinal injection is also known as intrathecal (into a sheath), subdural, subarachnoid, or lumbar injection. The technique is the same as that required for a lumbar puncture. Nurses do not administer drugs intraspinally.

In addition, drugs are occasionally administered by intracardiac, intrapericardial, intraperitoneal, and intraosseous injections; however, nurses do not administer drugs by these routes.

Specific techniques for geriatric, pediatric, and psychiatric patients

Geriatric patients. Geriatric patients may have slowed reflexes and display reduced understanding of treatment. It helps to organize the dispensing of medication so that enough time will be allowed for patients who require a great deal of attention and yet all patients will receive their medication on time. A nurse has roughly an hour's range in which to distribute all the medications during one administration period.

Some older patients may also have difficulty swallowing. They may find it easier to take oral medications by spoon when the medications are crushed, given in liquid form, or sprinkled on easy-to-swallow foods such as applesauce or Jell-O. If this approach is used, it is important that as much of the crushed drug as possible be taken with the first spoonfuls so that very little of the drug is wasted if the patient refuses the rest of the food. This approach cannot be used with enteric-coated medications or with medications in sustained-action form. Initiation of the mechanical act of swallowing may be facilitated by massaging the laryngeal prominence (Adam's apple) or the area just under the chin prominence; pressure here often creates a desire to swallow.

Selection of sites for injectable medications in elderly patients may present the nurse with a challenge. since muscle mass declines with age, suitable sites for intramuscular injection may be fewer than in younger patients and will require more skill and effort in palpating to detect muscles of adequate body and size. However, the decrease in sensory perception, including perception of pain, will make those injections less painful.

General loss in body weight of many elderly patients may make necessary the reevaluation of dosages used for them; the criterion for dosage should be shifted from age to weight. Some older patients weigh no more than the average large child, and some a lot less; yet they are prescribed the larger "adult" doses. For different reasons, however, stimulants are less effective in elderly patients, and large doses are often necessary. On the other hand, central nervous system depressants produce intensified effects in the elderly. Sedatives and hypnotics tend to produce paradoxical effects of irritability, incontinence, confusion, and disorientation. In view of these unfortunate effects, of the multiplicity of drugs prescribed for these patients, and of their propensity for adverse secondary effects, it is an important goal for nurses to make every attempt to simplify the drug therapy plan for their geriatric patient. Often what passes for senility is merely a drug-induced lethargy or confusion.

Probably the most important part of the nursing process of aging patients is the nurse's ability to communicate warmth and understanding and to treat them as persons with dignity and with the ability to reason, to feel, and to contribute.

Pediatric patients. The responsibility of drug administration to pediatric patients requires of nurses special knowledge and techniques. Physicians may prescribe the dosage of medication, but it is the nurse's responsibility to know the safe dosage range of any medication administered to children. A standard dosage of medication is nonexistent in pediatrics; medications are ordered according to the weight or body surface area of the child. Some pharmaceutical companies continue to supply medications in a standard adult dosage strength, and the nurse must be able to calculate the correct dosage before administering the medication. Following is a formula for calculating estimated safe dosages based on weight (Clark's rule):

$$\frac{\text{Average adult dose} \times \text{Weight of child in pounds}}{150} = \text{Estimated safe dose}$$

Example: How much aspirin should a 1-year-old child weighing 21 pounds receive if the average adult dose is 10 grains?

$$\text{Answer: } \frac{10 \text{ (grains)} \times 21 \text{ (weight in pounds)}}{150} = \text{gr } 1\frac{2}{5}$$

A nurse preparing calculated dosages of digitalis, insulin, barbiturates, and narcotics should have the calculations as well as the prepared medication dosage checked by another nurse before the drug is administered. Pediatric dosages are often minute, and a slight mistake in calculating the amount of medication to be administered results in greater proportional error.

Body surface area as a basis. More than 100 years ago, Hufeland suggested that drug doses should be calculated on size or a proportional amount of body surface area (BSA) to weight. Many physicians continue to use weight as the basis for calculating drug doses and body surface area for calculating fluid requirements. Most clinicians advocate using body surface area for determining drug dosage for adults as well as children. Physicians usually carry a simple slide rule or nomogram, such as the West nomogram (Fig. 6-13) to make rapid conversions from weight alone. It is believed that the larger amount of total body water (TBW) in children, as well as the percentage of water in body weight and the part of that percentage formed by extracellular water, accounts for the fact that children tolerate or require larger doses of some drugs on an mg/m² basis.

Although the previously stated rules have been devised for relating adult doses to infants and children, it must be emphasized that *no*

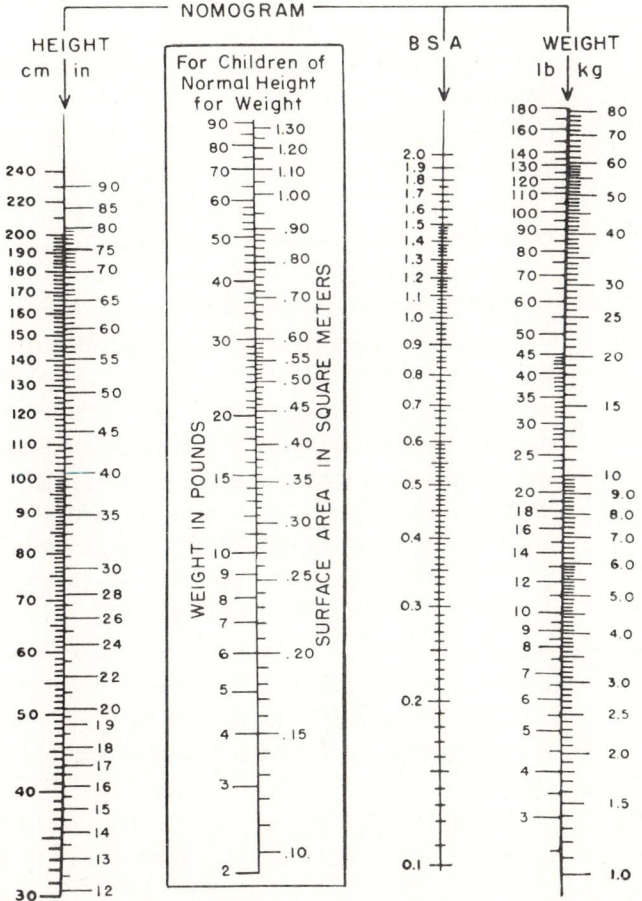

FIG. 6-13. BSA is indicated where straight line that connects height and weight levels intersects BSA column or, if patient is about average size, from weight alone (enclosed area). (Modified from data of E. Boyd by C.D. West. From Shirkey and Barba.)

rules or charts are adequate to guarantee safety of dosage at any age, particularly in the neonate. None of these methods takes into account all variables, partcularly individual tolerance differences. Astute, accurate nursing observations of the reactions of individual children to drugs can be of great assistance as the prescriber chooses drugs and regulates their dosage.

Nurses will find the administration of medications to infants and children challenging, as well as frustrating at times. The ability to give injections skillfully will enhance security and help to gain a child's cooperation when giving injections. A sound knowledge of growth and development will also provide the nurse with information as to how a child at a certain age might be approached, whether trying to reason with him will help or hinder the process, and also whether assistance will be needed in holding the child securely. Many of the principles of safe administration of medication apply to all age groups, but children are different from adults, and the nurse has certain added responsibilities.

Ideally, a nurse who has established a positive relationship with a child will find it easier to secure cooperation when administering medications. The child may also find it easier to accept the discomforts associated with injections and some oral medications from the nurse associated with daily hygiene, feeding, holding, play, and happy times. In addition, the nurse will experience fewer feelings of guilt when the child sees the nurse as someone who brings pleasure and comfort most of the time, as well as some discomfort necessary to getting well.

Regardless of what kinds of external stimuli produce fear or anxiety in a child, the natural response will be to strike out at the frustration or avoid it. By accepting this behavior as a natural response to some type of frustration or discomfort, the nurse will be able to deal with it and will be able to be honest with the child by telling him when a medication or procedure will be unpleasant or painful.

Honest explanations to children are essential, and the timing and type of explanation should be geared to their ability to perceive and understand. Each child has a right to some explanation of any procedure that concerns him. For the child 2 years of age or younger very simple explanations such as "I have some medicine for you to drink" or "I have an injection to give you, and it will hurt a little" will be sufficient. Long explanations to children up through 5 years of age do little more than delay his anticipated pain and increase his anxiety or fear. Telling a child of 4 to stop (when he has responded to being told that he is to receive a medication with kicking, hitting, or other avoidance behavior) only conveys to the child that he is not understood and that he will receive little or no help with his feelings of frustration.

Many children are courageous, or like to be considered so, and appealing to their courage is sometimes effective. Children 4 years old or over may choose to hold their own medicine cup, to drink unassisted, and to take pills from the container without any assistance from the nurse. Because of the sense of achievement that follows, they may want to save the medicine cups to show their mother and father.

Oral medications. Success in administering oral medications usually requires a kind but firm approach with a positive attitude. There should be no evidence of doubt in the nurse's choice of words or tone of voice that the child will take his medicines. The nurse might say: "Jimmy, it's time to take your yellow medicine" or "Do you want to take your pill now or with your Jell-O?" This is an indication that he is expected to cooperate and to do it willingly. An unwise approach that reveals doubt on the part of the nurse might be: "I have your yellow pill, Jimmy. Will you take it for me, please?"

Nurses should try to be aware of the taste of medicines they are giving to anyone, adult or child, so that they can answer such questions as: "Does it taste bad? Will it burn my mouth?" The nurse who knows what a medication tastes like might then reply: "It tastes like cherry to me. Tell me what it tastes like to you." Often the child will accept the suggestion to taste and find out. However, if the medication is bad tasting, attempting deceit or lying to the child is pointless.

Disagreeable-tasting medications should be disguised if at all possible. Small amounts of honey, syrup, jam, fruit, and some fruit juices are suitable sweet substances that might provide a vehicle for less palatable drugs. Pills can be crushed and suspended in small amounts of any of these as long as the two are not incompatible. Many liquid medications are more readily swallowed by infants and children if they are mixed with any of the suggested sweet substances or diluted with a small amount of water. If large amounts of water or other substances are used and the child refuses to take all of the mixture, it is difficult to estimate the amount of medication the child received. Fortunately, many drugs are available in the form of syrups or suspensions that are palatable and well suited for administration to infants and children. The following suggestions may be helpful:

1 Parents are frequently good sources of information about successful methods or vehicles for giving medications to their children.
2 Try to avoid the use of essential foods such as milk, cereal, or orange juice, since the child may become conditioned against future acceptance of that food in the diet.
3 Never underestimate the reaction of a child. He may not require that the taste of his medication be disguised.
4 A sip of fruit juice, a popsicle, or a mint-flavored substance before and after the administration of an unpalatable medicine may effectively dull its taste.
5 Sugarless vehicles such as those sweetened by saccharin should be used to disguise the taste of medications given to diabetic children or those on a ketogenic diet.
6 Honey and syrup are ideal for suspending drugs that do not dissolve easily in water.
7 Since fruit syrups are usually acid in reaction, they should not be used for medicines that react in an acid medium (for example, sodium bicarbonate, soluble barbiturates, and salicylates).
8 Elixirs have an alcohol base that, when undiluted, may cause the child to cough and choke or that may cause an interaction. Small amounts of water added to elixirs of phenobarbital, chloral hydrate, and the like will make them easier to swallow.
9 Much nursing time will be saved if the child's care plan is used to communicate the most successful method of administering medications or if pertinent nursing orders are written.

It is relatively easy to give oral medications to neonates and young infants, but caution must be exercised to prevent aspiration. It is important to give the medications slowly and in small amounts to avoid causing the infant to choke. Liquid medications may be administered by nipple, plastic medicine cup, plastic dropper, or a plastic syringe without the needle. Glass cups, droppers, or syringes should be avoided because of the obvious danger of breakage in the child's mouth. A dropper or syringe is best suited for placing a liquid medication along one side of the infant's tongue. Older infants and toddlers seem to prefer to take their medications from a plastic medicine cup. If children are held or placed in a sitting position, they will be less likely to aspirate the medication than if lying on their backs. When administering a medication with a dropper or syringe, the nurse may purse the infant's lips with one hand to keep the medicine from running out of his mouth.

If the child is still refusing to cooperate after explanations and encouragement, the nurse may have to ask the child whether he is going to take the medication himself or whether he would like the nurse to give it to him. Physical coercion is seldom necessary; but if and when it is, it should be a mild form used with dispatch and firmness, since there is danger of aspiration. It is important, however, not to combine force with anger, nor should force be resorted to because one nurse has been unable to administer the medication. Careful consideration should be given to such factors as: Why does the child resist? Does he/she disapprove only of this one nurse? Have past experiences with medications given at home or in the hospital frightened him/her? Will forcing a medication cause a struggle that will counteract the effects of the drug if the medication is intended to sedate the child? If mild force is necessary, the nurse should explain to the child that this form of treatment is necessary to well-being. The cooperation of the child cannot be gained if he/she feels that force was used as punishment for inability to cooperate, and often confidence in all personnel will be lost.

Intramuscular injections. The principles and techniques of the administration of injections are the same for children as they are for adults. There has been considerable concern, however, about the advisability of using the buttocks as a site for intramuscular injections for infants and children. Many authorities believe that the risk of sciatic nerve injury is too great to warrant the use of this site of administration. The sciatic nerve is the largest nerve in the body; its normal pathway is the hollow midway between the ischial tuberosity and the greater trochanter, covered by the gluteus maximus muscle. This, however, varies a great deal from individual to individual. In addition, the small size of the gluteal mass in the infant or neonate and the potential neurotoxicity of many drugs enhance the possibility of iatrogenic trauma secodary to intramuscular injections. According to some authorities, iatrogenic trauma of this kind is the leading cause of sciatic neuropathy in infancy. A lesion at this height of the sciatic nerve is usually tragically associated with marked permanent disability. The gluteal musculature develops more fully after the child begins to walk, so it is inadvisable to use this site for injection until he has at least reached the toddler stage.

The quadriceps muscle of the midanterolateral aspect of the thigh (vastus lateralis) is the site of choice for injections in infants, children, and adults. Injection sites should be rotated frequently, and if multiple injections over a long period of time necessitate the use of the gluteal region in older children, the nurse must be extremely cautious. A method that is relatively safe and adaptable for older children is to establish landmarks by placing the thumb on the trochanter and the middle finger on the iliac crest. The index finger is placed midway between the thumb and middle finger and above them to form a triangle. The index finger indicates the safe area for the injection site. Anatomic landmarks must always be felt, not arrived at by looking at the child, because of individual differences in body construction. Other sites that can be utilized are the deltoid area and the soft flesh inferior to the crest of the ilium.

As stated previously, injections should be given as rapidly as possible to avoid prolonging a fear-provoking experience. The child must be adequately restrained before the nurse attempts to give an injection. Children will often tell the nurse that they will "hold still" for an injection, but a wise pediatric nurse will be sure to have another person there to hold the patient so that the injection can be administered safely. Stabilizing a child over 4 years of age in order to give an injection in the thigh may require more than two persons.

Rectal administration. When oral administration is difficult or contraindicated, the rectal route is often advised. Many children perceive use of the rectal route as an extreme invasion of their bodies or anticipate pain as a result. It may help to let them insert the suppository. A number of drugs, such as sedatives, aspirin, and antiemetics, are available in suppository form. Suppositories made with a cocoa butter base will melt rapidly at normal body temperature, releasing the drug for absorption. After a suppository is inserted in an infant, the buttocks should be held or taped together for 5 to 10 minutes to relieve pressure on the anal sphincter and thereby help to ensure retention and absorption of the medication. Infants and children with diarrhea, however, may easily expel suppositories with explosive stools. Likewise, a suppository inserted into a child with a constipation problem or a rectum full of stool will be surrounded with stool and will have little chance for absorption of its contents.

Pharmacists and nurses often have to cut suppositories to obtain correct doses. This is a dangerous practice, since all the medication might be contained in one area of the suppository. If divided doses must be administered, the pharmacist should be the one to divide the suppository; it should be cut lengthwise and weighed in order to ensure as accurate a dosage as possible.

Nose drops, eardrops, and eyedrops. Aqueous preparations of nose drops are the only safe preparations to use, if it is deemed necessary to use them at all, because of the danger of aspiration. Many nose drop preparations contain vasoconstrictors, and prolonged or excessive use may be harmful. Infants are nose breathers, and nasal congestion will inhibit their sucking. For this reason, nose drops should be instilled 20 minutes to ½ hour before feedings.

To instill nose drops:

1 Hold the infant in your arm, allowing his head to fall back over the edge of your arm, or place a

small pillow under the shoulders and allow his head to fall back over the edge of the pillow.

2 Place your free arm so that the forearm is around the far side of the child's head, stabilizing his head between your forearm and your body. Use your hand to stabilize the arms and hands.

3 With your free hand you can then instill the prescribed drops with minimum struggle and maximum accuracy.

The instillation of eardrops requires a knowledge of anatomic structure, since the shape of the auditory canal of a young child is different from that of an adult. In children 3 years of age or younger the nurse must gently pull the pinna of the ear slightly down and straight back to properly instill eardrops. In older children and adults, the pinna should be held up and back. Gentle massage of the area immediately anterior to the ear will facilitate the entry of the drops into the ear canal.

Eyedrop instillation is done in the same way on children as with adults. The lower lid of the eye is gently pulled down and out so that it has a cup effect into which the correct number of drops is instilled. Many eyedrops cause a burning sensation in the eye for a few seconds, so if both eyes are to be medicated it is wise to do the second instillation quickly before the patient begins to blink and tear as a reaction to the burning sensation occurring in the first eye medicated.

Aqueous preparations of nose, ear, and eye drops may support the growth of bacteria and fungi. For this reason small volumes of such medications are ordered and should be used for only *one* individual (not shared by family members). Examination of these types of drops for clearness of fluid (hold the dropper up to the light) is a good method of checking for contamination. Contaminated fluid will appear cloudy when held up to the light.

Eyedrops and eardrops are more comfortably tolerated if they are warmed before instillation. This can be achieved by running warm water over the side of the bottle without the label or immersing the bottle in some warm water in a medicine cup. Even carrying the bottle in your pocket for half an hour or so will take the chill off the drops.

Intravenous medications. The use of IV drug therapy is widespread on most pediatric ser-

vices for several reasons. In children with vomiting and diarrhea, medications given by mouth may be vomited so that precious time is lost in drug management of disease processes. These same childrem may have poor absorption of drugs and fluids as a result of dehydration or peripheral vascular collapse, so that drugs administered via the intramuscular route may be ineffective. Before the now widespread use of the midanterolateral thigh muscle for intramuscular injections, there was a great danger of sciatic neuropathy and other neurologic sequelae associated with injections in the gluteal area. For these reasons, as well as the advantages associated with administering long-term drug therapy more accurately via a relatively simple vehicle, the use of IV therapy has increased greatly. Considering the dangers and contraindications of IV drug therapy, however, its use must be justifiable.

The pediatric nurse responsible for the administration of IV drugs may find the following suggestions helpful.

1 IV drug therapy should be used only when other channels of drug administration have failed. Pediatric nurses skilled in the administration of medications to children via other routes may greatly influence the physician's decisions regarding channels of drug administration.

2 Too rapid IV injection causes "speed shock": rapid fall in blood pressure, respiratory irregularity, incoagulability of the blood, and even death.

3 Once a drug is injected intravenously, it is impossible to exert further control except by specific antidote.

4 Drugs must be properly diluted. Too much emphasis cannot be placed on the caution: give the smallest possible dose at the slowest possible rate.

Most older children may be given fluids or drugs intravenously following the same principles and techniques used for adults. The younger and smaller the child, the greater the difficulty of administration and the greater the dangers associated with it.

Neonates, infants, and children must be adequately restrained so as not to dislodge or pull out an infusion needle once it is in place. Some of the following may be helpful hints to the nurse caring for a patient receiving IV therapy.

1 The needle should be fixed with plastic tape.

2 When a loop of tubing directly above the needle is

secured to the tape, it relieves some of the pressure on the needle.

3 Since most children move about or are restless, it will be necessary to support the limb and immobilize the site of IV therapy.

4 Support should extend to the joints above and below the site (with arm boards or IV boards).

5 Tape backed with gauze can be used to secure the limb to the support.

6 If the infusion bottle is too high, it will increase the pressure in the vein and may cause fluid seepage into the surrounding tissues.

Other conditions influencing the dosage of drugs in infants and children. Laboratory studies have shown that the same individual under almost identical situations at different time intervals will exhibit variations in measured drug responses. For example, frequent altering of drug dosage is often necessary in relation to insulin administration, digitalis administration, and oral enzyme therapy.

Some of the variables that influence drug dosage were mentioned briefly at the beginning of this section (such as age, size, weight, and immaturity of the child, routes and time of administration). A few other variables are considered here with some specific examples.

Tolerance to drugs exists in infants and children just as it does in adults, and the same principles are followed to handle such a problem. Either a larger dose of the drug is administered or a different drug is selected, preferably one without cross tolerance.

As previously discussed, the dosage of most agents is roughly proportional to the age, weight, and size of the child. Opiates, for example, can be given in dosages proportional to body weight, 0.15 to 0.2 mg of morphine sulfate per kilogram of body weight being a safe level. On the other hand, infants are more sensitive than adults to a few drugs, so that smaller dosages than those proportional to weight and size are recommended. Atropine sulfate is one of these drugs. For many years atropine was used in the medical treatment of pyloric stenosis as an antispasmodic to relax the pylorospasm. The reason for sensitivity to atropine in infants is not well known, but it may be contingent on the immaturity of the central nervous system. Products less toxic than atropine itself are being used with much greater success in the treatment of pylorospasm. Unfortunately, children have been termed "therapeutic orphans" because FDA regulations require full investigation as to the efficacy and safety of any drug labeled for use by children, and many drugs effective and safe for adults have not been tested for children's use because of the complex medicolegal issues involved in experimentation on children.

Presence of disease. The presence of disease or any basic abnormality in a child may alter his response to drugs. For example, in children with any of the metabolic diseases such as diabetes mellitus, melituria, galactosemia, or phenylketonuria, one can expect altered drug responses. Since the liver, kidneys, intestines, and lungs are the chief channels of drug elimination, the presence of disease in any of these organs will require that medications be administered with much knowledge and deliberation. It remains the nurse's responsibility in pediatrics to administer medications, to recognize and interpret the child's response to drug therapy, to teach parents about the drugs their children are receiving, and to foster compliant behavior. All ethical opportunities for learning about the pharmacodynamics of drugs should be maximally exploited by physicians and nurses alike so that children can benefit sooner from advances in medicine.

Summary of some pediatric pharmacokinetics influencing dosage. *

1 *Age.* Pharmacokinetic values are most unpredictably variable among neonates because of the different rate of development of systems.

2 *Form of drug. Liquids and suspensions* are more dispersible in gastrointestinal fluids and are therefore more readily absorbed. For example, absorption of digoxin in tablet form may be up to 85% complete; in elixir form it may be 100% complete. Percutaneous absorption of *topical preparations* is readily achieved in the preadolescent; therefore inadvertent systemic circulation can result in toxicity (for example, boric acid or steroids applied to inflamed, broken, or eczematous skin).

3 *Distribution.* Since most drugs are distributed in body water, increases in total body water and extracellular volume may also increase the volume of distribution of drugs. Compared with adults, neonates have proportionately higher vol-

*Adapted from Tso, Y.: Pharmacy update, Nurse Pract. **2:** Sept.-Oct. 1977.

umes of total body water and a higher ratio of extracellular fluid to intracellular fluid; so there is a greater possibility of toxicity in the newborn. The blood-brain barrier in the newborn is also fairly ineffective against drugs.

4 *Biotransformation.* Maturity of the various liver enzyme systems for metabolism generally proceeds unevenly. For example, acetylation is deficient in the newborn; yet sulfation is enhanced.

5 *Elimination.* Renal excretory mechanisms proceed to maturity after 1 year of age. Excretion of some substances (for example, aminoglycosides) through the renal system may be delayed because of immaturity before that age, resulting in higher circulation levels and longer duration of action than desirable.

Psychiatric patients. Giving medicines to a psychiatric patient may automatically assume symbolic meanings present in lesser degree on any hospital ward. All individuals need and seek meaningful interpersonal relationships; most individuals find such relationships outside medical situations. Psychiatric patients, however, are often starved for affection and yearn for some person to whom they may look for security and interest. Frequently, their emotional deprivation is concealed by an appearance of hostility or disdain.

In addition, the immediate personal needs of the patient and the current symptoms against which the patient is fighting must be considered. Overwhelming anxiety, depression to the point of suicide, pain of an uncanny nature, or distortions of thought that constantly separate the patient from others demand of the nurse much care in any contact, particularly that of medication. To the patient in a state of psychologic disequilibrium, that which is taken by mouth or given by injection may hold threats and symbolic meanings rarely felt by the medical or surgical patient. The fear of poisons or supernatural effects of capsules or the suggestions of witchcraft inherent in a needle often reach the degree of catastrophe unless the nurse is able to understand the thought processes of the patients. The psychiatric patient's tendency toward impulsiveness and increased emotional sensitivity must constantly be kept in mind.

No practical suggestions can take the place of the techniques practiced by the psychiatric nurse, but the following factors should be con-

sidered in the general handling of medications for the psychiatric patient:

1 Drugs used in emergencies must be anticipated, and such drugs must be made available.
2 Medicines should be given in paper, not glass, containers. The psychiatric patient is often so impulsive that all possible precautions must be taken to avoid accidents, and glass is always a potential weapon for suicide.
3 Precautions should be used whenever drugs are administered.
4 *The nurse must remain with the patient until oral medications have been swallowed.* This principle is basic in the giving of all medications but one of particular importance to the depressed and suicidal patient; such patients may conceal capsules in the mouth for long periods, only to hoard them until a lethal supply has been accumulated. Frequently, measures such as the piercing of the capsule case and staying with the patient until the drug is dissolved or the practice of using liquid preparations will ensure the actual ingestion of the drug.
5 It is often necessary not only to urge the psychiatric patient to take medication but also to insist on its acceptance. The psychiatric patient is frequently an indecisive, emotionally confused individual who tends to doubt everything. He/she often presses the nurse for detailed information about the drug prescribed and frequently rebels because of minor discrepancies in information. Paradoxically, however, he/she complies quickly if a positive yet interested attitude is presented without undue explanation.
6 It is of utmost importance to report all drug refusals to the physician in charge. But in the meantime it is frequently also of importance to persuade the patient to take the medicine. Omission of doses may cause the blood level of psychotropic drugs to be lowered so that larger doses than usual may eventually be needed. Intramuscular administration of pyschotropic drugs assists in calming the patient within a relatively short period of time, so that oral preparations may then be given. The oral route of administration is preferred and should be instituted as soon as possible.

RECORDING DRUG ADMINISTRATION

Recording the administration of each dose of medication as soon after it is given leaves a documented record that can be consulted if there is any question as to whether the patient received the dose. Otherwise the patient may inadvertently receive a second dose from another nurse or nursing student. The busy nurse who "double-pours" (prepares two doses at one time—an illegal technique) may also be tempted to record the second dose at the same time the first dose is recorded. Medications should not be recorded (charted) before they are actually given, because anything may come up to prevent that dose from being administered; then the medication record, which is a legal document, will have to be corrected carefully.

Several different forms are used to record medications for each patient. These forms usually include areas to note each medication name, dose, route, time, and the administering nurse's initial. Extra notations may be added in certain instances. For example, when digitalis is given, the apical and radial pulses taken just before administration may be noted ("AP, 48; RP, 46"). If the pulses are found to be outside the normal limits as established by that agency, the medication should not be given and the record should be marked "held" and initialed and the prescriber consulted. Patients also have the right to refuse treatment, including medications, and sometimes do, despite explanations. "Refused" is then noted in the appropriate spot on the medication record. Medication may also be recorded as "discarded" or "wasted" if only part of it was administered and the rest had to be thrown out (as in a prefilled syringe) or if the medication was dropped or contaminated. If the medication is a controlled substance, its disposal must be witnessed and initialed in the special record for this drug.

There are several kinds of medication recording forms in the charts or medication books in patient care areas. Routine (or continuous) daily medications usually are recorded on one type of form; once-only, loading dosages, p.r.n., and stat. medications go on another. Both look very similar. Both have places for the medication names, dose, and route to be transcribed; times of administration may be written in or checked off, and each dose is initialed by the administering nurse. Nurses' signatures identifying the initials are written in another area on the form. Administration of a controlled substance is recorded both on the p.r.n. medication sheet and on that particular drug's sheet (which includes a running tally of the balance of the controlled substance). A notation should be made on the patient's chart relating the administration of any p.r.n. medication and the patient's response to its effects.

Potential for error in drug administration is almost limitless. Some mistakes of significance can be rectified if discovered and acted upon quickly. Also, if the error was properly reported and appropriate actions were taken, courts tend to look more kindly upon the nurse than if these were not done. Courts generally recognize the humanness of people, including nurses, and recognize the potential for error in clinical practice.

PREVENTING AND REPORTING ERRORS

Perhaps it helps to be aware of some of the pitfalls with regard to medication administration. A selection of errors related to medication administration is presented here to call attention to some common but careless nursing acts.

1 Not knowing why a medication was to be administered caused one nurse to irrigate a patient's bladder with a topical antiinflammatant, Burow's solution, instead of the genitourinary antibiotic irrigant distributed by a manufacturer of a similar name. It caused another nurse to delay giving a dose of medication essential to recuperation after cancer chemotherapy because she believed it to be "just a vitamin" instead of folinic acid.
2 Not identifying patients by their armbands caused several nurses to give medication to the wrong patients in the right beds. One of the nurses even asked the patient his name, which turned out to be similar to her patient's. One called out her patient's name, and the wrong patient responded. The result was the same—they all got the wrong medication.
3 Not checking with the prescribing physician caused one nurse to give her patient 30 ml of milk of magnesia every hour rather than every night when she misinterpreted the "q.n." (an unacceptable abbreviation) order for "q.h." Another nurse gave 2.5 mg digoxin instead of 0.25 mg; although the order was wrong, the nurse did not recognize that it was excessive. The result was that the patient received a toxic dose of medication.

The current generation of computer programs for use in updating computational and evaluative skills is unwieldy at the present state-of-the-art and needs further refinement. For now, all personnel who as a part of their job must calculate dosages should at least be aware of their possibly tenuous grasp of mathematical competence and learn to rely on others to doublecheck calculations. This assumes another essential step: that all calculations are *written down* on paper to be checked.

To err is human, however, to admit its possibility and one's susceptibility is essential. Nursing process is an appropriate approach when a medication error is suspected. To safeguard one's patient as well as one's reputation and psyche, the first step is to backtrack to doublecheck one's actions or computations to see if an error occurred. Next is the step requiring the most accountability: to consult one's superior to inform her or him and to gain perspective and objective support. The patient's physician should also be informed. Actions to correct drug effects and to normalize the patient's condition follow. Concise, objective documentation of the event and the circumstances is made both in the patient's chart and on a special form, the incident report. This report is an intraagency communication that is filed to serve as legal evidence if a suit is instituted later by the patient.

PATIENT TEACHING

Although teaching-learning interactions between patient and nurse are among the most necessary and professionally demanding, teaching patients is not as visible as bathing them, taking their vital signs, or giving them injections. Thus it is not done as often as other nursing activities; when it is done it may not be seen as important enough to be noted in nursing progress notes. However, success in patient learning has a direct bearing on success in convalescence at home. Strong rationales for teaching patients come from the many state nurse practice acts that define teaching as a necessary part of nursing, thereby giving it the power of a state mandate: one could be sued for not teaching patients. Accreditation committees recognize the importance of patient teaching and look for documentation when they visit. Thus the resistance of other disciplines to patient teaching by nurses is becoming less of an issue than it was in the past.

Basic to any learning are the following tenets:

1 Patients must be ready to learn. If they are in pain, about to be discharged, or emotionally upset, they will be too distracted to assimilate information.

2 The atmosphere must be conducive to learning. Privacy, some quiet, and a rapport between the nurse and the patient that is facilitated by understanding of cultural or personal differences all aid the dynamics of learning.
3 Information must be presented at the level of patients' understanding. The nurse should find out what they already know and start there.
4 Information should be presented beginning with the simple and building to the complex. Too much too fast will overwhelm patients.
5 Learning and motivation will be enhanced by rewarding positive behavior. For example, relief of pain after patients put into use new learning will be its own reward; sometimes verbal rewards, such as a compliment on performing a procedure well, can be effective.
6 Active participation should be encouraged at each step.
7 Specific feedback from patients is necessary to evaluate if learning has taken place. It is not enough just to "tell" patients over and over again.

Patients need to learn the following about their medications: the names of the medications (write them down or print them on the labels), what they are for and how to recognize the proper effects (in very specific ways), some of the major secondary effects (expected and tolerable, and those representing toxicity) what to do if they miss a dose, how to store the medication, how to take it (for example, with meals), and whom to call if there is a problem. It can be expected that patients will forget many of the instructions; a printed fact sheet or checklist to take home will be helpful to many patients.

Evaluation

Evaluation of the effectiveness of a nursing process in pharmacotherapeutics relates directly to the goals. Clear and specifically stated goals make it easy to evaluate what has been done. When the time to evaluate arrives (as set by a properly stated goal), the patient's condition should be observed critically for a change attributable to the medication care given. If the goal was written, "The patient will have relief from headache by 11/27," then on 11/27 it should be determined if the drug is working as intended. In this case, one can ask the patient.

The effects of drugs are categorized by terms

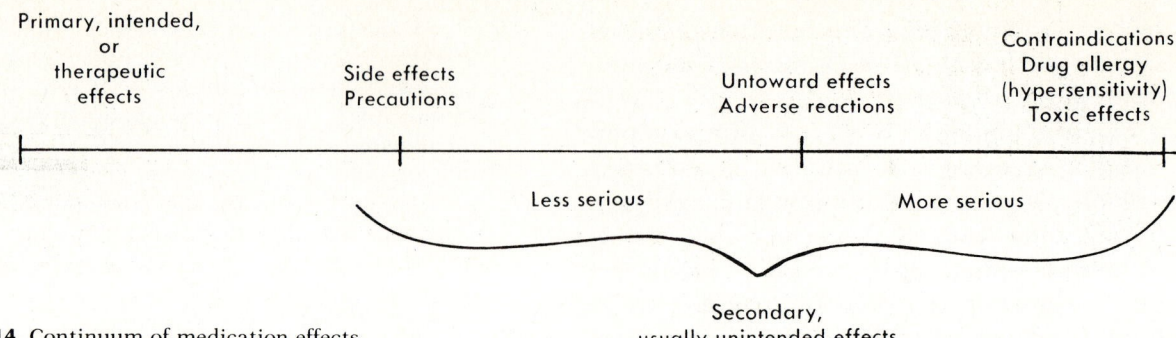

FIG. 6-14. Continuum of medication effects.

such as "untoward reactions," "side effects," and so forth. The meaning of these terms can be vague and confusing. To help clear up the confusion, Fig. 6-14 shows the relationships between some common terms on a continuum of relative significance or severity of effects.

Therapeutic or *primary effects* are those that are intended—the purpose for which the drug is prescribed and given. Secondary effects are defined, for this discussion, as "all other effects." Secondary effects are usually somewhat detrimental to the patient's well-being, but not always. In fact, a drug may be given deliberately to exploit its secondary effect.

Of the secondary effects, *side effects* and *precautions* are the least offensive and are often merely annoying mild reactions to drugs. The most common side effects are nausea, vomiting, and diarrhea; other common ones are drowsiness and sore throat. *Untoward effects* or *adverse reactions* are considered slightly more deleterious than side effects. The last effects on the continuum, *contraindications, drug allergy,* and *toxic effects* are cause for withholding or withdrawing the medication and treating the effects. Contraindications and drug allergy are so serious that drugs with these effects should not even be administered in the first place. Toxic effects, usually dose related, are nontherapeutic effects that are beyond acceptable limits; toxic effects may include coma and death.

In addition to the preceding categories, *idiosyncrasy* is an abnormal or peculiar response to a drug, such as an overresponse, an underresponse, or a paradoxically different effect from the one expected. Most are probably pharmacogenetic responses. That is, the patient may have a genetic enzyme deficiency that leads to abnormal metabolism of a drug or an inability to metabolize it. *Drug interactions* were includ-

ed under Assessment because they need to be recognized *before* administration of drugs. Neither idiosyncrasy nor drug interactions fits neatly on the continuum of effects, because the severity of response can vary so widely.

Noting whether a dose had the desired effect or whether there were also signs of secondary effects is the province of nursing. Patients should also be taught signs of secondary effects.

Any drug can be toxic if given in relatively high enough doses or if given within the usual range to someone who is allergic to it or who cannot metabolize or excrete it properly (see also Chapter 5). Unfortunately, the state of the art is not yet so developed that only the organ or system for which the drug is intended will react; the drug may also affect other tissue and give rise to secondary effects.

Signs of an aberrant response when the drug's effects are evaluated indicate that the cycle of the nursing process needs to begin again. That is, reassessment should be done. The drug's dosage must be changed, the drug should be withheld or discontinued, or the timing or type of drug must be changed. It may be necessary to change the mode or route of administration when a drug is found to be less than optimally effective. Nurses must develop greater awareness of drug effects if they are to give full-quality care. It is no longer enough simply to give out medications and assume that the medical personnel will follow up and observe for effects. Nurses are the ones at the bedside when the patient exhibits them.

Evaluation of the nursing process as applied to groups of patients is made by what is called a *nursing audit.* The nursing audit is a peer review process done by a quality assurance committee of a nursing administration. The committee is usually composed of a cross section of administration and staff members so that both points of view can be maintained. Standards of care, based on criteria of an accrediting body or on professional standards, are used as a rule against which to measure the nursing process.

The nursing audit committee gathers data in a variety of ways. Adequacy of care may be determined from direct patient interviews. Evidence of sufficient documentation of care may be examined by an audit of completed charts from the inactive records. Comparisons of treatment may be made from year to year. Charts of patients with a specific medical diagnosis may be selected to see if the nursing care in a given illness is consistent.

Whatever the focus, nurses acknowledge peer review objectively as a vehicle for professional growth, through accepting accountability for their actions. They see this as essential to patient welfare and their own professional status.

Summary of nursing considerations

Once the direction of the nursing process has been established in the assessment, the plan and implementation of nursing care easily follow.

The planning of care, based on carefully constructed behavioral objectives, establishes measurable goals for the patient to achieve. A time frame sets limits for activities, and the manner in which the goals will be demonstrated is stated. The activities are based on established principles in nursing science.

The implementation of the plan is the operational phase of the nursing process. The nurse draws on technical skills and nursing arts to assist the patient in the administration of his medications.

Evaluation is the final step of the nursing process. The nurse measures the achievements made against the criteria that were established in the plan. Collective evaluation of nursing care is possible in a nursing audit. Nursing audit is a peer review to determine the quality of care that is demonstrated.

QUESTIONS

FOR STUDY AND REVIEW

1 The most reliable method of identifying a patient before administering medication is to _____.
2 Medications should be charted *as soon as possible* _____ being given.
3 An intramuscular injection in the arm is given in the _____ muscle.
4 When a child asks if a medication is "bad," the nurse should _____.
5 Elixirs have a/an _____ base.

REFERENCES

Anderson, W.F.: Administration, labelling and general principles of drug prescription in the elderly, Gerontol. Clin. **16:**4, 1974.

Ballard, B.E., and Nelson, E.: Physicochemical properties of drugs that control absorption rate after subcutaneous implantation, J. Pharmacol. Exp. Ther. **135:**120, 1972.

Beaumont, E.: The new infusions pumps, Nursing '77 **7**(7):31, 1977.

Bender, A.D.: Pharmacodynamic principles of drug-therapy in the aged, American Geriatric Society **22:**296, 1974.

Bennett, C.R.: Monheim's local anesthesia and pain control in dental practice, ed. 6, St. Louis, 1978, The C.V. Mosby Co., pp. 102, 267.

Bivins, B.A., and others: Electronic flow control and roller clamp control in intravenous therapy, Arch. Surg. **115:**70, 1980.

Blackwell, B.: The drug defaulter, Clin. Pharmacol. Ther. **13:**841, 1972.

Borgen, L.: Total parenteral nutrition in adults, Am. J. Nurs. **78:**224, 1978.

Carr, J., and others: How to solve dosage problems in one easy lesson, Am. J. Nurs. **76:**1934, 1976.

Chezem, J.L.: Aspirating before I.M. injections, Nursing '74 **4:**87, 1974.

Dexter, P., and Applegate, M.: How to solve a math problem, J. Nurs. Ed. **19**(2):49, 1980.

Donn, R.: Intravenous admixture incompatibility, Am. J. Nurs. **71:**325, 1971.

Durgin, J., Hanan, Z.I., and Ward, C.O.: Pharmacy technician's manual, ed. 2, St. Louis, 1978, The C.V. Mosby Co.

Faulkner, H.M.: Medicine and metrication, ed. 2, Gorham, Me., 1977, International Informational Systems.

Freeman, J.T.: Some principles of medication in geriatrics, American Geriatric Society **22:**289, 1974.

Galton, L.: Drugs and the elderly, Nursing '76 **6**(6):39, 1976.

Geolot, D.H., and McKinney, N.P.: Administering parenteral drugs, Am. J. Nurs. **75**(5):788, 1975.

Gerald, M.C.: Pharmacology, an introduction to drugs, Englewood Cliffs, N.J., 1974, Prentice-Hall, Inc.

Gibbins, F.J.: Haematological problems in the older patient, Practitioner **215:**606, 1975.

Goodman, L.S., and Gilman, A., editors: The pharmacological basis of therapeutics, ed. 6, New York, 1980, The Macmillan Co.

Haggerty, R.J., and Roughmann, K.J.: Noncompliance and

self medication in pediatric practice, Pediatr. Clin. North Am. **21**:95, 1974.

Hall, M.R.P.: Drug therapy in the elderly, Br. Med. J. **4**:582, 1973.

Hansen, M.S. and Woods, S.L.: Nitroglycerin ointment—where and how to apply it, Am. J. Nurs. **80**:1122, 1980.

Hays, D.: Do it yourself the 2-track way, Am. J. Nurs. **74**:1070, l974.

Holloway, D.A.: Drug problems in the geriatric patient, Drug Intell. Clin. Pharmacy **8**:632, 1974.

Hymans, D.E.: Medicine in old age, gastrointestinal problems in the old—I, Br. Med. J. **1**:107, 1974.

Illingworth, R.S.: Drug dosage for children, Prescribers J. **13**:124, 1973.

The International Systems of Units (SI), U.S. Department of Commerce, National Bureau of Standards, Special Pub. no. 330, August 1977.

Keane, C.B., and Fletcher, S.M.: Drugs and solutions, ed. 4, Philadelphia, 1980, W.B. Saunders Co.

Kelleher, A., and others: Drug therapy by indwelling arterial catheter, Am. J. Nurs. **75**:1990, 1975.

Kurdi, W.J.: Refining your I.V. therapy technique, Nursing '75 **5**(11):41, 1975.

Kurdi, W.J.: Report on intravenous therapy national survey (Jan. 1979-1980), Nursing '81 **11**:80, 1981.

Lang, H.S., and others: Reducing discomfort from I.M. injections, Am. J. Nurs. **76**:800, 1976.

Little, D.E., and Carnevalli, D.L.: Nursing care planning, ed. 2, Philadelphia, 1976, J.B. Lippincott Co.

Lowenthal, W.: Factors affecting drug absorption, Am. J. Nurs. **73**:1391, 1973.

Maas, M., Specht, J., and Jacox, A.: Nurse autonomy, Am. J. Nurs. **75**:2201, 1975.

Maki, D.G.: Non-infective complications of infusion therapy, Infusion **2**(3):89, 1978.

Malassanos, L., and others: Health assessment, St. Louis, 1981, The C.V. Mosby Co.

Marriner, A.: The nursing process, ed. 2, St. Louis, 1979, The C.V. Mosby Co.

Maslow, A.: Motivation and personality, New York, 1970, Harper & Row, Publishers.

Mattar, M.E., and others: Inadequacies in the pharmacologic management of ambulatory children, J. Pediatr. **87**:137, 1975.

Modell, W.: Drugs of choice 1981-1982, St. Louis, 1982, The C.V. Mosby Co.

Monahan, J.J., and Webb, J.W.: Intravenous infusion pumps—an added dimension to parenteral therapy, Am. J. Hosp. Pharm. **29**:54, 1972.

Newton, D.W., and Newton M.: Needles, syringes and sites for administering injectable medication, Am. Pharmaceutical Assoc. J. **17**(11):685, 1977.

Newton, M., and Newton D.W.: Guidelines for handling drug errors, Nursing '79 **9**(7):62, 1979.

Ormond, E., and Caulfield, C.: A practical guide to giving oral medications to young children, Am. J. Maternal Child Nurs. **1**(5):320, 1976.

Parker, W.: Drug therapy; patient compliance, N. Engl. J. Med. **289**:249, 1973.

Parker, W.: Medication histories, Am. J. Nurs. **76**:1969, 1976.

Perlstein, P.H., and others: Errors in drug computation during newborn intensive care, Am. J. Dis. Child. **133**:376, 1979.

Rapp, R.P., and others: Effects of electronic infusion control on the efficacy, complications and cost of IV therapy, Hosp. Form. **14**(11):975, 1979.

Redman, B.K.: The process of patient teaching in nursing, ed. 4, St. Louis, 1980, The C.V. Mosby Co.

Rodman, M.J.: Adjusting medications for the needs of the elderly, R.N. **38**:65, 1975.

Route, site and technique, Nursing '79 **9**(7):18, 1979.

Ryan, P.B.: and others: In line filtration—a method of minimizing contamination in intravenous therapy, Bull. Parenter. Drug Assoc. **27**:1, 1973.

Sager, D.P. and Kovarovic, S.B.: Intravenous medications, Philadelphia, J.B. Lippincott Co., 1980.

Schwartz, D.: Safe self-medication for elderly outpatients, Am. J. Nurs. **75**:1808, 1975.

Shapiro, S., and others: Fatal drug reactions among medical inpatients, J.A.M.A. **216**:467, 1971.

Shields, E.M.: Introduction to drug therapy for older adults, Geriatric Nurs. **1**:8, March/April, 1975.

Shirkey, H.C., editor: Pediatric therapy, ed. 6, St. Louis, 1980, The C.V. Mosby Co.

Stewart, D.Y., and others: Unit dose medication: a nursing perspective, Am. J. Nurs. **76**:1308, 1976.

Stuart, D.M.: Unit dose medication, Pharmindex, April 1973.

Tso, Y.: Drug dosing for pediatric patients, pharmacy update, Nurse Pract. **2**(7):Sept.-Oct. 1977.

Turco, S. and Davis, N.M.: Preventing the injection of glass particles with furosemide injection, Hosp. Pharm. **7**(12):423, 1972.

Turco, S., and Davis, N.: Clinical significance of particulate matter: a review of the literature, Hosp. Pharm. **8**:137, 1973.

Turco, S., and King, R.E.: Sterile dosage forms: their preparation and clinical application, Philadelphia, 1974, Lea & Febiger.

Udkow, G.: Principles of pediatric clinical pharmacology, In Hoekelman, R.A., editor: *Principles of pediatrics; health care of the young*, New York, 1978, McGraw-Hill Inc.

Ungvarski, P.J.: Parenteral therapy, Am. J. Nurs. **76**:1974, 1976.

West, R.S., editor: Managing I.V. therapy, Nursing 80 Photobook, Horsham, Pa, 1980, Intermed Communications.

White, S.J.: IV fluids and electrolytes: how to head off the risks, RN, Nov. 1979, pp. 60-63.

Wilson, J.T.: Compliance with instructions in the evaluation of therapeutic efficacy: a common but frequently unrecognized major variable, Clin. Pediatr. **12**:333, 1973.

Wolff, L., and others: Fundamentals of nursing, ed. 6, Philadelphia, 1979, J.B. Lippincott, Co.

Yura, H. and Walsh, M.B.: The nursing process, ed. 3, New York, 1978, Appleton-Century-Crofts.

Ziser, M., Feezor, M., and Skolaut, M.W.: Regulating intravenous fluid flow: controller versus clamps. Am. J. Hosp. Pharm. **36**:1090, 1979.

CHAPTER 7

Psychologic aspects of drug therapy and self-medication

Psychologic aspects of drug therapy
  Placebo therapy
  Symbolic meaning of drugs
  Effects of drugs on the mind

Aspects of self-medication
  Self-administration of prescription drugs
  Self-treatment using nonprescription drugs
  Control of proprietary drugs

Summary of nursing considerations

Psychologic aspects of drug therapy

Every drug administered to a patient has a symbolic meaning and a potential psychologic effect in addition to its pharmacodynamic action. A drug not only alters in a useful way the function or structure of some part of the body, but it may also influence the behavior, sense of well-being, and mental state of the patient. Psychologic responses of patients to the symbol of medication may mimic pharmacologic reactions, adverse effects, or even allergic reactions to drugs. The most profound psychologic reactions may be observed in patients receiving placebos.

Medications tend to be more effective when patients believe in their capacity to get well, when they have a strong desire to get well, and when they believe that the health personnel expect the medication to be effective and say so. The patients' past and present conditioning to drugs, illness, hospitals, nurses, and other health personnel as well as their health goals are determinant factors in the response to drugs. Nurses must keep in mind that a major deterrent to successful drug therapy is divergent goals of the patient and the health personnel. An accurate appraisal of the patient's goal in seeking medical advice and therapy is important to planning and implementing an effective plan of care.

A patient's reaction to the symbolic meaning and pharmacologic action of drugs is extremely complex yet germane to his active participation in the therapeutic plan, as discussed in Chapter 5. Only an introduction to this aspect of drug therapy can be included here. For more detailed information, the student should consult the bibliography at the end of this chapter.

PLACEBO THERAPY

The term "placebo" is from a Latin word that means "I shall please." In medicine, placebos have two uses: (1) experimental drug studies and (2) a form of treatment for select patients. A placebo is either an inert substance such as lactose or sugar, distilled water, normal saline, and the like, or a relatively harmless medication, such as a subclinical dose of a vitamin.

In experimental drug studies, the placebo is

usually formulated to appear identical to the tablet, capsule, liquid, or solution of the drug being tested in an attempt to control bias and subjective drug effects. The placebo effects are compared with the effects produced by the drug being tested. Placebo effects are the psychologic and physiologic effects produced that are not related to specific pharmacologic action. For example, a subcutaneous injection of normal saline has no true pharmacologic action for pain control, yet a patient given such an injection may subjectively experience pain relief. The basic mechanism producing the placebo effect is not known, but it may be related to a psychologic phenomenon—the belief that an inert substance actually possesses pharmacologic action—or possibly to effects of endorphins or enkephalins. Patients, of course, are unaware that the substance administered is a placebo.

Placebos are given to soothe, comfort, satisfy, or meet a patient's desires. There are some individuals who believe that administration of a medication is essential to their well-being or to recovery from an illness. If the patient's condition does not warrant the administration of a pharmacologically active substance, a placebo may be prescribed to serve as a symbol of medical therapy to forestall narcotic analgesic overuse.

A major problem encountered with placebo therapy is whether or not the patient should eventually be told about the placebo therapy. The answer depends on the individual situation, trust, and the relationship existing between the patient and health team members. Placebo therapy should not be instituted unless the legal, moral, and ethical aspects have been taken into consideration. Placebo therapy should never be undertaken lightly.

SYMBOLIC MEANING OF DRUGS

Medications may be a symbol of *help* to the patient. This meaning is strengthened and drug effectiveness enhanced when physicians or nurses inform a patient that a particular drug will benefit or help him. Repeated suggestions to the patient that the drug is beneficial further reinforce the therapeutic value of the drug. This is similar to the relief a mother's kiss gives to the pain of her child; the assurance it gives makes the child feel better. Investigation of the effects of drugs on the mind has resulted in the conclusion that some drugs are effective only in the presence of an appropriate mental state.

Another important symbolic meaning of a drug is related to the *power* inherent in the drug. This symbolic power is united with the patient physically and emotionally. Although the emotional unity is most often unconscious, it provides the patient with *strength* and even a temporary sense of *security*. However, this symbolic power may propel an insecure and dependent individual into a state of drug dependence. When an individual's needs cannot be met independently, his incapacity can often be overcome with the help of an external factor such as a narcotic, drug, or alcohol. One of these might be the crutch that makes the patient feel the strength to meet the stresses with which he is confronted.

Drugs may also be viewed as symbols of *danger*. The patient may interpret the prospect of cure as a serious threat to his emotional security if he uses illness to meet a need for dependence. Taking medication may also be objectionable if there is a strong need to exhibit independence that will not allow the patient to feel reliant on anything for help. The result may be the occurrence of adverse symptoms from medications. The patient may complain of dry mouth, nausea, vomiting, palpitation, fatigue, and other vague feelings of discomfort. He may resist taking the medication, refuse to have the prescription refilled, or even throw the drug away. If the patient does take the medication to please the family, physician or nurse or because he can no longer withstand their pleading, he may immediately feel worse.

A patient may have ambivalent feelings about medications; there may be a wish to regain his health and an awareness of the importance of drug therapy in achieving this goal, but there may also be feelings that illness is essential for the gratification of needs. Drug therapy may then result in some of the symptoms being relieved while others are intensified.

Drug fantasies. Patients may harbor fantasies or irrational notions about medications. A patient may think a medication is too strong or that he does not need it any more, and he therefore may refuse to take the drug, decrease the amount of drug taken at any one time, or decrease the number of times the drug is taken. This type of fantasy may be suspected when a drug known to be effective for a specific condition is ineffective in a particular patient with that condition.

If a patient believes the drug is too weak, he may take the drug too often or request the drug more often than prescribed, or he may increase the amount of drug taken or continue drug therapy for a longer period of time than prescribed. A patient with this type of fantasy is quite likely to develop symptoms of overdosage.

Some fantasies may revolve around fear. Patients tend to fear radioactive drugs such as ^{32}P or ^{131}I and to fear dependence on drugs that have antidepressant, analgesic, or sedative effects. Although few people today believe in the claims of a cure-all remedy, there are some who believe that a certain medicament or combination of medicaments is essential to general good health and should, therefore, be taken habitually.

An honest presentation to the patient of the action of drugs and of his own responsibility in drug therapy will help alleviate the problem of drug fantasies. In addition, what the patient thinks and believes about drugs should be learned prior to instituting drug therapy; this information may be used as a basis for the teaching of realistic aspects of drug therapy.

Other reactions to drugs. Not only does a patient react to the symbol of medication but also to the pharmacodynamic properties of the drug and, if they occur, to the toxic, allergenic, or other adverse effects of the drug. A patient's reaction to the side effects of a particular drug may be somewhat reduced if he has been prepared in advance of their occurrence. Medical personnel may be reluctant to warn patients of ill effects from drugs, not wanting to cause unnecessary worry and anxiety or in an attempt to deflect time-consuming questions. On the whole, most patients prefer knowing the potential risks of drug therapy. Failure to prepare the patient for side effects may result in anxiety, panic, or rejection of therapy when

these effects occur. If a patient is harmed by a drug yet was not informed of the potential risk, litigation could ensue.

Patients who believe they are allergic to a certain drug, for real or imagined reasons, are likely to react with fear or panic when administration of that drug is contemplated. A detailed personal history and (if possible) tests for hypersensitivity should be used to corroborate or refute the patient's belief. Rejection of a patient's claim of hypersensitivity without evidence is unwise assessment of data and negligent, to say the least.

The route of administration of a drug and the financial cost of treatment as well as a patient's conscious and unconscious attitudes toward drugs, physician, nurse, illness, and so on influence the extent, duration, and intensity of the patient's response to medication. Studies indicate that when a patient is angry, resentful, or hostile, certain medications used in usual doses may not be effective.

A patient's illness may affect the emotional response to a drug. When a patient's illness is short and recovery is complete and medical and drug expense is not too great, he/she tends to have a positive reaction to drugs, hospitals, and medical and nursing personnel. Strong negative reactions toward drugs or medical personnel result when patients are led to believe that they will make a quick and complete recovery, and when drugs are both ineffective and expensive or symptoms of allergy, side or toxic effects, or overdosage occur. Preparing patients for limited beneficial effects of drugs, for side and toxic effects, and for drug expense tends to reduce or prevent negative reactions.

In any chronic illness a patient may suddenly rebel against ill health and may irrationally resist therapy with life-sustaining medications. When this occurs, the patient may be testing himself to see if he is really dependent on the drugs, or he may be attempting a real or symbolic act of self-destruction. Usually, the ill effects experienced from drug omission bring about reinstitution of drug therapy from which the patient does not deviate readily. The patient's denial of need for drug therapy is directly related to denial of illness. Rejection of medications is often associated with increase in stress. Such a patient usually needs supportive and reconstructive psychotherapy.

EFFECTS OF DRUGS ON THE MIND

Many common drugs have a secondary effect on the patient's mind. Drugs may interfere with judgment, mood, sense of values, motor ability, and coordination. Certain antihistaminics used to treat allergies may decrease the individual's alertness and cause him to be drowsy, depressed, or even accident prone. *Rauwolfia* compounds used to treat hypertension may cause depression. The barbiturates and tranquilizers may induce inattentiveness and confusion and reduce initiative and the ability to think creatively. Drug-induced depression calls for discontinuance of the offending drug. These patients should be watched for self-destructive tendencies, since pharmacologic literature has abundant examples of those with drug-induced depressions who have attempted suicide.

Aspects of self-medication

Public interest in self-care management is at an all-time high, as exemplified by the numerous self-care books and clinics that now abound. One of the most effective and inexpensive ways to stem the tide of rising health care costs may be through expanded, educated, self-care management. Studies show that half the people visiting a general practitioner have already started a self-treatment plan that helps more than 60% of the time. If these people were also helped to learn when to seek medical supervision and how to follow treatment advice wisely, they would have a still better potential for health.

Nursing, with its commitment to collaboration with the patient to further health, is in a position to educate. So are some other groups and federal agencies. Consumer information pamphlets printed by the FDA in large type for the visually impaired offer valuable advice about drug interactions, health foods, and non-prescription pain relievers.

Development of the science of public health has led to the realization that the state of a nation's health is not exclusively dependent on the interplay between professional medical practice on the one hand and bacteria, malignancy, and other causes of disease on the other. The influence on community health of the individual's personal attempts to relieve his ailments by self-medication or by changing lifestyle has frequently been ignored or underestimated. Here are a few of many varied aspects that affect self-medication either positively or negatively.

Drugs sold without prescription can induce sleep or wakefulness, relieve pain or tension, or supply the body with vitamins and minerals. Remedies can be purchased for any part of the body from head to toe. Sales of prescription and nonprescription (or over-the-counter) drugs have established the pharmaceutical industry as a multi–billion dollar industry that is still growing. Widespread use of self-medication (autotherapy) is primarily the result of advertising via mass communications media. Concern over the use of home remedies and self-medication is not new; self-medication continues to be a controversial subject. A critical assessment of the problem should include the investigation of the realistic and practical aspects of self-medication, so that the layperson's rights and obligations become apparent to the nursing student and the practicing nurse.

Autotherapy is based on the tradition of folk remedies. Among the many reasons given for the continuing popularity of autotherapy are convenience, fear or embarrassment with regard to medical consultation, disappointment with professional medical methods or results, and the fact that home remedies are more economical than medical consultation. That the locus of control and decision making remains with the individual may be another motivating force in self-medication.

SELF-ADMINISTRATION OF PRESCRIPTION DRUGS
Purchasing drugs

The elderly and the poor are the most likely to need prescription drugs and the least able to pay for them. Yet a Florida study[1] shows that these groups are less prone to take advantage of new laws in most states that allow consumers to purchase less expensive generic drug substitutes for brand name drugs. Two thirds of the people questioned answered "no" when asked if they would accept a generic substitute of the same chemical quality and amount as the prescribed trade name drug. The same study revealed that the poor and the elderly also had less general knowledge about drugs than other participants, and this was thought to be the reason for their heavy reliance on the prescriber's authority or on impressions gained from drug advertising. Despite this, where completely free substitution of generic for trade name drugs is permitted by law, the price of prescriptions is down by 20% to 30%. Education of the elderly and the poor regarding drug purchases is necessary if they are to be able to take advantage of hard-won legislation intended to help them cut drug costs.

Information regarding generic drugs for older Americans is available with membership in the American Association of Retired Persons (AARP). Members are also entitled to up to 50% discounts on generic drugs ordered by mail. For those who would find it valuable to be able to compare wholesale prices of many drugs in the United States, the Department of Health and Human Services has published a *Guide to Prescription Drug Costs.**

Practical information about prescription drugs in any of 10 common categories is available to consumers under a 3-year experimental program by the Department of Health and Human Services via package inserts produced by the pharmaceutical industry. Information includes the drug's purpose, possible side and toxic effects, and the best way to take the drug. It is claimed by some in the pharmaceutical industry that this service may add up to 18¢ to the consumer's cost of each prescription.

Additionally, some 500 common drugs are listed annually in the *U.S. Pharmacopeia Dispensing Information*, which is geared partly to inform those who dispense or administer prescription drugs and partly for those who take them. Section II, entitled "Advice to the Patient," offers jargon-free guidelines for safe

and informed self-administration of prescription drugs by generic name. The U.S.P.D.I. may be made available to the consumer by health practitioners or pharmacists who are permitted to reproduce for distribution a limited number of pages from the Advice section.*

Compliance

Why would a person go to all the trouble of visiting a physician's office for diagnosis and treatment of a bothersome condition and then not follow through on the suggested medication plan at home? The reasons why patients do not take their medication would fill volumes. But everyone is a potential "noncomplier," whether intentionally or not. Studies vary in their findings, showing that from 33% to 60% of prescription drugs purchased are never taken completely as directed. Some never fill the prescription, most take them at unscheduled times, and many stop taking the medication early.

The consequences include inexplicable medication failures with continuing symptoms or overdoses. Medication not used may be kept and taken inappropriately later when its potency and chemical activities may have changed. Prescribers tend simply to increase the drug dosage or change medications when confronted with apparent medication failures instead of investigating for noncompliance with the therapeutic plan.

Those persons who may not accept in toto and follow a medication plan can often be predicted when, for example:

1 The patient is chronically ill or on prolonged therapy. Chronic illness is marked by the oscillatory nature of symptoms, and patients do not often get to see any causal relationship between taking or not taking the prescribed medication methodically and the waxing and waning of symptoms. It has been shown that the routine action of reviewing medications with patients and inquiring about how they are taken at home dramatically increases compliance. It also needs to be reinforced that the medication will have to be taken for the rest of the patient's life and should not be precipitously discontinued.
2 The patient is relatively asymptomatic or feels

---

*Office of Pharmaceutical Reimbursement, Room 3076, Switzer Building, 330 C Street SW, Washington, D.C. 20201.

*The U.S.P.D.I. and its six bimonthly updates annually are available for purchase from: Secretary of the USPC Board of Trustees, 12601 Twinbrook Parkway, Rockville, Md. 20852.

better. Reasons for needing to complete taking the drug should be explained; many people just do not know that organisms mutate, for example, and that to assure their eradication in the first place antibiotic prescriptions should be finished.

3 The medication is expensive or inconvenient to obtain. Prescription by generic name and explanations may be effective in remotivating if this is the problem.

4 The medication instructions are complex and not easily understood. "Take with meals" means twice a day to the person who always skips breakfast, for example. Or it may mean before or after meals for some people. Written instructions with a sample of the drug taped to them help as a reminder when the patient is home and has forgotten what was heard in the office or when being discharged from the hospital.

5 The medication is unwieldy to take by virtue of bottle caps difficult for arthritic hands or complicated mixing or measuring directions. Measuring cups or droppers can be offered, and the patient can be told that easy-to-remove caps can be requested at the time of purchase.

6 The medication tastes unpleasant or must be taken at inconvenient times (during sleep hours, at work) or too many times a day to be feasible. Medication can be mixed with or taken with various liquids that are both pleasant and compatible. Medication prescriptions can often be changed after consultation with the prescriber to higher doses given less frequently or to a sustained-action form if available and if feasible.

7 The therapeutic plan contains many different medications, so the drug-taking schedule is complicated. Occasional systematic review of the medications by the prescriber or the nurse is necessary to ascertain the continuing need for all of them and to discern ways to reduce unnecessary complexity in the plan. Confrontation of the patient's habits is necessary when medication containers remain full when they should be empty. Written schedules with sample drugs attached are helpful. There are also for sale small medication boxes with separate compartments for each dosing time. It also helps to teach the patient to keep the medication near equipment used at a specific time each day (such as a coffee cup or toothbrush).

8 The usual waiting time in the physician's office is more than an hour. Waiting longer than this has been correlated with a distinct drop in concurrence with prescribers' medication instructions. Often the wait is unavoidable, but the situation can be ameliorated with an empathic expression by the practitioner.

9 There is lack of understanding or lack of acceptance of the fact of the illness or disorder, or the explanation of the illness or treatment plan does not fit the patient's concept of illness, health care, or system of beliefs about health. Typical of the patient beliefs that influence attitudes toward treatment are the extent to which patients believe (a) themselves to be susceptible to the illness, (b) the illness to be serious, (c) that they will benefit from taking action. *Giving information, therefore, is not the entire answer.* It helps to seek active participation of the patient in the medical and nursing process, to show interest in and respect for patient ideas, feelings, and beliefs.

10 The patient and health care practitioners perceive the patient's problems or goals in divergent ways, yet do not effectively communicate this.

11 The medication is seen as an artificial additive or contaminant to the body or a crutch on which dependence should be limited.

12 Side effects are severe or interfere with functioning in daily activities.

13 The patient has problems of memory or confusion.

SELF-TREATMENT USING NONPRESCRIPTION DRUGS
Advantages

Historical records and present-day surveys indicate that the individual has a desire and a right to practice self-medication. Throughout history the public has searched for medicines to relieve ailments and has tried almost every natural material known in the battle against pain, discomfort, and disease.

The public is health conscious; otherwise there would be no over-the-counter sales or use of nonprescribed drugs. Many ailments are minor and temporary, and the search is to alleviate these discomforts in the most expedient way possible. Minor ailments do not usually require the time or energy of a busy physician. The success with which minor complaints are treated by members of the public and nurse practitioners attests to this fact. Indeed, if individuals sought medical advice for every minor ailment (colds, headaches, slight wounds, temporary gastrointestinal upsets, or minor burns), health care providers would be unable to give attention to patients with illnesses requiring professional medical care. Although self-medication if misused or abused may harm an individual, available data indicate that there is a greater amount of harm caused by prescription drugs than by nonprescription drugs. Hazards of autotherapy can be minimized by educating the public about drugs.

Disadvantages

Most preparations available before the twentieth century were harmless vegetable concoctions. The advent of modern chemistry and pharmacology produced literally thousands of preparations for self-medication, some of which are worthless or even capable of causing harm.

Today, many drugs can be bought in supermarkets, restaurants, and vending machines, in addition to drugstores. The desire for self-medication can be easily gratified. Sales promotion via radio and television encourages self-medication for real or fancied ills. Since the hazards of medications are insufficiently outlined, persistent abuse of drugs may occur and toxic effects may result. Many drugs considered harmless by the general public, such as aspirin and vitamin tablets, can actually cause untoward reactions. Aspirin may upset the gastrointestinal tract and cause bleeding, while multiple-vitamin preparations containing iron, minerals, and salts may disturb gastrointestinal function and cause other more serious problems. Calcium preparations and excessive amounts of vitamin D may cause kidney damage. Persistent use of bromides may result in bromism, and habitual use of antihistaminics can cause cardiac irregularities. Habitual self-medication may also mask a serious condition, prevent diagnosis, endanger the individual's life, and create a need for prolonged and expensive medical therapy. The public's lack of knowledge of drugs and illness requires restriction of availability of potentially harmful drugs and education about the remainder.

Nursing interventions in patient self-medication

As has been noted, self-medication is very much a part of health care. If drug abuse and misuse by the public are to be prevented and if the potential benefits of self-medication are to be optimized, the self-medicating public must be taught to recognize the approximate boundaries of its therapeutic competence. That is, persons must be taught the potential benefits

and risks of self-medication, when to self-medicate, and when to seek professional health care.

Education of the public regarding nonprescription drugs is the responsibility of all health professionals. Nurses in both ambulatory health care settings and inpatient settings have a unique and distinct opportunity to fulfill this responsibility. All too often, unfortunately, consumer information regarding nonprescription drugs is derived from misleading advertising or reporting.

Prerequisite to the fulfillment of this nursing responsibility are specific knowledges and skills.

First, nurses need more information regarding the major categories of nonprescription drugs and the ingredients of those drugs. Antacids, internal and external analgesics, laxatives, sleep aids, cold medications, vitamins, corticosteroids, antihistaminics, and ophthalmic preparations are but a few of the categories of nonprescription drugs available. Drugs within each category may consist of many and varied ingredients, some of which may be harmful for some people. For example, aspirin is marketed under at least two dozen brand names and in combination with many other drugs such as caffeine, phenacetin, sodium bicarbonate, and aluminum hydroxide. Not only is the potential toxicity of aspirin greatly underestimated by the lay public, but combination forms of the drugs are used indiscriminately.

Second, nurses need to be skilled in interviewing techniques in order to obtain information regarding an individual's patterns of drug use. This is an especially significant skill for two reasons: (1) many laypersons do not recognize over-the-counter preparations as medications or drugs and do not always volunteer this relevant information for medical histories, and (2) symbolic investment in drug use should not be underestimated and should be assessed as part of a thorough patient-client evaluation. The nurse should understand that self-medication is complex, psychologically motivated behavior that, like all other behavior, persists when it either increases the individual's pleasure or reduces his discomfort. Practically speaking, then, interviewing regarding self-

TABLE 7-1   Medications useful for home treatment

Medication	Use
Analgesic balm or ointment	Muscular aches
Analgesic tablets (aspirin and aspirin combinations for adults and children)	Headaches, minor aches, pains, fever
Antacids	Indigestion or upset stomach
Antidiarrheal compounds	Mild or noncomplicated diarrhea
Antiseptics	
Liquid, cream, spray	Minor cuts and scrapes
Mouthwash	Mild sore throat
Throat lozenges	Mild sore throat
Calamine cream or lotion	Insect bites, minor itching, poison ivy
Cough syrup	Coughing caused by colds
Ipecac syrup	Accidental poisoning emergency
Laxatives, mild	Constipation
Motion or travel sickness remedies	Dizziness, nausea, vomiting from travel
Nasal decongestants	Nasal stuffiness resulting from colds or allergies
Skin creams or lotions	Chapped skin, diaper rash
Sunburn and other burn treatments	Sunburn, other minor burns
Vitamin preparations	Dietary supplement

medication should explore the individual's attitude toward self-medication as well as define the types of self-medication used including herbs, roots, poultices, as well as drugstore remedies.

After nurses have fulfilled these prerequisites, consumer education (or patient teaching) may proceed. Topics appropriate for health education regarding nonprescription drugs include the following:

1 Awareness that over-the-counter medications are truly drugs, just as are prescription drugs, and deserve the same discretion in use.
2 Identification of medications that can be considered useful for home treatment (see Table 7-1).
3 Safety precautions to prevent unnecessary accidents, such as:
  a Have all medications properly labeled (labels should be obvious and legible).
  b Follow instructions and heed warnings on labels (for example, Do not drive or operate machinery while taking this medication; discontinue use if rapid pulse, dizziness, or blurring of vision occurs) (see Fig. 7-1).
  c Check all medications periodically for expiration date and for deterioration by heat, light, or humidity and discard deteriorated and outdated medications.
  d Discard unused portions of prescription drugs and never "share" these drugs with friends or family even if they appear to manifest similar symptoms.
  e Keep all medications out of children's reach and never refer to medications as "candy" for the sake of inducement.
  f Do not take any medication in the dark.
  g Do not mix medications in one container. Always store drugs in the original container and keep tightly capped.
  h If you suspect an overdose or wrong medication has been taken, call your Poison Control Center, prescriber, or pharmacist with medication container in hand.
  i Learn both the generic and brand or trade names of all drugs used.
  j Tell the prescriber and pharmacist about any medical problems you have, allergies, previous unusual drug reactions, current pregnancy, or if you are breast-feeding.
  k Take the medication precisely as directed and for the duration of time prescribed.
4 Instruction that nonprescription drugs are not curative and offer only symptomatic relief, followed by instructions regarding the types of symptoms that can be treated with these drugs. Patients can also be referred to the *Physicians' Desk Reference for Nonprescription Drugs* for further information.
5 Counseling and instruction regarding alternative therapeutic regimens, if appropriate (such as the need for laxative drugs can be reduced with counseling regarding activity and food habits).
6 Instructions to seek professional health care if symptoms are chronic, persistent, unresponsive or frequently recurring or unusual reactions are noted.
7 Warning regarding drugs capable of producing physical and/or psychologic dependence (laxatives, nonprescription analgesics, stimulants).

Instruction sheet for the patient*

Medication warnings

☐   1. Avoid alcoholic beverages while taking this medication.

☐   2. Swallow these tablets. Do not chew them. Do not take if coating is cracked.

☐   3. Do not drive a car or operate machinery if this medication makes you drowsy. If you have to drive home, wait until you get home to take your first dose.

☐   4. Do not allow this medication to contact the skin, eyes, or clothing.

☐   5. Take this medication on an empty stomach either 1 hour before meals or 3 hours after meals. You may drink water.

☐   6. Do not take this medication with fruit juice.

☐   7. Take this medication _____ hour(s) before meals.

☐   8. Do not take this medication with milk or milk products. You may drink water or juice.

☐   9. Take this medication with plenty of water.

☐ 10. Take this medication immediately after meals.

☐ 11. This medication may color the urine or stools.

☐ 12. Do not take this medication with antacids.

☐ 13. Do not take aspirin with this medication.

☐ 14. Do not take mineral oil with this medication.

☐ 15. Take orange juice, bananas, and other foods high in potassium while taking this medication.

☐ 16. Avoid tyramine-rich food such as cheese, pickled herring, and wine while taking this medication.

Keep all medication out of reach of children

*You're welcome to reproduce this instruction sheet (by photocopy, mimeograph, etc.) for use with your patients.

FIG. 7-1. Instruction sheet for the patient: medication warnings. (Adapted from Martin, E.W.: Hazards of medication, Philadelphia, J.B. Lippincott Co.; from Nursing Update, Sept. 1972.)

CONTROL OF PROPRIETARY DRUGS

An important factor in determining the limits of autotherapy is governmental control of nonprescription drugs. Control of over-the-counter drugs has increased in Canada, the United States, and most European countries in the past few decades. Home remedies have existed from time immemorial, but their legislative history is of recent vintage. Drug laws in Canada and the United States were not intended to restrict the avilability of drugs for self-medication but were intended to make self-medication safer and more effective. As a result of these laws, the use of secret formulas and much deceptive advertising have disappeared.

Many nonprescription drugs available to the public have limitations of effectiveness. Thus analgesics such as aspirin are available for the relief of minor aches and pains, but agents such as morphine that relieve visceral pain are not available without a prescription. A nonprescription drug, like a prescription drug, must be proved safe and effective for the conditions for which it is recommended. It is this rule that has resulted in the withdrawal of many harmful and ineffective agents from the market. Nonprescription medicines must be made safe and effective within a wide range of dosage. This provides protection against misuse. Most drugs capable of causing dependence or addiction such as amphetamines and barbiturates are no longer available across the counter. Many nonprescription drugs are of low toxicity and pose no threat to the average consumer when directions are followed, but many do, especially if the consumer is allergic, pregnant, or breast-feeding, for example.

According to law, all nonprescription drugs must bear these seven points on their labels:

1 Name of the product
2 Name and address of the manufacturer, packer, or distributor
3 Net contents of the package
4 Active ingredients and the quantity of certain ingredients
5 Name of any habit-forming drug contained in the prescription
6 Cautions and warnings needed for the protection of the user
7 Adequate directions for safe and effective use

Labeling and warnings that accompany nonprescription drugs help to protect the public against misuse and potential harmful effects.

Retail sale of home remedies can also be important to proper use of autotherapy. Allowing drugs to be purchased in grocery stores or supermarkets, from mail-order houses, or from vending machines promotes the use of medications without benefit of the professional advice that can be given by the pharmacist. Restricting the sale of drugs to pharmacies or stores where a registered pharmacist is employed provides an opportunity for advice on the purchase of drugs and enables the pharmacist to observe which customers repeatedly buy the same medications to treat the same ailment, keep a drug profile, and advise these customers to see a physician as necessary.

Summary of nursing considerations

Medications tend to be more effective when the patient believes in his capacity to get well, when he has a strong desire to get well, and when he believes that the health personnel caring for him are sincerely interested in his health. Psychologic responses of patients to the symbol of medication (the placebo effect) may mimic pharmacologic reactions, adverse effects, or even allergic reactions to drugs. To the patient, medications may be a symbol of help, power, strength, security, and danger.

Autotherapy, or self-medication is continually popular because of convenience, fear or embarrassment with regard to medical consultation, disappointment with professional medical methods or results, and the fact that home remedies are more economical than medical consultation. In today's health-conscious society, there are advantages as well as disadvantages to self-medication. However, the key to minimizing the hazards of autotherapy lies in educating the public about drugs. Nurses in both ambulatory health care settings and impatient settings have a unique opportunity to fill this educational responsibility. Furthermore, the government can limit the hazards of autotherapy by regulating nonprescription drugs. Table 7-1 lists medications for home treatment and indicates their uses.

QUESTIONS

FOR STUDY AND REVIEW

1 For what effects are placebos most frequently used?

2 List some fantasies that an individual may have about taking medications.

3 Give some rules that an individual should follow regarding the taking of drugs.

REFERENCE

1. Lambert, Z.V., and others: Predispositions toward generic drug acceptance, J. Consumer Res. **7**:24, June 1980.

BIBLIOGRAPHY

Abernathy, J.D.: The problem of non-compliance in long-term antihypertensive therapy, Drug **11**:86, 1976.

Amarasingham, L.R.: Social and cultural perspectives on medication refusal, Am. J. Psychiatry **137**(3):353, 1980.

Becker, M., and Maiman, L.A.: Sociobehavioral determinants of compliance with health and medical care recommendations, Med. Care **13**:10, 1975.

Beecher, H.K.: The powerful placebo, J.A.M.A. **159**:1602, 1955.

Blackness, B.: Drug therapy; patient compliance, N. Engl. J. Med. **289**:249, 1973.

Consumer memos, H.E.W. Pub. Nos. (FDA) 79-2108 EV; (FDA) 78-3070 EV; (FDA) 78-3078 EV; Washington, D.C., 1978, U.S. Government Printing Office.

Dukes, M.N.G.: Patent medicines and autotherapy in society, Den Haag, The Netherlands, 1963, Drukkerij Pasmans.

Fischer, H.K.: Psychiatric progress and problems of drug therapy, GP **16**:92, 1957.

Fischer, H.K., and Olin, B.: The dynamics of placebo therapy, Am. J. Med. Sci. **232**:504, 1956.

Handbook of non-prescription drugs, Washington, D.C., 1978, American Pharmaceutical Association.

Hussar, D.A.: Your role in patient compliance, Nursing '79 **9**:48, 1979.

Jaco, E.G., editor: Patients, physicians, and illness, New York, 1970, The Free Press.

Kaufman, W.: Some psychological aspects of therapy with drugs, Parts I to IV, Conn. Med. **25**:300, 368, 438, 506, 1961.

Lasagna, L.: Placebos, Sci. Am. **193**:68, 1955.

Marston, M.V.: Compliance with medical regimens: a review of the literature, Nurs. Res. **19**:312, 1970.

Pennes, H.H., editor: Psychopharmacology, New York, 1958, Harper & Row, Publishers.

Rome, H.P.: Doctors: drugs: patients, Med. Clin. North Am. **34**:973, 1950.

Rosenstock, I.M.: Why people use health services, Milbank Mem. Fund Q. **44**:94, 1966.

Sacket, D.L.: The standardized compliance questionnaire, Hamilton, Ontario, 1976, McMaster University Health Sciences Center.

St. Whitelock, O.V., editor: Techniques for the study of behavioral effects of drugs, Ann. N.Y. Acad. Sci. **65**:247, 1956.

Spector, R., and others: Does intervention by a nurse improve medication compliance? Arch. Int. Med. **138**:36, 1978.

Spriet, A., and others: Adherence of elderly patients to treatment with pentoxifylline, Clin. Pharmacol. Ther. **27**(1):1, 1980.

Taylor, D.W.: Compliance with antihypertensive drug therapy, Ann. N.Y. Acad. Sci., 1978.

Wikler, A.: The relation of psychiatry to pharmacology, Baltimore, 1957, The Williams & Wilkins Co.

Wolf, S.: Effects of suggestion and conditioning on the action of chemical agents in human subjects—the pharmacology of placebos, J. Clin. Invest. **29**:110, 1950.

UNIT THREE

DRUGS ACTING ON THE CENTRAL NERVOUS SYSTEM AFFECTING THE SOMATIC MOTOR SYSTEMS AND NEUROEFFECTORS

CHAPTER 8

Central nervous system drugs

The central nervous system and drug action

Drugs act to increase or decrease the activity of nerve centers and conducting pathways. Stimulants and depressants of the brain, the spinal cord, or specific centers of each have been developed, and their effects, on the whole, are highly predictable.

The central nervous system is composed of the brain, spinal cord, and numerous nerve cells called neurons. It is often referred to as the somatic or cerebrospinal nervous system. Striated muscle (skeletal or voluntary muscle) con-trol and the unique functions of the brain (reasoning and memory) are primary concerns of the central nervous system.

The central nervous system of the human body functions much like a computer. Information from the external world (such as that related to sight, sound, touch, smell, and taste) and from the internal world (such as that related to oxygen or carbon dioxide blood levels, muscle tension, and body temperature) is sent to the appropriate part of the central nervous system. The information is integrated and instructions relayed to appropriate cells or tissues to

135

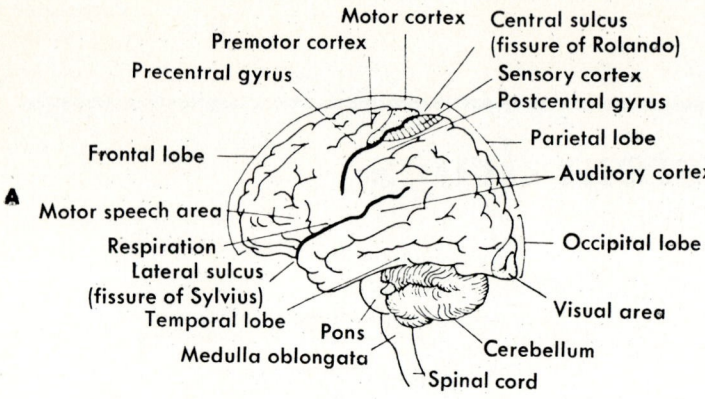

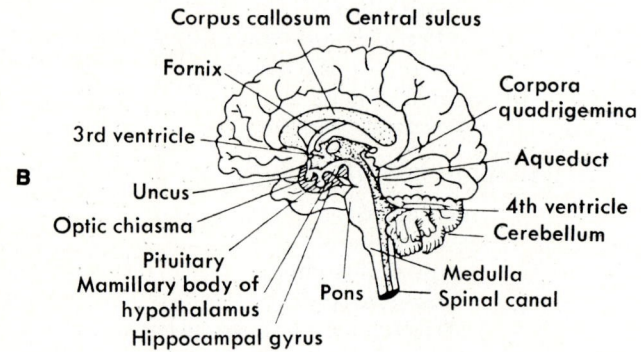

FIG. 8-1. The mature human brain viewed from the left side, **A,** showing the surface and **B,** the medial longitudinal section. (From Bowman, W.C., and Rand, M.J.: Textbook of pharmacology, ed. 2, London, 1980, Blackwell Scientific Publications.)

produce the necessary actions and environmental adjustments. Information concerning these actions and adjustments is again fed back into the central nervous system. The constant feeding of information into the central nervous system permits continuous adjustment to be made in the instructions sent to various tissues to ensure effective control of body functions.

Figs. 8-1 and 8-2 present the central nervous system digrammatically and show the major parts that will be discussed in the following paragraphs.

THE CENTRAL NERVOUS SYSTEM
Cerebral cortex

The *cerebral cortex* constitutes the outer layer of gray matter covering each of the two hemispheres of the brain and the four lobes into which each hemisphere is divided. These lobes are named for the bones of the skull under which they lie—frontal, parietal, occipital, and temporal. The frontal lobe contains the motor, and speech areas. The sensory cortex is located in the parietal lobe, the visual cortex in the occipital lobe, and the auditory cortex in the

temporal lobe. Association areas lie near these areas and act in conjunction with them. In addition, large parts of the cortex are concerned with higher mental activity—reasoning, creative thought, judgment, memory—those attributes that are unique to humans and separate them from other animals.

Drugs that depress cortical activity may decrease acuity of sensation and perception, inhibit motor activity, decrease alertness and concentration, and even promote drowsiness and sleep. Drugs that stimulate the cortical areas may cause more vivid impulses to be received and greater awareness of the surrounding environment. In addition increased muscle activity and reslessness may occur. The specific response brought forth by a drug depends to a large extent on the personality of the individual, his emotional and physiologic state, the specific attributes of the drug, and a host of other factors.

Limbic system

The limbic system is a group of paleocortical and subcortical structures that lie beneath

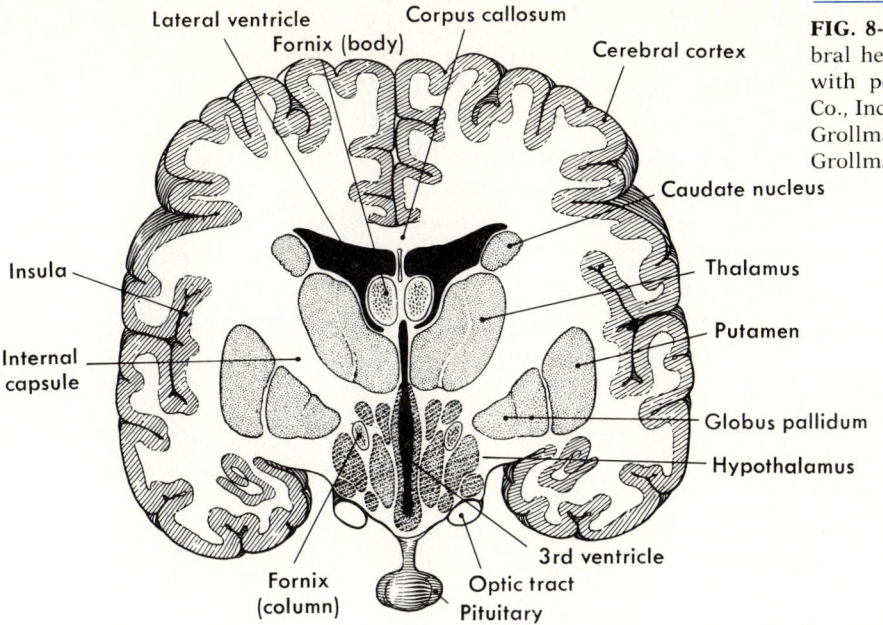

FIG. 8-2. Frontal section through the cerebral hemisphere (coronal slice). (Reprinted with permission of Macmillan Publishing Co., Inc. from The human body, ed. 2, by S. Grollman. Copyright © 1969 by Sigmund Grollman.)

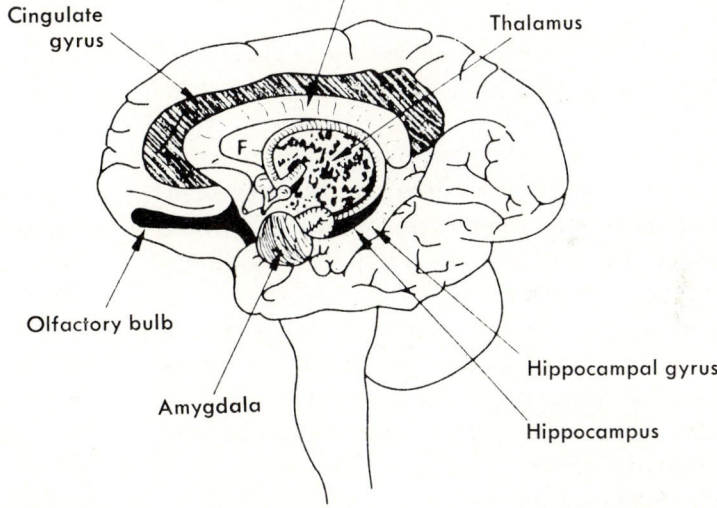

FIG. 8-3. Limbic system. (From Bowman, W.C., and Rand, M.J.: Textbook of pharmacology, ed. 2, London, 1980, Blackwell Scientific Publications.)

the cerebral cortex. These structures form a ring (limbus) around the top of the brainstem that consists of the portions of the brain remaining after the cerebral hemispheres and cerebellum have been removed. The subcortical structures of the limbic system include the preoptic area, septum, parolfactory area, amygdala, anterior nuclei of the thalamus, hypothalamic nuclei, caudate nucleus, and reticular formation of the brainstem. The paleocortical and related structures of the limbic system are the hippocampus, uncinate gyrus, hippocampal gyrus, cingulate gyrus, and olfactory bulb and tubercle. This last group forms a ring

around the subcortical structures and is known as the limbic cortex (Fig. 8-3).

The emotions of anger, fear, anxiety, sexual feelings, pleasure, and sorrow are related to this system. Learning and memory have been associated with the hippocampus.

The limbic system is extremely complex in its functioning. It may work with or inhibit other parts of the brain such as the cerebral cortex, brainstem, or hypothalamus to normalize expressions of emotions, influence their ultimate expression to other than normal, or affect the biologic rhythms, sexual behavior, and motivation of an individual.

Drugs that affect the limbic system are the benzodiazepines, meprobamate, and morphine. The benzodiazepines and meprobamate are believed to suppress the limbic system, preventing it from activating the reticular formation, thus resulting in drowsiness and sleep, especially in patients with anxiety. Morphine is thought to alter the subjective reactions of the patient to pain in addition to abolishing pain stimuli received by the amygdala and hippocampus.

Diencephalon

The diencephalon (between-brain) is composed of the thalamus, hypothalamus, and part of the third ventricle.

The *thalamus* is composed of sensory nuclei and serves as a relay center for impulses to and from the cerebral cortex. It also serves as a center of unlocalized sensations. It registers such sensations as pain, temperature, and touch.

The thalamus enables the individual to have impressions of the agreeableness or disagreeableness of a sensation. Drugs that depress cells in the various portions of the thalamus may interrupt the free flow of impulses to the cerebral cortex. This is one way pain is relieved.

The *hypothalamus* lies below the thalamus and contains centers that regulate body temperature, carbohydrate and fat metabolism, water balance, and autonomic function. There is evidence that there is also a center for sleep and wakefulness here. Some of the sleep-producing drugs are thought to depress centers in the hypothalamus.

The symptoms of depression are often diencephalic (relating the functions of the diencephalon)—weight loss, anorexia, decreased libido, and insomnia. The tricyclic antidepressants, (Chapter 11) often reverse these symptoms. Some psychotherapeutic drugs cause a number of hypothalamic side effects, including breast engorgement, lactation, amenorrhea, appetite stimulation, and alterations in temperature regulation.

Medulla oblongata

The *medulla oblongata* contains the so-called vital centers: the respiratory, vasomotor, and cardiac centers. If the respiratory center is stimulated, it will discharge an increased number of nerve impulses over nerve pathways to the muscles of respiration. If it is depressed, it will discharge fewer impulses, and respiration will be correspondingly affected. Other centers in the medulla that respond to certain drugs are the cough center and the vomiting center. The medulla, pons, and midbrain constitute the brainstem and contain many important correlation centers (gray matter) as well as ascending and descending pathways (white matter).

Reticular formation

The reticular formation is a part of the central nervous system that has been studied increasingly in recent years. Its importance is only beginning to be appreciated. It is made up of cells and fine bundles of nerve fibers that extend in many directions. The formation extends from the upper part of the spinal cord forward through the brainstem to the diencephalon. It exhibits both inhibitory and excitatory functions in relation to other parts of the nervous system. It receives afferent impulses from all parts of the body and relays impulses to the cortex to promote wakefulness and alertness, which affects many cerebral functions, such as consciousness and learning. It also inhibits or excites activity in motor neurons, promoting both reflex and voluntary movements. Its overall function is thought to be that of an integrating system that influences activities of other parts of the nervous system. Depression of the reticular formation produces sedation and loss of consciousness. Many drugs are believed to exert an effect on the reticular formation. It is particularly sensitive to certain depressant drugs, such as barbiturates and anesthetics.

Cerebellum

The cerebellum contains centers for muscle coordination, equilibrium, and muscle tone. It receives afferent impulses from the vestibular nuclei as well as the cerebrum and plays an important role in the maintenance of posture. Drugs that disturb the cerebellum or vestibular branch of the eighth cranial nerve cause loss of equilibrium and dizziness.

Spinal cord

The spinal cord, a center for reflex activity, also functions in the transmission of impulses to and from the higher centers in the brain and may be affected by the action of drugs. Ascending sensory tracts conduct up to the brain from peripheral nerves and descending motor tracts conduct down from the brain to peripheral nerves. Larger doses of spinal stimulants may cause convulsions; smaller doses may increase reflex excitability.

When a drug is described as having a central action, it means that it has an action on the brain or the spinal cord.

The blood-brain barrier prevents drug penetration to the brain and spinal cord. This has impeded both physiologic and pharmacologic research on the central nervous system. Therefore, less is known about the central nervous system than about the autonomic nervous system.

SYNAPTIC TRANSMISSION IN THE CENTRAL NERVOUS SYSTEM

There is evidence that transmission of impulses at synapses in the central nervous system is humoral. Many neurotransmitters are still to be identified. When released, they affect the postsynaptic neurons to stimulate or inhibit their activity. Fig. 8-4 illustrates some types of nerve synapses found in the central nervous system.

Inhibition of motor neuron activity may be presynaptic or postsynaptic. Studies indicate that presynaptic inhibition occurs in the brain and is widespread at the spinal level, affecting transmission in afferent fibers from skin and muscle. The function of presynaptic inhibition is probably to suppress weak inputs that would otherwise cause unnecessary responses. This modulation of nerve impulses results in less transmitter substance being liberated. The net effect is a limiting or "inhibiting" of impulses to postsynaptic nerve fibers. Inhibition is important for orderly function.

Postsynaptic inhibition may be the result of changes in the membrane permeability of the postsynaptic cells caused by release of chemical transmitters from presynaptic nerve endings.

Upper motor neurons are scattered throughout the cerebral cortex; a number of them are located in the motor cortex. About three fourths of the nerve fibers from these motor neurons cross to the opposite side at the level of the medulla, descend to the spinal cord, and synapse with interneurons, which in turn snyapse with the lower motor neurons. Almost all motor neurons of one side are controlled by the motor cortex of the other side. Therefore, injury to the motor cortex of the right side causes paralysis on the left side of the body (hemiplegia). Systems other than the upper and lower motor neuron systems are concerned with voluntary movement, but lower motor neurons form the common final pathway for stimuli for voluntary movement.

Some of the neurotransmitters that will be

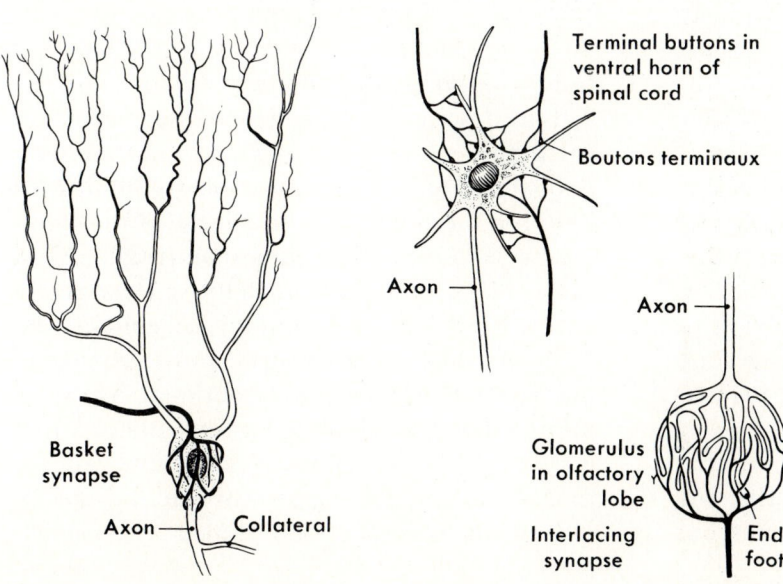

FIG. 8-4. Some types of synapses. (Reprinted with permission of Macmillan Publishing Co., Inc. from The human body, ed. 2, by S. Grollman. Copyright © 1969 by Sigmund Grollman.)

discussed are acetylcholine, the catecholamines (dopamine, norepinephrine, and epinephrine), serotonin, and neuroactive peptides (enkephalins and endorphins).

Acetylcholine

Acetylcholine is the best known chemical transmitter of nerve impulses. Not all parts of the central nervous system contain acetylcholine. Those areas that have high concentrations are the motor cortex, thalamus, hypothalamus, geniculate bodies, and anterior spinal roots; very low concentrations are found in the cerebellum, optic nerves, and dorsal roots of the spine. Acetylcholine can cause cardiac inhibition, vasodilation, gastrointestinal peristalsis, and other parasympathetic effects.

Lower motor neurons release acetylcholine at the neuromuscular junction, causing contraction in striated (voluntary) muscle. The concentration of acetylcholine must be high since a large number of muscle fibers must respond synchronously for striated muscle contraction to occur, and also because acetylcholine is very rapidly destroyed by the enzyme cholinesterase. In all likelihood this constitutes a protective mechanism for the body and prevents a person from being a constantly quivering organism.

Catecholamines and related substances

Catecholamines (dopamine, norepinephrine, and epinephrine) and the amine serotonin (5-hydroxytryptamine) are synthesized, stored, and metabolized in the brain. These substances do not easily penetrate the blood-brain barrier, but their precursors do. The effect of injected catecholamines on the central nervous system is slight in comparison to the effect on the autonomic nervous system. However, an increase in catecholamines and serotonin causes cerebral stimulation. Drugs, such as reserpine, that release catecholamines and reduce amine concentration in the brain have a depressing or sedative action. Methyldopa lowers the serotonin and norepinephrine levels and this, too, has a cerebral depressing effect.

Special staining techniques indicate that there are adrenergic (sympathomimetic) and serotoninergic tracts within the central nervous system. Dopamine, a catecholamine, is especially concentrated in the basal ganglia. The low level of dopamine at this site in individuals suffering from Parkinson's disease led to the new therapeutic approach of utilizing its precursor L-dopa with good results in many cases.

Neuroactive peptides

Neuroactive peptides may be considered neuromodulators, neurohormones, or neurotransmitters. Studies indicate that a peptide may affect neuronal activity by increasing or decreasing the synthesis, release, or breakdown of neurotransmitters, neurohormones, or neuromodulators. Basically, little is known of the catabolism, conservation, storage, or synthesis of the neuroactive peptides. Our knowledge is only beginning to uncover the neuroreceptor mechanisms of these substances.

The parenteral or intracerebral injection of these components causes potent behavioral effects. A number of these peptides exist in tissues other than the central nervous system, primarily in the gastrointestinal tract cells (myenteric plexus). Studies are being done to provide more information about the functions, sites of activity, and mechanisms of action of these peptides. A continual search to find additional neuroactive peptides and other substances having a role in neurotransmission is in progress.

Enkephalins and endorphins (peptides with endogenous opioid activity)

These endogenous pentapeptides have actions similar to the opiate alkaloids. The two isolated pentapeptides from the brain are methionine-enkephalin and leucine-enkephalin. Axon terminals releasing the enkephalins are found in the substantia gelatinosa of the spinal cord and in the thalamus and amygdala. These brain and spinal cord structures serve in the pathway for pain perception. Enkephalins behave as inhibitory neurotransmitters, decreasing the perception and emotional aspect of pain. Studies indicated that enkephalins may bind to the same neuroreceptor membranes as morphine, and the concept of internal opiates or natural pain killers developed. The enkephalins allow modification and control of the perception of pain.

Endorphins (from "endogenous morphine") is a general term that includes many peptides in the brain that suppress pain. These peptides are also found in the pituitary gland, intermediate lobe, and the corticotroph cells of the adenohypophysis. The discovery of the two opioid pentapeptides was less astounding than the fact that the complete structure of methionine-enkephalin is found within the pituitary hormone beta-lipoprotein. The first five amino acids of beta-endorphin (or "C" fragment with 31 amino acids) correspond to the pentapeptide methionine-enkephalin. Beta-endorphin's amino acid sequence is identical to a portion of the beta-lipoprotein, which is a peptide hormone from the pituitary gland.

Three endorphin peptides have been isolated and identified as alpha, gamma, and beta endorphin. Controversy exists over their exact roles as peptides or precursors. Technology has shown that the brain, pituitary gland, and gastrointestinal tract each have enkephalins and beta-endorphin. These peptides are not found in the same cells. Further, the brain cells containing beta-endorphin are different from those that contain enkephalins. The neurons containing beta-endorphin are in the basomedial and basolateral hypothalamus, with processes distributed to the anterior hypothalamic area, the septum, and the pons. The enkephalins are found in the globus pallidus, hippocampus, or spinal cord. Studies show that enkephalins and beta-endorphin influence naloxone-sensitive receptors in the central nervous system. The endorphins may be also responsible for the analgesic effect of the placebo.

Substance P

Isolated in 1931 from the brain and intestine, Substance P was found to be an undecapeptide (peptide containing 11 amino acids). Endorphins may act by suppressing the release in the spinal cord of a protein—Substance P—that apparently is involved in nerve impulse propagation by sensory nerves into the spinal cord and relayed to the brain. Substance P is found widely in the central and autonomic nervous system, with concentrations in the dorsal root (the nerve tract composed of nerve fibers with incoming sensory information from the body periphery to the spinal cord), in the myenteric plexus, and in the intestinal lining. The spinal cord dorsal horn has small-diameter pain fibers that contain the Substance P, as do tooth pulp pain fibers. Substance P has been proposed as the transmitter for primary afferent sensory fibers. In human neurologic disease, such as Huntington's chorea (degenerative disease characteristic of having profound movement disorders, progressive mental deterioration, and psychologic changes), Substance P levels in the brain's substantia nigra are reduced considerably, and there is loss of neurons with GABA neurotransmitter. Substance P is localized in the neurons, is released from neurons, and has an excitatory action on neurons.

Substance P was named because it was present in the dried acetone powder extract of brain and intestine. It is ironic that it is also a transmitter of pain impulses, by its presence in nerve fibers that carry pain signals. The possibility of Substance P being not a neurotransmitter but a neuromodulator (a chemical altering nerve responsiveness to neurotransmitters but that does not itself carry nerve signals) is also under investigation. A met⁵-enkephalin (a synthetic analog or endorphin) blocks the release of Substance P, and the effect of this synthetic enkephalin was blocked by naloxone. Further research suggests speculation that Substance P stimulates dopamine release, and overproduction of dopamine has implications in schizophrenia. In the autonomic nervous system it appears that Substance P may transmit sensory information from the periphery to the gut.

Somatostatin (somatotropin-releasing inhibiting factor)

Somatostatin is a tetradecapeptide (peptide containing 14 amino acids) secreted by the hypothalamus that has been demonstrated to stop the somatotropin production of the acidophils of the anterior pituitary gland. Somatostatin is widely distributed in the gastrointestinal tract and the delta cells of the pancreatic islets. Somatostatin appears to suppress the release of insulin and glucagon. In the diabetic individual, who is exogenous insulin dependent, the glucagon suppression is a determinant in daily insulin requirements. There is some evidence that somatostatin may share a similar pharmacologic profile with phenytoin, an anticonvulsant.

Dynorphin

Dynorphin (from the Greek for "power"), a brain peptide, was discovered in the posterior part of the pituitary gland. The first five amino acids of this peptide are identical to leucine-enkephalin, in the same manner as the first five amino acids of beta-endorphin are identical to methionine-enkephalin. Dynorphin is about 700 times more potent than leucine-enkephalin; in addition, the first 13 amino acids of dynorphin are about as potent as the whole molecule. So far this is the most potent pain-relieving substance discovered; dynorphin is 50 times more potent than beta-endorphin and 200 times more potent than morphine. From peptide research may come pain relievers with fewer side effects and minimal to no addiction potential, and we may also gain increased understanding of mental disorders and addiction mechanisms.

Neurobiologists are only now beginning to understand what these and other yet to be discovered peptides are doing in the brain and spinal cord. Only basic research will provide the answers to the peptide cascade and a understanding of the functions in the nervous system.

Central nervous system depressants

Mild drug-induced depression of the central nervous system is frequently characterized by lack of interest in surroundings, inability to focus attention on a subject, and lack of inclination to move or talk. The pulse and respiration may become slower than usual, and as the depression deepens, acuity of all sensations such as touch, vision, hearing, heat, cold, and pain diminish progressively. Psychic and motor activities decrease; reflexes become sluggish and finally are abolished. If the depression is not checked, it progresses to unconsciousness, stupor, coma, respiratory failure, and death. Some depressant drugs, such as the general anesthetics, act on the entire central nervous system; others, such as the anticonvulsant drugs, are more selective in their action. The depressants include the following: (1) analgesics, drugs that relieve pain; (2) hypnotics and sedatives, which produce sleep and rest; and (3) general anesthetics, which produce loss of sensation and unconsciousness (see Chapter 9).

Drugs used for relief of pain

Analgesics are drugs that relieve pain without producing loss of consciousness and reflex activity. Physical pain is a part of a larger experience called "pain experience," which includes, in addition to the sensation of pain, all the associated emotional sensations for a particular person under particular circumstances. This accounts for the wide variation in individual response to the sensation of pain. It is known that stimuli causing pain must be more intense than those evoking other sensations. Many times there is a link between pain and tissue damage.

In providing care to the patient, the nurse should assess the character of the pain the patient is undergoing from the causative disorder. The nurse's evaluation of the pain should include the location of pain, the onset of the pain symptoms, the factors leading to the pain, and the quality and duration of this pain symptom. This is accomplished through the nurse's interview with the patient or family. There are basically three types of pain: superficial (from skin or mucous membranes), visceral, (from the smooth musculature or organ systems, a deeper pain sensation with waxing and waning), and somatic (from skeletal muscles, facies, ligaments, vessels, or joints). The superficial and visceral pain may be relieved by narcotic-related analgesics, and the somatic pain may respond to nonnarcotic analgesics.

Pain perception and response are influenced by such psychologic factors as past experience, attention, and emotion. In addition, the intensity, duration, and location of harmful stimuli also influence pain perception and response.

Pain that increases rapidly in intensity (such as that accompanying acute myocardial infarction or extensive partial thickness burns) does not usually permit the individual to achieve any control over pain. Pain that is less severe with a slow rise in intensity permits the individual to exert some control over it. The latter may be achieved by the person thinking about something else or engaging in activity that diverts his attention.

There appears to be a relatively constant pain threshold for each individual. Although the pain threshold varies from individual to individual, tolerance to pain appears to be far more variable than pain threshold. For example, certain stimuli, such as heat applied to the skin at an intensity of 45° to 48° C, will initiate the sensation of pain in almost all individuals. Pain threshold is the minimum intensity of a harmful stimulus that produces the sensation of pain, while tolerance to pain refers to the point beyond which the pain can no longer be endured. There is evidence that some sensitization or adaptation to pain occurs, that is, there is a diminution of response with constant stimulation.

Action. Analgesics act in several ways: (1) by elevating the pain threshold, (2) by altering the attitude or mood of the patient from one of concern to one of detachment, promoting a sense of well-being or mild euphoria, and (3) by producing sedative and soporific effects.

Opium and its derivatives, related synthetic compounds, and the analgesic antipyretics, such as aspirin and phenacetin, belong to the analgesic group of drugs.

The search for an ideal analgesic continues, but it is difficult to find one that does all desired of it. It should (1) be potent, so that it will afford maximum relief of pain; (2) not cause dependence; (3) exhibit a minimum of side effects, such as constipation, respiratory depression, nausea, and vomiting; (4) not cause tolerance to develop; (5) act promptly and over a long period of time with a minimum amount of sedation, so that the patient is able to remain awake and be responsive; and (6) be relatively inexpensive. Needless to say, no present-day analgesic has all of these qualifications, and so the search continues.

NARCOTIC ANALGESICS—OPIATES

Opium is one of the oldest analgesics about which there is any record. Opium is described in Chinese literature written long before the time of Christ. The name comes from the Greek *opos*, meaning "juice of plants."

Opium is the hardened dried juice of the unripe seed capsules of *Papaver somniferum*, a species of poppy grown largely in China, India, Iran, Turkey, and Asia Minor. The poppy plant is indigenous to Asia Minor, and from there knowledge of opium spread to Greece and Arabia, where physicians became well versed in its use. Arabian traders were responsible for its introduction into the Orient, where it was known as "smoking dirt." The Chinese used it chiefly to control some of the symptoms of dysentery until its cultivation was exploited for commercial reasons by European powers, and the opium habit spread through many parts of the Orient.

Paracelsus is credited with compounding the preparation "laudanum." Paregoric was first used as an elixir for asthma and was prepared by a chemistry professor at Leyden. Thomas Dover, an English physician, used the powder as a sweating agent for gout in 1732.

Opium in the crude form was used until well into the nineteenth century, before the chief alkaloid, morphine, was isolated. The discovery of other alkaloids soon followed, and their use came to be preferred to that of the crude preparations.

Composition. The active principles of opium are alkaloids, of which there are some 20 in number, although only three are used widely in the practice of medicine—morphine, codeine, and papaverine.

The alkaloids of opium belong to two distinct classes. Morphine and codeine belong to the phenanthrene group, and papaverine is known as a benzylisoquinoline derivative. This helps to explain why papaverine has a much different effect in the body from other alkaloids. Papaverine has little effect on the nervous system but produces relaxation of certain smooth muscles in the body. (See Table 8-1.) Morphine and codeine act mainly on the central nervous system, where they produce a combination of depressing and stimulating effects. Both in-

T A B L E 8 - 1 **Selected effects of opiates**

	Morphine	Codeine	Dilaudid	Papaverine
Potency of analgesic action	Potent	One sixth to one tenth that of morphine	Ten times more potent than morphine	None
Effects				
Respiration	Markedly depressed Carbon dioxide retention	Depression one-fourth that of morphine	Like morphine	None or slight bronchial relaxation
Gastrointestinal	Decreased activity, spasm, and constipation	Like morphine but less prominent	Like morphine but less constipating	Relaxes
Biliary	Increased intrabiliary pressure Possibility of spasm	Less intense spasms than from morphine	Like codeine	Relaxes
Genitourinary				
Ureters	Possibility of spasms Increased tone, decreased motility	Increased tone, decreased motility	Like morphine	Relaxes
Bladder	Increased sphincter tone Retention of urine	Increased tone, decreased motility	Like morphine	Relaxes
Uterus	Tone increased Contractions decreased	Not significant	Like morphine	None
Eyes	Pupil constriction	Less than morphine	Like morphine	None
Cerebral	Stimulation of vomiting center—nausea and vomiting Depressed cough center Cortical sedation Rise in pain threshold Euphoria	Less than morphine Large doses required to produce euphoria	Less than morphine	None

crease smooth muscle tone and promote contraction of smooth muscle, especially muscle in organs of the gastrointestinal tract.

The alkaloids form 25% of the active constituents of opium; the rest are such substances as gums, oils, resins, and proteins.

Action and result of opium and morphine. The effects of opium result chiefly from the morphine that it contains; therefore, the two preparations will be considered together.

Of great research interest are recent discoveries that the brain contains peptides, such as endorphins and enkephalins, that act on the "opiate receptors" and mimic opiate effects. Many investigators believe that morphine and related compounds exert their remarkable effects because they act on the same receptors as the endogenous peptides.

Cerebrum. Morphine exerts a narcotic* action that results in analgesia and sleep. Morphine elevates the mood, causing euphoria in many patients, relieves fear, anxiety, and apprehension, and produces feelings of peace and tranquility. Its pronounced dependence liability is explained by its ability to cause a relatively intense euphoric state. Prolonged concentration becomes difficult, and the patient becomes apathetic, with a slowing of both mental and physical activities. The exact mode of action is still not known. The most outstanding effect of morphine is relief of pain. This is highly specific because pain may be effectively relieved without affecting other sensations appreciably. Continuous dull pain is more effectively relieved than sharp intermittent pain. It is especially effective for visceral pain,

---

*The word *"narcotic"* can be confusing because it is used in at least three different ways: (1) a central nervous system depressant, (2) a dependence-producing drug, and (3) a drug that may be neither of these but that may come under the restrictions of the federal narcotic law (Controlled Substances Act). In this chapter the term *"narcotic"* will be used to mean a depressant of the central nervous system with dependence-producing properties.

although when used in large enough doses it will abolish almost all forms of pain.

Morphine continues to be the most valuable analgesic in medicine, and ordinarily a nurse does not need to fear morphine dependence in a patient who is receiving the drug over a short period for severe pain.

In small doses morphine seems to have little or no effect on the motor areas of the brain. The diminished restlessness is probably caused by the drowsiness and sleep that is produced.

Brainstem and hypothalamus. Morphine has a highly selective action on the respiratory center. Doses that have little or no effect on other parts of the brain will depress respiration, causing a decrease in rate and minute volume, retention of carbon dioxide, and decreased sensitivity to carbon dioxide's stimulating effects. Toxic doses cause slow shallow respiration. Death from poisoning is caused by respiratory failure. Therapeutic doses of morphine and related alkaloids have little or no effect on the medullary centers concerned with blood pressure, heart rate, or rhythm.

Morphine acts as a miotic—it constricts the pupil of the eye. The exact mechanism or site of action is not clear, although there seems to be agreement that the action is central with an effect on the oculomotor nerve, since instillation of morphine in the eye does not cause miosis. Tolerance to this effect of morphine does not develop. In poisoning, pupils become pinpoint in size. It is believed that this is caused at least partly by increased sensitivity of the pupil to light, although pupil constriction occurs even in darkness.

After administration of morphine the cough center is depressed and coughing is relieved. Morphine and related compounds will abolish the cough reflex, but codeine is the drug of choice for this effect since it is less likely to cause respiratory depression and dependence.

The heat-regulating center is slightly depressed after therapeutic doses of morphine. Reduction of body temperature may be caused in part by this effect, but it is also caused by increased perspiration, decreased physical activity, and increased loss of heat because of peripheral vasodilation.

Nausea and vomiting may occur after administration of morphine and related alkaloids. This is thought to be caused by stimulation of a chemoreceptor emetic trigger zone in the medulla. Patients who remain in a recumbent position have nausea and vomiting less often than patients who are ambulatory.

Spinal cord. There is evidence that in laboratory animals morphine may stimulate the spinal cord to the extent that convulsive seizures result. In humans the action of morphine on the spinal cord is complex. There is some spinal stimulation, but the depressant action of morphine on higher centers prevents a convulsive reaction at the cord level. Morphine may also exert an indirect suppression of spinal reflexes.

Cardiovascular system. Hypotension and bradycardia occur. Toxic amounts of morphine or related alkaloids are required to produce significant changes in heart rate and blood pressure. With large doses of morphine, the T wave of the electrocardiogram may be depressed or inverted, which may interfere with electrocardiographic interpretations of patients with suspected myocardial infarctions. This is important to remember since these patients often receive large doses of morphine to reduce chest pain, anxiety, and restlessness. Morphine reduces the left ventricular work load, and this is a beneficial hemodynamic effect in the pain of myocardial infarction.

Changes that occur after therapeutic doses are believed to be the result of decreased physical activity and sleep. Toxic amounts will stimulate the vagal center and depress the vasomotor center, causing a lowering of blood pressure and a slowing of the heart rate. Diminished oxygen to the brain greatly contributes to the hypotension that develops in morphine intoxication. Therapeutic doses of morphine will produce relaxation of small blood vessels in the face, neck, and upper chest, making the patient feel flushed and warm. Sweating is common. Itching of the nose is frequently observed and is thought to be caused by histamine release. It indicates an allergic reaction and need for a different drug.

Gastrointestinal tract (smooth muscle and glands). Many of the effects of morphine on the gastrointestinal tract are probably the result of morphine's preventing the release of mediators from nerves innervating the smooth muscle of the gastrointestinal tract.

In general, glandular activity throughout the length of the alimentary tract is diminished. Gastric, biliary, and pancreatic secretions are decreased, and the digestion of food in the small intestine is hindered. The tone of smooth muscle in the sphincters is increased, and this delays the emptying of the stomach and small intestine. Although the nonpropulsive type of rhythmic contractions in the intestine are increased, propulsive peristalsis is decreased and a type of spasm has frequently been observed. The tendency to increased tone (biliary tract spasm) extends also to the biliary ducts and the sphincter of Oddi. The defecation reflex is depressed as a result of diminished sensitivity of the bowel and rectum and increased tone and spasticity of the muscle of the large bowel.

Many of the actions mentioned explain why patients receiving opiates, and especially morphine, are prone to develop gas pains, constipation, and sometimes abdominal distention. The stomach empties more slowly, peristalsis fails to keep the intestinal contents moving, water continues to be absorbed from the intestinal content, and the feces gradually become hardened. When the rectum does fill, there is little or no inclination to empty it. Decreased peristaltic activity may give rise to local accumulation of gas, which causes a painful stretching of the intestine. These effects are observed particularly in the postoperative patient who has had not only several doses of morphine but also an anesthetic and one or more doses of a sedative.

The effect of morphine on the smooth muscle of the gastrointestinal organs also explains why morphine does not always alleviate the pain and distress in these organs when, for some reason, the muscle already has become hypertonic. The presence of a stone in the common bile duct may cause the muscle of the duct to contract painfully, and this may be intensified rather than relieved by the effect of morphine, unless the dose of morphine is large enough to make the analgesic effect more pronounced than the effect on the smooth muscle.

These effects also help to explain the kind of diet that should be given to a patient who has had morphine. It is obvious that the patient is not likely to have either the inclination or ability to enjoy or digest a full meal. Tolerance to the effects of morphine on the gastrointestinal muscle develops slowly if at all.

The papaverine group of alkaloids differs in their effect on the muscle of the gastrointestinal tract in that they produce relaxation.

Genitourinary tract. The tone of the muscle in the ureters and the detrusor muscle of the urinary bladder is said to be affected much the same as the tone of the muscle in the gastrointestinal organs. Increased tone in the sphincter muscle of the bladder may contribute to difficulty in urination. In addition there is decreased perception of the stimulus to void. This sometimes explains a patient's inability to void and the need for catheterization. Morphine also stimulates the release of antidiuretic hormone and therefore has an antidiuretic effect. This is an important factor to keep in mind when checking the patient's urinary output.

Other smooth muscle. Morphine promotes contraction of the bronchial musculature, but this effect is significant only in persons subject to allergic reactions and asthma. Allergic reactions to morphine and related alkaloids are said to be rather common. Morphine may release histamine.

Although there seems to be no direct action of morphine on uterine muscle, normal labor may be delayed because of central depression, and the respiration of both the mother and the child will be depressed.

Therapeutic uses and the natural alkaloids. Morphine is used primarily as an analgesic for control of severe pain. It should not be used if other analgesics will suffice, but when pain is severe, the narcotic analgesics have no rival. When morphine is given to a patient who is already in severe pain, the chief effect seems to be that the patient's emotional reaction to the pain is altered. He is no longer afraid of the pain or thrown into a panic because of it. If the nurse asks such a patient about his condition half an hour or so after he has been given a hypodermic of morphine, he is likely to say: "I still have pain, but I can stand it."

If morphine is given before the patient begins to experience pain, its effect seems to be somewhat different; a better blocking of the pain impulses occurs and the patient may experience no pain. This explains why, on the first or possibly the second postoperative day, a patient should not be allowed to wait until he is in full pain if the greatest analgesic effect of morphine is to be achieved.

In surgical conditions in which the alleviation of severe pain may make diagnosis more difficult and lead to undue delay in operating, morphine should not be used or it should be employed only in very small doses and with great caution. It should not be used in chronic conditions in which there is pain, since prolonged administration is almost certain to result in dependence. Exceptions to this rule are to be found in cases of inoperable cancer in which the patient cannot recover and may be spared much unnecessary suffering by its use. The administration of a drug such as chlorpromazine or promethazine can be used to potentiate the action of morphine and reduce the amount of morphine needed. Morphine is not recommended for the relief of pain in persons of neurotic or hysteric temperaments unless its use is absolutely necessary.

Ordinarily, morphine or related alkaloids are not given to produce sleep unless sleeplessness is caused by pain or dyspnea. There are conditions in which the relief of restlessness and apprehension is essential, such as the patient suffering from a myocardial infarction.

Morphine is used to check peristalsis in conditions such as hemorrhage and severe diarrhea and after surgery on the stomach and bowel. Preparations of opium are prescribed more often than morphine to check diarrhea because of opium's slow absorption and effect on smooth muscle.

Morphine is frequently used as premedication prior to the administration of a general anesthetic to relieve apprehension and facilitate induction.

Codeine is the opiate of choice in relieving a cough because it effectively depresses the cough center and is less likely to produce dependence than morphine.

Tolerance. Different individuals require varying periods of time before the repeated administration of opium derivatives fails to have the effect that it originally produced. This condition is known as tolerance. A patient who suffers considerable pain may be relieved at first by 15 mg (gr ¼) of morphine, but if the painful condition persists, the time will come when he requires an ever-increasing dose to experience the same relief. The person who has developed tolerance may eventually take doses that would have caused death if given as an initial dose. Tolerance does not develop uniformly—tolerance is developed to the hypnotic, analgesic, and respiratory depressant effects of opiates but not to their effects on the pupil of the eye and on the gastrointestinal muscle. Tolerance develops faster when the dosage is administered regularly and is large and may occur after 2 weeks of repeated administration. The exact mechanism of action whereby tolerance develops is not known.

Side effects. Side effects may include one or more of the following.

Nausea and vomiting may be caused by pronounced stimulating effects on the vomiting center. These effects may be counteracted by some phenothiazine derivatives, but these drugs should not be given in the presence of hypotension, since they will augment it.

Constipation may outlast the analgesic effect. Laxatives, stool softeners, and enemas are frequently required. *Urinary retention* may require catheterization.

Postural hypotension with dizziness and faintness may occur. These patients should be instructed to arise or change positions slowly to allow compensatory mechanisms to become effective. These symptoms may not occur if the patient remains recumbent.

Depression of respiration and coughing tends to result in retained secretions and predisposition to atelectasis. Coughing and deep breathing should be encouraged in these patients. Mechanical assistance with intermittent positive pressure breathing (IPPB) may be necessary to promote adequate respiratory excursions.

Behavioral changes, such as increased restlessness and excitement, tremors, delirium, and insomnia, may occur. These usually require use of a different analgesic.

Allergic reactions, which include histamine release, urticaria, skin rash, itching (itching of the nose is common), or activation of other allergic phenomena such as asthma, may occur in the allergic individual. In these cases the drug should be discontinued and another analgesic substituted.

Contraindications. Because of its depressant effect on respiration, its tendency to increase intracranial pressure, to make the patient less responsive, and to cause miosis (masked diagnostic sign of pupil dilation or increased intracranial pressure), morphine is contraindicated or used cautiously for patients with head injuries, and for patients who have had a craniotomy performed. Other persons for whom it may not be indicated are those with bronchial asthma (decrease in ciliary activity and cough reflex and increased bronchomotor tone), hypertrophy of the prostate gland, or stricture of the urethra (because of the effect on smooth muscle). Morphine is also contraindicated in acute alcoholism and in convulsive disorders, and it must be used with caution for patients with inadequate oxygen–carbon dioxide exchange.

Acute poisoning. Poisoning with opium or a morphine is discussed in Chapter 12.

Opium

The following are the preparations of whole opium drugs.

Opium tincture, deodorized (laudanum). The usual dose is 0.6 ml (1.5 ml is equivalent to 6 to 15 mg of morphine). It is used to check intestinal peristalsis. It contains approximately 10 mg of morphine per milliliter in 18% alcohol.

Paregoric; camphorated opium tincture. The usual adult dose is 5 ml and range of dosage 5 to 10 ml (in children 0.25 to 0.5 ml/kg). This is a solution of opium together with benzoic acid, camphor, oil of anise, glycerin, and diluted alcohol. Paregoric is given to check intestinal peristalsis to relieve diarrhea. It contains approximately 0.4 mg of morphine per milliliter (2 mg/5 ml). It has a very bitter taste and an anise odor. It must be stored in light-resistant, air-tight containers away from heat.

The foregoing preparations of whole opium

must be given by mouth and are not suited to parenteral injection. This is partly because the two tinctures contain alcohol and because preparations of whole opium contain resins and other substances that are not readily soluble in water and tissue fluids.

Opium and belladonna suppositories. These are no longer official preparations, but they continue to be prescribed for the analgesic action of opium and the antispasmodic effect of belladonna. Some physicians prescribe them for relief of painful hemorrhoids and for patients who have had a transurethral resection. The usual dose is one suppository inserted rectally every 3 to 4 hours. Each suppository contains 30 or 65 mg (gr ½ or 1) of opium and 15 mg (gr ¼) of belladonna in a suitable base.

Morphine

Morphine sulfate. Morphine sulfate is available as tablets, capsules, an oral solution (10 mg/5 ml), and a solution for injection in vials or ampules. The injection form may also contain atropine or scopolamine. The usual dose is 10 mg (gr ⅙); the range of dosage is 5 to 20 mg (gr ¹⁄₁₂ to ¼) every 4 hours.

Morphine hydrochloride. The usual dose is 15 mg (gr ¼); the range of dosage is 8 to 20 mg (gr ⅛ to ⅓). However, investigators are of the opinion that 10 mg (gr ⅙) 70 kg of body weight comes closer to being an optimal dose for both morphine sulfate and morphine hydrochloride. Larger doses may be needed sometimes, but they are associated with a higher incidence of untoward effects. The action and uses of these two salts are the same.

Morphine is readily absorbed after subcutaneous or intramuscular injection; more than half the drug is absorbed within 30 minutes after injection. Onset of action occurs within 10 to 30 minutes, a euphoric action (pleasant drowsiness, freedom from anxiety and fear) occurs within 30 minutes, and peak action (rise in pain threshold) or maximum analgesic action occurs in 60 to 90 minutes. Actual increase in the pain threshold may last only a few hours, but the decreased subjective emotional reaction to pain may permit the patient to endure the pain for 4 to 6 hours or more. This depends on the patient's reaction to the drug, dosage given, and severity of pain. About 90% of the drug is excreted in the urine within 24 hours. The drug is inactivated by the liver. The oral route is not preferred because of the significant hepatic first-pass effect, which limits systemic absorption; morphine undergoes enterohepatic recirculation (biliary recycling).

Morphine may be given orally, and onset of action then occurs in 10 to 15 minutes. Since absorption from the gastrointestinal tract is highly variable, this route is less dependable for therapeutic effectiveness and is seldom used.

Morphine may be given intravenously (2.5 to 15 mg); peak action occurs in 5 minutes. The drug must be administered slowly and diluted to 4 or 5 ml with sterile water for injection to avoid severe reactions in patients with hypersensitivity to morphine.

Dosage for children is 0.1 to 0.2 mg/kg body weight given subcutaneously.

Morphine injection. This is a sterile solution of a suitable salt of morphine in water for injection. The oral to parenteral analgesic efficacy ratio is 6:1.

Codeine

Codeine phosphate injection; codeine phosphate tablets. The usual dose is 30 mg (gr ½); the range of dosage is 15 to 60 mg (gr ¼ to 1) every 4 hours. After subcutaneous injection peak effect is reached in 30 to 60 minutes; duration of effect is 3 to 4 hours. Codeine is a natural alkaloid of opium, but it is made from morphine. Codeine sulfate is like the phosphate except that it is less soluble in water. Codeine is about one sixth as potent an analgesic as morphine. It is also less constipating (although it does cause constipation) and less depressing to respiration. Codeine is less habit-forming than morphine, although drug dependence does occur. It is a preparation of choice in cough mixtures for the treatment of a dry, unproductive cough. As an antitussive the dose is 10 to 20 mg every 4 to 6 hours, not to exceed 120 mg/24 hours. Doses beyond 60 mg are thought to be inadvisable because if effect is not secured with 60 mg it will not be accomplished wth a higher dosage. Large doses of codeine tend to stimulate the brainstem. Codeine has a greater tendency to excite nerve centers than morphine.

Codeine is well absorbed from the gastrointestinal tract and metabolized primarily in the liver. The drug is excreted mainly in the urine as an inactive metabolite, norcodeine, and free and conjugated morphine. While the kidneys excrete the major portion of codeine, a small amount of the drug appears in the feces. Codeine may be removed by peritoneal dialysis and hemodialysis. Codeine does pass the blood-brain barrier and also may be found in the milk of nursing mothers. From a total oral dose of 60 mg the mean time of initial detection in the plasma is 15 minutes, the mean peak plasma level is 164.6 µg/ml, the mean time of peak plasma level is 66 minutes, and the mean elimination from plasma (half-life) is about 3 hours.

The central nervous system effects of codeine may be additive with those of other CNS depressants, such as other narcotic analgesics, antihistamines, general anesthetics, phenothiazines, other tranquilizers, sedative-hypnotics, and alcohol. If combined therapy is essential, the dose of one or both should be reduced to overcome these effects. It is recommended for relief of moderate to moderately severe pain and as an antitussive. Oral codeine is well absorbed from the gastrointestinal tract, and its approximate oral-to-parenteral analgesic efficacy ratio is 1:1.5, which is expressed more easily as 2:3.

Dosage for children for analgesia is 3 mg/kg body weight for a 24-hour period in six divided doses; for cough the antitussive dose is one third to one half that for analgesia (2.5 to 10 mg every 4 to 6 hours, not to exceed 60 mg/24 hours).

Codeine is available in a variety of forms as tablets or capsules, in solution for injection in vials and ampules, and in elixir and syrup form for coughs. Codeine is also prepared in combination with other drugs such as aspirin.

Terpin hydrate and codeine elixir. The usual dose is 5 ml, which contains 10 mg of codeine (gr ⅙) and contains 40% ethyl alcohol. This is used to relieve coughing.

Dihydrocodeinone bitartrate (Dicodid, Hycodan, Tussionex). This is similar in action to codeine sulfate (or phosphate) but more active and more likely to cause drug dependence. It is used to relieve cough. The dose is 5 to 15 mg (gr

$\frac{1}{12}$ to $\frac{1}{4}$). It is marketed in oral tablets and as liquid dosage forms.

Pantopon

Pantopon is an artificial mixture composed of the purified alkaloids of opium in the same proportion as they are found in opium but in about five times the concentration. It is free from gums, resins, and the like. Some think it is more valuable than opium itself; however, this is questionable. Pantopon has an advantage in that it can be injected and opium cannot. It is used for the same reasons as morphine (20 mg is equivalent to 15 mg morphine). Patients who are hypersensitive to morphine can sometimes tolerate pantopon satisfactorily. It may be administered intramuscularly or subcutaneously. The usual therapeutic dose is 5 to 20 mg intramuscularly or subcutaneously, available in in 20 mg/ml ampules.

Hydromorphone hydrochloride (Dilaudid)

Hydromorphone is prepared from morphine. The usual dose of hydromorphone is 2 mg (oral or parenteral), which is about five times as analgesic as morphine. It may be given orally, subcutaneously by slow intravenous injection or by suppository. The oral-to-parenteral analgesic efficacy ratio is about 1:1. The suppository allows for slower absorption and more prolonged effect, which is an advantage at bedtime because the duration of analgesic effect is shorter than that of morphine. Its analgesic effect is accompanied by minimal hypnotic effect, which is desirable when the drug is given to patients in whom it is important to relieve pain without producing a stupefying effect. It depresses respiration, but side actions such as euphoria, nausea, vomiting, and constipation seem to be less marked than with morphine. Both drug dependence and tolerance can occur. Hydromorphone is available in 1, 2, 3, and 4 mg/ml ampules; oral tablets containing 1, 2, 3, and 4 mg; and 3-mg suppositories.

SYNTHETIC NARCOTIC ANALGESICS

Mention has been made that morphine falls short of being an ideal analgesic, not because it is not sufficiently potent but because it depresses respiration, produces constipation, and may produce drug dependence. Consequently, there has been an almost continuous search for an analgesic with fewer of the disadvantages of morphine. Some newer agents have been found to exhibit some advantages over morphine. For a comparison of dosage and action time of various nonsynthetic and synthetic narcotic analgesics administered subcutaneously or intramuscularly, see Table 8-2.

Meperidine hydrochloride (Demerol Hydrochloride); pethidine hydrochloride

Meperidine hydrochloride is a synthetic substitute for morphine discovered by two German scientists who were searching for a substitute for atropine. It is a stable, white crystalline powder soluble in alcohol and very soluble in water.

Action and result. Meperidine depresses the central nervous system, probably at both the cortical and the subcortical levels. The mechanism of action is directed at the opiate receptors inhibiting ascending pain pathways. Its most outstanding effect is to produce analgesia. It is especially effective for visceral pain, although it also relieves pain in structures of the body wall. Its analgesic potency is said to be slightly greater than codeine and lasts 2 to 4 hours, depending on the dosage. The onset of action occurs in 15 minutes, and peak action occurs in 1 hour. It is about one eighth to one tenth as analgesic as morphine; hence, severe pain is not well controlled by meperidine. Euphoria is produced in some patients and lasts for an hour or so. Compared to morphine it is less likely to cause sleep and sedation unless large doses are given. There is little depression of the respiratory center with the usual therapeutic doses; however, toxic doses can produce marked depression. Compared to morphine, it is less likely to cause nausea and vomiting and it does not produce pupillary constriction or depress the cough center.

Meperidine in therapeutic doses has little or no effect on the cardiovascular system, particularly if the patient is in a recumbent position. When meperidine is given to patients who are up and about or is given by rapid intravenous

T A B L E   8 - 2   **Comparison of narcotic analgesics for subcutaneous or intramuscular administration**

Generic name	Trade name	Average adult dose (mg)	Usual range of single dose (mg)	Onset of action (minutes)	Peak action (hours)	Duration of action (hours)
Nonsynthetic narcotic analgesics						
Morphine	—	10 (gr ⅙)	5 to 15 (gr 1/12 to ¼)	5 to 10	1	4 to 6
Codeine	—	30 (gr ½)	15 to 60 (gr ¼ to 1)	15 to 30	½ to 1½	4 to 6
Hydromorphone	Dilaudid	2	1 to 4	15 to 30	½ to 1½	3 to 5
Pantopium	Pantopon	20 (gr ⅓)	5 to 20 (gr 1/12 to ⅓)	5 to 10	1	3 to 4
Synthetic narcotic analgesics						
Meperidine	Demerol Pethidine	50 to 100	50 to 150	10 to 15	½ to 1	2 to 4
Methadone	Dolophine	7.5	2.5 to 20	10	1 to 2	4 to 6
Levorphanol	Levo-Dromoran	2 to 3	1 to 3	15 to 45	1 to 1½	2 to 5

injection, postural hypotension and fainting may result. Like morphine it is prone to cause an elevation of intracranial pressure and must be used cautiously in patients with head injuries or conditions in which there is an elevation of cerebrospinal pressure.

Meperidine was formerly thought to be a useful agent to relieve the spasm of smooth muscle, but it has been found that it resembles morphine in some of its effects on smooth muscle; it has been found to promote spasm of muscle (spasmogenic) in the biliary tract. It exerts a rather weak antispasmodic effect on the bronchial musculature and can more safely be used than morphine for the asthmatic patient who needs an analgesic. The tendency to produce spasm in the smooth muscle of the gastrointestinal tract is said to be somewhere between that of morphine and codeine. It is rather mildly spasmogenic and does not produce constipation; therefore, it is of no value in the therapy of severe diarrhea. It has more effect on the small intestine than on the colon. The emptying of the stomach is somewhat retarded.

Uses. Meperidine is used primarily as a substitute for morphine to produce analgesia. When so used it has the advantage of producing much less sedation and constipation. However, it does not take the place of morphine for the relief of severe pain. It is quick acting and short acting. It is suited to the management of intermittent pain such as renal colic.

Meperidine is widely used as a preanesthetic agent and as a preoperative agent.

In obstetrics it may be combined with scopolamine, promethazine, or one of the short-acting barbiturates to produce obstetric amnesia. The dose of meperidine must be reduced proportionately (25% to 50%) when it is administered concomitantly with phenothiazines and other tranquilizers, since they potentiate the action of meperidine.

Preparation, dosage, and administration. Meperidine hydrochloride is available for oral use in 50- and 100-mg tablets and in ampules, vials, and disposable injection units for parenteral administration. The single oral or parenteral dose usually varies from 50 to 100 mg. For severe pain doses up to 150 mg may be given. The usual dosage for children is 6 mg/kg body weight for 24 hours, given in divided doses. It is also available as a syrup. Although meperidine can be given orally, it is more effective when given intramuscularly. The oral-to-parenteral efficacy ratio is 4:1. Occasionally it is given rectally, and it may be administered intravenously (slowly, diluted and reduced dosage). It may be given orally for relief of chronic pain. It is irritating to subcutaneous tissue. It is physically incompatible in solution with barbiturates.

Side effects and toxic effects. Side effects include dizziness, nausea and vomiting, dry mouth, sweating, headache, fainting, and drop in blood pressure. Toxic effects include dilated pupils, mental confusion, tremor, incoordination, convulsions, and respiratory depression. Death may result. Toxic effects are said to produce more physical impairment than that caused by other narcotic drugs.

Meperidine has a distinct capacity to produce drug dependence. Some physicians are of the opinion that dependence develops more rapidly than with morphine. Withdrawal symptoms develop more rapidly but are thought to be less severe. At one time tolerance was thought to develop more slowly than with morphine, but if pain is to be controlled, the drug must be given more often because of the short duration of action, and therefore tolerance develops more quickly. It is subject to provisions of the Controlled Substances Act.

Treatment of acute intoxication depends on severity of symptoms. If respiratory depression becomes severe it can be antagonized by the administration of nalorphine.

Contraindications. Meperidine is contraindicated in severe dysfunction of the liver (since the drug is inactivated in the liver), in certain conditions involving the gallbladder and the bile ducts (since meperidine causes contraction of these structures), and in cases in which there is increased intracranial pressure. Severe toxic reactions have occurred following use of meperidine in patients receiving monoamine oxidase inhibitors; hypotension, cyanosis, and respiratory depression occur.

Methadone hydrochloride (Dolophine)

Methadone was synthesized during World War II by German chemists. It occurs as a white crystalline substance that has a bitter taste; it is soluble in both alcohol and water.

Action and result. Methadone resembles morphine in a number of respects. It also depresses the central nervous system and acts as a potent analgesic, although it has a weaker sedative effect than morphine. Only in minimal doses does it cause less respiratory depression than morphine. Euphoria is less intense than that produced by morphine. the effects of methadone on smooth muscle are somewhat more variable than morphine, but on the whole the results are similar. Given parenterally it produces analgesia in 10 to 15 minutes; duration of action is 4 to 6 hours. Given orally analgesia occurs in 20 to 30 minutes. Cumulative effects are seen with repeated doses, and with long-term administration the half-life may extend up to 22 hours. The oral-to-parenteral analgesic efficacy ratio is 2:1.

Uses. Methadone is used primarily as an analgesic. The duration of its effect is about the same as for morphine. It is somewhat more satisfactory for the relief of chronic pain than morphine, but it is not as useful as a preanesthetic medication.

It is given to relieve cough because of its depressant effect on the cough center (antitussive effect).

Methadone can prevent or relieve acute withdrawal symptoms of morphine-like drugs and therefore it is used in the treatment of patients dependent on heroin or other morphine-like drugs. Methadone also produces withdrawal symptoms but dependence develops more slowly and the withdrawal symptoms are less severe than those associated with morphine or heroin. With addicts methadone is used as a substitute for the stronger narcotics. It is also widely used for withdrawal of persons who have been addicted to morphine or heroin (see Chapter 12).

Preparation, dosage, and administration. Methadone hydrochloride is available in 5- and 10-mg tablets, in oral solution containing 1 mg/ml, and in solutions dispensed in ampules or multiple-dose vials containing 10 mg/ml. The usual oral or parenteral dose is 2.5 to 10 mg every 3 or 4 hours as necessary; the range of dosage is 2.5 to 20 mg. It is more effective than morphine when given orally. It is also available in 2.5-, 5-, 10-, and 40-mg effervescent tablets for purposes of detoxification and maintenance treatment only.

Subcutaneous injections sometimes cause local irritation, in which case intramuscular injection is preferred. if it is given intravenously the patient should be in recumbent position.

Side effects and toxic effects. Methadone exhibits some of the same disadvantages as morphine. It causes nausea and vomiting, itching of the skin, constipation, light-headedness, and respiratory depression. Death results from respiratory failure.

TABLE 8-3 Selected effects of some synthetic narcotic analgesics

	Meperidine (Demerol)	Methadone	Levorphanol (Levo-Dromoran)
Analgesic potency	Between that of codeine (60 mg) and morphine (15 mg)	Like morphine	Four to eight times that of morphine Hypnotic effect similar to morphine
Action			
Onset	10 to 15 minutes	10 to 15 minutes	15 to 45 minutes (intramuscular)
Duration	2 to 4 hours (intramuscular)	4 to 6 hours	2 to 5 hours
Effects			
Respiratory	Mild depression Bronchodilation Sometimes bronchospasm	Depression—similar to morphine Bronchial constriction	Depression—like morphine Apnea caused by overdose
Gastrointestinal	Decreased motility Spasm No constipation effect	Increased tone Decreased motility Spasms—like morphine	Decreased motility Spasms Moderate constipation
Genitourinary			
Ureters	Decreased motility and tone	Spasms—like morphine	—
Bladder	Increased tone Retention uncommon	—	—
Kidney	Not significant Some decrease in urinary output	Antidiuretic action Reduced urinary output	Reduced urinary output
Uterus	Decreased tone and contractions	No relief of pain of labor or uterine contractions	Reduced motility
Eyes	No pupil change with therapeutic dose Blurred vision	Miosis with large dose	Miosis
Salivary glands	Moderate decrease in secretions Dryness of mouth	Stimulation Slight increase in secretions	—
Cerebral	Euphoria Mild depression Drowsiness Dizziness Giddiness	Not significant with therapeutic dose Cortical depression with large doses	—

Both tolerance and dependence occur following repeated doses of methadone. The same precautions need to be observed in the administration of methadone as for morphine. Nalorphine acts as an antagonist to methadone as it does for morphine and meperidine. The use and administration of methadone are subject to restrictions of the Controlled Substances Act.

Levorphanol tartrate (Levo-Dromoran Tartrate)

Levorphanol tartrate is a white, odorless crystalline powder. It has a bitter taste and is slightly soluble in water. It is a synthetic analgesic pharmacologically and chemically related to morphine.

Action and result. Its analgesic potency (intramuscular route) is four to eight times that of morphine but in smaller dosage. The analgesic effect is said to last somewhat longer than in the case of morphine (4 to 8 hours). Maximum analgesic effects are obtained 60 to 90 minutes after subcutaneous injection. In humans, 2 to 3 mg of levorphanol tartrate is said to relieve pain as effectively as 10 to 15 mg of morphine. It has less effect than morphine on the smooth muscle of the gastrointestinal tract. Tolerance develops slowly. (See Table 8-3.)

Uses. This drug is useful to relieve severe visceral pain, such as that associated with terminal carcinoma, renal and biliary colic, myocardial infarction, and gangrene. It is also used as a preanesthetic narcotic as well as for the relief of postoperative pain. It can be used for practically all the same conditions for which morphine is employed.

Preparation, dosage, and administration. Levorphanol tartrate is available in solution, dispensed in 1-ml ampules and 10-ml vials of solution containing 2 mg/ml. It is also available in scored 2-mg tablets for oral administration. Recommended average dose for adults is 2 to 3 mg. The initial dose should be as small as possible to delay the development of tolerance. This drug is usually given subcutaneously, but, unlike morphine, it is almost as effective after oral administration as when given subcutaneously. The oral to parenteral analgesic efficacy ratio is 2:1. This constitutes a possible advantage over morphine.

Side effects and toxic effects. The side effects are the same as those for morphine except for a lower incidence of constipation. As is true of most narcotics, dizziness and vomiting are observed more in ambulatory patients than in those who must remain in bed. The drug is capable of causing drug dependence and must be used with the same precautions that are observed in the use of other such drugs. It is subject to the restrictions of the Controlled Substances Act.

Oxycodone hydrochloride (Percodan, Tylox, Percocet)

Oxycodone is a derivative of morphine and related to codeine. It is five to six times more potent than codeine and also has a greater dependence potential than codeine, but it is less potent with less dependence potential than morphine. It is used as an analgesic for the treatment of moderate pain. Oxycodone has therapeutic side and toxic effects similar to the other narcotic analgesics. In the United States oxycodone is available only in combination with aspirin or acetaminophen. The usual oral dose is one tablet every 6 hours. The same precautions should be used when administering oxycodone as when giving other narcotics. Onset of action occurs in about 30 minutes and peak action in about 60 minutes, with duration of action lasting 3 to 6 hours.

Oxymorphone hydrochloride (Numorphan)

Oxymorphone is a semisynthetic narcotic with a pharmacologic action resembling that of morphine. It is a potent drug useful for treating severe pain. The dose of oxymorphone is about one tenth that of morphine. Oxymorphone is said to cause fewer untoward effects (constipation, nausea, and vomiting) than morphine. Precautions are necessary to prevent respirato-

TABLE 8-4 Comparison of analgesic (intramuscular or subcutaneous) dose of certain narcotic compounds to 10 mg morphine

Generic name	Trade name	Equivalent analgesic dose (mg)
Morphine		10
Codeine		120
Meperidine	Demerol	75-100
Methadone	Dolophine (and others)	7.5-10
Levorphanol	Levo-Dromoran	2-3
Hydromorphone	Dilaudid	1.5
Oxymorphone	Numorphan	1.0-1.5
Fentanyl	Sublimaze	0.1-0.2

ry depression and other toxic effects. It may be administered parenterally in 0.5- to 1.5-mg doses every 4 to 6 hours. Rectal suppositories are also available containing 5 mg of the drug (one tenth as potent rectally as by the intramuscular route). When given subcutaneously the drug acts in 5 to 10 minutes, peak action occurs in 10 to 20 minutes, and duration of action is 3 to 6 hours. Its margin of safety, dependence-producing potential, and duration of analgesic action are comparable to that of morphine.

NARCOTIC ANTAGONISTS

The term "agonist" means "to do" and the term "antagonist" means "to block." Opiates or drugs that act to relieve pain are agonists and opiates that block the effect of an agonist are the antagonists. In an opiate possessing both agonist and antagonist components, the antagonists portion acts to abate addiction and the agonist portion acts to relieve pain. Continuous contact with the receptor site causing addiction is essential for addiction.

Narcotic antagonists may be subdivided into three classifications based on receptor sites. None of these drugs has demonstrated a singular pure action and therefore the terms are relatively pure antagonists, mixed agonist-antagonists, and partial agonists of the morphine type. Three receptor sites are proposed to account for this effect: (1) mu receptors, which are identified with analgesic, euphoric, and other opiate-like effects, (2) kappa receptors, identified with sedative effects and miosis, and

T A B L E   8 - 5 **Comparison of narcotic agonist-antagonist analgesics with morphine and meperidine administered alone**

	Morphine	Meperidine	Nalbuphine	Butorphanol
Adult standard dose (range)				
Intramuscular	10 mg (5-20 mg)	60-80 mg (50-150 mg)	10 mg (10-20 mg)	2 mg (1-4 mg)
Intravenous	4-10 mg (2.5-15 mg)	100 mg (50-150 mg)	10 mg (10-20 mg)	1 mg (0.5-2 mg)
Subcutaneous	10 mg (5-20 mg)	100 mg* (50-100 mg)	10 mg (10-20 mg)	No recommendation
Onset of analgesia				
Intramuscular	<30 minutes	<30 minutes	<15 minutes	<30 minutes
Intravenous	Rapid	Rapid	2-3 minutes	Rapid
Subcutaneous	<30 minutes	<30 minutes	<15 minutes	Not used
Duration of analgesia	±4 hours	2-4 hours	3-6 hours	3-4 hours
Abuse potential	High	High	Low (with potential)	Low (with potential)
Effect of respiratory depression	High	High	Limited at higher doses†	Limited‡
Effect on cardiac work load	Lowered slightly	Lowered slightly	Lowered slightly	Increased
Indication for pain	Moderate to severe	Moderate to severe	Moderate to severe	Moderate to severe

*Suitable for occasional use.
†Nalbuphine at a dose of 10 mg/kg causes respiratory depression comparable to morphine, but higher dosages do not increase respiratory depression appreciably.
‡Butorphanol at a dose of 2 mg depresses respiration to a degree equal to 10 mg morphine. The magnitude of depression is not increased at 4 mg, but duration of depression is dose related.

(3) sigma receptors, identified with psychotomimetic effects.

Antagonists block the subjective and objective effects of the opiates and will precipitate withdrawal symptoms in patients receiving opiates or aggravate withdrawal symptoms in patients who have recently used opiates. Agonists produce opiate-like subjective and objective symptoms with a single dose. They can replace morphine or an opiate and suppress withdrawal symptoms in those patients discontinuing the opiate. They produce withdrawal symptoms of their own on abrupt discontinuation after long-term administration. The development of narcotic antagonists has provided drugs that may alleviate the effects of narcotic overdosage but also drugs that have potent analgesic properties. The two opposing properties described above are the narcotic agonist-antagonist. Table 8-5 compares some narcotic agonist-antagonist analgesics with morphine and meperidine.

Chemically the N-methyl group (like oxymorphine hydrochloride), an N-allyl (such as naloxone hydrochloride), or N-cyclopropylmethyl (such as nalbuphine hydrochloride) groups respectively exemplify the opiate agonist, antagonist, and mixed agonist-antagonist. Opiate antagonists bind to specific receptors without producing the biochemical changes associated with opiate narcotics. Naloxone, an opiate antagonist, does not relieve pain or cause euphoria but blocks the effects of other opiate-like narcotics. The medial section of the thalamus, which has high concentrations of opiate receptors, is concerned with deep, chronic, burning pain that is successfully relieved by opiate drugs. The discussion on central nervous system amine transmitters indicated their concentration in this same section of the hypothalamus.

Naloxone (Narcan)

Naloxone is a narcotic antagonist, a synthetic congener of oxymorphone where the methyl group in the nitrogen atom is replaced by an allyl group, thus creating an opiate antagonist from an opiate agonist. Naloxone antagonizes all actions of morphine. In the absence of narcotics or agonistic effects of other narcotic antagonists, naloxone demonstrates little activity, it is an essentially pure antagonist, and it does not possess the agonistic or morphine-like properties characteristic of other narcotic antagonists. Naloxone will produce withdrawal symptoms in a patient physically dependent on narcotics.

Uses. Naloxone is indicated for complete or partial reversal of narcotic depression and the respiratory depression induced by the natural and synthetic narcotics, propoxyphene and pentazocine. It may be used as a diagnostic agent in cases of suspected narcotic overdosage. An intravenous dose of 0.4 to 1.2 mg may be administered as a diagnostic test in patients presenting with apparent drug-induced coma.

Preparation, dosage, and administration. Naloxone may be administered by the intravenous, intramuscular, or subcutaneous routes. Onset occurs within 2 minutes after intravenous administration and slightly longer than 2 minutes after subcutaneous or intramuscular administration. Intramuscular administration has a more prolonged effect than intravenous administration. The need to repeat the dose (0.4 mg intravenously for two or three doses in 2- to 3-minute intervals) depends on the amount, type, and route of administration of the drug being antagonized. Failure of response may indicate nonopioid drugs or the presence of a disease process causing the depression.

In children in whom narcotic overdosage is known or suspected the initial dose is 0.01 mg/kg, which may be diluted with Sterile Water for Injection. For neonates with narcotic-induced depression the intial dose is also 0.01 mg/kg. Naloxone is available in ampule of 0.4 mg/ml and 1 ml, and there is also a neonatal strength of 0.02 mg/ml in 2-ml ampules.

Nursing implications. Nurses should observe patients carefully and administer naloxone cautiously if the patient is known or suspected to be physically dependent on opioids (narcotics, propoxyphene, or pentazocine), including newborns of dependent mothers, because abrupt and complete reversal of narcotic effects will produce an acute abstinence syndrome. Continued nursing observation is necessary for the patient who has responded to naloxone, and doses should be repeated as necessary, since the duration of action of some narcotics exceeds the duration of action of naloxone. The nurse should remember that naloxone

has no effect on respiratory depression caused by nonopiate drugs. Usage in pregnancy has not been established and it should be given only when the potential benefits outweigh the possible risks. Additional resuscitative measures should be available when necessary to counteract acute narcotic overdosage.

Levallorphan tartrate (Lorfan)

Levallorphan acts as a narcotic antagonist in the presence of narcotics and is similar to naloxone and chemically related to levorphanol. It relieves the respiratory depression caused by the action of narcotics but not the depression that may result from the action of anesthetics, barbiturates, nonnarcotic agents, or pathologic conditions. It is said to abolish respiratory depression without affecting the state of analgesia. When given alone (not in the presence of narcotics), however, it acts as a respiratory depressant and produces slight analgesia. If administered to a patient physically dependent on narcotics it will precipitate an acute abstinence syndrome. Levallorphan is indicated for the treatment of *significant* narcotic-induced respiratory depression and for parturient women to overcome narcotic-induced respiratory depression. It is available in injection form in 1 mg/ml concentrations, in 1-ml ampules, and 10-ml vials.

Preparation, dosage, and administration. To reverse respiratory depression from narcotic overdosage, 1 mg is given intravenously followed by one or two additional doses of 0.5 mg at 10- to 15-minute intervals. Maximum dose is 3 mg. Levallorphan is administered intravenously, as a rule, although it may be given subcutaneously and intramuscularly.

NARCOTIC AGONIST-ANTAGONISTS
Butorphanol tartrate (Stadol)

Butorphanol tartrate is a narcotic agonist-antagonist analgesic of the phenanthrene series (morphinan derivative). The indications are for relief of moderate to severe pain. Duration of analgesia is 3 to 4 hours, approximately that of morphine, onset time for analgesia is within 30 minutes for intramuscular administration and within 1 minute for intravenous administration, peak analgesia is 1 hour after the intramuscular administration and less than 30 minutes after the intravenous administration route. The narcotic antagonist activity is 30 times that of pentazocine and one fortieth that of naloxone. Because of this butorphanol should be considered capable of precipitating withdrawal symptoms in patients who have received narcotic analgesics for 10 days or longer or those physically dependent on narcotics (detoxification prior to butorphanol is required).

A dose of 2 mg depresses respiration equal to 10 mg of morphine but this is not increased in magnitude at 4-mg doses. The duration of respiratory depression is dose related and is reversible by naloxone, which is a specific antagonist. A lower dose is used in patients with respiratory depression, asthma, and obstructive pulmonary disease.

The cardiovascular effects are similar to those of pentazocine, but the nurse must remember that there may be an increase in pulmonary arterial pressure, pulmonary wedge pressure, and work load of the heart.

Butorphanol has been employed in relief of moderate to severe pain, postoperative pain, prepartum pain, and chronic pain of musculoskeletal origin. This drug can also be used for preoperative or preanesthetic medication and as a supplement to balanced anesthesia.

Preparation, dosage, and administration. Butorphanol is available in an injection of 1 mg/ml in 1-ml vials and 2 mg/ml in 1-, 2-, and 10-mg vials. It is not for use by the subcutaneous route.

Butorphanol is given to adults in dosages of 2 mg intramuscularly every 3 to 4 hours as necessary, with an effective dosage range of 1 to 4 mg every 3 to 4 hours depending on the severity of the pain; and 1 mg intravenously every 3 to 4 hours as necessary, with an effective dosage range of 0.5 to 2 mg every 3 to 4 hours. The dose is reduced when it is administered with phenothiazines, tranquilizers, or droperidol due to potentiation of butorphanol's action.

There is no clinical experience with butorphanol in children under 18; therefore it is not recommended for this age group.

Precautions. Special care is to be exercised when using this drug for emotionally unstable patients and for those with a history of drug abuse or misuse. The potential for physical addiction exists, since withdrawal symptoms are comparable to those from opiate derivatives. Evaluation in large groups over time will decide more fully the addiction liability of this drug.

Since increases in systolic blood pressure may occur with butorphanol's administration, the nurse should use caution when butorphanol is used for hypertensive patients. The use of this drug in patients with acute myocardial infarction, ventricular dysfunction, or coronary insufficiency is limited to those unable to tolerate other analgesics, because butorphanol may possibly increase pulmonary arterial pressure and work load on the heart.

Butorphanol may obscure the clinical course of head injuries in which there is increased intracranial pressure (by the elevation of cerebrospinal fluid pressure); therefore, it should be withheld from patients with such injuries.

Because butorphanol is metabolized in the liver, it should be given with caution to patients with compromised or impaired renal or hepatic function. Side effects and greater activity as a result of decreased metabolism of the drug in the liver may result.

The use of pancuronium in combination with butorphanol may cause an increase in conjunctival changes.

The safety of the use of butorphanol in pregnancy before the labor period has not been established, but the safety to the mother and fetus following the administration of butorphanol during labor has been established. The patients receiving butorphanol during labor have experienced no adverse effects other than those observed with commonly employed analgesics; however, this drug should be used with caution in women delivering premature infants.

Nalbuphine (Nubain)

Nalbuphine is a synthetic narcotic agonist-antagonist analgesic of the phenanthrene series. It is chemically related to both the narcotic antagonist naloxone and the narcotic analgesic oxymorphone. The analgesic potency is equivalent to that of morphine and is almost three times that of pentazocine on a milligram basis.

Action and result. The onset of action is

within 2 to 3 minutes after intravenous administration and within 14 minutes after an intramuscular or subcutaneous dose. Plasma half-life of nalbuphine is 5 hours and the duration of analgesic activity is from 3 to 6 hours. The narcotic antagonist activity is about 11 times that of pentazocine and 0.04 times that of naloxone.

The usual adult dose of 10 mg/70 kg causes some respiratory depression, similar to that of equal doses of morphine. In contrast to morphine, respiratory depression is not appreciably increased with higher doses of nalbuphine. This respiratory depression may be reversed by naloxone. The nurse should administer low doses with caution to patients with compromised respiration.

Uses. Nalbuphine can be used immediately in myocardial infarction, since it lowers the cardiac work load. However, it should be administered with caution in patients with myocardial infarction who have nausea or vomiting. Nalbuphine is used for relief of moderate to severe pain, preoperative analgesia, supplement to surgical anesthesia, and obstetric analgesia during labor.

Preparation, dosage, and administration. Nalbuphine is available in injection form at 10 mg/ml in 1- and 2-ml ampules and 10-ml vials.

The usual adult dose is 10 mg for a 70-kg individual by the subcutaneous, intramuscular, or intravenous route, repeated as necessary every 3 to 6 hours with individual adjustments according to severity of pain, physical status of the patient, and concurrent medications. In a patient who is nontolerant the recommended single maximum dose is 20 mg with a maximum total daily dose of 160 mg.

There is evidence that in a patient not dependent on narcotics, nalbuphine may not antagonize a narcotic analgesic if the narcotic is administered immediately, just before, concurrently with, or just after an injection of nalbuphine. An additive effect is exhibited with patients receiving a narcotic analgesic, general anesthetics, phenothiazines or other tranquilizers, sedatives, hypnotics, or other CNS depressants (such as alcohol) concomitantly with nalbuphine. Therefore the nurse should anticipate that when the combined therapy is contemplat-

ed the dose of one or both of the drugs should be reduced to overcome this additive effect.

Side effects and toxic effects. The most frequent adverse reaction is sedation. Less frequent are sweatiness, clamminess, nausea and vomiting, dizziness, vertigo, dry mouth, and headache. Fewer than 1% of the patients have experienced hallucinations, euphoria, floating, unusual dreams, confusion, and a sense of unreality.

Precautions. Patients with renal or hepatic dysfunction may overreact to usual adult doses of nalbuphine because the drug is metabolized in the liver and excreted by the kidneys with two inactive metabolites. Reduced doses in this case would be advised. Nalbuphine and all narcotic analgesics should be used cautiously in patients who are to have surgery of the biliary tract. Spasms of the sphincter of Oddi have often occurred in patients as a result of the narcotic analgesic's side effects.

Use of nalbuphine in ambulatory patients is not advised, since it may impair their mental or physical abilities and may be potentially dangerous if they are engaged in tasks that require their full physical and mental alertness. Use in pregnancy is not established, and use during labor and delivery may produce respiratory depression in the neonate.

The abuse potential of nalbuphine is comparable to that of pentazocine and may be less than that of codeine and propoxyphene. The nurse should be aware that psychologic and physical dependence and tolerance may follow the abuse and misuse of nalbuphine. Caution is needed in the emotionally unstable or substance abuse–prone individuals. Abrupt discontinuation following prolonged use may be followed by narcotic withdrawal symptoms (abdominal cramps, nausea, vomiting, rhinorrhea, lacrimation, restlessness, anxiety, elevated temperature, and piloerection). Patients given narcotics chronically may experience withdrawal symptoms if nalbuphine is administered. This may be controlled by the slow intravenous administration of small increments of morphine until relief occurs. If the previous analgesic was morphine, meperidine, codeine, or another narcotic with similar duration of activity, the nurse should administer only one fourth of the anticipated dose of nalbuphine initially and observe the patient for withdrawal signs. If these symptoms or signs of withdrawal do not occur, then progressively larger doses may be given in appropriate intervals until the desired level of analgesia is obtained. These withdrawal syndrome effects occur from the antagonistic aspect of this drug. Narcotic overdosage or overdosage of nalbuphine may be managed by the immediate intravenous use of naloxone (a specific antidote).

NONNARCOTIC ANALGESICS
Pentazocine (Talwin)

Pentazocine is a potent nonnarcotic analgesic for oral and parenteral use. It has agonistic and partial antagonistic properties because it usually antagonizes the respiratory depression and analgesia of morphine and meperidine. It is a synthetic compound that may be used in place of morphine and other narcotic analgesics. It is designated and classified as a controlled substance by the FDA. With repeated and frequent use, tolerance develops. Drug dependence potential seems likely. Precautions are the same as for other potent analgesics. (See Chapter 12.)

Uses. Pentazocine has been used for the relief of pain in connection with surgical procedures and in many medical disorders. It may cause respiratory depression in the fetus; therefore, use in obstetrics is limited.

Preparation, dosage, and administration. Pentazocine is supplied in parenteral forms with 1 ml containing 30 mg of the base. It is also available in disposable syringes and multiple-dose vials and in 50-mg tablets for oral use. Pentazocine should not be mixed in a syringe with soluble barbiturates because precipitation will occur.

Usual oral dose is 50 mg every 3 to 4 hours with an onset of 15 to 30 minutes, but because of relatively poor absorption, the dose may need to be 100 mg. Usual parenteral dose is 30 mg every 3 to 4 hours as necessary. Daily dose should not exceed 600 mg orally or 360 mg parenterally. Following subcutaneous or intramuscular administration, pentazocine acts in 10 to 30 minutes with a duration of effect of 2 to 3 hours. The duration of action is 3 to 4 hours, with an onset of 2 to 3 minutes with intravenous uses. For patients in labor a single intramuscular 30-mg dose may give adequate pain relief to some patients in labor when contractions become regular. This dose may be given two or three times at 2- to 3-hour intervals, as needed. Because of limited clinical experience, the use of pentazocine in children is not recommended. The oral-to-parenteral analgesic efficacy ratio is 3:1.

Side effects and toxic effects. Nausea, vertigo, dizziness, increase in cardiac work load, light headedness, vomiting, and euphoria may occur following the use of pentazocine. Psychologic and physiologic dependence are seen. Respiratory depression was reported in about 1% of the patients. The usual narcotic antagonist (naloxone) is effective in the treatment of respiratory depression produced by pentazocine. Repeated injections in one area produce abscess, scarring, and ulceration.

Propoxyphene hydrochloride (Darvon); dextropropoxyphene hydrochloride; propoxyphene napsylate (Darvon-N)

Propoxyphene hydrochloride is a synthetic analgesic compound structurally related to methadone with about two thirds to equal the potency of codeine; 65 mg may be equal to 650 mg aspirin or acetaminophen in analgesia. Like codeine, it does not depress respiration when given in ordinary therapeutic amounts, but unlike codeine, it produces little or no relief of cough. It may relieve mild to moderate pain. Onset of action and duration of effects are similar to codeine. Up to one third of the dose reaches systemic absorption after extensive first pass through the liver. The half-life of the parent is 6 to 12 hours, and its metabolite norpropoxyphene has a half-life of 30 to 36 hours. It does not act as an antipyretic. Next to aspirin and acetaminophen it is among the most widely prescribed analgesic.

Uses. It is used alone or along with certain other analgesics, such as acetaminophen or aspirin, for the relief of pain associated with chronic or recurring diseases like rheumatoid arthritis and migraine headache.

Preparation and dosage. Propoxyphene hydrocholoride is available in 32- and 65-mg capsules. The usual dose for adults is 65 mg four times a day (not more than 390 mg/day) with or without other medication for the relief of pain.

Dose for propoxyphene napsylate is 100 mg three or four times daily (not more than 600 mg/day).

Propoxyphene compound contains the following: propoxyphene hydrochloride, 32 mg (65 mg in propoxyphene Compound-65); phenacetin, 162 mg; aspirin, 227 mg; and caffeine, 32.4 mg. Dosage is one to two capsules three or four times a day. Propoxyphene hydrochloride is not suited to parenteral administration because of a local irritating action.

Side effects and toxic effects. Therapeutic doses do not produce euphoria, tolerance, or physical dependence. Abuse with morphine-like dependence has been reported, however. Sudden cessation of administration has not been known to produce withdrawal symptoms. It appears to have a low level of toxicity when used alone in therapeutic doses. Side effects of nausea, vomiting, and constipation are considered minimal. Large doses may cause drowsiness and dizziness. Patients are occasionally hypersensitive to this drug, and efficacy is reduced in cigarette smokers because liver enzymes must be induced for metabolism. There are no known contraindications except hypersensitivity. Alcohol and CNS depressants have an additive CNS depressant effect. It is subject to the restrictions of the Controlled Substances Act.

Overdosage may cause confusion, respiratory depression, coma, pupil constriction, and muscle fasciculations. Convulsions are prominent in most cases of propoxyphene poisoning, and arrhythmias and pulmonary edema have been reported. Apnea, cardiac arrest, and death have occurred. The narcotic antagonist naloxone may be used to overcome respiratory depression. Analeptics or other central nervous system stimulants should not be used because of their potential for precipitating fatal convulsions. Propoxyphene abuse is increasing, and deaths have resulted from ingestion of large doses of the drug alone and when taken with other CNS depressants. (See Chapter 12.)

Ethoheptazine citrate (Zactane)

Ethoheptazine is a synthetic nonnarcotic analgesic structurally similar to meperidine. It is without antipyretic and sedative effects and seemingly has no effect on cough and respira-tion. It is said to be more effective than aspirin when given alone. It is possibly effective when used for its analgesic effects for mild to moderate pain rather than for severe pain. Its greatest use seems to be for the control of pain associated with musculoskeletal disorders, for postpartum and postoperative patients, and for patients in the early stages of neoplastic diseases. It is not particularly effective for headaches. It has been combined with aspirin to enhance its effectiveness; this combination is called Zactirin.

Preparation, dosage, and administration. Ethoheptazine citrate is marketed in 75-mg tablets for oral administration. The dosage may be from 75 to 150 mg three or four times daily.

Ethoheptazine citrate with aspirin (Zactirin) contains 75 mg of ethoheptazine citrate and 325 mg (gr 5) of aspirin in each tablet. Dosage is one to two tablets three or four times a day. Zactirin compound-100 contains ethoheptazine, 100 mg; aspirin, 227 mg; phenacetin, 162 mg; and caffeine, 32.4 mg.

Side effects and toxic effects. Side effects are not often seen. Epigastric distress, nausea with and without vomiting, dizziness, and pruritus are effects that are observed occasionally. It does not cause dependence.

Methotrimeprazine (Levoprome)

Methotrimeprazine is a phenothiazine derivative with potent CNS depressant activity, having sites of action postulated in the thalamus, hypothalamus, and reticular and limbic systems. It produces sensory impulse suppression, motor activity reduction, sedation, and tranquilization; raises the pain threshold; and produces amnesia. As a phenothiazine it also possesses antihistamine, anticholinergic, and antiadrenergic effects coupled with the phenothiazine drug interactions. After parenteral administration this drug frequently produces orthostatic hypotension, sedation, fainting, or dizziness; therefore, ambulation of the patient should be carefully supervised for at least 6 hours following the initial dose. Tolerance to this effect usually develops with continued administration.

The analgesic effect is similar to morphine or meperidine, begins within 20 to 40 minutes after intramuscular injection, and lasts up to 4 hours. This drug also has a sedative effect. It is indicated for nonambulatory patients with pain of moderate to marked severity; in obstetric analgesia and sedation; and as a preanesthetic for producing sedation, somnolence, and relief of apprehension and anxiety. It may cause pain and inflammation at the injection site. Methotrimeprazine should not be mixed in the same syringe with any drug except atropine or scopolamine.

ANTIPYRETIC ANALGESICS

Antipyretics were more in demand when effort was made to cure fevers by antipyresis. Today many physicians look upon fever as a reaction of the body that helps the individual combat infection, and therefore reduction of the fever is not always desirable. Antipyretic drugs are still used for the relief of high fever, especially in children. Aspirin is probably used more than any other single agent for this purpose. Recently, however, the use of acetaminophen has increased to almost that of aspirin since studies have revealed that its antipyretic properties were equal to those of aspirin and that it has an added beneficial property of a lack of side effects affecting platelet adhesiveness. Because of this latter characteristic, acetaminophen is widely used over aspirin in the treatment of fever in myelosuppressed patients or patients with blood disorders that might be influenced by the side effects of aspirin.

This section will only discuss acetaminophen since it cannot be grouped with the antiinflammatory analgesics as aspirin is.

Acetaminophen (Tylenol, Tempra, Liquiprin, others)

Acetaminophen is a para-aminophenol derivative. Its primary use is as an analgesic and an antipyretic. Unlike aspirin, it lacks antiinflammatory or antirheumatic properties. The antipyretic and analgesic effects are mediated through the central nervous system. Analgesia is produced by elevation of the pain threshhold and antipyresis through action on the hypothalamic heat-regulating center.

With therapeutic doses, the peak plasma concentration occurs in ½ to 2 hours and is delayed up to 4 hours because of hepatic damage in an overdosed patient. The oral bioavailability is 100%, and 20% to 50% of the drug is protein bound at toxic serum concentrations, with the highest concentration in the liver. The elimination half-life is 1 to 3½ hours.

Uses. Acetaminophen is indicated in conditions involving musculoskeletal pain and for relief of pain of headache, dysmenorrhea, toothache, myalgias, and neuralgias. It is also used as an analgesic and antipyretic in diseases accompanied by discomfort and fever, such as the common cold and other viral infections. There is wide usage in patients with aspirin allergy, hemostatic disturbances (including anticoagulant therapy), bleeding diatheses (ulcer, gastritis, and hiatus hernia), and gouty arthritis.

Preparations, dosage, and administration. The current dosage forms available are chewable tablets of 20 and 80 mg); capsules and tablets of 325, 500, and 650 mg; and rectal suppositories of 120, 125, 130, 300, 325, 600 and 650 mg. The elixir has 120, 130, or 165 mg/5 ml, and a syrup is available with 160 mg/5 ml concentration. Oral drops are in 60 mg/0.6 ml and 120 mg/2.5 ml concentrations.

Acetaminophen is given to adults in a dosage of 300 to 650 mg three to four times daily, not exceeding 2.6 g/24 hours for long-term therapy and 4 g/24 hours in short-term therapy. Children from 7 to 12 years may be given 150 to 325 mg three to four times daily, not exceeding 1.3 g/24 hours. Children from 3 to 6 years may have a dosage of 120 to 200 mg three or four times daily, not exceeding 480 mg/24 hours.

Caution must be taken in those patients with glucose-6-phosphate dehydrogenase deficieny, continued anemia, or cardiac, pulmonary, or renal hepatic diseases. The nurse should caution patients not to exceed the dosage established for their therapy. Patients with impaired hepatic function should be monitored because of the potential for further hepatic damage. There is evidence that the acetaminophen half-life in patients with liver disease is increased; however, there is no evidence at this time that acetaminophen therapy causes increased risk to the patient.

Overdosage. Shortly after an acute overdose ingestion, there are signs of gastrointestinal irritability, loss of appetite, nausea, vomiting, cyanosis, tachycardia, anemia, jaundice, neutropenia, leukopenia, pancytopenia, CNS stimulation, sweating, fever, chills, and drowsiness. Following this, there is a latent period of 24 to 36 hours before the hepatotoxic symptoms (vomiting, abdominal pain, and signs of beginning hepatic coma) occur. Confirmation by laboratory tests may not reveal this liver toxicity for up to 7 days (liver failure with elevations of liver enzyme measurements); therefore serial hepatic enzyme determinations must be made.

The use of N-acetylcysteine (Mucomyst) has been successful in abating the liver damage by supplying the sulfhydryl groups to decrease liver injury from glutathione depletion and necrosos. Plasma acetaminophen levels of 300 mg/ml 4 hours after ingestion and over 50 mg/ml 12 hours after ingestion are associated with hepatic damage. After gastric emptying and emesis— regardless of how much was ingested in the previous 24 hours—the nurse administers a loading dose of N-acetylcysteine (140 mg/kg orally in a vehicle to mask the taste [grapefruit juice, carbonated beverage, or water] or a 5% concentration of acetylcysteine in the selected vehicle). This is followed by 70 mg/kg every 4 hours for 17 maintenance doses within the 68-hour treatment period. If vomiting occurs within 1 hour after a dose is given, it must be repeated immediately. Acetaminophen plasma levels should be monitored until at least 4 hours has elapsed after the overdose. If the plasma half-life exceeds 4 hours hepatic necrosis is probable, and if it is greater than 12 hours hepatic coma is probable. Liver function must be tested daily. If more than 24 hours has elapsed since the overdose, the condition should be in accordance with liver function studies and liver function tests.

Sedatives and hypnotics

Sleep can be defined as a recurrent, normal condition of inertia and unresponsiveness during which an individual's overt and covert responses to stimuli are markedly reduced.

During sleep a person is no longer in sensory contact with the immediate environment, and stimuli that have bombarded the senses of sight, hearing, touch, smell, and taste during waking hours will no longer attract attention or exert a controlling influence over the individual's voluntary and involuntary movements or functions. It certainly is not difficult to understand that everyone needs to escape from constant stimuli.

Present-day knowledge about sleep has been obtained from research on normal subjects using the electroencephalogram (EEG) and electrooculogram (EOG). The electroencephalogram provides graphic illustrations of brain waves, and this permits comparisons to be made between brain wave patterns of sleep and wakefulness. Brain waves are, of course, an indication of the electric activity occurring in the brain. The electric activity is greater during wakefulness than during sleep; during sleep the greatest electric activity occurs during dreaming sleep, with the least activity occurring in deep sleep. The electrooculogram provides graphic illustrations of eye movements. Electrodes placed near the outer canthus of each eye monitor the amount, rate, and size of eye movements. These are also recorded as wave patterns. Rapid eye movements during sleep are associated with dreaming sleep.

Sleep research has shown that sleep is not one level of unconsciousness; it actually consists of four main sleep stages that occur in regular cyclic patterns characterized by variations in depth of sleep and variations in brain waves and eye movements (see Fig. 8-5).

Onset of sleep is a drowsy period, and brain wave activity is similar to that seen in normal awake individuals, that is, the brain waves are relatively fast and frequent. As sleep gradually deepens to Stage II sleep, a change in brain waves is seen, with the waves becoming slower in frequency. Stages III and IV are deep sleep stages—the brain waves are slow and have

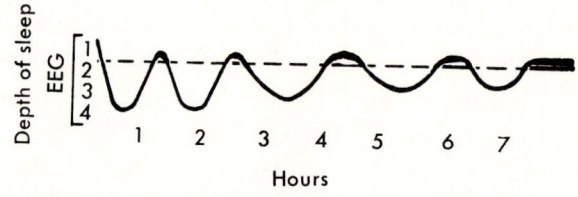

FIG. 8-5. Cyclic variation of a night of sleep.

great height and depth. In other words, large brain wave deflections are seen.

From the standpoint of dreaming, sleep consists of two main functional states. One is called "slow wave," nondreaming, or non–rapid eye movement (NREM) sleep. The other is referred to as "paradoxic," dreaming, or rapid eye movement (REM) sleep. It should be kept in mind that REM sleep is not synonymous with light sleep, since it takes a bigger stimulus to arouse an animal or person from REM sleep than from synchronous slow wave sleep.

Sleep research indicates that there is both a psychologic and physiologic need for the body to maintain an equilibrium between the various stages of sleep. Physiologic functions of the body tend to be depressed during nondreaming sleep. For example it is known that:

1 There is a fall in blood pressure (10 to 30 mm Hg).
2 Pulse rate is slowed.
3 Metabolic rate is decreased.
4 Activity of the gastrointestinal tract is slowed.
5 Urine formation slows.
6 Oxygen consumption and carbon dioxide production are lowered.
7 Body temperature decreases slightly.
8 Respirations are slower and more shallow.
9 Body movement is minimal.

Dreaming sleep tends to increase most of these parameters, and body movements are more noticeable—turning, jerking, arm and leg movements, talking, crying, or laughing—and of course, eye movements can be seen under the closed lids. The dynamic physiologic equilibrium of the body continues to be maintained even during sleep. Depression of physiologic functions occurs during deep sleep and an increase in functions occurs during dreaming. Repeated studies have shown that when individuals are deprived of deep sleep, they become physically uncomfortable, tend to withdraw from society and their friends, are less aggressive and outgoing, and manifest concern over vague physical complaints and changes in bodily feelings. The overall impression made by persons deprived of deep sleep is that of a depressive and hypochondriac reaction.

However, dreaming sleep is also important. From studies during which individuals were deprived of dreaming sleep (every time the subjects attempted to dream, as evidenced by rapid eye movements, they were awakened and not permitted to dream) the following results were observed. The individuals during their waking hours became less well integrated and less effective. They showed signs of confusion, suspicion, and withdrawal. They appeared anxious, insecure, and irritable, they had greater difficulty concentrating, they had a marked increase in appetite with a definite weight gain, and they were introspective and unable to derive support from other people.

It is the belief of many psychologists and psychiatrists that wish fulfillment finds expression in dreams, and potentially harmful thoughts, feelings, and impulses are released through the dream so as not to interfere in the functioning of the personality during waking hours.

It is also known that in dream deprivation studies, the longer dream deprivation continues, the greater the increase in attempts to dream, until the individual begins to dream almost upon falling asleep. When sujects are finally permitted to dream, a marked increase of dreaming is noted for the entire night, and as much as 75% of the night may be spent in dreaming. This amount diminishes for each succeeding recovery night until the individual has once again established his normal sleep pattern.

Research has shown that deep sleep takes priority over dreaming sleep when there has been prolonged sleep deprivation. In other words, deep sleep needs will be met first, after which dreaming sleep needs will be met. The body attempts to reestablish the normal equilibrium between the sleep stages.

Each individual establishes his own normal sleep pattern, which will vary somewhat from night to night and which is influenced by the individual's emotional and physical state. For most individuals, any alteration in sleeping habits will cause problems in falling asleep, staying asleep, or both. Since drugs affect an individual's physical or emotional state, they also influence his sleep pattern.

A hypnotic is a drug that produces sleep, and as a group these drugs have been widely used both for hospitalized patients and by the public at large. Sedatives are drugs that soothe and relieve anxiety.

Hospitalized patients often find it difficult to obtain rest and sleep for a variety of reasons. The surroundings are unfamiliar; they may be subjected to sensory overload or sensory deprivation, and their anxiety level is usually increased. In addition, pain or discomfort may prevent them from sleeping. Equally important as a deterrent to sleep are minor discomforts, such as cold feet, an aching back, a wrinkled bed, lack of sufficient ventilation, too few or too many blankets, a full bladder, or a distended rectum. Occasionally, a patient cannot sleep because he is hungry. It would be a poor nurse who would rely entirely on the effects of a hypnotic or sedative to remedy such discomforts.

The only difference between a hypnotic and a sedative action is one of degree. When a drug is given at the hour of retirement and in full dosage, producing sleep soon after administration, it is known as a hypnotic. When it is given in reduced dosage several times during the day and perhaps again at bedtime, it is called a sedative. Sedation is a calming, quieting effect, and the patient who is calm and relaxed during the day usually sleeps better at night. The terms "soporific" and "somnifacient" are synonymous with "hypnotic." Many of the drugs known as tranquilizers are used for some of the same effects as the sedatives. Hypnotics act much like general anesthetics if large enough doses are given. They characteristically spare the medullary centers until large doses have been given.

Sleep research has provided important knowledge about these drugs and their effects on sleep and dreaming. It has been found that they actually alter the occurrence and length of sleep stages. The stage particularly affected is Stage I, in which rapid eye movement occurs.

The drugs known to definitely affect the sleep pattern of humans are:

1 Sleeping medications—hypnotics or sedatives (such as glutethimide or pentobarbital)
2 Tranquilizers (such as chlorpromazine)
3 Amphetamines
4 Ethyl alcohol (such as that contained in whiskey or cocktails)

In no study reported in the literature up to the present time has any sleep medication failed to alter the individual's pattern of sleep, and these patterns continue to be disrupted long after the sleeping medication has been discontinued. Sleep research studies also show that it may take as long as 3 to 5 weeks after sleeping medications have been discontinued before the individual's sleep pattern returns to its predrug or normal pattern.

Since both the amphetamines and barbiturates reduce dreaming time, when both these drugs are administered to the same individual the effect on dreaming is an additive one; that is, dreaming sleep is more greatly reduced than when either drug is used alone. Some drugs, such as reserpine, increase dreaming time, which may account for the bizarre dreams reported by patients receiving this drug.

Side effects from alteration in sleep pattern include irritability, tremors, tenseness, agitation, confusion, decreased attentiveness, sluggishness or lethargy, and many other symptoms. A hypnotic, flurazepam (Dalmane), does not decrease dream time. However, it does decrease Stage IV sleep (deep sleep). The significance of this is yet to be determined.

Classification. The classification of sedative-hypnotic drugs is by the pharmacologic nature of the drug and the clinical indication (patient complaint) for which it is used. Sedative-hypnotic drugs may be grouped into three classes: barbiturates, nonbarbiturates, and anxiolytics. The barbiturates are those compounds synthesized from barbituric acid, including amobarbital, butabarbital, pentobarbital, phenobarbital, and secobarbital. The nonbarbiturates are grouped as the benzodiazepines (drugs with similar chemical structures such as chlordiazepoxide, clorazepate, diazepam, flurazepam, lorazepam, prazepam, and temazepam) and other nonbarbiturates synthesized from a variety of different pharmacologic agents (chloral hydrate, ethchlorvynol, glutethimide, meprobamate, methaqualone, and methyprylon). Another method of classifying these drugs is based on the clinical indication, such as hypnotics or anxiolytics. Hypnotics are those drugs used to treat insomnia and administered once daily at bedtime to induce sleep (for example, secobarbital, flurazepam, temazepam, and glutethimide). Anxiolytics are drugs used to treat anxiety and administered in divided doses daily to reduce tension or anxiety (for example, butabarbital, chlordiazepoxide, or meprobamate). Thus the same drug may be used as both a hypnotic and an anxiolytic, depending on dosage and frequency of administration.

The terms "sedatives" and "tranquilizers" are also used to describe these classes of drugs. Generally sedatives (barbiturates, ethchlorvynol, glutethimide, flurazepam, methyprylon, and methaqualone) are similar to the drugs classified as hypnotics. Generally the term "tranquilizers" is often used to describe and include chlordiazepoxide, diazepam, clorazepate, lorazepam, and prazepam), which are the drugs classed as anxiolytics.

Risks and benefits. The relative toxicity of various sedative-hypnotic agents deserves some attention in this chapter (see also Chapter 12). Certain groups of patients complaining of the symptom complex for which these drugs are used may demonstrate a significant degree of psychopathology, and, a large population of users, for example, the elderly, may be relatively more vulnerable to crises of life, making them a high-risk population for misusing these drugs for purposes of suicide.

The relative toxicity in terms of the amount of drug (or multiple of therapeutic dose) required to produce morbidity or mortality is a paramount consideration in the choice of a CNS depressant. The benzodiazepine group has a considerable margin of safety between the therapeutic dose and the dose required to produce serious overdose or death. The barbiturates and the nonbenzodiazepine sedative-hypnotics (chloral hydrate, paraldehyde, glutethimide, ethinamate, methylprylon, ethchlorvynol, methaqualone) possess a much narrower margin of safety. Doses as low as 10 to 15 times the therapeutic dose of these compounds have been related to severe respiratory compromise and death. Although the longer-acting barbiturates (such as phenobarbital and butabarbital) and meprobamate may have a more favorable therapeutic index, the margin of safety is clearly many magnitudes smaller than that observed with the benzodiazepines.

Tolerance develops to the therapeutic effects of these agents with long-term administration; only minimal tolerance appears to develop to the lethal effects. This factor favors long-term users who escalate the dose without medical supervision to achieve their personal desired effect.

Certain of the nonbarbiturate nonbenzodiazepines may present special difficulties in terms of the treatment of overdose (see Chapter 12). Glutethimide, because of its high lipid solubility* and anticholinergic activity, is notorious in this regard. Methaqualone presents difficulties in treating patients with overdoses. (see Chapter 12). The overdose problem is further complicated by the fact that multiple drug/substance abuse in suicide attempts is common. The intoxication with the benzodiazepines alone is not generally of life-threatening magnitude; the mixed overdose with compounds such as other CNS depressants, including alcohol, can prove fatal.

In addition to their acute lethality, these compounds have undesirable effects, such as drowsiness or sedation, when employed as anxiolytic agents. This is directly related to the slope of the dose response curve that a compound exhibits on the continuum of central nervous system depression. Simply stated, the dose-response curve is a graphic representation of the relationship between the dose administered and the biologic effect observed. The benzodiazepines have a flatter dose response curve along this continuum. Generally less sedation accompanies the use of the benzodiazepines as anxiolytics than comparable doses of other agents. This lack of sedation is even more evident with oxazepam, which is not metabolized to active metabolites, than with the benzodiazepines that are metabolized to active compounds.

The residual effects, commonly referred to as "hangover," depend on the dose level of drugs, variations in individual disposition, the pharmacokinetic profile (a time-dependent change in the amount of serum concentration of drugs and metabolites in the body), the sensi-

*It is stored in fat, and generally biologic membranes are much more permeable to unionized lipid-soluble molecules.

tivity of the measurements employed, and the individual patient's subjective behavioral measurement or interpretation of the feelings of drowsiness. Residual effects can be detected 15 to 18 hours after single doses of secobarbital, amobarbital, and pentobarbital when sensitive behavioral measures are utilized. There is evidence of residual effects for flurazepam and butabarbital as well.

Cumulative effects can be predicted by the dosing schedule and pharmacokinetic characteristics of the drug used. Long-term administration of CNS depressants is a more complex issue because of many factors. Metabolic and physiologic tolerance to barbiturates and many of the nonbarbiturate nonbenzodiazepines (glutethimide, meprobamate, methaqualone, and chloral hydrate) can be demonstrated to stimulate hepatic microsomal enzymes during long-term administration, thus decreasing their effective blood concentrations. A ceiling to this effect does exist. At high doses the benzodiazepines have been shown to stimulate microsomal enzymes in humans (but at doses of a higher magnitude than the barbiturates and the non-barbiturate nonbenzodiazepines). The clinical significance of this effect is less important with benzodiazepines than with the other drugs listed. Physiologic tolerance develops to all of the CNS depressants.

The barbiturates and the nonbarbiturate, nonbenzodiazepine sedative-hypnotics (except chloral hydrate) are metabolized to inactive metabolites. The benzodiazepines (except oxazepam, temazepam, or lorazepam and some of the newer agents) are converted to metabolites with fairly long half-lives. With long-term administration cumulation may result, as has been demonstrated for flurazepam, resulting in both increased clinical efficacy and at least some residual drowsiness. The biologic half-lives of the barbiturates (Table 8-7) are long. With any of the drugs employed as sedative-hypnotics, when the dosing schedule exceeds the rate of development of tolerance or the elimination rate, cumulation may be predicted. Therefore compounds with shorter half-lives (methyprylon [±4 hours], ethchlorvynol [±5 to 6 hours], or temazepam [±10 hours]) may in selected patients offer certain advantages when dosing is frequent.

Contraindications. Contraindications to the use of CNS depressants exist in certain patient populations. These include but are not limited to those with severe respiratory compromise or those with hypersensitivity to individual compounds. A confirmed contraindication is the use of barbiturates in the presence of acute intermittent porphyria. Limited exposure to barbiturates in such individuals has resulted in lethal outcomes, related in part to the effect of barbiturates on hepatic microsomal enzymes. Comparative effects of other agents could be toxic if stimulation of microsomal enzymes is involved.

A less understood phenomenon reported with CNS depressants in general is paradoxic excitement, commonly interpreted as a disinhibition reaction similar to that seen with alcohol. It has been reported particularly in children and the aged. Identifiable personality characteristics may predispose one to this paradoxic effect.

A subpopulation of elderly (over 60 years old) and debilitated persons is reported to respond differently to CNS depressants. Reports exist of increased sensitivity to the depressant properties and an increased number of paradoxic reactions to barbiturates and an increased incidence of side effects (mainly drowsiness with flurazepam, chlordiazepoxide, and diazepam), but these may be reversed by reduction in dose or cessation of drug use.

Individuals with impaired renal function (increase in BUN), those with longer hospital stays (more concomitant medications), debilitated persons, and those with decreases in serum albumin levels also report a higher incidence of complaints of CNS depression while taking benzodiazepines. There does exist the potential for danger to patients with hepatic, renal, pulmonary, metabolic, and cardiac insufficiency. For compounds that are eliminated only by the kidney, severe renal insufficiency has potential to prolong effects. Those patients with thyroid or adrenal gland hypofunction may be more susceptible to the sedative drugs, and caution is thus advised.

Drug interactions. There is ample information about the drug interactions of sedative-hypnotic drugs because of their widespread use and their opportunity in interact with other

TABLE 8-6 Drug interactions with barbiturates

Drug	Interaction effects
Acute alcohol intoxication	Enhanced CNS depression
Chronic alcohol use	Sedative effects of barbiturates lessened
Anticoagulants (coumarin derivatives)	Decreased anticoagulation
Tricyclic antidepressants	Decreased TAD effects
CNS depressants (antihistamines, sedatives, hypnotics, narcotics, phenothiazines, anxiolytics)	Enhanced CNS depression (dose related) Additive respiratory depression
Corticosteroids	Reduced corticosteroid effect
Cyclobenzaprine	Enhanced sedative effects
Griseofulvin	Reduced absorption
Phenmetrazine (anorexiant)	Reduced effectiveness of phenmetrazine
Procarbazine	Enhanced sedative effects of barbiturates
Valproic acid	Increased phenobarbital serum levels
Doxycycline	Decreased metabolism and half-life of antibiotic
Chloramphenicol	Inhibit metabolism of phenobarbital
Digitoxin	Increase digitoxin effect by inducing hepatic microsomal enzymes

drugs in polydrug users. The additive effects with other compounds that depress the central nervous system pose a definite hazard. The induction of hepatic microsomal enzymes by barbiturates and the nonbarbiturate nonbenzodiazepine is the most significant and clinically important drug interaction observed with this class of compounds. Long-term administration of certain of these drugs stimulates the metabolism of other drugs, such as the monoamine oxidase inhibitors, tricyclic antidepressants, phenytoin, and most notably the coumarin anticoagulants. A rebound rise in blood levels then follows discontinuation of these sedative-hypnotics, and this has been identified with exaggerated clinical response.

In addition to the sedative-hypnotics that induce metabolic enzymes, chloral hydrate and ethchlorvynol may also alter the response to coumarin drugs. Although the effect of ethchlorvynol is not entirely explained, the effects reported with chloral hydrate appear to be secondary to the displacement of coumarin drugs from plasma protein by trichloroacetic acid, a major metabolite.

There has been no major significant interaction between the benzodiazepines studied to date and the oral anticoagulants. Rarely chlordiazepoxide has variable effects on blood coagulation. The benzodiazepines appear to be benign both with respect to any interaction with anticoagulants and any shift in the activity of hepatic microsomal enzymes with limited periods of exposure. This may alter with more clinical experience with higher dose levels, longer treatment periods, and concomitant use of other benzodiazepines. Oxazepam, lorazepam, and temazepam are not metabolized in this manner and may be used with cimetidine. The half-life of some benzodiazepines (those metabolized by the microsomal enzyme system) may be increased in patients receiving cimetidine.

Table 8-6 outlines some of the potential interactions involving barbiturates.

Alterations in prescribing patterns. The FDA[1] published findings from the National Institute on Drug Abuse concerning an "update on sedative-hypnotics." Significant alterations in the prescribing patterns of these medications have been made because of the concerns about their safety and effectiveness in use. The objective of the study was to assess the health effects of sedative-hypnotic drugs, including benzodiazepines, and other sleeping pills.

The prescribing of sedative-hypnotics for insomnia (the primary use of these drugs) has decreased about 40% (25 million prescriptions) from 1971 to 1980. There has been a change of drug types used by physicians for sleep disturbances, shifting away from the barbiturates toward the benzodiazepines (for example, flurazepam [Dalmane]). The shift may be in response to drug abuse concerns, accidental deaths, suicides, and more rigid controls involving barbiturates (there was substantial

TABLE 8-7 Plasma half-life values (in hours) for some barbiturates in humans

Drug	Adult	Child	Newborn
Amobarbital	16-24		
Aprobarbital	14-34		
Butabarbital	62-138		
Hexabarbital	5		
Pentobarbital	21-48		
Phenobarbital	72-96	48-72	100-200
Secobarbital	20-28		

decrease in suicides involving barbiturates during this period). An additional reason for this shift is also the fact that the barbiturates suppress the REM stage of sleep while benzodiazepines do not.

The benzodiazepines used as hypnotics and the barbiturates are probably equally effective for short-term utilization, and neither of the two classes is an ideal hypnotic drug. Benzodiazepines suppress Stages III and IV of sleep, a possible disadvantage that may offset the apparent benefit of leaving the REM stage undisturbed.

The possible hazard associated with long-acting benzodiazepine metabolites does exist, and this aspect may require an every other night dosage regimen at a lower dose. Metabolites of flurazepam have a half-life of 50 to 100 hours, compared to the average half-life ranges of 14 to 48 hours for pentobarbital, secobarbital, and amobarbital, the barbiturates most often prescribed for sleep in the past.

There is a potential risk associated with the buildup of flurazepam in the body, since it may produce unwanted daytime carryover effects, resulting in poor coordination and drowsiness. This may be overcome by using lower doses every other evening. The nurse, physician, or pharmacist must warn the patient of this sustained effect; an unexpected toxic interaction may occur between the benzodiazepine used for nighttime sedation and alcohol consumed the following day because of the high blood levels of the active metabolites the following day and the sedative effects of the alcohol in synergism.

There is an increasing likelihood of adverse reactions in older persons and a greater propensity toward adverse reactions in patients with decreased kidney functions. Many of these

effects may be abated by more judicious use of the benzodiazepines, restricting them to short-term treatment for insomnia.

There is little evidence that sedative-hypnotics in general demonstrate continued effectiveness when administered nightly over long periods. Sleep laboratory research on most hypnotics has found that there is a loss in their sleep-promoting properties within 3 to 14 days of continuous use. This may prompt practitioners to discover and treat underlying disorders causing many patients' insomnia and to restrict even further the administration and prescribing of the hynotics.

Labeling changes. Labeling changes prompted by the FDA for sedative-hypnotic drugs include statements to indicate their duration of effectiveness, the duration of their efficacy, and key information for the patients, instructing them in proper use. Examples of this labeling are as follows:

Ethinamate (Valmid)—prolonged administration is not recommended since it has not been shown to be effective for a period of more than 7 days.

Methaqualone—prolonged administration is not recommended since it has not been shown to be effective for more than 14 days.

Sodium butabarbital (Butisol)—prolonged administration is not recommended since it has not been shown to be effective for more than 14 days; should insomnia persist, drug-free intervals of 1 week or more should elapse before retreatment is considered.

Triclofos sodium—has not been shown effective for more than 14 days except in persons over age 65; effective for up to 42 days in one inpatient study.

BARBITURATES

The barbiturates were among the first drugs to be synthesized. The first one was introduced into medicine by Emil Fischer and Joseph von Mehring in 1903 under the name of Veronal. Phenobarbital is the second oldest of the barbiturates. Since the time of their introduction, hundreds of similar compounds have been synthesized, but only a limited number have proved clinically useful. New compounds have resulted from slight changes in the basic barbiturate molecule, and these changes have resulted in compounds that vary from the earlier compounds mostly in speed and duration of action.

Some of the barbiturates have stood the test of time very well. Large amounts of these drugs are prescribed and used, as is evident from the fact that thousands of pounds are produced annually.

The barbiturates are all colorless, white crystalline powders that have a more or less bitter taste. They are sparingly soluble in water but freely soluble in alcohol. The sodium salts of these compounds are freely soluble in water.

Action and result. Important actions of the barbiturates are those of sedation and hypnotic effect. Barbiturates have been shown to depress the neurons and synapses of the ascending reticular formation of the brainstem, and this effect may be responsible for the reduction in electric activity of the cortex. Since the ascending reticular formation receives stimuli from all parts of the body and relays impulses to the cortex (thus promoting wakefulness and alertness), depression of the ascending reticular formation decreases cortical stimuli, reducing the need for wakefulness and alertness.

There is evidence that the barbiturates act at all levels of the central nervous system. The extent of effect varies from mild sedation to deep anesthesia, depending on the drug selected, method of administration, dosage, and the reaction of the individual's nervous system. The barbiturates are not usually regarded as analgesics and cannot be depended on to produce restful sleep when insomnia is caused by pain. However, when combined with an analgesic the sedative action seems to reinforce the action of the analgesic and to alter the patient's emotional reaction to pain. Therapeutic doses of the longer-acting barbiturates may result in depression and lowerd vitality on the following day ("hangover effect").

All of the barbiturates used clinically depress the motor cortex of the brain in large doses, but phenobarbital, mephobarbital, and metharbital exert a selective action on the motor cortex, even in small doses. This explains their use as anticonvulsants.

Ordinary therapeutic doses have little or no effect on medullary centers, but large doses, especially when administered intravenously, depress the respiratory and vasomotor centers. Death from overdosage is caused, as a rule, by respiratory failure accompanied by hypotension.

Smooth muscles of blood vessels and of the gastrointestinal organs are depressed after large amounts of barbiturates, but clinical doses do not usually produce untoward effects. Motility of the gastrointestinal organs may be reduced and emptying of the stomach delayed slightly, but there is apparently little interference with the ability to respond to normal stimuli. Uterine muscle is affected little by hypnotic doses of barbiturates, and the force of uterine contractions at the time of childbirth is not diminished unless anesthesia has been produced by one of these drugs.

Uses. The barbiturates have many uses and are very popular drugs.

Hypnotics. For best effects the barbiturates should be administered at such times as will coincide with the usual hour of retirement. Long-, short-, or intermediate-acting barbiturates are chosen to meet the needs of individual patients.

Sedatives. The barbiturates have, for purposes of sedation, a wide range of therapeutic uses. Although the tranquilizing drugs have come into a position of great prominence, the barbiturates are still used to calm and sedate the nervous patient and for patients who have physical illness in which there is usually an emotional factor, as in the case of hypertension, chronic ulcerative colitis, and gastric ulcer.

Anticonvulsants. Barbiturates are used to prevent or control convulsive seizures associated with tetanus, strychnine poisoning, cerebral pathology, and epilepsy. It may be prescribed alone or in conjunction with other anticonvulsant drugs. Mephobarbital and metharbital are also effective in the symptomatic treatment of certain types of epilepsy.

Anesthetics. For selected forms of surgical procedures, and especially for surgery of short duration, the rapid-acting barbiturates are employed. Thiopental sodium is the preparation most widely used in the United States. These barbiturates are further discussed under "Intravenous anesthetics."

Preanesthetic medications. The short-acting barbiturates, such as pentobarbital sodium, are selected for this effect. They are often ordered to be given the night before surgery to enable the patient to sleep and may also be ordered to be given the morning of the operation. They are frequently supplemented by other medications just before the patient is taken to the operating room.

Obstetric sedation and amnesia. For obstetric sedation and amnesia the barbiturates are used either alone or in conjunction with other drugs, such as scopolamine or meperidine. However, drugs that cause respiratory depression of the mother are likely to cause respiratory depression of the infant as well.

Psychiatry. Barbiturates are sometimes used in psychiatry to temporarily release a patient from strong inhibitions and enable him to cooperate more effectively with his therapist. Amobarbital, pentobarbital, and thiopental are the barbiturates likely to be chosen for this purpose.

Absorption and excretion. Barbiturates are readily absorbed after both oral and parenteral administration. The more soluble sodium salts are more rapidly absorbed than the free acids. Most of the barbiturates, with the exception of barbital, undergo change in the liver before they are excreted by the kidney. Some are excreted partly in an altered form and partly unchanged, and others are excreted in a com-

pletely altered form. The longer-acting barbiturates are said to be metabolized or chemically altered more slowly than the rapidly acting members. The more slowly a barbiturate is altered or excreted, the more prolonged is its action. If excretion is slow and administration prolonged, cumulative effects will result.

Classification. The barbiturates are classified according to the duration of their action as long-, intermediate-, short-, and ultrashort-acting drugs. This means that the short-acting drugs produce an effect or onset in a relatively short time (10 to 15 minutes) and have a peak over a relatively short period (3 to 4 hours). Short-acting barbiturates are used in the treatment of insomnia, for preanesthetic sedation, and in combination with other drugs for psychosomatic disorders. Long-acting barbiturates require over 60 minutes for onset and peak over a period of 10 to 12 hours. Long-acting barbiturates are used for treating epilepsy and other chronic neurologic disorders and for sedation in patients with high anxiety. Ultrashort-acting barbiturates are used as intravenous anesthetics. Thiopental sodium, which belongs to the ultrashort-acting group of barbiturates, acts rapidly and can produce a state of anesthesia in a few seconds. Intermediate act-

TABLE 8-8   Dosage, administration, and length of action of barbiturates

Preparation	Usual adult dose	Usual method of administration	Relative lengths of action
*Barbital; barbitone sodium	300 mg (gr 5)	Oral	Long
*Phenobarbital; phenobarbitone	30 to 100 mg (gr ½ to 1½)	Oral	Long
Mephobarbital (Mebaral)	400 to 600 mg (gr 6 to 10)	Oral	Long
Metharbital (Gemonil)	100 mg (gr 1½)	Oral	Long
*Amobarbital (Amytal)	100 mg (gr 1½)	Oral	Intermediate
Aprobarbital (Alurate)	60 to 120 mg (gr 1 to 2)	Oral	Intermediate
Butabarbital sodium (Butisol Sodium)	8 to 60 mg (gr ⅛ to 1)	Oral	Intermediate
Pentobarbital sodium (Nembutal Sodium); pentobarbitone sodium	100 mg (gr 1½)	Oral, rectal	Short
Secobarbital sodium (Seconal); quinalbarbitone sodium	100 to 200 mg (gr 1½ to 3)	Oral, rectal	Short
Sodium hexobarbital	2 to 4 ml 10%	Intravenous	Ultrashort
Thiopental sodium (Pentothal Sodium); thiopentone sodium	2 to 3 ml 2.5% in 10 to 15 seconds; repeated in 30 seconds as required	Intravenous	Ultrashort

*Sodium salts are available.

ing barbiturates have an onset of 45 to 60 minutes and a peak in 6 to 8 hours. See Table 8-8 for dosage, methods of administration, and length of action.

Administration. The oral channel of administration is preferred and should be used whenever possible. Certain preparations may be given subcutaneously, intramuscularly, intravenously, or rectally, depending on the purpose to be achieved and the general condition of the patient. The intravenous route is the most dangerous and used only for production of anesthesia or in emergencies. Parenteral administration is also used when a patient is too ill to take the drug orally or has nausea and vomiting or when it is important to have a rapid depressant action.

Contraindications. Barbiturates should be avoided for patients who manifest hypersensitivity toward them, patients with porphyria, elderly persons and children with paradoxic reactions, or those who have been previously dependent on them. If a patient tells the nurse that he is hypersensitive to this group of drugs, the statement should be recorded and the information made known to the physician. Seriously impaired hepatic or renal function may also constitute a contraindication for the use of these drugs, although only the physician can decide whether the degree of damage warrants the use of a different type of drug.

Side effects and toxic effects. Unusual effects or reactions may be exhibited as one or more of the following: (1) marked symptoms of hangover—listlessness, prolonged depression, nausea, and emotional disturbances; (2) skin rash, urticaria, swelling of the face, and asthmatic attack; and (3) bad dreams, restlessness, and delirium.

This last category of symptoms may be experienced especially by elderly or debilitated patients. Night nurses find that they need to watch older patients carefully when they have been given a hypnotic dose of a barbiturate. Such patients tend to go to the bathroom more frequently than younger adults and under the influence of a barbiturate may become confused and have difficulty orienting themselves. Barbital, amobarbital, and pentobarbital are said to exert this effect more often than phenobarbital.

Restlessness is also produced when barbiturates are administered to patients in severe pain. The drug, in this instance, does not relieve pain but depresses the higher centers that normally serve as control centers. Mental confusion and delirium may result. An analgesic is usually prescribed to be given with a barbiturate if the patient has pain.

Poisoning that may result from barbiturate use is discussed in Chapter 12.

Advantages and disadvantages encountered in the use of barbiturates. Barbiturates lend themselves to a variety of uses. They are anticonvulsants, anesthetics, hypnotics, and sedatives, although no one of them excels in all of these actions. They are easily administered in tablets or capsules and may be given rectally or parenterally. They have a reasonably wide margin of safety.

The main disadvantages are that in large doses they all depress the respiratory center and they are often used for suicide. In addition, they have a high dependence potential. These are drugs that should never be left at the bedside for the patient to take at will. Patients have been known to hoard barbiturates until they had enough to commit suicide.

In the past these drugs had wide use and were easily obtained, which resulted in indiscriminate use and use for suicidal purposes. State laws restrict the sale of hypnotic drugs and prohibit the sale or possession of barbiturates except under proper licensure. Barbiturates may not be purchased or dispensed without a physician's prescription, and the prescription may not be refilled without the physician's personal sanction.

Choice of barbiturate. In choosing barbiturate preparations, consideration is given primarily to the duration of effect produced by the drug and to individual needs of patients. Phenobarbital is an outstanding member of the group of barbiturates because of its anticonvulsant action. Secobarbital and pentobarbital are good examples of short-acting barbiturates, and the ultrashort-acting ones are described under anesthetics.

Barbiturates may be combined in the same capsule so that a long-acting and a short-acting or moderately long-acting preparation can be used to advantage for the patient who has difficulty both in getting to sleep and remaining asleep for the desired number of hours. Tuinal is an official combination of secobarbital sodium and amobarbital sodium. It is available in capsules containing gr ¾ (0.05 g) of each barbiturate (total 0.1 g, gr 1½) or gr 1½ of each (total 0.2 g, gr 3).

Phenobarbital

Phenobarbital has a long half-life (72 to 96 hours) and it can be administered once or twice daily. It is used when prolonged sedation is required. It is used as a hypnotic as well as a sedative for a variety of nervous conditions, such as chorea, gastrointestinal neuroses, and preoperative and postoperative states of tension. It is also used as a sedative for patients with hypertension and coronary artery disease. Because its action is rather slow, it is not the best drug for certain kinds of insomnia or for use as a preanesthetic medication. Adult hypnotic dose is 50 to 100 mg; sedative dose is 15 to 32 mg (gr ½). For children the daytime sedative dose is 2 mg/kg body weight in divided doses over 24 hours.

Phenobarbital has a selective depressant action on the motor cortex of the brain when given in sedative doses to epileptic patients. However, when effective anticonvulsant doses are given, some degree of central depression also results. (The patient feels tired, relaxed, and perhaps dull and sleepy.) In this respect phenobarbital is inferior to the anticonvulsant drug phenytoin (Dilantin). On the other hand, phenobarbital is regarded as one of the least, if not the least, toxic of the antiepileptic drugs. The dosage range for adults is 90 to 250 mg for convulsive disorders; for children the range is 3 to 5 mg/kg; for infants 8 mg/kg. The therapeutic plasma levels are 20 to 45 µg/ml. This may be given in one dose at bedtime or it may be given in divided doses throughout the day. Should it be necessary to discontinue the drug for an epileptic patient, it should be done gradually, never suddenly, or severe epileptic seizures may be precipitated. Phenobarbital is often given to patients after surgical operation on the brain to minimize the irritating effect of the procedure.

Patients may continue to take the drug for a year or more under medical supervision.

The action and uses of phenobarbital sodium are the same as those of phenobarbital except that it can be injected when phenobarbital either cannot be given by mouth or the desired effects are not being secured following oral administration.

Preparation, dosage, and administration. The following preparations are available.

Phenobarbital tablets; phenobarbitone tablets. Tablets containing 8, 15, 16, 32, 65, or 100 mg are available for oral administration.

Phenobarbital elixir. The elixir is for oral use only. Each 5 ml contains 20 mg of drug.

Phenobarbital sodium; phenobarbitone sodium. The usual dose is 100 mg (gr 1½). This is a powder dispensed in ampules for parenteral or oral administration.

Phenobarbital sodium injection. The usual parenteral dose is 100 mg (gr 1½). A sterile solution of phenobarbital sodium in a suitable solvent (50 mg in 1 ml, 125 mg in 1 or 5 ml, and 300 mg in 2 or 5 ml) may be used for intramuscular or subcutaneous injection. Aqueous solutions of phenobarbital sodium decompose on standing.

Phenobarbital sodium tablets; phenobarbitone sodium tablets. Tablets containing 30, 60, or 100 mg are available. The usual dose is 30 mg (gr ½) orally.

Phenobarbital is also available in 50-, 65-, and 100-mg sustained-release dosage forms.

Secobarbital sodium (Seconal)

Secobarbital sodium is a short-acting barbiturate, more active than barbital, and given in corresondingly smaller doses. Small doses produce a sedative effect and larger doses, a hypnotic effect.

Preparation, dosage, and administration. Dosage of secobarbital sodium is 100 mg (gr 1½) at bedtime for adults. As a preanesthetic agent, 100 to 200 mg is given 30 minutes to 1 hour before the patient goes to the operating room. Sedative dose for children is 6 mg/kg body weight daily divided into three doses; anticonvulsant dose is 3 to 5 mg/kg given intramuscularly or intravenously. It is available in

30-, 50-, and 100-mg capsules; 30-, 60-, 120-, and 200-mg rectal suppositories; 22 mg/5 ml; elixir and 50 mg/ml injection.

Pentobarbital sodium (Nembutal)

Pentobarbital sodium, the most widely used short-acting barbiturate, acts over a rather brief period of time (3 to 6 hours), which is sometimes an advantage, particularly if large doses have been given. It is used as a hypnotic and as a sedative prior to anesthesia.

Pentobarbital and pentobarbital calcium are similar in action and use to pentobarbital sodium. Pentobarbital calcium has no advantage except that it is better suited for making compressed tablets than sodium pentobarbital.

Preparation, dosage, and administration

Pentobarbital sodium elixir (Nembutal Sodium Elixir). The elixir contains 20 mg in 5 ml. It is used for sedation of children or elderly patients.

Pentobarbital sodium (Nembutal Sodium); pentobarbitone sodium. The usual hypnotic adult dose is 100 mg (gr 1½). Range of sedative dose for adults is 15 to 50 mg, which may be given three or four times daily. Sedative dose for children is 6 mg/kg body weight divided into three doses. Anticonvulsant dose is 3 to 5 mg/kg body weight. The preparation is available in capsules, ampules containing the drug in powder form or in solution for injection, suppositories for rectal administration, and sustained-release dosage forms for slow, continuous absorption. Pentobarbital sodium injection may be given intravenously if prompt action is essential to control convulsive seizures associated with some types of drug poisoning, rabies, tetanus, chorea, and eclampsia. Aqueous solutions of pentobarbital are not stable and decompose on standing or after boiling.

NONBARBITURATE SEDATIVES AND HYPNOTICS

Although several nonbarbiturate sedatives and hypnotics are available, it should be emphasized that all are habit forming, may cause physical dependence, and are subject to abuse.

Ethchlorvynol (Placidyl)

Ethchlorvynol (a tertiary acetylenic alcohol) is a colorless-to-yellow liquid with a pungent odor. It is a mild hypnotic somewhat less predictable than the barbiturates. It acts within 15 to 30 minutes after administration, and the duration of its effects is about 5 hours.

Uses. Ethchlorvynol is said to be useful in the treatment of insomnia if pain and anxiety are not complicating factors. It is also useful for patients who are unable to take barbiturates. It may be used as a daytime sedative. In addition it has anticonvulsant and muscle-relaxing actions.

Preparation, dosage, and administration. Ethchlorvynol is available in 100-, 200-, 500-, and 750-mg capsules. The usual adult hypnotic dose is 500 mg; sedative doses are correspondingly smaller. It is administered orally. Dosage for elderly and debilitated patients should be reduced to the smallest effective amount.

Side effects. This drug seems to have a wide margin of safety. Side effects include headache, fatigue, ataxia, dizziness, mental confusion, nightmares, and nausea and vomiting. Hypotension, mild hangover, and mild excitation have been reported.

Ethinamate (Valmid)

Ethinamate (a carbamate) exerts a mild sedative effect on the central nervous system. The duration of its effect is shorter than that produced by the barbiturates. It is effective within 15 to 25 minutes, and the duration of its effect is about 4 hours. It has not been known to cause habituation or dependence, and tolerance does not seem to develop. It is readily absorbed from the gastrointestinal tract and rapidly destroyed or excreted from the body.

Uses. It is used chiefly as a rapid-acting hypnotic for the treatment of simple insomnia. It can be used for patients with impaired function of the liver and kidney. It is not a hypnotic of choice for patients requiring heavy or continuous sedation.

Preparation, dosage, and administration. Ethinamate is available in 500-mg tablets. The minimal effective hypnotic dose for adults is 500 mg. Larger and repeated doses may be required to produce a full night's sleep. It is administered orally.

Side effects. Excitement in children, mild gastrointestinal symptoms, and skin rash have occurred with use of ethinamate. Use in children is not recommended. Patients who receive the drug over long periods of time should be carefully observed.

Glutethimide (Doriden)

Glutethimide (a piperidine derivative) is a hypnotic and sedative that depresses the central nervous system and produces effects similar to those produced by the short-acting barbiturates. The main advantage claimed for it is that it can be used for patients who do not tolerate the barbiturates. It is effective in 15 to 30 minutes and its effects last 4 to 8 hours. Hangover effects do not seem to be noticeable unless the drug is administered late at night or unless the dose is repeated in the course of the night. It is not considered an addicting agent in the same sense as morphine, but dependence has occurred. Its abuse has led to many cases of chronic and acute intoxication with a number of fatalities.

Uses. At present, the greatest use for glutethimide seems to be for relief of simple or nervous insomnia, provided it is uncomplicated by pain or severe agitation. It can be used both as a preoperative and as a daytime sedative.

Preparation, dosage, and administration. Gluthethimide is marketed in 125-, 250-, and 500-mg tablets. The usual hypnotic dose for adults is 500 mg given orally at bedtime. For daytime sedation, 125 to 250 mg may be given orally three times daily after meals. For preoperative sedation 500 mg the night before surgery and 500 to 1000 mg 1 hour before anesthesia may be given.

Side effects. The principal side effects seem to be nausea and, occasionally, skin rash. Toxic effects and treatment are much the same as those for poisoning with the barbiturates. Treatment of poisoning may be quite difficult.

Methyprylon (Noludar)

Methyprylon (a piperidine derivative) depresses the central nervous system in a manner similar to the barbiturates except that it has less tendency to depress the respiratory center. The onset of action is about 30 minutes and duration of action is about 7 hours. Its capacity to cause dependence is thought to be less than that of the barbiturates, although further study may prove otherwise.

Uses. Methyprylon is used in the treatment of simple and nervous insomnia.

Preparation, dosage, and administration. Methyprylon is marketed in 50- and 200-mg tablets and 300-mg capsules. Doses of 50 to 100 mg three or four times daily are prescribed to produce sedation, and 200 to 400 mg is the usual adult hypnotic dose given at bedtime.

Side effects. The incidence of side effects is thought to be low, although the following have been observed: nausea, vomiting, constipation, diarrhea, headache, itching, and skin rash. No serious toxic effects on the kidney, liver, or bone marrow have been reported.

Methaqualone hydrochloride (Mequin, Parest, Quaalude)

Methaqualone is a quiazolone-derivative, sedative-hypnotic acting in a site that is different from that of the barbiturates or glutethimide. It also has antitussive and antispasmodic activity. It is metabolized in the liver and excreted in the urine and feces.

Preparation, dosage, and administration. Usual adult dose for sleep is 150 to 300 mg (200 to 400 mg of the hydrochloride salt) at bedtime, since drowsiness is produced within 10 to 20 minutes. If the patient was using barbiturates or nonbarbiturate sedative-hypnotics immediately prior to therapy with methaqualone, then a dose given on consecutive evenings over a period of 1 week is needed to attain a satisfactory patient hypnotic response. The lowest possible individualized dose should be used in elderly, debilitated, or agitated patients and titrated to the desired response. Methaqualone is available in 150- and 300-mg base and 200 and 400 mg of the hydrochloride salt (175 mg base is equivalent to 200 mg of the hydrochloride salt).

Flurazepam (Dalmane)

Flurazepam is related to the benzodiazepine compounds such as chlordiazepoxide (Librium), which are widely used as tranquilizers. Numerous side effects have been reported. In elderly persons dizziness, staggering, ataxia, and falling have occurred. Flurazepam has become a very popular drug. It is claimed that flurazepam is useful in the therapy of all sleep disorders since it does not suppress dream or REM sleep. However, it does decrease deep sleep. It reduces sleep induction time and increases sleep duration time. Hypnotic effects occur in 20 to 45 minutes and sedative effects last 50 to 100 hours. It is available in 15- and 30-mg capsules. Usual adult dose is 30 mg at bedtime; for elderly patients initial dose is 15 mg every second or third night. Half-life for parent drug is 1 to 4 hours, and for metabolite 47 to 100 hours.

Flurazepam is becoming so popular as a hypnotic that it is replacing many of the barbiturates.

Temazepam (Restoril)

Temazepam, an oral benzodiazepine, is a 3-hydroxy derivative of diazepam that may be referred to as N-methyl oxazepam. It is used for relief of insomnia associated with difficulty in falling asleep and frequent or early awakenings. An advantage of this agent is its neglible accumulation of inactive metabolites. There are no active metabolites. A short biphasic half-life exists with a range of 9 to 12 hours. After total absorption from the gastrointestinal tract and complete hepatic metabolism occur, the drug is eliminated in the urine by the morning with a low incidence of behavioral impairment. The major metabolic pathway terminates with glucuronide conjugation and the minor metabolic pathway leads to oxazepam. Generally the glucuronide conjugation is affected by hepatic disease to a lesser degree than by the oxidative process. In hepatic disease the 3-hydroxylated derivatives such as temazepam, oxazepam, and lorazepam are more desirable. The rapid elimination with negligible accumulation decreases the incidence of residual hangover seen with long-acting benzodiazepines (those with an active intermediate metabolite as N-desmethyl diazepam).

The adult dose is individualized with 15 mg (in the elderly) and 30 mg before retiring pro-

ducing effective total sleep time for 7 to 8 hours. Peak concentration occurs in 2 to 3 hours after oral administration, with serum detection within 40 minutes.

The most reported common adverse effects include mild and transient drowsiness, dizziness, and lethargy. The patient information, contraindications, precautions, drug abuse, and dependence are similar to the other benzodiazepines. The patient should be told that after the first or second day of discontinuation sleep disturbances may be experienced.

OLDER HYPNOTICS

There are a number of hypnotics that were almost abandoned when the barbiturates became popular. They seem to be gradually regaining some of their lost popularity. They include chloral hydrate and paraldehyde as well as a number of others.

Chloral hydrate (Noctec)

Chloral hydrate was first synthesized in 1862. It is the oldest of the hypnotics and is still used. It is a chlorinated derivative of acetaldehyde, or it may be described as a hydrate of trichloracetaldehyde. It is a crystalline substance that has a bitter taste and a penetrating odor. It is readily soluble in water, alcohols, and oils such as olive oil.

Action and result. Locally, chloral hydrate is an irritant. Systemically, it depresses the central nervous system and decreases awareness of external stimuli. It acts promptly (10 to 15 minutes) and produces sleep that lasts 4 to 8 hours or more. It is metabolized to trichloroethanol (the active metabolite), which has a half-life of 8 to 10 hours, and inactivated by converson to trichloroacetic acid, which is excreted in the urine. The sleep produced greatly resembles natural sleep; the patient can be awakened without difficulty. It produces little or no analgesic effect, and it is neither an anesthetic nor an anticonvulsant.

In therapeutic doses there is little or no effect on the heart and respiratory center. The pulse and blood pressure are not lowered more than can be observed in ordinary sleep. In large doses chloral hydrate depresses the respiratory and vasomotor centers, resulting in slowed respiration and dilation of cutaneous blood vessels. Effect on the heart is said to be similar to that of chloroform. Overdoses will cause cardiac depression, especially in patients with heart disease.

Uses. Chloral hydrate is used as a sedative. It produces sedation similar to paraldehyde and the barbiturates. It is sometimes used to relieve symptoms during the withdrawal phase of drug dependence (alcoholism, opiate, or barbiturate).

Chloral hydrate is used as a hypnotic when insomnia is not the result of pain. Its chief disadvantage is that it can produce gastric irritation. It also has an unpleasant taste, but this problem is remedied by administering the drug in capsule form.

Preparation, dosage, and administration. The usual adult hypnotic dose of chloral hydrate is 500 mg to 1 g taken 15 to 30 minutes before bedtime. Larger doses may also be prescribed (up to 2 g). Adult sedative dose is 250 mg three times daily after meals. Hypnotic dose for children is 50 mg/kg; sedative dose is 25 mg/kg divided into three or four doses. It is marketed in soft gelatin capsules containing 250 and 500 mg; in suppository form containing 335, 500, 650, and 975 mg; in an elixir containing 500 mg; and as a syrup containing 250 or 500 mg/5 ml.

If the liquid solution is administered it should be well diluted with water or given in a syrup or milk to disguise the taste. It is sometimes given to children in the form of a retention enema (dissolved in oil). It is too irritating to be given parenterally. It should not be given with alcohol to avoid the additive effects of two depressant drugs. Such a combination is sometimes referred to as a "Mickey Finn" or knockout drops.

Side effects and toxic effects. Symptoms of both acute and chronic toxicity are sometimes observed. The local effects of the drug may cause nausea and vomiting when it is taken orally.

Although chloral hydrate has a wide safety range, acute poisoning can occur. Symptoms are similar to those of any central depressant and include deep sleep, stupor, coma, lowered blood pressure, slow weak pulse, slow respira-

tion, and cyanosis. Death is usually caused by respiratory depression or it may result from sudden heart failure in patients who have cardiac damage. If the patient survives, there is a possibility that damage may have been done to the liver and kidneys.

Treatment is essentially the same as that for acute poisoning with barbiturates.

Chloral hydrate habitues develop some tolerance to the drug, but habit formation is not common. It sometimes results in chronic poisoning, manifested by degenerative changes in the liver and kidneys, nervous disturbances, weakness, skin manifestations, and gastrointestinal disturbances. Treatment is gradual withdrawal of the drug and rehabilitative measures similar to those used in the treatment of the alcoholic.

Contraindications. Chloral hydrate is contraindicated for patients with serious heart disease or impaired function of the liver and kidney and sometimes for patients with gastric or duodenal ulcer.

Triclofos sodium (Triclos)

A phosphate ester of trichloroethanol, triclofos sodium is a derivative of chloral that exhibits a hypnotic and sedative action similar to chloral hydrate. It is better tolerated than the latter drug, because it has less odor and aftertaste, and it produces less gastric irritation. It has a wide margin of safety.

Preparation, dosage, and administration. Triclofos is available in 750-mg tablets and syrup containing 100 mg/ml. The usual hypnotic dose is 1500 mg.

Paraldehyde

Paraldehyde, a cyclic ether, has been used as a hypnotic since 1882, when it was introduced into medicine. It is a colorless, transparent liquid with a strong odor and a disagreeable taste. It is only slightly soluble in water but freely soluble in oils and in alcohol.

Paraldehyde is rapidly absorbed from the mucosa of the gastrointestinal tract and also from intramuscular sites of injection, although it may cause some irritation when given parenterally. A large part (70% to 80%) of it is metabolized in the liver. It is, therefore, contraindicated for patients who have serious impairment of liver function or slowed elimination rate from hepatic insufficiency. It is not contraindicated for patients with renal disease. A significant part (11% to 28%) of the drug is excreted unchanged by the lungs, where it tends to increase bronchial secretions; for this reason it is avoided for patients with bronchopulmonary disease.

Uses. Paraldehyde is employed for its hypnotic and sedative effects in treatment of conditions in which there is a threat of convulsive seizures or nervous hyperexcitability, eclampsia, status epilepticus, delirium tremens, and tetanus. It is sometimes used as a basal anesthetic, particularly for children; when so used it is given rectally.

Action and result. Paraldehyde depresses the central nervous system, producing onset of drowsiness and sleep in 10 to 15 minutes after a hypnotic oral dose. The sleep closely resembles a natural sleep and lasts for 4 to 8 hours. Therapeutic doses do not depress the medullary centers and do not affect the heart and respiration. It is less potent than chloral hydrate but also less toxic. It is not an analgesic, but it may compel sleep in spite of pain. After intramuscular administration the half-life is 3.4 to 9.8 hours.

Preparation, dosage, and administration. Paraldehyde is available as a plain liquid for oral administration or as a sterile solution, 1 g/ml in 2- 5-, and 10-ml ampules or 30-ml vials for parenteral use. The nurse must only use a glass syringe because the paraldehyde reacts with plastic syringes. The usual adult oral dose is 5 to 10 ml but may be increased to 15 or 30 ml. The dose for children is 0.15 to 0.3 ml/kg body weight. When paraldehyde is given orally it should be disguised in a suitable medium such as a flavored syrup, iced fruit juice, wine, or milk, and it should be very cold to minimize the odor and taste. It can also be given as a retention enema (mixed with vegetable or olive oil). When given intramuscularly (never subcutaneously) a pure sterile preparation should be used. The usual intramuscular dose of 5 ml is a transiently painful injection and should not be administered in the area of a nerve trunk because, like alcohol, paraldehyde causes nerve injury and paralysis. Intravenous administra-

tion is dangerous, because a toxic dose causes pulmonary hemorrhage, edema, dilation and failure of the right heart. The drug must be diluted in saline in a glass syringe for use. A rate of 0.5 ml of active drug per minute in IV push should not be exceeded. For intravenous administration the nurse must dilute 2 ml paraldehyde to a volume of 4 ml with saline and administer 1 ml of this diluted solution (0.5 ml of active drug) per minute slowly and cautiously over a 1-minute period. It is rarely (emergency only, as for convulsions) given intravenously (3 to 5 ml well diluted in normal saline). Paraldehyde must be stored in tight, light-resistant containers in a cold place. Paraldehyde from a container opened longer than 24 hours must be discarded since it can be completely converted to acetic acid, and fatality may occur if the converted drug is administered.

Side effects and toxic effects. The chief disadvantages of paraldehyde are its obnoxious odor, disagreeable taste, and irritating effect on the throat and stomach if the drug is not well diluted in a suitable medium. Because of the odor it is not suitable for patients who are up and about, for they will reek with the odor of the drug. Fortunately, if the patient is capable of noticing the odor, his sense of smell becomes dulled after a time. Paraldehyde is not as safe a drug as was once thought; it is now known that the margin between an anesthetic and a lethal dose is very narrow. Symptoms of overdosage resemble those of alcohol overdosage in that mild poisoning can usually be "slept off." The incidence of acute toxicity is low, although deaths from paraldehyde depression have been reported. The symptoms of poisoning and treatment are essentially the same as those for chloral hydrate. In spite of the taste and odor, some patients do become dependent on paraldehyde.

Bromides

The term "bromides" frequently refers to sodium bromide, although a number of bromide salts were popular. They have been used for their sedative, hypnotic, and anticonvulsant effects, but their range of usefulness has been narrowed because of the appearance of better drugs. They are slow-acting depressants of the nervous system. Bromide intoxication, by severe toxic psychoses, however, is still encountered.

NURSING IMPLICATIONS FOR SEDATIVES AND HYPNOTIC SLEEP MEDICATIONS

It is important for nurses to remember:

1 Sleeping medications (hypnotics or sedatives) cause dreaming sleep to be less than normal.
2 When sleeping medications or hypnotics are discontinued, a rebound occurs, and dreaming sleep increases markedly until the loss has been overcome.
3 Sleeping medications cause a prolonged alteration in the individual's normal sleep pattern, which may still be present 3 to 5 weeks after the sleeping medication has been discontinued.
4 Altering the sleep pattern affects the individual physically and emotionally.

Since nurses are in a strategic position to influence the sleep their patients receive, it cannot be stressed enough that nurses must exercise caution when making decisions about giving or repeating an h.s. or p.r.n. order for a sleeping medication, hypnotic, or sedative. Nurses who immediately resort to administering a sleeping medication when a patient complains of being unable to sleep may be doing the patient more harm than good. It is important for nurses to keep informed about the drugs they administer, since there continues to be new knowledge about drugs, and this includes the so-called old drugs.

Nurses must also teach patients and their families ways to promote good sleep without resorting to drugs—including over-the-counter drugs.

Nurses should find out from their patients what their sleep habits are and what they do to ensure good sleep at home. For example:

1 What do they do about environmental control, which includes ventilation, lighting, and noise?
2 What do they do about physical care? Do they shower before retiring or go for a walk?
3 What do they do about food? Do they ingest a snack before retiring?
4 What do they do about quiet recreation before sleep, such as reading?

The patient's sleep history and drug history can be valuable aids to help plan the nursing care for the patient that will best promote good sleep.

Another very important factor is that every effort should be made not to disrupt the patient while he is sleeping, if at all possible. Numerous interruptions for various aspects of care can do nothing but alter the patient's sleep pattern.

ALCOHOLS

Although there are many alcohols that vary physically from liquids to solids, the alcohol usually meant, unless otherwise specified, is ethyl alcohol. Methyl alcohol, propyl alcohol, butyl alcohol, and amyl alcohol are examples of other alcohols. Chemically speaking, they are hydroxy derivatives of aliphatic hydrocarbons.

Ethyl alcohol

Ethyl alcohol has been known in an impure form since earliest times, and it is the only alcohol used extensively in medicine. It was formerly thought to be a remedy for almost any disease or disorder. It is a colorless liquid and lighter than water, with which it mixes readily. It lowers surface tension and acts as a good solvent for a number of substances. In concentrations above 40% it is flammable. Ethyl alcohol, also referred to as grain alcohol, is the product of the fermentation of a sugar by yeast.

Action and result. Ethyl alcohol may have either a local or a systemic action.

Local. Ethyl alcohol denatures proteins by precipitation and dehydration. This is said to be the basis for its germicidal, irritant, and astringent effects. It irritates denuded skin, mucous membranes, and subcutaneous tissue. Considerable pain may be experienced from a subcutaneous injection of alcohol, and slough of the tissue may result. When it is injected into or near a nerve it may produce degeneration of the nerve and anesthesia. Alcohol evaporates readily from the skin, produces a cooling effect, and reduces the temperature of the skin. When rubbed on the surface of the body it acts as a mild counterirritant. It dries and hardens the epithelial layer of the skin and helps to prevent bed sores when used externally. However, its use on skin that is already dry and irritated is usually contraindicated. Solutions of ethyl alcohol that measure 70% by weight seem to exert the best bactericidal effects. High concentrations have a marked dehydrating effect but do not necessarily kill bacteria. Ethyl alcohol in proper concentration is considered an effective germicide for a number of uses, but it does not kill spores.

Systemic. According to modern scientific authorities alcohol is not considered a stimulant (popular ideas to the contrary). It is thought to interfere with the transmission of nerve impulses at synaptic connections, but how this is accomplished is not known. It exerts a progressive and continuous depression on the central nervous system (cerebrum, cerebellum, cord, and medulla). Its action is comparable to that of the general anesthetics. The excitement stage, however, is longer, and when the anesthetic stage is reached, definite toxic symptoms are present. Also, when alcohol is taken socially, attempts are usually made to stay in an early stage rather than to pass rapidly to unconsciousness. The margin between the anesthetic and fatal dose is a narrow one. What sometimes appears to be stimulation results from the depression of the higher faculties of the brain and represents the loss of learned inhibitions acquired by socialization.

The results of the action of alcohol vary with the individual, one's tolerance, the presence or absence of extraneous stimuli, and the rate of ingestion. Small or moderate quantities produce a feeling of well-being, talkativeness, greater vivacity, and increased confidence in one's mental and physical power. The personality becomes expansive, and there is a general loss of inhibitions. The finer powers of discrimination, concentration, insight, judgment, and memory are gradually dulled and lost. Large quantities of the drug may cause excitement, impulsive speech and behavior, laughter, hilarity, and, in some cases, pugnaciousness. Others may become melancholy or unduly sentimental. The individual usually becomes ataxic, mutters incoherently, has disturbance of the special senses, is often nauseated, may vomit, and eventually lapses into stupor or coma.

The respiratory center is not depressed except by large doses.

CARDIOVASCULAR. Alcohol depresses the vaso-motor center in the medulla and in this way brings about dilation of the peripheral blood vessels, especially those of the skin. This causes a feeling of warmth. Because of the dilation of the capillaries, heat is lost from the interior. This accounts for the fact that an intoxicated person may freeze to death more quickly than a normal person. Alcohol also depresses the heat-regulating mechanism in a manner similar to the antipyretics, and before the advent of the modern antipyretics it was used to reduce fever.

Small doses (10 to 25 ml) produce an insignificant increase in the pulse rate, caused mainly by the excitement and the reflex effect on the gastrointestinal tract. Larger doses produce the same effect but may be followed by lowered blood pressure caused by the effect on the vasoconstrictor center. Only high concentrations of alcohol depress the heart.

GASTROINTESTINAL. The effect of alcohol on the function of the digestive organs depends on the presence or absence of gastrointestinal disease, the degree of alcoholic tolerance, and the concentration of the beverage used as well as the type and amount of food present. Small doses in the patient who likes alcohol will stimulate the secretion of gastric juice rich in acid. Salivary secretion is also reflexly stimulated. Large and concentrated doses of alcohol tend to inhibit secretion and enzyme activity in the stomach, although the effect in the intestine seems to be negligible. However, when large quantities of alcohol are taken over a period of time, gastritis, nutritional deficiencies, and other untoward results have been observed.

Absorption and excretion. Since alcohol does not require digestion in the stomach or intestine it is readily absorbed from both organs. Ninety percent or more of the alcohol that is absorbed is metabolized, chiefly in the liver. It is oxidized first to acetaldehyde and eventually to carbon dioxide and water. It is oxidized at the rate of about 10 g/hour, which amounts to about 70 calories. Alcohol does not form glycogen and hence it cannot be stored, so that it is a food only in the sense that it contributes calories. It supplies no minerals or vitamins.

Alcohol that escapes oxidation is excreted

TABLE 8-9 Relation between clinical indications of alcoholic intoxication and concentration of alcohol of the blood and urine

Stage	Blood alcohol (%)	Urine alcohol (%)	Clinical observations
Subclinical	0 to 0.11	0 to 0.15	Normal by ordinary observations; slight changes detectable by special tests
Emotional instability	0.09 to 0.21	0.13 to 0.29	Decreased inhibitions; emotional instability; slight muscular incoordination; slowing of responses to stimuli
Confusion	0.18 to 0.33	0.26 to 0.45	Disturbance of sensation; decreased pain sense; staggering gait; slurred speech
Stupor	0.27 to 0.43	0.36 to 0.58	Marked decrease in response to stimuli; muscular incoordination approaching paralysis
Coma	0.36 to 0.56	0.48 to 0.72	Complete unconsciousness; depressed reflexes; subnormal temperature; anesthesia; impairment of circulation; possible death
Death (uncomplicated)	Over 0.44	Over 0.60	

by way of the lungs and kidneys, and some is found in a number of excretions such as sweat.

Alcohol produces an increased flow of urine because of increased fluid intake, which ordinarily accompanies the drinking of alcoholic beverages. It has been suggested that alcohol may also act as a diuretic through central nervous system depression and inhibition of ADH (antidiuretic hormone) release. If the patient has preexisting renal disease, there may be further damage to the kidney. Large and concentrated doses of alcohol are thought to injure the renal epithelium.

Since alcohol, after absorption, is distributed in the tissues of the body in approximately the same ratio as their water content, a rough estimate of the quantity taken may be obtained from an analysis of the blood and urine (Table 8-9).

The National Safety Council regards concentration of alcohol in the blood up to 0.05% as evidence of unquestioned sobriety. Concentrations between 0.051% and 0.149% are regarded as grounds for suspicion and for use of performance tests, and anything more than 0.15% is evidence of unquestionable intoxication. The states differ as to what is accepted as a legal limit.

Effects of alcohol that may not be discernible to the casual observer become apparent when the individual who has had a number of doses of alcohol attempts to operate a piece of power machinery such as an automobile.

Visual acuity (especially peripheral vision) is diminished, reaction time is slowed, judgment and self-control are impaired, and the individual tends to be complacent and pleased with himself. Many drivers will take chances when under the influence of alcohol that they would never take ordinarily. This leads to disaster, as statistics reveal.

Uses. Ethyl alcohol is used topically as an astringent and antiseptic. It is rubbed on the backs and buttocks of patients to prevent decubiti. It is used to cleanse the skin, and it is poured on dressings over wounds. It is a popular disinfectant for the skin.

It is an excellent solvent and preservative for many medicines and medicinal mixtures (spirits, elixirs, fluidextracts).

Alcohol sponges are given to lower the temperature of the patient with a high fever since it increases heat dissipation. Caution must be exercised when alcohol sponges are given, particularly to children, since alcohol intoxication can occur.

At times alcohol is injected into a nerve to destroy sensory nerve fibers and relieve pain associated with a severe and protracted neuralgia, such as trifacial neuralgia (tic douloureux) or inoperable cancer. An injection of 80% ethyl alcohol is used. Effects may persist for 1 to 3 years or until regeneration of the peripheral nerve fibers takes place.

Alcohol is used to produce vasodilation in peripheral vascular disease. Concentrated solutions often produce greater peripheral vasodilation than any other drug. The pain associated with Buerger's disease may be relieved with the use of ethyl alcohol administered orally. It may be prescribed to decrease the frequency of anginal attacks but effects are said to be unreliable. Benefits to the cardiac patient, if they occur, are believed to result from the rest and relaxation that the alcohol produces.

Alcohol is also used as an appetizer for patients with poor appetite during periods of convalescence and debility. From 5% to 10% solutions of alcohol have also been given in intravenous fluids (5% dextrose and isotonic saline solution) to supplement the caloric intake.

It may be used as a hypnotic for older persons who do not tolerate other hypnotics. It is used as a home remedy or for a hospitalized patient who requests it. It is occasionally given in intravenous fluids for its sedative effects—to reduce the amount of opiate or barbiturate needed to keep a patient comfortable.

Preparations and dosage. The following are various preparations of ethyl alcohol. Dosage varies with the purpose for which the alcohol is administered. When whiskey is prescribed as a vasodilator, 30 ml may be ordered to be given two or three times a day. When an alcoholic beverage is given for its effects as an appetizer, it should be given before meals. From 30 to 60 ml is usually given.

Alcohol (ethyl alcohol, ethanol). Alcohol contains not less than 92.3% by weight corresponding to approximately 94.9% by volume of C_2H_5OH.

Diluted alcohol. The diluted form contains not less than 41% and not more than 42% by weight of ethyl alcohol.

Whiskey (spiritus frumenti). Whiskey is an alcoholic liquid that is obtained by the distillation of the fermented mash of wholly or partly malted cereal grain and contains approximately 50% by volume of ethyl alcohol. It usually is stored in charred wood containers for a period of not less than 2 years.

Brandy (spiritus vini vitis). Brandy is an alcoholic liquid obtained by the distillation of the fermented juice of sound, ripe grapes. It contains approximately 50% by volume of ethyl alcohol. It is stored in wood containers, frequently as long as 2 years.

Other spirits are solutions of volatile substances in alcohol. In most cases the dissolved substance has a more important action than the alcohol, which is used merely as a solvent.

Wines. Wines are fermented liquors made from grapes or other fruit juices. Besides alcohol, wines may contain various acids, such as tartaric, tannic, or malic.

Dry wines are those that contain no added sugar. They contain about 10% alcohol.

Sweet wines are those to which sugar has been added. They contain about 15% alcohol.

Sparkling wines contain carbon dioxide, which makes them effervescent. Examples are champagne and sparkling burgundy.

Acute alcoholism. In states of acute intoxication the patient is stuporous or comatose, the skin is cold and clammy, respirations are noisy and slow, and pupils are dilated or normal. The breath is usually heavy with alcoholic fumes. Death may result if the coma is prolonged or if injury, hypostatic pneumonia, or infection complicates the picture.

Ordinary intoxication treats itself with time and sleep. In severe intoxication the stomach should be emptied. Emetics in cases of deep narcosis are inactive and worse than useless because they add to the depression. The stomach, therefore, should be emptied with a stomach tube. Difference of opinion exists as to the use of analeptic drugs, but if the depression is deep and the patient cannot be aroused, drugs such as amphetamine phosphate, pentylenetetrazol, methylphenidate hydrochloride, and others have been recommended. In case of threatened respiratory failure, artificial respiration and the inhalation of oxygen and carbon dioxide may be beneficial. The patient's position should be changed frequently to combat development of hypostatic pneumonia. As the patient emerges from a comatose state he may become acutely active and require the administration of a sedative. (Chlorpromazine should *not* be given; it potentiates the effects of alcohol.) Recovery is comparable to recovery from an anesthetic.

The headache, nervousness, and gastric irritability that frequently follow acute alcoholism are best relieved by antacids and demulcents, such as sodium bicarbonate and bismuth subcarbonate. The combined use of glucose and insulin therapy has been advocated by some because it promotes slightly the detoxication of alcohol. The administration of isotonic saline solution intravenously will help the dehydrated patient by reestablishing the electrolyte pattern of the blood.

Chronic alcoholism. The more common manifestations of chronic alcoholism are redness of the face, nose, and conjunctivae caused by the injection of the blood vessels, gastroenteritis, cirrhotic changes in the liver, nephritis, arteriosclerosis and chronic myocardial changes, amblyopia caused by orbital optic neuritis, dulling of the mental faculties, tremors caused by degeneration, and muscular weakness. Not infrequently, the prolonged use of alcohol leads to mental change, which may manifest itself in the gradual weakening of the mental powers, with hallucinations and delusions or other forms of psychosis. To be successfully treated the chronic alcoholic must want to be treated and must want to get well. Early establishment of rapport between the patient and the physician as well as with the nurse is very important. Treatment must include rehabilitation and help in making better adjustments to the patient's living conditions. The best results are probably obtained in a hospital.

Careful attention should be given to the patient's physical needs, such as diet, fluid balance, and general hygiene, since optimal physical fitness makes the patient feel better and increases his ability to deal with the problems that have contributed to his illness or have caused it to continue. Particular attention is given to supplying adequate amounts of vitamin B complex and ascorbic acid.

Sedatives and tranquilizing agents make the patient more comfortable, help him to sleep better, and relieve anxiety. The patient is also likely to eat better.

There is need for adequate medical supervision at all times as well as for good nursing care if good results are to be attained. Although relapses are frequent, fewer alcoholics relapse after treatment than those who are treated for morphine dependence.

In the treatment of chronic alcoholism, two additional aspects of treatment are deserving of mention because of the success that has been attained. The first is the psychologic approach to the problem or problems of the chronic alcoholic as made by Alcoholics Anonymous. This is an organization composed entirely of rehabilitated alcoholics who are, therefore, in a unique position to understand the problems of other alcoholics. The organization has its headquarters in New York and has many local groups in cities and towns throughout the United States. Frequent meetings, mutual assistance and understanding, and a definite program of constructive rehabilitation have resulted in the fact that approximately 50% of those who enter the organization with a sincere desire to stop drinking do so. Another 25% are reclaimed after one or more failures, and most of the remaining 25% are for one reason or another never successfully reclaimed. Another technique has involved the administration of a drug (disulfiram [Antabuse]) that the subject knows will produce unpleasant symptoms if he then takes alcohol.

Delirium tremens is a form of psychosis that sometimes develops in the chronic alcoholic. It usually occurs after prolonged excessive drinking followed by abstinence and can be viewed as a type of withdrawal syndrome comparable to that seen after withdrawal of barbiturates in persons addicted to them. In the alcoholic who has been drinking for some time it may be precipitated by exposure, surgical operation, or serious illness, especially pneumonia. There may be warning symptoms such as restlessness, insomnia, anorexia, anxiety, fear, and tremor. Chronic alcoholics refer to the first stage of delirium tremens as the "shakes." During the attack the patient continues to have tremor, insomnia, delirium, and terrifying hallucinations of such things as snakes and small animals creeping over him. The patient may have a temperature of 102° to 103° F. Death may result from collapse, traumatism, or infection.

Many methods of treatment have been tried. Sedatives such as paraldehyde, amobarbital sodium, mephobarbital, and some of the tranquilizing agents are tried when the patient is maniacal. Symptomatic treatment of the patient includes attention to fluids, nutrition, and vitamins. Some physicians have found ACTH and cortisone beneficial in promoting recovery.

Contraindications. Ethyl alcohol is contraindicated for certain persons and should be avoided by others. This includes the following:

1 Patients who have ulceration of the gastrointestinal tract, especially patients with hyperacidity and gastric or duodenal ulcers
2 Patients with acute infections of the genitourinary organs
3 Pregnant women
4 Epileptic persons
5 Patients with liver or kidney disease
6 Persons with personality problems, maladjusted persons, or those who have at one time been alcohol or drug dependent

Alcohol and life span. The effect of alcohol on resistance to infection and on the life span has been a subject of controversy for many years. It is believed that evidence is lacking to prove that moderate amounts of alcohol have much effect one way or the other. Statistics show, however, that chronic alcoholics and heavy drinkers have a shorter life span than those who abstain from alcohol. Some of the ill effects that have been attributed to alcohol have been found to be caused by general impairment of health, which in turn is caused by malnutrition and poor hygiene. Apparently, it often is not so much the direct effect of alcohol that injures the person as the inability of the alcoholic to take care of himself and others.

Ethanol has been implicated in inducing reproductive dysfunction from abuse and as a gonadal toxin, a teratogen, a mutagen, and an inhibitor of fertilization. The fetal alcohol syndrome is discussed in Chapter 12. Experiments have shown that the fetus is sensitive to alcohol during the period of organogenesis. In addition to the direct toxic effects ascribed to ethanol itself, acetaldehyde, the primary oxidation product of ethanol, is implicated in initiating birth defects and has been shown to cause an increase in the frequency of sister chromatid exchange. Acetaldehyde can be teratogenic and mutagenic and has been shown to inhibit testic-

ular production of testosterone. The nurse should discuss with the patient the risk of alcohol consumption during pregnancy and also the fact that alcohol enters breast milk and decreases mother's milk.

Methyl alcohol (wood alcohol)

Methyl alcohol is prepared on a large scale by the destructive distillation of wood. It has also been prepared synthetically. It is important in medicine chiefly because of the cases of poisoning that have resulted from its ingestion. The main effects are on the central nervous system. However, intoxication does not occur as readily as with ethyl alcohol unless large amounts are consumed. Methyl alcohol is oxidized in the tissues to formic acid, which is poorly metabolized. This is the basis for the development of a severe acidosis. Symptoms of poisoning include nausea and vomiting, abdominal pain, headache, dyspnea, blurred vision, and cold clammy skin. Symptoms may progress to delirium, convulsions, coma, and death. In nonfatal cases the patient may become blind or suffer from impaired vision. Treatment is directed toward the relief of acidosis since this seems to be related to the severity of the visual symptoms. Large amounts of sodium bicarbonate may be needed to treat acidosis successfully. Obviously, methyl alcohol is much more toxic than ethyl alcohol. One dose of 60 ml has been known to cause permanent blindness. Fluids containing methyl alcohol usually bear a "Poison" label.

Isopropyl alcohol

Isopropyl alcohol is a clear, colorless liquid with a characteristic odor and a bitter taste. It is miscible with water, chloroform, and ether but insoluble in salt solutions. It is a good solvent for creosote and compares favorably with ethyl alcohol in its antiseptic action. It has been recommended for disinfection of the skin and for rubbing compounds and lotions to be used on the skin. Its bactericidal effects are said to increase as its concentration approaches 100%. It differs in this respect from ethyl alcohol.

It is occasionally misused as a beverage. It can cause severe poisoning and death. The first symptoms are similar to intoxication from ethyl alcohol, but the symptoms progress to coma from which the patient may not recover.

Butyl and amyl alcohols

Butyl and amyl alcohols are said to be several times as toxic as ethyl alcohol.

DRUGS USED IN TREATMENT OF CHRONIC ALCOHOLISM
Disulfiram (Antabuse)

Action and result. Disulfiram is used to sensitize an individual to alcohol by bringing about an unpleasant alcohol-disulfiram reaction. This "disulfiram reaction" begins with flushing in the face, which develops into intense vasodilation of the face, neck, and upper part of the body. Hyperventilation and increased pulse rate may occur. Nausea may occur in 30 to 60 minutes along with facial pallor, hypotension, and copious vomiting. There is usually an intense feeling of discomfort, pulsating headache, palpitations, dyspnea, syncope, and a constrictive feeling in the neck. The reaction lasts from 30 to 60 minutes to several hours, as long as alcohol is being metabolized; it is then followed by drowsiness and sleep. This experience is so unpleasant that alcohol tends to repel the individual who does not wish to reexperience the discomforting symptoms.

In the body, alcohol is oxidized to acetaldehyde. Disulfiram inhibits the enzyme aldehyde dehydrogenase, which converts acetaldehyde to acetate. This permits acetaldehyde to accumulate and cause unpleasant toxic effects. Disulfiram has few effects unless the person ingests alcohol. A 50% success rate in the treatment of alcoholism has been reported by some study groups.

Preparations, dosage, and administration. Patients must be carefully selected, must be given a thorough explanation of the treatment and unpleasantness they will experience, and must give full consent for treatment. All signs of alcohol intoxication must be absent, and the patient should not have ingested alcohol for at least 12 hours prior to initiation of therapy. A daily dose of 500 mg disulfiram is given in the morning for a period of 1 to 2 weeks. Tablets may be crushed and mixed with a suitable liquid for those unable to swallow the tablet. The physician may then administer a dose of alcohol to produce the typical symptoms that will repel the individual from ingesting alcohol. The alcohol test may not be given at all, and it is usually omitted for patients over age 50. A maintenance dose of 250 mg (range of dosage is 125 to 500 mg) may then be given for months or years, depending on the individual. The act of taking the daily dose of disulfiram serves as a daily rededication to avoid use of alcohol. Effects persist for up to 2 weeks after discontinuance of therapy, because of slow absorption and elimination, and patients should be warned not to ingest any alcohol during this time. A patient receiving disulfiram can get a reaction from anything that has alcohol in it.

Alcohol is available in prescription drugs, over-the-counter drugs, liquid cough-cold analgesic products, foods, flavoring, mouthwashes, salad dressings, and the like, and the patient should be warned of possible interaction. Psychotherapy aimed at mental and social rehabilitation should accompany disulfiram therapy. Disulfiram is available in 250- and 500-mg tablets.

Side effects. During early weeks of therapy, drowsiness, impotence, headache, peripheral neuritis, and a metallic taste may occur. About 20% of patients experience fatigability. High doses may cause a confusional state and convulsions. Deaths have occurred following the "test drink." The abstinence from alcohol may cause anxiety, hostility, and even experimentation with other drugs.

Contraindications. Disulfiram is contraindicated if there is serious cardiovascular disease, diabetes, epilepsy, hypothyrodism, cirrhosis of the liver, nephritis, or pregnancy. It is contraindicated in patients receiving metronidazole, paraldehyde, and any alcohol or working with ethylene dibromide (leaded fuels).

Drug interactions. Disulfiram critically enhances the anticoagulant effects of coumarin anticoagulants. When taken with phenytoin it decreases phenytoin metabolism, resulting in increased anticonvulsant effect. When taken with isoniazid (INH) it may cause behavioral changes and coordination difficulties. Concomitant use with diazepam and chlordiazepoxide decreases the plasma clearance of these drugs. Disulfiram decreases the rate at which various drugs are metabolized and therefore may increase serum levels and ease the risk of toxic potential.

Drugs used for treatment of inflammation

When the cell membranes are distorted or damaged by physical trauma (inflammation, trauma, blood clots, etc.) or other injurious process, the prostaglandins release arachidonic acid from phospholipase. The prostaglandins are believed to cause inflammation, edema, and pain at the site of trauma and significantly contribute to the appearance of fever. When prostaglandin biosynthesis is reduced, the inflammation, edema, fever, and pain symptoms are decreased.

The prostaglandins are a unique group of 20-carbon essential fatty acids with a five-carbon ring having various modulating functions. Most cells can synthesize prostaglandins or other endoperoxides. They may be secreted into the bloodstream, where they undergo rapid metabolization and inactivation. They generally act by diffusing into neighboring cells to modulate their function, hence their name "tissue hormones." Their role as putative mediators of inflammation now has more meaning. The cell membrane's phospholipid fractions release arachidonic acid as a result of the enzymatic action of phospholipase A_2. This occurs when cell membranes are damaged or distorted during fever, inflammation, pain, and platelet aggregation. Cells do not store the prostaglandins, so continued prostaglandin release depends on immediate and continued prostaglandin synthesis. Prostaglandin synthetase, an enzyme complex, converts the arachidonic acid to other substances. An enzymatic action of cyclooxygenase (a term for prostaglandin synthetase) follows, producing the two cyclic endoperoxide intermediates, PGG_2 and PGH_2, which are capable of producing pain and vasoconstriction. It is thought that antiinflammatory drugs inhibit the release of cyclooxygenase and, therefore, in turn inhibit the release and synthesis of PGE_2 and PGF_2. PGH_2 is acted on by the isomerase and reductase within the prostaglandin synthetase complex, which results in the production of PGE_2 and PGF_2. These two prostaglandins have varied biologic actions such as the ability of PGE_2 to produce edema, erythema, fever, and pain and for PGF_2 to produce vasodilation and uterine contraction.

From PGG_2 and PGH_2 there are additional pathways leading to prostacyclin (PGI_2, formerly known as PGX), a potent vasodilator in blood vessel walls, and thromboxane (TXA_2 and TXB_2), a vasoconstrictor found in lung, spleen, and platelets. Thromboxane synthetase acts on PGG_2 and PGH_2 producing thromboxane A_2 (TXA_2), which has arterial vasoconstriction and platelet aggregation activity. The enzyme prostacylin synthetase acts on PGG_2 and PGH_2, forming PGI_2, which has vasodilation action and an antiaggregation effect on platelets.

Aspirin and the nonsteroidal antiinflammatory agents interfere with or inhibit the biosynthesis of cyclooxygenase to prevent the generation of PGG_2 and PGH_2 and thus reduce the levels of these endoperoxides to the prostaglandin cascade to PGE_2, PGF_2, and TXA_2. The cyclooxygenase inhibitors, which reduce the levels of the prostaglandin mediators, cause physiologic function alterations in the gastrointestinal tract, kidney, and uterus. Corticosteroids, on the other hand, are thought to inhibit prostaglandin production by limiting the substrate or inhibition of the phospholipase action, thus reducing the mediators of inflammation. In anaphylactic shock there is an explosive concurrent release of slow-reacting substance in anaphylaxis (SRS-A), TXA_2, PGE_2, and PGF_2.

Prostaglandins PGF_2 and PGE_2 have been reported to induce abortion and labor. The use of PGE_2 (Dinoprostone) vaginal suppositories (Prastin E_2, Upjohn Co.) for inducing abortion has been approved, and their use as an efficient method for managing midtrimester abortions has been well documented in intrauterine fetal death and missed abortion. PGF_2 (Dinoprost) has been available (Prostin F_2, alpha, Upjohn Co.) for intraamniotic administration to terminate pregnancy in the second trimester.

The uses of antiinflammatory agents are growing and include treatment of arthritis and rheumatic disease, thromboembolism, venous thrombosis, cerebrovascular disease, dysmenorrhea, pain, fever, dermal inflammation, premature infants with patent ductus arteriosus, ocular inflammation, acute and chronic glomerulonephritis, pericardial effusion, pleurisy, hypercalcemia, periodontal disease, sunburn, and Bartter's syndrome in early childhood, secondary prevention of myocardial infarction, and alterations of platelet function.

Drugs used for the treatment of inflammation include several group classifications. They are (1) the antiinflammatory analgesics, which include the salicylates, mefenamic acid, and salicylate combinations, (2) the antirheumatic agents, which include the nonsteroidal antiinflammatory agents of propionic acid derivatives (ibuprofen, fenoprofen, naproxen, and naproxen sodium), tolmetin, meclofenamate sodium, indomethacin, sulindac, the pyrazolone derivatives (phenylbutazone and oxyphenbutazone); and slow-acting nonsteroidal antiinflammatory drugs, which include the antimalarial hydroxychloroquine, penicillamine, the gold compounds, and the immunosuppressive drugs cyclophosphamide and azathioprine, and (3) the drugs used to treat gout, which include probenecid, sulfinpyrazone, allopurinol, and colchicine.

Antiinflammatory analgesics
SALICYLATES

The natural source of salicylic acid is willow bark, although it is now made synthetically from phenol. The cheaper snythetic product is identical with, and therefore as effective as, the natural product. Salicylic acid itself is irritating and can be used only externally, necessitating the synthesis of derivatives for systemic uses. All of these compounds will be referred to as "salicylates" and will be discussed as a group. Usefulness of the various members of the group depends upon their solubility, their salicylic acid content, and their tendency to cause local irritation.

Aspirin is by far the most widely used of all the salicylates. Americans spend millions of dollars for aspirin, for combinations of aspirin with other pain relievers, and for products to relieve arthritic and rheumatic pains.

Systemic action. These drugs are used systemically for their analgesic, antipyretic, and antiinflammatory actions.

Analgesic. The major use of salicylates (aspirin and sodium salicylate) is for the relief of pain (analgesia). When compared on the basis of weight, aspirin is said to be the more potent analgesic. These preparations are especially effective for headache, neuralgia, dysmenorrhea, myalgia, fibrositis, neuritis, rheumatoid arthritis, and rheumatic fever. Aspirin is probably more widely used than any other single therapeutic agent. The estimated amount used yearly in the United States is in excess of 10,500 tons.

Analgesic doses of the salicylates do not produce dulling of consciousness, mental sluggishness, or disturbances of memory. Unlike the opiates, analgesia produced by the salicylates is not accompanied by euphoria or sedation. They do not cause drug dependence.

Salicylates are effective in treating peripheral pain (musculoskeletal pain or muscle and joint pain) and in relieving headache. Salicylates are not effective in relieving visceral pain or severe traumatic pain. Their analgesic potency is less than that of codeine.

The preparations are somewhat helpful in the symptomatic treatment of gout. They are less valuable for this purpose than certain other agents, but they are also less toxic. They decrease the renal threshold of uric acid and promote its excretion. A uricosuric effect is seen with aspirin doses of 5 g/day and a decreased uric acid secretion is seen with 2 g/day or less.

Antipyretic. Little or no effect is observed in persons with a normal body temperature, but in the febrile patient, a marked fall in temperature may occur. The salicylates seem to reduce fever by increasing the elimination of heat. It is believed that they act upon the heat-regulating center in the hypothalamus. As a result of this action, peripheral blood vessels dilate, and heat is lost from the body by radiation and by evaporation of increased perspiration. There is evidently no effect on heat production.

However, care must be exercised to avoid giving any of these preparations if the patient is benefitting from the fever or if the cause of illness would be obscured by reduction of temperature.

Unpleasant symptoms associated with a cold or attack of influenza may be relieved by one or more of the salicylates since they relieve muscular aching, headache, and fever, but their use should be accompanied by rest in bed. They exert no effect on the progress of the infection. In other words, it is impossible to "break up" a cold with aspirin as is commonly believed.

Antiinflammatory. The relationship of prostaglandins and the antiinflammatory response is explained extensively at the beginning of this section. Salicylates intervene in this process by suppressing inflammation through the inhibition of prostaglandin biosynthesis. Aspirin in particular blocks the step of cyclooxygenase (also known as prostaglandin synthetase) from forming the two cyclic endoperoxides PGG_2 and PGH_2 from arachidonic acid, thereby decreasing the inflammation, edema, swelling, redness, fever, and the like that is mediated by the prostaglandins, PGF_2 and PGE_2.

Experiments indicate that aspirin also inhibits formation of excess prostaglandins in the brain. Since aspirin relieves headache, this suggests that aspirin has a central action. It has also been shown that some of these compounds elevate body temperature, and it is well known that in ordinary doses aspirin can reduce fever.

Respiratory. Therapeutic doses of aspirin and sodium salicylate do not affect respiration. Large or toxic doses at first stimulate the respiratory center, producing increased depth and rate of respiration, and can cause *respiratory alkalosis.* Later, toxic doses can cause respiratory acidosis and respiratory depression.

Cardiovascular. In patients receiving large doses of salicylates, the plasma volume of the blood increases as much as 20%, hematocrit falls, and cardiac output and work are increased. If the patient has cardiac insufficiency, these effects may lead to cardiac failure and pulmonary edema.

Gastrointestinal. Salicylates in large doses are prone to produce gastrointestinal irritation (gastric distress, nausea, and vomiting). This effect is attributed to both a local and a central action—the gastric mucosa may be affected and also the vomiting center in the brain. The administration of sodium bicarbonate with the oral doses of salicylates helps to prevent irritation, but it also promotes excretion via the kid-

ney. This is not an advantage when the maintenance of a definite blood level is desirable. It is claimed that gastric irritation is decreased appreciably when aspirin is buffered with aluminum glycinate and magnesium carbonate and that it is also absorbed more rapidly. A subsequent study fails to support this latter claim, however. Unlike sodium bicarbonate, these substances do not increase the sodium intake, which is an advantage in certain instances.

Gastric ulceration can occur and occult blood has been found in the stools of patients undergoing salicylate therapy. Extent of blood loss is dose related and may lead to iron deficiency anemia. The risk of gastric irritations increases when steroids, alcohol, phenylbutazone, or oxyphenbutazone is given concurrently. Gastric irritation may be reduced by taking the drug with milk, food, or large amounts of water and crushing the tablet.

Metabolic effects. Salicylates lower blood sugar levels in diabetic persons, and the drugs have been shown to deplete liver glycogen. However, normal doses of salicylates can be used by diabetic individuals without their interfering with the action of antidiabetic drugs or insulin. With very large doses of aspirin, adjustment in the dose of antidiabetic drugs and insulin may be necessary. Salicylates interfere with protein binding of thyroxine and can alter certain thyroid function tests (PBI).

Platelet aggregation and prothrombin synthesis. Aspirin inhibits platelet aggregation, weakly inhibits prothrombin synthesis, and prolongs bleeding time. For these reasons it is being investigated for the prevention of thrombosis. Aspirin displaces coumarin anticoagulants from protein-binding sites, which leads to higher concentrations of active anticoagulant drug, which in turn can result in active bleeding. Patients taking both drugs should have frequent prothrombin and bleeding time determinations to ascertain if anticoagulant dose needs to be reduced.

Local action. Salicylic acid is irritating to both skin and mucous membrane. It softens epidermis without producing inflammation. Salicylic acid is a constituent of some corn and callus removers, and it is used to remove warts and upper layers of the skin in the treatment of certain skin diseases. It is also used for the treatment of fungal infections. Whitfield's ointment contains benzoic acid and salicylic acid; it loosens the outer horny layers of the skin and is known as a *keratolytic*.

The salts of salicylic acid have no effect on skin, but after their oral ingestion the salicylic acid that is released is likely to cause gastric irritation, nausea, and vomiting. Methyl salicylate produces irritation of both skin and mucous membranes and at one time was used for its counterirritant effects. It was rubbed on sore and painful joints and muscles to produce some degree of redness and improved circulation. It now is rarely prescribed for this purpose. In solution the salicylates are weakly bacteriostatic and are capable of inhibiting certain fermentative and putrefactive processes. Sodium salicylate is sometimes used as a sclerosing agent in the treatment of varicose veins.

Side effects and toxic effects. In rare individuals hypersensitivity reactions to aspirin and other antiinflammatory drugs may produce rhinitis, angioneurotic edema, bronchial asthma, vasomotor collapse, and urticaria. Although this is often referred to as "aspirin allergy," its mechanism probably has no immunologic basis. It may be caused by inhibition of PGE induced by the aspirin and nonsteroidal antiinflammatory drug (related to bronchodilation). In any case, aspirin should never be given to an asthmatic patient with nasal polyps or allergy to tartrazine dyes or to one who claims that he has had an acute attack after taking aspirin. Sodium salicylate or choline salicylate are suitable alternatives if a salicylate is desired and aspirin hypersensitivity is present.

The safety range of the salicylates is wide (the usual toxic dose in children is 240 mg/kg), and most cases of poisoning are mild. However, the indiscriminate use of these drugs by lay persons for every kind of ache or pain has resulted in numerous instances of toxic reactions. Also, aspirin poisoning is common in children. Mild poisoning is called salicylism and consists of ringing in the ears, dizziness, disturbances of hearing and vision, sweating, nausea, vomiting, and diarrhea. The so-called salicylic jag results

from stimulation of the central nervous system and may progress to a state of delirium. Skin eruption and other allergic manifestations as well as deaths from salicylate poisoning have been reported. Intensive therapy with salicylates and massive doses can produce a decreased prothrombin level in the blood and hemorrhagic manifestations. This appears to accompany a deficiency or diminished intake of vitamin K. There is little likelihood of hemorrhage if the dosage is kept at 1 g or less a day. Other dangerous symptoms of salicylate poisoning include depression, coma, irregular pulse, first a rise and then a fall in blood pressure, and deep, labored respiration that become slower and slower until respiratory failure results. Hyperthermia may occur since salicylate can have a thermogenic effect. Hyperthermia should be treated vigorously with tepid sponges, ice packs, or hypothermal blanket. Poisoning and untoward reactions to the salicylates are frequently a matter of personal idiosyncrasy.

Salicylate overdosage and treatment. In overdose situations the patient's peak blood levels may not be evident for a period of 6 hours after ingestion. The nurse should ask if the aspirin was enteric coated because the absorption of this tablet may be erratic and a period of up to 28 hours may elapse before peak levels occur. If the suppository is employed this absorption is even more erratic. At high levels salicylates have zero order kinetics (doubling the dose may more than double plasma levels and half-life may be prolonged from 15 to 30 hours). The heat formation and increased cardiac output occur as the salicylates uncouple oxidative phosphorylation. The nurse should remember that hypoglycemia is seen in infants with chronic salicylism but hyperglycemia is seen in adult salicylism. Signs of aspirin toxicity can be seen with doses at or exceeding 3.5 to 5 g/day.

Salicylates producing a pK_a of 3.5 are excreted more readily by alkalinizing the urine where "trapping" the charged ions occurs. If the urine is acid only a small amount of salicylate is ionized and reabsorption continues.

If the patient's salicylate level shows a plateau for 24 hours, there may be an aspirin mass in the stomach. An abdominal flat plate should be used and contrast media instilled to confirm this. The enteric-coated tablets may be solubilized using isotonic (150 mEq/liter) sodium bicarbonate lavage. The enteric coating protects the aspirin in acid medium but not in an alkaline medium. As a last resort surgical removal of the mass may be indicated.

The symptoms of mild overdosage include tinnitus and deafness; severe overdosage is manifested by hyperventilation, severe vomiting, hyperthermia, coma, hypo- or hyperglycemia, and acidosis. Very severe overdosage causes pulmonary edema, convulsions, severe acidosis, and acute renal failure. Chronic salicylism may occur with prolonged salicylate ingestion when there is a decreased ability to excrete the drug as in chronic renal insufficiency. Normal use of salicylates near term has produced an intoxicated fetus with developing symptoms of salicylism soon after delivery (36 hours). Additionally, febrile dehydrated children are prone to salicylate intoxication.

There is no specific antidote for salicylate poisoning, hence treatment is largely symptomatic. All that is usually necessary in mild cases of poisoning is to stop administration of the drug and give plenty of fluids. If massive doses have been taken, it may be necessary and desirable to empty the stomach, preferably with gastric lavage, and then instill a saline evacuant. Hemodialysis or peritoneal dialysis may be useful in eliminating some of the salicylate from the body in severe symptom ranges.

Overdosage in children. Although aspirin and aspirin compounds are among the safest analgesics known, the ease with which they can be purchased has contributed to carelessness in their use. The so-called baby aspirin, which is available in 1¼-gr chewable flavored tablets, has been responsible for a high incidence of poisoning in young children. Children eat it thinking it is candy. This has produced severe and sometimes fatal poisoning. The younger the child, the more dangerous overdosage is likely to be. Methyl salicylate (1 ml = 1 g salicylate) should not be left where children can obtain it. Doses as small as 6 ml have caused death in

children. The fact that it is used as a wintergreen flavoring agent suggests to the child that it is good to eat.

All salicylates should be kept out of the hands of children and in child-resistant containers. Parents should be helped to understand that indiscriminate administration of these drugs to children, and particularly to young children, can be dangerous.

Drug interactions. Some drug interactions involving salicylates are as follows:

1 With probenecid and sulfinpyrazone: because of competition for renal tubular sites, there is a decrease in effect of uricosuric action
2 With anticoagulants: because of platelet inhibition and inhibition of prothrombin formation in high doses, there is an increase in risk of episodes of hemorrhage
3 With antacids: because of urinary alkalinization there is increases in salicylate excretion
4 With oral hypoglycemics: because of multiple mechanisms enhanced hypoglycemic effect may occur

Some drug-disease interactions of interest are:

1 In peptic ulcer disease the gastric irritant effect of salicylates produces irritation or reactivation of the ulcer
2 In gout, salicylates inhibit renal tubular secretion of uric acid, which increases uric acid levels (seen with 2.4 g/day of aspirin). Analgesic doses of salicylate cause uric acid retention leading to hyperuricemia. Large doses have a uricosuric effect, which may antagonize other uricosuric drugs. A patient with gout should avoid the use of salicylates.
3 Thrombocytopenia is effected because of inhibition of platelet aggregation resulting in an increased risk of hemorrhagic episodes
4 The diabetic patient using a copper reduction method of urine testing and using doses of 2.4 g salicylate daily may have a false positive reaction because the salicylate acts as a reducing agent; if the diabetic patient uses the glucose oxidase method a false negative reaction occurs because the salicylate inhibits the reaction

Aspirin

Aspirin or acetylsalicylic acid is the most common and most used of the salicylates. It has a bitter taste and is poorly soluble in water. In the presence of moisture, it hydrolyzes slowly to acetic acid and salicylic acid.

Action and result. Aspirin is absorbed from the gastrointestinal tract in the stomach and primarily in the small intestine. Aspirin is metabolized in the microsomal system and the mitochondria of the liver and is excreted mainly by the kidney. About 85% of the aspirin is eliminated unchanged in alkaline urine, and in acid urine about 5% may be eliminated unchanged. The major metabolites of aspirin include salicylic acid, phenolic glucuronide, and acyl glucuronide with gentisic acid as a minor metabolite. Therapeutic doses of aspirin can produce 50% to 90% of salicylate in the blood bound to plasma protein (most to albumin). After administration of a 650-mg dose of aspirin the mean time of initial detection in plasma is 10 minutes, the mean peak plasma level is 35 μg/ml, the mean time of peak plasma level is 102 minutes and the mean elimination from plasma (half-life) is 3.2 hours.

Besides being indicated in the use of the treatment of mild to moderate pain, fever, and various inflammatory conditions, aspirin is also indicated for reducing the risk of recurrent transient ischemic attacks or strokes in men who have had transient ischemia of the brain caused by fibrin platelet emboli.

Preparations, dosage, and administration. Aspirin is available in tablet and capsule forms in 150-, 325-, and 650-mg doses (gr2½, 5, and 10) for adults and 81-mg tablets for children. Enteric-coated tablets are available for patients who have gastric or duodenal ulcers and who do not tolerate the plain tablets. Chewable tablets are available for children for ease of administration.

Aspirin is available also in a chewable gum, 228 mg flavored with cherry or orange, and powders containing 842 mg/packet. Aspirin may also be found buffered with aluminum hydroxide, magnesium hydroxide, glycine, magnesium carbonate, or aluminum glycinate. Effervescent tablets contain 1.9 sodium bicarbonate per tablet, and this should be considered the medication is given to the hypertensive patient on sodium restriction.

Aspirin suppositories are also available in 65-, 130-, 150-, 195-, 300-, 325-, 600-, and 650-mg and 1.2-g strengths. Dosage for adults for minor pains and aches is 325 to 650 mg every 4 hours if necessary; for arthritis and rheumatic conditions, 2.6 to 5.2 g daily in divided dosages; for acute rheumatic fever, up to 7.8 g daily in divided dosages; for transient ischemic attacks in men, 1300 mg/day (as 375 mg four times a day or 650 mg twice daily). A timed release form (650 mg) may be used to provide 1.3 g every 8 hours. Children may have 65 mg/kg/24 hours in divided doses every 6 hours.

Choline salicylate (Arthropan). Choline salicylate is a liquid with 870 mg/5 ml in a mint-flavored vehicle. Each 5 ml is equivalent to 10 gr aspirin. The nurse should mix this with fruit juices, carbonated beverages, or water when administering. The liquid form makes this preparation useful for geriatric patients and other adult patients who have swallowing impairments or who refuse a solid dosage form. This product contains no sodium.

Choline magnesium trisalicylate, 500 mg (Trilisate). The dosage form is present as 293 mg choline salicylate combined with 362 mg magnesium salicylate to provide the 500-mg salicylate content. The salicylate is rapidly absorbed, reaching peak blood levels within 2 hours, and is excreted by the kidneys. At the recommended dosage (two to three 500-mg tablets every 12 hours for rheumatoid arthritis and more severe arthritis), the therapeutic range of 5 to 30 mg/ml is achieved and a steady-state concentration is reached after four to five doses. This means that each dose will maintain adequate blood levels throughout the 12-hour interval. This drug is used in relief of the signs and symptoms of rheumatoid arthritis, osteoarthritis, and other arthritides both for acute flareup and for long-term management. In salicylate content one tablet (500 mg) is equivalent to 10 gr aspirin. A cherry-flavored liquid (500 mg/5 ml) and a 750-mg tablet are also available.

Magnesium salicylate. This is a sodium-free salicylate derivative with a lower incidence of gastrointestinal upset. It is contraindicated in patients with renal insufficiency due to magnesium accumulation. It is available in 600- and 650-mg tablets.

Salsalate (Disalcid). After absorption the drug in this 500-mg tablet is slowly hydrolyzed to two molecules of free salicylic acid. It is insoluble in the stomach but is absorbed in the small intestine.

Sodium salicylate. This preparation is a white or pinkish powder with a sweetish saline taste. The usual dose is 325 to 650 mg (gr 10) every 2 to 4 hours as needed. It is relatively soluble in water and is absorbed more rapidly than aspirin. It is available in 325- and 650-mg tablets (gr 5 and 10), plain or enteric coated. It is also available in ampules of sterile solution for injection (1 and 1.5 g).

Both aspirin and sodium salicylate may be given in large doses to patients with acute rheumatic conditions every hour until untoward symptoms appear, such as ringing in the ears. The route of administration is usually oral, and both preparations should be accompanied by ample amounts of water. Sodium salicylate is occasionally given intravenously when high concentrations in the blood are desired and it is difficult to attain them with oral administration. It is not used by patients on sodium-restricted diets, since each 325-mg tablet is 14.6% sodium equal to 46 mg (2 mEq) sodium.

Salicylamide. Salicylamide, the amide of salicylic acid, shares the actions and uses of aspirin but is less effective. It is not hydrolyzed to salicylate and is metabolized before entering systemic circulation. Administration and dosage are essentially the same as for aspirin. Drowsiness may occur and may be found in some over-the-counter sleep products.

Salicylic acid. This form is too irritating for oral administration, but it is a component of many ointments and preparations for external use.

Methyl salicylate (Wintergreen Oil). This preparation is too irritating and toxic to be used internally except in low concentrations as a flavoring agent.

Aspirin and codeine. Frequently codeine is combined with aspirin or acetaminophen. Codeine contributes to the analgesia by action on the opiate receptors in the brain. Codeine and other narcotics do not produce the analgesic effect by inhibition of prostaglandin synthetase; rather, they act on the more subjective component of pain and decrease the psychologic impact by calming, soothing, and relieving fear about the pain. The combination (Empirin with Codeine) is beneficial for pain because the codeine acts centrally and the aspirin works peripherally (blocks generation of pain impulse). In theory this combination may produce more substantial pain relief than each of the drugs given alone.

Aspirin, phenacetin, and caffeine (APC). Each tablet or capsule contains 200 to 250 mg aspirin, 120 to 150 mg phenacetin, and 15 to 30 mg caffeine. These same drugs are found in combination and marketed as Aspirin Compound, APC, and a number of others. These three drugs are also combined with codeine or with one of the barbiturates. Phenacetin and caffeine have been found to have questionable value in these preparations and are being removed from many combination products that formerly contained them in their formulation. These preparations are preferably given orally.

Aspirin and para-aminobenzoic acid (PABA). Para-aminobenzoic acid, when administered with sodium salicylate, was found to raise the level of salicylate in the blood plasma. It acts by inhibiting the metabolism of the salicylates as well as their excretion from the kidney. Paraminobenzoic acid can be given orally for this purpose.

Side effects and toxic effects. Side effects are negligible, but the toxic effects are serious and have caused a number of deaths. Poisoning may occur from a single dose or overdose, but it is usually the result of the prolonged use of some proprietary headache remedy. Symptoms include profuse sweating, nausea and vomiting, skin eruption, weakness, cyanosis caused by the formation of methemoglobin, slow weak pulse, and slow respirations. Most severe cases of poisoning show subnormal temperature, leukopenia, and collapse.

Phenacetin may cause hemolytic anemia, renal papillary necrosis, and nephrotic states after prolonged use. Phenacetin produces allergic reactions. Considerable individual susceptibility to these drugs seems to exist; some persons are unharmed by them, whereas others develop severe reactions.

These drugs can damage the blood, bone marrow, kidneys (analgesic nephrotoxicity), and liver if the patient is adversely susceptible to the drug. This constitutes a strong point against prolonged self-medication. Dementia has also been reported after prolonged use of phenacetin.

In cases of mild poisoning it is usually sufficient simply to discontinue the drug and wait for its elimination from the body. In more severe cases gastic lavage may be indicated if the drug has been recently ingested. Blood transfusions and shock therapy may be necessary. Oxygen is sometimes indicated if the patient is cyanotic.

Mefenamic acid (Ponstel)

Mefenamic acid is an analgesic, antipyretic, and antiinflammatory drug that inhibits both prostaglandin synthesis and activity. It is indicated for relief of mild to moderate pain only when therapy does not exceed 1 week. The drug has recently been approved for use in dysmenorrhea.

Preparation, dosage, and administration. It is available in 250-mg capsules. It is given in dosages of 500 mg initially, followed by 250 mg every 6 hours as needed. Since the drug may upset the gastrointestinal tract, the nurse should administer it with food or milk.

Side effects and toxic effects. Adverse reactions include diarrhea, which may be severe and at times associated with inflammation of the bowel or hemorrhage. Severe autoimmune hemolytic anemia may occur in patients given this drug for prolonged time periods. Leukopenia, eosinophilia, thrombocytopenic purpura, agranulocytosis, pancytopenia, and bone marrow hypoplasia have also been reported in association with this drug.

Zomepirac sodium (Zomax)

Zomepirac is a chemical analog (pyrrole acetic acid derivative) of tolmetin with prominent titratable analgesic effects (mild to moderately severe pain) and some antipyretic and antiinflammatory effects. This agent is tried before a narcotic analgesic and after less than optimal results were achieved with acetylsalicylic acid and acetaminophen in conditions such as pain of oral surgery, orthopedic conditions, and postoperative and postpartum pain. Clinical relative equieffective analgesic doses of 50 to 100 mg are comparable to 650 mg acetylsalicylic acid, and 100 mg is compared to two APC tablets with a total of 60 mg codeine. The increased peripheral effectiveness over acetylsalicylic acid of this prostaglandin synthetase inhibitor has been proposed as resulting from the high lipid solubility (pK_a 4.73) in central nervous system penetration.

After rapid and complete gastrointestinal absorption a 100-mg dose reaches peak plasma concentration. The elimination half-life is about 4 hours, serum half-life is 60 minutes, and it is excreted as parent and metabolite in the urine. Consistent analgesic effects occur within 30 minutes, reach a maximum in 1 to 2 hours, and have a duration of 4 to 6 hours or more. Multiple repeated doses produce an increase in blood levels (33%), an increase in volume of distribution (75%), and a reduction in clearance culminating in a prolonged half-life (9 to 10 hours). Each 100-mg tablet contains 8 mg (0.34 mEq) sodium. Occult gastrointestinal blood loss equivalent to that produced by 4.8 g acetylsalicylic acid per day is seen with 600 mg/day zomepirac. Prolonged bleeding caused by decreasing platelet adhesion and aggregation occurs but returns to normal within 48 hours after discontinuing the drug. Neither the binding of warfarin to plasma protein nor prothrombin time is affected.

Dosage and administration. Dosage is titrated to severity of pain. Doses begin at 50 to 100 mg every 4 to 6 hours, and not more than 600 mg/day. In therapy exceeding 3 months the dosage should not exceed 400 mg/day. Concomitant administration with food decreases the rate and extent of absorption, but antacids do not affect its bioavailability.

Side effects and toxic effects. Adverse reactions are seen less often during short-term than during long-term therapy. Generally adverse effects are equivalent to those of other nonsteroidal antiinflammatory agents, including gastrointestinal effects (nausea, distress, diarrhea, abdominal pain, dyspepsia, constipation, gas, vomiting), vertigo, insomnia, edema, elevated blood pressure, rash, weakness, and urinary tract infections. Peptic ulceration and gastrointestinal bleeding have been reported. Treatment lasting over 6 months has produced adverse renal and urinary tract effects (cystitis, dysuria, urinary frequency, hematuria, pyuria, urinary infections). Mild peripheral edema is seen along with elevations in BUN and serum creatinine. Lower doses are needed in patients with impaired renal function.

Precautions. Demonstrated past sensitivity reactions (bronchospasm, rhinitis, urticaria, etc.) to acetylsalicylic acid or other nonsteroidal antiinflammatory agents prohibit the use of zomepirac. Use is not recommended during pregnancy or lactation.

Antirheumatic agents

Rheumatoid arthritis is a chronic systemic disease of unknown etiology with inflammation and connective tissue changes in articular and related structures. It tends to involve joints symmetrically, causing pain, limitation of motion, and joint deformity. This disease is chronic, progressive, and crippling, and it has no cure. Management has three objectives: (1) suppression of inflammation in the joints and other tissues, (2) maintenance of joint function and prevention of deformities, and (3) joint repair when relief of pain or improved functioning of the joint can be achieved.

Many times rheumatoid arthritis is treated only with a salicylate. Aspirin commonly causes gastric irritation in the dosages required for rheumatoid arthritis. Other salicylates that

have less gastric irritation, such as magnesium salicylate and choline salicylate (Arthropan Liquid), are often employed in its place.

Choline magnesium trisalicylate (Trilisate) and salsalate (Disalcid) have the advantages of longer serum half-lives, less frequent administration, and less gastric irritation than aspirin. Gastric irritation can be minimized by taking the salicylates after food or with an antacid.

Other nonsteroidal antiinflammatory drugs used to treat rheumatoid arthritis are the propionic acid derivatives, indole analogs (pyrroles), pyrazolones, and phenylanthranilic acid derivatives. They are as effective as aspirin but not *more* effective. Among their advantages over aspirin are that they have fewer gastrointestinal effects, less ototoxicity, and longer half-lives, resulting in less frequent administration. Their disadvantages are their expense, unpredictability, and variability in patient response. Patients sensitive to aspirin are also usually sensitive to these classes of drugs.

Other antirheumatic agents will be discussed individually. They are much more toxic than aspirin and the propionic acid derivatives (ibuprofen, fenoprofen, and naproxen) and are reserved primarily for advanced disease. Table 8-10 presents the most commonly used nonsteroidal antiinflammatory drugs and their dosage ranges for rheumatoid arthritis.

The glucocorticoids are not discussed in this chapter, but not to mention them here would be misleading. They are the most potent antiinflammatory drugs available. They are used in patients with rheumatoid arthritis who contin-

TABLE 8-10   Some nonsteroidal antiinflamatory agents

Generic name	Trade name	Dosage strengths (mg)	Usual adult divided dose range used in rheumatoid arthritis (mg)
Acetysalicylic acid (aspirin, ASA)	Various	325, 500, 650 (most commonly used)	2500-6000
Fenoprofen	Nalfon	200, 300, 600	1200-3200
Ibuprofen	Motrin	300, 400, 600	1200-2400
Indomethacin	Indocin	25, 50	50-200
Meclofenamate sodium	Meclomen	50, 100	200-400
Naproxen	Naprosyn	250, 375	500-750
Oxyphenbutazone	Oxalid, Tandearil	100	300-600
Phenylbutazone	Azolid, Butazolidin	100	300-600
Sulindac	Clinoril	150, 200	150-400
Tolmetin	Tolectin	200, 400	600-2000

ue to have synovitis in many joints. Glucocorticoids are injected into the joints only after the patient has had sufficient trials of the nonsteroidal antiinflammatory drugs, gold, penicillamine, or hydroxychloroquine. Patients who have had severe symptoms of fever, weight loss, anemia, vasculitis, and neuropathy also become candidates to receive glucocorticoid therapy. The smallest dose possible to relieve pain is usually used, since it is very difficult to stop glucocorticoid therapy after it has begun because of the great relief it brings to the patient. Also, using small doses delays the severe cumulative side effects that eventually appear.

Nonsteroidal antiinflammatory agents—rapid acting

Ibuprofen (Motrin)

Ibuprofen is a propionic acid derivative with antipyretic, analgesic, and antiinflammatory effects. It is an effective analgesic for mild to moderate pain (pain of primary dysmenorrhea, postextraction dental pain, postsurgical episiostomy pain and soft tissue athletic injury). It is used to reduce the pain, stiffness, swelling, and tenderness in patients with rheumatoid arthritis and osteoarthritis. Its chief advantage over aspirin is its lower incidence of adverse effects, including that of gastrointestinal bleeding. Ibuprofen's exact mode of action is unknown.

Ibuprofen is rapidly absorbed after oral administration; peak plasma level is reached in about 1 or 2 hours. However, if the drug is taken with food, absorption is slower and plasma levels lower. Plasma half-life is about 1½ to 2½ hours. It is excreted in the urine; it does not appear to be uricosuric, but there is no evidence of accumulation. Ibuprofen does not seem to affect the action of oral anticoagulants when it is administered at 2.4 g/day.

Preparation, dosage, and administration. Ibuprofen is available in 300-, 400- and 600-mg tablets. Dosage to adults with rheumatoid arthritis and osteoarthritis is 300, 400, or 600 mg three or four times daily, usually on arising, midmorning, midafternoon, and at bedtime. Dosage should not exceed 2.4 g/day. Therapeutic response may occur in a few days but most frequently occurs in 2 weeks. The optimal dose must be individually determined. For mild to moderate pain, 400 mg is given every 4 to 6 hours as necessary for relief.

Adverse and toxic effects. Most frequently noted adverse effects include nausea and vomiting; diarrhea, constipation, heartburn, and epigastric distress occur less frequently. To reduce gastrointestinal complaints ibuprofen should be administered with milk or meals. Other side effects include skin eruptions, pruritus, dizziness, blurred vision, fluid retention, and headache.

Toxic amblyopia has been reported, and patients experiencing visual difficulties (such as decreased visual acuity and problems with color discrimination) should have a complete eye examination, and the drug should be discontinued.

Precautions. Patients should be instructed to report any unfavorable reaction to their physician. It must be used cautiously in patients with a history of peptic ulcer, since a few cases of ibuprofen ulceration have been reported. Its safe use during pregnancy and in children under 14 years of age has not been established. Because of its affinity for serum albumin, ibuprofen may displace other drugs bound to albumin (sulfonamides, hydantoins, etc.).

Ibuprofen is contraindicated in patients

Chemical classification of the nonsteroidal antiinflammatory drugs (excluding aspirin)

1. Phenylpropionic acid derivatives
   A. Ibuprofen
   B. Fenoprofen
   C. Naproxen
2. Indole analogs (pyrroles)
   A. Indomethacin
   B. Sulindac
   C. Tolmetin
3. Pyrazolone drugs
   A. Phenylbutazone
   B. Oxyphenbutazone
4. Phenylanthranilic acid drugs
   A. Mefenamic acid
   B. Meclofenamate sodium

with a history of aspirin-induced broncho-spasm or those with symptoms of asthma, rhinitis, nasal polyps, angioedema and urti-caria.

No specific antidote to ibuprofen toxicity is known at the present time.

Fenoprofen calcium (Nalfon)

Like ibuprofen, fenoprofen is a propionic acid derivative with antiinflammatory, analge-sic, and antipyretic activity. Its therapeutic effect, adverse reactions, and precautions are similar to those for ibuprofen. It is indicated in rheumatoid arthritis, osteoarthritis, and mild to moderate pain.

Preparation, dosage, and administration. Fenoprofen is available in 200-mg capsules and 300- and 600-mg tablets for oral administra-tion. Initial dose for adults is 300 to 600 mg three to four times daily. For maximal effect the drug should be given ½ hour before or 2 hours after meals; if gastrointestinal symptoms oc-cur, the drug can be taken with meals, milk, or an antacid. Peak plasma level (50 μg/ml) occurs in about 60 minutes to 2 hours after ingestion of a 600-mg dose. Plasma half-life is about 3 hours. Administration with aspirin decreases its effects and increases its excretion. Maximum daily dose is about 3200 mg in adults at doses of 300 to 600 mg three or four times daily.

Precautions. Fenoprofen reduces platelet aggregation, increases bleeding time, and thus should not be used by patients with bleeding problems; it should be used cautiously for patients receiving coumarin-type anticoagu-lants. Fenoprofen, which is highly protein bound, may displace such drugs as hydantoin, sulfonamides, and sulfonylureas from binding sites and thus increase the likelihood of drug interaction and drug toxicity. Ninety percent is excreted in the urine within 24 hours as gluc-uronide, and 4-hydroxy metabolites.

The coadministration of aspirin decreases the biologic half-life of fenoprofen because of an increase in metabolic clearance that results in a greater amount of hydroxylated fenoprofen in the urine. Long-term administration of pheno-barbital (a known enzyme inducer) may be associated with a decrease in the plasma half-life of fenoprofen. Antacids (aluminum and magnesium hydroxide) do not interfere with the absorption of the drug; however, food inges-tion decreases the rate of and extent of absorp-tion. Therefore fenoprofen should be adminis-tered 30 minutes before or 2 hours after meals. The drug causes elevated serum transaminase levels and hepatocellular hypertrophy. Some patients developed elevated serum transami-nase, lactic dehydrogenase, and alkaline phos-phatase levels that persisted for some months. Therefore it is recommended that periodic liver function tests be performed and the drug dis-continued if abnormalities occur. It is not rec-ommended in pregnancy (in labor parturition is prolonged). Since peripheral edema has been observed, this drug is used with caution in those patients with compromised cardiac func-tion. Episodes of dysuria, cystitis, and hematu-ria are among the reported adverse renal effects.

Naproxen (Naprosyn)

Naproxen is a nonsteroidal, antiarthritic drug with therapeutic and adverse effects and precautions similar, but not identical to the other propionic acid derivative drugs in this classification. It is indicated for rheumatoid arthritis and osteoarthritis. It is well absorbed after oral administration; peak plasma levels occur in 2 to 4 hours; plasma half-life is about 13 hours.

It is available in 250- and 375-mg tablets. Dosage for adults is 500 to 750 mg daily in two divided doses (possible because of its long half-life). It crosses the placental barrier and is found in breast milk of lactating mothers.

Naproxen sodium (Anaprox)

Naproxen sodium is a nonsteroidal antiin-flammatory agent that was developed as an analgesic. It also possesses antipyretic proper-ties. It is indicated for relief of mild to moderate pain (acute or chronic), including musculoskel-etal pain from soft tissue injury, and for treat-ment of primary dysmenorrhea. Relief of pain is noticed in 1 hour and the analgesic effect may last up to 7 hours.

The pharmacology and related information are similar to those for naproxen.

Preparation, dosage, and administration. Each tablet of Anaprox contains 275 mg naproxen sodium, which is equivalent to 250 mg naproxen, and 25 mg (about 1 mEq) sodium. The dosage for mild to moderate pain is two tablets initially, followed by one tablet every 6 to 8 hours as needed, not exceeding five tablets (1375 mg). The dosage for rheumatoid arthritis and osteoarthritis is 500 to 750 mg daily in two divided doses.

Side effects. Naproxen sodium increases values for 17-ketogenic steroids. However, the 17-hydroxycorticosteroid measurements (Porter-Silber method) are not altered. Naproxen and naproxen sodium may interfere with some urinary assays of 5-hydroxyindoleacetic acid. Naproxen and naproxen sodium should be discontinued 72 hours before adrenal function tests because of interaction of the drugs or their metabolites and the *m*-nitrobenzene in the assay.

Naproxen and naproxen sodium should not be used concurrently because they both circulate in the plasma as the naproxen anion.

Tolmetin sodium (Tolectin)

Tolmetin is an indole analog (pyrrole) derivative and differs chemically from other nonsteroidal antiinflammatory agents but it has similar actions pharmacologically. After administration, it reaches peak serum levels in ½ to 1 hour, the peak absorption is in 1 hour, the half-life is 1 hour, and it is metabolized to an inactive metabolite. The drug is 99% protein bound and has a maximum daily dose of 200 mg.

Uses. Tolmetin is indicated for relief of signs and symptoms of osteoarthritis, for acute flare-ups and long-term management of rheumatoid arthritis and for juvenile rheumatoid arthritis. It is available in 200- and 400-mg tablets.

Dosage and administration. The recommended starting adult dose is 400 mg three times daily (1200 mg), with a dose in the morning and at bedtime, and it is then titrated on an individual basis to patient response. Control is seen at doses of 600 to 1800 mg daily in divided doses (three to four times daily), not to exceed 2000 mg/day. The recommended starting children's dose (2 years and older) is 20 mg/kg/day in divided doses three to four times daily. After

control is achieved the usual child's dose is in a range from 15 to 30 mg/kg/day, and a dose in excess of 30 mg/kg/day is not recommended. Therapeutic response is in a few days to a week. Antacids (not sodium bicarbonate), milk, or meals may overcome the gastrointestinal symptoms.

Drug interactions. There is a cross-sensitivity between tolmetin and aspirin or other nonsteroidal antiinflammatory agents. The combined use of these drugs has caused symptoms of asthma, rhinitis, or urticaria. Tolmetin is not to be used in patients with a history of upper gastrointestinal tract disease unless there is close supervision for signs of ulcer perforation or severe gastrointestinal bleeding. Tolmetin prolongs bleeding time. Tolmetin may induce edema and sodium retention leading to edema so it is used cautiously in patients with compromised cardiac function. This drug has not been studied in pregnancy and it may be excreted in the milk of lactating mothers. Tolmetin does displace protein-bound drugs to the same extent as the other nonsteroidal antiinflammatory agents. In patients receiving concomitant steroid therapy, any reduction in the steroid dose must be gradual to abate any possible complications of withdrawal.

Meclofenamate sodium (Meclomen)

Meclofenamate sodium is a phenylanthranilic acid derivative (a fenamate) with antiinflammatory, analgesic, and antipyretic activity. The antiinflammatory action may be achieved by inhibition of prostaglandin synthesis and competition for binding at the prostaglandin binding site. Peak plasma levels occur in ½ to 1 hour, the half-life is 2 hours (3⅓ hours after multiple doses), and excretion is by urine and feces. A dose of 300 mg daily produced fecal blood loss of 1 to 2 ml and 2 to 4 ml at 400 mg daily. (Aspirin at a daily dose of 3.6 g/day causes 6 ml/day fecal blood loss.) In comparison to aspirin and other nonsteroidal antiinflammatory agents, meclofenamate has a greater incidence of gastrointestinal reactions, specifically severe diarrhea (10% to 33%).

Uses. It is indicated for use in chronic rheumatoid arthritis and osteoarthritis but because of the gastrointestinal side effects (including severe diarrhea) it is not recommended as the initial drug. The major adverse reactions reported are gastrointestinal (dose-related diarrhea, nausea with or without vomiting, other gastrointestinal disorders, abdominal pain).

Precautions. Its use is contraindicated in patients who have exhibited prior hypersensitivity to it and to aspirin. Its use is also contraindicated in patients who experienced bronchospasm, allergic rhinitis, or urticaria from use of nonsteroidal antiinflammatory agents.

A history of upper gastrointestinal tract disease requires close supervision since peptic ulceration and sometimes severe gastrointestinal bleeding are reported to have occurred with this drug.

Decreases in hemoglobin and/or hematocrit levels occur, and these values need determination if anemia is suspected.

Patients should be told to discontinue the drug and notify the prescriber if gastrointestinal side effects occur due to the possible drug-related connection. Administration with meals or milk may alleviate gastrointestinal discomfort.

Drug interactions. Drug interactions reported are:

1 Warfarin effects are enhanced, so dosage needs reduction to prevent excessive prolongation of prothrombin time.
2 Aspirin may lower plasma levels by competing for protein-binding sites; combined use results in greater fecal blood loss.

It is not recommended for use during the first and third trimesters of pregnancy, or for nursing mothers. Use in children before 14 years is not established at this time.

Dosage and administration. Dosage is 200 mg daily in three or four equal doses, (not to exceed 400 mg daily). Improvement may be seen in a few days (or up to 3 weeks of therapy for optimum benefit). It is available in 50- and 100-mg tablets.

Indomethacin (Indocin)

Indomethacin has potent antiinflammatory, analgesic, and antipyretic activity of the indole analog (pyrrole) class, but it may cause serious adverse effects. It should not be used as a general antipyretic or analgesic. It is a potent inhibitor of prostaglandin synthesis.

Action and results. The drug is readily absorbed, achieving a peak plasma concentration of about 1 and 2 μg/ml following single oral doses of 25 and 50 mg respectively, and it is about 100% bioavailable. Elimination is by renal excretion, metabolism, and biliary excretion and the drug undergoes considerable enterohepatic circulation (biliary recycling). The mean half-life is about 4½ hours and with a therapeutic regimen of 25 or 50 mg three times daily the steady-state plasma concentrations average 1.4 times those following the first dose. In the plasma the parent drug and the 4 metabolites exist in the conjugated forms. From an oral dose 60% is recovered in the urine as the drug and metabolites (26% as indomethacin and its glucuronide), and 33% is in the feces (1.5% as indomethacin). About 90% is bound to plasma protein over the expected range or therapeutic plasma concentrations.

Because of its potential to cause adverse reactions, particularly at high dose levels, the use of this drug in adults with rheumatoid arthritis and osteoarthritis should be reserved and carefully considered for active disease unresponsive to adequate trial with salicylates and established measures of value and rest. Effectiveness has been observed in active stages of the following: moderate to severe rheumatoid arthritis, including acute flareups of chronic disease; moderate to severe ankylosing spondylitis; moderate to severe osteoarthritis of large joints (hips, knees, and shoulders); and acute gouty arthritis.

As an investigational drug indomethacin has been used in premature infants for pharmacologic closure of persistent patent ductus arteriosus (as an alternative to surgical ligation) and to suppress uterine activity in prevention of premature labor.

Preparation, dosage, and administration. Indomethacin is supplied in capsules of 25 and 50 mg each. The average dose for adults is 25 to 50 mg two or three times daily by mouth, not exceeding 200 mg daily.

The drug may enable a reduction of steroid

dosage in patients receiving steroids for more severe forms of rheumatoid arthritis. In such a case the steroid dosage is slowly titrated down and patients observed closely for possible adverse effects. The combined use of indomethacin and aspirin produces no superior effect to use of indomethacin alone since there may be an increase in gastrointestinal side effects.

Side effects and toxic effects. Because of its gastric toxicity indomethacin may cause peptic ulcer and hemorrhage, and it is contraindicated in patients who have peptic ulcer, gastritis, or ulcerative colitis. Other side effects that might be seen are headache, dizziness, nausea, vomiting, anorexia, tinnitus, skin rashes, edema, and, rarely, bone marrow depression. Indomethacin has also been reported to cause aggravation of psychiatric disturbances, epilepsy, and parkinsonism. Ocular changes have occurred, such as corneal deposits and retinal disturbances. Indomethacin can also mask the signs and symptoms of an infection and should be discontinued for 24 hours or more if an infection is suspected. About one half to one third of patients experience some side effects to indomethacin, and 20% have to discontinue its use altogether. The drug is contraindicated in patients with demonstrated allergic reactions to it or in those with nasal polyps associated with angioedema or bronchospastic reaction to aspirin or other of the nonsteroidal antiinflammatory agents.

Drug interactions. Some drug interactions of interest are as follows:

1 Aspirin, 3.6 g/day, along with indomethacin over long periods decreases the indomethacin blood levels by 20%.
2 Probenecid increases the plasma levels of indomethacin.
3 Patients on warfarin therapy or anticoagulant therapy should be observed closely for alterations of prothrombin time when indomethacin or any drug is added to their therapy.
4 There is a reduction in the natriuretic and antihypertensive effect of furosemide among some patients, and the furosemide-induced increases in plasma renin activity are blocked in hypertensive patients.
5 An elevation of plasma lithium levels and a decrease in renal lithium clearance may occur; patients should be observed for signs of lithium toxicity and lithium serum concentrations monitored to keep in a range of 0.6 to 1.4 mEq/liter.

6 Phenylpropanolamine found in over-the-counter cough/cold and anorexient products, when combined with indomethacin, causes an elevation in blood pressure.

Nursing implications. Indomethacin cannot be considered a simple analgesic and should not be used in conditions other than those recommended. Because of the variability in the potential for adverse reactions in individual patients, the following are strongly recommended to the nurse:

1 Titrate each dose to the lowest effective one prescribed. (Begin with 25 mg two or three times daily and increase the dose gradually.) An increased dosage (in excess of 150 to 200 mg daily) increases the potential for adverse effects with no appreciable increase in benefits.
2 The nurse should provide careful instructions to the patient about prevention of serious adverse reactions and signs of toxicity, especially to elderly persons who self-administer this drug and family members who administer to the patient.

Sulindac (Clinoril)

The molecular structure of sulindac, on indole analog (pyrrole), was designed to yield a drug with the antiinflammatory properties comparable to indomethacin but with less gastrointestinal activity, but this may not be the case. Sulindac may be termed a "prodrug" because its therapeutic effect depends on the sulfide metabolite that is readily produced by reduction and capable of reoxidation to the parent drug form, sulindac.

Action and result. This antiinflammatory, analgesic, antipyretic drug has a mode of action like that of other nonsteroidal antiinflammatory agents: the inhibition of prostaglandin synthesis by the sulfide metabolite. Absorption by the oral route is about 90%. Peak plasma levels appear in about 1 hour, and the pharmacologically active sulfide metabolite appears in 2 to 3 hours in the fasting state. Food will slightly delay the attainment of peaks (3 to 4 hours) with this drug. The mean effective half-life of sulindac is 7.8 hours and of the sulfide metabolite is 16.4 hours. Sulindac and the two metabolites undergo extensive enterohepatic circulation and, when coupled with the reversible metabolite (the sulfide), contribute to the sustained plasma levels. The sustained plasma levels of the sulfide metabolite are consistent with a prolonged antiinflammatory action, which is the rationale for twice-daily dosages. The sulindac is 93.1% and the sulfide is 97.9% bound to human plasma protein. Potentiation of warfarin's anticoagulant effect and prolongation of prothrombin time are reported. Excretion is 50% by the kidneys, 25% in the feces, and some biliary excretion.

Uses. Sulindac is indicated in osteoarthritis, rheumatoid arthritis, ankylosing spondylitis, acute painful shoulder, and acute gouty arthritis.

Preparation, dosage, and administration. Sulindac is available in 150- to 200-mg tablets. It is given with food orally twice daily with usual maximum dose of 400 mg daily. Titration of the dose is necessary in osteoarthritis, rheumatoid arthritis, and ankylosing spondylitis, beginning with 150 mg twice daily. For acute painful shoulder and acute gouty arthritis, the recommendation is 200 mg twice daily with therapy for 7 to 14 days needed. As observed with other nonsteroidal antiinflammatory agents, aspirin given concurrently significantly depressed the plasma levels of the active sulfide metabolite.

Side effects and toxic effects. Numerous adverse reactions are reported to indicate that sulindac has similar side effects to that of indomethacin, which may be predictable since sulindac is the isostere of indomethacin. A contraindication to sulindac is hypersensitivity to aspirin and other nonsteroidal antiinflammatory agents involving asthma, urticaria, nasal polyps, and rhinitis. The following adverse effects are seen: gastrointestinal disturbance, dermatologic rash and pruritus, and central nervous system effects such as dizziness, headache, nervousness, tinnitus, and edema. Congestive heart failure, Stevens-Johnson syndrome, toxic epidermal necrolysis, bone marrow depression, thrombocytopenia, leukopenia, gastrointestinal perforation, nephropathy, and pancreatitis have been reported. Adverse ophthalmic effects, such as diplopia, cloudy vision, eyeball swelling, noninflammatory ulceration of the cornea, retinal hemorrhage, blurred vision, and spots before the eyes, have also occurred.

PYRAZOLONE DERIVATIVES
Phenylbutazone (Butazolidin, Azolid)

Phenylbutazone is a pyrazolone derivative that exhibits analgesic and antipyretic actions. Phenylbutazone and its metabolite oxyphenbutazone are the oldest of the nonsteroidal antiinflammatory drugs. They are considered to be more effective in the treatment of ankylosing spondylitis, bursitis, traumatic tenosynovitis, and acute gout than of rheumatoid arthritis. When they are compared with other nonsteroidal antiinflammatory agents, their toxicity precludes them from long-term therapy.

Action and result. Phenylbutazone is absorbed rapidly and completely from the digestive tract. It is likely to cause some irritation to the gastrointestinal tract.

Renal excretion of sodium and chloride is reduced, causing retention of fluid. In patients with gout, the drug brings about a reduction of uric acid in the blood.

Uses. Phenylbutazone is regarded as a potent analgesic to relieve the pain of active rheumatoid arthritis and associated conditions (bursitis, peritendinitis, painful shoulder) and active ankylosing spondylitis. It is said to suppress inflammation, to relieve stiffness and swelling, and to shorten the period of disability. However, because of the high incidence of toxic effects, its use is recommended only for those patients who do not respond to less toxic drugs. It is used particularly to relieve symptoms of acute gouty arthritis, when the patient has an acute episode of this disease and does not respond well to conservative measures. It is also used for short-term treatment of degenerative joint disease of hips and knees unresponsive to other treatment.

Preparation, dosage, and administration. Phenylbutazone is available in 100-mg coated tablets. The initial daily dose for adults is 300 to 600 mg given in divided portions. The minimal effective dose is then determined and may be as low as 100 to 200 mg. It should not be used longer than a 7- to 10-day trial period. To avoid gastric irritation, it should be given at mealtime, just after a meal, or with a glass of milk.

Nonsodium antacids also help to minimize irritation without increasing the ingestion of sodium. A diet restricted in sodium chloride is recommended while the patient is receiving this drug.

Side effects and toxic effects. The administration of phenylbutazone is accompanied by a rather high incidence of side effects (approximately 40% of the patients). Side effects include gastric intolerance, edema (sodium and fluid retention), nausea, gastric distress, stomatitis, rash, and dizziness. Serious life-threatening toxic effects include hepatitis, hypertension, temporary psychosis, leukopenia, thrombocytopenia, agranulocytosis, and bone marrow depression. Chronic ingestion of the drug may be associated with acute leukemia and renal and liver necrosis. Some patients experience a reactivation of peptic ulcers with bleeding, and others complain of nervousness, confusion, visual disturbances, and fever and may develop cardiac arrhythmias.

Contraindications. Phenylbutazone is contraindicated in patients under 14 years, in senile patients, and for patients with aspirin hypersensitivity, hypertension, edema, gastrointestinal disorders, asthma, cardiac insufficiency, a history of peptic ulcer or blood dyscrasia, or hepatic or renal dysfunction. Patients receiving this drug should be under close medical supervision, and periodic examination of their blood is recommended to detect early indications of toxic effects even if the drug has only been given for 7 days.

Drug interactions. Phenylbutazone causes the following drug interactions:

1 Potentiates the action of warfarin; initially potentiates but later inhibits action of coumarin-type anticoagulants
2 Potentiates hypoglycemic action of sulfonylurea compounds and insulin; potentiates the action of penicillin, sulfonamides, and phenytoin
3 With barbiturates the activity of both drugs is inhibited
4 Inhibits action of steroids, sex hormones, aminopyrine, antipyrine, and dipyrone

Oxyphenbutazone (Tandearil, Oxalid)

Oxyphenbutazone is a hydroxylated metabolic product of phenylbutazone. Its uses and toxic effects are similar to those of the parent drug. It is reported to have less ulcerogenic effects than phenylbutazone. It is available in tablets containing 100 mg. The average daily dose for adults is 300 to 600 mg given in three to four equal portions. The administration of the drug after meals is preferable to minimize gastric irritation. Like phenylbutazone, oxyphenbutazone can cause liver damage and depression of the bone marrow.

Nonsteroidal antiinflammatory drugs—slow acting

The four classes of drugs to be discussed in this classification are gold compounds, antimalarials, D-penicillamine, and immunosuppressive agents. These drugs produce recognizable beneficial effects after weeks or months of therapy.

There is no absolute evidence that any of these drugs is able to induce remissions in rheumatoid arthritis. These drugs have shown the ability to interfere with the progression of this disease in many patients. This section briefly considers the four classes of drugs utilized to interrupt the progression of arthritis in patients with actively progressing disease (rheumatoid arthritis, juvenile rheumatoid arthritis, ankylosing spondylitis, psoriatic arthritis, discoid lupus erythematosus, and systemic lupus erythematosus) and in those who have failed to respond to the rapid-acting nonsteroidal antiinflammatory agents. The use of some of the immunosuppressive drugs (except azathioprine) in treating rheumatoid arthritis, juvenile rheumatoid arthritis, ankylosing spondylitis, and psoriatic arthritis is experimental and restricted to protocols of research and has not been approved by the Food and Drug Administration. These drugs will be covered briefly (azathioprine, chlorambucil, cyclophosphamide, and methotrexate).

The slow acting nonsteroidal antiinflammatory agents are effective but have serious, potentially hazardous effects. They appear to act by suppression of the underlying pathologic process rather than by providing transient symptomatic relief. The nurse should remember that this form of drug intervention may be needed before irreversible articular damage occurs. This is an objective that may be offset with these slow-acting drugs. This form of pharmacologic intervention has an unfavorable risk-to-benefit ratio, so use is limited to a truly demanding clinical picture unresponsive to more conservative measures (fast-acting nonsteroidal antiinflammatory agents or intraarticular corticosteroids).

GOLD COMPOUNDS (50% GOLD)
Gold sodium thiomalate (Myochrysine)
Aurothioglucose (Solganal)

The FDA-approved indications are for use in rheumatoid arthritis, both adult and juvenile. Chrysotherapy (gold) mechanism of action is not known; the disease progression is altered to prevent future structural damage to joints. There appears to be an effect of suppression of the synovitis of active rheumatoid disease. There is some evidence of antiviral activity, inhibition of the activity of lysosomal enzymes, reduction in lymphocyte proliferation, and lessening of enhancement in phagocytic activity of polymorphonuclear leukocytes and macrophages. Therapy should be started early in the disease course, since gold has no effect on damaged tissue.

Dosage and administration. An initial test dose of 10 mg intramuscularly (intragluteally) is administered for hypersensitivity, then followed in 1 or 2 weeks with 25 mg. This is followed by subsequent dosages of 25 to 50 mg/week. This 50-mg dosage is maintained at intervals of 1 week until the total cumulative dosage reaches 0.8 to 1.0 g (approximately 20 weeks). The simultaneous use of nonsteroidal antiinflammatory agents is effective until the patient achieves remission from the gold therapy. The therapy is discontinued if there is no significant improvement after a 1-g total dose. If the patient improves without signs of toxicity, then the 50-mg dose is continued at 3- to 4-week intervals for an indefinite time period. The dose for aurothioglucose in children 6 to 12 years old is 25% that of the adult dose, based on body weight. The dose in children for gold sodium thiomalate after the initial 10-mg test dose is 1

mg/kg body weight, not exceeding 50 mg per injection. To administer the intramuscular dose of aurothioglucose, the nurse must shake the vial vigorously and warm it to body temperature to ease drawing the suspension into the syringe. An 18-gauge, 1½-inch needle should be used to deposit the gold deep into the muscular tissue of the upper quadrant of the gluteal region. A 2-inch needle may be used for obese patients.

Side effects and toxic effects. About 40% of the patients experience adverse effects of relatively minor consequence. The most common side effects are transient localized dermatitis, metallic taste, and stomatitis. The side effects that would require discontinuing therapy are exfoliative dermatitis, agranulocytosis, proteinuria, liver damage, drug fever, nephritis, and other hematologic abnormalities associated with thrombocytopenia and marrow aplasia. These potentially fatal reactions require that blood and urine tests be performed before each injection.

D-Penicillamine, antimalarials, immunosuppressants, phenylbutazone, and oxyphenbutazone potentiate the hematologic effects of the gold. Because of this they are not to be concomitantly administered. Gold therapy is contraindicated in renal or hepatic dysfunctions, uncontrolled or severe diabetes, debilitation, marked hypertension, congestive heart failure, systemic lupus erythematosus, urticaria, eczema, colitis, and hematologic disorders and following radiation therapy.

The beneficial effects are noticed in 80% to 90% of patients when the dosage range of 200 to 400 mg has been achieved. An oral gold compound (auranofin) is currently under investigation for use in rheumatoid arthritis.

ANTIMALARIALS
Chloroquine phosphate
Hydroxychloroquine

Hydroxychloroquine is approved for use in rheumatoid arthritis, discoid lupus erythematosus, and systemic lupus erythematosus and to suppress acute attacks of malaria. It is also used for juvenile rheumatoid arthritis. Chloroquine is used in rheumatoid arthritis. Chloroquine was replaced by hydroxychloroquine because of the decreased risk of ophthalmologic (retinal) toxicity. This retinopathy and the relative lack of efficacy in severe rheumatoid arthritis assign this a more insignificant role in treatment. The ophthalmologic effects are dose related and necessitate eye examinations at 3- to 6-month intervals (fewer than 1% of patients have retinopathy). Other eye toxicity problems seen include reading difficulties, photophobia, blurry vision, and abnormal distant and peripheral visual fields. The visual problems, central nervous system reactions, neuromyopathy, blood dyscrasias, and bone marrow depression are significant enough to discontinue therapy, while the side effects of gastrointestinal upset and rash are tolerable. Alopecia, hyperpigmentation of skin, hair bleaching, skin lesions, and muscle weakness are also reported. The usual adult dose is 200 to 600 mg daily for rheumatoid arthritis, taken with meals or milk. Use of these drugs is avoided in patients with psoriasis, hepatic or renal disorders, and alcoholism.

The patient should have some beneficial effects within 3 to 6 months.

D-PENICILLAMINE (CUPRIMINE, DEPEN)

D-Penicillamine is indicated in Wilson's disease, cystinuria, and heavy metal (lead) poisoning. The FDA has also approved this drug for treatment of sustained and severe rheumatoid disease, often in patients who have not responded to chrysotherapy. Gold and D-penicillamine may not be given concomitantly. D-Penicillamine may be as clinically effective as gold and may be a choice before gold therapy. It has been effective in patients with extraarticular manifestations such as nodules, vasculitis, rheumatoid lung disease, and peripheral neuropathy. The use of D-penicillamine within 4 months of the gold therapy is contraindicated because the D-penicillamine has the potential for mobilizing the gold stores.

The mechanism of action is not entirely understood. It chelates copper, which is not important in rheumatoid arthritis, and it does not possess analgesic or antiinflammatory action. Cessation of therapy results in a return of symptoms within 3 to 4 weeks.

Preparations, dosage, and administration. The drug is available in 125- and 250-mg capsules and tablets. The recommended regimen currently used is to begin with low doses and slowly increase the dosage. Patients begin with one daily dose of 125 to 250 mg administered with water on an empty stomach at least 1 to 2 hours before or after meals or any other medication, food, or milk. This dose is administered for 3 months and if it is tolerated it is increased by 125 or 250 mg to 375 or 500 mg daily, although it may be necessary to raise the dose to 750 mg and rarely to 1.5 g daily. This go-low and go-very slowly regimen is necessary since it appears that the dosage rate increment is correlated to development of serious side effects. A reduction in the maintenance dose is begun when the patient's disease is under control, but if the disease is exacerbated then the dose may be increased. Clinically relevant changes in maintenance doses may not be noticed for 8 to 12 weeks (patience is essential), whether increased or decreased, and there is documentation of patients continuing D-pencillamine therapy for about 8 years. While initiating therapy with D-penicillamine rapid-acting nonsteroidal antiinflammatory agents, salicylates, or systemic corticosteroids should be used and then withdrawn gradually as improvement occurs with the D-penicillamine. This drug should not be used in patients receiving gold therapy, antimalarials, cytotoxic drugs, or the pyrazolones.

Precautions. A history of penicillin allergy should not be a contraindication to a cautious therapeutic trial with D-penicillamine (in theory a cross-sensitivity exists). If the patient with rheumatoid arthritis is nutritionally impaired, 25 mg pyridoxine should be given daily, since D-penicillamine increases the requirement for this vitamin. The source of pyridoxine should not be vitamins with minerals, since chelation may block the response to D-penicillamine.

Side effects and toxic effects. Although prolonged therapy may be tolerated, therapy is often discontinued because of the unpleasant adverse effects—frequently skin rash, taste impairment, oral ulcers, loss of appetite, nausea and gastrointestinal distress, skin odors, neuritis (pyridoxine should be administered), and bruises. More serious reactions include proteinuria (caused by an immune complex nephropathy similar to that seen with gold therapy), nephropathy, and hematologic abnormalities such as thrombocytopenia with sudden onset or aplastic anemia. This points up the importance of complete blood and platelet counts twice a month for the first 3 months and each month thereafter. Such testing is of major importance when dosage increases are made, since this is when hematologic toxicity most often develops. The drug is used cautiously in patients with hepatic or renal dysfunctions, since nephrotic syndrome and liver dysfunctions are seen. Infrequently seen are induction of autoimmune diseases such as systemic lupus erythematosus, membranous glomerulonephritis, myasthenia gravis, or pemphigus.

IMMUNOSUPPRESSIVE DRUGS
Azathioprine (Imuran)

Azathioprine appears to act by modifying the immune responsiveness in rheumatoid arthritis, juvenile rheumatoid synovitis, psoriatic arthritis, and ankylosing spondylitis. Azathioprine is approved by the FDA for use in rheumatoid arthritis to alleviate the pain, spasm, edema, and acute immobility. Azathioprine is approved and reserved for adult-onset rheumatoid arthritis patients with very severe, active, and erosive disease that has not responded to management including rest, aspirin, or nonsteroidal antiinflammatory drugs or to gold. The severity of adverse effects must be carefully considered before using these drugs. This is reserved for patients who develop relentlessly aggressive or life-threatening rheumatoid disease and are documented failures to adequate trials of the above mentioned management.

Action and result. The use of immunologic concepts in the pathogenesis of rheumatoid synovitis created the rationale for immunosuppressive drug use. The development of rheumatoid lesion is related to the production of immune complexes (associated with B cells) and the necrotizing pannus (associated with T cells), so it is reasonable to inhibit the process by pharmacologic intervention. It seems that the beneficial effects are produced not by suppression of immune response but rather by their functioning as cytostatic or cytotoxic agents by inhibiting the response or replication of cells, such as lymphocytes or macrophages, that may mediate rheumatoid joint inflammation and reduce rheumatoid synovitis. This action interferes with all lymphocyte functions, however, since they destroy or cripple all cells. The drug inhibits cell proliferation by interference with synthesis of RNA and DNA. A decrease in the quantity and immunologic responsiveness of circulating T and B lymphocytes is seen in rheumatoid arthritis. The dose is initially 1 mg/kg (50 to 100 mg) once or twice daily, increased in 6 to 8 weeks, and thereafter in 1-month intervals. Increments are 0.5 mg/kg/day up to a maximum of 2.5 mg/kg/day. The onset is gradual, with optimum effects seen within 3 to 4 months after therapy begins. If after 12 weeks there is no response, the patient may be refractory. Maintenance dose is incrementally lowered at 0.5 mg/kg (about 25 mg daily every month) and other drug therapy is not changed.

Side effects and toxic effects. The side effects are related to the interference with bone marrow function and risks of neutropenia, leukopenia, and thrombocytopenia, which may lead to sepsis and bleeding. There is an increase in the risk of neoplasm. Frequently seen side effects are gastrointestinal intolerance (nausea, vomiting, anorexia, jaundice), alopecia, hemorrhagic cystitis, increased incidence of infection, increased risk of neoplasia, and hematologic toxic complications. Since the drug interferes with nucleic acid function, it is contraindicated in pregnancy and used with extreme caution in patients of child-bearing age. Chromosomal abnormalities have been reported.

The drug should be used cautiously in patients with renal or hepatic impairment, those who have undergone previous x-ray or cytotoxic therapy, and those with hematologic complications. The dose must be decreased in those with renal impairment due to delayed clearance of azathioprine, and frequent blood tests must be performed. It is available in 25- and 50-mg tablets and injectable form containing 100 mg/20 ml.

Drug interactions. When a patient using

azathioprine (which is metabolized by xanthine oxidase) is also given allopurinol (an xanthine oxidase inhibitor), there is an increased risk of cytotoxicity (elevated blood levels). To prevent this initially it is necessary to decrease the azathioprine dosage to one third or one fourth of the usual dosage and to make subsequent dose adjustments based on the toxicity or observed response of the patient. This interaction is used to purposely decrease the dose of the azathioprine. Azathioprine is affected by drugs that induce liver microsomal enzymes (barbiturates, steroids).

Drugs used in gout

Gout is a metabolic disease of unknown origin. Heredity is thought to have a bearing on the incidence of the disease since it occurs more often in relatives of persons with gout than in the general population. It is seen mostly in males. It is characterized by defective purine metabolism and manifests itself by attacks of acute pain, swelling, and tenderness of joints such as those of the great toe, ankle, instep, knee, and elbow. The amount of uric acid in the blood becomes elevated, and tophi, which are deposits of uric acid or urates, form in the cartilage of various parts of the body. These deposits tend to increase in size. They are seen most often along the edge of the ear. Chronic arthritis, nephritis, and premature sclerosis of blood vessels may develop if gout is uncontrolled.

Colchicine is considered the drug of choice in the treatment of an acute gouty attack. Other nonsteroidal antiinflammatory agents can be used, such as phenylbutazone, indomethacin, sulindac, and ibuprofen. Their relief of the attack takes longer, however—12 to 24 hours compared to colchicine's 6 to 21 hours. Glucocorticoids may also be used in unusual acute attacks refractory to conventional therapy.

Gout may be treated prophylactically as well. Colchicine is the only drug that can be used for this purpose. Patients can also prevent attacks by maintaining normal uric acid levels by avoiding the use of aspirins, diuretics, a large alcohol intake, and foods high in purines (kidney, liver, sardines, sweetbreads, etc.).

Consistently high uric acid levels (hyperuri-

cemia) in gout patients is treated with the drug of choice, allopurinol. Uricosuric drugs, probenecid and sulfinpyrazone, are only used when allopurinol cannot be administered and when urinary uric acid is carefully monitored. Uricosuric drugs lower serum uric acid by interfering with uric acid renal tubular resorption. High fluid intake is required with their administration, and possibly alkalinization of the urine may be undertaken to minimize the risk of urate stone formation and gravel when they are given.

Colchicine

Colchicine is an alkaloid obtained from the seeds and corm (bulbous root) of the *Colchicum autumnale* (meadow saffron), which belongs to the lily family of plants. Extracts of this plant have been used for hundreds of years in the treatment of gout.

Action and result. Locally, colchicine is an irritant. The mechanism of its systemic action remains unknown. It does not affect the amount of uric acid in the blood or in the urine (thus it is not uricosuric) and it has no effect on the size of tophi. It does not effectively relieve pain other than that of acute gouty arthritis. It inhibits leukocyte migration and leukocyte lactic acid production, which leads to lower uric acid deposition, interference with kinin formation, and lowered phagocytosis, thus decreasing the inflammatory response. It is an interesting drug not only because of its potent analgesic effect in gout but also because of its ability to arrest mitotic division of cells when they are in metaphase. During this phase it prevents the development of the spindle. This occurs in both normal and cancer cells. Inflammation of synovial tissues is associated with lactic acid production, and this favors a local decrease in pH, which promotes uric acid deposition. Colchicine decreases lactic acid production and the inflammatory response. These effects are apparently caused by colchicine-inhibiting leukocyte mobility and phagocytoses.

Uses. Colchicine is used to prevent or relieve acute attacks of gout. The response is often dramatic, and pain may be relieved within a few hours, the fever and swelling often diminishing after the relief of pain. It frequently must be used in doses large enough to cause gastrointestinal irritation (80% of patients). Tolerance does not seem to develop. It is sometimes given every night or every other night to prevent the development of an acute attack.

Preparation, dosage, and administration. Colchicine is available in 0.5- and 0.6-mg tablets and in ampules containing 1 mg/2 ml solution for intravenous injection. The initial dose of 1 to 1.2 mg is usually followed by 0.5 to 1.2 mg every hour or every 2 hours until the pain is relieved or the patient begins to have diarrhea, nausea and vomiting, or abdominal pain. Opiates or other antidiarrheal agents may be required to control the diarrhea. Inflammatory symptoms usually subside in 12 hours and are completely gone in 48 to 72 hours. The drug should not be administered for the 3 days after the 10 tablets, to avoid toxic effects from accumulation. Occasionally, colchicine is given by intravenous injection (the dose is diluted to 30 ml with 0.9% normal saline prior to administration and given over 2 or 3 minutes or longer), when rapid relief is important, or when oral administration is not feasible. It is very irritating if injected outside a vein (necrosis and extravasation) and, therefore, cannot be given subcutaneously or intramuscularly.

To be effective, colchicine must be given promptly (it is rapidly absorbed) at the first indication of an oncoming attack, and dosage must be adequate. Once the dose that will cause diarrhea has been determined, it is often possible to reduce subsequent doses to prevent diarrhea and still achieve satisfactory relief of pain.

The amount of colchicine necessary to control the inflammation and pain in an acute episode ranges from 4 to 8 mg. The articular pain and swelling usually abate in 12 hours and disappear in 24 to 48 hours. If corticotropin (ACTH) is also administered, it is recommended that the colchicine be administered in doses of 1 mg/day and continued for a few days after the ACTH has been discontinued.

For prophylaxis during the intercritical periods, the drug is administered continuously, to reduce the number of paroxysms and lessen their severity. If the patient has one attack per year, then a dose of 0.5 to 0.6 mg taken each day for 3 or 4 days a week is necessary at the first sign of an acute episode. If more than one acute flareup is seen a year, then the dose of 0.5 to 0.6 mg daily is needed. Very severe cases require up to 1 or 1.8 mg daily with very close medical observation and supervision. Caution should be used when this drug is given to elderly or feeble persons and those with cardiac, renal, or gastrointestinal disease.

Side effects and toxic effects. Prolonged use can cause bone marrow depression, agranulocytosis, peripheral neuritis, and aplastic anemia. In acute poisoning the patient complains of abdominal pain, nausea, vomiting, and diarrhea, which may become bloody as poisoning advances. Excessive loss of fluid and electrolytes and the dilation of capillaries result in shock. Scanty urine and blood in the urine indicate damage to the kidney. The pulse becomes rapid and weak, and the patient becomes exhausted.

The main measures used in the treatment of poisoning depend on the patient and the symptoms presented. Treatment is directed toward removal of the poison if possible (hemodialysis, peritoneal dialysis, and gastric lavage) and the prevention of shock. Atropine and morphine will relieve abdominal pain. Artificial respiration and the administration of oxygen are indicated should there be symptoms of respiratory involvement.

Allopurinol (Zyloprim, Lopurin)

Allopurinol interrupts the process of purine degradation before uric acid is formed. This is an inhibitor of purine biosynthesis and of the activity of xanthine oxidase, because it blocks the last two steps involved in the synthesis of uric acid: the conversion of hypoxanthine to xanthine and xanthine to uric acid.

Action and result. Allopurinol is an effective medication for gout that guards against uric acid stone formation, inhibits production of uric acid, reduces the levels of uric acid in both serum and urine without kidney function involvement, and lessens the risk of uric acid lithiasis. Because of the long half-life (18 to 30 hours) of its active metabolite (oxypurinol), it can be given once daily in a dosage of 300 mg, which simplifies the therapeutic regimen. It may also be taken with salicylates. Allopurinol therapy is appropriate for patients with excessive uric acid synthesis measured as over 800 mg uric acid urinary excretion daily of a purine-free diet.

Peak plasma levels occur 2 to 6 hours after oral administration; the half-life is 2 to 3 hours and the half-life of the active metabolite xanthine analog, oxypurinol (an inhibiter of xanthine oxidase), is 18 to 30 hours. Plasma half-life depends on the renal excretion and the oxidation to oxypurinol; renal clearance of allopurinol is rapid and that of oxypurinol is slow. About 10% to 30% of the unchanged drug is excreted in the urine and 20% is excreted in the feces within 48 to 72 hours.

A high fluid intake (80 to 100 ounces daily to produce 1 liter of urine) and alkalinization of the urine are necessary to lessen the risk of stone formation and sludging of the tubules with urates.

Uses. Allopurinol is indicated and used in the following situations:

1 Treatment of gout, either primary or secondary to the hyperuricemia associated with blood dyscrasias and their therapy
2 Treatment of primary or secondary uric acid nephropathy, with or without accompanying symptoms of gout
3 Treatment of patients with recurrent uric acid stone formation
4 Prophylactic treatment to prevent tissue urate deposition, renal calculi, or uric acid nephropathy in patients with leukemias, lymphomas, and malignancies who are receiving cancer chemotherapy with its resultant elevating effect on serum uric acid levels

Preparation, dosage, and administration. Allopurinol is available in 100- and 300-mg scored tablets. It is commonly given in a dose of 200 to 300 mg/day for mild gout or 400 to 600 mg for severe tophaceous gout. It is adjusted every 2 to 4 weeks according to the serum uric acid levels in order to maintain levels of 6 mg/100 ml or less.

Side effects. Drug rashes have been reported in those patients using thiazides and/or ampicillin or allopurinol alone; bone marrow depression, reversible hepatotoxicity, and drowsiness have also been observed. The drug is not protein bound but because it has an

inhibitory effect on the hepatic microsomal system, which metabolizes the coumarin-type drugs, the anticoagulants must be used with care and at lower doses.

Drug interactions. Some drug interactions of interest are the following:

1 Azathioprine and mercaptopurine have increased cytotoxic effects when used with allopurinol, and it is necessary to reduce their dosage to approximately one fourth to one third of the usual dose (this may be beneficial since a lower dose of the cytotoxic agent is needed.
2 When used with allopurinol coumarin anticoagulants have enhanced effects due to prolonged half-life.
3 Iron salts may have increased hepatic iron stores.
4 Oral sulfonylureas, particularly chlorpropamide, have enhanced hypoglycemic effects.
5 Uricosurics such as probenecid and sulfinpyrazone have enhanced uricosuria.

URICOSURIC AGENTS
Probenecid (Benemid)

Probenecid is chemically related to the sulfonamides and it was first introduced as an agent to inhibit the excretion of penicillin by the kidney.

Action and result. Probenecid has been found to inhibit renal excretion of a number of other substances, including para-aminosalicylic acid (which is used in the treatment of tuberculosis) and uric acid. It inhibits the tubular reabsorption of urate in the kidney, and it increases the urinary excretion of uric acid. This results in reduction of uric acid in the blood. This uricosuric action helps to prevent or retard formation of tophi and joint changes in chronic gouty arthritis. Probenecid is not an analgesic. It is completely absorbed after oral administration. Peak concentration occurs in 2 to 4 hours. The serum half-life is 8 to 10 hours. It is excreted as metabolites in the urine. Probenecid is appropriate therapy in gouty arthritis and in patients with reduced urinary excretion of uric acid (less than 800 mg/day) on an unrestricted purine diet.

Uses. Probenecid is especially useful for the treatment of chronic gout and gouty arthritis. It is not effective in acute attacks of gout. Precipitation of urates in the kidney can be prevented by keeping the urine alkaline. It is also used in penicillin and cephalosporin therapy when it is desirable to maintain high levels (two to four times) of the antibiotic in the blood plasma by inhibiting tubular secretions.

Preparation, dosage, and administration. Probenecid is available in 500-mg tablets. The usual dose for treatment of gout is 250 mg twice daily for 1 week; then 500 mg twice daily. This may be increased to 500 mg four times daily.

From 3 to 7.5 g of sodium bicarbonate or 7.5 g/day of potassium citrate is administered orally to maintain alkalinity of the urine. Aspirin antagonizes the uricosuric effect of probenecid, and the two drugs should not be used simultaneously in gouty patients. A high fluid intake (10 glasses of water daily) to produce copious volumes of urine is recommended to minimize formation of uric acid stones and occurrence of renal colic and hematuria.

Side effects and toxic effects. Probenecid is well tolerated by most patients (except those with peptic ulcer disease, glucose-6-phosphate dehydrogenase deficiency, and acute intermittent porphyria). A few persons may experience headache, nausea, constipation, skin flushing, or skin rash. Blood dyscrasias, sore gums, liver necrosis, serious hypersensitive reactions, and nephrotic syndrome have been reported, but these are rare.

Drug interactions. Some drug interactions with probenecid include the following:

1 When used with probenecid allopurinol causes enhanced uricosuria but its other therapeutic effects are decreased because of the greater excretion of its active metabolite (oxypurinol).
2 Salicylates produce marked diminished uricosuric effect, so the nurse must warn the patient to use acetaminophen and not any salicylates.
3 Plasma levels of sulfonamides are increased.
4 Simultaneous use of para-aminosalicylic acid results in PAS toxicity.
5 Oral antidiabetic antihyperglycemic agents (such as chlorpropamide and possibly glyburide), have an enhanced hypoglycemic effect.
6 Thiazides and related diuretic (furosemide and ethacrynic acid, for example) decrease the uricosuric effect of the probenecid.
7 Plasma levels of cephalosporins, indomethacin, and penicillins may have increased plasma levels (penicillin up to four times).
8 Urinary excretion of phenolsulfonphthalein (PSP) is decreased which may interfere in the kidney function test.
9 Hepatic and renal excretion of sulfobromophthalein (BSP) is decreased which interferes with liver function tests.
10 Additionally probenecid inhibits the renal excretion and increases plasma levels of dapsone, indomethacin, methotrexate, naproxen, and rifampin.

Sulfinpyrazone (Anturane)

Sulfinpyrazone is indicated in treatment of chronic gouty arthritis and intermittent gouty arthritis and investigationally for the prophylactic treatment of recurrent myocardial infarctions, because of its ability to inhibit platelet aggregation. The drug is absorbed after oral administration, and the duration of effect by this route is up to 10 hours. It is almost completely protein bound. About 90% of the dose is excreted almost unchanged in the urine.

Sulfinpyrazone has minimal antiinflammatory effect and is not intended for the relief of an acute attack of gout, because in the initial stages of therapy there is a marked ability of this drug to mobilize urates, which may enhance the acute attack of gouty arthritis.

Preparation, dosage, and administration. The drug is available in 100-mg tablets and 200-mg capsules. It is administered in initial doses of 200 to 400 mg daily in two divided doses, preferably with meals. Maintenance dose is 200 to 800 mg daily, and reduced when blood urate levels are controlled. The dose may be gradually increased in 1 week to full maintenance dosage.

Patients should receive adequate fluid intake (10 to 12 glasses with 8 ounces each daily) and urinary alkalinization if necessary, since sulfinpyrazone is a potent uricosuric agent that may cause urolithiasis and renal colic, especially in the initial stages of therapy. Since salicylates antagonize the uricosuric action of this drug, concomitant use is contraindicated in gouty arthritis.

Side effects and toxic effects. The most frequently observed adverse reaction has been irritation of the upper gastrointestinal tract, which may be decreased by administration with milk, antacids or meals. Rash and blood dyscrasias have also been reported.

Sulfinpyrazone may provoke renal colic because of the precipitation of uric acid. It may

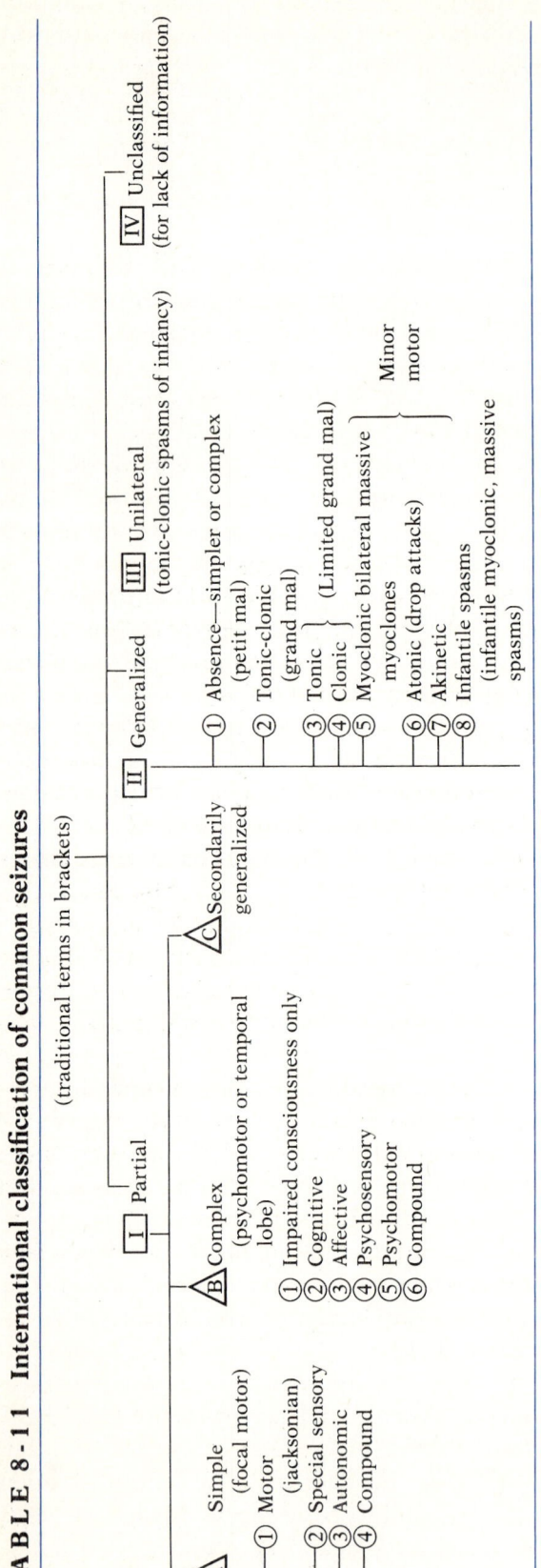

TABLE 8-11 International classification of common seizures
(traditional terms in brackets)

I Partial	
A Simple (focal motor)	① Motor (jacksonian)
	② Special sensory
	③ Autonomic
	④ Compound
B Complex (psychomotor or temporal lobe)	① Impaired consciousness only
	② Cognitive
	③ Affective
	④ Psychosensory
	⑤ Psychomotor
	⑥ Compound
C Secondarily generalized	
II Generalized	① Absence—simpler or complex (petit mal)
	② Tonic-clonic (grand mal)
	③ Tonic ⎱ (Limited grand mal)
	④ Clonic ⎰
	⑤ Myoclonic bilateral massive myoclones
	⑥ Atonic (drop attacks) ⎱ Minor motor
	⑦ Akinetic ⎰
	⑧ Infantile spasms (infantile myoclonic, massive spasms)
III Unilateral (tonic-clonic spasms of infancy)	
IV Unclassified (for lack of information)	

increase the incidence of acute attacks of gout in the early weeks of treatment. The drug may activate peptic ulcers, so patients with peptic ulcer or gastrointestinal inflammation or ulceration should not receive this drug. It should not be given to patients sensitive to other pyrazole derivatives (phenbutazone or oxyphenbutazone) or those with blood dyscrasias. It should be used with caution in pregnancy.

Drug interactions. Sulfinpyrazone potentiates sulfonamides, oral sulfonylureas, and insulin, and it may alter the activity of coumarin anticoagulants by depressing prothrombin activity. Periodic blood counts are recommended as is close medical supervision.

Anticonvulsant drugs

Epilepsy is regarded as a symptom of disease or disorder of the brain, rather than a disease in itself. It is associated with marked changes in the electric activity of the cerebral cortex, and these alterations are often detected in the electroencephalogram. Therefore the EEG is often a valuable aid to the physician in making a diagnosis.

The etiology and type of epilepsy are related to the age of onset. Neonatal seizures often are related to metabolic disorders, prenatal injury, severe hypoxia, or brain defects before birth; young adults may have focal seizures from head trauma. In the age group 6 years and older, brain tumors and vascular disease may cause seizures. Sometimes the convulsive seizure is associated with a brain infection, head trauma, fever, growth of scar tissue, cerebrovascular disease, the presence of a toxin or a poison, or drug withdrawal. A specific cause for seizures often will not be found in most patients. In addition to the EEG, other laboratory tests such as routine blood and urine series, calcium, blood sugar, electrolytes, phosphorus, and sometimes renal and hepatic function tests are done to assist in the determination of the diagnosis.

Epileptic seizures vary and are traditionally grouped according to grand mal seizures, petit mal seizures, jacksonian epilepsy, and psychomotor attacks. A new classification of seizures, however, has been implemented and is being more extensively used because it more adequately describes the seizure of the patient. It is called the International Classification of Seizures. Table 8-11 presents it with the traditional terms in brackets. For the purpose of this text, both seizure classifications will be used.

Grand mal (tonic-clonic generalized) epilepsy is the type most frequently seen. Such attacks are characterized by sudden loss of consciousness. The patient falls forcefully and experiences a series of tonic and clonic muscular contractions. The eyes roll upward, the arms are flexed, and the legs are extended. The force of the muscular contractions causes air to be forced out of the lungs, which accounts for the cry which the patient may make as he falls. Respiration is suspended temporarily, the skin becomes cyanotic, perspiration and saliva flow, and the patient may froth at the mouth and bite his tongue if it gets caught between his teeth. When the seizure subsides the patient regains partial consciousness and may complain of aching. He then tends to fall into a deep sleep.

Petit mal (generalized absence—simple or complex) seizures are most often seen in childhood and consist of temporary lapses of consciousness that last for a few seconds. Patients appear to be staring into space and may exhibit a few rhythmic movements of the eyes or head. They do not convulse. They may experience many attacks in a single day. Sometimes an attack of petit mal is followed by one of grand mal.

Jacksonian (partial simple motor) epilepsy is described by some authorities as a type of focal seizure; it is associated with irritation of a specific part of the brain. A single part, such as a finger or an extremity, may jerk and such movements may end spontaneously or spread over the whole musculature. Consciousness may not be lost unless the seizure develops into a generalized convulsion.

Psychomotor (partial complex) attacks are characterized by brief alterations in consciousness, unusual stereotyped movements (such as chewing or swallowing movements) repeated over and over, temperamental changes, confusion, and feelings of unreality. It is often associated with grand mal seizures and is likely to be resistant to therapy with drugs.

Status epilepticus. Status epilepticus is a recurrent seizure without an intervening stay of consciousness. There is a 10% to 20% mortality rate resulting from anoxia in this medical emergency. The major cause of status epilepticus is noncompliance with drug regimen, and other causes include cerebral infarction or cerebral infection.

Some patients have more than one type of seizure or have mixed seizures. This is significant because different types of seizures respond rather specifically to certain anticonvulsant drugs. The aim of therapy is to find the drug or drugs that will effectively control the seizures and will at the same time cause a minimum of undesirable side effects.

Mechanism of action of the anticonvulsant drugs. The effectiveness of anticonvulsant drugs is often measured by the amount of increased voltage necessary to provoke an electroconvulsion in an animal who has previously received the anticonvulsant to be tested or by the degree of their antagonism to chemical substances capable of producing convulsions. Pentylenetetrazol is a drug against which anticonvulsants are measured for effectiveness.

The mode and site of action of these drugs are still regarded as uncertain. The convulsive seizure may be effectively suppressed, but the abnormal brain waves may or may not be altered. All clinically useful drugs for epilepsy inhibit the seizure by depressing neural excitability by stabilization of cell membranes (transfer of sodium, calcium, and potassium ions across membranes) or by modifying synaptic transmission (by control of neurotransmitter release, uptake, or recycling). This prevents the spread of seizure discharges.

Although there is no ideal anticonvulsant drug, if one could be synthesized to order, a number of characteristics would be considered highly desirable:

1 The drug should be highly effective but exhibit a low incidence of toxicity.
2 It should be effective against more than one type of seizure and for mixed seizures.
3 It should be long acting and nonsedative so that the patient is not incapacitated with sleep or excessive drowsiness.
4 It should be well tolerated by the patient and inex-

T A B L E 8 - 1 2 **Indications and adverse effects of selected anticonvulsants**

Primary	International classification indications*	Some adverse effects most often encountered
Clonazepam (Clonopin)	c	Drowsiness, ataxia, behavior problems, increased secretions
Valproic acid (Depakene)	c	Gastrointestinal upset, elevation of SGOT and serum alkaline phosphate levels, thrombocytopenia
Phenytoin (Dilantin)	a,b,d (DC)	Nystagmus, ataxia, slurred speech, mental confusion, gastrointestinal upset, rashes, gingival hyperplasia, hirsutism, coarse facies
Primidone (Mysoline)	a,b,d	Ataxia, vertigo, gastrointestinal upset, hyperirritability, emotional disturbances, drowsiness
Phenobarbital	a,b,d (DC)	Excessive sedation, hyperkinetic behavior, nystagmus, ataxia, learning difficulties
Carbamazepine (Tegretol)	a,b,d	Dizziness, drowsiness, ataxia, gastrointestinal upset, skin rashes, visual disturbances
Ethosuximide (Zarontin)	c (DC)	Gastrointestinal upset, drowsiness, dizziness, irritability, hyperactivity, lethargy, fatigue, ataxia, skin rashes

*a, Generalized convulsive seizures.
b, All forms of partial seizures.
c, Generalized nonconvulsive seizures (absences).
d, Partial seizures with complex symptoms.
DC, Drug of choice.

pensive, since the patient may have to take it for years or for the rest of his life.

5 Tolerance to the therapeutic effects of the drug should not develop.

The present-day drugs that are considered especially satisfactory and safe are phenobarbital and phenytoin sodium. The bromides are among the oldest anticonvulsants known, but because they tend to cause states of chronic toxicity, they seldom are used. The barbiturates have been discussed but their use as anticonvulsants will be emphasized again. They are an important group of drugs for this purpose, especially the longer-acting members. Phenobarbital is effective against all types of epileptic seizures except certain petit mal types. It is considered one of the safest of the anticonvulsants. Its chief disadvantage is that it must often be given in doses that produce apathy and sleepiness.

The anticonvulsants may be classified into the following groups:

Barbiturates—phenobarbital, mephobarbital, metharbital, amobarbital, primidone
Hydantoins—phenytoin, mephytoin, ethotoin
Succinamides—ethosuximide, methsuximide, phensuximide
Oxazolidinediones—paramethadione, trimethadione

Benzodiazepines—clonazepam, diazepam, clorazepate
Miscellaneous—valproic acid (sodium valproate), carbamazepine, phenacemide, acetazolamide, bromides

Table 8-12 presents some of the most commonly used anticonvulsants in clinical practice along with their primary indications and the adverse effects most often encountered.

There are few parenteral forms of anticonvulsant drugs; anticonvulsants are usually given orally. There are, however, occasions when the parenteral form is the best choice for therapy. Table 8-13 lists these conditions or situations and the parenteral drugs indicated for the treatment of each.

Dosage adjustments. Anticonvulsant drugs may exhibit varying blood levels in different patients after each has received the same dose. This variation results from a complex of interrelated factors including individual patient compliance; individual absorption, metabolism, distribution, and excretion which may be caused by genetic and/or environmental factors; concomitant ailments, such as renal or hapatic dysfunctions; concurrent medication; diet; physical status; and a host of other variables. Certain drugs require an adjusted dosage

T A B L E 8 - 1 3 Parenteral use of anticonvulsant drugs

Parenteral drug	Use
Phenobarbital	Status epilepticus
	Severe recurrent seizures
Amobarbital	Status epilepticus
	Convulsant drug poisoning
	Other convulsive states
Secobarbital and so-	Status epilepticus
dium pentobarbital	Convulsant drug poisoning
Sodium thiopental	Other convulsive states
Phenytoin	Status epilepticus
	Seizure during neurosurgery
Diazepam	Status epilepticus and se-
	vere recurrent seizures
	(adjunctive use)
Magnesium sulfate	Eclampsia
Paraldehyde injection	Status epilepticus
	Tetanus, eclampsia

to obtain optimal therapeutic effects, and this dosage may have wide patient variation.

Therapeutic dosage ranges are intended to serve merely as rough guides to therapy and not firm as limits. They provide a point from which the dosage of a drug may be individualized to account for the extremes in variation to response and adverse effects. The patient beginning anticonvulsant therapy should have serum levels measured to establish his individual level/dose ratio. This level tends to be a constant measure for an individual, though it varies considerably among patients. The time required to reach a steady serum level is generally about four to five times the elimination half-life of a drug. A convenient time for serum level measurement is 1 month after initiating therapy, since levels measured much earlier may be lower than the steady state level finally achieved.

The serum half-life of a drug (the time required for the serum level to drop 50% when no additional drug is administered) is a measure of its rate of excretion and depends on the patient's age. Infants require about twice as high an administered dose as adolescents to maintain the same serum level.

One of the characteristics of the anticonvulsant drugs is that either the parent drug or the active metabolite has a long serum half-life, so the exact daily medication schedule is seldom critical. Administration of these drugs may be one to three times daily.

A loading dose is usually necessary to quickly attain a therapeutic steady-state serum drug concentration equal to the usual maintenance steady-state serum drug concentration.

This loading dose concept is based on a one-compartment, first-order kinetics model that predicts that steady-state serum concentrations of a drug are maintained by single doses administered intravenously at intervals equal to the drug's elimination half-life.

The first serum concentration after the first intravenous dose is half the peak value attained during long term administration. Therefore, under these conditions the patient can attain steady-state serum concentration quickly if the first dose is twice the maintenance dose for each elimination half-life. In adults, for example, a loading (intravenous) dose of phenytoin (1000 mg or 13 to 14 mg/kg, which is twice the usual maintenance dose of 300 to 400 mg per half-life of about 24 hours) will produce a therapeutic serum concentration of 10 to 20 µg/ml. The intravenous route is necessary because phenytoin is absorbed very slowly by intramuscular route because the water solubility of the drug decreases greatly and phenytoin crystals precipitate in the muscle.

Anticonvulsant drugs should not be administered intramuscularly in emergency situations (such as status epilepticus) because of the slowness of absorption from the injection site and the low peak serum levels achieved. The anticonvulsant drugs should be administered using as long an interval between doses as possible, depending on their half-life. The anticonvulsant drugs that have an elimination half-life of 24 hours or more generally need to be administered only once a day to maintain a therapeutic serum concentration. The daily dose may be administered at bedtime to overcome the sedation seen with peak levels of anticonvulsant drugs.

In a situation that is not an emergency, it is best to make changes in drug therapy with one drug at a time. The nurse and the patient must be aware, that each time a new anticonvulsant drug is started or the dose of a drug is increased or decreased, it takes four to five elimination half-life intervals (so the concentration of the drug has dropped by 95%) to know the new steady-state serum concentration and to achieve the total therapeutic effect of the new drug regimen.

Drugs that may precipitate seizures. There are drugs that increase the risk of epileptiform seizures (including drug-disease interactions), such as oral contraceptives, reserpine, and the tricyclic antidepressants. Oral contraceptives may cause fluid retention, which may precipitate seizures in epileptic individuals. Cases of this induced exacerbation of epilepsy by the oral contraceptives are reported. Anticonvulsant drugs cause liver enzyme induction and may reduce the efficacy of oral contraceptives. Reserpine lowers the convulsive threshold, and anticonvulsant dosage may have to be titrated to control epilepsy (to increase the dose). Very rarely the tricyclic antidepressants have produced epileptiform seizures in susceptible patients and high doses have created grand mal–type seizures even in nonepileptic patients.

Mephytoin is for patients whose trials with safer anticonvulsants have ended in failure and for those who are refractory to other anticonvulsants. It is also indicated in focal and jacksonian seizures.

Since the liver is the site of biotransformation of hydantoins, the patient with impaired liver function, the elderly, or those who are very ill may demonstrate early toxic signs. A small percentage of persons metabolize the drug slowly, because of limited enzyme availability that may be genetically determined. The metabolism of hydantoins is dose dependent at therapeutic doses.

HYDANTOINS

Phenytoin and some other hydantoins appear to inhibit the spread of seizure activity by possibly promoting sodium efflux from neurons, and they tend to stabilize the threshold against hyperexcitability caused by excess stimulation or environmental changes capable of reducing membrane sodium gradient. This includes the reduction of posttetanic potentiation at synapses. The loss of posttetanic potentiation prevents cortical seizure foci from detonating adjacent cortical areas. The hydantoins as a group act to reduce the maximal activity of brainstem centers responsible for the tonic phase of grand mal seizures.

The hydantoins are contraindicated in hypersensitivity, hepatic dysfunction, and hematologic disorders. Abrupt withdrawal may precipitate status epilepticus. There is an elevated incidence of birth defects in children born to mothers using anticonvulsants, though the majority deliver normal infants.

Phenytoin sodium extended (Dilantin)

Phenytoin is a synthetic agent chemically related to the barbiturates. It is an odorless white or cream-colored powder with a bitter taste.

Action and result. Phenytoin exerts a selective action on the cerebral motor cortex of the brain without appreciably affecting the sensory areas. It is an anticonvulsant but not a hypnotic. It is somewhat more effective in controlling grand mal seizures than phenobarbital, although patients vary in their response to these drugs. It is strongly alkaline in solution and may produce gastric irritation.

The time required to reach a peak plasma concentration after a single oral dose of phenytoin is 3 to 12 hours, the plasma half-life following oral administration is an average of 22 hours, with a range of 7 to 42 hours. Phenytoin half-life in children is shorter than for adults and is dose-dependent. The usual oral maintenance dose for adults is 300 to 400 mg/day and for children under 6 years old it is 4 to 8 mg/kg/day in two or three divided doses. Children over 6 years old may need the minimum adult dose of 300 mg/day. The therapeutic serum levels are 10 to 20 μg/ml. Toxic serum levels above 20 μg/ml result in nystagmus, above 30 μg/ml obvious side effects occur, while above 50 μg/ml coma results. Phenytoin is 70% to 95% protein bound. Steady-state therapeutic levels are reached at 7 to 10 days after therapy with a dose of 300 mg daily.

Uses. In the treatment of epilepsy it is more effective for grand mal than petit mal seizures. It may increase the attacks of petit mal. Psychomotor seizures are sometimes controlled. It does not cure the mental deterioration sometimes found in the epileptic individual. On the other hand, it does not cause mental deterioration. It is frequently prescribed in combination with phenobarbital. It may be prescribed for patients following surgical operations on the brain to prevent convulsive seizures and for status epilepticus. The effects of phenytoin on ventricular automaticity prohibit its use in sinus bradycardia, sinoatrial block, and second and third degree atrioventricular block and in patients with Adams-Stokes syndrome.

Preparation, dosage, and administration. Phenytoin is marketed in 30- and 100-mg capsules (delayed action or extended action, the only phenytoin that can be used for once daily dosing), in 50-mg scored tablets, and in an oral suspension of 30 and 125 mg/5 ml.* It is also available for parenteral administration in vials containing 100 to 250 mg of the drug. When used alone, the beginning daily dose for adults is 100 mg orally with one-half glass of water three times a day. The dosage may be gradually increased until optimum effects are obtained. Most adults seem to tolerate 300 to 400 mg daily without toxic effects. Dosage for younger children is 3 to 8 mg/kg (average 5 mg/kg/day). Increase in dosage is made slowly and with careful observation of the patient. When the drug is combined with one or more other anticonvulsants, the dosage of individual drugs is often reduced. The transition from phenobarbital, and other hypnotics to phenytoin is made gradually, with some overlapping of drugs to prevent the precipitation of convulsive seizures.

If intramuscular administration is required for a patient formerly stabilized on the oral drug, a compensating dosage adjustment is needed to maintain therapeutic plasma levels. The intramuscular dose is 50% greater than the oral dose to maintain these levels. When the patient is returned to the oral route, the dose should be reduced by 50% of the original oral dose for a 7-day period to compensate for the excessive plasma levels resulting from sustained release from the intramuscular site of injection.

For status epilepticus a 150- to 250-mg intravenous dose is administered slowly (50 mg over 1-minute period), then 100 to 150 mg is given in 30 minutes if needed. Higher doses may be needed. The dose for children is deter-

mined by weight in proportion to the dose of a 150-pound adult. Pediatric dose may also be calculated on the basis of 250 mg/m². This latter method is preferred. If the state of the patient is such that immobilization of an extremity is impossible because of convulsions or inaccessible veins, then the intramuscular route may be useful. If the administration does not terminate the seizure, the nurse must consider other anticonvulsants, intravenous barbiturates, general anesthesia, or other measures. The intramuscular route is not recommended for the treatment of status epilepticus, since the plasma levels of phenytoin in the therapeutic range cannot be readily achieved, and since pain and necrosis may occur at the injection site. Parenteral phenytoin should be used with caution in patients with hypotension and severe myocardial insufficiency.

Side effects and toxic effects. The incidence of toxic reactions with phenytoin is greater than with phenobarbital. The less serious side effects include apathy, nervousness, dizziness, ataxia, blurred vision, hyperplasia of the gums (excessive formation of gum tissues), and hirsutism (excessive growth of hair, especially on the face). Other reactions that sometimes occur are tremor, excitement, hallucinations, psychosis, nausea, and vomiting. If the patient is particularly sensitive to the drug he may develop skin rash, exfoliative dermatitis, fever, and difficult breathing. Hepatitis, blood dyscrasias, periarteritis nodosa, birth defects, and lupus erythematosus from phenytoin therapy have been reported.

The diverse signs of toxicity seen with intravenous phenytoin are cardiovascular collapse, central nervous system depression, and hypotension (seen with rapid intravenous administration). The rate of administration (50 mg over 1 minute) is important, since severe cardiotoxic reactions and fatal outcomes are reported in elderly or gravely ill patients. When the plasma concentration is over 20 μg/ml (above the usual therapeutic plasma concentration), parenteral phenytoin causes drowsiness, nystagmus, circumoral tingling, vertigo, nausea, and rarely vomiting.

Drug interactions. A serious interaction between phenytoin and alcohol is the development of cross-tolerance to phenytoin in patients

*Generic phenytoin (not Dilantin [Parke-Davis]) in *not* extended or delayed action but *is* prompt acting. Therefore it cannot be used for once-daily dosing and it is not generically equivalent to Parke-Davis' Dilantin capsules.

TABLE 8-14 Phenytoin drug interactions

Drugs that can potentiate the action of phenytoin

Aspirin	Griseofulvin
Phenylbutazone	Chlordiazepoxide
Chloramphenicol	Sulfonamides
Cycloserine	Anticoagulants
Isoniazid	Alcohol (acute intoxication)
Estrogens	

Drugs that inhibit the action of phenytoin*

Alcohol (chronic use)	Glutethimide
Antihistamines	Sedatives
Barbiturates	Hypnotics
CNS depressant effects may be additive	

Phenytoin potentiates the action of*

Antihypertensives	Propranolol
Folic acid antagonists	Quinidine
Methotrexate	Tubocurarine

Phenytoin inhibits the action of

Corticosteroids
Digitalis
Anticoagulants

*All of these drugs may enhance the metabolism of phenytoin, but CNS effects may be additive.

with epilepsy who are also heavy drinkers. Alcohol apparently speeds up the metabolism of phenytoin, causing accelerated removal of the drug and making normal doses inadequate. Other research has indicated that before this cross-tolerance develops in epileptic individuals, alcohol can delay the removal of phenytoin from the body. Such inhibition could increase the chances that patients will experience toxic side effects with otherwise appropriate dosages.

A critical drug interaction occurring with anticoagulants (oral coumarins) and phenytoin results in a decreased phenytoin metabolism, which leads to toxic effects (ataxia, nystagmus, vertigo). Initially a transient increase in anticoagulant effect is seen, which is followed by an enhancement of the metabolism of the anticoagulant and a resultant reduction in anticoagulant effect. The nurse must observe the patient and monitor with the necessary laboratory tests to adjust the dosage or one or both drugs if needed.

The interaction of phenytoin and isoniazid is also of critical significance, since a decrease in phenytoin metabolism results significantly in those patients who are slow acetylators (50% of American blacks and whites, 20% of Ameri-

can Indians, 5% of Eskimos, 13% of Japanese). Phenytoin plasma concentrations are increased when phenytoin is given with cimetidine. Table 8-14 summarizes other known phenytoin drug interactions.

Mephenytoin (Mesantoin); methoin

Mephenytoin is an anticonvulsant drug similar in chemical structure and activity to phenytoin. It is less potent as an anticonvulsant than phenytoin. It produces more sedation than phenytoin but less than phenobarbital. Tolerance develops with this drug.

Uses. Mephenytoin is effective for grand mal and focal, jacksonian, and psychomotor seizures (temporal lobe) refractory to other drugs. It is less effective for petit mal seizures, since it may provoke attacks of petit mal. Certain patients who do not respond favorably to phenytoin or to phenobarbital may benefit from this drug.

Preparation, dosage, and administration. Mephenytoin is available in 100-mg tablets for oral administration. The average daily dose for adults is 200 to 600 mg, up to 800 mg; for children, 100 to 400 mg. As with all anticonvulsants, the optimum daily dosage must be calculated to meet the needs of each patient.

Side effects and toxic effects. Side effects during initial therapy include nausea, vomiting, nervousness, sleeplessness, and dizziness. This is a drug that can produce serious toxic effects, and therefore caution in its use is recommended. In cases of hypersensitivity to the drug, destruction of blood cells can occur, which may vary from leukopenia to agranulocytosis and aplastic anemia. Some patients become jaundiced, indicating damage to the liver. Other symptoms of toxicity include fever and dermatitis.

Ethotoin (Peganone)

Ethotoin belongs to the hydantoin group of anticonvulsants.

Uses. Ethotoin is said to be less effective than phenytoin, but it is also less toxic. It is effective for grand mal epilepsy and psychomotor (temporal lobe) seizures but does not always bring about complete relief of seizures. To be satisfactory, it may need to be used with other anticonvulsants. Patients receiving ethotoin should have routine blood counts and urinalyses performed.

Preparation, dosage, and administration. The average daily adult dose of ethotoin is 2 to 3 g given orally after meals in four to six divided portions. Dosage for children is 500 mg to 1 g daily in divided doses, rarely up to 3 g daily. It is available in 250- and 500-mg tablets.

SUCCINIMIDES
Ethosuximide (Zarontin)

Ethosuximide is the drug of choice for treating petit mal (absence) epilepsy. It is as a rule ineffective for psychomotor or grand mal epilepsy. A single dose produces peak blood levels in 2 to 4 hours, which last for 24 hours. Large daily doses produce a peak on the fourth day, which is maintained until the drug is discontinued. It is eliminated from the blood 2 days after the drug is stopped.

Preparation and dosage. Ethosuximide is available in 250-mg capsules and a raspberry syrup containing 250 mg/5 ml. Dosage for adults and children over 6 years of age is 500 mg initially. The dose thereafter is individualized by increments of 250 mg every 4 to 7 days until seizures are controlled with minimal untoward effects. For children under 6 initial dose is 250 mg daily with gradual increase in dosage as above. Most children have an optimal dose range of 20 mg/kg/day.

Side effects. Side effects to ethosuximide include nausea, vomiting, drowsiness, vertigo, headache, diarrhea, and weight loss. Blood dyscrasias and neurologic and psychologic reactions have occurred rarely. Mental and physical abilities may be impaired, and patients should be cautioned about performing potentially hazardous tasks.

Other anticonvulsants. There are two other succinimides in current use. These include phensuximide (Milontin) and methsuximide (Celontin), which are effective for petit mal seizures.

OXAZOLIDINEDIONES
Trimethadione (Tridione)

Trimethadione belongs to a group of compounds known as the oxazolidinediones.

Action. Its primary action is on the central nervous system, although it is not restricted to the motor cortex. It exerts an analgesic effect in some instances as well as an anticonvulsant action. It is said to surpass all other anticonvulsants in raising the threshold to pentylenetetrazol-induced seizures. The precise mechanism of action, however, is unknown.

Uses. Trimethadione is used chiefly in the treatment of petit mal epilepsy. It appears to be more effective for petit mal in children than in adults. It is not effective for grand mal seizures. It is given with phenytoin or phenobarbital if the patient has attacks of both petit mal and grand mal seizures. It rarely seems to be adequate to control psychomotor seizures. Because of its toxicity it is recommended and warned that this drug be reserved for refractory cases when other less toxic drugs were ineffective in controlling petit mal seizures.

Preparation, dosage, and administration. Trimethadione is available in 150-mg tablets, 300-mg capsules, and in a solution containing 200 mg/5 ml for oral administration. The dose for children is 300 to 900 mg daily and for adults, 900 to 2400 mg daily, in three or four divided portions. Dosage may need to be increased.

Side effects and toxic effects. Symptoms of toxicity appear infrequently, but they may be serious and fatal. Nausea and vomiting, skin eruption, blurring of vision, and sensitivity to light are considered indications for reduction of dosage or temporary withdrawal of the drug. Careful medical supervision of the patient receiving the medication is essential. Rare instances of aplastic anemia explain why it is thought advisable for the patient to have periodic examinations of the blood to detect early signs of toxic effects.

The drug is not recommended for patients with hepatic or renal disease, with disease of the optic nerve, allergic reactions to drugs, or blood dyscrasias. Its use in pregnant women may cause malformation of the fetus.

Paramethadione (Paradione)

Action and uses. The action and uses of paramethadione are similar to those of trimethadione. It belongs to the same chemical group, and no significant pharmacologic difference between them is known. Some patients not benefited by trimethadione are benefited by paramethadione and vice versa.

Preparation, dosage, and administration. This drug is available as 150- and 800-mg capsules. The initial dose of paramethadione for adults is 900 mg given orally in divided doses. Thereafter, dosage is adjusted to the minimum effective dose. Initial dosage for children varies from 300 to 900 mg, depending on size. The solution of 300 mg/ml is 65% alcohol. This high alcohol content needs dilution with water prior to administration to small children.

Side effects. Side effects are similar to those of trimethadione, except the incidence of skin rash and photophobia is said to be less with paramethadione. Neutropenia has been reported.

BENZODIAZEPINES
Diazepam (Valium)

This benzodiazepine by the oral route is useful as an adjunctive drug in convulsive disorders but not as sole therapy. As with other anticonvulsant oral drugs, the possibility of an increase in frequency and/or severity of grand mal seizures may require an increased dosage of the standard anticonvulsant medication used prior to the addition of this agent. Further abrupt withdrawal of diazepam may also increase the risk of a temporary increase in frequency or severity of seizures.

Diazepam by the parenteral route is the drug of choice in status epilepticus and severe recurrent convulsive seizures. The uses of this drug as a muscle relaxant, antianxiety agent, and in acute alcohol withdrawal are discussed in Chapter 12.

Preparation, dosages, and administration. Dosages are individualized for each patient and are increased with caution to avoid adverse effects. Some patients require higher doses than indicated. In elderly or debilitated persons and those taking other sedative-hypnotic medications, a lower dose with slow increases is prudent. Usual dose for adults is 2 to 10 mg taken two to four times daily initially to abate ataxia or oversedation, and the dose is titrated upward slowly as necessary. In children over 6 months therapy is initiated with lower doses since there is a varied response to drugs acting on the central nervous system. A child is usually started with 1 to 2.5 mg three to four times daily, titrating to tolerated level slowly.

Parenteral route administration of diazepam is as follows. Because of the short-lived effect of intravenous diazepam administration, seizures, although brought under prompt control, may recur. The nurse should be ready to readminister the diazepam. Diazepam is not for maintenance; once siezure control is achieved, agents useful in long-term seizure control should be considered. Tonic status epilepticus has been precipitated in some patients treated with intravenous diazepam for petit mal status or petit mal variant status. The nurse must exercise extreme care in administering the parenteral diazepam (especially by the intravenous route) to elderly or very ill patients or those with compromised pulmonary reserve because of the possibility that apnea and/or cardiac arrest may occur. To reduce the chance of venous thrombosis, phlebitis, local irritation, swelling, and rarely vascular impairment the solution is injected, slowly—over a 1-minute period in 5-mg increments. It is not used in small veins such as on the dorsum of the hand or wrist, and care is taken to avoid intraarterial or extravasation injection. Diazepam absolutely must not be mixed or diluted with other solutions or drugs. If it is not possible to inject directly intravenously, diazepam may be injected slowly as above throughout the infusion tubing as close as possible to the vein insertion.

Diazepam is insoluble in water, therefore each milliliter of the parenteral form contains 40% propylene glycol, 10% ethyl alcohol, 5% sodium benzoate and benzoic acid as buffers, with 1.5% benzyl alcohol as a preservative. If this ratio is altered the diazepam is insoluble.

In the neonate (age 30 days or less) the efficacy and safety of parenteral diazepam are not established. Prolonged central nervous system depression has been reported in the neonate, probably resulting from the inability to biotransform diazepam into the inactive metabolites. The benzoate in the injectable form has been reported to displace other drugs and bilirubin from the plasma protein binding sites, causing jaundice. In pediatric use the drug is administered slowly over a 3-minute period in a dosage not exceeding 0.25 mg/kg. After this initial dose a 15- to 30-minute interval is allowed to elapse before a repeat dose is given. If after the third administration there is no symptom relief, other therapy is recommended and respiratory assistance should be readily available.

If intravenous administration is impossible in a convulsing patient, a deep intramuscular injection is useful.

Adults require 5 to 10 mg initially (intravenous route preferred) and repeated in 10- to 15-minute intervals (if needed) to 30 mg (in practice more may be necessary). Therapy may be repeated in 2 to 4 hours, but the residual active metabolite's persisting activity must be kept in mind.

For infants over 30 days and children under 5 years, a dose of 0.2 to 0.5 mg is given slowly every 2 to 5 minutes up to a maximum of 5 mg (intravenous route preferred). For children over 5 years a dose of 1 mg is given every 2 to 5 minutes up to a maximum of 10 mg, repeated in 2 to 4 hours if needed along with EEG monitoring of the seizure.

Diazepam is available in oral tablets of 2, 5, and 10 mg and in ampules, vials, and disposable syringes. The injectable forms contain 5 mg/ml diazepam.

Clorazepate dipotassium (Tranxene)

This benzodiazepine is indicated as adjunctive therapy in the management of partial seizures. For patients over 13 years, the maximum initial dose is 7.5 mg three times a day. This dose is increased by 7.5 mg weekly to a dosage not exceeding 90 mg/day. For patients 9 to 12 years, the maximum initital dose is 7.5 mg two times a day. This dose is increased by not more than 1.5 mg weekly and dosage should not exceed 60 mg/day.

Clonazepam (Clonopin)

Clonazepam is a benzodiazepine whose mechanism of action is presumed to involve activity on neurotransmitters or cell membranes, or both, but no specific mechanism has been established. Clonazepam may act by mimicking the effects of the neurotransmitter glycine or by increasing the serotonin concentration at synaptic sites. The drug is currently approved for use alone or as an adjunctive antiepileptic drug against Lennox-Gastaut syn-

drome (petit mal variant), akinetic and myoclonic seizures, and infantile spasms (infantile myoclonia, massive spasms). In patients with absence seizures (petit mal) who failed with succinimide therapy, this drug may be useful. Clonazepam is being tested for these and other indications: tonic-clonic (grand mal), complex partial (psychomotor, temporal lobe), or elementary partial (focal) seizures.

Action and result. The drug is largely nonionized in the physiologic pH range, and readily crosses the biologic membranes. The tablets are micronized, which aids in the dissolution in the gastrointestinal tract. Clonazepam passes rapidly from blood to brain and is about 50% protein bound. Five metabolites have been identified in humans. Less than 5% of clonazepam is excreted unchanged in the urine. Peak serum concentrations occur for clonazepam 1 in 3 hours after a single oral dose; the elimination half-life is 18 to 50 hours. Serum concentrations are variable and difficult to accurately predict from dosage. Most patients with seizures controlled with clonazepam have serum concentrations of 20 to 80 ng/ml. These are the same serum concentrations of those patients who do not respond to or have side effects with clonazepam. Therefore there is not a precise minimum serum concentration or usual toxic serum concentration. Clonazepam does not induce its own metabolism and addition of clonazepam does not appear to alter the steady state serum concentratons of phenytoin, phenobarbital (or primidone), or carbamazepine. The addition of phenytoin or phenobarbital may lower the steady state serum concentration for clonazepam when it is included in the therapy. Tolerance to the antiepileptic effect of clonazepam occurs in about 30% of the patients who initially responded well to this drug, and tolerance usually develops in 1 to 6 months of administration. When tolerance develops about 60% receive benefits with increased dosage and 30% do not show response to dosage increment adjustments.

Side effects and toxic effects. The effects in pregnancy and on nursing infants pose unknown risks. The drug is contraindicated in benzodiazepine sensitivity, those with evidence of liver or hepatic disease, and acute narrow angle glaucoma (may be used in open angle glaucoma patients receiving appropriate therapy).

The nurse should warn the patient of the CNS depressant effects and warn against the combined use of alcohol or other CNS depressants. The most common side effects are drowsiness, ataxia, and behavior changes. Other less common side effects include hypotonia, thick speech, hypersalivation, bronchial hypersecretion, anorexia, increased appetite, and neurologic, psychiatric, cardiovascular, dermatologic, genitourinary, musculoskeletal, hepatic, and hematopoietic reactions. With patients having several different types of coexisting seizure disorders, the clonazepam may increase the incidence or precipitate the onset of generalized tonic-clonic seizures (grand mal), which may necessitate the addition to or increase in their dosages. The concomitant use of valproic acid and clonazepam may produce absence status. Periodic blood counts and liver function tests are advisable during long-term therapy with clonazepam. The discontinuation of clonazepam must be gradual; abrupt withdrawal (particularly after administration in high doses or over a long time) may cause status epilepticus. Since the clonazepam metabolites are excreted by the kidneys, caution is needed in patients with impaired renal function.

Preparation, dosage, and administration. To minimize drowsiness, in infants and children up to 10 years old or 30 kg weight, the initial dose is between 0.01 to 0.03 mg/kg/day, not exceeding 0.05 mg/kg/day in two to three divided doses. This dose is increased by no more than 0.25 to 0.5 mg every third day until a daily maintenance dose of 0.1 to 0.2 mg/kg body weight is reached, unless seizures are controlled or side effects preclude further increases (three daily doses is the optimum therapy). If this is not possible the largest dose should be at bedtime. For adults the initial dose should not exceed 1.5 mg/day divided into three doses. Dose increments of 0.5 to 1.0 mg are made every 3 days until seizures are controlled or until side effects preclude any further upward increments. The maintenance dose is individualized; the maximum recommended daily dose is 20 mg.

The tablets are made in 0.5, 1, and 2 mg.

Drug interactions. The drug interactions of

interest center around the enhancement of CNS depression and are concerned with the following drugs: other anticonvulsants, antidepressants (tricyclic antidepressants and monoamine oxidase inhibitors), antipsychotic agents, and other CNS depressants (alcohol, antianxiety agents, barbiturates, hypnotics, and narcotics). The metabolism of clonazepam is increased through enzyme induction by carbamazepine.

MISCELLANEOUS ANTICONVULSANTS
Primidone (Mysoline)

Primidone per se has anticonvulsant activity as does its metabolites, phenobarbital and phenylethylmalonamide (PEMA). Studies based on clinical and laboratory observations have led to the discovery that primidone is a three-in-one anticonvulsant. Evidence indicates that the total anticonvulsant action of primidone exceeds that attributable to phenobarbital alone. It is indicated for control of grand mal, psychomotor (temporal-limbic), or focal epileptic seizures and may control grand mal seizures refractory to other anticonvulsant therapy.

Action and result. Absorption is relatively rapid after a single oral dose, a slower absorption times are expected in long-term administration. The three-in-one status evolved because at least two of its metabolites (PEMA and phenobarbital) have anticonvulsant activity, as does the unchanged (unmetabolized) primidone, thus interaction among the three compounds is extremely pertinent to the total therapeutic and toxic activity of the drug. The mechanism of primidone's antiepileptic action is not known. Animal studies have led to the conclusion that conversion of primidone to its active metabolites may be simultaneously influenced by the processes of metabolite induction (by phenobarbital) and metabolite inhibition (by PEMA), so a sequence of dose-related and time-related factors affects primidone metabolism and its clinical effectiveness. The rapid formation of PEMA (the major metabolite) and an increase in their serum concentration of primidone soon produce a proportionate increase in the serum concentration of PEMA.

It is difficult to determine the half-life of a

compound continually being formed but the half-life of PEMA appears to be significantly longer than primidone and is reflected by stable serum PEMA concentrations. About 15% to 20% of an oral dose of primidone is slowly converted to phenobarbital. The two known metabolites are themselves slowly metabolized and tend to maintain constant serum concentrations, and they appear to act synergistically as anticonvulsants.

About 60% to 80% of an oral dose of primidone is excreted in the urine within 24 hours in an unchanged form or as PEMA, and the balance may account for the phenobarbital metabolite. After long-term dosage, the rate of disposal of primidone is prolonged. There is considerable individual variation in the rate at which primidone is absorbed and excreted. After a single oral dose the time required for peak plasma concentration is an average of 3 to 24 hours for primidone, and for PEMA, 1 to 2 days. It may take several (3 to 5) days to achieve peak plasma concentration of the phenobarbital derived from the oxidation of primidone, and the plasma half-life of this phenobarbital in adults is 2 to 6 days and in children, 36 to 72 hours. Therapeutic serum levels for primidone is 5 to 15 μg/ml, not established for PEMA, and 10 to 40 μg/ml for the phenobarbital. Toxic serum levels for primidone are above 10 to 15 μg/ml (ataxia and lethargy), for PEMA not established, and for phenobarbital above 40 μg/ml (overt symptoms of toxicity); above 70 μg/ml of phenobarbital marked drowsiness and sometimes comatose states occur.

Preparation, dosage, and administration. Primidone is available in 250- and 50-mg tablets and in a suspension of 250 mg/5ml. The suspension is sugar free, has 13 mg of sodium per milliliter, and contains FDC Yellow No. 5 (a tartrazine), while the tablets both contain up to 60 μg of sodium per tablet.

The average adult dose is 0.75 to 1.5 g/day (comparable to 150 to 250 mg phenobarbital). The initial dose is 250 mg, with increments of 250 mg added usually at weekly intervals, to tolerance or therapeutic effect. The daily dose should not exceed 2.0 g. In children under 8 years of age the initial dose 125 mg, with gradual weekly increases of 125 mg to a total daily dose range of 500 to 750 mg. A pediatric dosage range has been suggested at 10 to 25 mg/kg/day.

In patients already being given other anticonvulsants, dosage of primidone is gradually increased as dosage of the other drug(s) is maintained or gradually decreased. A transition to primidone alone may be accomplished in about 2 weeks.

Valproic acid (Depakene)

Valproic acid is a carboxylic acid derivative also designated as 2-propylpentanoic acid or depropylacetic acid (pK$_a$ 4.8). This anticonvulsant is indicated for use as sole and adjunctive therapy in the treatment of simple and complex absence seizures, including petit mal, and as adjunctive therapy in patients with multiple seizure types including absence seizures. The International Classification of Seizures defines simple absence as a very brief clouding of the sensorium or loss of consciousness (lasting usually 2 to 15 seconds), with certain generalized epileptic discharges without other detectable clinical signs. Complex absence is the term used when other signs are also present. In Europe, valproic acid has been used to treat grand mal, simple and complex partial myoclonic, and mixed grand mal and petit mal seizures, because of its broad-spectrum anticonvulsant activity.

Action and results. The mechanism by which it exerts its anticonvulsant effects has not been fully established. It has been proposed that its activity is related to increased brain levels of the inhibitory neurotransmitter gamma-aminobutyric acid (GABA). By competitive inhibition it prevents the reuptake of GABA by glial cells and axonal terminals. The drug has a marked effect on the generalized spike wave discharges (3/second) in the EEG.

Valproic acid is rapidly and nearly completely absorbed after oral administration. The peak serum levels occur approximately 1 to 4 hours after a single oral dose, and the serum half-life of the parent compound is about 8 to 12 hours. There is a slight delay in initial absorption when it is administered with meals, which does not affect total absorption. A wide individual variation exists between daily dose and plasma levels, which may be caused by differences in absorption, biotransformation, or excretion. The drug is highly plasma protein bound (90% to 95%), and the percentage of binding decreases with increasing temperature. The binding of the drug influences the clearance of valproic acid; an increase in binding causes a decrease in clearance or elimination. Therapeutic plasma levels are generally 50 to 100 μg/ml, with some patients needing higher levels for optimal control. Elimination of the parent drug and its metabolites is principally in the urine, with minor amounts in the feces and expired air. Very little unmetabolized drug is found in the urine. The drug is primarily metabolized in the liver and is excreted as the glucuronide conjugate. It should not be administered to patients with preexisting hepatic disease. Other metabolites in the urine are products of beta and omega oxidation. Enterohepatic circulation has been demonstrated. The short half-life of valproic acid necessitates its administration in three divided doses. The diabetic patient should be made aware that a ketone-containing metabolite is excreted, since this may lead to a false interpretation (false positive) of the urine ketone test. Concurrent administration with phenobarbital may produce an elevated phenobarbital plasma concentration (increases of 30% to 40%), so phenobarbital (and primidone) dosage should be reduced to abate sedation. The reason for this increase in phenobarbital levels is not known for certain; it may be caused by hepatic enzyme inhibition. Various opinions exist as to the effect of phenytoin when it is administered along with valproic acid. Transient lower total phenytoin plasma levels may be caused by displacement of phenytoin from protein-binding sites and subsequent increase in phenytoin metabolism or subsequent enzyme inhibition. The decreased level returns in time to the level found prior to initiation of valproic acid therapy. Interaction of valproic acid and clonazepam may produce absence status epilepticus or drowsiness.

Preparation, dosage, and administration. The recommended initial oral dose is 15 mg/kg/day, increased in 1-week intervals by 5 to 10 mg/kg/day until control seizures is achieved or side effects preclude further increases. The maximum recommended dosage is 60 mg/kg/day, not exceeding 250 mg daily, in three divided doses. As levels are titrated upward, blood levels of phenobarbital, primidone, and/or phenytoin may be affected. Patients experiencing gastrointestinal irritation may benefit from administration with food or by slowly building up the dose from the intitial low level. The dose should be the lowest consistent with optimal seizure control.

Valproic acid is available in oral capsules of 250 mg and a syrup containing the equivalent of 250 mg valproic acid per 5 ml as the sodium salt.

Side effects. Deaths have occurred from hepatotoxicity; particularly at risk are children with severe seizure disorders, mental retardation, and organic brain syndrome. The deaths are not dose related, and the duration of onset of hepatic signs was from 3 days to 6 months, with the maximum risk found between 2 and 12 weeks after initiation of treatment. Those patients with irreversible hepatic dysfunction have elevated aminotransferases and serum bilirubin. Nonfatal hepatic dysfunction and depressed fibrinogen and other clotting factors have also been reported. A decreased serum albumin level has been seen and is important because the lowered albumin decreases the total valproated blood level. Liver function tests should be performed periodically during the first 6 months of treatment. The side effects generally associated with valproic acid include nausea, vomiting, abdominal cramps, and diarrhea occurring early in therapy. These are transient and minimized with administration of the drug with meals. Also reported are anorexia, weight gain, sedative effects (especially with combination therapy), central nervous system effects, alopecia, psychiatric effects, fine postural and resting tremor, mild thrombocytopenia, and an increase in hepatic enzymes. Nonspecific findings like loss of seizure control, malaise, loss of appetite, and vomiting may indicate impending irreversible hepatic damage. Platelet counts and liver function monitoring are to be completed during valproic acid therapy. The effects of valproic acid are unknown in pregnancy. It is excreted in breast milk. There is an increase in valproate plasma protein binding in anemic patients.

Drug interaction. In the patient receiving valproic acid the following drug interactions may occur.

1 With alcohol there is a potentiation of the CNS depressant acivity of the alcohol.
2 With aspirin there is a prolonged bleeding time.
3 With clonazepam absence status epilepticus may be induced.
4 With CNS depressants enhanced CNS depression may develop.
5 Phenobarbital serum levels may be increased.
6 With warfarin there is increased chance of bleeding resulting from platelet function inhibition.

Carbamazepine (Tegretol)

Carbamazepine is an iminostilbene derivative (structurally similar to the tricyclic antidepressants) indicated for the treatment of epilepsy in patients who have not responded to phenytoin, phenobarbital, or primidone, for partial seizures with complex symptomatology, for generalized tonic-clonic seizures, and for mixed seizure patterns. This is not the drug of choice but rather the third choice, used only after unresponsiveness to the first and second choices. It may be useful in combination with one or more other anticonvulsants. The drug is also indicated in the treatment of pain associated with true trigeminal neuralgia, which is characterized by intermittent sharp bursts of pain in the mandibular facial region.

Action and result. Its mechanism of action is obscure. It is metabolized in the liver; the epoxide metabolite also has anticonvulsant activity. The time required for peak plasma concentration after oral administration 2½ to 18 hours (mean 4 hours), initial half-life is 25 to 65 hours, the plasma half-life following repeated oral administration is 12 to 17 hours (carbamazepine may induce its own metabolism making half-life variable), the therapeutic serum level is 4 to 12 μg/ml, the toxic serum level is not established, and protein binding is about 80%.

Precautions. The drug is contraindicated in patients with a history of bone marrow depression, hypersensitivity, or sensitivity to the tricylic antidepressants. It has mild anticholinergic activity and should be used with caution in patients with increased intraocular pressure. It may activate latent psychosis. In elderly per-

sons confusion, agitation, or drowsiness may occur. It is contraindicated during pregnancy and lactation. Adverse reactions include dizziness, nausea, drowsiness, nystagmus, ataxia, hepatic and hematopoietic disorders, genitourinary disorders, and cardiovascular system disorders.

Dosage and administration. A low initial dose is advised with gradual increments. When adequate control is achieved, the dose may be reduced very gradually to minimum effective levels. For adults and children over 12 years old the initial dose is 200 mg (one tablet) twice daily on the first day. Up to 200 mg may be added daily in divided doses (every 6 to 8 hours) until the desired response is obtained. Generally dosage does not exceed 1000 mg daily in children 12 to 15 years and 1200 mg in patients over 15 years. Rarely doses over 1600 mg are used.

Side effects and toxic effects. Serious and sometimes fatal abnormalities of blood cells have been reported, necessitating complete pretreatment blood counts and repeated blood counts taken weekly during the first 3 months and monthly thereafter. The nurse should make the patient aware of the early toxic signs and symptoms of potential hematologic problems (fever, sore throat, mouth ulcers, easy bruising, petechial or purpuric hemorrhage). The drug should be discontinued if any evidence of bone marrow depression develops or if any of the preceding symptoms appear, and the prescriber should be notified immediately.

Drug interactions Some drug interactions of interest are as follows.

1 When the patient is being administered carbamazepine and oral anticoagulants, there is a decreased anticoagulant effect because of inducing hepatic microsomal enzymes and increasing warfarin metabolism by decreasing warfarin half-life.
2 Doxycycline metabolism may be increased.
3 Concurrent use with a monoamine oxidase inhibitor may cause enhancement of toxicity potentials of both drugs.
4 Concurrent use with propoxyphene may enhance CNS side effects from alteration of carbamazepine metabolism.
5 Women using oral contraceptives experience breakthrough bleeding, decreasing their birth control reliability.
6 Phenytoin, ethosuximide, and valproic acid have

their half-life decreased as a result of inducement of hepatic microsomal enzymes.

Phenacemide (Phenurone)

Uses and toxic effects. Phenacemide is a synthetic anticonvulsant that is often effective in absence seizures (petit mal) when other anticonvulsants are not, but it is one of the more toxic agents and may cause personality changes, liver damage, and depression of bone marrow. Deaths have been reported. Some physicians regard it as being too toxic for routine use.

Preparation, dosage, and administration. Phenacemide is available in 500-mg tablets for oral administration. It may be prescribed alone or with other anticonvulsants. The dosage recommended is as small as will permit control of seizures.

NURSING IMPLICATIONS

The nurse sometimes plays an important role in helping the patient with epilepsy to learn how to live with his handicap. The patient often needs encouragement and help to enable him to understand why strict adherence to the routine the physician has worked out for him is so important. The patient may never be cured, but with care he may experience minimal symptoms and be able to lead a full and useful life. The patient or a family member should be instructed to keep a record of the frequency, duration, and symptoms of attacks and to report signs and symptoms of undesirable drug effects. Urinalyses and blood counts should be performed every 1 to 3 months.

Central nervous system stimulants

Drugs included under the heading of stimulants will be limited, for the most part, to those whose major effect is on the central nervous system. There are drugs, such as atropine, cocaine, and ephedrine, that are central nervous system stimulants but, medically, they have more important actions on other systems of the body.

The central nervous system stimulants may produce dramatic effects, but their therapeutic usefulness is limited because of the multiplicity of their actions and side effects. Also, repeated administration and large doses are prone to precipitate convulsive seizures, coma, and exhaustion. The number of drugs that stimulate the central nervous system is large, but the number actually employed for this purpose is limited. Those having particular therapeutic value are the respiratory stimulants and the analeptics. Although analeptics restore consciousness and mental alertness, they are little used since they may cause convulsions.

Stimulants are classified on the basis of where in the nervous system they exert their major effects—on the cerebrum, on the medulla and brainstem, or on the hypothalamic limbic regions. Amphetamine is mainly a stimulant of the cerebral cortex; analeptics act mainly on the centers in the medulla and the brainstem; and anorexiants act to suppress the appetite, perhaps by a direct stimulant effect on the satiety center in the hypothalamic and limbic regions. These drugs may also affect other parts of the nervous system. The drugs that act primarily on the medullary centers are said to be the best analeptics.

Analeptics
XANTHINES

Caffeine, theobromine, and theophylline are known as methylated xanthines. Their actions are similar, although their effect on specific structures varies in intensity.

Caffeine is a trimethylxanthine (three methyl groups) and theobromine and theophylline are dimethylxanthines (two methyl groups). Caffeine, theophylline, and theobromine are alkaloids that all act on the central nervous system, the kidney, the heart, the skeletal muscle, and the smooth muscle, but the degree of their action on these structures varies considerably. Of the three xanthines, caffeine is the most effective stimulant of the central nervous system, theophylline is less effective, and theobromine has little effect. In regard to effects on the kidney, theophylline ranks first in effectiveness, (as a diuretic), theobromine second, and caffeine third. Aminophylline (a theophylline compound) is the xanthine preparation of choice to produce relaxation of the bronchial tubes.

Caffeine

Caffeine is a white crystalline powder commercially obtained from tea leaves. It is the active alkaloid occurring in a number of plants used as beverages—coffee, the seed of *Coffea arabica;* tea, the leaves of *Thea sinensis;* the kola nut of Central America; and guarana, derived from the seeds of a Brazilian plant and from yerba maté or Paraguay tea. Tea contains from 1% to 5% caffeine*; coffee, from 1% to 2%. Tea contains 10% to 24% tannin. Coffee contains a variable amount of caffetannic acid (average, about 12%), which is not very astringent.

Action and result
Cortical and medullary. Caffeine stimulates the central nervous system, especially the cerebral cortex. Its action is a descending one; small doses (100 to 150 mg) stimulate the cerebrum, and larger doses stimulate the medullary centers and the spinal cord. Doses large enough to stimulate the spinal cord are never ordered. As a result of the cortical stimulation the individual is more alert, thinks faster, has a better memory, forms judgments more quickly, learns faster (temporarily), and has a decreased reaction time. Drowsiness and fatigue disappear. The sense of touch may be more discriminating and the sense of pain more keen. Stimulation is not necessarily followed by depression, unless it exhausts natural reserves.

Caffeine, when taken orally in ordinary therapeutic doses, has little or no effect on medullary centers. Large doses given parenterally will stimulate the respiratory center, especially if it is moderately depressed. There is some stimulation of the vagus and vasoconstrictor centers of the medulla, although this is partially masked by the peripheral action on the heart and blood vessels.

Decreased susceptibility to fatigue has also been observed, but whether the action is a direct one on the striated muscle cells or wheth-

*Although tea contains more total methylated xanthines than coffee, less tea is usually used in preparing the beverage (at least in the United States), and it therefore usually contains less caffeine.

er the effect is produced by masking the sense of fatigue through cerebral stimulation is not fully understood. The half-life of caffeine is 3½ to 4 hours.

Large doses of caffeine stimulate the entire central nervous system, including the spinal cord. There is first an increased reflex excitability that may, with increasing dosage, result in muscle twitching, especially in the limbs and face.

Cardiovascular. Caffeine stimulates the myocardium, bringing about both an increased cardiac rate and an increased cardiac output. This effect is antagonistic to that produced on the vagus center; consequently, a slight slowing of the heart may be observed in some individuals and an increased rate in others. The latter effect usually predominates after large doses. Overstimulation may cause tachycardia and cardiac irregularities.

A slight and somewhat transitory elevation of blood pressure is sometimes notes. Some investigators are of the opinion that caffeine constricts the intracranial blood vessels and brings about some lowering of intracranial pressure.

Renal. Like the other xanthines, caffeine increases the flow of urine, but its action is relatively weak. The mode of action seems to be that of depressing the tubule cells and preventing reabsorption of fluid, although increase in glomerular filtration may be more important therapeutically.

Metabolic. The metabolic rate is slightly increased by caffeine. An appreciable tolerance to certain effects of caffeine is readily established, although apparently not to the cerebral effects. Caffeine is also used to relieve fatigue, depression, and headache.

Gastric. Caffeine stimulates the output of pepsin as well as hydrochloric acid in the gastric juice. Thus coffee is usually omitted from the diet of patients with gastic or duodenal ulcer.

Uses. Caffeine is used as a mild cerebral stimulant. It is used also occasionally as a respiratory stimulant, provided the depression of the medullary center is not severe. In cases of severe respiratory depression there are better respiratory stimulants. Caffeine is no longer used for the relief of narcotic depression unless more effective drugs are not available.

Caffeine is used with one or more analgesic drugs or with ergotamine tartrate for the relief of headache. Its effect in such cases is thought to be caused by its effect on cerebral blood vessels. Caffeine, as a cranial vasoconstrictor, enhances the ergotamine vasoconstriction and may enhance ergotamine absorption.

Preparation, dosage, and administration. The following are the preparations and dosages of caffeine.

Caffeine. The usual oral dose is 100 to 200 mg.

Caffeine and sodium benzoate injection. It is available in 2-ml ampules and 10-ml vials, 250 mg/ml. The usual dose is 0.5 g (500 mg) to 1 g.

Citrated caffeine. This is available in 60- and 120-mg tablets. The average dose is 60 to 120 mg orally.

Ergotamine tartrate with caffeine (Cafergot). Each tablet contains 1 mg ergotamine tartrate and 100 mg caffeine. The drug is given orally for migraine headache (two tablets at onset, then one tablet every ½ hour up tp six tablets per attack). A suppository form is also available.

Caffeine is usually prescribed as citrated caffeine or caffeine and sodium benzoate because they are more soluble than caffeine itself. Caffeine and sodium benzoate is usually given intramuscularly, whereas the citrated form is given orally. Caffeine may also be given in the form of a liquid, either orally or rectally. The caffeine content of an average cup of brewed coffee as made in the United States is between 100 and 150 mg. Instant coffee has 85 to 100 mg per cup. Twelve ounces of a cola drink contains 35 to 55 mg caffeine, while a cup of cocoa may contain as much as 50 mg caffeine. Caffeine sometimes exhibits a local irritant action on the gastic mucosa, resulting in nausea and vomiting or gastric distress. Sick persons often do not tolerate coffee well as a beverage, especially if they are slightly nauseated. Weak tea is often better tolerated.

Side effects and toxic effects. Fatal poisoning by caffeine is rare, partly because it is readily excreted. The fatal dose is presumably about 10 g. Toxic doses produce excessive irritability, restlessness, insomnia, nervousness, profuse flow of urine, nausea, vomiting, headache, and heart palpitation, particularly in susceptible individuals. The symptoms of chronic poisoning include insomnia, anxiety, and functional cardiac symptoms. Such signs are more commonly seen among workers such as night nurses, who use coffee to keep awake and continue to work when physically tired. The symptoms of nervousness disappear when the overuse of coffee is remedied. Stopping the intake of caffeine and providing rest and quiet are sufficient treatment measures. In certain individuals a short-acting sedative may be indicated. The use of coffee to combat fatigue is like a whip to a tired horse, and it would be better to get needed rest than to continue using coffee to keep going.

The question is sometimes raised as to whether or not caffeine causes physical and psychic dependence. Many persons note that if they do not have their usual cup or two of coffee in the morning, they feel irritable and nervous and develop a headache. This probably indicates psychic dependence.

A patient who is or may become pregnant should be advised to avoid or limit her consumption of caffeine-containing foods (coffee, tea, cola drinks, cocoa, milk chocolate, etc.) and drugs (over-the-counter stimulants, analgesic combinations, cold preparations, etc.), because there is evidence that caffeine may be an animal teratogen. Further studies are needed to establish a relationship between caffeine and human birth defects.

AMPHETAMINES

Amphetamines are synthetic sympathomimetic amines. Amphetamines are weak inhibitors of monoamine oxidase. However, their central nervous system stimulation is not thought to be a result of monoamine oxidase inhibition. They release catecholamines, which exert a stimulating effect on the cerebral cortex and probably on the reticular activating system. This effect produces feelings of wakefulness, alertness, and euphoria or elation.

Amphetamines used over long periods can produce psychological dependence and physical dependence. Prolonged use of amphetamines leads to tolerance. Amphetamines may be used to treat nonpsychotic, mild depressive states, but they are of little or no value in psychotic depressive states. They have been largely replaced by the tricyclic antidepressants. They are widely, but questionably, used for their ability to depress appetite and reduce obesity. Some state laws restrict their use and prohibit use in obesity.

Amphetamine

Amphetamine is prepared synthetically from ephedrine.

Action and result. Amphetamine stimulates the central nervous system, particularly the cerebral cortex. The effects depend on the personality and mental state of the individual and the amount of drug administered. The results of action seen after oral administration usually include an elevation of mood that may become a true euphoric exhilaration, decreased feeling of fatigue, increased willingness to work, increased confidence, alertness, power of concentration, and sometimes talkativeness. Continued use may cause irritability, sleeplessness, dizziness, and anorexia. Large doses tend to be followed by fatigue and mental depression. Amphetamine may fortify a person for prolonged physical and mental exertion, but the end result in terms of fatigue is correspondingly greater and requires a longer period for rest than usual. Amphetamine has a more pronounced effect on the cardiovascular system than dextroamphetamine or methamphetamine. When the respiratory center is depressed, amphetamine exerts a stimulating effect on it; this may be significant in treatment of poisoning from depressant drugs.

Uses. Currently, amphetamine has three principal uses: to treat narcolepsy (5 to 60 mg/ day in divided doses), hyperkinetic behavioral syndromes, and exogenous obesity (short-term, few weeks). Amphetamine is effective in controlling the symptoms of narcolepsy (such as the overpowering desire to sleep) but it is not curative. These patients do not appear to develop tolerance to amphetamine.

Behavioral syndrome, a manifestation of minimal brain dysfunction in children, is thought to be the result of faulty norepinephrine metabolism. Amphetamines may improve the behavior and performance of these children. A government-appointed panel of experts has concluded that amphetamines are safe and proper treatment for hyperkinesis and that no dangers (dependence, toxicity) exist with proper treatment.

As an anorexigenic (5 to 30 mg, divided doses, ½ to 1 hour before meals), amphetamine is less effective than dextroamphetamine, and the latter drug is usually preferred for this effect. Tolerance to the anorectic effect does occur, and the drug should not be used for periods longer than 6 to 10 weeks. Some clinicians advocate 2-week periods of amphetamine therapy alternating with 2-week periods without therapy rather than continuous treatment. The basic mechanism for depressing the appetite is not known.

Drug interactions. Amphetamine or its derivatives used during or within 14 days after administration of an monoamine oxidase inhibitor may result in hypertensive crisis. Concurrent use with general anesthetics may result in cardiac arrhythmias. Tricyclic antidepressants can potentiate the effects of amphetamine. Amphetamine blocks the uptake of guanethidine at nerve endings and loss of control of blood pressure may occur. The hypotensive action of methyldopa and of reserpine is also inhibited by amphetamines. Exogenous catecholamines have their pressor effects potentiated by amphetamines. Antidiabetic drug requirements are altered when used with amphetamines and diet restrictions.

Preparation, dosage, and administration. The drug is available with the hydrochloride, sulfate, or phosphate salt and in combination with barbiturates to depress excessive irritability and tension.

Amphetamine sulfate (Benzedrine). This drug is marketed in tablets of 5 and 10 mg, and in 15-mg sustained-release capsules. It is marketed under the trade name Benzedrine. Amphetamine sulfate is usually administered orally and given in divided doses—the total daily dose is divided into several smaller doses and distributed through the day. To prevent interference with sleep the final dose of the day should not be given after 4:00 PM.

Side effects and contraindications. There is danger in the promiscuous use of amphetamine to overcome sleepiness and lack of alertness, because the natural warning signs associated with fatigue may be eliminated. Furthermore, amphetamine has high drug abuse potential. It is to be avoided by persons with hypertension and cardiovascular disease and by persons who are unduly restless, anxious, agitated, and excited. Side effects include dryness of the mouth, headache, insomnia, irritability, a sense of intoxication, anxiety, and even paranoia.

Elevated blood pressure, tachycardia, and gastrointestinal disorders may occur. Abrupt withdrawal after prolonged use may cause depression and lethargy. Some clinicians advocate gradual withdrawal of the drug to avoid these effects. Despite the numerous side effects caused by these drugs, there is a wide margin of safety between therapeutic and toxic doses.

Large doses of amphetamine produce effects resembling those of schizophrenia. A high degree of abuse of these drugs continues to be so widespread that additional legal restrictions against them are being contemplated and restrictions on production are enforced.

Dextroamphetamine sulfate (Dexedrine)

Action and uses. Dextroamphetamine sulfate, for the most part, has the same action and uses as amphetamine sulfate, although it exhibits a greater stimulating effect on the central nervous system and causes euphoria. It is considered to be less toxic than amphetamine sulfate because of its diminished sympathomimetic activity it causes hyperinsulinemia. It seldom causes rapid pulse, changes in blood pressure, or tremor. However, the same dangers attend its indiscriminate use as is true of other amphetamines.

Preparation, dosage, and administration. Dextroamphetamine sulfate is available in 5- and 10-mg tablets, as an elixir (5 mg/5 ml), and in sustained-release capsules containing 5, 10, or 15 mg of drug. The usual dose of dextroamphetamine is 2.5 to 15 mg daily given orally.

It may be taken three times a day 30 minutes to 1 hour before meals. The last dose should be taken at least 6 hours before retiring to avoid insomnia. Sustained-release forms are taken once daily in the morning.

Methamphetamine hydrochloride (Desoxyephedrine Hydrochloride); methylamphetamine hydrochloride

Methamphetamine hydrochloride greatly resembles amphetamine sulfate; the two drugs differ in their action only in degree. The central stimulant action of this drug is slightly greater, and the cardiovascular action is slightly less than that of amphetamine. Like amphetamine, it is used in the treatment of narcolepsy, as part of the treatment of alcoholism or barbiturate poisoning, and for treatment of hyperkinesis. Because it allays hunger and depresses motility in the gastrointestinal tract, it has been used in the treatment of obesity.

It is contraindicated for patients with hypertension, cardiovascular disease, hyperthyroidism, anxiety states, or undue restlessness. Severe toxic psychoses have occurred in individuals who abuse methamphetamine, commonly referred to as "speed" (see Chapter 12).

Preparation, dosage, and administration. Methamphetamine hydrochloride is marketed in 5-mg tablets and sustained action forms (5, 10, and 15 mg). The beginning oral dose for exogenous obesity is 5 mg taken 30 minutes before each meal daily. The usual effective dose in behavioral syndrome in children is 20 to 25 mg/day.

NONAMPHETAMINES
Methylphenidate hydrochloride (Ritalin)

Methylphenidate is a piperidine derivative and a mild cortical stimulant and is less potent than amphetamine. It appreciably affects blood pressure, heart rate, and respiration.

The approved uses are in the treatment of hyperkinetic children and those with certain behavioral and learning problems. It has been found to significantly improve task performance in children in both groups probably because it improves mood, causes euphoria, and increases motor and mental activity, cognitive ability, and motor functions. It is approved for use in narcolepsy and is possibly effective for mild depression and apathetic or withdrawn senile behavior.

Preparation, dosage, and administration. Methylphenidate is available as tablets containing 5, 10, or 20 mg. Usual dose for adults varies with indication and patient response but may be 10 to 60 mg divided in doses two or three times daily given 30 to 45 minutes before meals. If the patient is unable to sleep at night, the last dose should be taken before 6 PM.

For children (over 6 years old) with behavioral syndrome, dose is 5 mg before breakfast and lunch; dosage may be increased gradually by 5 to 10 mg weekly. Dosage above 60 mg is not recommended. This treatment is usually stopped after puberty is reached.

Side effects. Nervousness and insomnia are common reactions that can usually be controlled by reducing dosage or omitting the afternoon or evening dose. Numerous other side effects can occur and include hypersensitivity, anorexia, nausea, dizziness, palpitations, headache, and skin rash. Hypertension, hypotension, and arrhythmias have occurred. Prolonged therapy has caused abdominal pain and weight loss, particularly in children.

Precautions. Methylphenidate must be used with caution in patients with epilepsy since the drug can lower the convulsive threshold. It should also be used cautiously in patients with hypertension. Long-term therapy should be accompanied by repeated medical examination and complete blood and platelet counts. Its use in pregnant or lactating women is not recommended. The symptoms of tension, anxiety, and agitation are seen. It is contraindicated in glaucoma.

Tolerance and psychic dependence have occurred with long-term use, and abnormal behavior and psychotic episodes have been observed. When the drug is withdrawn careful supervision is required since severe depression may result.

Methylphenidate must be used cautiously in emotionally unstable persons and in those with a history of drug dependence or alcoholism. It has been used as a substitute for amphetamines by drug abusers.

Overdosage. Signs and symptoms of acute intoxication are primarily the result of overstimulation of the central nervous system and sympathetic nervous system and include vomiting, agitation, tremors, muscle twitching, convulsions, euphoria, confusion, hallucinations, delirium, sweating, tachycardia, arrhythmias, hypertension, mydriasis, hyperpyrexia,

and dryness of mucous membranes.

Treatment consists of supportive measures, evacuation of gastric contents if possible, a short-acting barbiturate, cooling procedures for high body temperature, and adequate maintenance of circulation and respiration. The effectiveness of peritoneal dialysis or hemodialysis for methylphenidate overdosage has not been established.

Drug interactions. Methylphenidate can potentiate the action of many drugs including anticholinergics, anticonvulsants, anticoagulants, MAO drugs, pressor drugs, phenylbutazone, and tricyclic antidepressants. It decreases the hypotensive effect of guanethidine. Dosage of these drugs should be readjusted when given with methylphenidate.

Anorexiants

Phenmetrazine hydrochloride (Preludin)

Phenmetrazine hydrochloride, which is subject to the Controlled Substance Act, resembles amphetamine pharmacologically, especially in its ability to depress appetite. It should be used along with calorie restriction and moderate exercise when taken as an appetite depressant. It has dependency potential similar to dextroamphetamine. It is a mild stimulant of the central nervous system, and it rarely causes changes in pulse rate and blood pressure. Psychoses and electrocardiographic changes have been seen. It is administered orally in 25-mg doses two or three times a day, an hour before meals, or in an oral extended-release form containing 50 or 75 mg of the drug, which is taken once daily.

Other central nervous system stimulants used primarily as appetite suppressants are diethylpropion hydrochloride (Tenuate, Tepanil), phendimetrazine tartrate (Plegine), phentermine (Ionamin, Wilpo), chlorphentermine (Pre-Sate), and benzphetamine (Didrex).

Mazindol (Sanorex)
Fenfluramine (Pondimin)
Diethylpropion (Tepanil, Tenuate)
Phentermine (Fastin, Ionamin)

These are not structurally amphetamines but demonstrate amphetamine actions and side effects and are used as anorexiants. All of these drugs are scheduled under the Controlled Substances Act.

Fenfluramine produces diarrhea, sedation, and central nervous system depression rather than stimulation due to reduction of serotonin. Fenfluramine should not be prescribed for alcoholic patients because psychiatric symptoms (paranoia, depression, psychosis) have been reported. It may be preferred for the nervous patient.

Catecholamine depletion is seen with fenfluramine used over long periods. The action of fenfluramine on the central nervous system is mediated through sertonin metabolism and not norepinephrine or dopamine metabolism. Fenfluramine has some hallucinogenic qualities which may indicate abuse potential.

Mazindol has low abuse potential. Mazindol has greater central nervous system stimulation than diethylpropion, may increase heart rate, and may cause hyperinsulinemia and lower blood glucose levels.

Diethylpropion produces a lower incidence of side effects and may be used in mildly to moderately hypertensive patients. Phentermine hydrochloride causes more reported cases of insomnia than diethylpropion, causes an increase in blood pressure, and produces tachycardia.

The dependence liability is directly proportional to the stimulation effects. In descending order of high to low the agents with dependence potential are amphetamine, methamphetamine, dextroamphetamine, phenmetrazine, phentermine, phendimetrazine, mazindol, diethylpropion, and fenfluramine.

Summary of nursing considerations

The human central nervous system functions much like a computer, receiving and integrating information from external and internal environments, then relaying instructions to appropriate cells or tissues to produce necessary actions. The primary function of the central nervous system, which is composed of the brain and spinal cord, is to coordinate and control the activity of the various body systems so that they perform as an integrated whole.

The major brain regions with their associated functions are influenced by chemicals called neurotransmitters. The neurotransmitters that have been identified are acetylcholine, catecholamines (dopamine, norepinephrine, and epinephrine), and serotonin. Neuropeptides, known as enkephalins and endorphins, have been discovered in the central nervous system. Numerous experiments have shown that these endogenous hormones act as neuromodulators that have the capability of modifying and controlling the perception of pain.

Many drugs affecting the central nervous system are both depressants and stimulants. Central nervous system depressants include analgesics, antiinflammatory analgesics, sedative and hypnotics, and anticonvulsant drugs. The general anesthetics (Chapter 9) are also included in this category.

Analgesics relieve pain without loss of consciousness or reflex activity by (1) elevating the pain threshold, (2) altering the patient's attitude or mood, and (3) producing sedative or soporific effects.

Three *nonsynthetic narcotic analgesics* are used widely in the practice of medicine—the opiate alkaloids morphine, codeine, and papaverine. Morphine and codeine act principally on the nervous system, producing a combination of depressing and stimulating effects. Papaverine has little effect on the nervous system but relaxes certain smooth muscles. Effects of the opiates are compared in Table 8-1. All opiates (except papaverine) can produce drug dependency and poisoning if taken in sufficiently large doses.

The number of synthetic narcotic analgesics has increased in the search for an analgesic with fewer disadvantages than morphine. Among these synthetics are meperidine, methadone, alphaprodine, levorphanol, and oxymorphone.

Narcotic antagonists include nalorphine, levallorphan, butorphanol, nalbuphine, and naloxone. These drugs' antinarcotic action is to compete with stronger narcotics for central nervous system receptor sites.

Synthetic nonnarcotic analgesics include pentazocine, propoxyphene, and ethoheptazine. Of these, propoxyphene (Darvon) is a drug increasingly abused and cited as the cause of deaths by overdose.

Nonnarcotic analgesics that are also antipyretics include the salicylates (aspirin and sodium salicylate) and combinations of the salicylates with other drugs. For example, aspirin is frequently combined with codeine, phenacetin, and/or caffeine for more potent analgesic action. Analgesic dosages of salicylates do not dull consciousness, disturb memory, or cause euphoria, sedation, or drug dependence. The mechanism of their antiinflammatory action is associated with inhibition of prostaglandin synthesis, which accounts for the ability of some of these drugs to decrease inflammation.

Indiscriminate use of salicylates by laypersons can produce toxic reactions. Aspirin poisoning is common in children.

Other antiinflammatory analgesics currently used for rheumatoid arthritis and associated conditions include ibuprofen, phenylbutazone, oxyphenbutazone, indomethacin, and other agents. Like the salicylates they cause mild to severe gastric irritation.

Drugs used in the treatment of gout are given to relieve pain and increase elimination of uric acid. Probenecid, sulfinpyrazone, and colchicine are some current drugs of choice. Allopurinol represents a different approach to treatment in that it blocks the terminal steps in uric acid formation by inhibiting xanthine oxidase.

Hypnotic drugs produce sleep; sedatives soothe the patient and relieve anxiety. The only difference between their actions is one of degree.

Sleep consists of four main stages that occur in regular cyclic patterns characterized by variations in depth of sleep and variations in brain waves and eye movements. Dreaming occurs during REM (rapid eye movement) sleep; physiologic functions increase, and body movements are more noticeable. During nondreaming (deep) sleep, physiologic functions are depressed. Sleep research has shown that sleep deprivation in either stage causes serious side effects and that the body tries to maintain an equilibrium between the two stages.

Drugs commonly used to ensure a good night's sleep alter the occurrence and length of sleep stages, particularly REM sleep. Side effects from alteration in sleep patterns include irritability, tremors, confusion, lethargy, and many others. Reviewing the patient's sleep history and drug history and making an effort not to disturb the sleeping patient are valuable aids in promoting good sleep.

Barbiturates are some of the oldest, most popular hypnotic and sedative drugs. They are believed to act at all levels of the central nervous system with effects varying from mild sedation to deep anesthesia, depending on the drug selected, method of administration, dosage, and individual reaction. In addition to their sedative and hypnotic benefits, barbiturates are useful as anticonvulsants.

Barbiturates are classified according to length of action: long, intermediate, short, and ultrashort (Table 8-8). They can produce marked symptoms of hangover, skin rash, facial swelling, asthmatic attacks, bad dreams, and delirium. Acute poisoning and death can result from overdose; physical dependence on barbiturates is an increasing problem.

Nonbarbiturate sedatives and hypnotics are available, but all are habit forming, may cause physical dependence, and are subject to abuse. The most popular of these is flurazepam (Dalmane), which is replacing many of the barbiturates. Several older hypnotics seem to be regaining popularity. Among those are chloral hydrate, paraldehyde, and the bromides.

Ethyl alcohol is the only alcohol used extensively in medicine. It exerts a progressive, continuous depression on the central nervous system, comparable to general anesthesia, and the margin between an anesthetic dose and a fatal dose is narrow.

Alcohol is used topically as an astringent and antiseptic and as an antipyretic. It is also an excellent solvent and preservative for medicines and medicinal mixtures. Concentrated solutions of alcohol often produce greater peripheral vasodilation than any other drug. It is used as an appetite stimulant during convalescence and debility and to supplement caloric intake in intravenous fluids.

In acute alcoholic intoxication, the patient is comatose and may die if the coma is prolonged. Emptying the stomach with a stomach tube and inhalation of oxygen and carbon dioxide may prove effective. Changing the patient's position often will help prevent development of hypostatic pneumonia.

Chronic alcoholism presents multiple physical and mental problems, including *delirium tremens,* a psychosis producing tremors, insomnia, delirium, and hallucinations. Successful treatment must begin with the patient's desire for treatment and recovery. Physician-nurse-patient rapport is essential.

Alcoholics Anonymous has been instrumental in reclaiming many alcoholics through mutual assistance and constructive rehabilitation. The administration of Antabuse has proved successful in some cases of chronic alcoholism. This drug causes highly unpleasant reactions when alcohol is ingested, including hyperventilation, nausea, hypotension, and copious vomiting.

Other alcohols such as methyl alcohol (wood alcohol), isopropyl alcohol, and butyl and amyl alcohols are highly toxic, causing blindness and even death when ingested.

Anticonvulsant drugs are administered to control the various kinds of seizures produced by epilepsy. These are grouped as grand mal seizures, petit mal seizures, jacksonian epilepsy, and psychomotor attacks. Their mode and site of action are uncertain; brain waves may or may not be altered.

An ideal anticonvulsant would be highly effective in controlling more than one type of seizure, long acting, nonsedative, inexpensive, and unlikely to produce tolerance to its therapeutic effects and would have a low incidence of toxicity. There is no ideal anticonvulsant; however, there are six subgroups of drugs available for use.

Stimulants whose major effect is on the central nervous system may produce dramatic effects, but the multiplicity of their actions and side effects limits their therapeutic usefulness. The number of drugs that stimulate the central nervous system is large, but the number actually employed for this purpose is limited. Respiratory stimulants and analeptics have particular therapeutic value, but the latter are declining in use because of the potential danger of precipitating convulsions.

Stimulants are classified according to their major site of action: cerebrum, medulla, and brainstem, or hypothalamic limbic region. Xanthines (caffeine, theobromine, and theophylline) affect the entire central nervous system. Caffeine is the most effective of the three, theophylline the least. Amphetamines are synthetic sympathomimetic amines affecting mainly the cerebral cortex, producing feelings of wakefulness, alertness, and euphoria. Prolonged use leads to tolerance and possible emotional dependence. Abuse of amphetamines is a problem of such magnitude that additional legal restrictions against them are being contemplated.

QUESTIONS

FOR STUDY AND REVIEW

1 Explain the functional role of acetylcholine in the central nervous system. What areas of the brain contain a high concentration of acetylcholine?
2 Explain what is meant by the term "narcotic."
3 How should narcotics be stored in hospital clinical units?
4 Before administration of an analgesic drug, what information must the nurse obtain to determine if the patient is experiencing pain?
5 Survey several hospital clinical units (general surgical, orthopedic, intensive care, etc.) to determine the most commonly prescribed analgesics, range of dose, and frequency of administration. Determine the similarities and/or differences. Explain findings.
6 What side effects can morphine cause?
7 Name two specific antidotes for morphine poisoning. How do they aid in the recovery of the patient?
8 What indicates that a patient may be developing drug dependence?
9 What is the relationship between the prostaglandins and inflammation?
10 Explain the mechanism of action of salicylates.
11 Explain the antithrombotic effect of aspirin.
12 What are the signs of aspirin poisoning?
13 Which nonnarcotic analgesics do not have antiinflammatory effects?
14 What is the pharmacologic action of the uricosuric agents?
15 Identify the pros and cons of antipyretics versus tepid sponges to reduce body temperature.
16 Differentiate between the "short-acting," "ultra-short-acting," and "long-acting" barbiturates. Give five examples of each.
17 What rationale is used by some clinicians for not using analeptics for treatment of barbiturate poisoning?

18 Explain how a drug may be used as a sedative, a hypnotic, or an anesthetic.

19 Discuss the pros and cons of administration of sleeping medications.

20 Define alcoholism. What, if any, are the therapeutic uses of alcohol?

21 Explain the fetal alcohol syndrome.

22 Which drugs are used to treat grand mal convulsions; petit mal seizures?

23 Formulate a patient teaching plan for a specific anticonvulsant.

24 Describe the pharmacologic effects of caffeine.

25 Which drugs are used in the treatment of narcolepsy? Explain their mode of action.

26 Explain the following statement: "Drugs that decrease or release catecholamine concentration in the brain have a depressing or sedative action."

27 Why is weak tea better tolerated than coffee by a patient during an illness?

REFERENCE

1 FDA Drug Bull. **3:**Aug. 1979.

BIBLIOGRAPHY

GENERAL

A.M.A. drug evaluations, ed. 4, Acton, Mass., 1980, Publishing Sciences Group, Inc.

Barchas, J.D., and others: Behavioral neurochemistry: neuroregulators and behavior states, Science **200:**964, 1978.

Bumney, W.E., Jr., and others: Basic and clinical studies of endorphins, Ann. Intern. Med. **91:**239, 1979.

Cuthbert, M.F., editor: The prostaglandins, Philadelphia, 1973, J.B. Lippincott Co.

Drakontides, A.: Drugs to treat pain, Am. J. Nurs. **74:**508, 1974.

Goldstein, A.: Endorphins, The Sciences **18**(3):14, 1978.

Goodman, L.S., and Gilman, A., editors: The pharmacological basis of therapeutics, ed. 6, New York, 1980, Macmillan, Inc.

Goth, A.: Medical pharmacology, ed. 10, St. Louis, 1981, The C.V. Mosby Co.

Guillemin, R.: Beta lipotropin and endorphins: implications of current knowledge, Hosp. Pract. **18:**53, 1978.

Hughes, J., editor: Centrally acting peptides, Baltimore, 1978, University Park Press.

Johnson, M.: Pain—how do you know it's there and what do you do? Assessment, Nursing '76 **6**(9):48, 1976.

Meyers, F.H., Jarvetz, E., and Goldfien, A.: Review of medical pharmacology, ed. 4, Los Altos, Calif., 1974, Lange Medical Publications.

Modell, W.: Drugs of choice 1980-1981, St. Louis, 1980, The C.V. Mosby Co.

Pacel, J.B.: Helping patients overcome the disabling effects of chronic pain, Nursing '77 **7**(7):38, 1977.

Snyder, S.H., and Matthysse, S.: Opiate receptor mechanisms, Cambridge, 1975, The MIT Press.

Uhl, G.R., Childers, S.R., and Snyder, S.H.: Opioid peptides and the opiate receptor. In Ganong, W.F., and Martini, L., editors: Frontiers in neuroendocrinology, vol. 5, New York, 1978, Raven Press, p. 289.

ALCOHOL

Becker, C.E., and Scott, R.: The treatment of alcoholism, Ration. Drug Ther. **6:**1, 1972.

Franks, C.M.: Conditioning and conditioned aversion therapies in the treatment of the alcoholic, Int. J. Addict. **8:**451, 1973.

Freund, G.: Chronic central nervous system toxicity of alcohol, Annu. Rev. Pharmacol. **13:**217, 1973.

Heinemann, E., and Estes, N.: Assessing alcoholic patients, Am. J. Nurs. **76:**786, 1976.

Heinemann, E., and Estes, N.: Drugs and alcohol, Am. J. Nurs. **76:**65, 1976.

Rubin, E., and Lieber, C.S.: Alcoholism, alcohol and drugs, Science **172:**1097, 1971.

Seixas, F.A., and others: Medical consequences of alcoholism, Ann, N.Y. Acad. Sci. **252:**5, 1975.

Siegel, H.H.: Alcohol detoxification programs: treatment instead of jail, Springfield, Ill., 1973, Charles C Thomas, Publisher.

ANTICONVULSANTS

Atkinson, A.J.: Individualization of anticonvulsant therapy, Med. Clin. North Am. **58:**1037, 1974.

Bochner, R., and Eadie, M.J.: Treatment of seizure disorders, Ration. Drug Ther. **12:**1, 1978.

Browne, T.R.: Clinical pharmacology of antiepileptic drugs, Am. J. Hosp. Pharm. **35:**1048, 1978.

Browne, T.R.: Drug therapy of status epilepticus, Am. J. Hosp. Pharm. **35:**915, 1978.

Browne, T.R.: Clonazepam: review of new anticonvulsant drug, Arch. Neurol. **33:**326, 1976.

Bruni, J., and Wilder, B.J.: Valproic acid: review of new antiepileptic drug, Arch. Neurol. **36:**393, 1979.

Bruya, M., and Bolin, R.: Epilepsy: a controllable disease. Part II. Drug therapy and nursing care, Am. J. Nurs. **76:**393, 1976.

Cereghine, J.J., and others: Carbamazepine for epilepsy, Neurology **5:**401, 1974.

Cooper, C.: Anticonvulsant drugs and the epileptic's dilemma, Nursing '76 **6**(1):45, 1976.

Dreifuss, F.E.: Use of anticonvulsant drugs, J.A.M.A. **241:**607, 1979.

Drugs for epilepsy, Med. Letter **18:**25, 1976.

Eadie, M.J.: Plasma level monitoring of anticonvulsants, Clin, Pharmacokinet. **1:**52, 1976.

Harris, P., and Mawdsley, C.: Epilepsy, London, 1974, Churchill Livingstone.

Hepatotoxicity from depekene, FDA Drug. Bull. **11**(2):July 1981.

Hvidberg, E.F., and Dam, M.: Clinical pharmacokinetics of anticonvulsants, Clin. Pharmacokinet. **1:**161, 1976.

Kutt, H.: Interactions of antiepileptic drugs, Epilepsia **16:**393, 1975.

Kutt, H., and Louis, S.: Anticonvulsant drugs. Part 1. Pathophysiological and pharmacological aspects. Part 2. Clinical pharmacological and therapeutic aspects, Drugs **4:**227, 1972.

Lewis, J.R.: Valproic acid (Depakene): a new anticonvulsant agent, J.A.M.A. **240:**2190, 1978.

Livingston, S.: Medical treatment of epilepsy, parts I and II, South. Med. J. **71:**298,432, 1978.

Ludden, T.M., and others: Individualization of phenytoin dosage regimens, Clin. Pharmacol. Ther. **21:**287, 1977.

Meadow, S.R.: The teratogenicity of epilepsy, Dev. Med. Child Neurol. **16:**375, 1974.

Mullen, P.W.: Optimal phenytoin therapy: new technique for individualizing dosage, Clin. Pharmacol. Ther. **23:**228, 1978.

Penry, J.K., editor: Epilepsy: the Eighth International Symposium, New York, 1977, Raven Press.

Penry, J.K., and Newmark, M.E.: Use of antiepileptic drugs, Ann. Intern. Med. **90:**207, 1979.

Pinder, R.M., and others: Sodium valproate: a review of its pharmacological properties and therapeutic efficacy in epilepsy, Drugs **13:**81, 1977.

Reynolds, E.H.: Chronic antiepileptic toxicity: a review, Epilepsia **16:**319, 1975.

Richens, A.: Interactions with antiepileptic drugs, Drugs **13:**266, 1977.

Speidel, B.D., and Meadow, S.R.: Epilepsy, anticonvulsants and congenital malformations, Drugs **8:**354, 1974.

Vining, E.P.G., Botsford, E., and Freeman, J.M.: Sodium valproate in refractory seizures: a study of efficacy, Am. J. Dis. Child. **133:**274, 1979.

Woo, E., and Greenblatt, D.J.: Choosing right phenytoin dosage, Drug Ther. 7:131, 1977.

Woodbury, D.M., and others, editors: Antiepileptic drugs, New York, 1972, Raven Press.

HYPNOTICS AND SEDATIVES

Chambers, C.D., and others: Barbiturate use, misuse, and abuse, J. Drug Iss. **2:**15, 1972.

Clift, A.D.: Factors leading to dependence on hypnotic drugs, Br. Med. J. **3:**614, 1972.

Cooper, J.R., editors: Sedative-hypnotic drugs: risks and benefits, Rockville, Md., 1978, National Institute on Drug Abuse, National Clearinghouse for Drug Abuse Information.

Hartmann, E.: Drugs for insomnia, Ration. Drug Ther. **11:**1, 1977.

Johns, M.W.: Sleep and hypnotic drugs, Drugs **9:**488, 1975.

Johns, M.W.: Methods of assessing human sleep, Arch. Intern. Med. **127:**484, 1971.

Kales, A., and Kales, J.D.: Shortcomings in evaluation and promotion of hypnotic drugs, N. Engl. J. Med. **293:**826, 1975.

Kales, A., and others: Rebound insomnia: potential hazard following withdrawal of certain benzodiazepines, J.A.M.A. **241:**1692, 1979.

Kales, A., and others: Comparative effectiveness of nine hypnotic drugs: sleep laboratory studies, J. Clin. Pharmacol. **17:**207, 1977.

Kales, A., and others: Chronic hypnotic-drug use: ineffectiveness, drug-withdrawal insomnia, and dependence, J.A.M.A. **227:**513, 1974.

Koch-Weser, J., and Greenblatt, D.J.: The archaic barbiturate hypnotics, N. Engl. J. Med. **291:**790, 1974.

Morgan, A.: Minor tranquilizers, hypnotics, and sedatives, Am. J. Nurs. **73:**1220, 1973.

National Academy of Sciences, Institute of Medicine: Sleeping pills, insomnia and medical practice, Washington, D.C., 1979, The Academy.

Oswald, I.: Psychological medicine, sleep difficulties, Br. Med. J. **1:**557, 1975.

Soldatos, C.R., and others: Management of insomnia, Annu. Rev. Med. **30:**301, 1979.

Solomon, F., and others: Sleeping pills, insomnia and medical practice, N. Engl. J. Med. **300:**803, 1979.

NARCOTIC ANALGESICS

Berkowitz, B.A.: Relationship of pharmacokinetics to pharmacological activity: morphine, methadone and naloxone, Clin. Pharmacokinet. **1:**219, 1976.

Bloomfield, S.S., and others: Aspirin and codeine in two postpartum pain models, Clin. Pharmacol. Ther. **20:**499, 1976.

Bonica, J.J., editor: Symposium on pain, parts I and II, Arch. Surg. **112:**749,861, 1977.

Bonica, J.J.: International Symposium on Pain, Advances in neurology, vol. 4, New York, 1974, Raven Press.

Bonica, J.J., and Albe-fessaid, D.G., editors: Advances in pain research and therapy, vol. I, Proceedings of the First World Congress on Pain, New York, 1976, Raven Press.

Clouet, D.H., and Iwatsubo, K.: Mechanisms of tolerance to and dependence on narcotic analgesic drugs, Annu. Rev. Pharmacol. **15:**49, 1975.

Halpern, L.M.: Treating pain with drugs, Minn. Med. **57:**176, 1974.

Houde, R.W.: Systemic analgesics and related drugs: narcotic analgesics. In Bonica, J.J., and Ventafridda, V., editors: Advances in pain research and therapy, II. New York, 1979, Raven Press, p. 263.

Lewis, J.W., Bentley, K.W., and Cowan, A.: Narcotic analgesics and antagonists, Annu. Rev. Pharmacol. **11:**241, 1971.

Loan, W.B., and Morrison, J.D.: Strong analgesics, Drugs **5:**108, 1973.

McCafferty, M., and Hast, L.L.: Undertreatment of acute pain with narcotics, Am. J. Nurs. **76:**1586, 1976.

Miller, R.R., Feingold, A., and Pazinos, J.: Propoxyphene hydrochloride: a critical review, J.A.M.A. **213:**996, 1970.

Moertel, C.G., and others: A comparative evaluation of marketed analgesic drugs, N. Engl. J. Med. **286:**813, 1972.

Pert, C.B., and Snyder, S.H.: Opiate receptors: demonstration in nervous tissue, Science **179:**1011, 1973.

Rodman, M.J.: Drugs for pain problems, R.N. **34:**59, 1971.

Simon, E.J., and Hiller, J.M.: Opiate receptors, Annu. Rev. Pharmacol. Toxicol. **18:**371, 1978.

Sturner, W.Q., and Garriott, J.C.: Deaths involving propoxyphene: a study of 41 cases over a two-year period, J.A.M.A. **223:**1125, 1973.

Terenius, L.: Endogenous peptides and analgesia, Annu. Rev. Pharmacol. Toxicol. **18:**189, 1978.

Vandam, L.D.: The potent analgesics, N. Engl. J. Med. **286:**249, 1972.

Young, D.J.: Propoxyphene suicides, Arch. Intern. Med. **129:**62, 1972.

NARCOTIC ANTAGONISTS

Editorial: Naloxone, Lancet **1:**734, 1975.

Garrett, L. and others: Hemodynamic effects of morphine and nalbuphine in acute myocarbial infarction, Clin. Pharm. Ther. **29**(5):576, 1981.

Jasinski, D.R.: Effects in man of partial morphine agonists. In Kosterlitz, K.W., and others, editors: Agonist and antagonist actions of narcotic analgesic drugs, Baltimore, 1973, University Park Press, p. 94.

Martin, W.R.: History and development of mixed opioid agonists, partial agonists and antagonists, Br. J. Clin. Pharmacol. **7:**273S, 1979.

Martin, W.R.: Naloxone, Ann. Intern. Med. **85:**765, 1976.

Maugh, T.H.: Narcotic antagonists: the search accelerates, Science **177:**249, 1972.

Miller, R.R.: Evaluation of nalbuphine, Am. J. Hosp. Pharm. **37:**942, 1980.

Way, E.L., and Settle, A.A.: Uses of narcotic antagonists, Ration. Drug Ther. **9:**1, 1975.

NONNARCOTIC ANALGESICS

Analgesics and asthma, Br. Med. J. **3:**419, 1973.

Atkins, E., and Bodel, P.: Fever, N. Engl. J. Med. **286:**29, 1972.

Brogden, R.N., and others: Sulindac: review of its pharmacological properties and therapeutic efficacy in rheumatic diseases, Drugs **16:**97, 1978.

Brogden, R.N., and others: Tolmetin: review of its pharmacological properties and therapeutic efficacy in rheumatic diseases, Drugs **13:**241, 1977.

Constable, T.J., and others: Drug treatment of rheumatoid arthritis, Lancet **1:**1176, 1975.

Diamond, H.S., and Bankhurst, A.D.: Double-blind comparison of sulindac and phenylbutazone in acute gouty arthritis, Postgrad. Med. Comm. **75:**, 1979.

Emmerson, B.T.: Drug control of gout and hyperuricemia, Drugs **16:**158, 1978.

Ferreira, S.H., and Vane, J.R.: New aspects of mode of action of nonsteroid anti-inflammatory drugs, Annu. Rev. Pharmacol. Toxicol. **14:**57, 1974.

Flower, R.J.: Drugs which inhibit prostaglandin biosynthesis, Phamacol. Rev. **26:**33, 1974.

Gibson, T., and others: Kinetics of salicylate metabolism, Br. J. Clin. Pharmacol. **2:**233, 1975.

Hart, F.D.: The new antirheumatic drugs, Drugs **9:**321, 1975.

Heel, R.C., and others: Butorphanol: review of its pharmacological properties and therapeutic efficacy, Drugs **16:**473, 1978.

Hollingsworth, J.W.: Management of rheumatoid arthritis and its complications, Chicago, 1978, Year Book Medical Publishers, Inc.

Hunter, J.: Study of antipyretic therapy in current use, Arch. Dis. Child. **48:**313, 1973.

Huskisson, E.C.: Osteoarthritis: changing concepts in pathogenesis and treatment, Postgrad. Med. **65:**97, 1979.

Kingsley, D.P.E.:, and others: Analgesic nephropathy, Br. Med. J. **4:**656, 1972.

Krane, S.M.: Action of salicylates, N. Engl. J. Med. **286:**317, 1972.

Leonards, J.R., and others: Safe and effective therapy with aspirin, Drug Ther. **2:**78, 1972.

Lewis, J.R.: New antirheumatic agents: fenoprofen calcium (Nalfon), naproxen (Naprosyn), and tolmetin sodium (Tolectin), J.A.M.A. **237:**1260, 1977.

Mangini, R.J.: Pathogenesis and clinical management of hyperuricemia and gout, Am. J. Hosp. Pharm. **36:**497, 1979.

Mills, J.A.: Nonsteroidal anti-inflammatory drugs, N. Engl. J. Med. **290:**781, 1974.

New non-steroidal anti-inflammatory drugs, Bull. Rheum. Dis. **24:**8, 1973-1974.

Nickander, R., and others: Nonsteroidal anti-inflammatory agents, Annu. Rev. Pharmacol. Toxicol. **19:**469, 1979.

Paulus, H.E., and Whitehouse, M.W.: Nonsteroid anti-inflammatory agents, Annu. Rev. Pharmacol. **13:**107, 1973.

Penicillamine for rheumatoid arthritis, Med. Lett. Drugs Ther. **20:**73, 1978.

Pirofsky, B., and Baradana, E.J., Jr.: Immunosuppressive therapy in rheumatic disease, Med. Clin. North Am. **62:**419, 1977.

Plein, J.B.: Perspectives on aspirin: Part 1. Aspirin as an analgesic, Nurse Pract. **1(4):**34, 1976, Part 2. Aspirin as an anticoagulant—potentials for risk and benefit, Nurse Pract. **1(5):**31, 1976.

Popert, A.J.: Chloroquine: a review, Rheumatol. Rehabil. **15:**235, 1976.

Roe, R.L.: Drug therapy in rheumatic diseases, Med. Clin. North Am. **62:**405, 1977.

Scherbel, A.L.: Nonsteroidal anti-inflammatory drugs: new alternatives for rheumatic disease, Postgrad. Med. **36:**69, 1978.

Smyth, C.J., and Bravo, J.F.: Antirheumatic drugs: clinical pharmacological and therapeutic aspects, Drugs **10:**394, 1975.

Sokoloff, L.: Pathology of rheumatoid arthritis and allied disorders. In McCarty, D.J., editor: Arthritis and allied conditions, ed. 9, Philadelphia, 1979, Lea & Febiger, p. 429.

Vandam, L.D.: Analgesic drugs—the mild analgesics, N. Engl. J. Med. **286:**20, 1972.

Vane, J.R.: Inhibition of prostaglandin synthesis as a mechanism of action of aspirin-like drugs, Nature **231:**232, 1971.

Wilkens, R.F.: Use of nonsteroidal anti-inflammatory agents, J.A.M.A. **240:**1632, 1978.

Yu, T.F.: Milestones in treatment of gout, Am. J. Med. **56:**676, 1974.

Zvaitler, N.J.: Etiology and pathogenesis of rheumatoid arthritis. In McCarty, D.J., editor: Arthritis and allied conditions, ed. 9, Philadelphia, 1979, Lea & Febiger, pp. 417-428.

STIMULANTS

Albrink, M.J.: Obesity. In Beeson, P.B., and McDermott, W., editors: Textbook of medicine, ed. 14, Philadelphia, 1975, W.B. Saunders Co, p. 1375.

Craddock, D.: Anorectic drugs: use in general practice, Drugs **11:**378, 1978.

Craddock, D.: Obesity and its management, ed. 3, Edinburgh, 1978, Churchill Livingstone, p. 92.

Goldrick, R.B.: Management of obesity, Drugs **12:**301, 1976.

Griffith, J.D.: Dextroamphetamine: evaluation of psychomimetic properties in man, Arch. Gen. Psychiatry **26:**97, 1972.

Safer, D., Allen, R., and Barr, E.: Depression of growth in hyperactive children on stimulant drugs, N. Engl. J. Med. **287:**217, 1972.

Samuel, P.D., and Burland, W.L.: Drug treatment of obesity. In Obesity in perspective, part 2, Fogarty International Center Series on Preventive Medicine, vol. 2, Washington, D.C., 1975, U.S. Department of Health, Education and Welfare, p. 419.

Scoville, B.A.: Review of amphetamine-like drugs by Food and Drug Administration: clinical data and value judgments. In Obesity in perspective, part. 2, Fogarty International Center Series on Preventive Medicine, vol. 2, Washington, D.C., 1975, U.S. Department of Health, Education and Welfare, p. 441.

Sroute, L.A., and Stewart, M.A.: Treating problem children with stimulant drugs, N. Engl. J. Med. **289:**407, 1973.

Van Itallie, T.B., and Yang, M.-U.: Current concepts in nutrition: diet and weight loss, N. Engl. J. Med. **297:**1158, 1977.

CHAPTER 9

Anesthetic agents

Anesthetic drugs are central nervous system depressants that possess two characteristics: (1) they have an affinity for nervous tissue; and (2) their action is reversible, with cells returning to normal on elimination of the drug from the cells. There are two major classifications for these drugs. *General anesthetic agents* are capable of producing *narcosis*, that is, stupor or loss of consciousness, and thereby general loss of sensation. Loss of consciousness is preceded by analgesia and accompanied by varying degrees of muscular relaxation. *Local anesthetic agents* block nerve conduction when applied locally to any type of nerve tissue in any part of the nervous system and thereby abolish sensation in that region; they do not produce unconsciousness.

General anesthesia

General anesthesia is a drug-induced state in which the central nervous system is altered to produce varying degrees of analgesia, depression of consciousness, skeletal muscle relaxation, and reflex reduction in the body. It is an important mode of therapy, especially for surgical operations and procedures.

More than 100 years have passed since the first volatile anesthetics were used to produce anesthesia during a surgical operation. Prior to that, agents to relieve pain were limited to alcoholic beverages and opium. The psychic as well as physical trauma associated with surgery without a good anesthetic definitely limited what the surgeon could do for a patient. Surgical skill was equated with speed. An English physician, Sir Clifford Allbutt, is quoted as follows: "When I was a boy, surgeons operating upon the quick were pitted one against the other like runners on time. He was the best surgeon both for the patient and the onlooker, who broke the three minute record in an amputation or a lithotomy."*

Nitrous oxide was discovered in 1772 by Joseph Priestley, who did not realize that the gas had anesthetic properties. Sir Humphrey Davy in 1799 suggested that because of its pain-relieving property, it might be tried in connec-

*Beckman, H.: Pharmacology; the nature, action, and use of drugs, Philadelphia, 1961, W.B. Saunders Co., p. 272.

234

tion with surgery, but his suggestion passed unheeded for many years. Three hundred years elapsed from the time of the discovery of ether until it began to be used for the relief of pain during surgery. Dr. Crawford Long of Georgia in 1842 had a patient inhale ether while he removed a tumor from the neck. Dr. Long failed to publish a report of this administration in the medical literature and therefore failed to receive full credit for being the first to discover the value of ether as an anesthetic agent.

Horace Wells, a dentist, observed some of the properties of nitrous oxide and began to use it in connection with his dental practice. In 1845 he attempted to demonstrate its capacity to relieve pain during a surgical operation. The demonstration failed and his efforts were ridiculed, with the result that this useful agent received little attention for some time thereafter. It was not recognized in that day how difficult it is to produce a good level of anesthesia with nitrous oxide alone for the period of time required for a surgical operation.

In 1846 William Morton, another dentist, who later studied medicine, successfully anesthetized a patient with ether at the Massachusetts General Hospital in Boston. The success of this undertaking launched a new era in surgery.

Chloroform was discovered in 1831, and in 1847 James Simpson of England successfully demonstrated its usefulness. Queen Victoria knighted him for his contribution to the relief of pain.

More than 80 years elapsed before any other general anesthetic gained a permanent place in anesthesia. Since 1935 many new anesthetic agents have been introduced.

Action of general anesthetics

General anesthetics affect all excitable tissues of the body to produce anesthesia. They vary widely in chemical structure, and there is also great variation in the concentrations required of different anesthetics to produce a given state of anesthesia. There are a number of interesting theories to explain the mechanism whereby anesthetics act.

Theories of action. Although many theories of narcosis have been proposed, none satisfactorily explains the basic mechanisms of action. Indeed, it is possible that different anesthetics have different modes of action and that no one theory will suffice.

The Overton-Meyer theory stresses the relationship between the lipid solubility of an anesthetic agent and its potency; the greater the solubility in fat, the greater the narcotic power. Since the nervous system has a high lipid content because of the nerve cell membrane lipid bilayer, this theory explains why anesthetics are preferentially taken up by the brain. However, not all lipid-soluble substances possess anesthetic activity, and some narcotics are not fat soluble.

In 1939 Ferguson proposed that anesthetic potency is related not to action on receptors but to thermodynamic activity, which depends on the drug concentration necessary to give a biologic effect and on the drug's solubility. When the drug reaches a certain saturation at the cellular level, it interferes with or impedes some metabolic function.

In 1961 Miller and Pauling put forth the theory that anesthetic action is essentially a physical event whereby an anesthetic reacts with the water in brain tissue to form microcrystals of ice, which then form an *ice cover* at nerve cell membranes. This blocks the passage of ions across the membranes, reducing their excitability and interfering with synaptic transmission. This event results in narcosis. It is also hypothesized that an ice cover is always present, even in the absence of an anesthetic, and that the ice cover increases as the body temperature falls. This theory provides an explanation for anesthesia caused solely by hypothermia and the need for less anesthetic drug with hypothermia.

Biochemical theories of anesthesia have also been proposed. These theories claim that various biochemical processes are interfered with, such as oxidation, phosphate uptake, and synthesis of adenosine triphosphate (ATP) and acetylcholine (ACh), causing impaired synaptic transmission in the brain. Although there is some experimental support for these theories, there is also evidence against them.

When anesthesia is first induced, the concentration gradient from alveolar air to blood is steep and therefore absorption of the gas into the blood is rapid. With time the concentration of gas in alveolar air, blood, and tissues approaches equilibrium and absorption of the gas slows. When the anesthetic is stopped, the reverse process occurs. Elimination is very rapid at first and then slower. Equilibrium of anesthetics in the fat depots of the body is more slowly reached than in other tissues and is more slowly eliminated. This effect is probably caused by the relatively small blood supply to fat depots. Alveolar walls are highly permeable to anesthetics, and free diffusion occurs between the alveoli and capillary membranes. A great deal of investigational work is being done, but regardless of the ultimate explanation, anesthesia is produced by progressively increasing the amount of the anesthetic agent, first in the blood and subsequently in the nervous system.

Unlike many other drugs, the anesthetics that can be given by inhalation were thought to be absorbed, transported, and excreted by the body without undergoing significant chemical change. There is evidence, however, for some quantitative hepatic metabolism of many anesthetics. For the most part, they are exhaled and excreted by the lungs, except for small amounts metabolized by the liver and excreted by kidneys and skin. Associations have been made between biotransformation of inhalation anesthetics and toxicity. The metabolic rate of inhaled anesthetics may be modified by the concentration being inhaled (for example, halothane metabolism is modified in a dose-dependent manner). An inhaled anesthetic may inhibit metabolism of other drugs. Anesthetics are relatively safe agents with skilled supervision, since their anesthetic effect can be rapidly reversed by elimination from the lungs, provided respiration is maintained satisfactorily. This possibility of rapid removal by breathing permits the safe use of drugs in which there is a surprisingly small difference between an anesthetic dose and a fatal dose.

The pattern of depression is similar for all anesthetics—irregular descending depression. The medullary centers are depressed last. It is fortunate that the medulla is spared temporarily, since it contains the vital centers concerned with heart action, blood pressure, and respiration.

Stages of general anesthesia

Anesthetists have learned to observe the reaction of a patient under anesthesia and have come to know when conditions are satisfactory for surgical procedure and when a reaction constitutes a danger signal.

The stages of anesthesia vary with the choice of anesthetic, speed of induction, and skill of the anesthetist. Present-day practice of inducing anesthesia with an intravenously administered anesthetic prior to inhalation anesthesia promotes rapid transition from consciousness to surgical anesthesia, and the early stages of anesthesia are not seen. However, if the drug is given slowly enough, usually all stages can be observed. They are most easily seen when ether is used as the only anesthetic. Not all stages may be seen with all anesthetics. (See Table 9-1.)

Stage 1: analgesia. This stage begins with onset of anesthetic administration and lasts until loss of consciousness. Smell and pain are abolished before consciousness is lost. Vivid dreams and auditory or visual hallucinations may be experienced. Speech becomes difficult and indistinct. Numbness spreads gradually over the body. The body feels stiff and unmanageable. When ether is used alone, its irritating effects may cause choking, coughing, a feeling of asphyxia, and increased secretions.

Stage 2: excitement. This stage varies greatly with individuals but begins with loss of consciousness. Reflexes are still present and may be exaggerated, particularly with sensory stimulation such as noise. The patient may struggle, shout, laugh, swear, or sing. There is an increase in autonomic activity, muscle tone, eye movement, and rapid and irregular breathing. Irregular respiration may cause uneven absorption of anesthetic; a period of apnea followed by a few deep breaths may produce a toxic concentration of anesthetic in the blood. Most anesthetic deaths have occurred in this stage.

The variability in this stage results from (1)

T A B L E   9 - 1   **Stages and planes of ether anesthesia and selected central nervous system effects**

Central nervous system effects	Stage 1	Stage 2	Stage 3 planes				Stage 4
			1	2	3	4	
Consciousness	Maintained Analgesia Euphoria Some distortion of perceptions Variable amnesia	Lost	Absent	Absent	Absent	Absent	Absent
Respiration	No alteration or increased rate with some irregularity	Rapid, irregular	Regular	Regular but expirations longer than inspirations	Diaphragmatic	Thoracic ceased Diaphragmatic depressed	No respiratory movement Respiratory paralysis
Skeletal muscles	Normal tone	Tone increased	Small muscles relaxed	Large muscles relaxed	Complete relaxation	Complete relaxation	Diaphragm paralyzed
Eyes							
Pupils	Reaction to light	Dilated	Constriction	Mid-dilation		Dilated	Dilated
Movements	Unchanged	Increased	Increased	None	None	None	None
Tear secretion				Decreased	Decreased	Absent	
Reflexes							
Lid	Present	Present	Absent	Absent	Absent	Absent	Absent
Corneal	Present	Present	Present	Absent	Absent	Absent	Absent
Pharyngeal or "gag"			Absent				
Laryngeal				Absent			
Cough					Absent in large bronchi	Absent in small bronchi	
Heart rate		Increased	Decreased				
Blood pressure	Unchanged	Increased	Normal	Normal	Decreased	Decreased	Decreased
Venous pressure	Unchanged	Increased	Unchanged				Increased

the amount and type of premedication, (2) the anesthetic agent used, and (3) the degree of external sensory stimuli. Since the advent of balanced anesthesia, excitement during induction is rare. However, this stage is important for classifying and analyzing drug effects in investigational studies.

Stages 1 and 2 constitute the *stage of induction.*

Stage 3: surgical anesthesia. The third stage is divided into four planes of increasing depth of anesthesia. Whether a patient is in one or the other of these four planes is determined by the character of the respirations, eyeball movement, pupil size, and degree to which reflexes are present or absent. Most operations are done in plane 2 or in the upper part of plane 3. (See Table 9-1.) As the patient moves into plane 1, the respiratory irregularities of the second

stage have usually disappeared and respiration becomes full and regular. As anesthesia deepens, respiration becomes more shallow and also more rapid. Paralysis of the intercostal muscles is followed by increased abdominal breathing; finally, only the diaphragm is active. The eyeballs, which exhibit a rolling type of movement at first, gradually move less and then cease to move at all. Normally, if the pupils were reflexly dilated in the second stage, they now constrict to about the size they are in natural sleep. The reaction to light becomes sluggish. The pupils dilate as plane 4 is approached.

The face is calm and expressionless and may be flushed or even cyanotic. The musculature becomes increasingly relaxed as reflexes are progressively abolished. Most abdominal operations cannot be performed until the abdominal reflexes are absent and the abdominal wall

T A B L E 9 - 2   Preanesthetic agents

| Drug classification | Agent most frequently used | | Desired effect |
	Generic name	Trade name	
Narcotic analgesics	Morphine Meperidine	Demerol	Sedation to decrease tension, anxiety, and provide analgesia
Barbiturates	Pentobarbital Secobarbital	Nembutal Seconal	Decreased apprehension Sedation Rapid induction
Phenothiazines	Promethazine	Phenergan	Sedation Antihistaminic Antiemetic Decreased motor activity
Anticholinergics	Atropine Scopolamine	— —	Inhibition of secretions, vomiting, and laryngospasms Sedation (with scopolamine)
Skeletal muscle relaxants	Succinylcholine (depolarizing) d-Tubocurarine (nondepolarizing)	Anectine Quelicin Sucostrin Sux-cert	Promotion of muscular relaxation
Intravenous barbiturate	Thiopental	Pentothal	Rapid induction

is soft. The body temperature is lowered as the anesthetic state continues. The pulse remains full and strong. Blood pressure may be slightly elevated, but in plane 4 the blood pressure drops and the pulse becomes weak. The skin, which was warm, now becomes cold, wet, and pale.

With an anesthetic such as ether the third stage (upper planes) may be maintained for hours with little change by the repeated administration of small amounts of the drug.

Stage 4: medullary paralysis (toxic stage). The fourth stage is characterized by respiratory arrest and vasomotor collapse. Respiration ceases before the heart action, so artificial respiration may lighten the anesthetic state (if a gaseous agent has been used) and save the patient's life.

Combination anesthesia

In combination anesthesia two or more drugs are combined to produce the desired general anesthetic effect. There are two methods of combined anesthesia: balanced anesthesia and neuroleptanesthesia.

Balanced anesthesia. Balanced anesthesia should provide not only sleep but also analge-

sia, elimination of certain reflexes, and good muscular relaxation. Following is an example of how these goals can be achieved:

1 Premedication with a barbiturate, a narcotic analgesic (meperidine, morphine, fentanyl), and a parasympathetic inhibitor (atropine) (Table 9-2)
2 Induction with an intravenous or ultra short-acting barbiturate anesthetic (thiopental)
3 Maintenance of general anesthesia with an anesthetic gas (nitrous oxide), possibly in conjunction with an intravenous barbiturate or narcotic analgesic (meperidine, morphine, fentanyl)
4 Maintenance of muscle relaxation with a curare-type drug or neuromuscular blocking agent (succinylcholine) with controlled ventilation

The advantages of this procedure are (1) rapid induction, (2) reduction in amount of drug required to maintain a desired state of anesthesia, (3) minimal adverse effects (postoperative nausea, excitement, and pain), (4) minimal disturbance of physiologic functions and of organs of detoxification and excretion, and (5) deep state of anesthesia unnecessary for optimal muscle relaxation.

Factors influencing drug choice, dose, and frequency are the patient's physical condition and previous drug therapy, the operative procedure to be performed, and the estimated length of the operation.

TABLE 9-3 Properties of some inhalation anesthetics

Properties	Ether (diethyl)	Chloroform	Halothane
Inflammable and explosive	Yes	No	No
Induction	Slow—unpleasant	Rapid—pleasant	More rapid than ether—pleasant
Recovery	Slow	Rapid	More rapid than ether
Mucous membrane irritant	Yes—coughing, laryngeal spasms, profuse mucous secretions	Less than ether	No
Sympathetic stimulant	Yes	No	No
Increased capillary bleeding	Yes	No	No
Cardiovascular effects			
Sensitization of myocardium to epinephrine	No	Yes—may cause arrhythmia	Yes
Heart rate	Decreased in plane 3	Decreased	Bradycardia
Blood pressure	Decreased in plane 3	Decreased	Hypotension
Skeletal muscle relaxation	Excellent	Good	Not adequate when used alone
Postoperative effects	Nausea, vomiting	Nausea, vomiting, possibly permanent liver and kidney damage	Rare (a few cases of severe liver damage have been reported)
Use	Major and prolonged operations Obstetric labor	Not common	Widely used, often used with nitrous oxide

Neuroleptanesthesia. Neuroleptanesthesia is a general anesthesia produced by a combination of a neuroleptic (antipsychotic) such as droperidol; diazepam (Valium), or ketamine (Ketaject, Ketalar) and a narcotic analgesic, most commonly fentanyl but sometimes meperidine (Demerol), morphine, or pentazocine (Talwin). It is used primarily for procedures that require the patient's cooperation.

General anesthetics

General anesthetics are usually divided into two groups: (1) the inhalation anesthestics, which include gases, nonhalogenated volatile liquids, and halogenated volatile liquids; and (2) the intravenous anesthetics, which include barbiturates and nonbarbiturates.

Inhalation anesthetics

Inhalation or *volatile anesthetics* are gases or liquids that can be administered by inhalation when mixed with oxygen and can effect a concentration in the blood and brain to depress the central nervous system and cause anesthesia or narcosis. (See Table 9-3.) They have the following characteristics:

1 They are complete anesthetics and thus can abolish superficial and deep reflexes.
2 They provide for controllable anesthesia, since depth of anesthesia is easily varied by changing the inhaled concentration.
3 Allergic reactions to these agents are uncommon.
4 Rapid recovery can occur as soon as administration ceases, since the anesthetic is excreted in expired air.

They are administered by the semiclosed or the closed method.

Semiclosed method. The semiclosed method involves the use of some means to decrease the escape of the anesthetic vapor. A mixture containing gases or vapors and air or oxygen is inhaled from a closed mask that communicates with a reservoir or breathing bag. Recirculation of expired gases is prevented by valves. Exhalations pass through a valve on the top of the mask. There is greater retention of carbon dioxide than with the open method, but a higher concentration of anesthetic vapor is provided. This method sacrifices simplicity, and the exhaled gases may be a fire hazard.

T A B L E 9 - 4 Properties of gaseous anesthetics

Properties	Cyclopropane	Nitrous oxide
Inflammable and explosive	Yes	No—but supports combustion
Induction	Rapid	Rapid
Recovery	Rapid	Rapid
Results in increased capillary bleeding	Yes	No
Sensitization of myocardium to epinephrine	Yes—may cause arrhythmia	No
Skeletal muscle relaxation	Adequate at deep levels of anesthesia	Poor when used alone
Postoperative effects	Nausea and vomiting Excitement and laryngospasm may occur	Anoxia if oxygen supply inadequate (should be prevented)
Use	Widely used	To induce anesthesia For brief anesthesia (dental extraction) Principal agent in balanced anesthesia

Closed method. The closed method can be used for both gases and volatile liquids. An anesthetic machine is used; an apparatus that fits over the nose and face of the patient or an endotracheal tube connects the respiratory tract of the patient with the anesthetic machine, thus forming a closed system. Provision is made for removal of carbon dioxide, absorption of moisture, and regulation of the intake of the anesthetic agent or agents as well as oxygen. The anesthetist regulates respiration by periodic and rhythmic compression of the breathing bag. The closed method affords better control of the anesthetic state, as well as greater economy of the anesthetic, since rebreathing of the mixture occurs. Minimal waste of drug makes it more economical, and the fire hazard is decreased.

GASES
Nitrous oxide (Nitrogen Monoxide)

Nitrous oxide, one of the oldest and safest anesthetics, is a colorless gas somewhat heavier than air, with a slight odor and a sweetish taste. It long has been known as "laughing gas." It is unique among volatile anesthetics in that it is an inorganic compound (contains no carbon atoms) and is made from ammonium nitrate. It is nonflammable and nonexplosive, but at sufficiently high temperatures it will dissociate, release oxygen, and support combustion. (See Table 9-4.)

Action and result. The central nervous system is the only part of the body that seems to react to nitrous oxide. When the gas is mixed with air and inhaled, it produces an effect similar to that of a mild intoxicant. The patient feels merry, laughs, and talks but does not go to sleep.

When the pure gas is inhaled, the patient first feels warm, numb, dizzy, and confused. Vivid dreams and hallucinations may be experienced. After a few deep inspirations the patient becomes pale and soon loses consciousness. If administration is continued, the patient becomes cyanotic and death results from asphyxia. The upper planes of surgical anesthesia are reached in 1 or 2 minutes, but by this time the patient is already becoming seriously depleted of oxygen. Respirations are deep and rapid, later becoming irregular and shallow. If administration is stopped before cyanosis is marked, consciousness is regained rapidly. Because many untoward effects are associated with anoxia, administration of undiluted nitrous oxide is not recommended. Anesthesia can be safely prolonged when a mixture of 35% oxygen and 65% nitrous oxide is used, but this combination is insufficiently potent to produce satisfactory surgical anesthesia without premedication for many operations. Higher concentrations may be used during induction or for brief intermittent use during labor. Nitrous oxide has no untoward effects on circulation, respiration, and the liver or kidneys unless oxygen deficiency (at least 20%) is allowed to develop and persist. Nitrous oxide does not irritate the respiratory mucous membrane. Skeletal muscular relaxation is not as complete as it is with ether or cyclopropane, and a neuromuscular blocking agent must be used for procedures requiring muscular relaxation. It does produce excellent analgesia. Oxygen should be administered during emergence.

Uses. If nitrous oxide were more potent, it would probably be regarded as an ideal anesthetic. Owing to its excellent analgesia, 25% to 50% nitrous oxide can be given with 75% to 50% oxygen to produce analgesia in dental procedures, surgical procedures that are brief and do not require muscular relaxation, and obstetrics (second stage of labor). It is also used as an agent for induction prior to the use of other anesthetics. Its greatest use is as a component of balanced anesthesia for prolonged or complicated surgery.

Preparation and administration. Nitrous oxide is available in the compressed state in blue steel cylinders for closed system administration. It is also available for self-administration during childbirth. Brief use of 100% nitrous oxide during contractions and 100% oxygen between contractions can produce analgesia without decreasing uterine contractions or maternal oxygen saturation.

Side effects and toxic effects. Nitrous oxide itself has low side and toxic effects, but hypoxia is dangerous. It can cause bone marrow depression and leukopenia with prolonged administration. If anoxia occurs, it is probably the result of poor technique and not the gas itself. The disadvantage of nitrous oxide is its low anesthetic potency, although this can be remedied by proper use of supplemental agents.

Ethylene

Ethylene is a colorless, highly volatile gas with a slightly sweet taste and an unpleasant but not intolerable odor. When mixed with a certain amount of oxygen, it is highly explosive and flammable. However, it is believed to be no more explosive than ether-oxygen or ether-oxygen–nitrous oxide mixtures when comparable precautions are taken. Ethylene was first used for clinical surgery in 1923.

Action and result. Induction is smooth and rapid. Ethylene is less powerful as an anesthetic than either ether or cyclopropane but slightly more potent than nitrous oxide. It is difficult to reach more than plane 1 or possibly plane 2 of surgical anesthesia with ethylene and it has poor muscle relaxant properties.

Ethylene does not irritate the respiratory mucosa, and it does not increase salivary secretion. The patient awakens readily when administration of ethylene is stopped. Respiratory depression and vasomotor depression are uncommon, and postoperative complications are rare but hypoxia is a complication.

Uses. Because of its explosiveness, the availability of more potent anesthetics, and its slight increase in potency over nitrous oxide, the use of ethylene has been almost abandoned.

Preparation and administration. Ethylene is available in red steel tanks in which the gas is kept under pressure. It is administered with oxygen in a closed system technique with a gas machine. It is important for the patient to receive a preliminary medication so that adequate oxygen (80%) may be given during anesthesia to prevent hypoxia.

Disadvantages. The chief disadvantage associated with the use of ethylene is the hazard of fire and explosion. As is true of certain other anesthetics, the time of greatest danger is at the end of the operation, when the mask is lifted from the patient's face. For this reason no one should touch the anesthetist or the anesthetic machine other than those constantly working with the patient or with the machine. A small spark of static electricity may set off an explosion. This precaution applies to all explosive mixtures.

Cyclopropane

Cyclopropane is a colorless gas, heavier than air, flammable, and explosive in all anesthetic concentrations when mixed with air or oxygen. It has a mildly pungent but not unpleasant odor. It is stable and is stored in metal cylinders where, under pressure, it liquefies easily.

Action and result. Cyclopropane is a rarely used potent anesthetic. Adequate amounts of oxygen can be given with it, to the extent of 20% or more, and it will still produce satisfactory anesthesia. A wide margin of safety exists between the anesthetic and the toxic dose. Induction is pleasant and rapid (1 to 2 minutes).

The drug does not irritate the respiratory mucous membrane. There is little change in respiration until deep depression is produced. Laryngospasm occasionally develops; therefore atropine or scopolamine is likely to be prescribed as a preliminary medication. Cyclopropane in full anesthetic doses produces a fair amount of muscle relaxation, although the supplemental effect of a nondepolarizing neuromuscular blocking agent may be required, but at reduced doses. Uterine and intestinal muscles are not affected unless the patient is in the lower planes of surgical anesthesia.

Uses. Cyclopropane in closed systems has been used successfully as a general anesthetic for a wide variety of operations. It has been approved as an anesthetic for chest surgery in which quiet respirations and absence of bronchial irritation are important. It is also used in obstetrics, since it can be administered in amounts that do not affect uterine activity or the respirations of the child. Its explosiveness has limited its use in favor of newer, nonflammable agents. However, it is still often selected for patients in shock or impending shock.

Preparation and administration. Stored in orange steel cylinders, cyclopropane is administered by inhalation, preferably with 80% oxygen in a closed system because it is both expensive and explosive.

Side effects and toxic effects. As anesthesia with cyclopropane deepens, disturbance of cardiac rhythm (arrhythmias) may occur. Sudden death has been known to result. This effect seems to be related to the development of hypoxia and the retention of carbon dioxide. It can be prevented by maintaining adequate ventilation. The incidence of postanesthetic nausea, vomiting, headache, and postoperative distention is more than that seen after anesthesia with nitrous oxide or ethylene. Postanesthetic delirium may occur.

NONHALOGENATED VOLATILE LIQUID
Ether (diethyl ether)

Ether is a clear, colorless liquid with a pungent odor and a bitter, burning taste. It is formed by the action of sulfuric acid on ethyl alcohol. It is highly volatile and very flammable. Mixtures of ether and air or ether and oxygen are explosive. It is decomposed by light, air, and moisture and should therefore be kept in sealed metal containers. Ether is a good solvent for fats, oils, resins, and adhesive plaster.

Action and result. Ether may have either a local or systemic action.

Local. When applied to the skin and allowed to evaporate, ether has a cooling effect. If it is not allowed to evaporate, it reddens the skin and acts as a rubefacient. Ether irritates mucous membranes and causes increased secretion of mucus, saliva, and tears. When moderately dilute, it acts as a carminative in the digestive tract. Nausea and vomiting may result from gastric irritation or from central stimulation of the vomiting center.

Systemic. The systemic action of ether has been described in the presentation of the stages of anesthesia. Ether has an action similar to that of curare at the myoneural junctions (relaxes skeletal muscles). It is said to be the only anesthetic to possess this action. Therefore when ether and a nondepolarizing neuromuscular blocking agent (curariform drug) are used together, their dose must be reduced. The induction period is comparatively slow, and the period of recovery is longer than for a number of other general anesthetics. Nausea and vomiting are common in the recovery phase.

For a time, ether increases cardiac output (makes the heart beat faster and stronger). In the deeper planes of surgical anesthesia the myocardium is directly depressed, but the sympathetic nervous system is stimulated. Ether produces peripheral vasodilation. As a result there may be oozing of blood from the cut edges of skin during and after surgery. Blood pressure is lowered as anesthesia deepens. The skin feels warm, and the face is frequently flushed. Sudden, marked pupil dilation is regarded as a danger signal, since it may mean the beginning of respiratory failure. Of course, the size of the pupils may be modified by the action of the preanesthetic drugs such as morphine and atropine.

Some reversible effect on the kidney is indicated by the presence of albumin in the urine and scanty urine formation for several hours after anesthesia. Postoperative urinary retention may result from poor tone in the bladder. There is no evidence that ether causes any damage to the liver.

Contractions of the uterus are not much affected by moderate degrees of anesthesia, but they are slowed and decreased by deep anesthesia. Ether is not an entirely satisfactory anesthetic to relieve the pain of childbirth because its analgesic effect cannot be obtained fast enough. There are better analgesics for this purpose.

In the early stages of anesthesia there may be sufficient stimulation of smooth muscle of the gastrointestinal tract to cause nausea and vomiting. During moderate or deep surgical anesthesia ether produces diminished peristalsis and tone of smooth muscle of the gastrointestinal organs. This is sometimes responsible for the development of distention. Early ambulation is helpful in preventing local accumulation of gas.

Recovery from ether anesthesia proceeds in reverse order; the patient goes from the stage of surgical anesthesia through the stage of excitement and on through the stage of analgesia before becoming fully conscious. The nurse must make sure that the patient's face is turned to the side to prevent aspiration of mucus or vomitus. No patient who is not fully conscious should ever be left alone.

The sense of hearing returns comparatively early. This is a fact worth noting by attendants, who might discuss the patient's medical status, assuming that he is still unconscious. Postanesthetic doses of morphine or similar narcotics should be withheld until the gagging, swallowing, and coughing reflexes have fully returned. Return of function of these reflexes coincides with the return of consciousness.

Uses. Ether is obsolete and now infrequently used as a general anesthetic. A combination of nitrous oxide gas, oxygen, and ether (G-O-E) is used for surgical anesthesia (10% to 30% ether for induction and 5% to 15% ether for maintenance). Nitrous oxide is used for induction to avoid the unpleasant suffocating effects of ether and the excitement of the second stage. Ether can be used to check convulsive seizures associated with tetanus and strychnine poisoning. It

Preparation, dosage, and administration. is used as a fat solvent to cleanse the skin prior to surgical procedures.

The dose of ether depends on the patient, the length of operation, and the depth of anesthesia to be maintained. Only unopened sealed containers of ether should be used for anesthesia.

Ether is administered in any of the ways mentioned under administration of anesthetics in this chapter. The closed system is employed, especially if ether is combined with other agents.

Side effects and toxic effects. Acute toxicity caused by overdosage may occur during administration. If induction occurs too rapidly, there may be a temporary respiratory arrest. (Aside from patient variability, the anesthetic dose is generally half the dose that can lead to respiratory arrest.) Removal of the mask or facepiece is usually all that needs to be done. Respiration is usually resumed at the normal rate. Prolonged administration of ether may result in respiratory depression and respiratory failure. The pulse becomes feeble and irregular, and the blood pressure drops. The skin becomes cold, clammy, and gray. The pupils dilate widely and do not react to light. Other dangers associated with ether anesthesia are those which arise from aspiration of mucus or vomitus or from some other form of airway obstruction.

Overdosage is prevented by keeping the patient in the lighter planes of surgical anesthesia. Oxygen and artificial respiration will hasten elimination of the ether and lighten the anesthesia.

Advantages. Ether is considered to be a relatively safe anesthetic. There is a wide margin of safety between the anesthetic and toxic dose. It brings about excellent muscular relaxation.

Disadvantages. Ether is flammable and potentially explosive. It is irritating to mucous membranes and unpleasant to inhale; atrophine should be used to reduce respiratory secretions. The slow recovery period from ether anesthesia may be unpleasant because of nausea and vomiting.

Contraindications. Although ether has long been thought to be contraindicated in pulmonary disease, this opinion has, to some extent, been reversed. Ether depresses activity of the vagus nerve, a desirable effect in thoracic surgery. When ether is administered in a closed system with adequate amounts of oxygen and continual removal of carbon dioxide and when steps are taken to prevent accumulation of secretions in the bronchial tubes and trachea, this anesthetic seems to serve satisfactorily for thoracic surgery even when pulmonary disease is present. Because ether dilates the bronchioles, it is useful in asthmatic patients. Its use is not recommended for patients in acidosis or for those who have advanced renal disease. Unless special precautions are taken, it should not be administered when an open flame or cautery must be used.

Drug interactions. Certain antibiotics such as neomycin and polymyxin B have neuromuscular blocking action. Ether may intensify this block in patients taking these antibiotics preoperatively. This potentiation may cause respiratory arrest. Patients receiving adrenergic blocking drugs such as phenoxybenzamine (an alpha blocker) or propranolol (a beta blocker) preoperatively may not be able to maintain optimal level of blood pressure or cardiac output during anesthesia. A risk of convulsions in epilepsy also exists.

HALOGENATED VOLATILE LIQUIDS
Halothane (Fluothane)

Halothane is a volatile, nonflammable, nonirritating general anesthetic whose potency is said to be about twice that of chloroform and four times that of ether. Induction with this agent is made rapidly and smoothly with little excitement, and during recovery the return of consciousness is also rapid. Pharyngeal and laryngeal reflexes are easily suppressed; therefore there is little likelihood of complications such as laryngospasm, coughing, or bronchospasm. Since the agent is nonirritating and because it depresses salivary and mucous secretions and dilates bronchioles, there is little or no increase in bronchial and salivary secretions, which makes it useful in asthmatics. Muscular relaxation is moderately satisfactory; muscle relaxants are sometimes needed to promote adequate relaxation. There is a low inci-

dence of postoperative nausea and vomiting.

Uses. Halothane is widely used. It can be used alone or with nitrous oxide and neuromuscular relaxants for a wide variety of operations; it has no analgesic property.

Advantages. Halothane is nonexplosive, does not burn, provides rapid induction and rapid recovery, is nonirritating, has a relatively pleasant odor, depresses salivary and bronchial secretions, and is easy to administer. It is potent and can be given with adequate amounts of oxygen. Patients may need respiratory assistance, but completely controlled respiration is easily achieved.

Disadvantages. Halothane is a strong respiratory and circulatory depressant. It causes vasodilation, hypotension, hypoxia, apnea, acidosis, and tachypnea (rapid, shallow respirations) in the upper planes of anesthesia. In addition, the drug is expensive. It is destructive to steel, rubber, and plastic materials if the liquid drug is permitted to come in contact with them.

Preparation, dosage, and administration. Halothane is available in 125- and 250-ml containers. It is administered by closed inhalation. The drug is usually vaporized with oxygen or an oxygen–nitrous oxide mixture; 0.5% to 1.5% halothane concentration will maintain surgical anesthesia.

Side effects and toxic effects. Some degree of hypotension has been noted with most patients. Severe hypotension may result from a suddenly increased concentration of the anesthetic or when deep planes of anesthesia are attempted. Alterations in the cardiac rate and rhythm are frequently produced by halothane, the most common of which is a slow pulse. This can usually be prevented by the administration of atropine or a related type of drug. Halothane sensitizes the cardiac muscle (myocardium) to epinephrine and levarterenol; therefore the administration of these catecholamine drugs during anesthesia with halothane is avoided. Anesthetists use ephedrine, phenylephrine, or methoxamine to combat hypotension.

Respiration is frequently depressed, and the depression progresses with increasing depth of anesthesia. Uterine contractions during labor cease. Halothane apparently does not harm the kidneys. However, patients who develop jaundice after exposure to halothane should not be reexposed to this drug. Severe, even fatal, hepatic failure has occurred in a few individuals following halothane anesthesia. It is difficult to deny a causal role of the anesthetic in some of these cases. Halothane is such a potent anesthetic that the margin of safety between the toxic dose and the therapeutic dose is not great. Malignant hyperpyrexia may occur in muscular disorders. Because of depressed liver blood flow, phenytoin toxicity may occur. There is significant interpatient variation in the hepatic metabolism.

Contraindications. Halothane is contraindicated in most obstetric deliveries and in patients with known hepatic or biliary disease.

Methoxyflurane (Penthrane)

Methoxyflurane is an inhalation anesthetic suitable for both induction (about 2%) and maintenance (0.1% to 2% with oxygen and 50% nitrous oxide) of anesthesia for analgesia (0.3% to 0.8%). It is not flammable or explosive in any concentration mixed with air or oxygen at operating room temperatures. It is a colorless liquid with a boiling point of 104.65° C, and it has a fruity odor. It is stable in light and in the presence of oxygen, moisture, and carbon dioxide absorbers. Methoxyflurane can be administered by any of the usual techniques—closed or semiclosed. It is highly soluble in fat and blood. Induction is slow, and emergence or recovery prolonged. It produces as good muscle relaxation as does diethyl ether but with slower onset and less intensity. When muscle relaxants are used with it, they should be administered in less than the usual dose. It depresses the cardiovascular system similar to halothane. Methoxyflurane, unlike halothane, does not significantly sensitize the myocardium to catecholamines but lowers the blood pressure. Since it is a halogenated compound that is metabolized to a free fluoride ion, it may possibly cause acute or delayed hepatic and renal damage such as polyuric renal failure; its administration in the presence of liver disease or with other nephro-

toxic drugs (for example, tetracycline, polypeptide antibiotics, aminoglycosides, and cephaloridine) is contraindicated. It is available in 15-ml and 125-ml containers.

Enflurane (Ēthrane)

Enflurane is a relatively new, nonflammable, and very stable anesthetic that has gained widespread popularity. Clinical anesthesia with enflurane resembles that of halothane and methoxyflurane; induction (3.5 to 4.5%) and recovery are rapid (7 to 10 minutes), but muscular relaxation is more pronounced, and tachypnea is uncommon. Surgical anesthesia is attained at 1.5% to 3% concentration but not more than 3% is used for maintenance. Enflurane is thus superior to halothane for intraabdominal surgery. Small doses of neuromuscular blocking agents may be used in conjunction with enflurane. It is generally administered with nitrous oxide.

Enflurane, when used alone, mildly stimulates bronchial secretions. Laryngeal and pharyngeal reflexes are readily obtained with its use. Enflurane sensitizes the myocardium to catecholamines. Some cardiovascular depression is seen in higher doses, and this depression is enhanced by beta adrenergic blockers (for example, metoprolol, propranolol, nadolol and timolol). When the patient's anesthesia is increased, there is an increase in arterial hypotension. Renal and hepatic toxicity and convulsions have been reported with enflurane. Its biotransformation to fluoride ions is less than that of methoxyflurane; however, precautions should still be taken in patients with renal disease. It is available in 125- and 250-ml containers.

Isoflurane (Forane)

Isoflurane, like enflurane, is an isomer of methoxyflurane and has some similarities to halothane. It is a volatile, nonflammable liquid with a rapid onset of action. When premedication and nitrous oxide are given with it, there is a smooth induction with little excitement. Isoflurane is used for both induction and maintenance of general anesthesia.

Isoflurane can cause respiratory depression

that requires controlled ventilation. Its cardiovascular effects cause fewer dysrhythmias than halothane. Isoflurane is primarily eliminated by the lungs with minimal metabolism.

Isoflurane potentiates the action of nondepolarizing muscular relaxants. Their dose must be reduced by at least one third before isoflurane administration. It is available in 125- and 250-ml containers.

Intravenous anesthetics

Intravenous or *nonvolatile anesthetics* (also called basal anesthetics) include organic solids or liquids that are water soluble and lend themselves to intravenous or intramuscular injection or rectal instillation. Although they can produce loss of consciousness, cortical activity is not completely interrupted, a number of reflexes remain active, and patients respond to painful stimuli. These are not controllable anesthetics. Nonvolatile anesthetics are suitable only for basal narcosis (a reversible condition characterized by complete unconsciousness and analgesia). Intravenous anesthetics are valuable to allay emotional distress, since many patients dread having a tight mask placed over the face while they are fully conscious. These anesthetics reduce the amount of an inhalation anesthetic required. The principal drug used for this purpose is thiopental sodium.

The intravenous anesthetics most commonly used are the ultrashort-acting barbiturates. These drugs are rapidly taken up by brain tissue because of their high oil-water solubility. For example, equilibrium between brain and blood occurs within 1 minute after injection of thiopental. Shortness of action results from the drug being quickly redistributed into the fat depots of the body. Amount of body fat affects drug action; the greater the amount of body fat, the briefer the effect of a single intravenous dose. However, with prolonged administration or large doses there is prolonged drug action resulting in delayed recovery; this is caused by saturation of fat depots and the slow rate of drug release (10% to 15% per hour).

Advantages for using intravenous anesthetics include the rapidity with which unconsciousness is induced, amnesic effects, prompt recovery with minimal doses, and simplicity of administration. They are nonirritating to mucous membranes, and use is not accompanied by the hazard of fire or explosion.

Disadvantages of using this type of anesthetic include swelling, pain, ulceration, tissue sloughing, and necrosis if drug infiltrates into tissue; thrombosis and gangrene if arterial injection occurs; and hypotension, laryngospasm, and respiratory failure from overdosage or prolonged administration. Muscle relaxation and analgesic effects are minimal.

Barbiturates
Thiopental sodium (Pentothal sodium); thiopentone

Barbiturates are used both as general anesthetics and as basal anesthetics. Thiopental sodium is an ultrashort-acting barbiturate and seems to be the most popular.

Action and result. Thiopental sodium produces loss of consciousness in 30 to 60 seconds. Induction is smooth, easy, and pleasant for the patient. Recovery is uneventful and rapid, and complications are rare. Opinion has been expressed that the experienced, skillful anesthetist finds the control of anesthesia with this agent as easy or easier than with many of the anesthetics given by inhalation. Abdominal relaxation is likely to be inadequate even with deep anesthesia; and if used as a general anesthetic, thiopental is frequently supplemented with one of the curariform drugs. Due attention must be given to the possible dangers of hypoxia, obstruction of air passages, and respiratory depression.

Uses. Thiopental sodium is used as a basal anesthetic to carry the patient through the period of induction prior to the use of an anesthetic given by inhalation or injection. It is also used in combination with a number of other drugs for many kinds of minor and major surgery. It may be given by intermittent intravenous injection along with a muscle relaxant and nitrous oxide and oxygen.

Preparation, dosage, and administration.

Thiopental sodium is marketed in 250-, 400-, and 500-mg syringes; 500-mg and 1-g vials with diluent; 1-, 2-, and 5-g kits; and as a rectal suspension (400 mg/g) in a 2-g disposable syringe with rectal applicator. The powder has anhydrous sodium carbonate, which acts as a buffer and makes the resulting solution less irritating to tissues. Thiopental sodium is unstable when in solution and must be freshly made. The dose is determined by each person's age, sex, and body weight; it is given intravenously in about 10 to 15 seconds and is repeated in 30 to 60 seconds as required until the desired effect is obtained. A 40% suspension is sometimes given rectally as a basal anesthetic (onset 8 to 10 minutes) for children (30 mg/kg body weight), not exceeding a total dose of 1 to 1.5 g for children weighing 34 kg (75 pounds) or more or 3 to 4 g for adults weighing 90 kg (200 pounds). Basal narcosis dose for active healthy patients is up to 45 mg/kg, and this is the safe upper limit dose.

Side effects and toxic effects. The rapid onset of action of this barbiturate is both a desirable effect and a potential danger. Medullary paralysis may develop rapidly when an overdose is given. The drug also has a tendency to produce laryngospasm. This can be prevented or handled successfully with the use of atropine or succinylcholine or by the use of endotracheal intubation. Although some difference of opinion exists as to how thiopental is metabolized, there seems to be agreement that it is detoxified chiefly in the liver and the metabolic products are excreted by the kidney. This accounts for the prolonged emergence phase associated with this drug. Its use is not recommended for patients with severe heart disease, hepatic disease, anemia, or respiratory difficulties. Its use is absolutely contraindicated in patients hypersensitive to barbiturates and those with porphyria. The absence of veins suitable for intravenous administration also prohibits its use.

Thiamylal sodium (Surital Sodium); methohexital sodium (Brevital Sodium)

Thiamylal sodium and methohexital sodium are ultrashort-acting barbiturates with properties similar to those of thiopental.

Nonbarbiturates
Ketamine hydrochloride (Ketalar, Ketaject)

Ketamine is a rapid-acting nonbarbiturate intravenous anesthetic. It is a derivative of the psychotomimetic drug of abuse phencyclidine. Ketamine acts on the midbrain within the reticular formation, as do the barbiturates. It produces analgesia and amnesia but not muscular relaxation. Ketamine has been called a "dissociative anesthetic"; that is, it produces a cataleptic state in which the patient appears to be awake but detached from his environment and unresponsive to pain. The patient's eyelids usually do not close, nystagmus is common, and there may be slight involuntary and purposeless movements. After recovery the patient does not recall the experience. Since ketamine causes hypertonus, muscle tone in the oropharynx is maintained and airway obstruction caused by relaxation of soft tissues seldom occurs; mechanical stimulation may cause laryngospasm. Respiration is usually not depressed. Ketamine is a potent cerebral vasodilator; it increases both cerebral blood flow and cerebrospinal fluid pressure.

Uses. Ketamine has its greatest usefulness for diagnostic studies in infants and children and for repeated anesthesia in burned children. It is best suited for short diagnostic or surgical procedures not requiring skeletal muscle relaxation. Ketamine is also recommended for induction of anesthesia when a barbiturate is contraindicated. Its adverse effects limit its usefulness in adults.

Preparation and dosage. Ketamine is prepared in concentrations of 10, 50, and 100 mg/ml. It is usually administered intravenously over a period of 60 seconds in doses ranging from 1 to 4.5 mg/kg body weight for induction of anesthesia. Onset of action is rapid, occurring in less than 1 minute; duration of anesthetic action is 5 to 10 minutes. When given intramuscularly, the usual induction dose is 6.5 to 13 mg/kg body weight. Onset of anesthetic action is about 5 minutes; duration of action from 12 to 25 minutes.

Side effects and precautions. Ketamine can cause numerous side effects, and therefore a number of precautions are necessary with this drug.

Psychologic. Emergence from ketamine anesthesia may be accompanied by unpleasant dreams, hallucinations, and emergence delirium. Patients may show irrational behavior, excitement, confusion, or euphoria. These reactions occur more frequently in adults than in children or the elderly. These effects are less likely to occur with intramuscular administration of the drug. These psychic reactions (a reason for ketamine drug abuse) usually last only a few hours; however, recurrences may occur up to 24 hours postoperatively. If nurses and recovery room personnel protect the patient from visual, tactile, and auditory stimuli during recovery, the incidence of psychic effects may be reduced. Ketamine should not be given to neurotic or psychotic patients.

Cardiovascular. Ketamine has pressor effects, which may result from liberation of catecholamines. It increases heart rate and cardiac output and elevates systolic and diastolic blood pressures. This necessitates caution when ketamine is given to elderly patients with arteriosclerosis; and ketamine is contraindicated in patients with severe hypertension. Bradycardia and hypotension may also occur. Severe arrhythmias occur rarely.

Respiratory. Although respirations are usually not depressed by ketamine, severe respiratory depression and apnea may occur with high doses given rapidly by intravenous injection.

Neurologic. Ketamine enhances skeletal muscle tone, and this may cause fasciculations and tremors. Convulsions have also been reported. Ketamine also increases cerebrospinal fluid pressure. It should not be used in patients with convulsive disorders or in those in whom an increase in cerebrospinal fluid pressure could be disastrous.

Gastrointestinal. Nausea and vomiting may occur but are usually not severe; patients are able to take liquids shortly after regaining consciousness.

General. Local pain and redness (exanthema) at injection site have been reported.

Drug interactions. Ketamine is formulated in slightly acid (pH 3.5 to 5.5) solutions and should not be injected in the same syringe with a barbiturate. The latter is alkaline, and the mixture will form a precipitate. Diazepam inhibits ketamine biotransformation, prolonging half-life and increasing sleep time.

Ketamine appears to be clinically compatible with commonly used general and local anesthetics. It is available in 10, 50, and 100 mg/ml concentrations and is subject to regulation by the Controlled Substances Act.

Droperidol (Inapsine)

Droperidol is related to haloperidol, which is pharmacologically similar to the phenothiazine psychotherapeutic drugs. Droperidol was first synthesized in Belgium after a long period of research for a potent, short-acting, well-tolerated neuroleptic drug for use in anesthesiology.

A parenteral injection of droperidol produces tranquility and detachment without loss of consciousness, although the patient may experience considerable drowsiness. Voluntary movements are markedly decreased. As a preoperative medication, droperidol significantly decreases the incidence of postoperative nausea and vomiting in patients given strong opiate analgesics. It may cause a moderate degree of tachycardia; in large doses it may cause hypotension because of a vasodilating effect. When administered alone, it has *no* analgesic effect.

After intravenous or intramuscular administration onset of action occurs in 3 to 10 minutes; full effect is seen within 30 minutes; sedative and tranquilizing effects last 2 to 4 hours; but consciousness is altered for 12 hours. Most of the drug is metabolized in the liver and excreted via the urinary and intestinal tracts.

Uses. Droperidol is used preoperatively and during induction and maintenance of anesthesia as an adjunct to general or regional anesthesia.

Dosage. Adult preoperative dose (reduced in the poor risk, debilitated, or elderly patient and in those patients taking depressant drugs) intravenous or intramuscular, is 2.5 to 10 mg given 30 to 60 minutes before induction of anesthesia. In children 2 to 12 years old it is 1 to 1.5 mg/9.1 to 11.25 kg (20 to 25 lb) for premedication or induction of anesthesia. To reduce incidence of postoperative nausea and vomiting, 1.25 to 2.5 mg may be given. The drug is available in 2.5 mg/ml concentration.

Side effects. Common side effects of droperidol are extrapyramidal symptoms (tremors, flexed arms, extended neck, upward rotation of eyes, etc.) and hypotension. Mild to moderate hypotension and tachycardia may occur immediately after administration; severe hypotension may occur postoperatively. Patients have also experienced hallucinations and nightmares when given droperidol postoperatively. Other reported side effects include dizziness, chills, facial sweating, and restlessness.

Cautions. Droperidol should be used with extreme caution in elderly or debilitated patients, in those who have received depressant drugs, and in those with cardiovascular disorders.

Drug interactions. Droperidol can potentiate the action of narcotics, barbiturates, anesthetics, tranquilizers, alcohol, and other CNS depressants. When droperidol is used with other depressants, dosage of each drug should be reduced.

Fentanyl citrate (Sublimaze)

Fentanyl is a strong narcotic analgesic (0.1 mg is equivalent to 10 mg morphine) that has morphinelike action. It has a faster onset but shorter duration of action than morphine. After intramuscular injection, onset of action occurs in 5 to 15 minutes; the peak occurs in 30 minutes; duration of action is 1 to 2 hours. After intravenous injection, peak action occurs in 3 to 5 minutes; duration of action is 30 to 60 minutes. Most of the drug is metabolized in the liver.

Because of its short duration of action, fentanyl is not recommended for the same uses as morphine. It is used preoperatively for minor and major surgery, urologic procedures, and gastroscopy.

Dosage. Fentanyl is available in 0.05 mg/ml concentration in 2- and 5-ml ampules. Preoperative (30 to 60 minutes before surgery) adult dose is 0.05 to 0.1 mg (1 to 2 ml) given intramuscularly; the same dose can be given postoperatively every 1 to 2 hours. As an adjunct to regional anesthesia and induction of general anesthesia 0.05 to 0.1 mg is used. For poor-risk patients half this dose is used. A dose of 0.02 to 0.03 mg/9.1 to 11.25 kg is the child's (2 to 12

years) dose for maintenance and induction.

Side effects. A variety of side effects can be produced by fentanyl, including euphoria, miosis, nausea, vomiting, pruritus, constipation, hypotension, and respiratory depression. Rapid intravenous injection or large doses may cause muscle rigidity and apnea. Succinylcholine may be used to counteract these effects. Naloxone can be used to counteract respiratory depression; it must be remembered, however, that this drug will also overcome the analgesic effect of fentanyl. The duration of action of naloxone is shorter than that of fentanyl, necessitating repeated doses of naloxone.

Precautions. The patient must be closely observed for signs of respiratory depression and muscle rigidity. Drugs for counteracting adverse effects as well as equipment to support respiration should be immediately available. This has become a drug of abuse for social and recreational purposes.

Drug interactions. CNS depressants (sedatives, hypnotics, tranquilizers, alcohol) potentiate the respiratory and sedative effects of fentanyl. If any of these drugs are used with fentanyl, dosage of each drug should be reduced one fourth to one third.

Droperidol and fentanyl (Innovar)

The preparation of droperidol and fentanyl, Innovar, consists of 1 part fentanyl to 50 parts droperidol: 0.05 mg of fentanyl to 2.5 mg droperidol per milliliter. It is available in 2- and 5-ml ampules.

Innovar is used to produce neuroleptic anesthesia. Droperidol is a neuroleptic drug with prolonged action; fentanyl is a narcotic analgesic with a very short duration of action. This combination produces quiescence, reduced response to painful stimuli, and decreased motor activity. This state permits the patient to undergo short procedures requiring a conscious and cooperative patient, such as bronchoscopy and cystoscopy, without pain. Innovar is also used as a premedication for anesthesia and as an adjunct for induction and maintenance of anesthesia.

Innovar has lost some of its earlier popularity, since clinical investigation has demonstrated that the depression of respiratory rate and alveolar ventilation may persist longer than the analgesic effect. Additional narcotic analgesics may further increase respiratory depression, and apnea may result. Patients given Innovar should be closely and carefully monitored, and appropriate resuscitative equipment and a narcotic antagonist (naloxone) should be readily available for use if apnea occurs.

Dosage. Both an intravenous injection or an intravenous drop (10 ml/250 ml 5% dextrose in water) may be used for induction of anesthesia. Recommended dosage for preoperative medication is 0.5 to 2.0 ml given intramuscularly 45 to 60 minutes preoperatively depending on the patient's weight, age, physical status, pathologic state, concomitant drugs, type of anesthesia, and surgical procedure. The first two or three doses postoperatively may be half the preoperative dose.

Side effects. The fentanyl component of Innovar may cause severe respiratory depression, and extrapyramidal symptoms (tremor, akathisia, etc.) may be caused by the droperidol component. Apnea, laryngospasm, bronchospasm, bradycardia, and hallucinations may also occur.

Cautions. Innovar should be used cautiously in children; in patients with impaired liver, kidney, or pulmonary function; and in those who are poor surgical risks. It probably should not be used for patients with parkinsonism.

Innovar should not be administered with other psychosedatives, hypnotics, or strong analgesics because of possible additive or potentiating effects increasing the risk of hypotension and respiratory depression.

The fixed dose combination of droperidol (2.5 mg/ml) and fentanyl (0.05 mg/ml) is controversial and disapproved of by some authorities. Repeated injections of Innovar after induction can result in droperidol overdosage.

Reactions to general anesthetics

Treatment of disease with a variety of drugs having varying degrees of potency and diverse effects on body systems establishes a propensity for drug-induced reactions to anesthetics. Interactions between drugs and anesthetics may be responsible for anesthetic morbidity and mortality. Certain drugs and anesthetic agents are hepatotoxic, and their concurrent administration to the same patient can result in severe additive effects and even fatal liver damage. Drugs that have depressant effects on cardiac function in conjunction with the depressant action of anesthetics can cause decreased cardiac output and hypotension, which may result in ventricular fibrillation or cardiac arrest. Drug-induced reactions to anesthetics are not uncommon and not decreasing; indeed, this problem appears to be rapidly increasing. Table 9-5 summarizes some of the common drug-induced reactions to anesthetics. Not all drug interactions occur during anesthesia; some reactions are delayed or latent. The nurse needs to closely observe postoperative patients for undesirable signs and symptoms. Early detection and treatment of drug interactions may be vital.

Geriatric patients. In the elderly patient there is the potential for undesirable interactions between the anesthetic drug employed and the patient's physiology. The elderly patient may have lean muscle replaced by fat, changes in enzyme activity, and diminished glucose tolerance; in addition, reduction in renal blood flow and glomerular filtration rate occurs even in the absence of renal disease. Other aspects of the aging process must also be considered in the selection of an anesthetic. The declining physiologic state is reflected in alterations in the central nervous system, cardiac function, respiratory system, gastrointestinal system, hepatic system, and renal system. In addition, the elderly are reported to experience exaggerated effects to many drugs, including analgesics, anticonvulsants, cardiac drugs, narcotic analgesics, sedatives, hypnotics, and tranquilizers.

The loss of brain cells and a reduction in neuron reserve may be responsible for the reduced tolerance to CNS depressants and anesthetics and for the confusion that elderly patients often experience during the period after anesthesia recovery. The respiratory alterations result in increased residual capacity, lowered vital capacity, and decreased small airways with larger lung volumes. The aim of postanesthetic management is to minimize the risk of pneumonia, which often occurs in the elderly. The reduced coronary circulation results in

TABLE 9-5 Some drug-induced reactions to anesthetics

| Type of drug | Example of drug | | Reaction | Prevention |
	Generic name	Trade name		
Antihypertensives	Bretylium Reserpine Guanethidine	Bretylol Ismelin	Circulatory depession Reduced cardiac output Hypotension Bradycardia	Use vasopressors during anesthesia
Antidepressants (monoamine oxidase inhibitors)	Isocarboxazid Pargyline Furazolidone Tranylcypromine Phenelzine Procarbazine	Marplan Eutonyl Furokone Parnate Nardil Matulane	Hypotension, depressive effect Potentiation of action of narcotics, hypnotics	Discontinue monoamine oxidase inhibitor 7 to 14 days before anesthesia and be fully aware of drug interaction effect Avoid use of narcotics and barbiturates with these drugs
Adrenergics	Epinephrine Norepinephrine		Cardiac arrhythmias Tissue slough when used with local anesthetics	Avoid use with anesthetics that sensitize myocardium to catecholamines (halothane, cyclopropane)
Antibiotics (parenteral) (aminoglycosides, polymyxin B)	Amikacin Gentamicin Neomycin Kanamycin Streptomycin Tobramycin Polymyxin B		Enhancement of neuromuscular blockade Muscle paralysis, apnea, bradycardia, hypotension	
Adrenal steroids	Cortisone Cortisol		Adrenal insufficiency and hypotension during stress of surgery after prolonged use Circulatory collapse	Administer steroids preoperatively and if necessary during surgery and postoperatively
Tranquilizers (phenothiazines)	Chlorpromazine Promazine	Thorazine Sparine	Potentiation of action of narcotics, hypnotics Central nervous system depression Hypotension Respiratory depression	Use minor tranquilizers with no adrenergic blocking effect Reduce dosages of drugs and anesthetics
Pituitary hormones	Oxytocin Vasopressin	Pitocin Syntocinon Pitressin	Coronary vasoconstriction Myocardial ischemia Hypotension	
Ergot alkaloids	Ergonovine Methylergonovine	Ergotrate Methergine	Potentiation of effects of vasopressors used to overcome hypotension caused by spinal anesthesia Severe hypertension during third stage of labor	Use pressor drugs sparingly in obstetric patient

a lowered ability to increase cardiac output because the anesthetics generally act to depress myocardial contraction. Fluid management in the elderly is complicated by the decline in renal function, the decline in ability to concentrate urine, a gradual loss of nephrons, and the increased renal tubular necrosis that follows a period of anesthetic-induced hypotension in the elderly. Selection of an anesthetic is further complicated by the multiple chronic diseases often seen in the elderly and the medications used to treat these states. Following are some examples of possible interactions: thiazides may deplete the serum potassium; clonidine produces hypotension; guanethidine reduces myocardial contractility and the response to indirect sympathomimetics (alpha and beta agonists) and therefore should be discontinued about 2 weeks prior to surgery in a nonemergency situation; because beta adrenergic blocking drugs depress the myocardium, the morning dose before surgery should be omitted; phenothiazines potentiate anesthetics; tricyclic antidepressants with their anticholinergic and cardiovascular effects should be discontinued 2 weeks prior to elective surgery because of their long half-lives; monoamine oxidase inhibitors and meperidine may create hyperpyrexia, hypotension, coma, death, metabolic interference with other drugs, catecholamine effects, and intensification of the action of barbiturates and narcotics. Therefore monoamine oxidase inhibitors should be discontinued 1 to 3 weeks prior to elective surgery. In addition, it has been proved that a myocardial infarction within 2 years increases the chance of an infarction during or just after anesthesia and surgery. Because of the many variables in the elderly patient, the nurse should participate actively in the selection of an anesthetic that is not contraindicated by the patient's physical condition and current medication and should titrate the anesthetic to the individual patient's response based on blood pressure, pulse, and cardiac monitoring of vital signs.

Nursing implications for general anesthesia

Preoperative preparations. Satisfactory anesthesia is partly dependent on the preparation of the patient. Preanesthetic medications are administered for the following several reasons: (1) sedative and amnesic effects to decrease anxiety (barbiturates and narcotic analgesics), (2) inhibition of salivary and mucous secretion for anticipated undesirable side effects such as vagal stimulation (abolished by atropine) and spasms (relieved by succinylcholine), (3) increase of effectiveness of an incomplete anesthetic (nitrous oxide), and (4) decrease of the amount of anesthetic required.

A frequent preoperative order is morphine or meperidine, hydroxyzine, and atropine. Atropine is used to block the action of acetylcholine at parasympathetic nerve endings, to overcome vagal effects of anesthesia, and to dry secretions. (It may cause tachycardia in addition to the mild cerebral stimulation.) A dose of 0.4 or 0.6 mg is most useful in adults, but as high as 2 mg is needed to produce palpitations and cardiac effects such as a rapid heart rate.

Barbiturates may be administered the night before the operation to ensure a sound and restful sleep. Narcotics, barbiturates, or tranquilizers administered prior to the patient being taken to the operating room promote serenity, amnesia, and smooth induction. It is important that the nurse administer the medications at the exact time they are ordered to be given, since a narcotic given too close to the time of administration of the general anesthetic may achieve its full effect during anesthesia and cause severe respiratory depression.

Patients have been known to faint after receiving promethazine along with morphine or meperidine. Ambulatory patients receiving these drugs should be carefully watched.

Preparation of the patient for general anesthesia is very important. Vital signs should be carefully checked before the patient is taken to the operating room, and any alteration from normal should be recorded and immediately reported. The mental state of the patient should be noted, and any undue anxiety or expressions of fear of death should be reported immediately. Severe anxiety or fear, unless allayed, affects both the autonomic and central nervous systems and may cause reactions that are detrimental physiologically and psychologically. These patients may resist relaxation and fight the anesthetic. A greater amount of anesthetic is therefore required, and toxic levels of drugs may be administered inadvertently. Preparation for surgical procedures should be carefully explained to patients. It may be helpful to highlight the safety factors incorporated in today's modern operative procedures.

Food is usually withheld after the evening meal, and standard procedure is to give the patient nothing to eat or drink after midnight. This procedure helps prevent aspiration if nausea and vomiting occur.

Patients may complain of dry mouth caused by the use of atropine or scopolamine to minimize secretions of saliva and mucus. Frequent rinsing of the mouth may be helpful. The necessity for coughing, deep breathing, and frequent turning during the postoperative period should be taught to the patient preoperatively. This promotes patient cooperation postoperatively when he is asked to perform procedures that often induce pain.

Common postoperative complications. A wide variety of signs and symptoms may be observed in the postoperative patient. Nurses should be aware of the more common postoperative complications and the possible causative factors to enable them to determine effective modes of intervention.

Hypotension may result from an excess of nonvolatile drugs that depress the vasomotor center. Narcotics are to be avoided because they may increase the hypotension. However, severe pain can cause hypotension; in these cases a narcotic may both alleviate pain and increase the blood pressure.

Nausea and vomiting may be caused by stimulation of the vomiting center as a result of anoxia during anesthesia.

Hypoventilation may result from excess or cumulative effects of drugs administered during anesthesia. It may be a lingering effect of neuromuscular blocking agents.

Oliguria caused by anesthesia is very common, as are *atony and urinary retention* after perineal and genital operations.

Nerve injury may follow spinal anesthesia or malpositioning during general anesthesia. Brachial, radial, ulnar, and perineal nerves are most likely to be injured.

Intestinal distention and at times paralytic ileus may occur from the anesthetic agent, postoperative sedation, or a combination of both. *Thrombosis* may also be observed.

Important in the postoperative period are protection of the patient from injury until he has fully responded and maintenance of a patent airway. Patients should be closely observed for signs and symptoms of shock, a not uncommon postoperative complication. Early detection of impending shock and institution of proper therapy may prevent or at least modify its severity. Rate, volume, and rhythm of the pulse should be noted as well as the patient's color and skin temperature. A rapid, thready, weak pulse, cyanosis or extreme pallor, cold and clammy skin, and low blood pressure are characteristic signs of shock. The patient should be checked for bleeding at the operative site; if he continues to lose blood postoperatively, hemorrhagic shock may occur. Postoperative shock may also result from extensive surgical trauma, prolonged operating time, prolonged deep anesthesia, or even inadequate anesthesia. Patients should be adequately ven-

tilated postoperatively to prevent atelectasis. Heavy smokers in particular are likely to have postoperative chest complications.

Other important factors to keep in mind are the following:

1 Patients on steroid therapy have depressed ability to respond to stress in the immediate postoperative period, an increased risk of infection, and possible delay in wound healing. Asepsis is particularly important with these patients.
2 Antihypertensive drugs can cause the blood pressure to be erratic when certain other drugs are given. For example, an overshoot can occur with vasopressors, and a precipitous fall may occur with narcotics or depressants. If antihypertensive therapy was discontinued preoperatively, hypertensive crisis might occur postoperatively.
3 Phenothiazine drugs given in large doses over a long period of time prior to surgery may cause the patient in the immediate postoperative period to have a prolonged recovery owing to potentiation.
4 Antibiotics (tetracycline, clindamycin, lincomycin, aminoglycosides, streptomycin, neomycin, polymyxin) in large doses can have a curariform (neuromuscular blocking) effect.
5 Patients who have been on long-term anticoagulant therapy have a high hemorrhage risk during surgery. Blood and vitamin K should be available, the patient should be closely observed for any bleeding tendency, and the use of barbiturates should be avoided. Interruption of anticoagulant therapy may precipitate thromboembolism; conversely, if anticoagulants are maintained at full doses, some patients may hemorrhage excessively. If it is elected to administer anticoagulants prior to, during, or immediately following the procedure, the dosage of the anticoagulant should be adjusted to maintain the prothrombin time at approximately 1½ to 2 times the control level. The operative site should be limited to allow the effective use of local hemostasis procedures, including the use of absorbable hemostatic agents.
6 Patients who have had ketamine anesthesia should be protected from unnecessary visual, tactile, and auditory stimuli to help prevent excitement and psychic reactions during emergence from anesthesia.
7 If droperidol is given to control nausea and vomiting, the nurse should remember that it has *no analgesic effect*. An analgesic will be needed to control pain. However, since droperidol potentiates the action of narcotics, the narcotic dose should be reduced. The nurse's judgment in these cases is important.
8 Succinylcholine may cause postoperative muscle pains. This is more likely to occur if the patient is ambulated within 24 hours after the drug has been administered. Several studies indicate that confin-

ing the patient to bed for the first 24 hours postoperatively decreases the incidence of muscle pains. This pain is believed to be caused by the initial muscle fasciculations.

9 Succinylcholine can cause prolonged muscle weakness, particularly in the respiratory muscles.

Local anesthesia
Surface, or topical, anesthesia

Surface, or topical, anesthesia is restricted to mucous membranes, damaged skin surfaces, wounds, and burns. The local anesthetic is applied in the form of a solution, ointment, gel, cream, or powder to produce loss of sensation by paralyzing afferent nerve endings. Local anesthetics do not penetrate unbroken skin. Topical anesthesia is used to relieve pain and itching and to anesthetize mucous membranes of the eye, nose, throat, or urethra for minor surgical procedures. Cocaine in a 4% to 10% solution continues to be one of the most widely used agents for topical anesthesia.

Local anesthesia may also be achieved by freezing. Low temperatures in living tissues produce diminished sensation. This form of anesthesia is sometimes employed for minor operative procedures. Packing an extremity in ice may be used for the major operative procedure of amputation of part of an extremity, particularly in elderly and debilitated persons or in patients considered to be at "high risk" if given a general anesthetic. Tissues that are frozen too intensely and over too long a time may be destroyed.

Ethyl chloride is a local anesthetic that can be used to produce this effect, although it is not employed extensively.

Anesthesia by injection

Anesthesia by injection is accomplished by infiltration, conduction, spinal, caudal, and saddle block.

Infiltration anesthesia is produced by injecting dilute solutions (0.1%) of the agent into the skin and then subcutaneously into the region to be anesthetized. Epinephrine is often added to the solution to intensify the anesthesia in a limited region and to prevent excessive bleeding

and systemic effects. Repeated injection will prolong the anesthesia as long as it may be needed. The sensory nerve endings are anesthetized. This method of administration is used for minor operations such as incision and drainage or excision of a cyst.

Conduction, or block, anesthesia means that the anesthetic is injected into the vicinity of a nerve trunk that supplies the region of the operative site. The injection may be made at some distance from the site of surgical procedure. A single nerve may be blocked, or the anesthetic may be injected in a location where several nerve trunks emerge from the spinal cord (paravertebral block). A more concentrated solution (2%) is required because of the thickness of nerve trunk fibers. This method of anesthesia is often used for operations on the foot and hand.

Spinal anesthesia is a type of extensive nerve block, sometimes called a subarachnoid block. The anesthetic solution is injected into the subarachnoid space and affects the lower part of the spinal cord and nerve roots.

Spinal anesthesia

For *low spinal anesthesia* the patient is placed in a flat or Fowler position. A solution with a specific gravity greater than that of spinal fluid is used, since it tends to diffuse downward. For *high spinal anesthesia* the Trendelenburg position with the head sharply flexed is used in conjunction with an anesthetic solution of lower specific gravity than that of spinal fluid (which tends to diffuse upward) or a solution with the same specific gravity as spinal fluid (which may diffuse upward or downward, depending on position used). Solutions with the same specific gravity as spinal fluid act primarily at the site of injection.

Onset of anesthesia usually occurs within 1 to 2 minutes after injection. Duration of anesthesia is 60 to 180 minutes, depending on the anesthetic used. Spinal anesthesia is used for surgical procedures on the lower abdomen, inguinal area, or lower extremities; it may be the method of choice for patients with severe respiratory problems or with liver, kidney, or metabolic disease. Marked hypotension, decreased cardiac output, and respiratory inadequacy tend to occur during anesthesia and are considered to be disadvantages of this method of anesthesia.

Postoperatively, headache is the most common complaint; this may be accompanied by difficulty in hearing or seeing. Headache may be postural and occur only in the head-up or sitting or standing position. This symptom is the result of the opening in the dura made by the large spinal needle, which may persist for days or weeks, permitting loss of cerebrospinal fluid. Headache and auditory and visual problems following lumbar puncture result from decreased intracranial pressure. These symptoms are usually alleviated when spinal fluid pressure returns to normal. Paresthesias such as numbness and tingling may occur after spinal anesthesia; they are usually located in the lumbar or sacral areas and disappear within a relatively short time. The success and safety of spinal anesthesia depend primarily on the anesthetist's skill and knowledge.

Caudal anesthesia is produced by injecting an anesthetic solution into the caudal canal, the sacral part of the vertebral canal containing the caudal equina, or bundle of spinal nerves that innervates the pelvic viscera. It is used in obstetrics and for operations on pelvic or genital organs. Its advantage over spinal anesthesia is that the anesthetic does not have direct access to the spinal cord and medullary centers. Thus the respiratory muscles and blood pressure are not directly affected, and undesirable effects are less likely to occur.

Saddle block is sometimes used in obstetrics and for surgery involving the perineum, rectum, genitalia, and upper parts of the thighs. The patient sits upright while the anesthetic is injected, after a lumbar puncture has been done. The patient remains upright for a short time, until the anesthetic has had a chance to be effective. The parts that would contact a saddle when riding become anesthetized, hence the name.

Local anesthetics

Local anesthetics are drugs used to abolish pain sensation in a particular part of the body (Table 9-6). Basic mechanism of action of these drugs is unknown, but most of these drugs act by stabilizing or elevating the threshold of excitation of the nerve cell membrane without affecting resting potential. This action is a result of reduction of membrane permeability to all ions; thus depolarization and transmission of nerve impulses are prevented. Local anesthetics are capable of abolishing all sensa-

TABLE 9-6 Local anesthetics—administration and use

Method	Tissue affected	Preparation used	Examples of drugs used	Therapeutic use
Topical	Sensory nerve of mucous membranes and dermis	Solution Ointment Cream Powder	Cocaine Benzocaine Ethyl aminobenzoate Lidocaine Tetracaine	Relief of pain or itching Examination of conjunctiva
Infiltration	Sensory nerve endings in subcutaneous tissues or dermis	Injection	Etidocaine Procaine Prilocaine Lidocaine Chloroprocaine Mepivacaine	Minor operations
Block	Nerve trunk	Injection	Etidocaine Procaine Prilocaine Lidocaine Chloroprocaine Mepivacaine	Dental and limb operations Muscle relaxation
Spinal (subarachnoid block)	Spinal roots	Injection	Dibucaine Procaine Tetracaine Lidocaine	Abdominal operations Muscle relaxation

tion, but pain fibers are affected first, probably since they are thinner, unmyelinated, and more easily penetrated by these drugs. Loss of pain is followed in sequence by loss of response to cold, warmth, touch, and pressure. Most motor fibers can also be anesthetized when there is sufficient concentration of the drug over a long enough time.

The concentration of local anesthetic needed to block conduction of nerve impulses is much less than the concentration of local anesthetic in the blood that would cause death, but even relatively small doses of local anesthetics reaching the heart or brain may cause serious reactions. For this reason effort is made to confine the local anesthetic to a limited region or small area near a nerve or among nerve endings. The action of the local anesthetic is reversible; it is followed by complete recovery and, as a rule, produces no damage to the nerve cells.

The categories of local anesthetics are alcohols, esters of benzoic acid, esters of para-aminobenzoic acid, and amides. Each has an aromatic portion (lipophilic determinant), amine portion (hydrophilic determinant), and an intermediate chain. Table 9-7 presents some commonly used local anesthetics and their properties. The alcohols (phenol, cresol, menthol, and benzyl alcohol) are seldom employed today. Benzyl alcohol, an aromatic alcohol of low potency, is used topically with procaine to extend its duration of action. Examples of benzoic acid esters are cocaine, hexylcaine, and piperocaine. Examples of the esters of para-aminobenzoic acid are procaine, chloroprocaine, and tetracaine, which are all metabolized by plasma cholinesterase. Examples of the amides are dibucaine, etidocaine, lidocaine, prilocaine, mepivacaine, and bupivacaine, which are not metabolized by plasma cholinesterase but excreted in the urine and metabolized in the liver.

Vasoconstrictors (epinephrine) are used with the local anesthetic to decrease the systemic absorption and prolong the anesthetic's duration of action. They are not used for nerve blocks in areas with end-arteries (fingers, toes, ears, nose, penis) because ischemia may develop, resulting in gangrene.

Local anesthetics may also be classified as

T A B L E 9 - 7 Properties of commonly used local anesthetics

	Cocaine	Procaine	Benzocaine
Trade names	—	Novocain	Americaine Hurricaine
Potency	Two to three times that of procaine		Very low
Onset of action	1 minute	2 to 5 minutes	Immediate
Duration of action	1 hour	1 hour	During contact only
Dose	1% to 4% topically 5% to 10% for anesthe- sia of nose and throat	0.25% to 2%, depend- ing upon method of administration 10% for spinal anes- thesia Not used topically	Variable 5% to 10% ointment topically
Toxicity	Four times more toxic than procaine when injected subcutane- ously	Least toxic of all lo- cal anesthetics	Relatively nontoxic
Precautions	Not recommended for infiltration, nerve block, or spinal anes- thesia Repeated use causes psychic dependence Repeated use in eye may cause clouding, pitting, ulceration of cornea, and mydriasis	Overdose or rapid in- jection may cause stimulation	Suitable for topical use only Sensitization may develop

injectable or topical, according to the way they are primarily used and administered, even though some can be included in both groups. The drugs in each classification are presented below.

Injectable local anesthetics

SHORT DURATION OF ACTION
Procaine hydrochloride (Novocain)

Procaine is a synthetic local anesthetic. It is a white powder that is readily soluble in water and has low lipid solubility. In solution it withstands sterilization with heat, although a precipitate may form when the solution stands for a long time.

Procaine is less potent than cocaine but also less toxic. It is rapidly destroyed by plasma enzymes in the blood and other tissues. It does not constrict blood vessels and does not dilate the pupil of the eye. It produces no particular central action like cocaine, and it is not dependence producing. The 1-hour duration of action is prolonged by use of epinephrine.

Uses. Procaine is the best known of the local anesthetics, and it is said to be the safest for both nerve block and infiltration. Reactions occur comparatively seldom and tend to be mild; elimination is rapid, and tissue damage is seldom produced. Procaine is not well absorbed from mucous membranes; hence it is not suited for topical administration. It is useful for many

---

Injectable local anesthetics

Amides
  Long duration of action
    Bupivacaine
    Dibucaine
    Etidocaine
  Intermediate duration of action
    Lidocaine
    Mepivacaine
    Prilocaine
Para-aminobenzoic acid esters
  Long duration of action
    Tetracaine
  Short duration of action
    Chloroprocaine
    Procaine

Lidocaine	Tetracaine	Mepivacaine	Dibucaine
Xylocaine Lignocaine	Pontocaine	Carbocaine	Nupercaine
Two times that of procaine	Ten times that of procaine	Two times that of procaine	Ten to twenty times that of procaine
Immediate	5 to 10 minutes	Less rapid than procaine	10 minutes
1 to 2 hours	1½ to 2 hours	More prolonged than procaine or lidocaine	2½ to 3 hours
0.5% to 4% for injection 2% and 5% topically	0.5% to 2% topically 0.15% to 0.25% for injection	1% to 2% solution	0.25% to 2% for injection or topical application
Like that of procaine	More toxic than procaine, but toxic effects rare because of low dosage used	Two times that of procaine—less than lidocaine	Ten or twenty times that of procaine
When administered rapidly or in large doses may cause convulsions and hypotension	May cause vasodepressor effects	Has vasoconstrictor action	Tissue sloughs when injected subcutaneously

---

Topical local anesthetics

Amides
  Lidocaine (Xylocaine, Anestacon)
  Dibucaine (Nupercainal)
Esters
  Benzoic acid type
    Cocaine
    Hexylcaine (Cyclaine)
    Piperocaine (Metycaine)
    Proparacaine (Ophthaine, Alcaine, Ophthetic)
  Para-aminobenzoic acid type
    Benzocaine (Americaine, Hurricaine)
    Benoxinate (Dorsacaine)
    Butamben Picrate (Butesin Picrate)
    Tetracaine (Pontocaine)
Miscellaneous
  Cyclomethycaine (Surfacaine)
  Dimethisoquin (Quotane)
  Diperodon (Diothane)
  Dyclonine (Dyclone)
  Pramoxine (Tronothane)

---

types of local anesthesia when given by injection. Procaine hydrochloride has been used to overcome cardiac arrhythmias, although procainamide is used more often for this purpose. Lidocaine has greatly displaced its use.

Preparation and dosage. The following are the procaine preparations available.

Procaine hydrochloride. This is available as a white crystalline powder intended for parenteral solutions.

Procaine hydrochloride injection; procaine and epinephrine injection. The procaine hydrochloride preparation is available in concentrations of 1%, 2%, and 10% procaine hydrochloride. It may or may not contain epinephrine.

The dosage of procaine used for anesthesia varies with the technique of administration employed. Concentrations of 1% or 2% are adequate for most purposes of nerve block, although concentrations of 0.25% to 0.5% may be used for extensive field block and infiltration. The duration of anesthesia for a nerve block is about 45 minutes and for spinal anesthesia about 1 hour. The 10% solution is used for spinal anesthesia.

Chloroprocaine hydrochloride (Nesacaine)

Chloroprocaine is more potent and rapid acting than procaine. It has relatively low toxicity.

The drug is not a potent surface anesthetic. It apparently can be given in all the ways that procaine can be given by injection, although its use for spinal anesthesia has not been fully evaluated. It is indicated in infiltration and nerve block (1% and 2% solution) and for caudal and epidural block (2% and 3% solution without preservatives).

Toxic effects. Chloroprocaine's toxic effects are said to be less or similar to those produced by procaine. Several cases of thrombophlebitis have been reported after intravenous injection of chloroprocaine. Since it does not produce vasoconstriction, its toxicity can be decreased by giving it with epinephrine to delay absorption.

INTERMEDIATE DURATION OF ACTION
Lidocaine hydrochloride (Xylocaine Hydrochloride); lignocaine

Lidocaine hydrochloride is another synthetic local anesthetic. It is becoming more popular than procaine. It has average lipid solubility, is 65% plasma protein bound, and has about the same anesthetic potency as cocaine. It is said to produce effects more promptly (within 5 minutes) and with greater intensity (60 to 90 minutes) than those produced by an equal amount of procaine. Lidocaine is suited for topical anesthesia as well as for spinal, infiltration, and nerve block anesthesia. Common side effects are sedation, sleepiness, and dizziness. Metabolism is in the liver to active metabolites.

Preparation and dosage. Solutions are available in 0.5% to 4% concentration for injection, with or without epinephrine hydrochloride. A 2% jelly is used for mucous membranes of the urethra, and 2.5% and 5% ointment is available for application to burns and skin lesions.

A 4% solution is used for topical anesthesia of accessible mucous membranes of oral and nasal cavities and the upper digestive tract. A "viscous" 2% product is used for the production of topical anesthesia of irritated or inflamed mucous membranes of mouth and pharynx.

Toxic effects. In low concentrations lidocaine's toxicity is thought to be about the same as that of procaine. It has an advantage of being effective in small amounts of low concentrations. Overdosage may result in many of the toxic symptoms associated with local anesthetics. A biphasic action on the central nervous system is stimulation followed by depression, such as drop in blood pressure, nausea, vomiting, pallor, apprehension, muscular twitching, and convulsions. Lidocaine is contraindicated in patients with blood dyscrasias. Lidocaine has a cardiovascular depressant effect.

Drug interactions. Lidocaine enhances the neuromuscular blocking action of succinylcholine, decamethonium, and tubocurarine. The reason for this interaction is not known.

Mepivacaine hydrochloride (Carbocaine Hydrochloride)

Mepivacaine is a nonirritating potent local anesthetic similar in action to lidocaine. Its action is less rapid and slightly more prolonged than that of lidocaine. It is 80% plasma protein bound and metabolized in the liver. It can be used for infiltration, regional nerve block, caudal, and peridural anesthesia. It is not effective topically except in large doses and thus should not be used topically. It exerts its effect without the use of a vasoconstrictor, thereby eliminating the necessity to use agents such as epinephrine. Thus mepivacaine has a definite advantage over other local anesthetics for use with elderly patients or patients with cardiovascular disease, diabetes mellitus, or thyrotoxicosis. Mepivacaine may cause adverse reactions similar to those noted for lidocaine, but the drowsiness, lassitude, and amnesia observed with lidocaine do not occur. It is available in solutions of 1%, 1.5%, and 2% and in a dental cartridge 3% injection.

Prilocaine hydrochloride (Citanest Hydrochloride) Prilocaine has properties similar to lidocaine but is less toxic. It is used in infiltration, peripheral nerve blocks, central neural blocks (epidural and caudal), and for local anesthesia by nerve block or infiltration in dental procedures. It is of average lipid solubility and is 50% plasma protein bound at an anesthetic concentration equal to that of cocaine. It is liver metabolized, with an onset in 4 minutes and a duration of action of 98 minutes. After large doses (600 to 800 mg) methemoglobinemia has been reported. The methemoglobinemia is treated with and reversed by oxygen and methylene blue (1% solution, 1 to 2 mg/kg body weight) by the intravenous route over 5 minutes.

LONG DURATION OF ACTION
Bupivacaine (Marcaine)

Bupivacaine, an amide, is related chemically to mepivacaine but is four times more potent than that drug. It is highly lipid soluble, 95% protein bound in plasma, and metabolized in the liver. Onset of action is comparable to that of mepivacaine and lidocaine. Duration of anesthesia with bupivacaine is two to three times longer than that of mepivacaine or lidocaine and 20% to 30% longer than that of tetracaine. The addition of epinephrine increases its duration of action; some nerve blocks may last 12 hours or more. Its long duration of anesthesia makes it a desirable drug for nerve block peripheral, epidural, or caudal anesthesia for long surgical or obstetric procedures, relief of pain during labor, local infiltration, and sympathetic block.

Preparation and dosage. Bupivacaine is available as a 0.25%, 0.5%, and 0.75% solution for injection with or without epinephrine. Maximal single dose for adults should not exceed 175 mg without epinephrine and 225 mg with epinephrine. Dose should not be repeated at intervals of less than 3 hours, and a total dose of 400 mg/24 hours should not be exceeded.

Toxic effects. Bupivacaine may cause hypotension, tremors, fainting, bradycardia, nausea, vomiting, headache, and paresthesias. The same precautions should be followed as for other local anesthetics.

Dibucaine hydrochloride (Nupercaine Hydrochloride)

Dibucaine hydrochloride is not only one of the more potent local anesthetics but also one of the most toxic. It is 15 to 20 times more toxic and potent than procaine when injected and 10 to 15 times more potent than cocaine when applied topically. Onset of action is slow and may be delayed for 15 minutes, but its effects may last 2½ to 3 hours.

It is used to produce surface anesthesia but can be used for all types of local anesthesia and for spinal anesthesia (mixed with spinal fluid) in 1:200 solution. It can be given with epinephrine.

Preparation and dosage. Dibucaine hydrochloride is marketed in ampules and vials containing various amounts of the drug. The drug is used in concentrations of 1:1500 for hypobaric spinal anesthesia without use of spinal fluid to 1:200 for isobaric spinal anesthesia with use of spinal fluid, for injection and topical application. It is a constituent of certain creams (0.5%) and ointments (1%) used to relieve the discomfort of burns and hemorrhoids. It is also available in suppository form and 0.25% aerosol spray.

Toxic effects. Caution in its use is recommended because of its potential toxicity.

Etidocaine (Duranest)

Etidocaine is a derivative of lidocaine but is four times more potent and four times more toxic than lidocaine. The analgesia is accompanied by motor blockade. The drug is used for regional nerve blocks and epidural block anesthesia with low fetal blood levels. Onset of action occurs in 3 to 5 minutes; duration of action may be 5 to 10 hours. This prolonged action even without the use of epinephrine reduces the need for repeated injections, decreases the potential for undesirable effects, and makes the drug suitable for percutaneous infiltration. Dosage is highly variable. It is available as 0.5%, 1%, and 1.5% with or without epinephrine.

Tetracaine hydrochloride (Pontocaine Hydrochloride); amethocaine hydrochloride

Tetracaine hydrochloride is a synthetic local anesthetic with slow onset of action that is metabolized in plasma; its effects are 10 times more potent and more than twice as prolonged than those of procaine. It is highly lipid soluble and is also more toxic than procaine. Its ability to penetrate mucous membranes far exceeds that of procaine; it approaches that of cocaine.

It can be employed in dilute concentrations and serves as a useful anesthetic for a number of purposes. It can be used to produce surface anesthesia of the eye, nose, and throat, as well as for infiltration and spinal and caudal anesthesia. It is the most widely used drug for spinal anesthesia.

Preparation and dosage. Tetracaine hydrochloride is available in solutions of various concentrations. An official ophthalmic ointment, 0.5% in white petrolatum, is also available. The concentration used varies with the part to be anesthetized; a 0.5% solution is commonly employed for the eye, a 1% or 2% solution for mucous membranes of the nose and throat, 1% and 0.2% or 0.3% dextrose is used for spinal anesthesia in operations of 2 to 3 hours. It can be given with epinephrine.

Topical anesthetics

A number of local anesthetic agents cannot be injected. Because they are absorbed slowly, they can be used safely on open wounds, ulcers, and mucous surfaces. They occasionally cause dermatitis and allergic sensitization, which necessitate discontinuation of their use.

Topical anesthetics for skin disorders are used primarily to relieve pruritus, discomfort, pain, and soreness; indications for mucous membranes are similar. The anesthetics are poorly absorbed through the intact skin, but from mucous membranes and skin breaks and sores (abrasions, trauma, ulcers, etc.) absorption is increased, involving the possibility of systemic involvement. When employed in the oral cavity (mouth and pharynx), there may be interference with swallowing. The nurse should be aware of this because aspiration may occur if food is ingested within 1 hour after use of an oral topical anesthetic, particularly in children.

Cocaine; cocaine hydrochloride

Cocaine, one of the oldest local anesthetics, is the prototype of all local anesthetics. This naturally occurring alkaloid is derived from the leaves of the *Erythroxylon coca* shrub, which grows in Peru, other parts of South America, and the Far East. The native people have been known to chew the leaves to give them added energy and ability to endure fatigue. In medicine, cocaine is used chiefly in the form of cocaine hydrochloride, which occurs as a white crystalline powder that is freely soluble in water and alcohol.

Action and result. Cocaine has both local and systemic actions.

Local. Cocaine is unrivaled in its power to penetrate mucous membranes to produce surface anesthesia of the ear, nose, and throat. It is two to three times more potent than procaine. It is of average lipid solubility. Onset of action is immediate, occurring within 60 seconds; duration of action is about 1 hour. Cocaine also causes local vasoconstrictor actions. Applied to the eye it causes pupil dilation; applied to the tongue it removes the taste of bitter substances; applied to nasal mucosa it paralyzes the sense of smell. It is usually not used with epinephrine, since cocaine possesses vasoconstrictor action and shrinks mucous membranes.

Systemic. Today it is not recommended that cocaine be injected for anesthetic effects because of its toxicity. Therefore it is used topically. However, its systemic effects are of interest, since it is one of the drugs often abused. Cocaine potentiates the effects of norepinephrine (a catecholamine) by inhibiting its uptake into the sympathetic (adrenergic) nerve terminals from which it is liberated. This effect causes a higher concentration of norepinephrine and increased sympathetic stimulation. In addition, cocaine has a direct stimulant action on the central nervous system and autonomic centers in the brain.

As a result of its stimulant action, there is a feeling of euphoria, increased mental and muscular power, and increased resistance to fatigue. The individual is more talkative and active. The pulse is stronger and faster, blood pressure is elevated, respirations are faster and deeper, and vomiting may occur.

Toxic effects. Toxic doses of cocaine cause hyperexcitability and convulsions. Depression of the central and autonomic nervous systems follows stimulation.

Body temperature may increase 3° to 5° C as a result of increased muscular activity, decreased heat loss as a result of vasoconstriction, and direct action of cocaine on the temperature-regulating center. Death is usually caused by respiratory failure, but circulatory failure may also occur.

Uses. Cocaine is used chiefly for surface anesthesia of the nose and throat. Since cocaine causes opacity of the cornea and retards corneal epithelial regeneration, its use in ophthalmology has been virtually abandoned.

It is also injected in low concentrations for the removal of tonsils and similar procedures, although some authorities do not recommend its administration by injection.

Preparation and dosage. Concentrations of 1% to 4% are used for surface anesthesia of the eye (also causing mydriasis and corneal clouding), 1% to 2% for mucous membranes of vagina, rectum, ear, nose and throat, and up to 20% for mucous membranes of the nose and throat. Cocaine crystals moistened in epinephrine hydrochloride solution for placement on the nasal mucosa prior to surgical operation in the nose is considered a dangerous procedure. A 0.2% concentration is the strength usually used for injection.

Cocaine dependence. See chapter on drug abuse.

Hexylcaine hydrochloride (Cyclaine)

Hexylcaine hydrochloride is used in a concentration of 5% for topical anesthesia. For surface anesthesia it is said to be as effective as cocaine. It is *effective* for topical anesthesia of intact mucous membranes, urinary tract, upper gastrointestinal tract, and respiratory tract and for dental procedures.

Toxic effects. It exhibits toxic effects similar to other local anesthetics and must be employed with the same precautions.

Piperocaine hydrochloride (Metycaine Hydrochloride)

Piperocaine hydrochloride is chemically related to cocaine but produces effects similar to procaine. It differs from procaine in that it is suited to topical application for surface anesthesia as well as for injection. It is slightly more potent and more toxic than procaine, and effects last about the same length of time. It is compatible with epinephrine and is used for anything for which procaine can be used unless the patient is hypersensitive to the agent. It is *not* used for spinal anesthesia.

Preparation, dosage, and administration. Solutions from the 2% dosage form can be made to various concentrations for injection. The drug is used in concentrations that vary, depending on the route of administration. For example, a 0.5% to 1% solution is used for infiltration, and a 0.5% to 2% solution is used for nerve block.

Benzocaine (Americaine, Hurricaine)

Benzocaine acts as a local anesthetic when applied to painful wounds and ulcers of the skin and mucous membranes. It is widely used for relief of sunburn and pruritus. It may be applied as a dusting powder or as an ointment to denuded areas of the skin and to mucous membranes. It is used to relieve itching and discomfort associated with hemorrhoids and rectal fissures. It is also available in the form of rectal and vaginal suppositories, and as anesthetic gel lubricants (Americaine) for use with intratracheal catheters, pharyngeal and nasal airways, etc. Benzocaine is also available as 5% to 20% preparations of the drug in ointments, liquids, lotions, creams, or aerosols.

Butamben Picrate (Butesin Picrate)

This preparation is used as an anesthetic ointment (1%).

Cyclomethycaine sulfate (Surfacaine)

Cyclomethycaine sulfate is used as a topical anesthetic for certain types of skin lesions and abrasions in which discomfort is caused by pain and itching. It is also used on vaginal, urethral, and rectal mucous membranes to reduce pain from fissures and ulcerations.

Preparation and administration. Cyclomethycaine sulfate is available in preparations that include a topical cream and ointment, a urethral jelly for clinical examination or instrumentation, topical solutions, and suppositories. The concentration of the drug in various preparations varies from 0.5% cream to 1% ointment to 5% jelly. Suppositories contain 10 mg of the drug.

Dimethisoquin hydrochloride (Quotane Hydrochloride)

Dimethisoquin is a local anesthetic applied topically to the skin to relieve itching, irritation, burning, or pain of various dermatoses. It may also be used to relieve pain of sutured surgical wounds. It is available as a 0.5% ointment. Onset of action occurs in a few minutes, and duration of effect lasts from 2 to 4 hours.

Diperodon (Diothane)

Diperodon is used for surface anesthesia of the skin and mucous membranes. It is as potent as cocaine with a longer duration of action. It can be irritating, and it can cause allergic reactions. It is available as a 1% ointment.

Dyclonine hydrochloride (Dyclone)

Dyclonine is a ketone. It does not contain the esters or amides of other local anesthetics. Thus cross-sensitization with other local anesthetics does not occur, making it useful for patients hypersensitive to other agents. Its potency is like that of cocaine, and its toxicity is low. It is applied topically to the skin or mucous membranes as a 0.5% or 1% solution; it is not injected. Onset of action occurs in 10 minutes; duration of effect is 45 to 60 minutes. For anesthetizing accessible mucous membranes prior to endoscopic examination the 0.5% solution is used to block the gag reflex and relieve oral or anogenital lesion pain.

Pramoxine hydrochloride (Tronothane Hydrochloride)

Pramoxine is used primarily to relieve itching and pain of skin conditions, to anesthetize laryngopharyngeal surfaces prior to instrumentation, and to facilitate sigmoidoscopic examination. Pramoxine should not be injected or applied to the eye or nasal mucosa, since it may irritate these tissues. It is used in a 1% cream or jelly.

Reactions to local anesthetics

Local anesthetics produce vasodilation by direct action on blood vessels and by anesthetizing sympathetic vasoconstrictor fibers. This action can cause rapid absorption of the drug; when rate of absorption exceeds rate of elimination, toxic effects can occur. To decrease rate of absorption and incidence of toxic effects by allowing more time for metabolic degradation and to prolong local anesthetic effects, epinephrine or other vasoconstrictor drugs are used. Dosage of the latter drugs must be carefully determined to prevent ischemic necrosis at the injection site. Since local anesthetics are potentially toxic drugs, a patient's age, weight, physical condition, and liver function must be taken into account in determining drug dosage. Caution is advised with the use of amide anesthetics in patients with compromised livers, since the liver is the site of their metabolism.

Most reactions to local anesthetics result from overdosage, rapid absorption into systemic circulation, and individual hypersensitivity or allergic response.

Central nervous system. At first the central nervous system may be stimulated and cause anxiety, restlessness, confusion, dizziness, tremors, and even convulsions. Then depression may occur, and unconsciousness and death may ensue.

Cardiovascular system. Myocardial depression, bradycardia, and hypotension can occur because of smooth muscle relaxation and inhibition of neuromuscular conduction. The patient suddenly becomes pale, feels faint, and has a drop in blood pressure. Cardiac arrest can be the end result of a cardiovascular reaction.

Anesthetics containing a vasoconstrictor are employed with caution in patients receiving drugs that may change blood pressure, such as monoamine oxidase inhibitors, phenothiazines, and tricyclic antidepressants. The combination may produce severe hypotension or hypertension. Cardiac arrhythmias occur when catecholamine vasoconstrictors (for example, epinephrine) are used with patients receiving cyclopropane, halothane, or trichloroethylene.

Allergic reaction. True allergic reactions are said to be uncommon. Sometimes a reaction is thought to be allergic when it is really caused by overdosage. However, allergic reactions can occur. They may be relatively mild (hives, itching, skin rash) or they may be of an acute anaphylactic nature.

The allergic reactions are characteristically manifested by cutaneous lesions, urticaria, or edema. They may be due to various factors such as hypersensitivity, idiosyncrasy, or diminished tolerance. These rare hypersensitivity reactions are usually limited to the ester type of anesthetics. The most important risk of local anesthetics is a dose-related central nervous system toxicity, which may progress from sleepiness to convulsion. Patients from families that exhibit malignant hyperthermia (hyperpyrexia) should be administered only the ester type of local anesthetics because the amide-type anesthetics are known for this reaction. Skin testing for sensitivity is of doubtful value. Allergy to the derivatives of para-aminobenzoic acid derivatives have not demonstrated a cross-sensitivity to the amide type (lidocaine).

Small test doses are frequently given by the physician to gauge the extent of the patient's sensitivity to the anesthetic agent. The anesthetic agent chosen, its concentration, the rate of injection, and physical and emotional factors in the patient all influence reactions to local anesthetics.

Nursing implications for local anesthesia

Preparation of patient. Preliminary medication is frequently prescribed prior to the use of a local anesthetic, much the same as before a general anesthetic. Use of a barbiturate is believed to prevent or decrease toxic reactions.

Methods of administration of local anesthetics. Some local anesthetics are suited only for surface anesthesia, some must be injected, and some are suitable for both topical administration and injection. See Table 9-6. To minimize toxicity from local anesthetics, the smallest amount of the lowest effective concentration should be used.

Summary of nursing considerations

Anesthetics are central nervous system drugs characterized by (1) an affinity for nervous tissue and (2) reversible action (cells return to normal when drug is eliminated from the cells). *Local anesthetic agents* abolish sensation in a specific region without producing unconsciousness; *general anesthetic agents* produce loss of consciousness and, thereby, loss of sensation.

Anesthesia is produced by progressively increasing the amount of the anesthetic agent, first in the blood and subsequently in the nervous system. Inhalation anesthetics are absorbed, transported, and excreted by the body without undergoing significant chemical change. All anesthetics produce a similar pattern of irregular descending depression.

Balanced anesthesia should provide not only sleep, but also analgesia, elimination of certain reflexes, and good muscular relaxation. Factors influencing drug choice are the patient's physical condition, previous drug therapy, operative procedure to be performed, and estimated length of the operation.

An ideal general anesthetic would fulfill all the following requirements:

1 A wide safety range—considerable difference between therapeutic and toxic dosages
2 Rapid effect and not unpleasant to take
3 Rapid, comfortable recovery
4 Readily excreted without damage to body tissues
5 Maximal muscular relaxation without increased capillary bleeding
6 Potency that permits easily controlled levels of anesthesia and simultaneous oxygen administration
7 Stable and nonexplosive
8 Nonirritating and free from side effects
9 Nondepressing to the cardiovascular system
10 Compatible with catecholamines

No agent meets all these criteria, but these standards are useful in evaluating the properties of various anesthetic agents.

Preparation of the patient is important to satisfactory anesthesia. Preanesthetic medications are administered for sedative and amnesic effects, inhibition of salivary and mucous secretions, and inhibition of anticipated undesirable side effects. The time of administration is critically important, as are the patient's vital signs and mental state. Preoperative preparation by the nurse should be carefully explained to patients, as should the necessity for coughing, deep breathing, and frequent turning during the postoperative period.

The four stages of general anesthesia are analgesia, excitement, surgical anesthesia, and medullary paralysis (toxic stage). These stages are summarized in Table 9-1. The excitement stage is rarely seen, and the toxic stage should be prevented.

Methods of administering anesthetics by inhalation include the semiclosed method and the closed method. Of these two, the closed method affords best control of the anesthetic state, greater economy, and safety.

Inhalation (volatile) anesthetics have the following advantages:

1 They are complete anesthetics, abolishing superficial and deep reflexes.
2 They provide for controllable anesthesia.
3 Allergic reactions to them are uncommon.
4 Rapid recovery can occur as soon as administration ceases.

The nurse needs to monitor postoperative patients closely for signs and symptoms of drug-induced reactions to anesthesia. These include depressed cardiac function, hypotension, and cardiac arrhythmias. Common postoperative complications requiring nursing care are nausea and vomiting, hypoventilation, oliguria, atony, urinary retention, nerve injury, intestinal distention, and thrombosis.

Local anesthetics are used to eliminate pain sensation in a particular part of the body. Even relatively small doses of local anesthetics may cause serious reactions if they reach the heart or brain. Thus these agents should be confined to a small area near a nerve or among nerve endings. Most reactions result from overdosage, rapid absorption into systemic circulation, or individual hypersensitivity. These reactions can affect the central nervous system and the cardiovascular system; mild or severe anaphylactic reactions may also occur. Use of a barbiturate before administering a local anesthetic is thought to prevent or decrease toxic reactions.

Some local anesthetics are suited only for surface (topical) anesthesia and are applied in the form of a solution, ointment, cream, or powder to relieve pain and itching and to anesthetize mucous membranes of the eye, nose, throat, or urethra for minor surgical procedures.

Local anesthesia by injection is accomplished by infiltration, conduction, spinal, caudal, and saddle block. (See Table 9-6.)

QUESTIONS

FOR STUDY AND REVIEW

1 Define balanced anesthesia.
2 What are the advantages of balanced anesthesia?
3 What is the desired pharmacologic effect obtained from the administration of atropine when employed as a preoperative drug?
4 What is the difference between a volatile anesthetic and a nonvolatile anesthetic?
5 What is meant by "dissociative anesthesia"?
6 How should preoperative patients be evaluated for surgery?
7 What specific observations and precautions should be taken if an anesthetic produces catecholamine sensitivity?
8 Obtain data (for 1 or more days) on the preoperative medications given on a surgical unit. Analyze the findings.
9 Obtain data on the anesthetics used on any single day in a hospital to which you have access.
   a What anesthetics were used for which operative procedures? Why?
   b What was the length of time the anesthetic was administered?
   c Did any adverse reactions occur from the anesthesia? If yes, what action was taken?
   d What was the period of time from discontinuation of the anesthetic to patient emergence?
   e How soon after emergence did the patient require an analgesic?
   f Interpret the above findings.
10 In the elderly, what are some of the physiologic changes that must be considered in the selection of an anesthetic drug?
11 Explain the use of a vasoconstrictor with a local anesthetic.
12 What is the nurse's responsibility concerning topical anesthetics?
13 What are some important nursing care aspects for the postanesthetic patient?

BIBLIOGRAPHY

Ad Hoc Committee, American Society of Anesthesiologists: Occupational disease among operating room personnel: a national study, Anesthesiology **41:**321, 1974.

AMA drug evaluations, ed. 4, New York, 1980, John Wiley & Sons, Inc.

Anderson, W.G.: Respiratory aspects of the preoperative examination, Br. J. Anaesth. **46:**549, 1974.

Avery, G.S.: Drug treatment, ed. 2, New York and Australia, 1980, ADIS Press.

Britt, B.A.: Malignant hyperthermia, Clin. Anesth. **11:**61, 1975.

Brogden, R.N., and others: Alfathesin: a review, Drugs **8:**87, 1974.

Brown, E.B., Jr.: Drugs and respiratory control, Annu. Rev. Pharmacol. **11:**271, 1971.

Brown, E.B., Jr., and others: Mechanisms of acute hepatic toxicity: chloroform, halothane, and glutathione, Anesthesiology **41:**554, 1974.

Brown, T.C.K.: Pediatric pharmacology, Anaesth. Intensive Care **1:**473, 1973.

Brown, W.U., and others: Newborn blood levels of lidocaine and mepivacaine in the first postnatal day following maternal epidural anesthesia, Anesthesiology **42:**698, 1975.

Cascorbi, H.F.: Biotransformation of drugs used in anesthesia, Anesthesiology **39:**115, 1973.

Clarke, R.S.J., and others: Adverse reactions to intravenous anesthetics, Br. J. Anaesth. **47:**575, 1975.

Cohen, E.N.: Metabolism of volatile anesthetics, Anesthesiology **35:**193, 1971.

Cohen, E.N.: Toxicity of inhalation anesthetic agents, Br. J. Anaesth. **50:**665, 1978.

Cook, D.R.: Neonatal anesthetic pharmacology: a review, Anesth. Analg. (Cleve.) **53:**544, 1974.

Cousins, M.J., and Mazze, R.I.: Methoxyflurane nephrotoxicity: a study of dose response in man, J.A.M.A. **225:**1611, 1973.

Covino, B.G.: Local anesthesia, N. Engl. J. Med. **286:**975 (Part 1); 1035 (Part 2), 1972.

Cullen, S.C., and Larson, C.P., Jr.: Essentials of anesthetic practice, Chicago, 1974, Year Book Medical Publishers, Inc.

de Jong, R.H.: Toxic effects of local anesthetics, J.A.M.A. **239:**1166, 1978.

Diamond, B.I., and others: Differential membrane effects of general and local anesthetics, Anesthesiology **43:**651, 1975.

Dundee, J.W., Knox, J.W., and Black, G.W.: Ketamine as an induction agent in anesthetics, Lancet **1:**1370, 1970.

Dundee, J.W., and Pandit, S.K.: Anterograde amnesic effects of pethidine, hyoscine, and diazepam in adults, Br. J. Pharmacol. **44:**140, 1972.

Dundee, J.W., and others: Sensitivity to local anaesthetics, Br. Med. J. **1:**63, 1974.

Editorial: Halothane, Lancet **1:**841, 1975.

Editorial: The pulmonary toxicity of oxygen, Br. J. Anaesth. **46:**325, 1974.

Evans, D.E.: Anaesthesia and the epileptic patient, Anaesthesia **30:**34, 1975.

Evans, T.I.: The physiological basis of geriatric general anaesthesia, Anaesth. Intensive Care **1:**319, 1973.

Fleming, P.R.: Cardiological aspects of the preoperative examination, Br. J. Anaesth. **46:**555, 1974.

Foëx, P., and Prys-Roberts, C.: Anaesthesia and the hypertensive patient, Br. J. Anaesth. **46:**575, 1974.

Goldstein, A., and Keats, A.S.: The risk of anesthesia, Anesthesiology **33:**130, 1970.

Goodman, L.S., and Gilman, A.: The pharmacological basis of therapeutics, ed. 6, New York, 1980, Macmillan Publishing Co., Inc.

Goth, A.: Medical pharmacology: principles and concepts, ed. 10, St. Louis, 1981, The C.V. Mosby Co.

Grad, R.K., and Woodside, J.: Obstetrical analgesics and anesthesia, Am. J. Nurs. **77:**242, 1977.

Innovar: a followup, Med. Letter **23**(17):Aug. 21, 1981.

Kaufman, R.D.: Biophysical mechanisms of anesthetic action: historical perspectives and review of current concepts, Anesthesiology **46:**49, 1977.

McPeek, B., and Gilbert, J.P.: Onset of postoperative jaundice related to anaesthetic history, Br. Med. J. **2:**615, 1974.

Merin, R.G.: Effect of anesthetic drugs on myocardial performance in man, Annu. Rev. Med. **28:**75, 1977.

Modell, W.: Drugs of choice 1980-1981, St. Louis, 1980, The C.V. Mosby Co.

Moult, P.J.A., and Sherlock, S.: Halothane-related hepatitis, Q. J. Med. **44**(NS):99, 1975.

Ostlere, G., and Bryce-Smith, R.: Anaesthetics for medical students, ed. 7, London, 1974, Churchill-Livingstone.

Pontoppidan, H., and others: Acute respiratory failure in the adult, N. Engl. J. Med. **287:**690 (Part 1); 743 (Part 2); 799 (Part 3), 1972.

Proceedings of a symposium on local anaesthesia, Br. J. Anaesth. **47:**163, 1975.

Seeman, P.: The membrane actions of anesthetics and tranquilizers, Pharmacol. Rev. **24:**583, 1972.

Simpson, B.R., and others: Halothane and jaundice, Br. J. Hosp. Med. **13:**433, 1975.

Smith, B.J.: After anesthesia, Nursing 1974 **4:**28, 1974.

Stanton-Hicks, M., and others: Effects of peridural block: properties, circulatory effects, and blood levels of etidocaine and lidocaine, Anesthesiology **42:**398, 1975.

Steen, P.A., Tinker, J., and Tarhens, S.: Myocardial reinfarction after anesthesia and surgery, J.A.M.A. **239:**2566, 1978.

Tweed, W.A., Mimick, M., and Mymin, D.: Circulatory responses to ketamine anesthesia, Anesthesiology **37:**613, 1972.

Waud, B.E., and Waud, D.R.: The effects of diethyl ether, enflurane, and isoflurane at the neuromuscular junction, Anesthesiology **42:**275, 1975.

Wright, R., and others: Controlled prospective study of the effect on liver function of multiple exposures to halothane, Lancet **1:**817, 1975.

CHAPTER 10

Skeletal muscle relaxants and agents used in myasthenia gravis and Parkinson's disease

Neuromuscular junction

Skeletal muscles are striated or striped muscles attached to the skeleton that are usually under voluntary control. These muscles function to produce body movements, maintain body position against the force of gravity, and counteract environmental stresses such as wind. A muscle is composed of numerous muscle cells or muscle fibers. Each muscle cell is connected to only one motor nerve fiber, but each of the nerve fibers is connected to several muscle cells. Therefore stimulation of one nerve fiber will cause stimulation and activation of a group of muscle cells.

Motor nerves originate in the anterior horn cells in the gray matter of the spinal cord. Each anterior horn cell has a single axon that leaves the horn cell by way of the spinal nerve root. When this axon, or motor neuron, reaches the muscle it innervates, it branches to innervate a group of muscle fibers. The motor neuron and all the muscle fibers innervated by the same anterior horn cell constitute a motor unit. A particular muscle may contain thousands of these units. When the motor nerve is stimulated, every muscle fiber in the motor unit contracts. Individual fibers do not react on their own unless the motor nerve is nonfunctional; then individual fibers may twitch and cause *fasciculation.*

Muscle cells or fibers are long and thin with cross striations (Fig. 10-1). When nerve impulses pass along motor nerves, the muscle fibers shorten and the muscle contracts; in the absence of nerve impulses the muscle relaxes. This relaxed, or weak, state is called flaccid paralysis.

The region where a motor nerve fiber makes functional contact with a skeletal muscle fiber (synaptic contact) is known as the neuromuscular junction (Fig. 10-2). The end-plate of the muscle cell is chemically excitable; the rest of the muscle fiber is not but is electrically excitable. Acetylcholine (ACh) is the neurohormonal

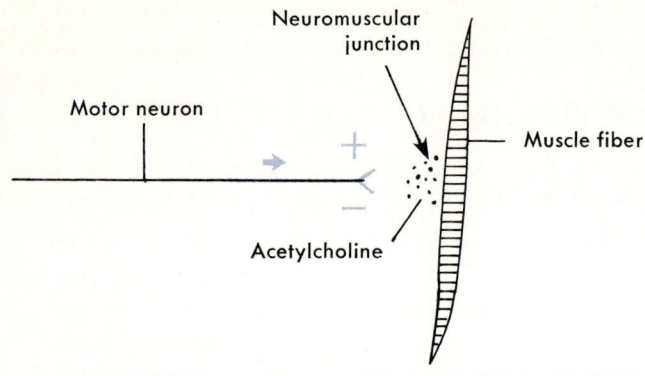

FIG. 10-1. Striated muscle fiber with a single excitatory nerve supply.

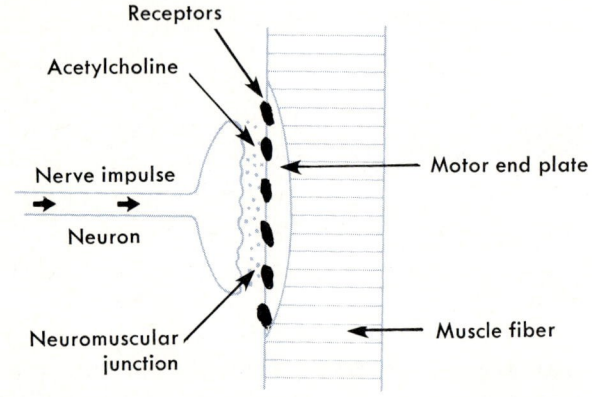

FIG. 10-2. Neuromuscular junction where the motor nerve makes functional contact with a muscle fiber. Acetylcholine bridges the gap between the neuron and muscle fiber until it is destroyed or hydrolyzed.

transmitter that chemically excites the muscle fibers. ACh is formed in the motor nerve cell or in the axon of the motor nerve and stored in vesicles in the motor nerve. Depolarization of the presynaptic membrane is followed by release of ACh, which is taken up by receptors on the motor end-plate of the muscle fiber. ACh alters the membrane permeability of the motor end-plate, allowing sodium to diffuse, thereby producing a change in voltage known as an end-plate potential. Depolarization spreads from the motor end-plate to the whole of the muscle fiber, a propagated action potential; calcium ions are released, and the muscle contracts. ACh is destroyed shortly after its release by the enzyme cholinesterase, enabling the next nerve impulse to be effective (Fig. 10-3).

SKELETAL MUSCLE HYPERACTIVITY

Skeletal muscle hyperactivity is characterized by skeletal muscle *spasticity* or *spasm*. Skeletal muscle spasticity happens when gamma motor neurons, which tonically control muscle spindle contractile activity, become hyperactive. There are two primary types of muscle spasticity, spinal and cerebral. Spinal spasticity can be identified by a marked loss of inhibitory influences with hyperactive tendon stretch reflexes, hyperactive stretch reflexes, clonus, primitive flexion withdrawal reflexes, and a flexed posture. Varying degrees of spasticity of the bladder and bowel can also be seen.

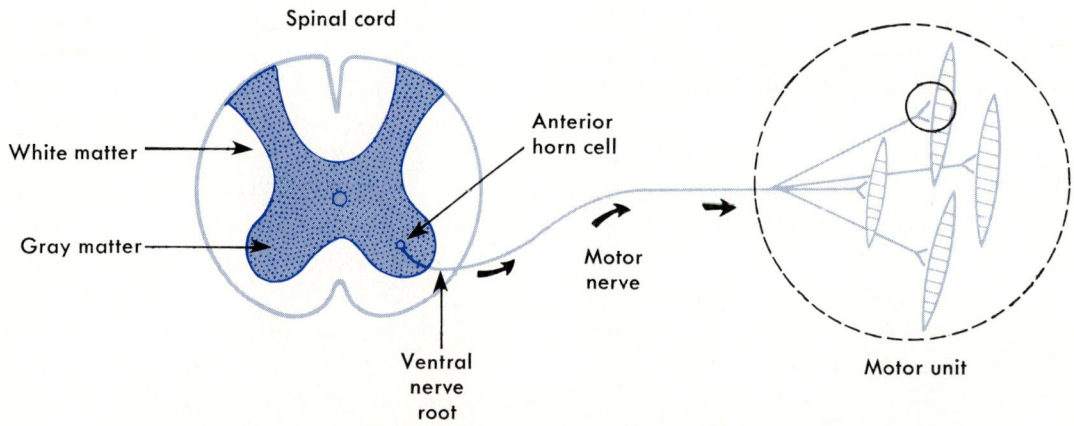

FIG. 10-3. Anterior cell and motor unit. Motor nerves originate in anterior horn cells and leave via the ventral or spinal nerve root. When the axon of the nerve reaches the muscle supplied, it branches to supply a group of striated muscle fibers. The motor nerve and all the muscle fibers supplied by the same anterior horn cell are a motor unit. The circle within the motor unit illustrates the neuromuscular junction, which is enlarged in Fig. 10-2.

Cerebral spasticity has less reflex excitability, increased muscle tone, and no primitive flexion withdrawal reflexes or flexed posture. Dystonia may also be present in such patients.

Muscle spasticity is most commonly seen in patients with central nervous system injuries and strokes. Moderate to severe spasticity can be seen in two thirds of patients with multiple sclerosis. Patients with cerebral palsy and rare neurologic disorders can also have muscle spasticity, but it is seen less frequently in these patients.

Centrally and direct acting skeletal muscle relaxants are the drugs of choice in the treatment of muscle spasticity. These drugs include baclofen, diazepam, and dantrolene sodium. They are more effective in the treatment of spinal spasticity than cerebral spasticity. However, optimal therapy cannot be achieved in the treatment of either unless physical therapy is given concurrently.

Skeletal muscle spasms result when there is an involuntary contraction of a muscle or group of muscles that is accompanied by pain or limited function. Most are caused by local injuries, but some may be due to low calcium levels or epileptic myoclonic spasms. Each type of spasm is treated according to its etiology.

Skeletal muscle injuries are usually self-limiting and can be treated with rest; physical therapy; immobility such as that brought about by casts, neck collars, crutches, or arm slings; or whirlpool baths without the use of skeletal muscle relaxants. With tissue damage and edema, antiinflammatory drugs may be used, however.

Central skeletal muscle relaxants are used primarily for conditions in which muscles spasms are not readily responsive to other measures of therapy, such as musculoskeletal strains and sprains, trauma, and cervical or lumbar radiculopathy as a result of degenerative osteoarthritis, herniated disc, spondylolysis, or laminectomy. The centrally acting drug, baclofen, which is used for skeletal muscle spasticity, has not been found useful in the treatment of muscle spasms, as has diazepam. All centrally acting skeletal muscle relaxants except diazepam are more effective when given parenterally than orally.

Skeletal muscle relaxants
Centrally acting skeletal muscle relaxants

Action and uses. The most beneficial results from the administration of centrally acting skeletal muscle relaxants seem to be associated with their ability to relieve acute muscle spasm of local origin. They are used as adjuncts to rest and physiotherapy in the treatment of sprains, strains, or trauma to ligaments. They often accompany the administration of other drugs (salicylates, adrenal coricosteroids) in the treatment of myositis, fibrositis, spondylitis, bursitis, and arthritis. These agents have been used effectively to lessen motor activity in certain neurologic disorders (e.g., cerebral palsy) and in other dyskinesias characterized by abnormal reflex activity, increased muscle tonus, involuntary movements, and incoordination. Many physicians believe that benefits from their administration come from the sedative effects produced rather than from actual muscle relaxation.

The exact mechanism of action of the central skeletal muscle relaxants is not known at present. Action may result from general central nervous system depression. The drugs do not seem to affect muscles, myoneural junctions, monosynaptic pathways, or motor nerves. However, they do affect the central pathways and neuronal systems that control tone and movement of muscles. These drugs are known to produce relaxation of striated muscle spasm by depression of the central nervous system (brainstem, thalamus, and basal ganglia). Skeletal muscle relaxants exert a selective action on internuncial neurons of the spinal cord, thereby reducing polysynaptic spinal and supraspinal reflex pathways.

Central skeletal muscle relaxants most commonly used are diazepam, baclofen, carisoprodol, chlorphenesin carbamate, chlorzoxazone, cyclobenzaprine, metaxalone, methocarbamol, and orphenadrine.

Side effects and precautions. Usually the side effects associated with the centrally acting skeletal muscle relaxants have been mild and transient. Mild symptoms such as drowsiness, dizziness, blurred vision, light-headedness, headache, feelings of weakness, lassitude, and lethargy occur during initial phases of drug therapy. Physicians and nursing personnel should caution patients taking these agents to avoid activities that require mental alertness, judgment, and physical coordination—such as operating dangerous machinery or driving an automobile. After a sufficient time, when it is known that the drug no longer causes drowsiness or vertigo, these activities are possible. Large oral dosages have caused nausea, vomiting, heartburn, abdominal distress, constipation, and diarrhea. With the occurrence of other signs or symptoms of drug incompatibility, administration of these agents should be discontinued. Some of the centrally acting skeletal muscle relaxants (chlorzoxazone and metaxalone) have been reported to cause jaundice. Periodic liver function tests and blood counts are recommended to avoid complications. This group of muscle relaxants is contraindicated in patients with myasthenia gravis or muscular dystrophy, since their effects may reduce the strength of remaining active muscle fibers and produce further impairment and/or debilitation. Patients with a history of liver disease should not be given these drugs because of their metabolism in the liver, and the therapeutic effect should be weighed against the possible side effects in their administration during pregnancy.

Since most of these drugs were introduced between 1938 and 1962, they have been subjected to evaluation by the National Academy of Sciences–National Research Council panel. Many of the drugs in this category received an *ineffective* rating for claims relating to organic diseases of the nervous system, and a rating of *possibly effective* for other claims. These drugs will probably be acceptable for the treatment of muscle spasticity of brief duration such as in bursitis, myositis, and fibrositis. The FDA disapproves of prolonged administration of these drugs and discourages their use for periods longer than 3 weeks. This is a precautionary stand taken because fatalities had occurred after prolonged use of one of these drugs (zoxazolamine), which is no longer available. The usefulness of these drugs appears to be the result of their sedative effect and ability to relieve anxiety.

Baclofen (Lioresal)

Baclofen is useful in alleviating spasticity resulting from multiple sclerosis, mainly for the flexor spasms with concomitant pain, clonus, and muscular rigidity. Baclofen may be of some value in spinal cord injuries and diseases and cerebrovascular lesions. It is not indicated in skeletal muscle spasm from rheumatic disorders, stroke, cerebral palsy, and Parkinson's disease.

Baclofen is analogous to the putative inhibitory neurotransmitter gamma-aminobutyric acid (GABA). Baclofen may act at a spinal level, where it has an inhibitory effect on monosynaptic and polysynaptic transmission. The drug is rapidly and extensively absorbed and eliminated. Absorption may be dose dependent (absorption decreases with increase in dosage). Peak serum levels occur in about 2 hours, half-life is 3 to 4 hours, biotransformation is not extensive, three fourths of the drug is excreted by the kidney in unchanged form (therefore reduced doses are necessary in impaired renal function), large individual variation in absorption and elimination exists, and about 30% is protein bound.

Side effects and precautions. The nurse should be aware that hallucinations occur with the abrupt withdrawal (discontinued use) of this drug; thus gradually reduced dosages are required. In pregnant women the drug is used only when the benefits to the mother outweigh potential risks to the fetus. Alcohol and other CNS depressants cause additive CNS depressant effects. In epilepsy there is a deterioration in seizure control.

The most common adverse effects are transient drowsiness (10% to 63%), dizziness (5% to 15%), weakness (5% to 15%), fatigue (2% to 4%), confusion (1% to 11%), headache (4% to 8%), insomnia (2% to 7%), hypotension (up to 9%), nausea (4% to 12%), constipation (2% to 6%), and urinary frequency (2% to 6%). The nurse should strongly remind the patient to anticipate the vivid and colorful hallucinations experienced on abrupt withdrawal of this drug.

Preparation and dosage. The dosage is 5 mg three times daily, increased by 5 mg three times daily every 3 days, not to exceed a maximum of 80 mg (20 mg four times daily). Optimal effect is usually at 40 to 80 mg daily. The drug is available in 10- and 20-mg tablets.

Diazepam (Valium)

The use of this benzodiazepine (see Chapter 11) is described here because of its adjunctive use in relief of skeletal muscle spasm caused by reflex spasm to a local pathologic condition (inflammation of muscle and joints or secondary to trauma) and spasticity caused by upper motor neuron disorders (cerebral palsy and paraplegia), athetosis, and the stiff-man syndrome (to overcome the widespread chronic muscular rigidity, pain, and skeletal muscle spasm).

Dosage. As an adjunct in skeletal muscle spasm the dose is 2 to 10 mg three to four times daily. In the geriatric or debilitated patient the initial dose is reduced to 2 to 2.5 mg one or two times daily and is increased as needed and tolerated on an individual basis. For muscle spasm in adults the parenteral dose is 5 to 10 mg deep intramuscularly or slow intravenously initially, then 5 to 10 mg in 3 to 4 hours if necessary. (Spasms caused by tetanus may require larger doses.)

Action. The major muscle relaxant actions of benzodiazepines occur in the central nervous system, relieving spasticity by suppression of activity in spinal and intraneuronal pathways. Two sites have been suggested. The first site is the spinal level, where gamma-aminobutyric acid–mediated presynaptic activity is enhanced. The second is neurons at supraspinal sites, which may be in the brainstem or descending lateral reticular facilitatory system. Diazepam additionally has an action at the neuromuscular synapse, which may involve direct muscle depression.

Carisoprodol (Rela, Soma)

Carisoprodol is related to meprobamate and has approximately the same actions and limited degree of effectiveness as other centrally acting skeletal muscle relaxants. Its muscle relaxant action is eight times greater than that of mephenesin.

Preparation, dosage, and administration. Carisoprodol is administered orally in tablets of 350 mg. The average daily adult dose is 350 mg given four times a day with the last dose at bedtime. Onset of action occurs in 30 minutes, and duration of action is about 4 to 6 hours.

Side effects. On rare occasions the initial dose has caused an idiosyncratic reaction that includes transient quadriplegia, ataxia, extreme weakness, diplopia, loss of vision, agitation, and confusion. These symptoms usually subside in a few hours. The patient should receive supportive and symptomatic therapy during this frightening experience. Drowsiness, which may occur with high dosages, indicates a need for dosage reduction.

To avoid excess accumulation, caution should be used in patients with compromised liver or kidney function. The patient taking carisoprodol should be told by the nurse to avoid other CNS depressants, including alcohol and psychotropic drugs, because an additive, dose-related, CNS depressant effect will occur. The drug may be administered with food or meals if a gastrointestinal upset occurs. If dizziness caused by postural hypotension is evident, the patient should avoid sudden changes in posture and climbing stairs.

Chlorphenesin carbamate (Maolate)

Chlorphenesin carbamate is chemically and pharmacologically related to mephenesin and produces similar actions and side effects. It is used to treat muscle spasms caused by sprains, strains, and trauma to tendons and ligaments. It is not effective for the treatment of spastic disorders involving the central nervous system.

Preparation, dosage, and administration. Chlorphenesin carbamate is administered orally initially as 800 mg three times daily. The average daily maintenance dose for adults is 400 mg four times daily or less.

Chorphenesin is rapidly absorbed from the gastrointestinal tract, with a maximal serum concentration in 1 to 3 hours and a biologic half-life of 3.5 ± 0.2 hours. It is rapidly excreted in the urine in three metabolites.

Side effects and precautions. The most frequently encountered side effects are drowsiness and dizziness. Other side effects include hematopoietic reactions, gastrointestinal disturbances, headache, insomnia, and weakness. Side effects generally will subside if dosage is reduced or stopped. Allergic phenomena, hypersensitivity, anaphylactic reactions, and drug fever are indications to discontinue this drug. Patients taking chlorphenesin should not engage in hazardous activities or those requiring keen mental alertness or muscle coordination until it is known that the drug is not causing drowsiness.

Chlorphenesin should be used with caution or not at all in patients with renal or liver damage. Duration of therapy should not exceed 8 weeks.

Chlorzoxazone (Paraflex)

The actions and effects of chlorzoxazone are similar to those of the other centrally acting skeletal muscle relaxants.

Preparation, dosage, and administration. Chlorzoxazone is administered orally in tablets of 250 mg. The average adult daily dose is 250 to 750 mg three to four times a day. Peak action occurs within 2 to 3 hours; duration of action is about 6 hours. Dose for children is 20 mg/kg body weight daily divided into three or four doses.

The tablets may be crushed and mixed with food or other suitable vehicle. Blood levels are detected in the first hour after administration and peak in the third or fourth hour; chlorzoxazone is rapidly metabolized in the liver and excreted in the urine.

Side effects and precautions. Adverse reactions include nausea, vomiting, diarrhea, abdominal distress, drowsiness, vertigo, and headache. A few cases of jaundice have been reported, and chlorzoxazone should not be given to patients with a history of liver disease. It is chemically related to zoxazolamine, which was withdrawn from the market following fatalities resulting from drug-induced liver damage. Patients taking chlorzoxazone should be observed closely for signs of liver damage.

If a sensitivity reaction such as urticaria, redness, or itching of the skin occurs, chlorzoxazone should be discontinued. This drug may discolor the urine to orange or purple red. The nurse needs to alert the patient to the possibility of such a color change.

Cyclobenzaprine hydrochloride (Flexeril)

Cyclobenzaprine is a tricyclic amine derivative indicated for short-term (up to 2 or 3 weeks) treatment of skeletal muscle spasm of local origin associated with acute painful musculoskeletal conditions. Relief of muscle spasm is not effective in treatment of spasticity associated with cerebral or spinal cord disease or in children with cerebral palsy. There is no interference with muscle function, and the drug acts within the central nervous system at the brainstem, not spinal cord, level. Evidence indicates that a net effect is a decrease in tonic somatic motor activity, influencing the gamma and alpha motor systems. Effects are similar to those seen with the tricyclic antidepressants (reserpine antagonism, potentiation of norepinephrine, peripheral and central anticholinergic effects, sedation, and increase in heart rate).

Cyclobenzaprine is highly protein bound (93%) to plasma proteins and is absorbed well after oral administration (with individual variation in plasma levels). It is extensively metabolized, primarily to glucuronide-like conjugates, and because of the first-pass effect through the liver and/or gut wall, about half the drug reaches systemic circulation. Its slow elimination through the kidneys results in a half-life ranging from 1 to 3 days.

Side effects and precautions. The contraindications and drug interactions are similar to those seen with the tricyclic antidepressants (for example, imipramine and amitriptyline): interaction with monoamine oxidase inhibitors (circulatory collapse, hypertensive crisis, fever convulsions, coma); enhancement of alcohol, barbiturates, and CNS depressants; and atropine-like action. Cyclobenzaprine is used cautiously in patients taking anticholinergic-like medications. It blocks the antihypertensive action of guanethidine and similarly acting compounds. It is contraindicated in the acute recovery phase of myocardial infarction (prolongs conduction time) and in patients with arrhythmias, heart block, conduction disturbances, stroke, congestive heart failure, or hyperthyroidism. Use for more than 2 to 3 weeks is not recommended because impairment of mental and/or physical abilities may result. Because of its atropine-like effect, it is used with caution in patients with urinary retention, narrow-angle closure glaucoma, or increased intraocular pressure.

Adverse reactions most frequently seen are drowsiness (40%), dry mouth (28%), and dizziness (11%). Many other adverse effects occur less frequently and exhibit similarity to those caused by tricyclic antidepressants. During the short duration of therapy the nurse should warn the patient of the possible drowsiness, dizziness, dry mouth, blurred vision, impairment of mental and physical abilities, and additive effects of alcohol and CNS depressants.

Preparation and dosage. The usual adult dosage is 10 mg administered three times daily with a range of 20 to 40 mg daily in divided doses, not to exceed 60 mg/24 hours and not for more than 2 to 3 weeks. Flexeril is available in 10-mg pentagonal (five-sided) tablets.

Metaxalone (Skelaxin)

Metaxalone blocks neural transmission through polysynaptic pathways in the spinal cord. There is some evidence that metaxalone is effective in reducing neurogenic spasticity. However, because its side effects are numerous and serious, its potential toxicity may outweigh potential benefits of therapy.

Preparation and dosage. Metaxalone is available in 400-mg tablets. The dose for adults and children over 12 years is 800 mg three or four times daily.

Side effects and precautions. Nausea and gastrointestinal disturbances are the most common side effects. Metaxalone has caused leukopenia, skin rash, jaundice, hemoglobin depression, and liver damage. (Thus several liver function studies are required when it is used.) It is not recommended for pregnant patients, epileptics, or those with kidney or liver disease. Metaxalone should not be administered for more than 10 days. The nurse should caution the patient to notify the prescriber if skin rash or yellowish discoloration of skin or eyes occurs (signs of liver-related jaundice).

Methocarbamol (Robaxin, others)

Methocarbamol is chemically related to mephenesin carbamate and has similar actions and effectiveness. Methocarbamol has a longer duration of action than mephenesin.

Methocarbamol may have a beneficial effect in controlling the neuromuscular manifestations of tetanus. Its use does not replace the usual procedure of debridement, tetanus antitoxin, penicillin, tracheotomy, attention to fluid balance, and supportive care.

Preparation, dosage, and administration. Routes of administration of methocarbamol are oral, intramuscular, and intravenous. Initial daily dose for adults is 1.5 g given four times a day for 2 or 3 days; 1 g four times a day may be given as a maintenance dose. When given intramuscularly, the dosage should not exceed 500 mg. Intramuscular injection should be given in divided doses in each buttock (gluteal region) at 8-hour intervals. Oral administration should be initiated as soon as possible. Intravenous solutions are highly irritating (hypertonic) and should be injected slowly at no more than 3 ml/minute. Infusions with normal saline or 5% dextrose may be prepared from one vial diluted to a maximum of 250 ml. The patient is left in the recumbent position for 10 to 15 minutes after infusion, with care taken to avoid vascular extravasation. Average dose per injection is 1 to 3 g and should not exceed 3 g daily for 3 consecutive days (except in treatment of tetanus). Solutions are available for injection in 100 mg/ml with polyethylene glycol in 10-ml containers. Tablets are available in 500- and 750-mg strengths. The tablets may be crushed and suspended in water or saline for administration via a nasogastric tube.

Side effects and precautions. Side effects from oral administration are similar to those of other centrally acting muscle relaxants. Side effects from parenteral administration include metallic taste, thrombophlebitis (from vascular extravasation), urticaria, sloughing at site of injection, anaphylactic reactions, and convulsions.

Methocarbamol is not recommended for pregnant women, children under 12 years of age, or epileptics. Parenteral administration is contraindicated in patients with renal disease, since the polyethylene glycol 300 vehicle has the potential of being nephrotoxic (i.e., it may increase preexisting acidosis and urea retention in patients with renal impairment). Patients' urine may darken on standing.

Among the adverse reactions (some of which result from overly rapid rate of injection) of the parenteral route, syncope is reported. In most cases of syncope, recovery is hastened with epinephrine, injectable steroids, and/or injectable antihistamines, which should be available in cases of too rapid injection rates. A case is reported of methocarbamol impairing the effect of pyridostigmine in a patient with myasthenia gravis. This is consistent with the anticholinergic action of methocarbamol. The nurse should advise the patient to notify the prescriber if skin rash, itching, fever, or nasal congestion occurs—all are adverse reactions to this drug.

Orphenadrine citrate (Norflex)

Orphenadrine citrate is an analog of diphenhydramine with more anticholinergic activity and less antihistaminic activity. It is used in the management of muscle spasm and supportive treatment of Parkinson's disease. Most benefit is received by relaxation of muscle stiffness and increase in muscle strength. This citrate form (the hydrochloride form is discussed in the section on Parkinson's disease) is a slow-release form and may be combined with analgesics (such as aspirin). It is metabolized in the liver and excreted in the urine and feces. Urinary excretion of this basic drug depends on the pH and flow of the urine.

It is contraindicated in glaucoma, pyloric or duodenal obstruction, prostate problems, obstruction of the bladder neck, cardiospasm (megaesophagus), and myasthenia gravis.

Preparation and dosage. The normal oral dosage is 100 mg every 12 hours. Injection dosage (intramuscular or intravenous) is 60 mg every 12 hours. The drug is available in 100-mg tablets and injection concentration of 30 mg/ml.

Side effects and precautions. The adverse effects are mainly from the anticholinergic action and are seen more frequently with higher doses. Evidence of a possible interaction between this drug and propoxyphene, producing confusion, anxiety, and tremors, is not clinically significant and no longer considered meaningful. Orphenadrine is used with caution in patients with cardiac decompensation, coronary insufficiency, cardiac arrhythmias, or tachycardia.

Dry mouth, drowsiness, dizziness, and blurred vision or fainting are observed side effects. These side effects as well as the potential for urinary retention, constipation, headache, gastrointestinal upset, nervousness and trembling, skin rash, mental confusion, rapid heart rate, and palpitations should be discussed with the patient by the nurse.

Direct acting skeletal muscle relaxant

Dantrolene (Dantrium)

Dantrolene in oral form produces skeletal muscle relaxation by acting directly on skeletal muscles. It probably acts by inhibiting the release of calcium from the sarcoplasmic reticulum to the myoplasm, resulting in decreased muscle response to the action potential and decreased muscle contraction. Muscle fiber cells contain a systematic network of sacs and tubules, which are the sarcoplasmic reticulum. Nerve impulses arriving at muscle fibers trigger release of calcium. When calcium is released from these sacs, the muscle contraction begins. When calcium withdraws back into the sacs, muscle contraction stops and muscle relaxation begins. Dantrolene has no apparent effect on peripheral nerve conduction or neuromuscular transmission. Central nervous system side effects may be caused indirectly by the decreased skeletal muscle activity. Clinical studies show that dantrolene produces generalized mild weakness of skeletal muscles and decreases the force of reflex muscle contractions, hyperreflexia, clonus, muscle stiffness, spasticity, and involuntary movements.

Dantrolene has serious potential for hepatotoxicity. Symptomatic hepatitis (fatal and nonfatal) is reported, and the incidence in patients needing 400 mg daily is less than those needing 800 mg or more per day, including short courses of therapy. Liver dysfunction or overt hepatitis are observed between the third and twelfth month of therapy. The risk of hepatic injury appears to be greater in females, in patients over 35 years of age, and in patients taking other medication in addition to dantrolene, such as estrogens or tranquilizing agents. Estrogen therapy may enhance the hepatotoxicity, particularly in women over 35 years of age. CNS depressants enhance the muscle relaxation property. This drug demands careful monitoring of hepatic function, including frequent evaluations of SGOT or SGPT, with available baseline determination for comparison with future test results.

Absorption of dantrolene after oral administration is slow and incomplete, about 35% of the drug being absorbed from the gastrointestinal tract. Biologic half-life after intravenous administration of the drug is about 5 hours. Biologic half-life in adults averages about 8.7 hours after a single 100-mg oral dose; in children the half-life averages about 7.3 hours. Dantrolene is excreted mainly in the urine. Dantrolene is metabolized in the liver by hepatic microsomal enzymes, and enhancement of metabolism by other drugs is possible. Binding to plasma protein (albumin) is reduced by warfarin and clofibrate but increased with tolbutamide.

Preparation and dosage. Dantrolene is available in 25-, 50-, and 100-mg capsules for oral administration and powder for intravenous injection as 20 mg/70 ml vials.

Recommended oral dosage for adults is 25 mg daily initially, which may be increased to 25 mg two to four times daily at 4- to 7-day intervals, and then by 25-mg increments up to 100 mg two to four times daily. Most patients respond to 400 mg or less daily.

Oral dosage for children is initially 0.5 mg/kg body weight twice daily, which is gradually increased to 0.5 mg/kg of body weight three or four times daily, and up to 3 mg/kg two to four times daily if necessary. Dosages greater then 100 mg four times daily should not be given to children.

For the treatment of malignant hyperthermia the initial intravenous adult and child's dose of 1 mg/kg is administered rapidly. This dose may be repeated (up to a cumulative dose of 10 mg/kg) if the metabolic and physiologic abnormalities reappear or persist. Reversal of these abnormalities may be achieved with an average cumulative dose of 2.5 mg/kg. An oral dosage of 1 to 2 mg/kg four times daily for 1 to 3 days may prevent recurrence of the manifestations of malignant hyperthermia. In the preparation of this solution only Sterile Water for Injection, U.S.P. (60 ml), without a bacterio-static agent should be used. The nurse should shake the solution until it is clear, protect it from direct light and from temperatures above 86° F (30° C) and below 59° F (15° C), and use it within 6 hours.

Uses. Dantrolene in oral form is used for the symptomatic treatment of clinical skeletal muscle spasm resulting from upper motor neuron disorders such as multiple sclerosis, spinal cord injury, cerebral palsy, and stroke. It is not indicated for the treatment of muscle spasms caused by rheumatic disorders. It benefits patients whose functional rehabilitation is retarded by spasticity.

A therapeutic trial is necessary to determine whether or not a patient will benefit from the drug. Tolerance to dantrolene apparently does not occur. The safety of long-term treatment with dantrolene has not been established, but its use is considered justifiable if the drug produces a significant reduction in painful and/or disabling spasticity such as clonus, if it reduces the intensity of nursing care required, or if it relieves the patient of subjective annoying manifestations of muscle spasms. The potential for liver toxicity in long-term use dictates discontinuance of the drug if no benefit is evident in 45 days.

The intravenous form is indicated for use in malignant hyperthermia along with appropriate supportive measures (discontinuance of the triggering agent [anesthetic agents], attention to increasing oxygen needs of the patient, metabolic acidosis management, cooling of the patient, measurement of urinary output, and fluid and electrolyte management in the management of fulminant hypermetabolism of skeletal muscle characteristic of malignant hyperthermia crisis). Dantrolene is administered as soon as the malignant hyperthermia reaction is evident (tachycardia, tachypnea, central venous desaturation, hypercapnia, metabolic acidosis, skeletal muscle rigidity, increased use of anesthesia circuit carbon dioxide absorber, cyanosis, mottling of the skin, and, in many instances, fever.

Side effects and toxic effects. Aside from the important hepatotoxic potential (fatal and nonfatal hepatitis), the common side effects from dantrolene therapy (not seen in short-term intravenous therapy for malignant hyperthermia) include muscle weakness, drowsiness, malaise, nausea, dizziness, diarrhea, and lightheadedness. These side effects are usually transient, occur early in treatment, and may be prevented by initiating therapy with a low dose and increasing it by gradual increments until the desired therapeutic effect is obtained. Side effects are usually related to the rate of increase in dosage, total daily dose, and duration of therapy. If the diarrhea or weakness is severe, the dosage should be decreased or even discontinued. If diarrhea recurs after dantrolene therapy is restarted, the drug should probably be discontinued permanently. Other side effects include anorexia, constipation, gastric irritation, gastrointestinal bleeding, and hepatitis.

Neurologic side effects include difficulty in swallowing, speech and visual disturbances, alteration of taste, mental depression, confusion, increased nervousness, and insomnia.

Urogenital side effects include urinary frequency, incontinence, nocturia, difficult urination, urinary retention, orange-red urine, crystalluria, and difficulty in attaining erection.

Additional side effects include tachycardia, erratic blood pressure, phlebitis, abnormal hair growth, dermatitis, backache, excessive tearing, chills and fever, and a feeling of suffocation. Alterations in laboratory tests have also been reported and include increased or decreased white blood cell count, increased serum bilirubin level, decreased serum phosphate level, and proteinuria.

Precautions. Caution should be exercised when dantrolene is given to patients with impaired pulmonary function, impaired myocardial function, or liver disease. Hepatic function monitoring (frequent tests for SGOT or SGPT, alkaline phosphate, and total bilirubin levels) is necessary because of the hepatotoxic potential. These tests also should be done prior to initiation of therapy for baseline determination and to rule out existing liver disease. Dantrolene's safe use in pregnancy or in children younger than 5 years of age has not been determined; it should not be given to nursing mothers. Its possible carcinogenic potential has not been established. Hepatotoxicity has occurred

in women over 35 years of age who received concomitant estrogen therapy.

The nurse should caution patients undergoing dantrolene therapy about engaging in activities requiring alertness and skill, such as operating hazardous equipment, particularly if central nervous system depression occurs. All alcohol and CNS depressants should be avoided. Since drug-induced photosensitivity may occur, patients taking dantrolene should refrain from excessive or unnecessary exposure to sunlight. The prescribing physician should be notified if any of the following symptoms occur: skin rash, itching, tarry stools, yellowing of skin or eyes. Dantrolene should be used with caution in patients taking tranquilizers because it may cause weakness, malaise, fatigue, nausea, and diarrhea.

Contraindications. Dantrolene is contraindicated for patients with active hepatic disease (acute hepatitis and active cirrhosis) and for patients whose spasticity is used to obtain or maintain upright posture, balance, or increased body function.

Neuromuscular blocking agents (adjuncts to anesthesia)

Neuromuscular blocking agents are important muscle relaxants. These drugs can be classified as (1) *nondepolarizing*, or *competitive, neuromuscular blocking agents* (they may also be referred to as *stabilizing agents*) (for example, curare, tubocurarine chloride, metocurine, gallamine triethiodide, and pancuronium bromide) and (2) *depolarizing blocking agents* (for example, decamethonium bromide and succinylcholine chloride).

These drugs are used to (1) produce adequate muscle relaxation during anesthesia and reduce excessive use of general anesthetics, (2) facilitate endotracheal intubation and prevent laryngospasm, (3) aid in the management of tetanus, and (4) decrease muscular activity in electroshock therapy. They do not affect pain or other sensory perception. Nondepolarizing agents are preferred in long procedures, and depolarizing agents in brief procedures.

Neuromuscular blocking agents are usually given intravenously but may be given intramuscularly. The intravenous route is preferred, since onset of action is faster and more predictable than with the intramuscular route. All neuromuscular blocking drugs are poorly absorbed from the gastrointestinal tract.

Side effects shared by all neuromuscular blocking agents are (1) interference with respiratory function, even progressing to respiratory paralysis, (2) residual muscle weakness, and (3) hypersensitivity reactions. Many, but not all, neuromuscular blocking agents can cause hypotension, bronchospasm, and cardiac disturbances. The hypotension is believed to be caused by sympathetic ganglionic blockade and histamine release, both of which cause peripheral vasodilation. Bronchospasm is probably caused by the histamine release.

Since these are potent drugs, not without danger, it is recommended that they be used only by persons thoroughly familiar with their effects and under conditions where the patient can receive constant, close attention for signs of respiratory embarassment. Adequate equipment for artificial respiration, antidotes, and other measures for prompt treatment of toxicity must be readily available.

In addition, there are centrally acting muscle relaxants that exert their effects by action on the central nervous system, thereby decreasing voluntary muscle hyperactivity. These drugs exert a selective action on internuncial neurons of the spinal cord and reduce multisynaptic but not monosynaptic spinal reflexes. Actually, these drugs can be classified as sedatives. In large doses these drugs may cause depression similar to that of the sedative-hypnotics.

Muscle spasm is a symptom associated with many conditions and is the result of several processes. These processes include injury to the muscle itself, presence of an inflammatory process of the tissues around the muscle that precipitates muscular contraction, and damage to the nerve fibers of the central nervous system responsible for the control of motor activity of muscles. Skeletal muscle relaxants are advocat-

ed for the management of almost every musculoskeletal and neuromuscular condition associated with muscle pain or spasticity.

Nondepolarizing (competitive) neuromuscular blocking agents

Competitive neuromuscular blocking agents produce skeletal muscle relaxation by occupying the cholinergic receptor sites at the myoneural junction, thereby preventing acetylcholine from acting on these receptors. Consequently, depolarization of the postsynaptic membrane does not occur, the muscle fibers are not stimulated, and skeletal muscle contraction does not take place. These drugs may also interfere with the movement of potassium and sodium ions responsible for depolarization and repolarization of the membranes involved in muscle contraction.

Neuromuscular blockade by nondepolarizing drugs is (1) antagonized by depolarizing agents, (2) reversed by anticholinesterases (physostigmine, neostigmine, edrophonium), which increase acetylcholine concentration at the end-plate, and (3) intensified or prolonged by ether anesthesia. These drugs are also referred to as curariform blocking agents. Table 10-1 summarizes common drug interactions with these agents.

Repeated doses of curare-type drugs may accumulate, especially in patients with renal impairment, because these drugs are excreted by the kidneys. Hypotension results from prolonged usage. It also occurs following ganglionic blockade or as a complication of positive pressure breathing. Acidosis, electrolyte imbalance, and neuromuscular disease may potentiate the activity of these drugs. If the injection is too rapid (a sustained intravenous injection over a period of 1 to 1½ minutes is recommended), an increased release of histamine may develop, with resultant decreased respiratory capacity because of bronchospasm and respiratory muscle paralysis. The action of these drugs is altered also in hypothermia (doses may have to be increased), hyperthermia (doses may have to be decreased), dehydration, and renal disease.

TABLE 10-1 Drug interactions of nondepolarizing (competitive) drugs (curare, tubocurarine, gallamine, pancuronium, and metocurine)

Drug(s)	Drug interaction effects	Comments
Inhalation anesthetics (diethyl ether, enflurane, halothane, and methoxyflurane)	Increased intensity of blockade and duration of action of curare-type drug	No increase is seen with droperidol, narcotic analgesics, nitrous oxide, or thiobarbiturates
Parenteral aminoglycoside antibiotics (gentamicin, kanamycin, tobramycin, etc.)	Increased intensity of curare-type drugs	
Polypeptide antibiotics (colistimethate, bacitracin, and polymyxin)	Increased neuromuscular blockade and apnea	
Lincomycins (clindamycin and lincomycin)	Increased neuromuscular blockade	
Thiazide diuretics	Increased sensitivity to neuromuscular blocking agents	Adequate serum potassium levels must be maintained to avoid interaction or thiazides must be discontinued 4 days before surgery
Amphotericin B	Increased sensitivity to neuromuscular blocking agents	Interaction is secondary to amphotericin B–induced hypokalemia
Succinylcholine	Increased relaxant effects of curare-type agents	Curare-type drug should be withheld until the succinylcholine effects diminish
Quinidine	Enhanced postoperative effects of curare-type drugs	Respiratory depression or paralysis may occur
Acetylcholine	Antagonization of curare effects	
Calcium salts, benzodiazepines, quinine, magnesium salts, beta blockers, and trimethaphan	Potentiation of curare effects	
Lithium	Increased neuromuscular blockade	

TABLE 10-2 Nondepolarizing (competitive) blocking drugs

	Tubocurarine	Metocurine iodide (Metubine)	Pancuronium (Pavulon)
Maximal action			
Intravenous	3 to 5 minutes	3 to 5 minutes	2 to 3 minutes
Intramuscular	Unpredictable	5 to 10 minutes	—
Oral	No effect	No effect	No effect
Duration of action	Variable; 25 to 90 minutes with large single dose or multiple doses; action may last 24 hours	15 to 90 minutes	35 to 45 minutes
Mode of action	Competitive blocker of acetylcholine	Competitive blocker of acetylcholine	Comeptitive blocker of acetylcholine
Effects			
Central	None	None	None
Cardiovascular	N.S.*	N.S.*	Tachycardia
Respiratory	Hypoventilation, apnea from cumulative effects	Hypoventilation, apnea	
Antagonists	Neostigmine Edrophonium	Neostigmine Edrophonium	Neostigmine Edrophonium

*Not significant when administered slowly. Rapid induction may cause a precipitous fall in blood pressure.

Apnea or prolonged curarization is treated with controlled respiratory support. Edrophonium or neostigmine may antagonize skeletal muscle relaxant action. The neostigmine injection should be preceded by an injection of atropine (both by the intravenous route). The atropine is used to antagonize muscarinic actions. The edrophonium adjunct/antagonist effect lasts up to 5 minutes, and the effects of neostigmine are seen for ½ to 1½ hours. The hypotension caused by ganglionic blockade is treated with fluids and elevation of the foot of the bed; vasopressors are used only if hypotension continues and fails to respond to anticholinesterase drugs (preferably neostigmine with atropine).

Curare

Curare is a generic name for a number of arrow poisons obtained from tropical vines and used by South American Indians. A number of separate alkaloids are extracted from the plant genus *Strychnos* and certain species of *Chondodendron*. *Chondodendron tomentosum* is a source of *d*-tubocurarine. Previously, curare was obtained from a variety of plants, resulting in variability in strength and composition, and it gained a reputation for unreliability. The isolation of *d*-tubocurarine by King in 1935, the development of an assay method, and standardization of the drug produced a pure crystalline compound with pure curare action.

Action and result. In therapeutic doses curare blocks transmission at the myoneural junctions of skeletal muscle (see Table 10-2). When an appropriate dose of curare is injected intravenously in man, the first effects of flaccid paralysis occur in the short muscles such as those found in the eyes, eyelids, fingers, and toes. Within 2 to 3 minutes haziness of vision, difficulty in talking and swallowing, ptosis of the eyelids, and weakness of the muscles of the jaw, neck, and legs occur; then follow relaxation and, finally, paralysis of the muscles of the neck, spine, legs, arms, and abdomen. The last muscles to be affected are the intercostals and the diaphragm. In recovery after the ordinary clinical dose the paralysis disappears in reverse order and may require 25 to 90 minutes.

An undesirable action of curare is that of blockage of transmission in the autonomic ganglia. This action may cause lowering of blood pressure.

Absorption and excretion. Because of its poor absorption, curare may be swallowed (ordinary doses) without ill effect, provided there are no wounds or abrasions along the digestive tract. It is rapidly excreted by the kidney and also rapidly destroyed by the liver.

Uses. Curare was formerly used to enhance muscular relaxation during anesthesia to permit adequate relaxation without subjecting patients to deep planes of anesthesia that border on medullary paralysis. However, the margin of safety between the dose that produced good relaxation of voluntary muscle and the one producing paralysis of respiratory muscles was small.

It was formerly used also to prevent trauma and excessive muscular contraction in electroshock therapy and to provide muscular relaxation during endoscopy and the reduction of fractures and dislocations. It has been replaced to a great extent by succinylcholine.

Other former uses of curare include relief of spasticity of muscles in certain convulsive states and neuromuscular conditions. It was also used as a diagnostic agent for myasthenia gravis. (It may still be used for this purpose when tests with neostigmine or edrophonium are inconclusive.) (An injection of one fifteenth to one fifth of the average adult dose will produce profound exaggeration of symptoms if the patient has myasthenia gravis.)

Patients receiving curare had to be closely observed for respiratory failure. If this occurred, artificial respiration was instituted and an injection of neostigmine was given as an antidote.

The clinical use of curare from natural sources has been supplanted by use of tubocurarine and synthetic curarimimetic drugs.

Tubocurarine chloride (*d*-tubocurarine)

Tubocurarine is the active principle of curare. It produces a paralytic effect on neuromuscular transmission. Its pharmacologic effects are similar to those of other nondepolarizing neuromuscular blocking agents.

A single intravenous dose of tubocurarine

produces muscle relaxation in 3 to 5 minutes, which may persist for approximately 20 to 40 minutes. Muscles are affected in the following order: (1) those innervated by the cranial nerves (for example, facial muscles, (2) muscles of the trunk and extremities, and (3) muscles of respiration, with the diaphragm being affected last. After intramuscular injection paralysis is unpredictable. Additional doses will have longer durations of action than the initial dose owing to cumulative effects. A large single dose or multiple small doses can saturate the body tissues; the residual effects of the drug may persist in the tissues for 8 to 12 or more hours after the last dose has been given. Duration of action is dependent on the rate of urinary excretion. From 33% to 75% of the drug is eliminated unchanged in urine; some of the drug is eliminated through the intestinal tract via the bile. Thus its actions may be prolonged because of delayed drug excretion in patients with renal or liver disease and in the elderly or debilitated.

Tubocurarine does not readily cross the blood-brain barrier and thus in therapeutic doses does not cause central nervous system effects. Significant amounts do not cross the placental barrier, and therefore it can be used in obstetric anesthesia.

Uses. Tubocurarine is used for the following purposes: (1) as an adjunct to anesthesia to induce skeletal muscle relaxation, (2) to decrease the intensity of muscle contraction in electroshock therapy, and (3) as a diagnostic agent for myasthenia gravis when results with anticholinesterases have been inconclusive.

Side effects, toxic effects, and precautions. Tubocurarine can cause hypotension because of its sympathetic ganglionic blocking ability and its capacity to release histamine from storage sites. The resulting peripheral vasodilation produces a drop in blood pressure. The diminished venous return caused by loss of skeletal muscle tone also contributes to the hypotension. The histamine release may cause bronchospasm.

Since myasthenia gravis patients are particularly sensitive to tubocurarine blocking effects, this drug should be used with extreme caution in these patients. The blocking effect of tubocurarine is enhanced by acidosis and decreased by alkalosis.

Depression of the muscles of respiration can cause hypoxia and even death. Treatment includes establishing an open airway (endotracheal tube) and positive pressure artificial respiration with oxygen.

Neostigmine methylsulfate (Prostigmin Methylsulfate) and edrophonium chloride (Tensilon Chloride) are used as antidotes under certain conditions but only as supplements to artificial respiration with oxygen. These antidotes inactivate cholinesterase and permit acetylcholine to be built up, and unless large overdoses of curare have been given, this increased level of acetylcholine tends to overcome the paralysis. However, overdosage with the antidote can also produce untoward effects. Effective doses of neostigmine are likely to produce increased flow of saliva, slowing of the heart, hypotension, and increased motility of the intestine. Atropine to antagonize muscarinic actions is sometimes given to counteract the latter effects. The anticurare drugs are said to be most safely used when employed in small and, if necessary, repeated doses.

Preparation, dosage, and administration. The drug is available in ampules containing 3 mg, (20 units) of tubocurarine/ml and in 10- and 20-ml vials.

The following is used for conversions and calculations: 3 mg (20 units)/ml, 1 mg (7 units)/0.33 ml, and 1 unit (0.15 mg)/0.05 ml. No accurate dose-response relationship is established for adults or children. A sustained intravenous injection is administered over a period of 1 to 1½ minutes. As a precaution the initial dose is reduced by 3 mg (20 units) below the calculated dose. The dose is calculated on the basis of 0.075 mg (0.5 unit)/pound. This is administered only by or under the supervision of experienced anesthesia clinicians. Thorough patient evaluation necessitates individualized doses.

The following doses are offered only as a guide for average patients without sensitivity, receiving preanesthetic medications, and under light surgical anesthesia. When using inhalation anesthetics that enhance the action of such curariform drugs, the initial dose is reduced and the patient response is a guide to incremental doses.

Surgery: at time of incision 6 mg (40 units) to 9 mg (60 units) intravenously and for further relaxation 3 mg (20 units) to 4.5 mg (30 units) in 3 to 5 minutes is used. This 50% reduction of the initial dose prevents summation.

Electroshock therapy: to reduce convulsive severity and abate fractures, the dose is 0.075 mg (0.5 unit)/pound given sustained over a 1- to 1½-minute period and reducing the initial dose by 3 mg (20 units).

Diagnosis of myasthenia gravis: the dose is one fifteenth to one fifth of the average intravenous adult dose for electroshock therapy. This small dose produces a profound exaggeration of the myasthenia gravis syndrome.

Metocurine iodide (Metubine)

This preparation is chemically similar to the parent compound tubocurarine but it is about three to nine times as potent. Dosage must be individualized, and the drug must be administered slowly over 30 to 60 seconds. Maximal effect occurs in 3 to 5 minutes; duration of blockade ranges from 25 to 90 (average 60) minutes depending on the dose and general anesthetic used. Side effects, toxic effects, and precautions are the same as those for tubocurarine. This low-pH product will precipitate in high-pH solutions (for example, barbiturates, methohexital, thiopental).

The iodide preparation should not be used in patients sensitive to iodides.

The drug is available in 2 mg/ml solution in 20-ml containers.

Gallamine triethiodide (Flaxedil)

Gallamine triethiodide is a synthetic compound whose action, uses, drug interactions, and contraindications are similar to those of the curare drugs. It is not chemically a curare drug but pharmacologically it acts like curare. It is about one fifth as potent as tubocurarine. Advantages claimed for this preparation include the following: (1) it has no effect on autonomic ganglia, (2) it does not cause bronchospasm from histamine release, and (3) it affords a high degree of flexibility because of rapid onset and short duration of action lasting two to four times the neuromuscular blocking effect. Its major disadvantage is that it

TABLE 10-3 Drug interactions of gallamine

Drug(s)	Drug interaction effects
Drugs with anticholinergic activity (phenothiazines, tricyclic antidepressants, atropine-like drugs)	Enhanced cardiac effects (tachycardia)
Anesthetic agents (ether, methoxyflurane, fluroxene)	Potentiation of effects of gallamine
Antibiotics (aminoglycosides, polypeptides)	Potentiation of effects of gallamine

produces vagal blockade similar to that of atropine and thus can cause tachycardia and blood pressure elevation. It is antagonized by neostigmine and edrophonium.

Uses. Gallamine is used as an adjunct to anesthesia for muscle relaxation and in management of mechanical ventilation. It is not approved for electroshock therapy because of its side effects and short duration of action.

Preparation, dosage, and administration. Gallamine triethiodide is administered intravenously in an aqueous solution. It may be mixed with a 2.5% thiopental sodium solution. Body weight is the main factor in determining dosage. Muscularity, age, sex, and pathologic conditions are also considered. At 1 mg/kg a 30% reduction in respiratory minute volume is seen, and at 1.5 mg/kg a 75% decrease is seen.

Not more than 100 mg is injected at any one time. Muscular relaxation begins immediately after intravenous injection and reaches a maximum in about 3 to 5 minutes; duration of action is 15 to 35 minutes. Dosage must be individually adjusted for each patient. Gallamine triethiodide is available in 20 and 100 mg/ml solutions.

Side effects and toxic effects. This drug may produce an allergic reaction in patients sensitive to iodine. It may also produce a marked tachycardia, which occurs within 3 minutes after administration of a dose equal to 0.5 mg/kg body weight. It crosses the placental barrier, and although no perceptible effect on newborns has been reported, it should be used with extreme caution for cesarean section. It is excreted unchanged by the kidneys and should not be administered to patients with impaired renal function because it may accumulate. It must be used with the same precautions as other potent skeletal muscle relaxants. It is not the relaxant of choice for patients with cardiovascular disease, and it is absolutely contraindicated in myasthenia gravis. Table 10-3 summarizes common drug interactions of gallamine.

Pancuronium bromide (Pavulon)

Pancuronium is a synthetic nondepolarizing neuromuscular blocking agent. It is about five times more potent than tubocurarine, and it has a slightly more rapid onset of action. Pancuronium has some advantages over tubocurarine: (1) it does not cause ganglionic blockade and thus does not cause hypotension (only a slight rise in blood pressure) and (2) it causes little or no histamine release and therefore does not cause bronchospasm. It causes varying degrees of an increase in heart rate (chronotropic effect) by blocking the ACh receptors of the heart, but this is minimal with usual doses and less than that produced by gallamine. Although it has a steroidal structure, the drug appears to have no hormonal activity.

Uses. Pancuronium is used primarily to produce skeletal muscle relaxation during surgery after general anesthesia has been induced. It is compatible with all currently used general anesthetics. It has been used to facilitate mechanical respiration in patients with status asthmaticus and to facilitate endotracheal intubation.

After intravenous injection muscle relaxation takes place in 2 to 3 minutes; duration of action is 35 to 40 minutes. The drug is metabolized in the liver and excreted by the kidneys. It is highly protein bound.

Dosage and preparation. Dosage of pancuronium must be individually determined. However, usual initial dose as an adjunct to anesthesia is 0.04 to 0.1 mg/kg body weight. Additional doses of 0.01 mg/kg may be administered at 25- to 60-minute intervals during prolonged surgery or assisted respiration.

It is available in 2-ml ampules containing 2 mg of pancuronium/ml and in 10-ml vials containing 1 mg of drug/ml.

Side effects, toxic effects, and precautions. Pancuronium has the same toxic potentials as other nondepolarizing neuromuscular blocking agents and is antagonized by pyridostigmine and neostigmine with atropine. It should not be used in patients with a history of tachycardia or in patients in whom an increase in heart rate is undesirable. It is contraindicated in patients sensitive to bromides.

Pancuronium has caused excessive salivation and sweating in children. Its use is not recommended for children under the age of 10. It should be used cautiously in children, since only limited data on its use in this age group are available at this time.

Transient skin rashes, wheezing, and a burning sensation at the site of injection have been reported. Accumulation is seen with repeated doses in patients with renal disease.

Depolarizing neuromuscular blocking agents

Depolarizing agents resemble acetylcholine in structure, have a high affinity for ACh receptor sites, and, like acetylcholine, produce depolarization of the motor end-plate at the myoneural junction. These drugs produce a more prolonged depolarization of the motor end-plate than ACh because of their high affinity for ACh receptors and their slower inactivation by cholinesterase. During depolarization the end-plate is incapable of responding to motor nerve stimulation. These drugs are associated with phase I and phase II blocks. Succinylcholine is an example of a depolarizing drug.

Phase I block is the initial depolarization block, during which paralysis may be preceded by signs of stimulation (e.g., fasciculations). This type of block is potentiated by anticholinesterase drugs and reversed by nondepolarizing agents.

Phase II block, or desensitization block of the receptors, follows the use of a depolarizing drug for a prolonged time; that is, it is a block that develops with time. It is similar to a competitive block. Since the end-plate does not remain depolarized for an indefinite period, a state probably occurs whereby depolarization is no longer present but the neuromuscular block persists. During phase II block, drugs that antagonize competitive blocking agents (anticholinesterase drugs such as neostigmine) are effective for reversing the block even though they are not effective for reversing phase I block.

The phase II block is not well understood, and a variety of factors are probably involved. There is evidence that depolarization causes a considerable shift in ions. Muscle cells with greatly altered ionic distribution may be blocked more easily. There are reports that phase II block seems to occur sooner in patients with decreased potassium levels.

Succinylcholine chloride (Anectine Chloride, Quelicin, Sucostrin, Sux-Cert); suxamethonium chloride

Action and result. Succinylcholine is an ultrashort-acting myoneural blocking agent. Although the end result of its action is similar to that of curare, its mode of action is the same as that of decamethonium—it intensifies the depolarizing effect to such an extent that repolarization of the end-plate, which is necessary for muscle contraction, does not occur.

Its action is of shorter duration than that of decamethonium. The concentration gradient of succinylcholine is largely controlled by enzymatic destruction. Succinylcholine is easily hydrolyzed by destruction by cholinesterase to form choline and succinic acid. Alkaline solutions of the drug undergo rapid hydrolysis; therefore succinylcholine chloride should not be mixed with alkaline solutions of anesthetics such as thiopental sodium. The intensity of its effect can be modified readily by varying the rate of administration.

Clinical doses do not seem to produce significant effects on the circulatory system and autonomic ganglia, and they cause no significant liberation of histamine.

Uses. Some authorities are of the opinion that succinylcholine approaches the ideal muscle relaxant. It is the relaxant of choice whenever it is important to have rapid skeletal muscle relaxation.

It is used to produce muscular relaxation during anesthesia and in conjunction with electroshock therapy. Because of its short action, it is particularly well suited to procedures of short duration such as endotracheal intubation and endoscopy. In part because of its low lipid solubility and high ionization, it does not readily cross the placenta.

Preparation, dosage, and administration. Succinylcholine chloride is available as succinylcholine chloride injection and is administered intravenously, either in repeated injections or as a continuous drip infusion. After a 10-mg test dose the dose range is 20 to 80 mg for an adult when used for short procedures. Relaxation occurs in about 1 minute with peak action in 1 to 3 minutes, after which there is rapid recovery in 5 to 10 minutes. Sustained relaxation for prolonged procedures is obtained by continuous drip infusion (dextrose in normal saline, 0.1% to 0.2%) in which approximately 2.5 mg is given per minute. Administration of succinylcholine is said to require closer attention than administration of other muscle relaxants, but there is also greater ease of control.

Side effects and toxic effects. Succinylcholine exhibits a low level of toxicity. However, large doses produce respiratory depression, and facilities to combat respiratory paralysis must be at hand. There is no effective antagonist. Anticholinesterase drugs such as physostigmine, neostigmine, and edrophonium chloride prolong the effect of succinylcholine by interfering with metabolism by cholinesterase and therefore are contraindicated as antidotes in case of overdosage. However, because it loses its potency rapidly (up to 90% in 5 minutes) when administration is discontinued, succinylcholine is a relatively safe drug. The patient must be observed closely to prevent undue respiratory depression.

Since succinylcholine can cause autonomic (vaqomimetic) stimulation, bradycardia, salivation, hypotension, cardiac arrhythmias, and cardiac arrest may occur with its use. Tachycardia and hypertension have also been reported; these symptoms are the result of sympathetic ganglion stimulation. A rise in serum potassium level is also seen.

Precautions. Patients with a deficiency of plasma cholinesterase resulting from a genetic variant defect, liver disease, occupational exposure to organophosphorous insecticides, severe anemia, uremia, severe dehydration, or malnutrition should not be given succinylcholine.

T A B L E   1 0 - 4   **Drug interactions of succinylcholine**

Drug(s)	Drug interaction effects
Diazepam	Reduction of duration of action of succinylcholine
Quinine, quinidine, magnesium salts	Potentiation of succinylcholine
Acetylcholine, anticholinesterases, other nondepolarizing or depolarizing relaxants, aminoglycosides, tetracyclines, polypeptides, lincomycin, clindamycin, and local anesthetics	Alteration of succinylcholine action
Procaine	Enhanced neuromuscular blocking action of succinylcholine

Such persons tend to be highly sensitive to even small doses of the drug, and there is a risk of prolonged postoperative apnea in these patients. Cholinesterase levels can also be decreased by topical administration of long-acting anticholinesterases such as echothiophate, which is used in the treatment of wide-angle glaucoma. These drugs should be discontinued 2 to 4 weeks before surgery if succinylcholine is to be given. Succinylcholine causes a rise in intraocular pressure, which is hazardous to patients with glaucoma, those undergoing eye surgery, and patients with penetrating wounds of the eye. It may also increase intragastric pressure, particularly if the patient was unable to fast prior to surgery. Patients with neuromuscular disorders may have an abnormal response to depolarizing agents.

Particular caution should be used when administering this drug to patients with cardiovascular, hepatic, pulmonary, metabolic, or renal disorders; severe burns; severe trauma; cardiac complications; hyperkalemia; or spinal cord injuries; or to digitalized patients.

A dual block effect develops when the drug is administered over a prolonged period; the characteristic depolarization block of the myoneural junction may change to a nondepolarizing block (competitive type), which may lead to prolonged respiratory depression and apnea. Under these conditions small repeated doses of neostigmine or edrophonium preceded by atro-

pine may act as antagonists. Table 10-4 summarizes some drug interactions of succinylcholine.

Decamethonium bromide (Syncurine)

Action. Decamethonium bromide is a very potent depolarizing skeletal muscle relaxant with a rapid onset of action but rather short duration of effect.

The duration of its effect (15 minutes) is said to be intermediate between that of tubocurarine and succinylcholine. It does not produce a ganglionic blocking action, and it does not cause bronchospasm from a liberation of histamine. It has no cumulative effect even after repeated dosage, it does not increase intraocular pressure, and it has no direct effect on myocardium.

Decamethonium bromide mimics acetylcholine for the cholinergic receptors of the motor end-plate, and, like acetylcholine, its union with these receptors produces depolarization followed by an initial, transient muscle contraction, often visible as fasciculations. In this mechanism the neuromuscular transmission is inhibited and remains so as long as adequate concentrations of decamethonium are present at these sites, causing flaccid paralysis.

Decamethonium is not altered by serum cholinesterase, is not metabolized by the liver or at the end-plate, and is excreted by the kidneys with no apparent metabolic degradation. The drug will not readily cross the placenta, in part because the drug is highly ionized and has a low lipid solubility.

A dual block (depolarization followed by nondepolarization blockade) rarely occurs except with repeated and prolonged administration. If the primary depolarizing block has become a nondepolarizing block, then edrophonium (10 mg intravenously) or neostigmine (adults: 1 to 3 mg; children: 0.5 mg) preceded by atropine (adults: 1 to 1.5 mg; children: 0.08 mg/kg) may be used as adjunctive treatment in association with good patient monitoring. Neostigmine is preferred over edrophonium because edrophonium has a very brief duration of action.

Uses. Decamethonium bromide has been

used to produce marked but short-term relaxation in connection with brief procedures such as endoscopy, endotracheal intubation, and closure of the peritoneum during surgery. However, the drug is seldom used because tachyphylaxis occurs frequently with repeated doses, a satisfactory antidote is not available, and its effects are rather unpredictable.

Preparation, dosage, and administration. The usual initial dose varies from 2 to 2.5 mg, depending on the response of the patient and the degree of relaxation desired. It is administered by a single intravenous injection (1 mg/minute); additional doses of 0.5 to 1 mg may be given at intervals of 10 to 30 minutes. Muscle relaxation occurs in 2 to 4 minutes; muscle activity begins to return in about 10 minutes and is back to normal in about 30 minutes. The drug is available in a concentration of 1 mg/ml in 10-ml vials.

Side effects. Despite its relatively short duration of action, this drug may cause respiratory depression. Anticholinesterases (neostigmine and edrophonium chloride) are of no value as inhibitors, antidotes, or antagonists except in the instance of dual block; therefore facilities for controlled artificial respiration with oxygen are essential in case respiratory depression occurs.

Plasma cholinesterase inhibitor

Hexafluorenium bromide (Mylaxen)

Hexafluorenium is a plasma cholinesterase inhibitor used only to prolong the action of succinylcholine. It delays the enzymatic hydrolysis of succinylcholine, thereby increasing the intensity and duration of succinylcholine action. Hexafluorenium is used to prevent the muscle fasciculations and pain associated with succinylcholine administration.

Bronchospasm has been caused by the combined use of succinylcholine and hexafluorenium, so these drugs should not be given concomitantly to patients with bronchial asthma.

If used with other relaxants, hexafluorenium holds the potential for synergistic or antagonistic effects. The following adverse reactions are reported with hexafluorenium: bradycardia, tachycardia, hypertension, hypo-

tension, cardiac arrest, hyperthermia, and increased intraocular pressure. Pronounced and prolonged muscle paralysis may occur, leading to respiratory depression or apnea. Hexafluorenium is administered in a ratio of 2 mg of hexafluorenium for each 1 mg of succinylcholine. The duration of effect is about 20 to 30 minutes; to avoid distress to the patient, this drug is administered only after unconsciousness is induced. The drug is available in 20 mg/ml concentration in 10-ml vials; dosage is calculated on a mg/kg body weight basis.

Agents used in myasthenia gravis

Myasthenia gravis is a disorder characterized by weakness and easy fatigability of voluntary skeletal muscles, especially of muscles innervated by the bulbar nuclei. Lid ptosis, diplopia, and facial weakness may also be seen. The etiology of myasthenia gravis is unknown, but it has been suggested that rapid splitting and inactivation of acetylcholine at the myoneural junction may be the cause. Some believe that myasthenia gravis may be an autoimmune disease, since autoantibodies have been found in blood sera of patients. The disease usually appears in women 20 to 30 years of age. Along with the previously mentioned signs and symptoms, positive neostigmine (Prostigmin) and endrophonium chloride (Tensilon) tests are diagnostic of the presence of the disease.

The agents used to diagnose and treat myasthenia gravis are also used as antagonists of curariform drugs to reverse their effects. The following discussion presents these agents and how they are used. They are often referred to as cholinergic muscle stimulants.

Neostigmine methylsulfate (Prostigmin Methylsulfate); neostigmine bromide (Prostigmin Bromide)

Neostigmine is capable of functioning as an antagonist to curare-type drugs such as tubocurarine, which are used for skeletal muscle relaxation during surgical anesthesia. These relaxants inhibit acetylcholine depolarization at the neuromuscular junction. Neostigmine inhibits cholinesterase and permits sufficient acetylcholine to accumulate and overcome the curare action. It does not antagonize decamethonium or succinylcholine.

Its primary use is for the symptomatic control of myasthenia gravis. Its greatest usefulness is in prolonged therapy where no difficulty in swallowing is present. It has also been used in acute myasthenic crises.

The usual dose as a curare antagonist is 0.5 to 2 mg given by slow intravenous injection; this may be repeated. Total dose should not exceed 5 mg. It is recommended that atropine sulfate, 0.6 to 1.2 mg, be given intravenously when neostigmine is given intravenously.

The usual dose in the treatment of myasthenia gravis is 150 mg of *neostigmine bromide* given orally over 24 hours. The interval between doses is established by trial and error. The parenteral form used for symptomatic control of myasthenia gravis is given subcutaneously or intramuscularly in a 1-ml volume of the 1:2000 solution (0.5 mg) of *neostigmine methylsulfate*. Subsequent doses are based on the patient's response.

Neostigmine is available in 1:1000, 1:2000, and 1:4000 solutions and 15-mg tablets in the bromide salt.

Edrophonium chloride (Tensilon)

Edrophonium is an antagonist of skeletal muscle relaxants such as tubocurarine and similar preparations that act by competing with acetylcholine for end-plate receptors at the myoneural junction. Edrophonium is an anticholinesterase muscle stimulant agent; it inactivates or inhibits acetylcholinesterase at sites of cholinergic transmission, permitting accumulation of acetylcholine to overcome the curare effects. It may also have direct excitatory effects on skeletal muscle.

Uses. Edrophonium can be used to terminate the effects of curariform agents when muscular relaxation is no longer desired or to reverse respiratory muscle paralysis produced by overdosage. It is used as a differential diagnostic test agent for myasthenia gravis. This is based on its ability to increase muscle strength in myasthenia gravis; improvement in muscle strength occurs in 30 seconds to 5 minutes. It is also used for emergency treatment of myasthenic crises. Since its action is brief, it cannot be used for maintenance therapy. It is not effective when used as an antidote for succinylcholine or decamethonium.

Preparation, dosage, and administration. Edrophonium is administered intravenously. The dosage employed for antagonism of appropriate curariform drugs, 10 mg up to 40 mg, is slowly injected over 30 to 45 seconds. It is not recommended if apnea is present. To counteract overdosage of appropriate muscle relaxants, therefore, it is used along with artificial respiration and oxygen therapy and only when some definite sign of voluntary respiration can be observed.

Side effects and toxic effects. Side effects of edrophonium include increased flow of saliva (salivation), bronchiolar spasm (especially in asthmatic patients), slow pulse, disturbance of cardiac rhythm (especially in elderly patients), central nervous system effects, skeletal muscle effects, and effects on the eye. When edrophonium is used in large doses, it intensifies the peripheral effects of the curariform drugs instead of antagonizing them. Furthermore, it does not combat circulatory collapse that is associated with respiratory depression. The drug is available in 10 mg/ml concentration in 1-ml ampules or 10-ml vials.

Pyridostigmine bromide (Mestinon, Regonal)

This anticholinesterase muscle stimulant is useful in the treatment of myasthenia gravis; the injectable form is also indicated as a reversal agent or antagonist to nondepolarizing muscle relaxants such as curariform drugs and gallamine. When pyridostigmine is administered intravenously to reverse the nondepolarizing muscle relaxants, it is recommended that atropine sulfate (0.6 to 1.2 mg) be administered intravenously immediately prior to the pyridostigmine, (about 10 to 20 mg) to reduce the excessive secretions and bradycardia. Recovery is seen in 15 to 30 minutes or more. Skin rash has been reported, and thrombophlebitis is seen after intravenous administration. Failure of pyridostigmine to provide prompt (within 30 minutes) reversal may occur in the presence of extreme debilitation, carcinomatosis, or concomitant use of certain broad-spectrum antibiotics or anesthetic agents such as ether. It is necessary to use artificial ventilatory support until the patient has resumed control of his respiration.

Preparation, dosage, and administration. Pyridostigmine is available in 5 mg/ml concentration in 2-ml ampules, in a sustained-action tablet of 180 mg, in a tablet of 60 mg (not a sustained-action form), and in a raspberry syrup of 60 mg/5 ml concentration.

When given for myasthenia gravis, the oral doses are titrated by both the amount and frequency to the individual patient needs. An average dose of 600 mg/day is separated over the periods when maximum strength is needed. Mild cases may need 60 to 360 mg/day, but up to 1500 mg/day or more may be needed for more severe cases. The sustained-release tablets are used in 6-hour periods, and supplemental doses of the regular rapid-acting tablets or syrup may also be required.The sustained-action tablets have been used in a dose range of 180 to 540 mg once or twice daily.

Agents used in Parkinson's disease

Parkinson's disease, also called paralysis agitans, is a chronic disorder of the central nervous system. It is characterized by muscle tremors, rigidity, slowness of movement, and muscle weakness with alterations in posture and equilibrium. The exact cause of parkinsonism remains unknown, but it currently believed that it reflects an imbalance between cholinergic and dopaminergic mechanisms in the central nervous system.

Dopamine, a catecholamine, is the precursor of norepinephrine. Dopamine is normally present in the corpus striatum. However, in patients with idiopathic or postencephalitic parkinsonism there is a depletion of dopamine. It has been postulated that the cholinergic and dopaminergic mechanisms are antagonistic; the cholinergic mechanisms innervated by acetylcholine are excitory; the dopaminergic mechanisms innervated by dopamine are inhibitory. The symptoms of parkinsonism thus reflect cholinergic dominance resulting from low levels of dopamine in the brain.

Treatment of parkinsonism remains pallia-tive rather than curative, with the goals of therapy being (1) to provide maximal relief of symptoms and (2) to maintain some independence of movement and activity. Drug therapy consists of (1) anticholinergic drugs to inhibit the cholinergic mechanisms, (2) antihistaminic drugs, which also have anticholinergic action, and (3) levodopa to replenish dopamine levels and enhance the dopaminergic mechanisms.

Drugs with central anticholinergic activity

Three groups of drugs with central anticholinergic activity are used in Parkinson's disease: anticholinergic agents, antihistamines, and the phenothiazine ethopropazine.

These agents are less active than drugs affecting brain dopamine and are therefore used in the treatment of mild Parkinson's disease where age or glaucoma is not contraindicative. They are also used as adjuncts to the more potent agents used to treat Parkinson's disease.

ANTICHOLINERGIC AGENTS

The belladonna alkaloids atropine and scopalamine were the first centrally active anticholinergics used to treat parkinsonism and for many years were the only drugs available for such treatment. These drugs have been supplanted by other anitcholinergics, which were developed in an effort to produce drugs as effective as the belladonna drugs in treating parkinsonism but with fewer disturbing side effects.

The anticholinergics that readily cross the blood-brain barrier can produce slight to moderate improvement in functional capacity. The usefulness of these drugs is limited by their side effects and their tendency to be less effective with continued use. Anticholinergics are also used to control the extrapyramidal reactions (rigidity, akinesia, tremor, akathisia) caused by antipsychotic drugs (for example, phenothiazines).

The anticholinergics are used alone or in conjunction with other antiparkinsonism drugs such as levodopa. All produce "atropine-like" side effects such as dryness of the mouth, blurred vision, dizziness, and dysuria. All have the potential of causing constipation, drowsiness, urinary hesitancy or retention, tachycardia, dilation of the pupil, increased intraocular tension, and intestinal obstruction.

Benztropine mesylate (Cogentin)

Benztropine is a synthetic drug chemically related to atropine and diphenhydramine. Its anticholinergic activity is almost equal to that of atropine; its antihistaminic action is like that of pyrilamine maleate. It is assumed that benztropine acts by depressing synaptic transmission in cholinergic neurons in the central nervous system. It is used primarily in small doses to supplement levodopa or other antiparkinsonism drugs. In full dosage it causes intense side effects that are rarely tolerated. It is also used to control extrapyramidal disorders (not tardive dyskinesia) caused by neuroleptic drugs.

Benztropine is considered by some physicians to be one of the best drugs available for treating parkinsonism, particularly for the control of rigidity, contracture, tremor, and insomnia. Other symptoms may also be relieved. The drug's effects are cumulative and may take 2 or 3 days to occur.

Preparation and dosage. Benztropine is available in 0.5-, 1-, and 2-mg tablets and in 2-ml ampules containing 1 mg of drug/ml for intravenous or intramuscular injection. Range of total daily parkinsonism oral dose is 0.5 to 6.0 mg and usual daily dose is 1 to 2 mg.

Side effects and precautions. The side effects of benztropine are manifestations of its anticholinergic and antihistaminic action. Sedation, hypnosis, and dryness of the mouth are common. Because of its long duration of action, a bedtime dosage regimen is rational. It may produce mydriasis and thus can produce or aggravate glaucoma. Patients sensitive to the drug may develop weakness and inability to move certain muscle groups. Contraindications are the same as for other anticholinergics.

Trihexyphenidyl hydrochloride (Artane, Tremin)

Trihexyphenidyl is considered the anticholinergic of choice in therapy in patients with moderate or severe parkinsonism. It is also used to treat extrapyramidal reactions to phenothiazines. It has an antispasmodic effect on smooth muscle and an inhibitory effect on the parasympathetic system. Thus it relieves smooth muscle spasm by both direct action and parasympathetic inhibition. It relieves spasticity of voluntary muscles by a cholinergic blocking action and by acting on the cerebral motor center. Trihexyphenidyl's antispasmodic action is half that of atropine, its mydriatic effect about one third, its antisialagogic (counteracting dryness of the mouth) effect about one eighth, and its cardiovagal inhibitory action about one hundredth that of atropine.

Preparation and dosage. Trihexyphenidyl is available in 2- and 5-mg tablets, as an elixir containing 2 mg in 5 ml, and as a sustained-release capsule (for maintenance after stabilization) containing 5 mg. Initial dosage is 1 to 2 mg two or three times daily before or after meals. Dosage is gradually increased until the therapeutic effect is obtained (usually 6 to 10 mg daily) or severe reactions occur precluding further increase. For extrapyramidal reactions the usual daily dose is 5 to 15 mg. Onset of action occurs in 1 hour, peak action in 2 to 3 hours; duration of action is 6 to 12 hours.

Side effects and precautions. The most common side effects are dry mouth, blurred vision, dizziness, nausea, and nervousness. Overdosage causes cerebral excitement, hallucinations, and delirium. This drug should not be given to patients with glaucoma.

Biperiden (Akineton)

Biperiden is a derivative of trihexyphenidyl and has similar actions, uses, and adverse effects. It is a weak visceral anticholinergic agent that reduces akinesia and rigidity and, to a lesser extent, tremor. Biperiden may also elevate the mood. It is *effective* for all forms of parkinsonism and for reserpine or phenothiazine-induced extrapyramidal reactions.

It is available in 2-mg tablets and in a lactate solution in 1-ml ampules containing 5 mg/ml for injection. Initial parkinsonism dose is 2 mg three or four times daily orally. For drug-induced extrapyramidal reactions the dose for adults is 2 mg one to three times daily.

Cycrimine hydrochloride (Pagitane Hydrochloride)

Cycrimine is another derivative of trihexyphenidyl with similar actions, uses, and adverse reactions. It is slightly more potent than trihexyphenidyl. It is more effective in the treatment of rigidity, akinesia, and oculogyric crises than in the reduction of tremor. It is *effective* for parkinsonism but *ineffective* for extrapyramidal reactions to phenothiazines. Cycrimine is available in 1.25-and 2.5-mg tablets. Dosage must be individualized but ranges from 1.25 to 5 mg three or four times daily.

Procyclidine hydrochloride (Kemadrin)

Procyclidine is also a derivative of trihexyphenidyl with similar actions, uses, and adverse effects. It is *effective* for parkinsonism (12 to 15 mg daily) and drug-induced extrapyramidal reactions (10 to 20 mg daily). It is available in 2-and 5-mg tablets. Daily parkinsonism dosage initially is 2 to 2.5 mg three times daily, after meals, and may be increased to 4 to 5 mg three times daily. The atropine-like action exerts an antispasmodic effect on smooth muscle.

ANTIHISTAMINES

Antihistamines are used primarily as adjuncts to other more potent antiparkinsonism drugs. However, they may be used alone for initial therapy in patients with mild parkinsonism or for elderly patients, since they are less likely to cause mental disturbances such as confusion and disorientation. In addition to having anticholinergic effects, antihistamines have a sedative effect that helps to counteract the insomnia that can be caused by potent anticholinergics.

Diphenhydramine hydrochloride (Benadryl Hydrochloride)

Diphenhydramine was the first antihistaminic drug available in the United States and the first antihistamine to be used in the treatment of parkinsonism. It has served as a comparison in the development of many other antihistamines. Diphenhydramine has many therapeutic effects; it is an antiemetic, anticholinergic (antispasmodic), and antitussive, and it has local anesthetic and sedative actions. Its use in parkinsonism is based on its central cholinergic blocking action. It decreases rigidity and improves voluntary movement and speech. It is most commonly used with levodopa or one of the more potent anticholinergics. It is also used

to treat drug-induced extrapyramidal reactions.

Preparation and dosage. Diphenhydramine is available in 25- and 50-mg capsules; 25-mg enteric-coated tablets; an elixir containing 2.5 mg/ml; and in solutions for injection containing 10 mg/ml in 10- and 30-ml vials, and 50 mg/ml in 1- and 10-ml containers. Dose for adults is 25 to 50 mg three to four times daily. The maximal parenteral dose is 100 mg, and total daily parenteral dose should not exceed 400 mg. For children the usual dose is 5 mg/kg of body weight divided into four doses over 24 hours or 150 mg/m^2/24 hours; maximal daily child's dose is 300 mg. When taken orally, the drug is readily absorbed from the gastrointestinal tract; peak tissue concentration occurs in 1 hour; duration of action is 4 to 6 hours.

Side effects and precautions. Diphenhydramine causes a high incidence of side effects. Fortunately, most of these are minor, and most disappear with continued therapy. Sedation and drowsiness are the most common side effects. Other side effects are nausea, headache, vertigo, epigastric distress, dry mouth, blurred vision, hypotension, rash, and urticaria.

Diphenhydramine should not be given to patients with narrow-angle glaucoma, prostatic hypertrophy, or obstruction of the intestinal or urinary tract. Persons taking diphenhydramine should be extremely cautious around hazardous machinery. If the drug causes drowsiness, they should not drive motor vehicles.

Drug interactions. Diphenhydramine may potentiate the action of alcohol, hypnotics, sedatives, tranquilizers, and other CNS depressants.

Monoamine oxidase inhibitors may potentiate the action of diphenhydramine.

Diphenhydramine may enhance the action of atropine and other anticholinergic drugs.

Orphenadrine hydrochloride (Disipal)

Orphenadrine, as reviewed earlier, is a derivative of diphenhydramine with similar actions and uses. It is used alone or with other drugs in the treatment of Parkinson's disease. It relieves muscle rigidity more than tremor, and it has a slight euphoriant action that helps to counteract depression and fatigue. Its anticholinergic action helps to control sialorrhea, diaphoresis, and oculogyria. Orphenadrine's effectiveness tends to diminish with use. Unlike diphenhydramine, it does not cause drowsiness. Side effects are relatively few and mild and similar to those caused by diphenhydramine. Orphenadrine may cause mild excitation and mental clouding in the elderly.

Orphenadrine should not be given to patients with glaucoma, obstructions, or myasthenia gravis. Extreme caution is required if given to patients with a history of tachycardia.

Preparation and dosage. Orphenadrine is available in 50-mg tablets. Oral dosage for adults initially is 50 mg three times daily, which may be increased to 250 mg daily depending on the patient's response.

Drug interactions. Use of orphenadrine with propoxyphene (Darvon) may result in mental confusion, anxiety, and tremors. Orphenadrine plus chlorpromazine has caused hypoglycemic coma. Orphenadrine may inhibit the action of griseofulvin, hexobarbital, and phenylbutazone.

Chlorphenoxamine hydrochloride (Phenoxene)

Chlorphenoxamine is a derivative of diphenhydramine possessing antihistaminic and anticholinergic properties. Its actions and side effects are like those of diphenhydramine. Chlorphenoxamine is effective for all forms of parkinsonism. It is available in 50-mg tablets. Dosage initially is 50 mg three times a day; this may be increased to 100 mg two to four times daily. This antihistamine reduces rigidity of parkinsonism with little effect on tremor. It may depress motor nerve centers of the brainstem and spinal cord. The patient may experience increased muscle power and endurance.

PHENOTHIAZINE
Ethopropazine hydrochloride (Parsidol Hydrochloride)

Ethopropazine is a phenothiazine derivative used to treat parkinsonism, usually in conjunction with other drugs, and to treat drug-induced extrapyramidal reactions. Like some other phenothiazines, ethopropazine has antihistaminic, ganglionic-blocking, adrenergic-blocking, and local anesthetic action. It usually produces central nervous system depression. Ethopropazine helps control tremor and rigidity and improves the patient's posture, gait, and speech. It also promotes better sleep.

Preparation and dosage. Ethopropazine is available in 10- and 50-mg tablets. Dosage is variable and dependent on patient response. Initial dosage of 50 mg once to twice daily is increased gradually to 100 to 400 mg in mild or moderate cases of parkinsonism; severe cases may require 500 to 600 mg or more daily.

Side effects and precautions. Ethopropazine causes numerous side effects, and many patients, particularly the elderly, cannot tolerate therapeutic dosages. EEG slowing, seizures, ECG abnormality, drowsiness, dizziness, inability to concentrate, and confusion are the most common side effects. Muscle cramps, paresthesia, epigastric distress, and hypotension may also occur. Ethopropazine should be used with caution in patients with glaucoma, cardiac disease, or prostatic hypertrophy.

Drugs affecting brain dopamine

Three classifications of drugs affect brain dopamine: that which releases dopamine, those which increase brain levels of dopamine, and the dopaminergic agonist. The drugs of choice in the treatment of Parkinson's disease are those which increase the brain levels of dopamine. The other two classifications are used as adjuncts or when the therapy normally used is contraindicated.

DOPAMINE-RELEASING DRUG
Amantadine hydrochloride (Symmetrel)

Amantadine is a synthetic antiviral compound used in the prophylaxis and symptomatic management of influenza A and in the treatment of parkinsonism. Its exact mechanism in reducing symptoms of parkinsonism and improving functional capacity is not known. It has been postulated that amantadine releases dopamine and other catecholamines from neuronal storage sites. It may also block the reuptake of dopamine into presynaptic neurons, thus permitting peripheral and central accumulation of dopamine.

Although amantadine is less effective than levodopa in the treatment of parkinsonism, it produces more rapid clinical improvement and causes fewer untoward reactions. Amantadine relieves akinesia, rigidity, tremor, salivation, gait disturbances, and functional disability. It may also give the patient a sense of well-being and elevation of mood. Improvement in symptoms occurs within 4 to 48 hours after initiation of therapy; optimal results occur within 2 weeks to 3 months. Improvement may last up to 30 months. In some patients a reduction in beneficial effects occurs after 4 to 12 weeks of therapy. Amantadine is usually used along with other antiparkinsonism drugs.

There is complete absorption after oral administration. A 100-mg dose results in peak serum blood levels of 0.2 mg/ml within 1 to 8 hours. Serum half-life values range from 9 to 37 hours (average 20 hours). Ninety percent of the drug is excreted unchanged in the urine (27% to 74% is excreted within 24 hours). The elimination half-life is about 20 hours. The excretion of amantadine is about five times the glomerular filtration rate and is pH dependent. Since this is a basic amine, the administration of urine-acidifying agents increases the rate of excretion from the body.

Amantadine enhances the anticholinergic effects of anticholinergic drugs (for example, atropine and scopolamine). Patients receiving large doses of anticholinergics exhibit such central nervous system effects as stimulation, delirium, extrapyramidal symptoms, tachycardia, and hypotension.

Dosage. Amantadine is available in 100-mg capsules and as a syrup containing 50 mg in 5 ml. Dosage initially is 100-mg once daily after breakfast for 5 to 7 days. If side effects do not occur, an additional 100 mg is given after lunch. Increasing the dosage beyond this level increases the severity of side effects without significantly increasing beneficial effects. Amantadine therapy should be discontinued gradually; abrupt cessation of the drug has been associated with exacerbations of parkinsonism symptoms within 24 hours and onset of parkinsonian crises within 3 days.

Side effects and precautions. Many of the side effects of amantadine are central nervous system disturbances such as nervousness, mental depression, congestive heart failure, psychoses, slurred speech, blurred vision, feeling of drunkenness, inability to concentrate, detachment, insomnia, confusion, halucinations, and ataxia. The drug may accumulate in patients with inadequate renal function. Other side effects include edema, orthostatic hypotension, skin rash, nausea, vomiting, abdominal discomfort, constipation, urinary retention, and increased frequency of urination.

Amantadine should be used cautiously (if at all) in elderly patients, epileptics, psychotics, those with liver, renal, or cardiac disease, pregnant women, and those with cerebrovascular disease. Amantadine is contraindicated in nursing mothers. There have been reports of it being embryotoxic and teratogenic in rats.

DRUGS THAT INCREASE BRAIN LEVELS OF DOPAMINE
Levodopa (L-dopa, Dopar, Larodopa)

Levodopa is the drug of choice and the most effective drug available for treating parkinsonism. All major symptoms of parkinsonism may be relieved by levodopa therapy. Most patients show a marked reduction in akinesia and rigidity. Tremors may increase in severity during initial therapy before improving. Improvements have occurred in balance, posture, gait, speech, and handwriting. Drooling may be completely abolished, and oculogyric crisis is reduced in both severity and frequency. There may also be improved intellectual function and an elevation in mood.

Levodopa is not effective in counteracting extrapyramidal reactions induced by antipsychotic agents such as phenothiazines.

Preparation, dosage, and administration. Levodopa is available in 100-, 250-, and 500-mg capsules and in 100-, 250-, and 500-mg tablets. Dosage must be individualized, and optimal dosage may not be achieved before 6 to 8 weeks of therapy. Average daily dosage range appears to be 4 to 8 g in three or more divided doses given with food. Constant observation and dosage adjustment are needed.

Side effects and toxic effects. Numerous side effects occur in almost all patients receiving levodopa. *Gastrointestinal* side effects range from nausea, vomiting, and anorexia to bleeding, constipation, diarrhea, and abdominal distress.

Cardiovascular side effects include a variety of arrhythmias, orthostatic hypotension, palpitation, hypertension, and phlebitis.

Musculoskeletal side effects are numerous and include various involuntary muscular movements such as grimacing, jerky movements of the shoulders or pelvis, and rhythmic movements of the neck, hands, feet, mouth, and head. Opisthotonos may also occur.

A host of *psychologic* and *neurologic* side effects can occur. These include anxiety, confusion, depression, hallucinations, insomnia, paranoia, and suicidal tendencies. Ataxia, convulsions, headaches, tremors, weakness, and numbness also occur.

Respiratory, urinary, ocular, and *hematologic* disorders have also been reported.

Although many of the side effects are dose related and disappear after reduction of dosage, neurologic and psychologic side effects may persist for several months after reduction or discontinuance of the drug.

Precautions. Levadopa should be administered only with great caution to patients with almost any physiologic disorder with an organic basis. Evaluations of most body system functions (hepatic, cardiovascular, and so on) should be performed periodically. Levodopa is *not* recommended for children under 12 years of age, pregnant women, or nursing mothers.

Drug interactions. Monoamine oxidase inhibitors and other sympathomimetic drugs will increase the adrenergic effect of levodopa. Antihypertensive and antianxiety drugs that block adrenergic receptors will decrease the therapeutic effect of levodopa. Pyridoxine also decreases the effects of levodopa by promoting its peripheral decarboxylation.

Levodopa carbidopa combination (Sinemet)

When levodopa is administered, most of it is decarboxylated to dopamine by extracerebral tissues, and dopamine does not penetrate into the central nervous system. To prevent this wasteful peripheral metabolism, levodopa has been combined with a decarboxylase inhibitor, carbidopa, under the trade name Sinemet. Carbidopa does not cross the blood-brain barrier,

so it does not interfere with the intracerebral transformation of levopoda to dopamine.

Carbidopa administered alone has no pharmacodynamic effects; it is indicated only in combination with levodopa. When a patient has been maintained with levodopa alone and carbidopa is to be added, the following directions must be followed. The levodopa should be discontinued 8 hours before the combined therapy is initiated. The two drugs are then administered at the same time, with the dosage of levodopa reduced to 20% to 25% of the previous dosage. This simultaneous administration produces greater urinary levodopa excretion in proportion to the dopamine excretion than would administration of the two drugs at separate times. The maximal daily dose of carbidopa generally does not exceed 200 mg. Titration with carbidopa alone is useful in reducing nausea and vomiting in patients receiving fixed combinations of carbidopa and levodopa.

Levodopa is the metabolic precursor of dopamine. It does cross the blood-brain barrier and presumably is converted to dopamine in the basal ganglia. It is thought that levodopa relieves the symptoms of Parkinson's disease by this mechanism.

Administered orally, levodopa is rapidly converted to dopamine in extracerebral tissues, and a small amount is transported unchanged to the central nervous system. The large doses needed for adequate effects produce nausea and other adverse reactions attributable to dopamine formation in extracerebral tissues. Carbidopa inhibits decarboxylation of levodopa in extracerebral tissues, making more levodopa available for transport to the brain. Carbidopa reduces the amount of levodopa needed by 75% to 80%, and when the two drugs are administered together, the plasma levels and plasma half-life of levodopa increase and the plasma and urinary dopamine and homovanillic acid levels decrease.

Pyridoxine hydrochloride (vitamin B_6) in oral doses of 10 to 25 mg may reverse the effects of levodopa by increasing the rate of aromatic acid decarboxylation. Carbidopa, however, inhibits this action of pyridoxine.

This combination of levodopa and carbidopa is indicated in the treatment of symptoms of idiopathic Parkinson's disease, postencephalitic parkinsonism, and symptomatic parkinsonism from injury to the nervous system by carbon monoxide intoxication and manganese intoxication; in reducing doses of levodopa that may cause nausea and vomiting; in providing a more rapid individual drug dosage titration with a smoother response; and for use with supplemental pyridoxine. Patients with markedly irregular ("on-off") responses to levodopa have not been shown to benefit from the combination.

The nurse need not be as concerned about pyridoxine-containing foods with this combination drug as with levodopa alone because carbidopa prevents the reversal of levodopa effects caused by pyridoxine. The combination drug can therefore be administered to patients receiving supplemental pyridoxine. The most common side effect is nausea; other adverse effects include cardiac irregularities, palpitations, orthostatic hypotensive episodes, bradykinetic episodes (the "on-off" phenomenon, described later), anorexia, vomiting, and dizziness. Carbidopa does not lower adverse reaction to the central nervous system effects of levodopa. Because more levodopa is allowed to reach the brain, certain central nervous system effects (involuntary movements or dyskinesias owing to increased formation of dopamine in brain) may occur at lower dosages and faster during therapy with this combination than with levodopa alone, particularly when nausea and vomiting are not dose-limiting factors. A dosage reduction may be needed if dyskinesias occur. Blepharospasm (tonic spasm almost closing the eyelids) is a useful early sign of excess dosage.

This combination must not be given to a patient receiving monoamine oxidase inhibitors because of a potential substantial increase in blood pressure; the monoanine oxidase inhibitors must be discontinued at least 14 days before therapy. Since levodopa may activate a malignant melanoma, it should be avoided in patients with undiagnosed skin lesions or melanoma history. Mental changes observed include paranoid ideation, psychotic episodes, depression, and dementia. Laboratory values are affected depending on the test used. During long-term therapy a positive Coombs test may occur. Elevated uric acid levels are seen with a colorimetric test and not with uricase methods. Using a copper reduction method a false-positive test occurs and a false-negative with glucose oxidase when testing for urine glucose. Additionally, lower levels of blood urea nitrogen, creatinine and uric acid levels are seen with the carbidopa levodopa combination therapy than with levodopa alone.

The "on-off" phenomenon is seen in patients previously controlled with levodopa for sustained periods who suddenly experience rigidity, akinesia, and tremor, most frequently in lower extremities and thus affecting walking. This is an extremely distressing change to the patient, and its possibility should be described to the patient who is receiving this therapy. This effect may last from an hour to almost all the patient's waking hours, as though the patient had received no therapy at all. This unpredictable "off" response is followed by the "on" period at equally abrupt and unpredictable times. Various explanations have been offered for this "on-off" phenomenon: alterations in intestinal absorption, peripheral decarboxylation of dopa, changes in dopamine receptor sensitivity, and lower plasma levels of levodopa. Long-term levodopa therapy is characterized by increasingly frequent "on-off" episodes.

Preparation, dosage, and administration. Sinemet 10/100 tablets contain 10 mg of carbidopa and 100 mg of levodopa (1:10 ratio); Sinemet 25/250 tablets contain 25 mg of carbidopa and 250 mg of levodopa; and Sinemet 25/100 tablets contain 25 mg of carbidopa and 100 mg of levodopa (1:4 ratio). Carbidopa is available in 25-mg tablets (Lodosyn). The optimal dosage must be determined by careful trial. When the patient is being treated with levodopa, the drug must be discontinued at least 8 hours before Sinemet treatment is started in the morning. Dosage may be initiated with one tablet of Sinemet 10/100 three times a day. Dosage may be increased by one tablet every day or every other day until a total daily dose of six tablets is reached. For patients who have been receiving levodopa, a dosage of Sinemet may be chosen that contains 25% of the total daily dose of levodopa. Although it may be necessary to increase the dose of Sinemet gradually, a total daily dose of eight 25/250 or 25/100 tablets should not be exceeded due to limited clinical experiences with larger doses of carbidopa.

Side effects and precautions. The most common adverse reaction that follows the administration of Sinemet is related to involuntary movements, which may be choreiform or dystonic. Mental changes that include paranoidal ideas, suicidal tendencies, depression, and dementia have also been encountered. Nausea, cardiac irregularities, anorexia, hypotension, and dizziness may also occur. Sinemet should be used cautiously for patients receiving antihypertensive therapy or for those with narrow-angle glaucoma. Phenothiazines and butyrophenones may reduce the therapeutic effectiveness of levodopa. Levodopa's therapeutic effect may be reversed by phenytoin and papaverine.

DOPAMINERGIC AGONIST
Bromocriptine (Parlodel)

The approved uses of this drug are in amenorrhea, galactorrhea, and prevention of postpartum lactation (secretion, congestion, and engorgement). Published data indicate the effectiveness of this drug in Parkinson's disease and acromegaly.

Bromocriptine's action as a dopamine agonist is the focus of its use in parkinsonism. It reduces tremor and rigidity, and slightly reduces bradykinesia. It decreases the severity and frequency of fluctuations in the "on-off" phenomenon but not the continuation of such episodes. The abnormal involuntary movements are reduced. Mental alterations (visual and auditory hallucinations and delusions with personality changes) and orthostatic hypotension are more intense than seen with levodopa and carbidopa combinations. The role of bromocriptine in parkinsonism needs additional extensive and well-controlled studies. As an adjunct (in doses of 60 to 100 mg/day) to the treatment, it permits a reduced dosage or withdrawal of levodopa and some improvement in some patients.

Bromocriptine is a peptide ergot alkaloid derivative marketed as the first agonist of dopamine receptor activity. It activates postsynaptic dopamine receptors. Bromocriptine has been approved for use in short-term (6 months) treatment of amenorrhea/galactorrhea associated with hyperprolactinemia. It presumably acts as a dopamine receptor to inhibit prolactin secretion by the anterior pituitary acidophils.

Bromocriptine is highly (90% to 96%) protein bound and poorly absorbed (28%) from the gastrointestinal tract because of the first-pass effect of the liver (6% reaches systemic circulation); hepatic metabolism renders it inactive.

The major route of excretion of the absorbed portion of the drug is the bile; less than 5.5% is excreted in the urine, whereas about 85% of the total dose is found in the feces within 120 hours.

Side effects and precautions. Adverse reactions include nausea, headache, dizziness, fatigue, abdominal cramps, light-headedness, vomiting, nasal congestion, painful vasospasm in extremities, constipation, diarrhea, diuresis, altered behavior, and hallucinations. These dose-related reactions are generally mild to moderate. Since this drug may result in a restoration of fertility, the use of a contraceptive measure should be included in the nurse's cautions to patients; a mechanical barrier device should be suggested rather than oral contraceptives because estrogen oral contraceptives increase the risk of stimulating prolactin-secreting cells. Contraceptive measures may be coupled with pregnancy tests not less than every 4 weeks during therapy. The indication for female infertility is 2.5 mg twice daily up to three or four times daily, based on prolactin levels. The hypotensive effect may be decreased with a reduced dosage, and bromocriptine should be used cautiously with patients receiving drugs known to have hypotensive action. Additionally, diuretics and phenothiazines should be avoided during therapy with bromocriptine.

Dosage. The 2.5-mg tablet(s) are administered with meals two to three times daily, with a low initial dosage (2.5 mg daily) that is increased to the therapeutic range within the first week of therapy to ameliorate the adverse reactions.

Summary of nursing considerations

Skeletal muscle cells or fibers are long and thin with cross striations. Nerve impulses passing along motor nerves cause the muscle fibers to shorten, and the muscle contracts. In the absence of nerve impulses the muscle relaxes. This state is called *flaccidity*. When the motor nerve is nonfunctional, individual muscle fibers may twitch and cause *fasciculation*.

The area where a motor nerve fiber makes functional contact with a skeletal muscle fiber is called the neuromuscular junction. Acetylcholine (ACh) bridges the gap between the neuron and the motor end-plate of the muscle fiber. ACh is formed in the motor nerve cell and released after depolarization of the presynaptic membrane. Depolarization spreads from the motor end-plate to the entire muscle fiber, and the muscle contracts. Shortly after its release ACh is destroyed by the enzyme cholinesterase, allowing the next nerve impulse to be effective.

Skeletal muscle relaxants are of three types: (1) centrally acting relaxants, (2) direct acting muscle relaxants, and (3) neuromuscular blocking agents.

Centrally acting skeletal muscle relaxants are of the greatest benefit in relieving acute muscle spasm of local origin. Used as adjuncts to physiotherapy in sprains, strains, or trauma to ligaments, they often accompany the administration of salicylates and adrenal corticosteroids in the treatment of inflammatory joint disorders. Their exact mechanism of action is not known; however, they affect central pathways and neuronal systems that control tone and movement of muscles, producing relaxation of striated muscle spasm by depression of the central nervous system.

The most common centrally acting skeletal muscle relaxants are baclofen, diazepam, carisoprodol, chlorphenesin carbamate, chlorzoxazone, metaxalone, methocarbamol, and cyclobenzaprine. The side effects, usually mild and transient, are drowsiness, dizziness, blurred vision, headache, and feelings of weakness, lassitude, and lethargy. Large doses have caused nausea, vomiting, and other gastrointestinal complications. Chlorzoxazone and metaxalone have been reported to cause jaundice.

The *direct acting skeletal muscle relaxant* dantrolene is used for the symptomatic treatment of skeletal muscle spasm caused by multiple sclerosis, spinal cord injury, cerebral palsy, and

stroke. The injectable form of dantrolene is available for use in malignant hyperthermia. Its exact mechanism of action is not fully understood; however, it does produce generalized mild weakness of skeletal muscles and decreases the force of reflex muscle contractions, clonus, muscle stiffness, spasticity, and involuntary movements. Side effects include drowsiness, malaise, nausea, dizziness, diarrhea, and light-headedness. Its safety in pregnancy or in children under 5 years of age has not been established.

Neuromuscular blocking agents are classified as (1) nondepolarizing, or competitive, and (2) depolarizing. These potent drugs are used to produce adequate muscle relaxation during anesthesia, facilitate endotracheal intubation, aid in the management of tetanus, and decrease muscular activity in electroshock therapy. Side effects include interference with respiratory function, residual muscle weakness, and hypersensitivity reactions. Many of these drugs cause hypotension.

Nondepolarizing neuromuscular blocking agents, also referred to as the curariform drugs, cause skeletal muscle relaxation by occupying the cholinergic receptor sites and preventing ACh from acting on these receptors. Their blockade of receptor sites is (1) antagonized by depolarizing agents, (2) reversed by anticholinesterase, and (3) intensified or prolonged by ether anesthesia. Their actions, effects, and antagonists are summarized in Table 10-2. These drugs include tubocurarine, metocurine iodide, and pancuronium. Gallamine triethiodide is a synthetic compound whose action, uses, drug interactions, and contraindications resemble those of the curare drugs. However, it has no effect on autonomic ganglia, does not cause bronchospasm, and affords great flexibility because of its rapid onset and short duration of action. *Antagonists of curariform drugs* are used to terminate the effects of curariform agents when muscular relaxation is no longer desired or to reverse respiratory muscle paralysis caused by overdosage. These include edrophonium and neostigmine.

Depolarizing neuromuscular blocking agents produce more prolonged depolarization of the motor end-plate than ACh because of their high affinity for ACh receptors and their slower inactivation by cholinesterase. These drugs include succinylcholine, hexafluorenium bromide, and decamethonium bromide. Succinylcholine is believed to be an almost ideal muscle relaxant, ultrashort acting, with low toxicity. Large doses produce respiratory depression, and there is no effective antagonist. Hexafluorenium is used only to prolong the action of succinylcholine, but it should not be used for patients with bronchial asthma. Decamethonium is a potent, short-acting drug that is seldom used because tachyphylaxis frequently occurs and no satisfactory antidote is known.

Myasthenia gravis is a neuromuscular disease that is characterized by a defect in transmission of impulses at the neuromuscular junction. It has been suggested that this disorder is caused by an autoimmune mechanism whereby the plasma antibodies reduce the number of receptors needed for acetylcholine to act on the muscle. In this instance the receptor acts as the antigen. Symptomatic control of myasthenia gravis involves the use of *anticholinesterase drugs* that permit sufficient acetylcholine to accumulate at the receptors of the motor endplate to activate muscle contraction. Neostigmine, edrophonium, and pyridostigmine are anticholinesterase agents used for the symptomatic relief of myasthenia gravis.

Antiparkinsonism drugs are administered to provide maximal relief of symptoms and to maintain some independence of movement. Parkinsonism is believed to result from an imbalance between cholinergic and dopaminergic mechanisms in the central nervous system. Drug therapy consists of (1) anticholinergic drugs to inhibit the cholinergic mechanisms, (2) antihistaminic drugs that also have anticholinergic action, and (3) levodopa to replenish dopamine levels and enhance the dopaminergic mechanisms.

Levodopa is the most effective drug available for relieving all major symptoms of parkinsonism. However, its multiple physical and psychologic side effects mandate caution in its administration and long-term use. It is *not* recommended for children under 12 years of age, pregnant women, or nursing mothers.

Amantadine is a synthetic antiviral drug, producing more rapid clinical improvement than levodopa in the treatment of parkinsonism with fewer untoward reactions. Its side effects are many, particularly in elderly patients; epileptics; psychotics; those with liver, kidney, cerebrovascular or cardiac disease; and pregnant women.

QUESTIONS

FOR STUDY AND REVIEW

1 Explain the differences in action and uses between the centrally acting skeletal muscle relaxants and the neuromuscular blocking agents.
2 What drugs potentiate the action of tubocurarine?
3 What drugs inhibit the action of tubocurarine?
4 Compare the pharmacologic action of tubocurarine with that of succinylcholine.
5 Through library research do a historical study of curare.
6 What group of drugs is used for the symptomatic relief of myasthenia gravis? How does it improve muscle contraction?
7 Name the classes of drugs used to treat Parkinson's disease.
8 What advantage does the use of Sinemet have over levodopa?
9 What instructions concerning diet should the nurse give to a patient who is taking levodopa?

BIBLIOGRAPHY

AMA drug evaluations, ed. 4, New York, 1980, John Wiley & Sons, Inc.
Baily, E.V., and Stone, T.W.: The mechanism of action of amantadine in parkinsonism: a review, Arch. Int. Pharmacol. **216:**246, 1975.
Barbeau, A.: Long-term assessment of levodopa therapy in Parkinson's disease, Can. Med. Assoc. J. **112:**1379, 1975.
Colquhoun, D.: Mechanisms of drug action at the voluntary muscle endplate, Annu. Rev. Pharmacol. **15:**307, 1975.
Editoral: Dopa decarboxylate inhibitors, Br. Med. J. **4:**250, 1974.
Feldman, S.A.: Muscle relaxants, Philadelphia, 1973, W.B. Saunders Co.
Galindo, A.: Depolarizing neuromuscular block, J. Pharmacol. Exp. Ther. **178:**339, 1971.
Goodman, L.S., and Gilman, A.: Pharmacological basis of therapeutics, ed. 6, New York, 1980, Macmillan Publishing Co., Inc.
Goth, A.: Medical pharmacology: principles and concepts, ed. 10, St. Louis, 1981, The C.V. Mosby Co.
Greenblatt, D.J., and Shader, R.I.: Anticholinergics, N. Engl. J. Med. **288:**1215, 1973.
Markham, C.H., and others: Parkinson's disease and levodopa: a five-year follow-up and review, West. J. Med. **121:**188, 1974.
Modell, W.: Drugs of choice, 1980-1981, St. Louis, 1980, The C.V. Mosby Co.
Monks, P.S.: The reversal of non-depolarizing relaxants, Anesthesia, **27:**313, 1972.

Sweet, R.D., and McDowell, F.H.: Five years' treatment of Parkinson's disease with levodopa, Ann. Intern. Med. **83:**456, 1975.

Wagner, S.L.: The management of Parkinson's syndrome, Med. Clin. North Am. **56:**693, 1972.

Walker, J.E., and others: Amantadine and levodopa in the treatment of Parkinson's disease, Clin. Pharmacol. Ther. **13:**28, 1972.

Yahr, M.D.: The treatment of parkinsonism, Med. Clin. North Am. **56:**1377, 1972.

Yahr, M.D.: Levodopa, Ann. Intern. Med. **83;**677, 1975.

Young, R.R., and Delwaide: Drug therapy spasity, N. Engl. J. Med. **308:**28, 1981.

UNIT FOUR

DRUGS ACTING ON THE CENTRAL NERVOUS SYSTEM AFFECTING MOOD AND BEHAVIOR

CHAPTER 11

Psychotherapeutic drugs

Anatomy and physiology of emotions

To understand the action of drugs in alleviating the symptoms of mental illness, the nurse must have knowledge of the functioning of the nervous system. The trend in nursing toward a holistic view of human beings and their phenomenologic experience no longer allows the practitioner to separate the functions of the mind from the body. Neurophysiologists have traditionally identified each part of the nervous system by a specific function or made tentative architectonic maps of the cerebral cortex, allocating specific functions to various areas of the brain. Recent research has indicated a change in this perspective. The brain is considered to be a single organ composed of various structures that produce a final unified effect when they react on each other in a normal fashion. The interrelationship of various structures is extremely intricate, and it is difficult to allo-

cate special functions to each structure. Papez in 1937 was one of the first to suggest the function of a reverberating circuit in the brain as an explanation of emotional experience. Research has revealed methods for measuring certain types of brain activity, and such information has made it possible to speculate in some detail on the physiologic substrates of emotional activity. For purposes of clarity in the discussion of the neuroanatomic and neurophysiologic bases of emotions, the various aspects of the nervous system are discussed under the following headings:
1. Central nervous system
2. Autonomic regulation
3. Biochemical mechanisms

CENTRAL NERVOUS SYSTEM

The central nervous system functions in the coordination and direction of activities in the tissues and organs of the body. The various parts and levels of the central nervous system form a closely related and integrated series of mechanisms and systems through which the human being achieves adjustment and adaptation to the environment. The central nervous system is responsible for consciousness, behavior, memory, recognition, learning, and the more highly developed attributes of human beings such as imagination, abstract reasoning, and creative thought. In addition, it serves to coordinate such vital regulatory functions as blood pressure, heart rate, respiration, salivary, and gastric secretions, muscular activity, and body temperature. Discussion is limited to consideration of the functions of the central nervous system that are believed to affect the emotions and behavior.

The cerebrum, the largest part of the brain, is divided into two hemispheres. The outer surface of the cerebral hemispheres is composed of gray matter known as the cerebral cortex. It is believed to be the site of consciousness and is divided into sensory, motor, and association areas. These areas receive sensations from organs of special sense (sight, hearing, smell, and taste) as well as from the skin, muscles, joints, and tendons (touch, pain, and temperature). Large parts of the cortex now appear to function as a whole in providing the anatomic basis for such mental attributes as recognition, memory, intelligence, imagination, and creative thought.

Beneath the cortex are tracts of fibers comprising the white matter, which connect the lower centers of the brain, spinal cord, and associated areas of the cortex with each other. The basal ganglia (corpus striatum, claustrum, and amygdaloid nucleus) are located near the lateral ventricle of the cerebrum. The hippocampus, a mass of gray matter lying close to the lateral ventricle, is connected by a tract of fibers (the fornix) to the mamillary bodies in the hypothalamus. The hippocampus, the fornix, the amygdaloid nucleus, the hippocampal gyrus, and the uncus are collectively referred to as the limbic system. This system is believed to be concerned with the conscious experience of emotion.

The midbrain, pons, and medulla form the part of the brain below the cerebrum. The midbrain contains the nuclei of cranial nerves III and IV. The pons is mainly a pathway for ascending and descending tracts of the fibers. The medulla oblongata is continuous with the spinal cord. It contains vital groups of synapses that are concerned with the reflex control of blood pressure (vasomotor center), heart rate and force (cardiac center), respiration (respiratory center), and vomiting (vomiting center). The reticular formation consists of a complex network of cell bodies and interlacing fibers in the medulla, pons, midbrain, and diencephalon. The reticular activating system (Fig. 11-1) is believed to function in alerting the cortex to sensory stimuli and in originating the emotional reactions associated with somatic sensory experiences (pain, touch, hearing, sight). Experimental stimulation of this system produces alertness in behavior, whereas a decrease in its activity leads to relaxation and drowsiness. The reticular activating system has its upper end in the posterior hypothalamus and lower thalamus.

The cerebellum lies on the dorsal side of the pons and is attached to the brainstem. It functions as part of the feedback mechanisms concerned with subconscious control of equilibrium, posture, and movement.

The thalamus and hypothalamus are located in the region of the brain that is called the diencephalon (the "between-brain"). Most sensations are relayed through the thalamus to the cerebral cortex. The conscious appreciation of pain is said to be located in the thalamus. In recent years there has been a gradual increase of knowledge relative to the functions of the hypothalamus. Despite extensive research and experimentation there still seems to be some question of its specific mode of function. It has been conjectured that the hypothalamus contains integrative mechanisms that, in addition to their effect on behavior patterns, also aid in regulating the basic human life functions (control of water excretion, appetite, sleep-wake mechanisms, temperature, and blood pressure). The hypothalamus seems to function through its relationships with other parts of the

FIG. 11-1. Reticular activating system.

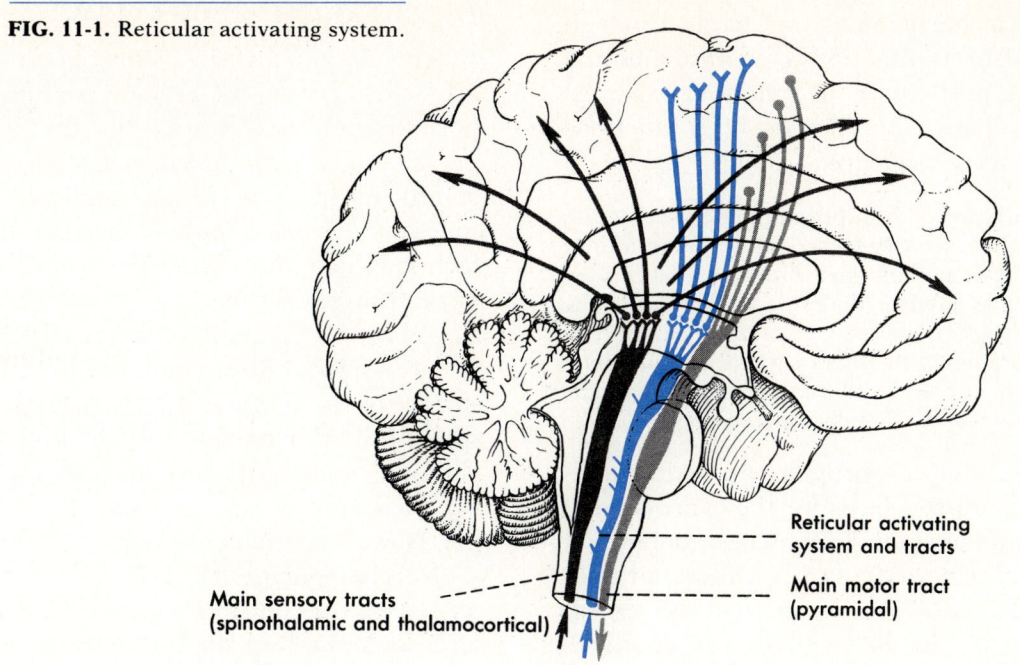

Reticular activating
system and tracts

Main motor tract
(pyramidal)

Main sensory tracts
(spinothalamic and thalamocortical)

FIG. 11-2. Papez circuit and the limbic system.

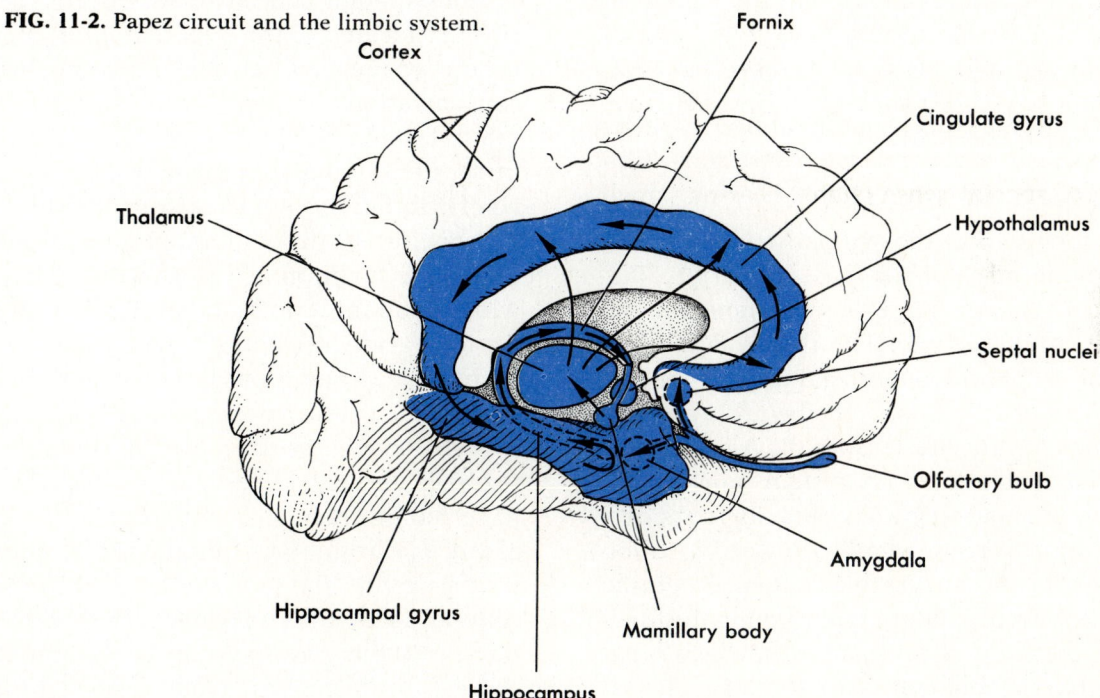

Cortex

Fornix

Cingulate gyrus

Thalamus

Hypothalamus

Septal nuclei

Olfactory bulb

Amygdala

Hippocampal gyrus

Mamillary body

Hippocampus

nervous system and endocrine system. It is part of a system of complex circuits within the brain so strategically placed that its derangement may have profound effects. These interrelationships between cerebral cortex, thalamus, hypothalamus, and various other circuits in the brain produce patterns of behavior that are modifiable by situations and autonomic adjustments to adapt the individual to changes in both external and internal environments.

Papez proposed that "the hypothalamus, the anterior thalamic nuclei, the gyrus cingulum, the hippocampus, and their interconnections constitute a harmonious mechanism which may elaborate the functions of central emotion as well as participate in emotional expression."* The Papez circuit (Fig. 11-2) functions in the following sequence:

> On stimulation of the hippocampus this structure relays impulses via the fornix to the mammillary bodies of the hypothalamus. From that area they continue to the anterior thalamic nuclei and to the cingulate gyrus of the cerebral cortex. The functional circuit is completed by fibers leaving the cingulate gyrus by way of the cingulum and returning to the hippocampus via the hippocampal gyrus.*

This proposed circuit provides an understanding of the anatomic basis for the expression of emotion and behavior. The intricate balance of positive and negative controls leads to a better conceptualization of the function of the central nervous system in the regulation of emotions and behavioral patterns in human beings. There is increasing evidence that these areas of the central nervous system have some control over behavior and emotions; however, at best, these data have been superficial, inconclusive, and merely theoretical.

AUTONOMIC REGULATIONS

The functions of the sympathetic and parasympathetic visceral nervous system are discussed in Chapter 13. The importance of the reactions of these systems in the production of behavior is paramount in gaining an understanding of drug action or the behavioral manifestations of side effects from the use of drugs. Since the central nervous system functions in the regulation of integrated behavior, considerable effort has been extended toward locating and defining the integrative centers. Scientific evidence is accumulating for grouping the functions of the subcortical systems into two separate and antagonistic divisions. Two such systems have been identified in the hypothalamus and have been labeled the "ergotropic division" and the "trophotropic system." Much of the work in defining and locating these divisions is based on the behavioral and physiologic responses elicited by their stimulation.

*Marks, J.: Scientific basis of drug therapy, New York, 1965, Pergamon Press, Inc., p. 5.

BIOCHEMICAL MECHANISMS

The functions of the central nervous system are dependent on the actions of certain neurohormonal agents located in the brain and peripheral tissues. These neurohormones are stored in inactive forms, and at the right moment nerve impulses release their free forms, which then stimulate transmission of appropriate reactions.

There is evidence that acetylcholine is released from central neural tissue, such as the surface of the cerebral cortex, into the cerebrospinal fluid during activity. The rate of release is proportional to the level of activity. Thus it is known that some central synapses are cholinergic. However, others are not.

Norepinephrine has also been found to be present in the central nervous system. Tyrosine and dopamine are normal constituents of the brain and known precursors of norepinephrine synthesis. High concentrations of norepinephrine are located in the hypothalamus, medulla, limbic system, and cranial nerve nuclei. Low concentrations of norepinephrine are found in the striatum and caudate nucleus where dopamine, the immediate precursor of norepinephrine, is found in high concentration (Fig. 11-3). It is believed that both norepinephrine and dopamine function as transmitters. They have widespread inhibitory and excitatory effects on a wide variety of centrally mediated functions such as sleep and arousal, affect, and memory. Thus some central synapses are adrenergic.

Serotonin is another transmitter substance found in the central nervous system. Areas rich in serotonin include the hypothalamus, pineal gland, midbrain, and spinal cord. Serotonin is synthesized in the brain and stored in the subcellular particles. Alteration of the level of serotonin in the nervous system is associated with changes in behavior. Many drugs mimic or block the action of serotonin on peripheral tissues and produce changes in mood and behavior, which suggests that they interfere with the action of serotonin and norepinephrine in the brain.

Other proposed central neurotransmitters include histamine, amino acids (such as glutamate, glycine, excitatory transmitters, aspartate, and GABA), Substance P (a polypeptide

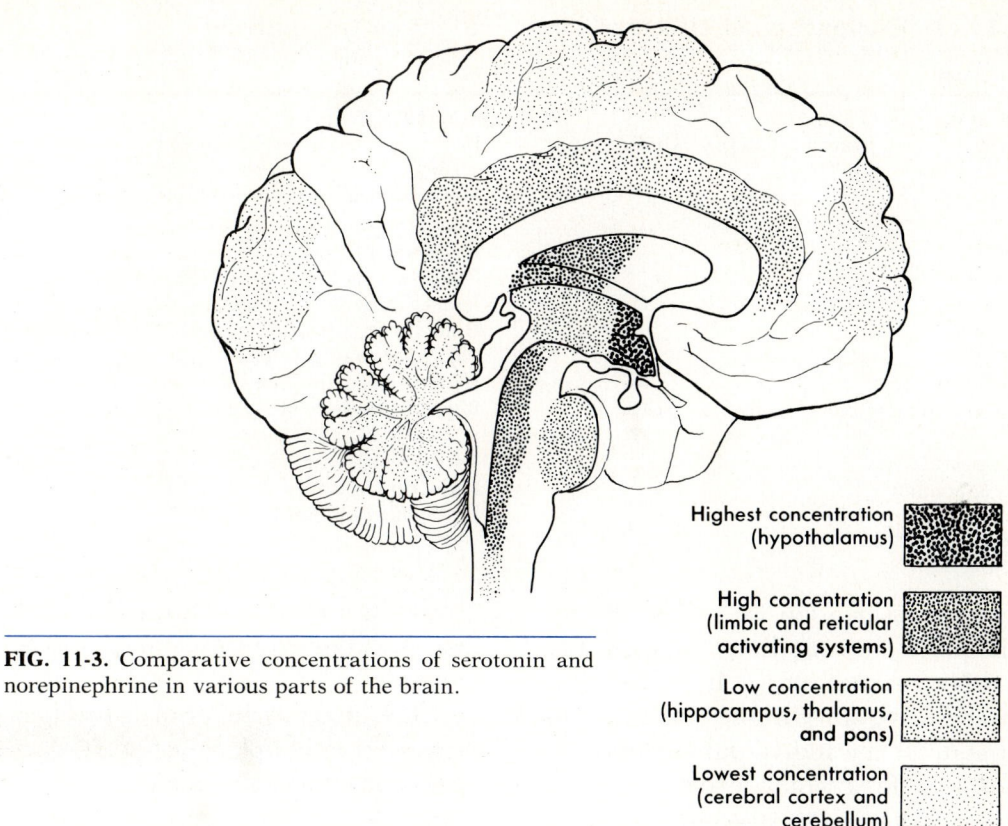

Highest concentration
(hypothalamus)

High concentration
(limbic and reticular
activating systems)

Low concentration
(hippocampus, thalamus,
and pons)

Lowest concentration
(cerebral cortex and
cerebellum)

FIG. 11-3. Comparative concentrations of serotonin and norepinephrine in various parts of the brain.

composed of 13 different amino acids), prostaglandins, and the endorphins. The relationship of dopamine to major psychoses is receiving much attention. Drugs such as the phenothiazines block the effects of dopamine and function as antipsychotic agents.

Role of drug therapy in psychiatry

Drugs play an important role in contemporary approaches to psychiatric care. The development of the tranquilizing drugs opened many avenues of treatment that were not available before. Although emphasis in therapy is placed on milieu factors by many workers in the field, drug therapy is a valuable adjunct to providing comprehensive psychiatric care. The effect of drug therapy in psychiatric illness can be neither ignored nor overestimated. Because the use of the psychotropic drugs is not presently thought of as a "cure," consideration is given to the patient's total life situation as an important determinant of his health status. The use of drugs alleviates symptoms and allows the

patient an opportunity to participate more easily in other forms of treatment. Drugs temporarily modify behavior, whereas other therapies, such as psychotherapy, can shape behavior and produce a permanent change. Some drugs disrupt patterns of behavior or modify the electric patterns or fields within the brain that produce changes. However, any enduring effects on behavior are more likely to result from the individual's concurrent interaction with the environment. Since incoming information must be translated into biochemical changes before it can affect the nervous system function, environmental transactions, like drugs, may affect similar pathways before influencing behavior. Their effects can be additive, potentiating, or antagonistic, depending on their nature and direction. The milieu may potentiate the effectiveness of the drug or detract from it.

In the treatment of emotional disorders two major drug groups discussed in this chapter that comprise the classification of psychotherapeutic drugs are the *tranquilizers* and the *mood modifiers*. The drugs used in psychotherapeu-

TABLE 11-1 Comparison of effects of major and minor tranquilizers

Major tranquilizers	Minor tranquilizers
Antipsychotic effect	Antianxiety effect
Depress activity of lower brain centers (e.g., vomiting center): antiemetic effect	Do not depress lower brain centers; significance antiemetic effect
Extrapyramidal effects (e.g., tremors and spasticity)	No extrapyramidal effects: tend to produce general muscular relaxation
Autonomic effects	No autonomic effects
Monophasic effect	Biphasic effect: small doses tend to produce a euphoric state; large doses tend to produce a sedative effect
Low abuse potential	High abuse potential
No tolerance	Tolerance may develop
No withdrawal syndrome	Withdrawal symptoms can occur
Suppress active avoidance behavior but not escape response	Suppress both avoidance behavior and escape response
No anticonvulsive activity	Anticonvulsive activity
No reduction of conflict	Reduction of conflict
Depress general motor activity	Little effect on motor activity

tics and their classification are presented on p. 307. The term "tranquilizer" reflects the action of this group of drugs in effecting a change toward tranquility in the affective and behavioral state of the individual. Tranquilizers have a direct effect on the levels of anxiety that create a pathologic adjustment to intrapersonal and interpersonal experiences. Anxiety is reduced without subsequent impairment of consciousness, and overt behavior, perception, mood, and hyperactivity are controlled. The delusions, hallucinations, and confusion associated with psychopathology are decreased to a tolerable level. The tranquilizers were commonly classified as *major* and *minor* tranquilizers. The major tranquilizers are now referred to as "neuroleptics" or "ataractics" (from the Greek word *ataraktos* meaning "undisturbed" or "peace of mind"). The neuroleptics (major tranquilizers, ataractics) or "antipsychotic" agents are substances that affect psychotic symptoms and autonomic regulations. The anxiolytics (minor tranquilizers), or "antineurotic" agents, are substances that are characterized by their action in the relief of mild or moderate anxiety and that are not usually known to be effective as antipsychotic agents. The main therapeutic action of the anxiolytics seems to be in treatment of anxiety that accompanies neurotic symptoms. The anxiolytics do not evoke extrapyramidal symptoms such as tremor, rigidity, or dystonic reactions; they produce few autonomic symptoms and tend to

raise the convulsive threshold. Table 11-1 compares major and minor tranquilizers with one another.

The mood modifier drug group has led to an effective psychopharmacologic treatment of depression states. The mood modifiers, also called "psychostimulants" or "psychic energizers" because of their stimulating and energy-producing action, have replaced some of the older drugs (amphetamine, caffeine) in the treatment of depressive states. The older drugs were found to cause a rise in blood pressure, increase in heart rate, and loss of appetite. Drugs such as the amphetamines are high-risk drugs for causing psychic dependency, which reduces their effectiveness for long-term treatment.

Another group of drugs, the psychotomimetics (hallucinogens and psychodysleptics) are included in this psychotherapeutic drug classification. This group of drugs is not given consideration in this discussion of the psychotherapeutic drugs since mechanism of action is not understood and their usefulness in the treatment of mental illness is still in the experimental stages. The action of these drugs has been known to mimic or produce psychotic states, and therefore they are sometimes called *hallucinogenic drugs*. The most publicized and best known of these drugs is lysergic acid diethylamide (LSD). These drugs cause initial autonomic disturbances (tachycardia, dilation of the pupil, tightness in the chest and abdomen,

Psychotherapeutic drugs

Tranquilizers
Antianxiety (anxiolytic) agents—minor tranquilizers
Benzodiazepines
Chlordiazepoxide hydrochloride (Librium, others)
Clorazepate dipotassium (Tranxene)
Clorazepate monopotassium (Azene)
Diazepam (Valium)
Lorazepam (Ativan)
Oxazepam (Serax)
Temazepam (Restoril)
Prazepam (Centrax)
Nonbenzodiazepines
Meprobamate
Tybamate (Tybatran)
Hydroxyzine hydrochloride (Atarax, Vistaril)
Doxepin hydrochloride (Adapin, Sinequan)
Chlormezanone (Trancopal Caplets)
Droperidol (Inapsine)
Antipsychotic (neuroleptic) agents—major tranquilizers
Phenothiazines
Aliphatic compounds
Chlorpromazine hydrochloride (Thorazine)
Triflupromazine hydrochloride (Vesprin)
Piperidine compounds
Thioridazine hydrochloride (Mellaril)
Mesoridazine besylate (Serentil)
Piperacetazine (Quide)
Trifluoperazine hydrochloride (Stelazine)
Acetophenazine dimaleate (Tindal)
Butaperazine dimaleate (Repoise)
Carphenazine dimaleate (Proketazine)
Fluphenazine hydrochloride (Permitil, Prolixin)
Perphenazine (Trilafon)
Prochlorperazine dimaleate (Compazine, various)
Thioxanthene derivatives
Chlorprothixene (Taractan)
Thiothixene hydrochloride (Navane)
Butyrophenone derivative
Haloperidol (Haldol)
Dibenzoxazepine derivative
Loxapine succinate (Daxolin, Loxitane)
Dihydroindolone derivative
Molindone hydrochloride
Diphenylbutylpiperidine derivative
Pimozide (Orap)
Mood modifiers
Antidepressants
Tricyclic antidepressants
Imipramine hydrochloride (Tofranil, others)
Amitriptyline hydrochloride (Elavil, others)
Desipramine hydrochloride (Norpramin, Pertofrane)
Doxepin hydrochloride (Adapin, Sinequan)
Nortriptyline hydrochloride (Aventyl, Pamelor)
Protriptyline hydrochloride (Vivactil)
Trimipramine maleate (Surmontil)
Monoamine oxidase inhibitors
Phenelzine (Nardil)
Isocarboxazid (Marplan)
Tranylcypromine sulfate (Parnate)
Antimanic agent
Lithium carbonate, citrate (Eskalith, others)
Drugs used in nonpsychotic mental disorders
Stimulants
Methylphenidate hydrochloride (Ritalin)
Pemoline (Cylert)
Amphetamines

and nausea) followed by vivid visual hallucinations, severe anxiety, and delusions. Use of these drugs is restricted to controlled experimental research because of the grave danger of irreversible sequelae.

SELECTION AND USE OF PSYCHOTHERAPEUTIC DRUGS

In the past, physicians selected psychotherapeutic agents on the basis of the diagnostic category—schizophrenia, manic-depressive syndrome, or psychoneurosis. More recent proposals have indicated a radical change in the physician's approach to selecting drugs for the mentally ill person. The pharmacologic treatment of psychiatric disorders would appear to be similar to that of somatic disorders—modifications of the most disabling components of the patient's behavior so that the patient may more effectively cope with his environment and take advantage of the therapeutic milieu available. It would seem more rational to deemphasize the diagnostic classifications of psychiatric disorders as a basis for drug selectivity and to consider instead the most disabling behavioral manifestations that can be observed. This implies a thorough assessment of the patient before the administration of drugs. This assessment should include the specific disabling features of the patient's behavior, a decision as to the goals of therapy, the dynamics involved, and the specific directional changes sought. Other factors helpful in making an accurate assessment of the patient's need for drug therapy are as follows:

1. Degree of agitation or behavioral arousal
2. Degree of overactivity or underactivity
3. Patterns of affective response to stress (avoidance or escape, aggression, fear, inhibited withdrawal)
4. Degree of social withdrawal
5. Nature and dynamics of depressive elements present
6. Sleep problems
7. Need for environmental control
8. Medical complaints
9. Possible drug dependence
10. Past drug history—effectiveness of response to drugs

When the physician establishes the need for drug therapy, it must be decided what agent or combination of agents is best suited for the behavioral and medical needs of the patient. Since there are many drugs available, it is judicious for the physician to become familiar with a few drugs rather than make a haphazard selection of several agents. This requires an intimate knowledge of the behavioral actions, the pharmacologic effects, and the potential adverse reactions of the agents used, as well as an awareness of the many individual and environment-related factors present. After selection of the agent or agents to be used, the dosage is increased until the desired and expected effects are produced. Continuous reevaluation based on observation of the effects of the drug selected is needed. Increase or reduction of dosage may be indicated to gain the desired effects. The nurse plays an important role in the evaluation and reassessment of a patient's response to drug therapy. It is important to be aware of the criteria the physician uses in selecting psychotherapeutic drugs and the expected effects so that the patient's progress may be observed and reported. Knowledge of the action of drugs also assists the nurse in understanding the interpersonal responses that take place in the therapeutic nurse-patient relationship.

Tranquilizers
Antianxiety (anxiolytic) agents— minor tranquilizers

Anxiolytics (minor tranquilizers), also known as antianxiety drugs, have been recommended for the treatment of symptoms associated with psychoneurotic and psychosomatic conditions. The advantage of their use in these conditions is their effect in allaying moderate anxiety states and the muscle tension associated with psychomotor agitation. Psychoneurotic conditions with severe disabling symptoms are treated more effectively with the stronger phenothiazine derivatives. In milder forms of psychoneuroses, the anxiolytics act as a valuable adjunct to psychotherapy by diminishing anxiety and tension associated with the treatment process. The anxiolytics are not recommended for the long-term treatment of psychotic conditions; however, large doses have been effective in controlling the psychomotor hyperexcitability of acute psychotic episodes. Chlordiazepoxide has been especially effective in treating hyperactive alcoholic patients with withdrawal reactions or delirium tremens. Most of the compounds in this group can be given alone or in conjunction with antispasmodics, analgesics, vasodilators, adrenal corticosteroids, and estrogens. They have been effective in relieving the symptoms of certain gastrointestinal, musculoskeletal, and cardiovascular disorders as well as menopausal discomforts. They differ in their sedative effects from barbiturates in that they do not produce a significant loss of mental acuity.

Chemical structure, site, and mechanism of action. The anxiolytics share similar central depressant action, but their secondary central and peripheral effects vary. They can be divided according to the following subgroups: (1)

TABLE 11-2 Secondary effects of some antianxiety agents

Generic name	Trade name	Side effects*
Benzodiazepine group		
Chlordiazepoxide	Librium, Libritabs	1-3, 6, 7, 9-11, 14, 16, 20, 22, 23, 25
Diazepam	Valium	1-3, 5, 7, 9-11, 16, 23, 27
Oxazepam	Serax	2, 3, 8-10, 16, 21
Lorazepam	Ativan	1-3, 5, 7, 8, 9, 11, 14, 16, 18, 20, 21, 23, 26, 27
Prazepam	Verstran	1-3, 4, 5, 7, 8, 11, 14, 15, 16, 18, 22
Clorazepate		
dipotassium	Tranxene	1-7, 16, 21-23
monopotassium	Azene	
Nonbenzodiazepine group		
Hydroxyzine	Atarax, Vistaril	2-5, 8, 13, 14, 17, 18
Meprobamate	Equanil, Miltown	1-4, 7, 8, 10, 11, 13, 15, 16, 18, 19, 22-24

Key to table

1. Anxiety or agitation	10. Jaundice	19. Activation of peptic ulcer
2. Sedation and sleep	11. Convulsive seizures	20. Decreased libido
3. Ataxia	12. Hypothermia	21. Depressive symptoms
4. Dry mouth	13. Antiemetic	22. Mental confusion
5. Blurred vision	14. Increased appetite	23. Dependence
6. Constipation	15. Edema	24. Hyperthermia
7. Dermatitis	16. Nausea or vomiting, or both	25. Menstrual irregularities
8. Hypotension	17. Bradycardia	26. Mydriasis
9. Blood dyscrasias	18. Increased gastric motility or diarrhea	27. Hallucinations

*Side effects here are not intended to be a complete account of all possible adverse reactions.

benzodiazepines and (2) nonbenzodiazepines. One action of these drugs that accounts for their anxiolytic response is their depressive effect on the polysynaptic reflexes of the spinal cord. This effect suggests that their main mode of action is that of reducing skeletal muscle tension, which indirectly reduces the number of afferent proprioceptive impulses aggravating existing anxiety.

These drugs are believed to exert very little effect, if any, on the neocortex and neurotransmitter centers. However, their anxiolytic action seems to parallel their depressant action on the limbic system structures (septum, amygdala, and hippocampus). Since it has been postulated that the amygdala and the hippocampus influence behavior, the action of anxiolytics may inhibit their stimulation and thus inhibit the subsequent behavioral responses that these organs regulate. A similar reduction of sensitivity brought about by the depressant effect of these drugs reduces reactions to stressful influences and stimuli. They have the ability to produce mild sedation without adversely affecting the level of consciousness or the quality of psychomotor performance.

Side effects and precautions. The anxiolytics are relatively safe when used in small dosages. Table 11-2 summarizes some of the most common side effects with antianxiety agents. They have fewer disabling side effects than the phenothiazine derivatives; however, numerous reports of untoward effects have appeared. Drowsiness, ataxia, dizziness, and headache occur occasionally after initial doses. Patients should be cautioned against driving an automobile, operating dangerous machinery, or performing tasks that require absolute precision, motor coordination, and mental alertness. Drowsiness, ataxia, and confusion are more commonly seen in the elderly. These reactions can be avoided when the dosage is gradually increased until the desired effects are produced. Some patients have been known to exhibit mild forms of inappropriate behavior that were not related to their current condition after initial doses. Other signs of drug hypersensitivity have been noted such as rash, fever, chills, nausea, vomiting, and dry mouth. Blood dyscrasias and jaundice have been reported occasionally. Some of these drugs are habit-forming, and withdrawal of the drug may cause mild to severe withdrawal reactions including delirium and convulsions. Caution should be taken to avoid dependence on these drugs. Physicians and nurses should maintain close supervision of individuals who are taking these drugs for prolonged periods, especially individuals who have a history of alcoholism, drug addiction, or severe dependency problems. Overdosage with massive amounts of these drugs produces coma, shock, and death. Patients with a history of blood dyscrasias, impaired renal function, hepatic disease, or allergies should be evaluated carefully before the administration of these drugs is initiated, even though there have been relatively few reports of adverse effects in these conditions. Use of any drug in pregnancy or lactation requires that the potential benefit of the drug be weighed against its possible hazards to mother and child.

Phenothiazine compounds and antidepressant drugs that potentiate the action of other drugs should not be used concomitantly with the anxiolytic agents.

Paradoxic reactions of rage, excitement, stimulation, hostility, confusion, and depersonalization have occurred when these agents have been administered to severely disturbed or psychotic patients.

BENZODIAZEPINES

Benzodiazepines are among the most widely prescribed drugs in clinical medicine. The popularity of these drugs probably results from the fact that their anxiolytic effects occur at nontoxic doses. Drowsiness and undesirable central nervous system depression occur less frequently with benzodiazepine agents than with comparable doses of meprobamate or barbiturates.

Effects. The site of anxiolytic activity appears to be the limbic system. Electrical discharges and transmission in the limbic system are inhibited by low doses of benzodiazepines that do not depress the rest of the brain and probably stimulate or antagonize the GABA (gamma-aminobutyric acid) effects in the central nervous system. Benzodiazepines have a disinhibiting effect; major tranquilizers do not produce disinhibition at any dosage level.

The limbic system, associated with the regulation of emotional behavior, contains a highly dense area of benzodiazepine receptors in the amygdala that may correspond to specific antianxiety action of certain drugs. These proposed benzodiazepine receptors may share some sites

of action with other drugs such as alcohol, meprobamate, and barbiturates and may further explain cross-tolerance to these drugs. The benzodiazepines' receptor concentration in the dorsal spinal cord may account for their muscle relaxant effect; there may also be an endogenous benzodiazepine-like substance. GABA, an inhibitory neurotransmitter, affects benzodiazepine receptors, and a benzodiazepine receptor may be a portion of a GABA receptor. Benzodiazepines enhance the action of GABA at its receptors. The identification of psychotropic drug receptors is leading to the discovery and understanding of the time and course of receptor site occupancy. This knowledge will allow more effective therapeutic use of the agents affecting mood and behavior and will further explain how the drugs exert their action in the neurotransmitter interaction within the central nervous system.

Benzodiazepines can precipitate hostility, rage, and physical violence. This paradoxic reaction may represent a disinhibition or release of "anxiety-bound" hostility. Fig. 11-4 shows shared metabolic routes of some selected parent benzodiazepines and metabolites.

Other effects of benzodiazepines include the following.

Muscle relaxation. The exact mechanism for this is unknown. The benzodiazepines probably have more than one site of muscle-relaxant activity.

Anticonvulsant effect. Benzodiazepines prevent or arrest generalized seizure activity caused by electric shock, systemic administration of analeptics, or local anesthetics. How the action occurs has not been established.

Circulation and respiration. Benzodiazepines even in large doses produce only minor circulatory and respiratory depression. Rapid intravenous injection of diazepam can cause transient bradycardia, hypotension, and apnea.

Clinical uses. Chlordiazepoxide, diazepam, and prazepam are long-acting compounds with pharmacologically active metabolites. More than two daily doses are seldom necessary. Clorazepate's metabolite, nordiazepam, also has a long duration of action. Many patients need only a single dose at bedtime for promotion of sleep at night and reduced anxiety during the day. If necessary, a second smaller dose can be

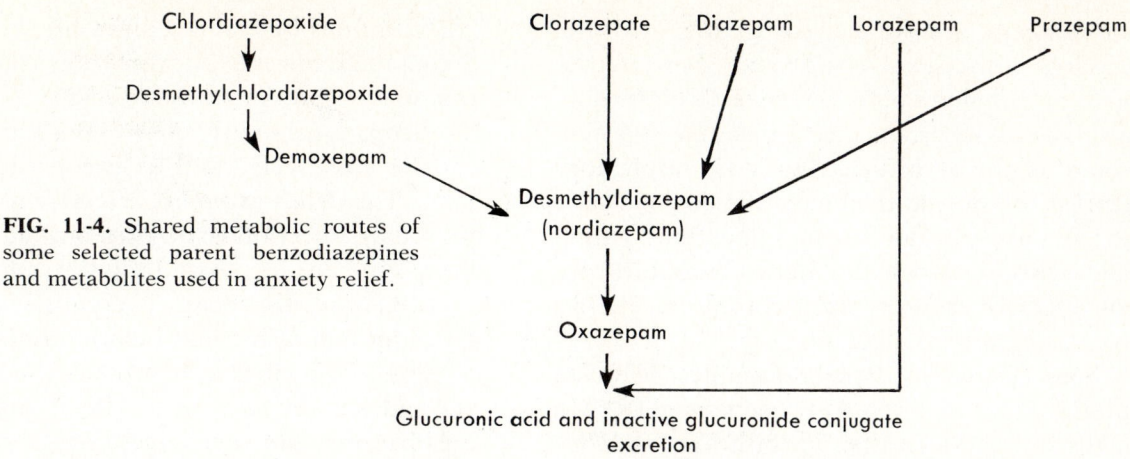

FIG. 11-4. Shared metabolic routes of some selected parent benzodiazepines and metabolites used in anxiety relief.

added during the day. This schedule is particularly useful for patients with sleep disturbances associated with anxiety.

Nurses need to know that even with single daily doses, the drugs or their metabolites can accumulate in the body after several days of therapy; therapeutic effects may not appear for 5 to 10 days after initiation of therapy, and clinical effects may persist for several days after termination of therapy. Oxazepam and lorazepam are more rapidly converted to inactive metabolites and therefore are short acting and nonaccumulating. Most patients need three or four daily doses of oxazepam.

The nurse should enforce compliance by having the patient adhere rigidly to the physician's dosing instructions.

Antianxiety drugs are most effective during short-term use, such as for periodic anxiety, but are ineffective or unnecessary when given continuously for months.

The anxiolytics are not to be prescribed for the management of anxiety or tension associated with the stress of daily life. Their indication is for the management of anxiety disorders or for short-term relief of the symptoms of anxiety. The concern that the benzodiazepines can cause psychologic or physical dependence in some patients when taken in higher than therapeutic doses and for long periods should be kept in mind.

The abrupt discontinuance of a benzodiazepine (5 to 10 mg two to four times daily for several months to years) may result in hallucinations, confusion, and seizures. It is prudent to gradually discontinue this drug under such circumstances after several months of therapy.

Emotional disorders. Benzodiazepines are used for patients with neurotic anxiety. They are also beneficial for patients with neurotic or reactive depression. They are not of value for treatment of schizophrenia; they have no specific effect in disordered thought of psychotic patients, and some schizophrenics appear to deteriorate from chronic treatment with chlordiazepoxide or diazepam.

Neuromuscular disease. Benzodiazepines produce partial relief of spasticity in patients with cerebral palsy, multiple sclerosis, parkinsonism, amyotrophic lateral sclerosis, cerebrovascular accident, or traumatic spinal cord lesions. Effective muscle-relaxant doses are relatively high for these conditions, and many patients experience drowsiness or sedation.

Diazepam is used extensively for acute, reversible musculoskeletal disorders, such as back strain and "slipped disk." It does not supplant the need for analgesics, local heat, and rest, but it is superior to other muscle-relaxant drugs such as methocarbamol and carisoprodol. It has also been used in treatment of tetanus.

Seizures. When intractable, repetitive seizures occur (status epilepticus), intravenous diazepam appears to be the drug of choice. It is effective for grand mal, petit mal, psychomotor, and myoclonic seizures. Diazepam given orally is of no value in the treatment of grand mal epilepsy. Clonazepam is useful in preventing petit mal seizures.

Alcohol withdrawal. Chlordiazepoxide and

chlorazopate are popular for treatment of the alcohol withdrawal syndrome. Benzodiazepines do not share potential hazards of the phenothiazines to produce seizures and hypotension or of the barbiturates to cause respiratory depression; nor do they have the noxious odor and serious injection site complications associated with paraldehyde. Benzodiazepines are not effective in preventing chronic alcoholics from returning to alcoholism.

Sleep disorders. Benzodiazepines seem to interfere less with rapid eye movement (REM), or dreaming, sleep than barbiturates and certain other hypnotics. REM rebound does not occur when the benzodiazepines are discontinued.

Benzodiazepines inhibit slow-wave, or deep, sleep and are being tested for their effectiveness to control somnambulism (sleep-walking), enuresis, and night terrors that occur during slow-wave sleep.

Flurazepam (Dalmane) is a benzodiazepine marketed specifically for use as a hypnotic. Metabolites of flurazepam remain in the patient for several days. When alcohol is consumed a day after this drug is ingested, driving skills are impaired.

Benzodiazepines are metabolized largely in the liver and metabolites are excreted in the urine.

Cardioversion. Diazepam can be given intravenously for cardioversion. If countershock is performed within 5 minutes of the injection, patients are in a state of light sleep and will not remember the shock. Adverse cardiovascular and respiratory effects are less frequent with diazepam than with thiopental or methohexital. However, full recovery is delayed because of diazepam's long duration of action.

Labor and delivery. Diazepam and chlordiazepoxide given parenterally are suitable adjuncts to local and systemic analgesics used during labor and delivery. They enhance analgesia, reduce opiate requirements, enhance amnesia, and with adequate precautions have no serious adverse effects on the infant. However, diazepam readily crosses the placenta and reaches higher concentrations in fetal circulation than in maternal blood. High doses of diazepam may produce lethargy, hypothermia, and respiratory depression in the newborn.

Lactation. Benzodiazepines are excreted in breast milk and cause adverse effects in nursing infants.

Preoperative medication. Benzodiazepines can be effectively used as preoperative sedatives. The drugs are more effective after intramuscular injection than after oral administration. They are less toxic than the opiates.

Induction. Diazepam is commonly used as an induction agent just before administration of general anesthesia. It produces more amnesia and has fewer adverse effects than do the barbiturates. However, recovery from general anesthesia is more delayed with diazepam than with barbiturates.

Geriatric patients. In the elderly or debilitated, the incidence of drowsiness and central nervous system depression may be related to low serum albumin, and therefore a greater amount of the active drug remains unbound to protein, giving an extended depressant effect. In the elderly the volume of distribution and elimination half-life increase. Thus a larger volume of distribution makes less drug available for liver metabolism and elimination. Liver disease will increase the half-life of the drug. Smoking and decreased serum albumin will also prolong the half-life. The usual recommended dosage in elderly or debilitated persons must be reduced from the normal dose; a low dose is used and titrated to the effective response in the individual patient to avoid accumulation and sedation. This reduction may be one-fourth to one-half of the usual adult recommended dose.

These agents are useful in treating elderly patients who are suffering from anxiety, tension, and the accompanying somatic disturbances and who are intellectually intact and neither psychotic nor depressed. Individual susceptibility to the sedative effects of these drugs varies and general guidelines for dosage in younger adults may not be applicable.

Adverse effects. Like all drugs, the benzodiazepines are not without their adverse effects and hazards and are contraindicated in acute narrow angle glaucoma but may be used by patients with adequately controlled chronic open angle glaucoma.

Neurologic. The central nervous system depressant effects include fatigue, drowsiness, somnolence, muscle weakness, nystagmus, ataxia, and dysarthria. The effects are dose dependent and subside when dosage is decreased or discontinued. These effects are more likely to occur in elderly patients and less likely to occur in heavy cigarette smokers. Impairment of motor and cognitive performance may also occur. Patients should be cautioned about automobile driving and working with hazardous equipment.

Psychiatric. Benzodiazepines can cause sleep disturbances and nightmares. There are two reports in the literature of self-destructive ideation leading to successful suicide by patients undergoing diazepam therapy.

Benzodiazepines may produce paradoxic excitement, hostility, rage, and violent, destructive behavior. The frequency of these reactions is not established.

Injection-site complications. Intravenous injection of diazepam causes local pain and irritation in many patients, which may lead to phlebitis. Intramuscular administration of diazepam is also painful.

Abuse, dependence, overdosage, and tolerance. Any drug can be abused and this is true for benzodiazepines. Dependence may occur if large doses are taken over a long period of time.

Addiction to benzodiazepines is not severe, habituation is encountered, and danger from overdosage of only benzodiazepines is minimal. The combined use of benzodiazepines and alcohol or other central nervous system depressants may produce serious and dangerous complications. The benzodiazepines are the most frequently prescribed anxiolytics and sleep medication. Recent studies have shown that there is increased impairment from combined use of alcohol and benzodiazepines. The nurse should caution the patient on concurrent use of alcoholic beverages and drugs with potential for synergism of central nervous system depression, such as over-the-counter sleep medications (doxylamine, pyrilamine), antihistamines, sedatives, tranquilizers, and alcohol contained in over-the-counter drugs (cough syrups). Cross-tolerance to alcohol and barbiturates may occur.

Some disease states may also alter responses to benzodiazepines. Blood levels of these drugs in alcoholic individuals may be lower than those in normal or nonalcoholic persons. The alcoholic malabsorption syndrome contributes to this or there may be an increased metabolism attributable to enzyme induction. The alcoholic person may be tolerant of high doses of benzodiazepines since less of the drug is absorbed because of gastrointestinal disorders.

The phenomenon of receptor-site tolerance (pharmacodynamic or cellular) or adaptation to benzodiazepines complicates interpretation of blood levels and pharmacokinetics in relation to clinical effect. A given blood level may elicit one clinical effect at one time (such as sedation or ataxia) and differ at a second attempt after a period of drug exposure. Receptor-site tolerance refers to the effect that duration of exposure of the central nervous system receptor site to any given drug concentration may have on the clinical and physiologic manifestations of the drug-receptor interaction. A given central nervous system receptor-site drug concentration may have different effects, depending on the duration and the concentration of the drug to which the receptor has been exposed. This tolerance may reduce clinical drug effects as the duration of drug exposure increases. This is not to be confused with pharmacokinetic or metabolic tolerance (hepatic enzyme induction), which is the effect of prolonged drug exposure on its own pharmacokinetic properties.

Others. Patients being given benzodiazepines should be cautioned by the nurse against engaging in hazardous occupations requiring mental alertness. The benzodiazepines are known for a central nervous system depressant effect, so the nurse should strongly advise against the simultaneous use of other CNS depressant drugs, including the phenothiazines, alcohol, narcotics, barbiturates, monoamine oxidase inhibitors, and other antidepressants. Physical and psychologic dependence manifested as withdrawal symptoms similar in character to those noted with barbiturates and alcohol have occurred after the abrupt cessation of the benzodiazepines that were taken continuously at therapeutic levels for several months. These symptoms include convulsions, tremor, abdominal and muscle cramps, vomiting, and sweating. Addiction-prone individuals (drug addicts and alcoholics) should be under cautious surveillance when receiving benzodiazepines because these patients are predisposed to habituation and dependence.

Precautions. An increased risk of congenital malformations has been observed with the use of anxiolytics. The use of these drugs is rarely considered a matter of utmost urgency. Their use during pregnancy should almost always be avoided. The possibility that a woman of childbearing potential may be pregnant should be considered at the time of initiating therapy. The nurse should advise patients that if they become pregnant during anxiolytic therapy or intend to become pregnant they should immediately notify all the physicians giving them care about the desirability of conception and the discontinuance of the drug. In view of their molecular size, the benzodiazepines and their metabolites are probably excreted in breast milk and therefore should not be given to a nursing mother.

In those patients in whom a degree of depression accompanies the anxiety, the incidence of suicidal tendencies is significant, and this may necessitate further protective measures to avoid precipitation of self-destructive acts such as multi-drug overdosage. The least amount of the drug that is feasible should be available to such a patient at any one time. This would require accurate medical office data about prescriptions and their refill dates; these will ensure a higher degree of control by the prescriber.

Patients receiving benzodiazepines for prolonged periods should have periodic blood counts (neutropenia) and liver function tests (jaundice). The usual precautions in treating patients with impaired renal or hepatic function should also be observed. In animal studies hepatomegaly and cholestasis were observed.

In elderly or debilitated patients, the initial dose should be small and increments should be made gradually, based on the response of the individual patient, to preclude ataxia or excessive sedation. Doses of benzodiazepines sufficient to control anxiety cause unwanted drowsiness less frequently than equivalent doses of barbiturates or meprobamate. The benzodiazepines have high therapeutic effectiveness and low addiction potential and lethality; they are generally desirable agents for use in anxious elderly patients. These drugs occasionally cause paradoxic reactions such as agitation and confusion, but these occur to a lesser degree than with barbiturates.

Frequently multiple physical and psychiatric problems occur concurrently, and these must be treated with multiple drugs (polypharmacy). It is challenging to the nurse to distinguish the intended effect of the drugs, side effects, placebo effects, and outward manifestations of the patient's initial symptoms. Patients undergoing polypharmacy require continual close observations and any undesirable effects should be reported for the well-being of the patient. A patient may benefit diagnostically and therapeutically from a drug-free baseline so that evaluation can be made accurately.

Chlordiazepoxide hydrochloride (Librium, Libritabs)

Action and uses. The actions and uses are similar to all antianxiety agents. Chlordiazepoxide has been effective in controlling the acute withdrawal symptoms of chronic alcoholic conditions (delirium tremens and agitation). However, since alcoholic persons in general are addiction prone, caution should be exerted in its use for these patients over prolonged periods. Chlordiazepoxide is known to have a muscle-relaxant effect and has been beneficial in treating musculoskeletal conditions in which anxiety and tension intensify the symptoms. Its direct action in these instances is unknown and may well be the result of its sedative effect. It has found a wide range of uses as an antianxiety agent in nonpsychiatric settings, mainly for the control of mild to moderate anxiety associated with psychosomatic conditions. This drug should be limited to small dosages in elderly patients.

Chlordiazepoxide is slightly more effective than meprobamate, but in comparison to diazepam it is less potent as an antianxiety agent, has less anticonvulsant action, and produces less drowsiness.

Preparation, dosage, and administration. This drug can be administered orally, intramuscularly, or intravenously. It is prepared as capsules and tablets of 5, 10, and 25 mg and as a powder for injection of 100 mg per ampule. The diluent provided in the commercial package should not be used for intravenous use. This diluent is for intramuscular use only. The average daily dosage should not exceed 300 mg. The usual daily adult dosage for relief of mild to moderate anxiety is 15 to 40 mg and 10 to 20 mg for elderly or debilitated patients. For children over 6 years of age, dosage is 0.5 mg/kg body weight daily in divided doses. It is well absorbed after oral administration, and peak blood concentration is reached in about 4 hours. Absorption by the intramuscular route is slow and erratic. For rapid and reliable sedative effects the oral or intravenous route should be used. Repeated dosages of chlordiazepoxide can produce cumulative effects because of accumulation in the body of the drug and its two active metabolites. The half-life of the drug is from 20 to 24 hours. In the patient with alcoholic agitation or delirium tremens, intramuscular or intravenous injections initially may be as high as 50 to 100 mg.

Side effects and toxic effects. Paradoxic reactions of rage, excitement, stimulation, hostility, confusion, and depersonalization have resulted from the administration of this drug to severely disturbed psychotic patients.

Drowsiness, ataxia, and lethargy occur frequently. Rash, nausea, headache, increased or decreased libido, an increase in vivid dreams, agranulocytosis, and jaundice occur less frequently.

Clorazepate dipotassium (Tranxene)

Its actions and uses are similar to those of the other benzodiazepine derivatives and it is approved for adjunctive management of partial seizures. Controlled studies indicate that it is an effective antianxiety drug. It is rapidly hydrolyzed in the body to nordiazepam, which is very slowly biotransformed, and thus long-lasting (up to 200 hours) cumulative effects occur with clorazepate. Peak plasma levels of nordiazepam occur within 1 hour after oral administration; the half-life of nordiazepam is about 24 hours. Clorazepate and diazepam appear to be equally effective. Most common side effects are sedation and ataxia. Adverse effects are the same as for other benzodiazepine compounds.

Preparation, dosage, and administration. Clorazepate is available in 3.75-, 7.5-, and 15-mg tablets and capsules and 11.25- and 22.5-mg tablets. For anxiety the 30-mg dose is administered in divided doses. Patients respond to gradual dosage adjustments up to 15 to 60 mg/day. In elderly or debilitated patients an initial dose of 7.5 to 15 mg is recommended or a single daily bedtime dose. As an adjunct to antiepileptic drugs the following schedules for clorazepate are used: Children over age 12, 7.5 mg three times daily increased by 7.5 mg/week and up to 90 mg/day; children age 9 to 12, a maximum initial dose of 7.5 mg twice daily increased by 7.5 mg/week and up to 60 mg/day. The approved use of clorazepate dipotassium for symptomatic relief of acute alcohol withdrawal has the following recommended dosage schedule: day 1 (first 24 hours), 30 mg initially followed by 30 to 60 mg in divided doses; day 2 (second 24 hours), 45 to 90 mg in divided doses; day 3 (third 24 hours), 22.5 to 45 mg in divided doses; day 4 (fourth 24 hours), 15 to 30 mg in divided doses; thereafter the dose is gradually reduced to a range of 7.5 to 15 mg daily. The maximum recommended dose is 90 mg daily. Nordiazepam is metabolized in the liver to oxazepam and parahydroxynordiazepam. Thus clorazepate may be considered a "pro-drug" or drug precursor. It is hydrolized in the acid pH of the stomach or on absorption to desmethyldiazepam (nordiazepam), the active metabolic agent. Recent studies indicate that administration of an antacid does not alter this process in a clinically significant manner.

Prolonged administration of single daily doses (up to 120 mg) resulted in no toxic effects; abrupt cessation of high doses may be followed by nervousness, insomnia, restlessness, irritability, diarrhea, muscle aches, or memory impairments.

Clorazepate monopotassium (Azene)

There exists no apparent significant difference between this salt of clorazepate and that of the dipotassium form (Tranxene).

Preparation, dosage and administration. The strengths available are 3.25-, 6.5-, and 13-mg capsules. The usual oral dose of 26 mg is administered in divided doses. Drowsiness may occur at treatment initiation and with dosage increments. In elderly or debilitated patients a lower daily dose of 6.5 to 13 mg is recommended in divided doses. For symptomatic relief of acute alcohol withdrawal the recommendation is day 1 (first 24 hours), 26 mg initially followed by 26 to 52 mg in divided doses; day 2 (second 24 hours), 39 to 78 mg in divided doses; day 3 (third 24 hours), 19.5 to 39 mg divided doses; day 4 (fourth 24 hours), 13 to 26 mg in divided doses; thereafter the daily dose is gradually reduced to a range of 6.3 to 13 mg and the drug therapy discontinued when the patient's condition is stable. The maximum dose is 78 mg.

Diazepam (Valium)

Diazepam is effective in the treatment of anxiety and tension related to organic or functional conditions. Diazepam is more effective than meprobamate and five times more potent than chlordiazepoxide. Long-term use may result in psychic and physical dependence. Sudden cessation of the drug can result in withdrawal symptoms. It has been found to be useful in treating mild to moderate depression with anxiety and tension. Because of its muscle-relaxant properties, it is a useful adjunct in the treatment of muscle spasms. It is becoming the drug of choice for status epilepticus.

Preparation, dosage, and administration. This drug is available in tablets of 2, 5, and 10 mg and in 2- and 10-ml containers, 5 mg/ml, for injection. Daily doses for adults range from 4 to 40 mg. When given intramuscularly, diazepam is absorbed slowly, erratically, and probably incompletely. Given orally, diazepam is rapidly and completely absorbed; peak blood concentrations are reached in 2 hours. Thus this drug should be given either orally or intravenously.

After a single oral or intravenous dose, clinical effects may seem to "wear off" rapidly because of rapid and extensive tissue distribution. Diazepam is metabolized slowly and has a biphasic half-life between 20 and 40 hours in most patients, but it may be as long as 50 hours in some individuals. Repeated dosage leads to cumulative effects. Steady-state concentrations are usually obtained after 5 to 10 days of therapy. Diazepam or its metabolite can still be detected in the blood a week or more after termination of therapy. Diazepam should not be mixed or diluted with other solutions or drugs, or added to intravenous fluids.

An intravenous dose of diazepam administered for an epileptic seizure rapidly loses effectiveness because the diazepam diffuses away from the site of action in the central nervous system. For use in status epilepticus and severe recurrent convulsion seizures, the intravenous route is preferred in the convulsing patient. The injection is made slowly, with 5 to 10 mg being initially recommended at 10- to 15- minute intervals or less since residual active metabolites persist; this may be more often as the situation necessitates because epileptic seizures are suppressed when the plasma level of diazepam is in excess of 600 mg/ml.

Caution is observed in patients with chronic lung disease or unstable cardiovascular status. Some severe cardiovascular and respiratory problems have been associated with diazepam given intravenously and may be attributed to rapid injection of the propylene glycol (40%) vehicle of the diazepam injection.

The intravenous dose should be administered slowly over a 1-minute elapsed period. The first phase of the biphasic half-life (1 to 6 hours) is the distribution phase; the second phase (20 to 50 hours) is the slow biotransformation and excretion phase, which lasts up to 200 hours. The resurgence of the drug at 6 hours may be attributable to diazepam and its active metabolites from the enterohepatic circulation.

Flurazepam (Dalmane)

Actions and uses. A benzodiazepine indicated as a hypnotic agent, flurazepam is one of the most often prescribed drugs in the United States and is frequently used as floor stock in hospitals and extended care facilities. REM rebound does not occur with chronic use and it is effective through consecutive nights for at least a month. Since insomnia may be transient and intermittent, the prolonged use of hypnotics should only be considered with individual patient evaluation. The risks of developing oversedation, dizziness, confusion, or ataxia increase markedly with larger doses in the elderly and debilitated patient. The dose should be initiated at 15 mg in these circumstances. It may be further desirable to limit prescription quantities and refills to only a 1-month supply to maintain adequate medical supervision and assessment of the patient's changing needs.

Flurazepam is rapidly absorbed from the gastrointestinal tract, metabolized in the liver, and excreted in the urine. The onset of action is 15 to 30 minutes and the duration of action may be 8 hours. The pharmacokinetics of the drug indicate the following clinical observations: flurazepam is increasingly effective on the second or third night of consecutive use because of slow accumulation of the active metabolite, and for 1 or 2 nights after the drug is discontinued, both sleep latency and total time awake may still be decreased because of active metabolites. The major metabolite remains active and has a half-life of 47 to 100 hours. The patient should avoid combined use of alcohol and other CNS depressants. This must be emphasized by the nurse to the patient. The abrupt withdrawal may produce rebound insomnia.

Preparation, dosage, and administration. Flurazepam is administered orally in 15- to 30-mg capsules. Dosage is individualized; the usual adult dose is 15 to 30 mg before retiring. In elderly or debilitated persons the dose is initiated at 15 mg and titrated to individual responses.

Side effects. Dizziness, drowsiness, lightheadedness, staggering, ataxia, and falling (particularly in elderly or debilitated persons) are common adverse effects. Severe sedation, lethargy, disorientation, and coma may be indicative of intolerance to the drug or overdosage. The other reported adverse reactions are similar to those of the benzodiazepines in general.

Lorazepam (Ativan)

The indications for use of lorazepam are similar to other benzodiazepines with slight variation. It is used for symptomatic relief of anxiety, tension, agitation, irritability, and insomnia associated with anxiety neuroses and transient situational disturbances, anxiety associated with depressive symptoms, and symptoms of anxiety associated with functional or organic disorders (gastrointestinal or cardiovascular); it is also hypnotic. The effectiveness in long-term use (for over 4 months) has not been assessed by systematic clinical studies. The injectable form is indicated in adults for preanesthetic (0.05 mg/kg up to a total of 4 mg) medication (duration 6 to 8 hours) for sedation, to reduce anxiety, and diminish recall of events of the day of surgery.

A substantial portion (75%) of lorazepam is metabolized to inactive glucuronide metabolites with minor metabolites. During a 5-day interval 95% of a single 5-mg dose is excreted in the urine and feces. The extent of accumulation appears to be less than other of the longer acting benzodiazepines.

Preparation, dosage, and administration. Lorazepam is currently available in the oral dosage forms of 1- and 2-mg tablets and for injection (intramuscular or intravenous) as 2 or 4 mg/ml. The usual oral dose is 2 to 6 mg/day in divided doses, with the largest dose administered before bedtime. A daily dosage range is 1 to 10 mg/day. In anxiety the initial dosage is 2 to 3 mg twice to three times daily, and as a hypnotic (onset 20 to 30 minutes and duration 8 hours) it is given as a single dose at bedtime. For the geriatric or debilitated patient an initial dosage of 1 to 2 mg/day in divided doses, and as with other benzodiazepines the dose is adjusted and titrated as needed and tolerated to avoid oversedation. Elderly persons may experience hangover effects. A dose of 2 to 4 mg was found to be equivalent to a 30-mg dose of flurazepam. Hallucinations were reported in a 6-year-old child who accidentally ingested lorazepam. Research with the intravenous form of lorazepam (4 mg) as a preanesthetic medication produced postoperative disorientation, restlessness, agitation, inappropriate behavior dreams, hallucinations, and relative dose-related impairment of memory recall. As with other benzodiazepines it is contraindicated in narrow angle glaucoma. The drug's pharmacokinetic characteristics differ from those discussed with the benzodiazepines, since lorazepam's elimination half-life is only 10 to 15 hours and it does not have active metabolites.

Pain, burning, and reddening are reported at the injection site. Immediately before intravenous use this drug must be diluted with an equal volume of compatible solution (Sterile Water for Injection, sodium chloride injection, or 5% dextrose injection). The rate of injection should not exceed 2 mg/minute. The injectable form contains the diluents polyethylene and propylene glycol, and other medications should not be mixed in the same syringe.

Oxazepam (Serax)

Oxazepam is closely related in its effects to chlordiazepoxide. It has been effective in the treatment of patients with anxiety, tension, and irritability associated with psychoneurotic conditions. It is said to be particularly valuable in the management of anxiety in elderly patients; however, scientific data have not validated this belief as yet. Oxazepam has a lower incidence of adverse reactions than chlordiazepoxide or diazepam. Its half-life in normal persons ranges between 3 and 21 hours. Oxazepam is relatively rapidly metabolized to a psychopharmacologically inactive substance, and therefore cumulative effects are less important during prolonged therapy than is true for chlordiazepoxide or diazepam.

Preparation, dosage, and administration. This drug is administered orally in capsules of 10, 15, and 30 mg or 15-mg tablets. Daily doses range from 30 to 120 mg for adults. Parenteral preparations are not available.

Temazepam (Restoril)

Temazepam, a benzodiazepine that is given orally, is a 3-hydroxy derivative of diazepam and may be referred to as N-methyl oxazepam. Indications are for relief of insomnia associated with difficulty in falling asleep and frequent or early awakenings. An advantage of this agent is negligible accumulation of active metabolites. A short biphasic half-life exists with a range of 9 to 12 hours. After total absorption from the gastrointestinal tract and complete hepatic metabolism occur, the drug is eliminated in the urine by the next morning with a low incidence of behavorial impairment. The major metabolic pathway terminates with glucuronide conjugation and the minor metabolic pathway becomes oxazepam. Generally the glucuronide conjugation is affected to a lesser degree by hepatic disease than by the oxidative process. In hepatic disease the 3-hydroxylated derivative, such as temazepam, oxazepam, and lorazepam, is more desirable. The rapid elimination with negligible accumulation decreases the incidence of residual hangover, as seen with long-acting benzodiazepines (those with an active intermediate metabolite such as N-desmethyldiazepam). Before the patient retires, the adult dose is individualized with 15 and 30 mg, producing effective total sleep time for 7 to 8 hours. Peak concentration occurs in 2 to 3 hours after oral administration with serum detection within 40 minutes. The most reported common adverse effects include mild and transient drowsiness, dizziness, and lethargy. The patient information, contraindications, precautions, drug abuse, and dependence is similar to the other benzodiazepines. The patient should be told that after the first or second day of discontinuation sleep disturbances may be experienced.

Prazepam (Centrax)

Actions and uses. Prazepam is indicated for symptomatic relief of anxiety associated with an anxiety neurosis, in other psychoneuroses in which anxiety symptoms are prominent characteristics, and as an adjunct in disease states in which anxiety is manifested.

Negligible amounts of the parent compound appear in blood since prazepam has a substantial "first pass" removal of the large side chain yielding desmethyldiazepam. Desmethyldiazepam is the only active unconjugated benzodiazepine found in the blood in measurable and important amounts. After single doses unconjugated metabolites of prazepam are reported to have half-life in the 30- to 120-hour range, and the glucuronide metabolites are reported to have a half-life of 36 hours. This may substantiate the once-daily anxiolytic dosing, as also seen in clorazepate. The large alkyl side chain provides resistance to metabolic degradation, which imparts a longer action to this benzodiazepine (up to 200 hours).

Preparation, dosage, and administration. The dosage form is a 10-mg tablet or capsule. The usual daily oral dose is 30 mg, with a range of 20 to 60 mg daily. Once-daily dosing is possible because of long half-lives. The recommended usual starting nightly dose is 20 mg with a range of 20 to 40 mg. The usual recommended dose in the elderly or debilitated patient is 10 to 15 mg in divided doses.

NONBENZODIAZEPINES
Meprobamate (Equanil, Miltown)
Tybamate (Tybatran)

Meprobamate is a synthetic drug that is chemically related to mephenesin, a skeletal muscle relaxant. The chemical structure differs greatly from that of reserpine or the phenothiazine derivatives. Meprobamate is a straight-chain aliphatic compound. It is a crystalline white powder with a bitter taste.

Action and result. The effects of meprobamate depend on the dosage employed. When used in large doses, as in animal experiments, the drug is not only an anxiolytic agent but also a muscle relaxant and anticonvulsant. It acts as an interneuronal blocking agent and causes relaxation of skeletal muscle. It is also referred to as a centrally acting muscle relaxant. Some investigators believe, however, that meprobamate as employed in ordinary doses acts mainly as a sedative. Some even believe that its action under these circumstances does not differ significantly from that of phenobarbital.

Uses. Meprobamate has been effective in bringing about relief of anxiety and tension, abnormal fears, psychosomatic disorders, behavior disorders, and insomnia. It is not a potent hypnotic, but the relief of tension that it produces is conducive to sleep. Improvement after administration of this drug is usually characterized by decreased irritability, improved sense of well-being, and greater relaxation. It may also be used to treat musculoskeletal disorders and petit mal epilepsy.

Precautions. Meprobamate possesses less sedative effect than the benzodiazepines; however, 400 to 800 mg may be administered as a hypnotic. This propanediol may be useful in managing anxiety and mild agitation in the elderly because mental functions are not significantly impaired and muscular instability is not intolerable. Meprobamate has a pronounced addiction potential and overdosage produces serious poisoning. Suicidal attempts have resulted in drowsiness, lethargy, stupor, ataxia, shock, convulsions, respiratory depression, and coma. The effectiveness of tybamate needs further clinical study, and the greater efficacy and less addiction potential may make it more suitable than meprobamate. The propanediols do not cause clinically significant hepatic enzyme induction in humans, but propanediols potentiate monoamine oxidate inhibitors and may have an effect on oral anticoagulants. False elevation of transaminase, alkaline phosphatase, and bilirubin have been reported.

In animal studies, effects at multiple sites in the central nervous system, including the thalamus and limbic system, have been observed.

Meprobamate is contraindicated in acute intermittent porphyria as well as allergic or idiosyncratic reactions to related compounds such as carisoprodol, tybamate (seldom used), or carbromal.

The physical and psychologic dependence that results as well as the possibility of abuses require that the nurse monitor the dose amounts prescribed and used and the length of time of administration, especially in alcoholic persons and patients with a known propensity for abusive self-administration of excessive amounts of drugs. Abrupt cessation of meprobamate may precipitate the onset of withdrawal symptoms within 12 to 48 hours, which usually subside in the next 24 to 48 hours. The nurse should advise a period of 1 to 2 weeks of gradual withdrawal to abate the withdrawal symptoms caused by excessive dosage over months of use. Meprobamate has an additive effect with other psychotropic drugs and alcohol.

There is an increased risk of congenital malformations during the first trimester in pregnancy. The drug passes the placental barrier and is present in the breast milk of lactating mothers.

The precaution of giving the lowest effective dose in elderly and debilitated patients to prevent oversedation should be observed. The possibility of suicidal attempts creates the need to encourage dispensing at nonexcessive amounts of the drug on each prescription and to monitor the refills.

Meprobamate is metabolized in the liver and excreted in the urine (10% to 20%). In patients with renal failure the dose intervals may be altered to the following: mild renal failure every 6 hours, moderate renal failure 9 to 12 hours, and severe renal failure 12 to 18 hours. Patients with hepatic insufficiency, liver disease, cirrhosis, or hepatitis may have a prolonged half-life (18 to 24 hours), and to prevent accumulation, one should adjust successive doses. Meprobamate has precipitated seizures in patients with seizure disorders.

A single oral dose of 800 mg reaches peak blood levels (10 to 11 mg/ml) in about 3 hours, and the dose-dependent half-life is in a range of 6.5 to 18 hours (for tybamate the half-life is about 3 hours). The adverse reactions affect the central nervous system, gastrointestinal tract, and cardiovascular system and cause allergic, idiosyncratic, and hematologic reactions.

Preparation, dosage, and administration. Meprobamate is marketed in sustained-release capsules of 200 mg and in tablets of 200, 400, plus 600 mg. The usual adult dose is 400 mg three or four times daily. Initial dose for children over 6 years of age is 100 to 200 mg two or three times daily. Older children may tolerate doses as high as 2.4 g.

Side effects and toxic effects. Meprobamate is considered a potentially toxic drug. It has been known to cause a number of side effects, untoward reaction, and fatal outcomes. The more common reactions are drowsiness and allergic manifestations, such as skin rash, itching, and urticaria. The allergic reaction is sometimes sufficiently severe to require the administration of a corticosteroid and cessation of administration, but the symptoms usually respond well to administration of one of the antihistaminic drugs. Evidence exists that both psychic dependence and physical dependence can develop. Some patients seem to develop tolerance as well. Withdrawal symptoms, including convulsions, have been observed. Such symptoms are seen only after prolonged administration and abrupt discontinuance of administration.

Gradual withdrawal of meprobamate therapy is essential in the event that physical or psychic dependence develops.

Hydroxyzine hydrochloride (Atarax); hydroxyzine pamoate (Vistaril)

Hydroxyzine has been efficacious in the treatment of anxiety and pruritic dermatoses.

This agent has significant anticholinergic properties and has the potential for anticholinergic toxicity in elderly persons.

Action and result. Hydroxyzine induces a calming effect in anxious, tense, psychoneurotic adults and anxious hyperkinetic children, without impairing mental alertness. The action may be attributable to activity suppression in subcortical areas of the central nervous system. Furthermore, the drug has antihistaminic and antiemetic effects.

Hydroxyzine is absorbed from the gastrointestinal tract with effects noticed in 15 to 30 minutes. The pamoate salt is converted to the hydrochloride salt in the stomach. The efficacy of hydroxyzine is an adjunct to preoperative and postoperative sedation, and it is clinically established because it allays anxiety, controls emesis, can potentiate effects of narcotics used concurrently, and thus reduces the dose of the narcotic required (such as meperidine, central nervous system depressants, and barbiturates). A reduced dosage of the other agents is necessary. Hydroxyzine is contraindicated in early pregnancy.

Preparation, dosage, and administration. Both drugs may be administered orally and intramuscularly. The usual dosage for adults is 25 to 100 mg given three or four times daily. Parenteral administration should be reserved for emergency situations only, and oral dosages should be substituted as soon as possible. Dosage for sedation of children is 1 mg/kg body weight.

Hydroxyzine hydrochloride. It comes in 10-, 25-, 50-, and 100-mg tablets and in syrup, 10 mg/5 ml. It is also prepared in solution for injection, 25 and 50 mg/ml.

Hydroxyzine pamoate. This is available in capsules of 25, 50, and 100 mg; as a suspension of 25 mg/5 ml; and in solutions for injection of 25 and 50 mg/ml.

Antipsychotic (neuroleptic) agents—major tranquilizers

The first of the drugs to play an important part in the pharmacologic treatment of mental illness were the rauwolfia alkaloids. These drugs came into prominence around 1953, though they have been used in India for many years for the treatment of mental disorders. The most widely used of these compounds is reserpine. The principal use of the rauwolfia alkaloid compounds today is in the treatment of hypertension. The rauwolfia alkaloids are still considered as neuroleptic agents; however, they are not widely used because of the discovery of newer agents. As a tranquilizer, reserpine produces many of the same effects as the phenothiazine drug groups; however, its use is now restricted to those patients who do not respond to phenothiazine treatment. Since the phenothiazine drugs achieve the same tranquilizing effects, the rauwolfia compounds have been replaced by these drugs.

PHENOTHIAZINE DERIVATIVES

Discovery of the phenothiazine derivatives arose out of resrach in the area of the antihistamines. Chlorpromazine hydrochloride was introduced in 1951 and has found wide acceptance in the treatment of mental illness. Additional investigation of the action of chloropromazine in producing undesirable side effects led to the development of numerous derivatives, which now comprise the largest group of psychotropic agents.

About two thirds of all antipsychotic drugs are phenothiazine derivatives. They are commonly divided chemically into the following three subgroups: (1) the aliphatic compounds (chlorpromazine and triflupromazine), (2) the piperidine compounds (thioridazine, mesoridazine, and piperacetazine), and (3) the piperazine compounds (acetophenazine, fluphenazine, perphenazine, prochlorperazine, trifluoperazine, carphenazine, and butaperazine). Although a close structural similarity exists thioxanthene derivatives (thiothixene and chlorprothixene) are not phenothiazine derivatives. The chemical structure of these compounds and specific information regarding their action, effects, and adverse reactions are presented separately after the general discussion of similarities that have been identified. The type of action is essentially similar with all phenothiazine derivatives; individual compounds vary chiefly in their potency and in the nature and severity of their side effects.

Pharmacokinetics. The phenothiazines are highly lipid soluble and are highly (90%) protein bound. Their therapeutic half-life is in a range of 2 to 30 hours, with 6 hours or less encountered in most patients; this is prolonged in overdose situations. The acute fatal dose is found in the range of 15 to 150 mg/kg, depending on the individual agent involved. The list (Table 11-3) of phenothiazine-equivalent doses expressed in milligrams may assist the nurse in evaluating this range as equivalent to 50 mg of chlorpromazine. The nonphenothiazine types are as follows: the butyrophenone class (haloperidol, 1 mg), thioxanthene class (Table 11-4), dihydroindolone class (such as molidone 5 mg), and the dibenzoazepine class (loxapine 5 mg).

The phenothiazines are almost completely absorbed from the gut after oral administration. The liver (on first pass) removes about 65% of the drug from the plasma from enterohepatic circulation. Urinary metabolites have been found after 18 hours. Most of the 30 to 40 metabolites from the liver are inert except for the glucuronide, which has antipsychotic effects. It is stored in body fat and can be found in the circulation 18 months after long-term dosages have been discontinued.

Chemical structure–activity relationships. The potency, expected therapeutic efficacy, and the nature of the side effects of the phenothiazines can be predicted from the type of chemical substitutions on the phenothiazine nucleus and the side-chain variations (Fig. 11-5).

Substitution on the R_2 position is a determinant of side effects and potency, particularly in the aliphatics (dimethylamine). Promazine (Sparine) has hydrogen in this position and is an agent of minimal potency (position-2 hydrogen). If this hydrogen atom is replaced or substituted with a halogen atom, the potency of the drug will increase. When the atomic weight of

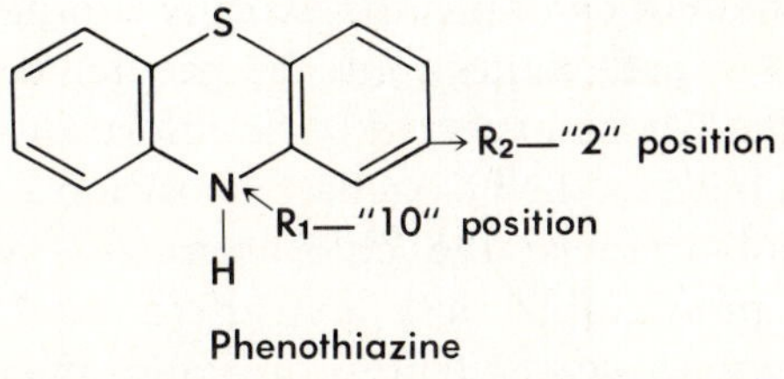

FIG. 11-5. Phenothiazine nucleus structure.

T A B L E 1 1 - 3   Side effects and dose equivalents of phenothiazines and thioxanthene derivatives

Generic name	Trade name	Side effects*	Dosage range† per 24-hour period (mg)	Chlorpromazine oral dose equivalent (mg)
Aliphatic dimethylamine subgroup				
Chlorpromazine hydrochloride	Thorazine	1-9, 11, 12-15, 23	30 to 1200	50
Triflupromazine	Vesprin	1-12	60 to 150	12.5 to 15
Piperidine subgroup				
Thioridazine hydrochloride	Mellaril	1-3, 6, 7, 12, 13, 17-19	30 to 800	50
Mesoridazine besylate	Serentil	1-7, 13, 19, 21	100 to 400	25
Piperacetazine	Quide	1, 6, 7, 10, 11, 19, 20, 23, 29	20 to 160	5
Piperazine subgroup				
Acetophenazine dimaleate	Tindal	1, 6	40 to 80	10
Carphenazine dimaleate	Proketazine	1, 6, 8, 9	75 to 400	12.5 to 15
Fluphenazine hydrochloride	Permitil, Prolixin	1-9, 11, 12, 15, 18	1 to 20	1
Perphenazine	Trilafon	1-9, 11, 12	6 to 64	4
Prochlorperazine dimaleate	Compazine	1-7, 9, 11, 12, 15, 20	15 to 150	5 to 10
Trifluoperazine hydrochloride	Stelazine	1, 2, 4-9, 11, 12, 15, 18	2 to 20	2
Thioxanthene subgroup				
Thiothixene hydrochloride	Navane	1, 3, 5-7, 10, 12-14, 18, 23	6 to 60	2 to 4
Chlorprothixene	Taractan	1-10, 14, 15, 18, 20, 21, 23	30 to 600	50

Key to table

1. Sedation or sleep
2. Ataxia
3. Dry mouth
4. Constipation
5. Dermatitis
6. Extrapyramidal symptoms
7. Orthostatic hypotension
8. Blood dyscrasia (usually agranulocytosis)

9. Jaundice
10. Convulsions
11. Antiemetic
12. Blurred vision
13. Hypothermia
14. Tachycardia
15. Nasal congestion
16. Menstrual irregularities

17. Nausea and vomiting
18. Edema
19. Impotence
20. Increased appetite
21. Bradycardia
22. Increased gastric secretions
23. Photosensitivity

*Side effects here are not intended to be a complete account of all possible adverse reactions reported.
†Drug dosage varies with the patient's response and the severity of the disease.

this substituted halogen atom increases, there is a corresponding increase in drug potency. The potency therefore increases progressively when the position-2 hydrogen is replaced by chlorine (chlorpromazine) and by fluorine (triflupromazine) respectively. Therefore the atom substitution going from chloride to fluoride increases the potency of the drug. In using this structure-activity relationship the nurse is able to determine potency relative to another phenothiazine. For example, the extrapyramidal side effects of promazine could be predicted to be less than those expected with chlorpromazine on the basis of the halogenated position 2 at R_2, and furthermore the chlorpromazine would have predictably less extrapyramidal side effects than would triflupromazine. It can be

seen how the degree of antiemetic properties, potency, and side effects may be relative to the halogenation of the R_2 position.

Substitution on the side chain at the position R_1 (position 10) increases the potency of these compounds with antipsychotic potency and decreases the sedative effects. Three phenothiazine subfamilies (aliphatic, piperidine, and piperazine) may be distinguished on the basis of substitutions at R_1 (position 10).

The aliphatic phenothiazines include the compounds promethazine, chlorpromazine, and triflupromazine. This group of phenothiazines has fewer extrapyriamidal reactions (except tardive dyskinesia) and dystonic reactions and is more sedative than some of the other phenothiazine groups. The aliphatic derivatives, however, also have the highest incidence of agranulocytosis and obstructive jaundice. This group has the R_1 side chain (at position 10) consist of three straight-chain carbon atoms. The effect decreases greatly when the number of carbon atoms is decreased or increased. To illustrate this, promethazine has a two-carbon side chain attached to the amine at position R_1 (before the tertiary amine of the side chain). This aliphatic phenothiazine drug has a sedative and antihistaminic effect instead of the antipsychotic effects.

Piperidine phenothiazines (mesoridazine and thioridazine) have a piperidine-like "tail" in the R_1 position. The piperidine phenothiazines have a milligram potency approximately equal to that of the aliphatic group; however, the extrapyramidal effects are less prominent than those of the aliphatic subfamily. In addition they cause sedative effects similar to those of the aliphatics. Modifications in structure at position R_2 alter the potency, as with the aliphatics. The 2-methylthio group of thioridazine produces the least extrapyramidal effects of the piperidines, and these effects increase with halogenation or with the 2-acetyl group on piperacetazine.

The piperazine phenothiazines have the highest incidence of extrapyramidal reactions. Predictably they are also more potent than both their ring-substituted analogs in the aliphatic series and the piperidine phenothiazines. This group causes less sedation than the aliphatics and piperidines, but this is offset by the degree of side effects and extrapyramidal effects, especially acute dystonic reactions. The R_1 position relates to the sedative effects, and the R_2 position relates to the antiemetic and side effects. The more halogenated the position becomes, the higher the incidence of side effects and the greater the potency. Acetophenazine with the R_2 position having a 2-acetyl group is less potent than the halogenated agents of this piperazine group.

Site and mechanism of action of phenothiazine derivatives. It has been suggested that the cause of schizophrenia may be related to an excess of dopamine in the central nervous system. The phenothiazines block dopamine-mediated transmission. Although this leads to increased synthesis of dopamine as a compensatory phenomenon, the mediator is also more rapidly destroyed. The net effect is blockade of dopamine-mediated response. These actions could also account for the extrapyramidal side effects (parkinsonism-like effects) of the phenothiazines.

Phenothiazines depress lower levels of the central nervous system. Depression of the vomiting center accounts for the antiemetic effect of these drugs. Alteration of the temperature-regulating center results in a minor fall in body temperature except in the extremities where vasodilation occurs. Shivering is also suppressed. Thus chlorpromazine and related drugs can be used when it is desirable to induce hypothermia. The phenothiazines are believed to act centrally as antinorepinephrine drugs, blocking the adrenergic synapses.

The administration of phenothiazines to human beings leads to a widespread reduction of sympathetic tone in the body. There is vasodilation and hypotension with compensatory tachycardia, relaxation of smooth muscle, alteration of pupillary size, and decreased salivary and gastric secretions. Because the phenothiazines act to suppress central sympathetic activity without significantly depressing the reticular activating system, their use is favored in the control of psychomotor agitation, since this effect is produced without significant loss of cortical functioning or consciousness. The hallucinations and delusions associated with psychosis are mitigated or eliminated by the action of the phenothiazines.

Pharmacologic characteristics and uses. The most important pharmacologic characteristics of these substances are (1) antipsychotic activity (an ability to calm aggressive, overactive, disturbed patients), (2) failure of large doses to produce deep coma and anesthesia (patients show both behavioral and electroencephalographic arousal when stimulated), (3) production of reversible and irreversible effects on the extrapyramidal system, leading to the development of related signs and symptoms, and (4) lack of any notable tendency to cause psychogenic or physical dependence.

In addition to the antipsychotic or neuroleptic use these drugs are also used as antiemetics, antihistamines, antipruritics, and analgesics and for antiserotonin activity and antiparkinson activity.

Behavioral effects. The phenothiazine derivatives are used to reduce psychotic symptoms and therefore are useful in the treatment of acute and chronic psychoses. Control of deeply disturbed patients is achieved without causing depression of vital centers. Psychotic conditions characterized by excessive psychomotor activity, panic, fear, and hostility respond well to the administration of the phenothiazines. Relief of emotional tension, excitement, and agitation lessens the patient's response to hallucinations and delusions. Destructive and combative behaviors are notably reduced. On the other hand, some of the piperazine compounds are useful in stimulating the withdrawn apathetic patient so that he becomes more alert, sociable, and communicative. The phenothiazines may make some depressive reactions worse and do not seem to be of value in treating hysteria or obsessive-compulsive reactions. However, phenothiazines seem to be helpful in allaying the agitation and anxiety that occurs before electroconvulsive treatments.

Small doses of the phenothiazines are sometimes used to control the anxiety, tension and emotional disturbance in the psychoneurotic patient. Anxiety that often accompanies diseases with psychogenic components is easily controlled with small doses of the phenothiazine derivatives. However, the risk involved from the side effects does not seen to warrant their use in these instances. The minor tranquilizers appear to be more useful in these conditions.

Some of the phenothiazine derivatives have been used in nonpsychiatric settings because of their secondary actions (antiemesis; potentiation of hypnotic, analgesic, and anesthetic agents).

Adverse behavioral effects. Phenothiazines can cause unpleasant effects. For the most part, phenothiazine therapy is not a subjectively pleasant experience. The feelings of lassitude and fatigability limit the patient's ability to engage in many otherwise normal and nonexhausting activities. The depressing effects may decrease the patient's willingness to take medication. Depression may also account for the greater incidence of suicide in psychotic persons undergoing drug therapy than in those receiving only institutional care.

Some patients experience feelings of excitement and restlessness. These reactions are more likely to occur early in treatment and after administration of piperazine derivatives.

All antipsychotics affect sleep. Chlorpromazine may inhibit or enhance REM sleep, depending on dosage. Lithium carbonate is a REM suppressant, and REM rebound may occur after withdrawal.

Side effects. The phenothiazine derivatives produce a wide variety of untoward effects (see Table 11-4). Individuals vary in their ability to tolerate these compounds, and difficulty with side effects may determine the effectiveness of the compound. The pattern of adverse reactions is one of the important factors that the physician considers in choosing among the compounds. Some of these side effects result from the secondary action of the drugs on the central and autonomic nervous systems, whereas others are idiosyncratic or allergic in nature.

Quinidine-like effect. Phenothiazines have effects on the heart similar to those of quinidine. ECG findings show T-wave changes and a prolonged PR interval and QRS complex, reflecting slowed conduction. Ventricular ectopic pacemaker activity may occur and can lead to ventricular fibrillation and death. Thioridazine (Mellaril) is particularly hazardous in this regard.

Autonomic (peripheral) effects. The autonomic effects are as follows.

Anticholinergic effects—Tranquilizers have atropine-like properties that can be very prominent with large doses. Manifestations of this effect include dry mouth, failure of accommodation for near vision, constipation, and urinary retention.
Antiadrenergic (beta-adrenergic) effects—Phenothiazines and related drugs intensify beta-adrenergic effects of sympathetic nerve stimulation. This action accounts for the vasodilating and orthostatic hypotensive effects.
Convulsant effect—Extremely high doses of tranquilizers may cause convulsions, though this is rare clinically. Epileptic individuals are more susceptible to this effect.

Patients should be cautioned against driving an automobile, operating dangerous machinery, or performing tasks that require absolute precision, motor coordination, and mental alertness.

Decreased libido may be a troublesome side effect for patients on a maintenance dosage of these drugs. Careful explanation of the cause of this side effect may alleviate the patient's anxiety. Some patients refuse medications before home visits for this reason.

Liver. Cholestatic hepatitis with obstructive jaundice is the most frequent form of liver disorder observed. This reaction of cholestatic jaundice may occur more frequently than clinically observed. This reaction may be attributable to precipitation of the protein and glycoprotein components of bile. This type of reaction has also been demonstrated in vitro for some of the tricyclic antidepressants. This reaction has some similarity to an allergic reaction. The sudden occurrence with fever, eosinophilia, and rashes or other allergic reactions is often exacerbated by challenge doses of the drug.

Cholestatic hepatitis with obstructive jaundice usually develops within the first 5 weeks of treatment. If bilirubinuria and icterus are detected in liver function tests, the drug should be withdrawn immediately. Since the subsequent changes in the liver persist for a much longer time, it is not advisable to change treatment to another phenothiazine compound. Fatality is rare, and recovery from phenothiazine jaundice usually occurs within a few weeks. It is undesirable to use these drugs in patients who have known liver disease. Such patients are probably no more susceptible to such reactions than other patients, but the consequences might be more serious should they occur.

Hematologic complications. Leukopenia, granulocytopenia, agranulocytosis, purpura, and pancytopenia are hematologic complications that occur. The incidence of their occurrence is low; however, the mortality is high. Physicians and nurses should be alert to the appearance of such signs as sore throat, fever, or weakness in patients taking these drugs. With the apperance of these symptoms the drug is usually discontinued and a white blood cell and differential count are made to determine the cause of the disturbance. Some physicians order routine monthly or bimonthly laboratory tests to avoid such complications. However, most physicians believe that this precaution is of little value, since blood dyscrasias occur so rapidly that it is impractical to do blood counts frequently enough to protect the patient.

Orthostatic hypotension. Orthostatic (postural) hypotension is usually mild and occurs with the initial dose of the phenothiazines. Compensatory adjustment usually takes place in a few days. It can be especially serious, though, with patients in whom a sudden drop in blood pressure would be undesirable (elderly patients with evidence of arteriosclerosis or patients with cardiovascular disease). If this side effect is causing an unusual amount of difficulty or serious hazards, the following remedial measures may be instituted: (1) a change of medication to one of the phenothiazine derivatives that is not known to produce this side effect with such frequency, (2) reduction of dosage, or (3) discontinuation of medication for a 24-hour period with a gradual buildup of dosage as tolerated. The patient who complains of dizziness, light-headedness, or palpitation may be experiencing orthostatic hypotension. This can easily be confirmed when the patient's blood pressure is compared in the prone and standing positions. The nurse may instruct the patient to rise slowly from the recumbent position and to sit on the edge of the bed for a few minutes before attempting to stand. Support and reassurance may be necessary to allay the patient's anxiety. Explanation of this phenomenon may also aid in the patient's understanding of this experience and reduce his anxiety. Patients should be encouraged to remain in a recumbent position for 1 hour after initial doses, parenterally administered doses, or large oral doses of the phenothiazines.

Allergic reactions. These usually are mild urticarial reactions and can be controlled by discontinuance of the drug. It is often possible to resume treatment later with another compound, or even the same one, without recurrence of the allergic skin reaction. If photosensitivity develops, the patient should stay out of the sunlight or wear protective clothing to prevent solar erythema. Nurses should instruct patients regarding this side effect or assist them in providing the necessary protective measures to avoid exposure. A dark purplish brown skin pigmentation induced by light (photosensitivity) has been reported in hospitalized psychiatric patients who were given large dosages of phenothiazines for 3 to 10 years.

Ocular changes. The occurrence of ocular changes exceeds skin pigmentation reactions. This is most dramatic in patients receiving chlorpromazine in dosages of 300 mg daily and higher for 2 or more years. The characteristic eye changes are deposition of fine particulate matter in both the lens and the cornea. In more advanced cases, star-shaped opacities have been observed in the anterior portion of the lens. The nature of these eye deposits has not been determined. A small number of patients with severe ocular changes have some visual impairment. The corneal and lenticular changes have also been associated with observations of epithelial keratopathy and pigmentary retinopathy. Some reports indicate that after withdrawal of the drug the eye lesions may regress. The nurse should indicate to the patient that the eye-change occurrence may be related to dosage levels or therapy duration; therefore the patient with a long-term regimen or moderate- to high-dose therapy should have periodic ophthamologic examinations.

The cause of dermatologic and ocular reactions appears to be associated with dosage levels or duration of therapy along with exposure to sunlight.

Endocrine imbalance. Endocrine imbalance is caused by depression of hypothalamic functions. These symptoms have been reported infrequently and include delayed ovulation and menstruation, amenorrhea with false-positive results from pregnancy tests, lactogenic response in female patients, and weight gain. These symptoms may cause unwarranted anxiety and compound the patient's problems. After ordinary steps are initiated to determine other possible causative factors for these symptoms without positive results, the patient should be reassured that the medication she is receiving is the causative factor. Depending on the patient's current pattern of symptoms, reinforcement of these facts may be necessary.

In pregnancy the risk of administration of these drugs should be weighed against the expected therapeutic outcome.

Extrapyramidal symptoms. Extrapyramidal symptoms may appear after the administration of a single dose of phenothiazines or after prolonged usage. Extrapyramidal symptoms are considered to be a rather normal consequence of drug action. The extrapyramidal effects of the phenothiazines and thioxanthenes are probably caused by diminished dopaminergic stimulation in basal ganglia at the corpus striatum. These reactions are of four general types: pseudoparkinsonism, dystonias, akathisia, and dyskinesia. Pseudoparkinsonism resembles true parkinsonism and manifests symptoms such as tremor, masklike facial expression, rigidity, drooling, loss of associated movements of the arms, and some restlessness. Occurence of dystonia (in the form of acute torsion dystonia) in less than hours or a few days is seen after parenteral administration in a younger patient (under 30 years), and becomes evident to medical personnel when the patient complains of fatigue, muscle rigidity, abnormal posturing, perioral spasms (with protrusion of the tongue), mandibular movements, dysphagia, dysphasia, oculogyric crisis, and weakness of the arms and legs.

Akathisia (motor restlessness) becomes apparent when the patient is observed to be extremely restless, continually moving his hands, mouth, and body and being unable to sit or lie quietly. Dyskinesia is a less common disturbance that takes many forms such as torsion spasm, opisthotonos, oculogyric crises, drooping of the head, protrusion of the tongue, and other facial disturbances (Fig. 11-6). Patients complain of stiff neck and inability to swallow and usually become very frightened with the onset of these symptoms. The dramatic suddenness of onset is often frightening to nursing personnel as well. Recognition of the cause of this combination of symptoms is helpful in allaying the anxiety of both nurse and patient. Immediate action should be instituted to reverse this extrapyramidal reaction. The administration of an antiparkinsonian agent orally (when possible) or parenterally will produce a reversal of

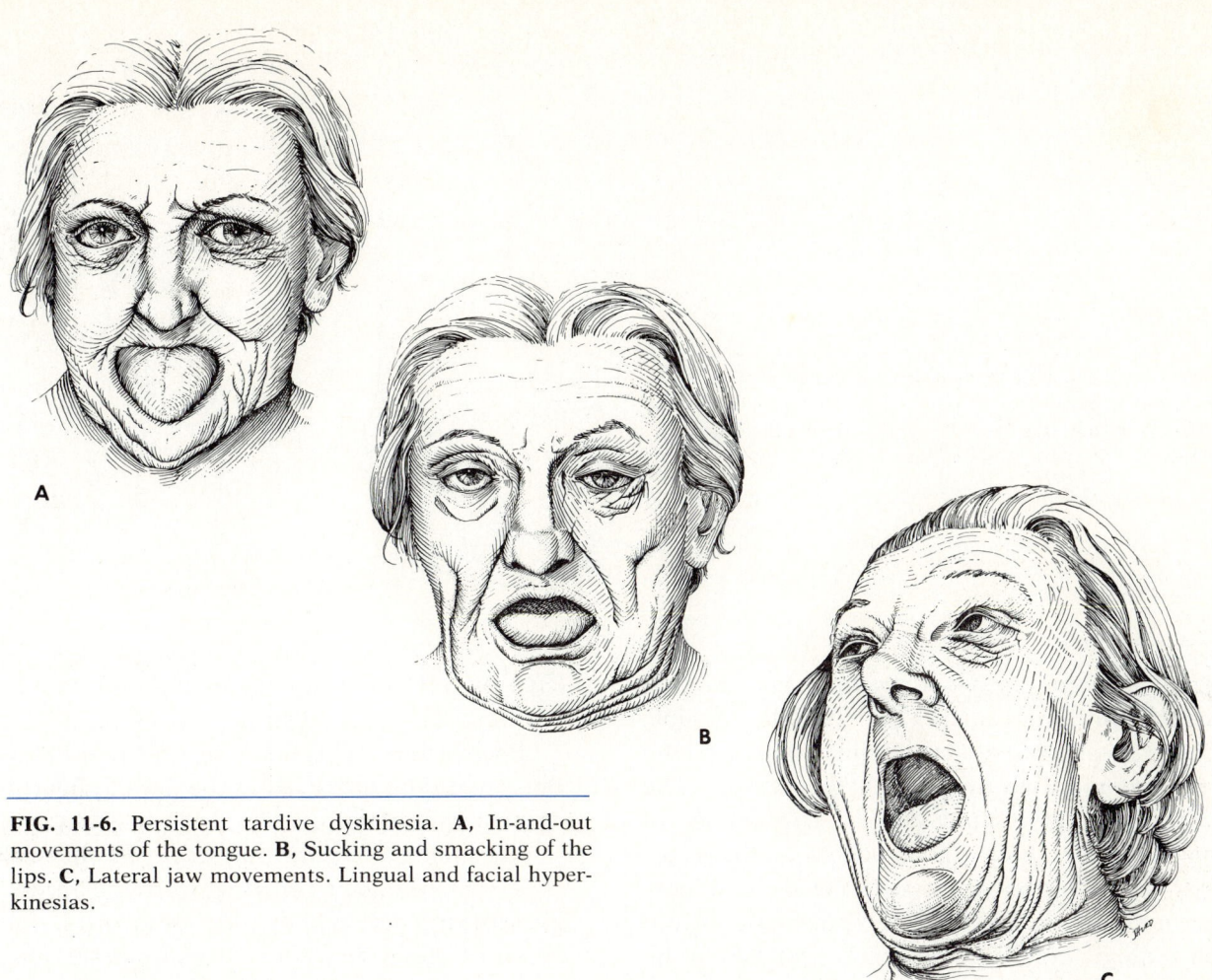

FIG. 11-6. Persistent tardive dyskinesia. **A,** In-and-out movements of the tongue. **B,** Sucking and smacking of the lips. **C,** Lateral jaw movements. Lingual and facial hyperkinesias.

symptoms in as dramatic a fashion as the onset of the symptoms. The nurse should stay with the patient and reassure him that the symptoms will subside; this also gives the nurse an opportunity to observe the patient closely. Pseudoparkinsonism, akathisia, and dystonias may have a more gradual onset than dyskinesia; however, they may be just as troublesome to patients. Generally these extrapyramidal symptoms, except for tardive dyskinesia, are easily controlled when one lowers the dosage, discontinues the medication, uses a compound that has a low incidence of these reactions, or allows short drug-free periods (Table 11-4). Those drugs having the fewest extrapyramidal effects are almost always less effective therapeutically than those that produce extrapyramidal activity.

Persistent tardive dyskinesia. As with all antipsychotic agents, tardive dyskinesia may ap-

TABLE 11-4 Frequency of incidence of extrapyramidal symptoms of phenothiazines

	Generic name	Trade name
Highest incidence	Fluphenazine	Permitil; Prolixin
	Trifluoperazine	Stelazine
	Perphenazine	Trilafon
	Prochlorperazine	Compazine
	Acetophenazine	Tindal
	Carphenazine	Proketazine
	Triflupromazine	Vesprin
	Chlorpromazine	Thorazine
	Piperacetazine	Quide
Lowest incidence	Thioridazine	Mellaril
	Mesoridazine	Serentil

pear in some patients during long-term therapy or may appear after drug therapy is discontinued. This may appear in patients of all ages, but there appears to be a greater incidence in elderly females and patients with organic brain syndrome who are undergoing high-dose therapy.

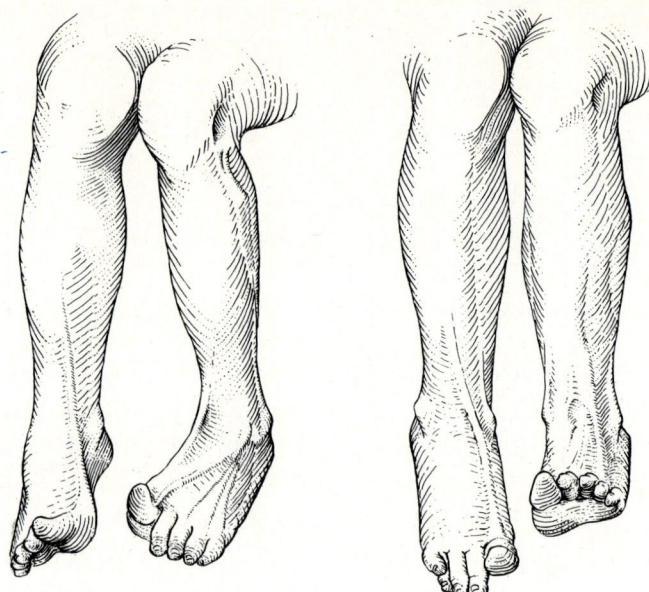

FIG. 11-7. Persistent tardive dyskinesia (abnormal movements of extremities). Complication of long-term therapy with antipsychotics (neuroleptics). Choreoathetoid movements.

The symptoms consist of rhythmic coordinated involuntary movements of muscle groups, which most often affect the musculature of the faciolinguobuccal area and the hands. The symptoms persist and may be irreversible in some patients. This syndrome may be the result of this long-term therapy with dopamine-blocking neuroleptic agents. The underlying pathophysiologic condition has been proposed to be attributed to a dopamine-receptor supersensitivity in the extrapyramidal system. The overt symptoms are characteristic (Fig. 11-6) of the following: movements of the tongue, face, mouth, and jaw (such as protrusion of the tongue, chewing of the cheeks (the inside of the patient's mouth should be checked for this on admission), puckering of the mouth, and chewing movements; these may be coupled with movements of an involuntary nature of the extremities (Fig. 11-7). It is suggested that all antipsychotic agents be discontinued if these symptoms appear.

There is no known effective treatment for tardive dyskinesia; antiparkinsonism drugs usually do not alleviate the symptoms of this syndrome. There is a belief that the addition of an anticholinergic to a neuroleptic regimen may promote the induction of tardive dyskinesia because the anticholinergic may promote neuroleptic-induced dopamine-receptor hypersensitivity.

The efficacy of amantadine hydrochloride

(Symmetrel) in relieving neuroleptic-induced parkinsonism is recognized.

Precautions. There are several precautions that should be observed in the use of phenothiazine compounds.

Autonomic blockade may occur as one of the most serious effects resulting from the adrenergic blocking action of the phenothiazines. If circulatory collapse occurs, a vasopressor agent such as levaretrenol should be given. *Epinephrine* should *never* be used, since its administration to a patient with partial adrenergic blockade may result in a further fall of blood pressure.

Potentiation of other drugs is a common effect produced by the phenothiazine derivatives. They should be used cautiously in patients who are under the influence of alcohol, barbiturates, or morphine-like analgesics. The phenothiazines in combination with alcohol produce severe, possibly fatal, depression of the respiratory center and impaired hepatic functions that result in toxic manifestations. Use of phenothiazines to control alcohol withdrawal can be hazardous because phenothiazines increase seizure susceptibility. Furthermore, hypotension, a side effect of these drugs, can be exacerbated by alcohol. Several studies in humans indicate strongly, but not conclusively, that alcohol in combination with any of the neuroleptics impairs driving skills.

The dosage of anesthetics should be reduced. These drugs should also be used with care in patients who are taking antihypertensive drugs. They should be used cautiously in patients receiving atropine or related drugs because of the additive anticholinergic effects.

Antiemetic effects of these agents may complicate the diagnosis of nausea and vomiting related to organic disorders.

Other adverse reactions that have been observed are melanosis of internal organs such as the heart, liver, and kidneys after the administration of chlorpromazine in large doses. The hepatolenticular degenerative syndrome with pigmentation in deposit areas occurs with long-term aliphatic phenothiazine therapy caused by the oxidative and methylated derivatives, which also deposit on the skin and cornea and retina of the eye. Each of the specific phenothiazines varies with the amount of the dose excreted as metabolites in the urine and the portion that passes through the bile and into fecal excretion. Electrocardiographic alterations resembling those caused by quinidine or by hypokalemia and pigmentary retinopathy have been noted, especially when large doses of thioridazine have been administered. These drugs should be administered cautiously to patients with suspected heart disease. Because of the pronounced anticholinergic action of these agents, they should not be administered to patients with a history of glaucoma or prostatic hypertrophy. During the summer months, instances of hyperthermia and heat prostration have been reported. The phenothiazines should be used cautiously and in small doses in patients with a history of convulsive disorders because of their action in reducing the convulsive threshold. These drugs are contraindicated in comatose patients because of their central nervous system depressive effect.

Cardiac findings in sudden death after prolonged use of the phenothiazines have been inconclusive. Patients have been known to die suddenly and unexpectedly. Postmortem examinations of these patients have revealed the presence of a brown granular pigment in the heart and other viscera. It has been hypothesized that death is caused by ventricular arrhythmia or asphyxia attributable to failure of the cough reflex during a convulsive seizure.

ALIPHATIC COMPOUNDS
Chlorpromazine hydrochloride (Thorazine Hydrochloride)

Chlorpromazine was introduced for clinical trial in 1951. It is a grayish white, crystalline powder that is soluble in water. It is chemically related to the antihistaminic promethazine (Phenergan) but in comparison chlorpromazine has little antihistaminic activity. It was introduced in Europe under the name of Largactil.

Preparation, dosage, and administration. Chlorpromazine hydrochloride is marketed in sustained-release capsules (30, 75, 150, 200, and 300 mg); in solution, in ampules and multiple-dose vials (25 mg/ml); in syrup (2 mg/ml); in tablets (10, 25, 50, 100, and 200 mg); and as a concentrate (30 mg/ml). Chlorpromazine is available also in suppository form (25 and 100 mg).

The smallest effective dose is the one recommended. Oral adult dosage varies from 10 mg to 1 g or more per day. Total daily amounts are usually given in three evenly spaced doses. For children the oral dose is 2 mg/kg body weight daily in divided doses. Intramuscular dose is 0.5 mg/kg every 6 to 8 hours.

Chlorpromazine hydrochloride is administered orally, intramuscularly, and intravenously. It is usually given orally unless for some reason the patient is unable to take the dose by mouth. Often patients will conceal tablets in the back of their mouth or around the teeth and lip area. The concentrate may be used effectively in this case. The taste of chlorpromazine hydrochloride concentrate can become more palatable when given in fruit juice; however, the patient should be told there is medication in the juice. If chlorpromazine concentrate is used for long periods of time, close attention must be given to proper oral hygiene. The concentrate is a highly irritating substance on contact with skin and eyes. Care should be taken to immediately wash areas of the body that come into contact with this substance. Nurses have been known to contract very uncomfortable contact dermatologic conditions as a result of their contact with this substance.

Chlorpromazine hydrochloride is considered too irritating to be given subcutaneously. When given intramuscularly, it should be injected deeply and slowly in divided doses of not more than 1 ml per injection site. Massage of the site of injection helps to reduce local irritation. Some patients have been known to develop abscesses at the injection site, which are believed to result from large doses of this substance in one area. Use of the intramuscular route of administration of chlorpromazine is usually indicated when the patient refuses the tablet or concentrate form or when the most immediate effect of the drug is desired. If the patient is severely agitated, combative, or struggling, care should be taken to follow safe administration technique. This technique usually requires enough well-trained personnel to adequately restrain the patient while the medication is being given.

Triflupromazine hydrochloride (Vesprin)

Action and uses. This compound is at least twice as active as chlorpromazine but otherwise is similar to chlorpromazine in its spectrum. It has been found to be useful in the management of pernicious vomiting of pregnancy, postoperative emesis, and the nausea and vomiting occurring after encephalograms or ventriculograms.

Preparation, dosage, and administration. Triflupromazine hydrochloride can be administered orally in tablets of 10, 25, and 50 mg, in a suspension of 50 mg/5 ml, and intramuscularly in solutions of 10 and 20 mg/ml. Oral therapy should be substituted for parenteral administration as soon as possible. The usual dose for hospitalized psychotic adults is 100 to 150 mg daily. Dosage for children is 30 to 150 mg daily in divided doses. The initial daily dosage for elderly patients with psychoses is 10 mg three times a day. For prevention and treatment of nausea and vomiting in adults, the oral dose is 20 to 30 mg daily.

PIPERIDINE COMPOUNDS
Thioridazine hydrochloride (Mellaril)

This phenothiazine derivative is not a highly potent tranquilizer. It does not exert an antiemetic effect, and it seems to have no effect on temperature regulation. It has a broad spectrum of useful antipsychotic activity and is considered by many to be a good all-around tranquilizer. It is believed to have the advantage of

producing minimal extra-pyramidal effects.

The presence of a thiomethyl radical (S—CH_3) in position 2, conventionally occupied by a halogen, is unique and could account for the greater toleration obtained with thioridazine.

Cardiotoxicity from overdoses of thioridazine may be as frequent and dangerous as that observed with the overdose of the tricyclic antidepressants; therefore, the same precautions and observations should be taken as done for the tricyclic antidepressants.

Patients taking large doses also have been known to develop pigmentary retinopathy. Sudden death has been reported after prolonged usage of this drug.

Preparation, dosage, and administration. Thioridazine hydrochloride is available in 10-, 25-, 50-, 100-, 150-, and 200-mg tablets, as a concentrate (30 and 100 mg/ml) for oral administration and as an oral suspension at 25 and 100 mg/5 ml with a buttermint flavor. Adult dosage varies from 20 to 800 mg daily. Dosage for children 2 years of age or over is 1 mg/kg body weight in three or four divided doses. Dosage for this preparation as well as for other tranquilizers is adjusted to meet the needs of the individual.

Side effects and toxic effects. Drowsiness is a frequent side effect, especially after large doses. Many other side effects associated with therapy with the phenothiazine compounds have been seen after the administration of this drug, but on the whole, toxic effects are said to occur less often than after the administration of chlorpromazine. Visual impairment and blindness have occurred. Therefore, patients should be closely observed for signs of diminished visual acuity, impaired night vision, and brown discoloration of objects. (For other side effects, see the discussion of phenothiazine derivatives, pp. 324-328.)

Mesoridazine besylate (Serentil)

Mesoridazine is a metabolite of thioridazine. It was introduced in 1970 and is used for treating acute and chronic schizophrenia, the manic phase of manic-depressive psychosis, and involutional, senile, organic, or toxic psychosis with the exception of delirium tremens. Its actions, side effects, precautions, and drug interactions are the same as for thioridazine and the antipsychotic phenothiazines (see chlorpromazine).

Preparation and dosage. It is available in oral tablets of 10, 25, 50, and 100 mg and as a solution for injection containing 25 mg/ml. Oral dosage for adults and for children over 12 years is 100 to 400 mg daily in divided doses. For elderly patients dosage is one fourth to one half the usual dose. Intramuscular dosage is 25 to 200 mg daily in divided doses.

Piperacetazine (Quide)

Piperacetazine is an antipsychotic drug of the piperidyl group of the phenothiazines. It is closely related to acetophenazine. It is used for the control of hyperactivity, agitation, and anxiety states associated with acute and chronic schizophrenic reactions in adult patients under adequate medical supervision. It is more effective in acute than chronic schizophrenia. Piperacetazine causes a higher incidence of extrapyramidal effects than other piperedine compounds do and resembles the piperazine drugs in this respect. Side effects and precautions are the same as for the phenothiazines and chlorpromazine.

Contraindications. Piperacetazine is contraindicated for pregnant women or those who may become pregnant, for patients who are comatose or greatly depressed, and for patients with blood dyscrasias or liver disease.

Preparation and dosage. Piperacetazine is available in 10- and 25-mg tablets. Dosage for adults and children over 12 years of age is 20 to 40 mg daily in divided doses initially. Maintenance dose is up to 160 mg daily in divided doses. Elderly patients should receive one fourth to one half the usual dose.

PIPERAZINE COMPOUNDS
Acetophenazine dimaleate (Tindal)

Action and uses. Acetophenazine dimaleate is a member of the piperazine group of phenothiazine derivatives and may be effective in the management of patients with chronic brain syndrome. Large doses have been effective in the treatment of psychotic patients. It has limited usefulness in the treatment of patients whose anxiety is associated with psychosomat-

ic conditions (peptic ulcer, hypertension). It is much less potent than other derivatives. It is more sedative and produces fewer extrapyramidal phenomena.

Preparation, dosage, and administration. Acetophenazine dimaleate is available for administration in tablets of 20 mg only. It is not available for parenteral administration. The usual oral dosage is 40 to 80 mg/day. In patients who have insomnia, the last tablet should be taken 1 hour before retiring. Dosage for hospitalized patients ranges from 80 to 120 mg/day in divided doses; patients with severe schizophrenia have received doses as high as 400 to 600 mg/day.

Fluphenazine hydrochloride (Permitil, Prolixin)

In terms of potency fluphenazine hydrochloride is one of the most active compounds and is considered more than 20 times as potent as chlorpromazine. It offers the advantage of sustained and prolonged action as an antipsychotic agent. It is the prototype of the piperazine compounds.

Preparation, dosage, and administration. Fluphenazine hydrochloride can be administered either orally or intramuscularly. The oral dose is about two to three times greater than the parenteral dose. An initial daily dose of 0.5 to 10 mg is suggested for adults with psychotic conditions. The dosage may be gradually increased to 20 mg/day or as high as 40 mg/day; however, the usual maintenance dose is 1 to 5 mg. Elderly patients may require much less than the average amounts. Oral preparations include a concentrate of 5 mg/ml (Permitil); an elixir of 2.5 mg/5 ml (Prolixin); 0.25-, 1-, 2.5-, 5-, and 10-mg tablets (Permitil or Prolixin); and repeat-action tablets of 1 mg (Permitil Chronotab). The intramuscular preparation is in a solution of 2.5 mg/ml in 10-ml containers. Parenteral injection has an average duration of action of 2 weeks.

Fluphenazine enanthate (Prolixin Enanthate); fluphenazine decanoate (Prolixin Decanoate)

Fluphenazine enanthate is an esterified derivative of fluphenazine hydrochloride. It maintains all the properties and actions of the phenothiazines; however, it has gained increasing popularity because of its prolonged action. One injection of 12.5 to 25 mg/ml solution maintains its action and effects for 1 to 3 weeks or longer for the enanthate form and up to 4 weeks or longer for the decanoate form. This effect seems to facilitate its use with outpatients or individuals who might not otherwise be disposed to taking medication on a daily basis. Because of its potency and the high incidence of extrapyramidal symptoms, some physicians believe concomitant treatment with antiparkinsonian agents is necessary. The risk of irreversible extrapyramidal symptoms seems to be the greatest in elderly female patients with organic brain disease or damage who have received fairly high dosages of phenothiazines for prolonged periods. Dosage should not exceed 100 mg.

Perphenazine (Trilafon)

Perphenazine is similar to chlorpromazine in action and clinical uses. Milligram for milligram it is said to be 12 times more potent than chlorpromazine. It has an antiemetic effect.

Preparation, dosage, and administration. Administration of perphenazine may be oral, intramuscular, and occasionally intravenous. The oral dosage for psychotic adults varies from 16 to 64 mg daily given in two to four divided doses. It is marketed in solution for injection, 5 mg/ml in 1- and 10-ml containers; as a liquid concentrate, 16 mg/5 ml; and in tablets of 2, 4, 8, and 16 mg. Perphenazine should not be administered intravenously (1 mg over 1 minute) except during surgery to counteract retching, hiccups, and vomiting; this route is not recommended for psychiatric conditions.

Prochlorperazine dimaleate (Compazine)

Prochlorperazine is approximately 10 times more potent than chlorpromazine on a milligram-for-milligram basis. It has a rapid and stimulating effect, which makes it useful in the treatment of psychomotor retardation, apathy, and withdrawal. It shares all the additional effects of the phenothiazines in antipsychotic activity. In small doses it has been effective in controlling nausea and vomiting associated with some somatic conditions.

Preparation, dosage, and administration

Prochlorperazine suppositories (Compazine). Prochlorperazine is administered rectally. The suggested dose for adults is one 25-mg suppository twice daily. Suppositories are available in 2.5, 5, and 25 mg.

Prochlorperazine edisylate (Compazine Edisylate). Administration may be oral in doses similar to those given for the dimaleate salt. Intramuscular injection is given of 10 to 20 mg, repeated at intervals of 1 to 6 hours, for control of psychotic symptoms. Intramuscular dose for adults with nonpsychiatric conditions is 5 to 10 mg, repeated once if necessary. It is available in solution for injection, 5 mg/ml in 2- (ampule and syringe) and 10-ml containers; the solution concentrate contains 10 mg/ml and the syrup contains 5 mg/5 ml.

Prochlorperazine dimaleate (Compazine). This preparation, when administered orally to psychotic adults is given initially in divided doses that range from 30 to 40 mg daily. Dosage is gradually increased to 75 to 150 mg a day. Tablets come in 5-, 10-, and 25-mg strengths and sustained-release capsules of 10, 15, 30, and 75 mg.

Trifluoperazine hydrochloride (Stelazine)

Trifluoperazine is fast acting and approximately 25 times more potent on a milligram-for-milligram basis than chlorpromazine. It has been successful in stimulating patients with symptoms of psychomotor retardation, apathy, and withdrawal. Its use in psychoneurotic and psychosomatic conditions has not been established. It has been proved to be an effective anti-psychotic agent.

Preparation, dosage, and administration. Trifluoperazine hydrochloride is available in concentrate solution of 10 mg/ml and in 1-, 2-, 5-, and 10-mg tablets for oral administration. A solution is also available for intramuscular injection, 2 mg/ml in 10-ml containers.

Dosage varies considerably, depending on the severity of symptoms to be controlled. For mild anxiety reactions, the oral dosage may range from 1 to 4 mg daily. The dosage for patients with major psychosis may start at 2 to 5 mg twice daily, but the optimal dosage may become 15 to 20 mg daily. Some patients require as much as 40 mg daily. For children 6 to 12 years of age the dosage is 1 mg once or twice daily, which may be increased up to 15 mg daily.

Carphenazine dimaleate (Proketazine)

Carphenazine has a spectrum of activity similar to that of other piperazine phenothiazines. Uses, side effects, precautions, and drug interactions are like those of other phenothiazines. It is available in 25- and 50-mg tablets. Initial oral dose for adults is 50 to 150 mg daily in divided doses. Dosage may be increased by 25 to 50 mg daily every 7 to 14 days. Maximal dosage is 400 mg daily. For elderly patients the dose is one fourth to one half the usual dose and is adjusted according to response.

THIOXANTHENE DERIVATIVES
Thiothixene hydrochloride (Navane)

The difference between the phenothiazine and the thioxanthene nucleus is that the nitrogen atom in the middle ring (position 10) of the phenothiazine is replaced by a carbon atom (position 9) in the thioxanthene nucleus. Neuroleptic activity occurs when the side chain at R_1 is attached to the carbon atom of the ring by a double bond. There is a lower rate of skin pigmentation and photosensitivity with the thioxanthenes than the phenothiazines because of the different metabolites.

Thiothixene, a thioxanthene derivative, resembles the piperazine phenothiazines in its tranquilizing and antiemetic actions and to a lesser degree in its spasmolytic and hypotensive effects. Its indications for use, side effects, precautions, and drug interactions are the same as those for the phenothiazines. Extrapyramidal symptoms and insomnia occur frequently with this drug. It is available in 1-, 2-, 5-, 10-, and 20-mg capsules; as a liquid concentrate, 5 mg/ml; and as a solution for injection containing 2 and 5 mg/ml in 2-ml ampules and vials and for intramuscular injection in 10-mg vials.

Preparation, dosage, and administration. Oral dosage for adults and for children over 12 years of age is 6 to 15 mg daily in divided doses initially, which may be gradually increased to a maximum dosage of 60 mg daily. Intramuscular dosage is 8 to 16 mg daily in divided doses, which may be increased to a maximum dosage of 30 mg daily.

Chlorprothixene (Taractan)

Action and uses. Although chlorprothixene is not a phenothiazine, its action and effects are very similar to the phenothiazine compounds. It is used in similar conditions, and adverse reactions associated with phenothiazine therapy should be borne in mind when this agent is used. This compound is believed to be less likely to produce troublesome side effects such as extrapyramidal symptoms, agranulocytosis, and cholestatic hepatitis. However, a few incidences of these effects have been reported. This agent has also been reported to be useful as an antiemetic.

Preparation, dosage, and administration. Chlorprothixene is administered orally and intramuscularly. Oral dosages range from 30 to 600 mg/day. The drug is administered orally in tablets of 10, 25, 50, and 100 mg; a concentrate of 100 mg/5 ml is also available. Dosage for children over 6 years of age is 30 to 100 mg daily in divided doses. Intramuscular dosage for the acutely agitated patient with a psychotic condition is 75 to 200 mg/day. Children over age 6 or elderly and debilitated patients receive lower initial doses of 10 to 25 mg three or four times daily. Preparations for injection come in a solution of 12.5 mg/ml in 2-ml containers.

BUTYROPHENONE DERIVATIVE
Haloperidol (Haldol)

The butyrophenones are structurally different from the phenothiazines and the thioxanthines but have similar properties in terms of antipsychotic efficacy. The receptor-blockade activity in the central nervous system may be at the level of the dopamine receptors. They have relatively less effect on the norepinephrine and epinephrine receptors and are probably more potent than most of the phenothiazine agents in their dopaminergic effects and possess a significant degree of extrapyramidal effects. The drug has both antiemetic and antipsychotic effects.

After oral administration, rapid absorption

occurs, with blood levels of the drug seen within 1 hour; the drug is concentrated in extravascular space; with 2 to 3 hours after administration the drug appears in the urine; but after 5 days about 40% of the drug is recovered in the urine and may be significantly tissue bound.

Action and uses. Haloperidol was introduced in the United States as an antipsychotic agent in 1967. Research conducted in Europe in the area of anesthesia brought this compound into view as a possible antipsychotic agent. Subsequent use indicated its effectiveness in the control of hyperactivity associated with the manic phase. Extrapyramidal symptoms occur frequently and, as the manic phase becomes controlled, severe depressive elements may be seen in some patients, precipitating a suicide risk. Adverse reactions discussed earlier in regard to the phenothiazines also apply to this compound.

Haloperidol is indicated in management of schizophrenic patients with acute manic symptoms, social withdrawal, and paranoid behavior; in the manic phase of manic-depressive psychosis; and to control emotionally disturbed aggressive behavior in children, Gilles de la Tourette's disease, and delirium tremens. It has been used in the treatment of stuttering, persistent hiccups, and antiemetic applications. The drug may act by inhibiting specific areas in the extrapyramidal system by forming a film on membranes in the central nervous system that contain gamma-aminobutyric acid and dopamine.

Preparation, dosage, and administration. Haloperidol is administered orally in tablets of 0.5, 1, 2.5, and 10 mg and as haloperidol concentrate of 2 mg/ml. A solution for injection contains 5 mg/ml in 1-ml ampules. Initial dosages should be gradually increased in increments of 0.5 to 1 mg every 3 days until the desired effects are attained. Daily doses greater than 15 mg are not recommended. Maintenance dose is usually 2 to 8 mg daily. Dosage is the same for adults and children over 12 years of age. The safety of doses exceeding 100 mg/day for prolonged periods has not been established.

DIBENZOXAPINE DERIVATIVE
Loxapine (Loxitane, Daxolin)

Loxapine is a member of a distinct chemical class of antipsychotic drugs: a dibenzoxapine. There is no significant advantage of this drug over other antipsychotic drugs. It has structural similarity to phenothiazines because it contains a piperazine side chain. It has a rapid and complete absorption.

Loxitane is indicated in psychosis particularly schizophrenic manifestations, because it has a calming effect and supresses aggressive behavior. Signs of sedation occur within 20 to 30 minutes after administration and are pronounced in 1½ to 3 hours, with a duration of 12 hours.

Preparation, dosage, and administration. Administration is in divided doses two to four times daily. The initial dose is 10 mg twice daily; in the severely depressed person up to 50 mg is used, with the dose being increased rapidly over a 7- to 10-day period for effective control of psychiatric symptoms. The daily dose range is 150 to 225 mg, with a maintenance dose of 40 to 100 mg. The usual therapeutic dose and maintenance dose are 60 to 100 mg; exceeding 250 mg is not recommended. It is emphasized that doses should be absolutely the lowest compatible with symptom control.

The nurse should administer the oral concentrate loxapine hydrochloride, known as Loxitan or Daxolin C Oral Concentrate, with the calibrated dropper, which has 1 ml equal to 25 mg only. The drug should be mixed with fruit juice such as orange or grapefruit juice shortly before administration to the patient.

It is available in capsules of 5, 10, 25, and 50 mg in the succinate form and for injection of 50 mg/ml in the hydrochloride form.

Side effects and toxic effects. Adverse effects are described as extrapyramidal symptoms of all types, anticholinergic effects, and orthostatic hypotension. The last is seen more often in the elderly females who have been taking high doses over longer periods.

Safety in pregnancy and lactation is not established. Loxitane lowers the convulsive threshold. The drug is contraindicated in comatose or severe drug-induced depressed states as in those caused by alcohol, barbiturates, narcotics, and reserpine.

DIHYDROINDOLONE DERIVATIVE
Molindone (Lidone, Moban)

Molindone is an antipsychotic, chemically an oxygenated indole (dihydroindolone), and is a new chemical class having a chemical resemblance to reserpine. In theory molindone acts on the ascending reticular activating system, with activity similar to major tranquilizers such as phenothiazines.

Uses. It is used to treat psychosis, particularly schizophrenia since it activates the previously withdrawn schizophrenic person. It has demonstrated efficacy in acute and chronic schizophrenia and paranoid schizophrenia, and in younger adults with acute psychotic episodes with a short history it may be used where alternatives yielded no response or an allergy.

Preparation, dosage, and administration. Molindone is clinically half as potent on a milligram-for-milligram basis as trifluoperazine (Stelazine) (3 to 5 mg of molindone is dose equated to 50 mg of chlorpromazine or 2 mg trifluoperazine). No changes in dose may be necessary in renal or hepatic failure. Elderly or debilitated patients should be started with low doses (one-third to one-half the usual adult dose), such as 5 mg three times daily, and titrated to individual patient response as with other patients. The daily dose in acute psychotic episodes may be from 150 to 225 mg, with a maintenance range of 40 to 100 mg daily in divided doses. Mild symptoms require 5 to 15 mg three to four times daily; moderate symptoms require 10 to 25 mg three to four times daily; severe symptoms show response up to 225 mg (with 300 to 400 mg/day being reported). A once-daily dosage may be possible because peak plasma levels occur shortly after ingestion and gradually decline over the next 20 hours, and if it is administered at bedtime, it may be advantageous over divided doses for increased compliance and reduction of adverse effects.

Molindone has a short half-life (1.5 hours) for divided doses; the effect lasts up to 36 hours.

Molindone is available in 5-, 10-, 25-, 50-, and 100-mg capsules and tablets and as an oral cherry flavored concentrate of 20 mg/ml.

Side effects and toxic effects. The adverse effects parallel those of the piperazine phenothiazines: low incidence of anticholinergic effects (dry mouth, blurred vision, constipation), high incidence of extrapyramidal effects (rigidity, dysphagia, akathisia, dystonia, and tonic spasm), and minimal sedation. Precautions are to be exercised when molindone is used during pregnancy (benefits anticipated must outweigh unknown fetal risks) or lactation or in patients with epilepsy or seizure disorders (since convulsive seizures have been reported), leukopenia, orthostatic hypotension, and tachycardia. Molindone will aggravate tardive dyskinesia and a dose reduction or an antiparkinsonian drug may be used. Transient drowsiness, central nervous system stimulation, weight gain or loss, menstrual irregularities, and gastrointestinal effects (xerostomia) have been reported. Depression, hyperactivity, and euphoria all have been shown to occur with this drug.

The nurse should encourage the patient to adhere to the regimen. The patient is to avoid alcohol and central nervous system depressants, including over-the-counter drugs with CNS depressant effects. It is suggested that fine vermicular movements of the tongue may be an early sign of the syndrome (persistent tardive dyskinesia), and if the medication is stopped at that time, the syndrome may not develop. It is necessary for the nurse to discuss this syndrome with the patient and family. The drug is contraindicated in severe central nervous system depression, drug related conditions (alcohol, barbiturates, and narcotics), a comatose patient, and hypersensitivity to the drug. The tablet form contains the excipient calcium sulfate; since calcium ions impair the absorption of tetracycline and phenytoin, the patient must remember this interaction.

Antidepressants

Interest in psychotherapeutic agents useful for alleviating depressions has brought about a significant change in the treatment of these conditions. Depressive states appear to be unique to the human being and have been classified by psychiatrists as endogenous psychotic depressions and reactive depressions. Endogenous psychotic depressions are characterized by the absence of external causes for depression (death of a loved one, loss of employment, or debilitating illness), and the apparent grief and depression are of psychopathologic origin. Reactive depressions usually are abnormal depressive responses to environmental factors and are associated with emotional tension and instability. Psychomotor hyperexcitability (agitation) often occurs. Other behavioral manifestations characterizing depression are the expression of feelings of worthlessness, inadequacy, hopelessness, ambivalence, dependence, guilt, and suicidal tendencies. Delusions are common, the content of which express self-accusatory and guilt feelings. Initiative is lost and the patient is apathetic. The eyes are often directed downward, the corners of the mouth sag, lower eyelids droop, and the skin on the forehead may be furrowed. Depression is usually accompanied by poor appetite, loss of weight, sleep disturbances, coated tongue, foul breath, and constipation. About 30 years ago depressed patients were treated with analeptic drugs, such as pentylenetetrazole, to induce convulsions, which seemed to improve their condition. Later insulin was used to produce convulsions resulting from hypoglycemia. Electroconvulsive therapy (ECT) was developed and found to be much safer than the aforementioned treatments. Electroconvulsive therapy is still used today, specifically for the depressed patient with manifestations of agitation.

Short-acting neuromuscular blocking agents and barbiturates are used before these treatments to prevent damage to the patient's limbs during the convulsions. These convulsions are induced by passing an AC current, for a fraction of a second, through electrodes fixed to the scalp. It is assumed that the cycle of events leading to the depressive symptoms is broken by the electric charge that allows neuronal activity to return to normal. Electroconvulsive therapy has also been known to increase the free amines in the brain. The psychoactive

drugs used in the treatment of depression have not replaced electroconvulsive treatment; however, they have occasionally been a valuable adjunct to this form of treatment. Other measures such as psychotherapy, reduction of environmental stresses, and milieu therapy should also accompany electroconvulsive therapy. The psychotherapeutic drugs most commonly used in the treatment of unipolar affective disorders are the tricyclic compounds and the monoamine oxidase inhibitors. All these drugs appear to be most therapeutic in the treatment of endogenous depression. The monoamine oxidase inhibitors have produced favorable results in both endogenous and reactive depressions. Favorable responses to these drugs include elevation of mood, increased physical activity and mental alertness, and improved appetite and sleep patterns, accompanied by a reduction of premorbid preoccupation and delusions.

The tricyclic compounds, the monoamine oxidase inhibitors, and the amphetamines provide relief for some of the symptoms related to depression. However, they do not treat the underlying causes of depression. They may relieve the depressive effects of temporary situational stress, but caution should be exerted to avoid using these drugs without a thorough evaluation of causative factors. The amphetamines act to stimulate the nervous system directly with little or no monoamine oxidase inhibition. Their action is brief (3 to 4 hours) and is frequently followed by a letdown. Hypertensive effect and reduced appetite are additional effects. Dependency can result from prolonged use of amphetamines. The difficulties involved with the use of these drugs should be weighed against the expected therapeutic results.

The major psychostimulants in use today are the amphetamines. Their official use for depression may be altered by FDA regulations limiting their use. The amphetamines possess powerful effects on all the amine systems. They may operate primarily on noradrenergic and dopaminergic neurons. The amphetamines can selectively release neurotransmitters from these nerve endings and also stimulate the postsynaptic receptors. Dextroamphetamine has about 10 times the potency of levoamphetamine on norepinephrine neurons, but it has approximately the same potency of action on dopaminergic neurons as levoamphetamine doses. Amphetamines in large doses have been found to cause a state similar to acute paranoid schizophrenia, with the excitation and arousal being mediated by catecholamine neurons.

Since the amphetamines are not widely used for the treatment of depression, further discussion of antidepressant drugs is confined to the tricyclic compounds and monoamine oxidase inhibitors.

Tricyclic antidepressants

Tricyclic antidepressants (TCAs) may be used to treat endogenous depression characterized by inactivity and regression. The second indication approved by the U.S. Food and Drug Administration is for childhood and adolescent enuresis (a use for imipramine). Imipramine is also used in treating phobic anxiety (such as agoraphobia characterized by spontaneous panic attacks with depression and anxiety). Amitriptyline and imipramine are being investigated for use in constant central pain syndrome; amitriptyline is being studied for use in migraine headache. Imipramine, its demethylated derivative desipramine, and trimipramine are dibenzapine derivatives; amitriptyline, nortriptyline, and protriptyline are dibenzocycloheptadiene derivatives; and doxepin is a dibenzoxazepine derivative. The tricyclic antidepressants are presented as a class, since they possess close structural similarities, similar physiochemical properties, and some indistinguishable pharmacologic actions.

The structural relationships of the tricyclic antidepressants can be seen from their basic structure. The three-ring nucleus characteristic of this group of drugs has given rise to the expression "tricyclics." The TCAs have a close chemical resemblance to the phenothiazines but less of a pharmacologic similarity. TCAs share with variation some of the phenothiazine-associated anticholinergics, alpha adrenergic receptor–blocking and alpha adrenergic properties. The dibenzapine class has a nucleus that most closely resembles that of the phenothiazines.

Imipramine, trimipramine, and amitriptyline are classified as tertiary amines because the nitrogen atom on their aminopropyl side chain has three substituents. Doxepin is also a tertiary amine. The monodemethylated (N-desmethyl) side-chain metabolite of imipramine is desipramine, and the metabolite of amitriptyline is nortriptyline. Desipramine, protriptyline, and nortriptyline are classified as secondary amines because the side-chain nitrogen atom has only two substituents.

Pharmacokinetics. The TCAs are absorbed rapidly by the gastrointestinal tract, rapidly distributed, lipophilic, and highly bound to plasma, protein, and tissue. The TCAs are metabolized (genetically determined variations) through the hepatic microsomal enzyme systems. The two metabolic routes most often used are (1) transformation of the "tricyclic" nucleus by ring hydroxylation and conjugation to form glucuronides and (2) alteration of the aliphatic side chain by demethylation of the nitrogen. It is obvious that when the tertiary amines (amitriptyline, imipramine) are administered to the patient two active drugs (the metabolites nortriptyline and desipramine, respectively) are present in the plasma concentrations when measurements are taken. The wide variation in interpretation in steady-state plasma levels may be attributable to the extensive first-pass metabolism in the liver and the rate of individual genetic differences. Plasma concentration levels may be of value in the suspected noncompliant patient, or in the determination of inadequacies in dosage, or during the recovery phases in the overdose situations (to be described later). The TCAs are highly bound to plasma protein, with individual differences that may be caused by individual genetic differences. Plasma concentrations may also be of use in calculating the dosage for elderly or the very young persons. Elderly patients may have lower hydroxylase levels, and there is a tendency to develop toxic levels because of this slowed metabolism. After the TCAs enter the plasma, the TCAs of the tissue levels are bound to endoplasmic reticulum, mitochondria, and the cellular sites.

When TCAs are administered to patients having endogenous depression, the therapeutic effects (mood elevation) of all the TCAs become evident within a lag period only after 2 to 3 weeks of treatment. This period may be required for steady-state blood levels to be obtained. The TCAs possess the pharmacologic properties of mood elevation, sedation, and peripheral and central anticholinergic action, by blocking the reuptake of norepinephrine by adrenergic nerve terminals (blockage of the "amine pump," an active-transport system in the presynaptic nerve endings that recaptures released amine neurotransmitters). They have quinidine-like myocardial effects and also block animal reserpine-induced sedative or "depressive" patterns. The metabolic alteration of norepinephrine is believed to be responsible for the changes in mood.

Site and mechanism of action. This group of antidepressant drugs does not inhibit monoamine oxidase or change the concentration of serotonin or other amines in the brain. Their mechanism of action is not known. However, it is hypothesized that the action of the drugs may be to affect brain amine levels by interfering with their reuptake into nerves; thus they potentiate the action of catecholamines. The drugs have atropine-like, antihistamine, antiepinephrine, and antiserotonin actions. Autonomic side effects associated with these actions occur but are not serious and usually subside as treatment continues. They have only a slight depressant effect on the central nervous system. They antagonize the antihypertensive action of guanethid and similar agents.

Therapeutic doses have obvious anticholinergic responses and cause orthostatic hypotension. A broad discussion of the adverse reactions is described later in this chapter.

The TCAs are more effective than the monoamine oxidase inhibitors in treatment of depression (both act by increasing availability of centralmonoamines), the former by blocking their reuptake and the latter by inhibition of their deamination. There is speculation that the greater efficiency is attributable to the greater selective action on norepinephrine and serotonin neurons. The inhibition of central monoamines by their deamination as seen with the monoamine oxidase inhibitors can be best described as the following: monoamine oxidase inhibitors block a major degradative pathway for the amine neurotransmitters, which presumably permits more amines to accumulate presynaptically and more to be released. The sympathomimetic amines also block the amine pump; however, the action is primarily by increase in the release of catecholaminergic neurotransmitters.

Research has demonstrated that the tertiary amines (such as amitriptyline) may strongly block the amine pump for serotonin (thus not effective in norepinephrine depletion), and the secondary amines (such as desipramine) more selectively block the amine pump for norepinephrine (thus not effective in serotonin depletion).

Selection. There are investigations in the literature to determine by biochemical tests a speculative definition of subtypes of depression and to predict the most efficacious TCA. There are many norepinephrine metabolites excreted in the urine that result more from peripheral than from central adrenergic activity. In the periphery, the major products of norepinephrine are vanillylmandelic acid (VMA) and a secondary product, 3-methoxy-4-hydroxyphenylglycol (MHPG); in the brain the major metabolite is the MHPG, from central adrenergic activity. When the urine contains little MHPG, the biochemical defect is assumed to be a deficiency of noradrenergic neurotransmission; a drug selected in blocking uptake of norepinephrine would be nortriptyline or desipramine. If the urine has normal or high excretion of MHPG, it is assumed to indicate a deficiency of serotonin, and a drug selected to blocking the uptake of serotonin would be amitriptyline. Further investigation of urine excretion of MHPG may provide a useful guide when one selects a drug to use in a particular patient subtype (high or low MHPG).

In selecting a TCA there are several criteria to consider. A thorough understanding of the adverse effects is essential. All the TCAs are relatively effective as antidepressants; the sedation effect of the TCAs may result in an anxious, restless, or insomnious depression wherein amitriptyline, doxepin, or trimipramine would be the drug of choice. If the sedative and anticholinergic effects are great, then desipramine, which has the least of these effects, may be used. In addition to the sedative and anticholinergic criteria, the patient's individual past experience with a TCA, such as any adverse reactions, will play an important role in the selection. Some patients will respond better to a TCA effective in norepinephrine depletion, and others respond to the TCA effective in serotonin depletion. Table 11-5 presents a comparison of the tricyclic antidepressants and provides assistance in the selection of them.

Side effects and toxic effects. The possibility of suicide is inherent in any severely depressed patient and persists until a significant remission occurs. When a patient presents with a serious overt suicidal potential and is not hospitalized, the quantity of the prescription of the TCA should not exceed 1 week's supply because the suicidal risks of this drug class are high and suicidal attempts with TCAs are frequently seen in many emergency rooms. In schizophrenic patients activation of the psychosis may occur and require reduction of the dosage or the addition of a major tranquilizer to the therapeutic regimen. Manic or hypomanic episodes may occur in patients with the cyclic type of disorders. If this occurs, the TCA should be discontinued until the episode is relieved and then the TCA may be reinstituted but at a lowered dosage if the TCA is still needed in the therapy. Concurrent administration of a TCA and electroconvulsive therapy may increase the hazards of therapy; therefore, when possible, the TCA should be discontinued for several days before the electroconvulsive therapy.

The literature is filled with reports that TCAs can potentiate the effects of catecholamines. Similarly, atropine-like effects may be more pronounced in patients receiving anticholinergic or antihistamine therapy. Particular care must be exercised when it is necessary to administer TCAs with sympathomimetic amines, local decongestants, local anesthetics containing epinephrine, atropine, or drugs with an anticholinergic effect.

In resistant cases of depression in adults a dose of 2.5 mg/kg/day may have to be exceeded in the hospital. If such a dose or higher is necessitated, the use of EGG monitoring should be maintained during the initiation of therapy and at appropriate intervals during stabilization of the dose. For use in pregnancy the potential benefits must justify the potential fetal risks.

Each of the following reactions must be considered when one administers a TCA. The significant differences are described separately. Table 11-6 summarizes the common reversible side effects of all tricyclic antidepressants.

Cardiovascular reactions. Cardiovascular reactions include hypotension, hypertension, tachycardia (the conduction and repolarization abnormalities produce prolongations of the QT interval, T-wave changes, and ST-segment changes), palpitation, myocardial infarction, arrhythmia, heart block, stroke, and falls.

The orthostatic hypotension may be caused by a combination of peripheral adrenergic blocking actions as well as a decreased inotropic action on the heart. Cardiac effects may be related to the fact that these drugs prevent reuptake of catecholamines. This blockade of reuptake results in higher concentrations of norepinephrine in cardiac tissues. Both bradycardia and tachycardia occur, and the latter may be related to the anticholinergic effects of TCAs.

Cardiotoxicity is attributed to the quinidine-like or membrane-stabilizing effect, direct myocardial depressant effects, and alpha adrenergic blocking effects.

Psychiatric reactions. Confusional states, especially seen in elderly persons include hallucinations, disorientation, delusions, anxiety, restlessness, agitation, insomnia, nightmares, hypomania, and exacerbation of psychosis.

Neurologic manifestations. Numbness, tingling, paresthesia of extremities, incoordination, ataxia, tremors, peripheral neuropathy, extrapyramidal symptoms, seizures, alterations in EEG patterns, and tinnitus may occur.

Anticholinergic reactions. Dry mouth may be relieved by sugarless candy containing sorbitol, because the sorbitol, as a result of its osmotic effect, may cause laxation. Rarely does sublingual adenitis, blurred vision, disturbance of accommodation, mydriasis, constipation, paralytic ileus, delayed micturition, and dilation of the urinary tract occur.

Constipation may be effectively and effi-

TABLE 11-5   Comparison of some tricyclic antidepressants

	Amitriptyline	Desipramine	Doxepin	Imipramine	Nortriptyline	Protriptyline	Trimipramine	Amoxapine
Effective in depletion of norepinephrine	0	++++	0	++	++	++	++	++
Effective in depletion of serotonin	++++	0	++++	++	++	++	++	+
Stimulating effect	0	+++	0	+	++	+++	0	0
Anticholinergic effect	++++++	+	++	++	++	++	++	+
Sedative effect	+++	+	++	++	++	0-+	+++	++
Amine type	Tertiary	Secondary	Tertiary	Tertiary	Secondary	Secondary	Tertiary	Secondary
Therapeutic* range daily dose in mg after 2 weeks of therapy	50 to 300	75 to 300	75 to 300	50 to 300	20 to 150	15 to 60	50 to 300	150 to 300
Steady-state plasma level	1 to 2 weeks	1 to 2 weeks	1 to 2 weeks	1 to 2 weeks	1 to 2 weeks	5 days	1 to 2 weeks	1 to 2 weeks
Adolescent and elderly daily dose	50 mg	25 to 100 mg	25 to 50 mg	30 to 100 mg	30 to 50 mg	15 to 20 mg	50 to 100 mg	75 to 150 mg

0, indicates Insignificant or none; ++, twice as great as −; +++, three times greater than +, and so on.
*Individual dosages vary for inpatients and outpatients.

TABLE 11-6 Common reversible side effects of tricyclic antidepressants*

Muscular hypertension	Dizziness
Drowsiness	Excitement
Dry mouth	Headache
Tremor	Numbness and tingling
Fatigue	of extremities
Weakness	Epigastric distress
Blurring of vision	Nausea, vomiting
Constipation	Insomnia
Urinary retention	Headache
Tachycardia	Flushing
Orthostatic hypotension	Impotence
Anorexia	Mild extrapyramidal
Generalized convulsions	stimulation
Excessive perspiration	

*These reactions can be relieved or controlled by reduction of drug dosage.

ciently relieved by lactulose (Chronolac), a colon-specific laxative.

Allergic reactions. Skin rash, petechiae, urticaria, itching, photosensitization, and edema of face and tongue may be found.

Hematologic reactions. Bone-marrow depression including agranulocytosis, eosinophilia, purpura, and thrombocytopenia may occur. Leukocyte and differential counts should be performed in any patient who develops a fever and sore throat during therapy. The drug should be discontinued if there is evidence of pathologic neutrophil depression.

Gastrointestinal reactions. There may be nausea, vomiting, anorexia, epigastric distress, diarrhea, peculiar taste, stomatitis, abdominal cramps, and black tongue.

Endocrine reactions. Breast enlargement, galactorrhea, increased or decreased libido, impotence, testicular swelling, and elevation or depression of blood-glucose levels may occur.

Miscellaneous reactions. Jaundice (simulating obstructive hepatic necrosis), altered liver function, weight gain or loss, perspiration, flushing, urinary frequency, drowsiness, dizziness, weakness, fatigue, headache, parotid swelling, and alopecia are also found on occasion.

Abrupt cessation of treatment after prolonged therapy may produce nausea, headache, and malaise, a form of withdrawal symptom but not addiction.

Contraindications. TCAs should not be given in conjunction with drugs of the monoamine

TABLE 11-7 Conditions that contraindicate administration of tricyclic antidepressants

Glaucoma	Angina pectoris
Kidney disease	Congestive heart failure
Pyloric stenosis	Paroxysmal tachycardia
Epilepsy	Benign prostatic hyper-
Overactivity, overstimula-	trophy
tion, or agitation	Before surgery
Impaired liver function	Pregnancy (risks to fetus)
Myocardial infarction (re-	
cent)	

oxidase inhibitor class, such as isocarboxazid, phenelzine, or tranylcypromine. The concomitant use of monoamine oxidase inhibitors and tricyclic antidepressants has caused severe hyperpyretic reactions, hypotension, coma, convulsive drives, and death in some patients. These results have not precluded use of TCAs together in an inpatient setting where sophisticated medical observations are routinely employed. At least 2 weeks should elapse after cessation of therapy with monoamine oxidase inhibitors before one begins therapy with the TCA. The initial dosage should be low and be titrated gradually upward with caution and careful observations. The TCAs are contraindicated during the acute recovery period after a myocardial infarction. Extreme caution (monitoring and nursing observations) should be employed when the TCAs are administered to patients with any evidence of cardiovascular disease because of the possibility of conduction defects, arrhythmias, myocardial infarction, strokes, and tachycardia. The quinidine-like cardiac effects are well documented in the literature.

Tricyclic antidepressants are contraindicative in patients with increased intraocular pressure, history of urinary retention, or history of narrow angle glaucoma, because the TCAs possess significant anticholinergic properties; hyperthyroid patients or those patients taking thyroid medication, because of the possibility of cardiovascular toxicity; patients with a past history of seizure disorders, because this class of drugs have been demonstrated to lower the seizure threshold; patients receiving guanethidine, methyldopa, clonidine, or similar agents, because the TCAs block the pharmacologic effects of these drugs. Table 11-7 summarizes the conditions that contraindicate administration of tricyclic antidepressants.

Overdosage and treatment. The signs and symptoms of overdosage may vary in severity, depending on many factors, including but not limited to the amount of the tricyclic antidepressant ingested and absorbed, age of the patient, and interval between ingestion and initiation of treatment modality. Any acute overdosage or unwarranted ingestion of any amount must be considered as serious and potentially fatal.

The central nervous system abnormalities caused by overdosage may be agitation, ataxia, athetoid and choreiform movements, coma, convulsions, drowsiness, hyperactive reflexes, muscle rigidity, restlessness, and stupor.

Cardiac abnormalities may include the following: arrhythmia, electrocardiographic evidence of impaired conduction, signs of congestive heart failure, and tachycardia. Quinidine-like effects are common in poisonings with TCAs.

These additional conditions may also be present: cyanosis, diaphoresis, hyperpyrexia, hypotension, mydriasis, respiratory shock, and vomiting.

Since no specific antidote is known, the treatment for tricyclic overdose is supportive and symptomatic. It necessitates hospitalization and close medical attention for the central nervous system involvement, respiratory depression, and cardiac arrhythmias of sudden onset. This is suggested at all times even when the quantity ingested is alleged to be small or the initial degree of intoxication apparently is minor or moderate. Each patient having ECG abnormalities must have continuous cardiac monitoring for not less than 72 hours coupled with close observations until well after the cardiac status has returned to normal because after the apparent recovery period a relapse may occur. Cardiac arrhythmias have occurred up to 6 days after massive doses of TCAs and may be treated with lidocaine (phenytoin for those arrhythmias retractory to lidocaine). The reported greater sensitivity of children to acute TCA overdosage necessitates hospital cardiac monitoring for at least 4 days or more.

If the patient is not comatose and is alert, his stomach should be promptly emptied by inducing emesis and follow with lavage. If the patient is obtunded, the airway should be secured with a cuffed endotracheal tube before beginning the lavage and emesis should be induced. The lavage is continued for 24 hours or longer, based on the degree of intoxication. In children and adults the use of 0.9% or 0.45% saline solution avoids water intoxication. The use of activated charcoal instilled as a slurry may reduce absorption; however, this is done only after ipecac-induced emesis has occurred. If these two agents (activated charcoal and syrup of ipecac) are used, the charcoal will adsorb the ipecac and therefore reduce substantially its emetic effect.

The use of physostigmine is directed at patients with life-threatening signs (coma with respiratory depression, severe hypertension, or uncontrollable seizures). There are reports of very slow (over 2 minutes) administration of physostigmine salicylate to reverse some of the central nervous system and cardiovascular effects of TCA. The adult dose should start with 1 to 2 mg (slow intravenous injection at 1 mg over 1 minute). This initial dose may be repeated in 10 to 15 minutes, not exceeding a total of 4 mg. In children, the initial dose is 0.5 mg slowly intravenously and repeated at 10-minute intervals to arrive at the minimum effective dose; the dose should not exceed 2 mg. The minimum effective dose may be repeated as necessary in 30- 60-minute intervals because the duration of action of physostigmine is short. Slow intravenous use of physostigmine is mandatory because rapid injections may possibly cause physostigmine-induced convulsions. Physostigmine can increase conduction blocks, causing cardiac arrest, and can aggravate TCA- or phenothiazine-induced conduction abnormalities. It may also cause bronchospasm, muscle weakness, an increase in respiratory secretions, and bradycardia.

Adequate respiratory exchanges must be maintained without the use of respiratory stimulants. Shock may be treated with supportive measures, such as intravenous fluids, oxygen, and corticosteroids. The use of digitalis may induce further conduction abnormalities and thus aggravate a previously sensitized myocardium. Extreme care must be exercised if rapid digitalization is required because of congestive heart failure.

The tendency to convulsions may be reduced by the minimization of external stimulation. If anticonvulsants are necessary, diazepam, short-acting barbiturates, paraldehyde, or methocarbamol may be useful. Barbiturates should be avoided because monoamine oxidase inhibitors may have been ingested recently. Hyperpyrexia may be controlled by ice packs and cooling sponge baths.

Since the TCAs are rapidly fixed in the tissues, hemodialysis, peritoneal dialysis, exchange transfusions, and forced diuresis have been generally unsuccessful and ineffective. The level of TCAs in the blood and urine may not correlate with the degree of intoxication or reflect the severity of the poisoning and is thus an unreliable index in the clinical management of this TCA-overdosage syndrome, but it does have diagnostic value.

Indications. The depressions for which the TCAs are indicated are characterized by severe depressive affects with manifested diencephalic signs (anorexia, decreased energy, diminished libido, insomnia, and weight reduction). when the physical signs of endogenous depression are coupled with a significant affective component, TCA administration may yield satisfactory results. TCAs are not indicated for normal reactions precipitated by grief or situational reactive depression. Relief of anxiety and anorexia may be achieved near the second week of therapy, an increase in energy may be noticed near the third week of therapy, and the antidepressant and normal sleep effects are recognized by the third or fourth week of therapy.

Drug interactions. The Department of Health and Human Services has given support to education of the alcohol-drug interactions described as follows. The tricyclic antidepressants produce either synergistic or antagonistic interactions with alcohol, depending on the ratio of sedative activity or stimulant activity of the individual drug: Desipramine, a predominantly stimulant variety, tends to antagonize the depressant effects of alcohol, but amitripty-

TABLE 11-8 Drug interactions with administration of tricyclic antidepressants

Tricyclic compounds		Interacting drugs
Generic name	**Trade name**	
Imipramine	Tofranil	Monoamine oxidase inhibitors
Desipramine	Norpramin	
	Pertofrane	Alcohol
Nortriptyline	Aventyl	Barbiturates
	Pamelor	Central nervous system depressants
Amitriptyline	Elavil	
Protriptyline	Vivactil	Thiazide diuretics
Doxepin	Sinequan	Vasodilators
	Adapin	Anticholinergic agents
Trimipramine	Surmontil	Thyroid
Amoxapine	Asendin	Guanethidine-like agents
		Sympathomimetic amine
		Narcotics
		Antihistamines
		Anxiolytics
		Anticonvulsants
		Antiparkinsonian agents
		Alpha and beta adrenergic agonists
		Alpha and beta adrenergic blockers
		Phenothiazines
		Methylphenidate
		Physostigmine

line, a depressant variety, may potentiate alcohol's sedative effects. The tricyclic antidepressants increase the potential of convulsions and should be administered cautiously to patients undergoing alcohol withdrawal. These drugs cause hypotension and must be carefully monitored when administered to alcoholic patients.

An emerging significant public health problem is that of tricyclic antidepressant poisoning or overdoses in children. Doses in excess of 10 mg/kg body weight are potentially dangerous. The incidents are characterized as accidental because most occur when the drug is made available to a household member being treated with the TCA for depression or to the enuretic child in the home. The adult family member should be alerted to the possibility of accidental overdosage and to the need for security and administrative responsibility over the medication.

Table 11-8 gives other drug interactions of tricyclic compounds.

Imipramine hydrochloride (Tofranil)

Imipramine hydrochloride is an effective antidepressant drug that has found wide acceptance in the treatment of endogenous and reactive depressions. Initial improvement in depressive symptoms may be noted within the first few days; however, maximal benefit is usually achieved in 1 to 2 weeks.

Preparation, dosage, and administration. Imipramine hydrochloride is administered orally in tablets of 10, 25, and 50 mg, an oral concentrate of 10 mg/ml, and intramuscularly in solution for injection of 12.5 mg/ml. The initial dosage for hospitalized patients is 100 to 150 mg daily in divided doses. Gradual increment of dosage is suggested until the desired effects are observed; however, these doses should not exceed 300 mg/day. Outpatients may receive 75 mg initial daily dosages in divided amounts and with gradual increments not exceeding 200 mg/day. Reduction of dosage to a maintenance level of 50 to 150 mg/day may be indicated as soon as desirable effects are noted. High dosages are not recommended for the elderly or adolescent patient. The therapeutic range in plasma is 150 to 300 ng/ml. The plasma half-life is 9 to 24 hours, and the drug in the plasma is 76% to 96% protein bound.

Imipramine pamoate (Tofranil-PM)

Milligram for milligram imipramine pamoate is equivalent to the hydrochloride salt. It is available in 75-, 100-, 125-, and 150-mg capsules.

Amitriptyline hydrochloride (Elavil Hydrochloride, Endep)

Amitriptyline hydrochloride produces antidepressant and mild tranquilizing effects. Its uses and actions are as effective as imipramine in the treatment of endogenous depression. Reports indicate that this drug is effective in neurotic patients with excessive ruminative tendencies related to their depression; however, it has not been successful with other neurotic depressive conditions.

Preparation, dosage, and administration. Amitriptyline hydrochloride is marketed for oral administration in tablets of 10, 25, 50, 75,

100, and 150 mg and for intramuscular uses in solution for injection, 10 mg/ml. The usual initial dosage range is 50 to 100 mg/day in divided doses with gradual increments to 150 mg/day. Additional doses may be added to the bedtime dosage in 25-mg increments if this is necessary. Elderly and adolescent patients may find 10 mg three tims a day with 20 mg at bedtime a satisfactory regimen. The dosage range per day is 75 to 300 mg. The therapeutic range in plasma is 125 to 250 ng/ml. The plasma half-life is 17 to 40 hours, and the drug in the plasma is 82% to 96% protein bound.

Desipramine hydrochloride (Norpramin, Pertofrane)

Desipramine hydrochloride is believed to be as useful as imipramine in the treatment of endogenous and reactive depressions. It is believe to selectively block the reuptake of norepinephrine in the central nervous system. Desipramine hydrochloride has been identified as the primary active metabolite of imipramine, and it is thought that the antidepressive action of imipramine is caused by desipramine. The effectiveness of this drug may be reduced after a few weeks in some patients.

Preparation, dosage, and administration. Desipramine hydrochloride is only administered orally in 25- to 50-mg capsules (Pertofrane) and in 25- to 50-mg tablets (Norpramin). The average initial daily dosage is 50 to 150 mg given in divided doses. When the desired results are achieved, the average daily maintenance dose is 50 to 100 mg in divided doses. Daily doses should not exceed 200 mg. The dosage range is 75 to 300 mg/day, and the therapeutic range in plasma is 150 to 300 ng/ml. The plasma half-life is 14 to 76 hours, and the drug in the plasma is 73% to 92% protein bound.

Nortriptyline hydrochloride (Aventyl Hydrochloride, Pamelor)

Nortriptyline hydrochloride is as effective as amitriptyline in the treatment of endogenous and reactive depressions and produces similar results. Patients who respond to this drug ordinarily indicate a change in behavior within the first week of therapy. The effectiveness of nortriptyline as an adjunct to electroconvulsive treatment is unpredictable. It is used as an antidepressant and has some tranquilizing action.

Preparation, dosage, and administration. Nortriptyline hydrochloride is administered orally in 10-, 25-, 50-, and 75-mg capsules and as a liquid of 10 mg/5 ml. The average initial daily dosage is 20 to 40 mg given in divided dosages. This dosage may be continued for 5 to 7 days or until the desired results are attained. Reduction of dosage may then be necessary for maintenance therapy. Usual maintenance doses are from 30 to 75 mg/day. Daily dosages should not exceed 100 mg because adverse side effects may occur. For elderly and adolescent patients 30 to 50 mg/day may be sufficient in either divided doses or once a day. The therapeutic range in plasma is 50 to 150 ng/ml, and the drug in the plasma is 93% to 95% protein bound. The plasma half-life is 18 to 93 hours.

Protriptyline hydrochloride (Vivactil)

Protriptyline is a tricyclic antidepressant related structurally to amitriptyline and nortriptyline. Like these other drugs its mechanism of action is unknown. It is useful for the treatment of endogenous and exogenous depression. Its psychomotor activating action makes it particularly suitable for treating withdrawn, apathetic, and lethargic patients. Depressed patients with agitation, tension, and anxiety may become more disturbed when treated with protriptyline. Side effects and precautions are the same as for other tricyclics.

Protriptyline is well absorbed from the gastrointestinal tract. Plasma levels of the drug appear in 2 hours; peak levels occur in 8 to 12 hours and then gradually decline. The rate of excretion is slow; about 50% of the drug is excreted in 16 days. The therapeutic range in plasma is 50 to 150 ng/ml, and the plasma half-life is 54 to 198 hours.

Preparation and dosage. Protriptyline is available in 5- and 10-mg tablets. Oral dosage for adults is 15 to 60 mg daily in three or four divided doses; for adolescents and elderly patients the dosage is 15 mg daily in three divided doses. Any increase in the dose should be made in the morning. The cardiovascular

system of elderly patients should be monitored.

Doxepin hydrochloride (Sinequan, Adapin)

Doxepin is a tricyclic drug with pharmacologic action similar to that of amitriptyline. It has anticholinergic, antihistaminic, and antiserotonin effects. Doxepin is reported to be as effective as, and in some cases more effective than, amitriptyline in relieving symptoms of depression in psychoneurotic patients.

Preparation and dosage. Doxepin is available in 10-, 25-, 50-, and 75-mg capsules. The oral concentrate has 1 ml equaling 10 mg. The oral dose for adults is 75 mg daily in three divided doses initially, with an increase or decrease in dose depending on the response of the patient. For severely depressed patients 150 to 300 mg daily may be required. The dose range is 75 to 300 mg daily. The therapeutic range in plasma is 75 to 200 ng/ml.

Trimipramine (Surmontil)

Trimipramine is indicated for the relief of symptoms of depression. Endogenous depression is more likely alleviated than other depressive states. Studies with neurotic outpatients indicate that the drug appeared to be of equivalent effectiveness to amitriptyline in less depressed patients and somewhat less effective than amitriptyline in more severely depressed patients. Studies of hospitalized depressed patients show equal effectiveness with imipramine for relieving depression. Reported side effects, warnings, precautions, and adverse reactions are typical of other TCAs. Most of the antidepressant drugs have a lag period of 10 days to 4 weeks before a therapeutic response is noted; increasing a dose will not shorten this lag period but rather increase the incidence of adverse reactions.

Trimipramine is supplied as 25- and 50-mg capsules. The recommended dosages are as follows: For adult outpatients, initially 75 mg/day is given in divided doses, increased to 150 mg/day. Dosages over 200 mg/day are not recommended. Maintenance therapy is in the range of 50 to 150 mg/day. Since sedation is pronounced (greater than that from imipramine) and for convenient therapy to facilitate patient compliance, the total dosage required may be given at bedtime. For hospitalized patients: initially, 100 mg/day is given in divided doses, increased gradually in a few days to 200 mg/day depending on individual response and tolerance. For adolescent and geriatric patients; an initial dose of 50 mg/day is recommended, with gradual increments up to 100 mg/day depending on patient response and tolerance. This is an antidepressant with an anxiety-reducing sedative component to its action. The mode of action on the central nervous system is not known; however it is implicated in the inhibition of reuptake of norepinephrine and serotonin.

Amoxapine (Asendin)

This tricyclic antidepressant is similar to loxapine and is referred to as desmethylloxapine. In structure and activity it is similar to imipramine. This antidepressant has a mild sedative component. In animals it reduces the uptake of norepinephrine and serotonin and blocks response to dopamine receptors. Peak blood levels are reached in 90 minutes; it is excreted in the urine and bound to human serum (90%).

Serum concentrations decline with a half-life of 8 hours, whereas the major metabolite (8-hydroxyamoxapine) has a half-life of 30 hours. A more rapid onset of action is seen than that of amitriptyline or imipramine. The antidepressant effects are seen within 4 to 7 days, and 80% of the patients within 14 days display these effects.

The pharmacology, contraindications, precautions, and adverse reactions are similar to those seen with the other tricyclic antidepressants. The most frequent adverse reactions reported are sedation, anticholinergic effect, drowsiness, dry mouth, and constipation.

The available forms are heptagonal scored tablets of 50, 100, and 150 mg. Effective dose range is 200 to 300 mg, with gradual increases of 100 mg three times daily over 3-day periods up to a maximum of 600 mg. A dose of 300 mg is given once daily at bedtime; a dose of 600 mg is given in divided doses.

Commercially available fixed combinations containing TCAs. The TCAs are combined with antipsychotics (a fixed combination of perphenazine and amitriptyline under the trade names Etrafon, Triavil, and others). TCAs are also manufactured in combination with chlordiazepoxide under the name Limbitrol.

Tetracyclic antidepressant
Maprotiline (Ludiomil)

This tetracyclic antidepressant is a secondary amine chemically composed of a tricylic antidepressant with an ethylene ring bridge across the central ring of a tricyclic structure formation.

In addition to the comparable tricyclic antidepressant pharmacologic characteristics, this drug also demonstrates psychosedative, anxiolytic, antiaggressive, and weak anticholinergic action. The exact mechanism of action is unknown. It is theorized that the ethylene type of ring may be responsible for the highly selective inhibition of norepinephrine reuptake from nerve endings in the peripheral and central neurons, thus potentiating the central adrenergic synapse. No inhibition of the monoamine serotonin central metabolism or uptake was reported. Because of serotonin's role in endogenous depression, it is theorized that maprotiline may then be more effective in neurotic depression types.

Depressed patients demonstrate both a reduction in time to fall asleep and a shorter duration of episodic awakenings. Most of the clinical studies compared maprotiline to imipramine or amitriptyline. The oral route produces a linear related dose-dependent steady state within 2 weeks of repeated administration. This may account for the suggestions that it is more rapid acting than imipramine and amitriptyline.

Hepatic detoxification by biotransformation (N-demethylation, deamination, and hydroxylation) produces primarily slowly eliminated glucuronide metabolites, which are excreted in the urine (two thirds of the drug) and the feces (one third of the drug). The profile of contraindications, warnings, adverse reactions, precautions, drug interactions, and overdose treatment is similar to that of the tricyclic antidepressants. A more prominent increased incidence of skin reactions is reported with maprotiline.

The oral dose is titrated to individual patient response, usually commencing with 75 mg daily in single or divided doses and not exceeding 300 mg daily. Patients over 60 years old may begin with doses of 50 to 75 mg daily. It is available in 25- and 50-mg tablets.

Monoamine oxidase inhibitors

The monoamines (norepinephrine, dopamine, and serotonin) are transmitters in the central nervous system. Norepinephrine is also a peripheral transmitter at the sympathetic neuroeffector junction. Epinephrine and histamine may also be considered monoamine transmitters.

Monoamine oxidase (MAO) is a flavoprotein that catalyzes the deamination of a number of amines to their corresponding aldehydes. The monoamine oxidases are complex enzymes responsible for the oxidative deamination of a wide number and types of amines, including the indole derivative serotonin and the catecholamine dopamine, norepinephrine, and epinephrine. The monoamine oxidase enzymes are present within cells of many tissues (brain, blood platelets, liver, spleen, and kidneys).

The monoamine oxidase inhibitors (MAOIs) are diverse chemical compounds with capability of blocking or diminishing the activity of MAO. The common biochemical property of MAO inhibition confers certain pharmacologic actions on these pharmaceutical products. Thus the result of MAOIs is blockade of intracellular deamination of biogenic amines in the nerve terminal resulting in a net increase in brain amine levels. MAOIs also block amine uptake, and this may account for their clinical usefulness. Potentiation of indirect-acting amines (amphetamine and tyramine) and the reversal of the norepinephrine-depleting effect of reserpine (reserpine decreases the concentration of norepinephrine in the central and peripheral nervous system) have been associated with the antidepressant effects of these drugs in humans.

During early clinical trials of MAOIs as antidepressants, orthostatic hypotension was encountered as a common but inconsistent side effect, and a large number of MAOIs were then produced and studied specifically as antidepressants and antihypertensive agents.

MAOIs encompass a variety of activities: as antidepressants, as an antineoplastic agent (procarbazine use in Hodgkin's disease), and as an antibiotic (furazolidone). Pargyline hydrochloride (Eutonyl) is seldom used in control of some types of hypertension. The MAOIs to be discussed in this section are the agents used as antidepressants; isocarboxazid (Marplan), phenelzine (Nardil), and tranylcypromine (Parnate). There is evidence that the primary properties seem to have special relevance to their psychiatric (mood-modification) activity—reserpine reversal and potentiation of indirect-acting pressor amines. The MAOIs are indicated primarily in particularly resistant depressions (to tricyclic antidepressant effects), anxious and hostile depressions, atypical nondepressions, mixed anxiety, and depression with phobic or hypochondriac features.

The MAOIs found intraneuronally and extraneuronally and primarily at the level of the mitochondria (localized in the mitochondria and the mitochondral membrane) in the nerve endings prevent the destruction of the cytoplasmic monoamines. This therefore increases the concentration of these amines with the nerve terminal, and as a result they are released in greater concentration during nerve transmissions. MAOIs can increase the concentration of all central amines, though it is possible that there are different effects on the individual amines. For example, some of the MAOIs may increase dopamine or norepinephrine concentrations to a more extensive degree than serotonin concentrations, whereas other MAOIs may raise the level of serotonins to a greater degree than those of norepinephrine and dopamine. The increase in amine concentration is associated with behavioral hyperactivity (amphetamine-like psychomotor stimulation with large doses) produced by the MAOIs and, in some cases, with the exacerbation of psychotic symptoms. In lower doses the antiphobic and antidepressant activities are seen. In general, these compounds are most effective in reversing the dysphoric state and its attendant vegetative

TABLE 11-9 Drugs whose metabolism is inhibited by MAOIs

Barbiturates	Anticholinergics
Aminopyrine	Disulfiram
Indirect-acting adrenergic agents (including over-the-counter sympathomimetics)	Alcohol
	Levodopa
Methyldopa	Antiparkinsonian drugs
Thiazide diuretics	Insulin
Meperidine	Cocaine
Morphine derivatives	Ether
Reserpine	Procaine
	Tryptophan
	Phenothiazines

disturbances in patients with depressive syndromes.

The therapeutic doses of the MAOIs require days to weeks to attain a maximum therapeutic effect. MAOIs produce an irreversible inactivation of MAO by forming a stable complex with the enzyme; thus degradation of biologic amines by this route is prevented and as such does not inhibit MAO production. Recovery from the effect of MAOIs thus depends on enzyme regeneration, which may occur over several weeks. MAOIs inhibit enzymes other than MAO; such as dopamine-β-oxidase, diamine oxidase, amino acid decarboxylases, and choline dehydrogenase. Inhibition occurs only in very high doses and may be responsible for some of the toxic effects of MAOIs. MAOIs potentiate a number of other drugs by inhibiting their metabolism. Table 11-9 lists these drugs. The reduced dosage of each agent is essential if the drugs must be used concurrently. MAOIs are to be discontinued for at least 1 week before guanethidine is started. Fatal hypertensive crises have been reported when sympathomimetics or tyramine was administered to patients receiving therapeutic doses of MAOIs; these occurred within several hours of ingestion of the contraindicated substances.

Side effects and toxic effects. The MAOIs affect many enzyme systems, and a wide variety of adverse affects may be anticipated. These adverse effects may be described as follows:

Central nervous system effects: stimulation such as insomnia, increased reflexes (hyperflexia), con-

vulsions, hypomania, hallucinations, schizophrenic symptoms, tremor, twitching, dizziness, fatigue, drowsiness, and weakness.

Autonomic effects: perspiration, dry mouth, blurred vision.

Cardiovascular effects: changes in blood pressure, orthostatic hypotension (by blockade in vascular bed response), paradoxic hypertension, hypertensive crisis (occipital headache, neck stiffness or soreness, palpitations, sweating, fever, photophobia, edema, nausea, vomiting, excitement, delirium, tachycardia, or bradycardia associated with constricting chest pain, dilated pupils), possible increase of intracranial or subarachnoid bleeding because of increase in blood pressure, and finally circulatory collapse, or death. (These effects may be precipitated by disregard of dietary precautions and drug interactions.)

Gastrointestinal effects: hepatocellular damage, constipation, diarrhea, and nausea.

It is imperative that the nurse teach the patient and family to recognize the adverse effects of this drug, to know the dietary precautions, and to understand drug reactions that precipitate adverse reactions. This knowledge by the patient and family may avert the cardiovascular effects.

Dietary precautions. MAOIs potentiate the action of sympathomimetic drugs (amphetamines, methyldopa, L-dopa, dopamine, ephedrine, epinephrine, norepinephrine, phenylpropanolamine, and so on, and this may result in a hypertensive crisis. Sympathomimetic amines (vasoconstrictors) are often encountered in proprietary or over-the-counter drugs such as cold, allergy, hay-fever, cough, and diet products. The patient should avoid excessive alcohol (a depressant) and codeine found in many cough syrups and prescription drugs. Chocolate and excessive amounts of caffeine should be avoided. Tryptophan, tyramine, and tryptamine may be found in natural and health food products, and this must be pointed out to the patient. Tryptamine- or tyramine-containing substances are found in high amounts in the following food products: organ meats, chicken livers, yeast products, sharp aged cheeses, beer, sherry, Chianti wines, sour cream, yogurt, pickled herring, broad bean pods (fava), canned figs, raisins, bananas, avocados (particularly if overripe), meat extracts, and soy sauce, and in foods in which aging or protein breakdown is used to enhance flavor (such as meat-product tenderizing).

The previous list of examples and the following discussion will assist the nurse to demonstrate the value of a thoroughly understood diet for the compliant patient and family. A patient treated with MAOIs becomes sensitive to cheeses because the cheese contains tyramine formed from tyrosine, tyramine normally is destroyed by MAO. When the MAOI drug inhibits MAO, a large rise in blood pressure occurs, and an intracranial hemorrhage may develop. A patient treated with MAOIs also should avoid broad beans because they have dopa in their bean pods, and when these are cooked and eaten, the dopamine is formed. The dopamine is not destroyed by MAO because of the MAOI drug being used, and the dopa may be converted to norepinephrine.

Drug interactions. The use of MAOIs and the tricyclic antidepressants (particularly the dibenzapines) together offers value to patients refractory to other therapy. This combined therapy requires conservative dosages under close knowledgeable medical supervision.

The MAOIs are divided into the hydrazines and the nonhydrazines. The MAOIs that contain a hydrazine moiety (phenelzine and isocarboxazid) are slow to evoke a response (2 to 3 weeks), and the MAOIs without a hydrazine group (propargylamine derivatives such as pargyline used in hypertension and cyclopropylamine derivatives such as tranylcypromine) act more promptly (7 days).

A 10-day elapsed period (medication-free interval) should follow when one MAOI is used immediately after another. A 14-day period should elapse between use of an MAOI and a tricyclic antidepressant, because such a combination may produce a hypertensive crisis. A 10-day period should also elapse before elective surgery is performed because while the excretion of the MAOI is rapid, the inhibition of MAO may persist for several days. The 10-day period provides for recovery of enzyme activity before elective surgery is performed. The blocking agents of general and spinal anesthesia when combined with the MAOI may produce hypo-

TABLE 11-10 Contraindicated conditions for administration of monoamine oxidase inhibitors

Cardiovascular disease
Cardiac decompensation
Congestive heart failure
Cerebrovascular disorders
Pheochromocytoma
Hepatic disease
Blood dyscrasias—anemia, hepatitis
Pregnancy
Angina pectoris*
Epilepsy
Kidney dysfunction
Depressions accompanying:
   Chronic brain syndromes
   Schizophrenia
   Alcoholism
   Drug addiction
Conditions manifesting:
   Overactivity
   Overstimulation
   Agitation

*May suppress the warning signal of pain. Should be used with caution.

tensive effects. Local anesthetics may contain sympathomimetic vasoconstrictors (epinephrine), which are not to be used with MAOIs.

Contraindications. Contraindications to the use of MAOIs (Table 11-10) are for patients with cerebrovascular defects, cardiovascular disease, hypertension, congestive heart failure, history of liver disease or abnormal liver function tests, and pheochromocytoma (since the tumors secrete pressor substances).

Periodic liver function tests (bilirubins, alkaline phosphatase or transaminase) should be performed. The nurse should encourage the patient to have his blood pressure checked to detect evidence of pressor amine response and orthostatic hypotension. In patients with impaired renal function, the MAOIs should be used with caution to prevent accumulation.

Nursing implications. The nurse should read the current literature (such as professional journals) to keep current with adverse drug reactions, drug interactions, and diet-drug interactions that affect the patient population being treated. These areas are in constant flux because of the sophisticated data retrieval, collecting devices, and reports that are becoming more accessible as a result of wide distribution

TABLE 11-11   Some frequent adverse effects from monoamine oxidase inhibitors*

Orthostatic hypertension	Nausea	Tachycardia
Dizziness	Vomiting	Edema
Restlessness	Diarrhea	Palpitation
Insomnia	Abdominal pain	Impotence
Weakness	Constipation	Headaches
Drowsiness	Anorexia	(not from
Anxiety	Dryness of mouth	rise in
Agitation	Blurred vision	blood
Manic episodes	Chills	pressure)

*These side effects can usually be relieved with reduction of dosage. Most of the side effects reported are related to failure to recognize the cumulative action of these drugs with subsequent incorrect dosage. It is important to reduce dosage as soon as improvement of symptoms is observed to avoid precipitating side effects caused by the cumulative action of the drug.

TABLE 11-12   Drug incompatibility with administration of monoamine oxidase inhibitors used as antidepressants

Monoamine oxidase inhibitors		
Generic name	Trade name	Some incompatible drugs
Isocarboxazid	Marplan	Combination of any mono-
Phenelzine	Nardil	amine oxidase inhibitor
Tranylcypromine	Parnate	Other antidepressants
		Amphetamines
		Alcohol
		Barbiturates
		Morphine-like analgesics
		Meperidine
		Cocaine, procaine, ether
		Phenothiazine compounds
		Methyldopa, dopamine
		Tryptophan
		Antihypertensives
		Antiparkinsonian drugs
		Insulin
		Thiazide diuretics
		Sympathomimetic amines—phenylephrine

and publication. The MAOIs are an example of drugs with potential and fatal adverse affects (Table 11-11) caused by diet and drug therapy (Table 11-12). The MAOIs also slow the metabolism of alcohol, causing intoxication to be greater than expected.

During hospitalization, the depressed patient's anorexia may prompt well-meaning family members or friends to bring supplementary foods to the patient or a little wine to stim-ulate his appetite. Careful nursing observation during visiting hours and instruction of the family regarding these restrictions can avoid serious consequences. Communication with the hospital dietitian may also prevent these foods from appearing on the patient's hospital menu. As the patient's depression lifts or if electroconvulsive therapy is used concomitantly with drug therapy, reinstruction of the patient may be necessary. These foods and beverages should not be ingested for at least 2 to 3 weeks after discontinuance of drug therapy.

Discontinuation of the drug immediately is recommended when any adverse signs and symptoms occur. Fever is managed by external cooling and either phentolamine mesylate (5 mg slowly intravenously to avoid hypotensive effect) or pentolinium tartrate (3 mg intravenously) is used to control severe hypertension reactions.

Overactive, overstimulated, or agitated patients usually do not respond well to MAOIs. These drugs are also contraindicated in many other conditions (Table 11-11).

The suicidal tendencies present in the patient's condition may compound his nursing care problem because of the delayed effect of these drugs in relieving suicidal tendencies. This effect presents an additional risk to the patient during initial phases of drug therapy. The nurse should be alert to the possibility of any impulsive ingestion of these substances.

Since the risk of suicide is frequently higher near the end of the depressive cycle, attention should be given to the possibility of suicidal attempts during this period. Overt patient behavior may indicate a remission of depressive symptoms; however, this may be caused by drug action and not by alleviation of pathologic processes. Antidepressants should generally be continued for several months after the remission of symptoms and should never be discontinued abruptly, since a relapse may occur.

Tranylcypromine sulfate (Parnate)

Tranylcypromine sulfate should be reserved for use in patients with severe reactive or endogenous depressive conditions who have not responded to electroconvulsive treatment or in whom such therapy is contraindicated and for patients who do not respond to other antidepressant therapy.

Preparation, dosage, and administration. Tranylcypromine sulfate is administered orally in 10-mg tablets. Initial dosage per day is 20 mg in divided doses with gradual increments not to exceed 30 mg. It is recommended that the lowest effective dosage be used. Improvement may be seen 48 hours to 3 weeks after therapy begins.

Isocarboxazid (Marplan)

Isocarboxazid is administered to patients with symptoms of depression and withdrawal and seems to be an effective antidepressant in selected psychiatric conditions. It is useful in treating the depressed phases of anxiety or the depression of manic-depressive syndromes, as well as certain involutional, obsessive, and dissociative reactions. It does not appear to be as effective as electroconvulsive therapy in the treatment of severe psychiatric disorders. Its effects are cumulative and require 3 to 4 weeks of therapy before improvement is noted.

Preparation, dosage, and administration. Isocarboxazid is administered orally in 10-mg tablets. The proposed initial dosage is 20 to 30 mg daily given in single or divided doses. The average daily dosage should not exceed 30 mg, and the suggested maintenance dosage is 10 to 20 mg a day or less.

Phenelzine sulfate (Nardil)

Phenelzine sulfate is useful in the treatment of both endogenous and reactive depressions. There is a latent period before onset of action, and the maximal effect occurs within 2 to 3 weeks or more.

Preparation, dosage, and administration. Phenelzine sulfate is administered orally in 15-mg tablets. The initial daily dosage is 15 mg three times a day. The average daily dosage should not exceed 90 mg, and effective maintenance dosages as low as 15 mg every other day have been reported.

Antimanic agent

Mania symptoms are characterized by pressure of speech, motor hyperactivity, reduced sleep requirement, flight of ideas, grandiosity, elation, poor judgment, agressiveness, and possible hostility. There are three types of manic-depressive illnesses: (1) the *manic form*, with recurrent manic symptoms with little or no depression, (2) the *depressed type* (unipolar depression), which is essentially endogenous depression previously discussed, and (3) the *circular form* (bipolar depression), in which there is alternating episodes of mania and depression.

Lithium carbonate (Lithane, Lithobid, Eskalith, Lithotabs), lithium citrate (Lithonate-S)

Lithium is the preferred specific (antimanic) treatment for maintenance therapy to prevent or diminish the intensity of manic episodes of bipolar or affective disorders (circular manic-depressive disorders), with a success rate in a range of 60% to 80% in remission. Other indications for disorders seen in the literature are unrelated to this approved use. Such indications will be determined in the future based on successful, repeated, documented applications of the drug. Some of these indications of applied lithium therapy are decreasing incidence of depressive episodes in bipolar affective disorders, acute or cyclic recurrent endogenous depression (unipolar) with imipramine, failure of response to TCAs and electroconvulsive therapy, uncontrollable aggressive behavior (institutionalized patients), cluster headaches, chronic maladaptive behavior, blocking of amphetamine effects in nonmanic patients, syndrome of inappropriate antidiuretic hormone, organic brain syndrome, granulopoiesis, and impaired immune function (cancer chemotherapy and radiation therapy result in myelosuppression, and reduction of white blood cell count and lithium will ameliorate this to elevate white blood cell count).

Mechanism of action. A specific biochemical mechanism for therapeutic effects of lithium in mania has not been totally accepted. It is proposed that lithium alters sodium transport in nerve and muscle cells and effects a shift toward intraneuronal metabolism of catecholamines. It is theorized that lithium accelerates the presynaptic destruction of catecholamines (which may be opposite to the action of MAOIs), inhibits transmitter release at the synapse, and decreases postsynaptic receptor sensitivity, with the result that the presumed overactive catecholamine systems in mania are corrected. This may be achieved by inhibition of membrane adenylcyclase, which regulates transmitter and metabolic transport across neuroendocrine cells. Futhermore, serotonin has been implicated because patients undergoing lithium therapy for manic episodes have greater increases in cerebrospinal fluid of serotonin metabolite than of the major metabolite of dopamine. A hypothesis to explain the stabilizing action of lithium in depression and mania is as follows: during depression the cell sodium is high, with a restricted flow out of the cell. Extracellular lithium acts like potassium and encourages sodium efflux from the cell, either by cation exchange or stimulation of the sodium-pump mechanism. The opposite would apply in mania, where lithium enters the cells and retards efflux of sodium.

Pharmacokinetics. Lithium is a cation and is distributed more evenly in body water than sodium or potassium and may easily substitute for either cation. Absorption of lithium is rapid after oral doses and completed within 6 to 8 hours. Lithium is excreted in the urine (95%) and, of this, one third to two thirds appears in the urine for 6 to 12 hours, and the balance is excreted slowly over 10 to 14 days. Renal excretion is proportional to its plasma concentration. The elimination half-time is approximately 24 hours.

A patient on long-term diuretic therapy (thiazides, ethacrynic acid, furosemide, and xanthine diuretics) may experience a reduced clearance of lithium (of about a 24% decrease in lithium clearance), which produces elevations in serum lithium with possible toxicity; a compensating increase in sodium reabsorption occurs in the kidney proximal tubules. The thiazides exert little effect in proximal tubules where lithium and sodium are absorbed. Lithium may be reabsorbed more rapidly with a consequent decrease in its clearance. The opposite effect will be achieved when the patient's dietary sodium is increased, lithium levels fall, and mania symptoms return. If an elevated

temperature caused by infection occurs, a temporary reduction or cessation of therapy may be desirable under medical supervision. There is no protein binding, no metabolism occurs, and almost all the lithium is excreted by the kidney.

Preparation, dosage, and administration. Lithium is available in the carbonate salt in 300-mg capsules and the citrate salt 8 mEq/5 ml (300 mg) in a raspberry-flavored syrup. The dosage and administration are based on individual serum level monitoring and clinical and judgmental response.

For acute mania, 600 mg given three times daily may produce a serum lithium level of 1 to 1.5 mEq/liter; the levels should be determined twice a week in the acute phase until stabilization occurs. Range of dosage is 600 to 2100 mg.

For long-term management, levels should be obtained not less than every 2 months. Desirable levels of 0.6 to 1.2 mEq/liter are usually attained at a dose of 300 mg three to four times daily. Range of dosage is 900 to 1200 mg.

After the administration of lithium during manic episodes normalization of symptoms may be evident in 1 to 3 weeks. This slow onset or threshold level in tissues must be achieved before lithium is effective. This time lapse occurs because the lithium ion slowly enters the cells over a time span of 1 to 3 weeks and is dependent on the lithium rate of entry.

Clinical observations and judgments are the key to successful therapy because lithium levels are secondary to this expertise. The risk of lithium toxicity is significantly higher in patients with renal disorders, cardiovascular disease, debilitation, dehydration, and sodium depletion and in those receiving diuretic therapy. If a life-threatening psychiatric indication occurs in patients in these patients at risk and they fail to adequately respond to other therapy (potential benefits then outweigh the risks), the cautious institution of lithium therapy must include hospitalization, checking of daily serum lithium levels, and titration beginning with the lowest tolerable dose. Blood samples for lithium must be drawn 10 to 12 hours after the last dose when levels are tolerated.

Side effects and toxic effects. Adverse reac-

T A B L E 1 1 - 1 3 Toxic reactions related to serum levels

Neuromuscular	Fine tremor
	Chronic whole-limb movements
	Choreoathetoid movements
Central nervous system	Epileptiform seizure
	Coma
	Vertigo
	Drowsiness
Cardiovascular	Cardiac arrhythmias
	Hypotension
	Peripheral circulatory collapse
Gastrointestinal	Anorexia
	Nausea
	Vomiting
	Diarrhea
Genitourinary	Albuminuria
	Oliguria
	Polyuria
	Glycosuria
	Nephrogenic diabetes insipidus
Dermatologic	Dry and thin hair
	Skin anesthesia
Autonomic nervous system	Blurred vision
	Dry mouth
Miscellaneous	Fatigue
	Lethargy
	Sleep
	Dehydration
	Thyroid abnormalities
	EEG changes
	ECG irregularities

tions are encountered at serum lithium levels with narrow limits. These levels are all based on individual patient response and sensitivity to lithium. Lithium-sensitive individuals exhibit toxicity at 1 to 1.5 mEq/liter. Elderly patients may respond to reduced doses and exhibit toxicity at the levels ordinarily tolerated by other patients. Generally, at a level over 1.5 mEq/liter, adverse reactions may be expected. Mild to moderate toxicity may occur at levels ranging from 1.5 to 2.5 mEq/liter, and moderate to severe toxicity reactions are observed from 2 to 2.5 mEq/liter. Table 11-13 gives some toxic reactions related to serum levels.

Some miscellaneous reactions unrelated to dosage are the following: transient electroencephalographic and electrocardiographic changes, leukocytosis, hyperglycemia, headache, pruritus, cutaneous ulcers, albuminuria,

worsening of organic brain syndrome, weight gain, ankle and wrist swelling, thirst, and polyuria.

During the manic phase there appears to be a greater ability to tolerate lithium than when the manic phase subsides.

There is conflict in the literature concerning the combined use of lithium and haloperidol. The manufacturers state that patients being administered both drugs concomitantly should be monitored for early signs of neurologic toxicity, culminating in irreversible brain damage. Haloperidol, electroconvulsive therapy, or other drugs may be desirable in severely manic patients because of the slow onset of complete therapeutic effects of lithium. Haloperidol administered parenterally is discontinued when the manic episode is managed with lithium. It has been suggested that imipramine may aggravate the manic phase of the illness, and some investigators have a higher degree of response with the tricyclic antidepressants added to the maintenance therapy for the breakthrough depressive episode. Lithium should not be used during the first trimester unless the potential benefits far outweigh the risks to the fetus. Lithium is excreted in the breast milk of lactating mothers in quantities sufficient to affect the child with lithium toxicity, prohibiting its use in breast-feeding mothers. Lithium is also secreted in the saliva and the plasma concentration–to–salivary concentration ratio is fairly constant; thus salivary lithium levels can be monitored.

Nursing implications. The nurse should relate to the patient and family the inconveniences of initial therapy (often existing over the duration of therapy): fine hand tremor, polyuria, and mild thirst. During the first few days transient mild nausea and general malaise exist. This may subside with continuation of therapy, reduced therapy, or cessation of therapy (if they persist).

The nurse should inform the patient and family that lithium taken with or immediately after meals may lessen the incidence of gastrointestinal distress and not to confuse the distress with symptoms of toxicity.

For implementation of maintenance therapy several factors are considered necessary.

First, the patient compliance, cooperation, and commitment to adhere strictly to all the therapy considerations are essential. The family of the patient should be fully apprised of all the ramifications of this therapy. Second, the history of manic episodes, occurrence, and degree of severity must be assessed, along with the cyclic appearance of pattern. Family intervention for treatment when manic-depressive symptoms appear is essential. Finally the patient must accept and recognize fully that lithium is not intended to abate the exhilaration, elation, and feelings of limitless energy; instead, it is used to enable the patient to negotiate life more effectively within his environment so that he and those with whom he interacts have a more meaningful relationship.

The nurse should discuss with the potential outpatient, patient's family, or closest companion about what the overt clinical signs of lithium toxicity are. Some of these symptoms are diarrhea, vomiting, tremors, mild ataxia, lack of coordination, drowsiness, and muscular weakness. If any of these signs appear, the patient is to discontinue therapy and promptly notify the prescriber. The acute treatment phase should have lithium levels below 2 mEq/liter. At levels of greater than 2 mEq/liter giddiness, ataxia, blurred vision, tinnitus, and large outputs of dilute urine are seen. At levels above 3 mEq/liter a complex clinical picture involving multiple organ and organ systems develops. This demonstrates the narrow range between therapeutic levels and levels with toxic manifestations.

The outpatient should be aware of facilities where prompt and accurate serum lithium determinations may be obtained.

Finally lithium decreases sodium reabsorption by the renal tubules, which may produce sodium depletion, and the nurse should discuss with the patient and family the importance of a normal diet including salt (NaCl) and an intake of 2500 to 3000 ml of liquid daily during the initial stabilization period. If any condition that precipitates sodium depletion (low-sodium diets, dehydration, dieting, diuretics, protracted sweating, vomiting, diarrhea, and electrolyte loss) occurs, a decreased tolerance to lithium may begin. The patient should be instructed to supplement fluid, electrolyte solutions, and sodium chloride.

Drugs used in nonpsychotic mental disorders

STIMULANTS
Methylphenidate hydrochloride (Ritalin)

Methylphenidate is a central nervous system stimulant that is less potent than amphetamine but more potent than caffeine. It does not appreciably affect blood pressure, heart rate, circulation time, or respiration.

Its most important use is in the treatment of hyperkinetic children and those with certain behavioral and learning problems. It has been found to significantly improve task performance in children in both groups probably because it improves mood, causes euphoria, and increases motor and mental activity, cognitive ability, and motor functions.

Preparation, dosage, and administration. Methylphenidate is available as tablets containing 5, 10, or 20 mg. The usual dose for adults is 10 to 60 mg two or three times daily given 30 to 45 minutes before meals. If the patient is unable to sleep at night, the last dose should be taken before 6 PM.

For children with the behavioral syndrome the dose is 5 mg before breakfast and before lunch; the dosage may be increased gradually by 5 to 10 mg weekly. A dosage above 60 mg is not recommended.

Side effects. Nervousness and insomnia are common reactions, which can usually be controlled by reducing the dosage or omitting the afternoon or evening dose. Numerous other side effects can occur and include anorexia, nausea, dizziness, palpitations, headache, and skin rash. Hypertension, hypotension, and arrhythmias have occurred. Prolonged therapy has caused abdominal pain and weight loss, particularly in children.

Precautions. Methylphenidate must be used with caution in patients with epilepsy since the drug can lower the convulsive threshold. It should also be used cautiously in patients with hypertension. Long-term therapy should be accompanied by repeated medical examination and complete blood and platelet counts. Its use in pregnant or lactating women is not recommended.

Tolerance and psychic dependence has occurred with long-term use, and abnormal behavior and psychotic episodes have been observed. When the drug is withdrawn, careful supervision is required, since severe depression may result.

Methylphenidate must be used cautiously in emotionally unstable persons and in those with a history of drug dependence or alcoholism. It has been used as a substitute for amphetamines by drug abusers.

Overdosage and treatment. Signs and symptoms of acute intoxication are primarily the result of overstimulation of the central nervous system and sympathetic nervous system and include vomiting, agitation, tremors, muscle twitching, convulsions, euphoria, confusion, hallucinations, delirium, sweating, tachycardia, arrhythmias, hypertension, mydriasis, hyperpyrexia, and dryness of mucous membranes.

Treatment consists of supportive measures, evacuation of gastric contents if possible, a shortacting barbiturate, cooling procedures for high body temperature, and adequate maintenance of circulation and respiration. The effectiveness of dialysis for methylphenidate overdosage has not been established.

Drug interactions. Methylphenidate can potentiate the action of many drugs including angiotensin, anticholinergics, anticonvulsants, anticoagulants, monoamine oxidase drugs, pressor drugs, phenylbutazone, and tricyclic antidepressants. It decreases the hypotensive effect of guanethidine. Dosage of these drugs should be readjusted when given with methylphenidate.

Pemoline (Cylert)

A central nervous system stimulant structurally different from amphetamine but closer to methylphenidate, pemoline has minimal sympathomimetic effects. It is indicated in behavioral syndromes with developmentally inappropriate symptoms of children (such as attention deficit disorders and the hyperkinetic syndrome). The mechanism or site of action is not known. The serum half-life is 12 hours, with a steady state reached in 2 to 3 days. The onset of action is gradual, and effects may not be seen for 3 to 4 weeks of administration. A common adverse effect is insomnia and anorexia. Misuse of the drug in adults has resulted in a psychotic reaction. It is available in oral tablets of 18.75, 37.5, and 75 mg and a chewable tablet of 37.5 mg.

Summary of nursing considerations

The parts of the central nervous system believed to affect emotions and behavior include the cerebrum, composed of the cerebral cortex, basal ganglia, hippocampus, fornix, amygdaloid nucleus, hippocampal gyrus, and uncus; the midbrain, pons, and medulla; the cerebullum; and the thalamus and hypothalamus. Papex in 1937 was one of the first researchers to suggest the function of a reverberating circuit in the brain as an explanation for emotional experiences.

Central nervous system functions depend on the action of neurohormonal transmitter substances, such as acetylcholine, norepinephrine, tyrosine, dopamine, and serotonin. Research suggests that histamine, amino acids (GABA), endorphins, and prostaglandins may also be transmitters.

The use of drugs in psychiatric care can alleviate symptoms, making it possible for the patient to participate in other forms of treatment. The effects of psychotherapeutic drugs may be potentiated or diluted by the patient's environmental transactions.

Tranquilizers and mood modifiers are the two primary groups of psychotherapeutic drugs. Neuroleptics (major tranquilizers) affect psychotic symptoms and autonomic regulations. Anxiolytics (minor tranquilizers) relieve mild or moderate anxiety. Mood modifiers (tricyclic antidepressants and Monoamine oxidase inhibitors) have replaced drugs such as amphetamines in the treatment of depression states.

Psychotomimetics (hallucinogens) are a group of drugs whose mechanism of action is still unknown; their use in the treatment of mental illness is in the experimental stages.

Selection of psychotherapeutic drugs now deemphasizes the diagnostic classifications of psychiatric disorders, and treatment with drugs now attempts to modify the most disabling behavioral manifestations so that the patient can take advantage of the therapeutic milieu available. This demands careful assessment of the patient by the physician and subsequent evaluation and reassessment of the patient's response by both physician and nurse.

Anxiolytics (minor tranquilizers) are used to allay moderate anxiety and muscle tension. This group of drugs shares similar central nervous system depressant action, but their secondary central and peripheral effects vary. They are divided into two subgroups: benzodiazepines and nonbenzodiazepines. The secondary effects of both types are listed in Table 11-3. Although these drugs produce fewer disabling side effects than do major tranquilizers, some of them are habit forming. Withdrawal of the drug may cause mild to severe reactions including delirium and convulsions. Individuals taking these drugs for prolonged periods, especially those with a history of alcoholism or severe drug dependency problems, should be carefully monitored. Patients with a history of blood dyscrasias, impaired renal function, hepatic disease, or allergies should be evaluated carefully before these drugs are administered.

Neuroleptics (major tranquilizers) are drugs that have an important role in psychiatric treatment. They are divided into six subgroups: (1) phenothiazines, (2) thioxanthene derivatives, (3) butyrophenone derivatives, (4) dibenzoxazepine derivatives, (5) dihydroindolone derivatives, and (6) diphenylbutylpiperidine derivatives. The secondary effects of the drugs listed under the first and second subgroups are summarized in Table 11-4.

Neureleptics block dopamine-mediated transmission, depress lower levels of the central nervous system, and reduce sympathetic tone in the body without significant loss of cortical function or consciousness. Their use can produce both reversible and irreversible extrapyramidal side effects but no notable psy-chogenic or physical dependence. In comparison to the other subgroups, phenothiazines have a higher potency but lower sedative and autonomic blocking effects; however, they may produce more extrapyramidal effects. As potency decreases (with some exceptions), the reverse is seen.

Precautions to be observed in the use of phenothiazine compounds include monitoring the patient for signs of autonomic blockade; potentiation of other drugs such as alcohol, barbiturates, or morphine-like analgesics; and quinidine-like electrocardiographic alterations. Patients should also be monitored for adverse behavioral effects, dermatoses, orthostatic hypotension, and blood dyscrasias. These drugs are contraindicated for comatose patients and patients with a history of glaucoma, prostatic hypertrophy, or convulsive disorders.

Depressive states have been classified as endogenous psychotic depressions (characterized by absence of external causes for depression, such as death of a loved one) and reactive depressions (abnormal depressive responses to environmental factors). Psychotherapeutic drugs commonly used to treat the depressed patient are the tricyclic compounds and the monoamine oxidase inhibitors, all of which appear most effective in treatment of endogenous depression.

The nurse needs to be alert for the possibility of suicidal attempts by the patient, even though his overt behavior may indicate a remission of depressive symptoms. Antidepressants should generally be continued for several months after the remission of symptoms. Sudden withdrawal may cause a relapse.

Tricyclic antidepressants produce potent antidepressant and mild tranquilizing effects, but with fewer side effects than the monoamine oxidase inhibitors. Their mechanism of action is not known. It is theorized that an increase in amounts of norepinephrine and serotonin is achieved by inhibition of the neurotransmitter reuptake in the brain. They have atropine-like, antihistamine, antiepinephrine, and antiserotonin actions. The most common side effects are summarized in Table 11-6. The tricyclic antidepressants should not be given in the late afternoon or evening because their stimulating effect can cause insomnia.

Monoamine oxidase inhibitors act to increase psychomotor activity, increase appetite, and potentiate other drugs. They also prevent the release of norepinephrine from storage sites in the adrenergic neurons.

The wide variety of side effects produced by monoamine oxidase inhibitors has been cause for concern among most authorities. The most frequent effects are summarized in Table 11-11. Paradoxic hypertension and hepatic toxicity are two of the most common.

The monoamine oxidase inhibitors are contraindicated in hypertension, impaired kidney function, or epilepsy, as well as in many other conditions summarized in Table 11-10. They have a great interaction potential as indicated in Table 11-12.

Salts of lithium have been used successfully in mania and in manic-depressive disorders. It has been proposed that this drug stabilizes the nerve cell membrane by the influx of lithium instead of sodium into the cell. This possibly accelerates destruction of norepinephrine, inhibiting transmitter release at the synapse, with resultant correction of overactive catecholamine systems in mania. Toxic reactions associated with the administration of lithium depletion of sodium and water, the nurse should discuss with the patient and family the importance of a normal diet that includes salt and intake of 2 to 3 liters of liquid daily during the initial stabilization period of lithium administration.

QUESTIONS

FOR STUDY AND REVIEW

1 Differentiate between neuroleptic and anxiolytic drugs.
2 Define "drug-induced, extrapyramidal symptoms."
3 How is the "risk versus benefit" of treatment with neuroleptic drugs determined?
4 Why do schizophrenic patients refuse to take their drugs?
5 How can the nurse facilitate "intelligent drug compliance?"
6 How effective is prophylactic drug treatment of schizophrenia?
7 Do chronic schizophrenics undergo relapse when medication is discontinued?
8 How does lithium produce its psychotherapeutic effects?

9 Why is it necessary to monitor lithium serum levels?
10 What effect does sodium and fluid intake have on lithium therapy?
11 What additional medication may be needed to treat acute mania before lithium therapy becomes effective?
12 How do mood modifiers exert their effects?
13 Why are tricyclic antidepressants more widely used than monoamine oxidase inhibitors in the treatment of depression?
14 What common side effects are produced by the tricyclic antidepressants?
15 Give the clinical use for the administration of ritalin. What precautions are observed during therapy?

BIBLIOGRAPHY
SCHIZOPHRENIA

American College of Neuropsychopharmacology: Neurologic syndromes associated with antipsychotic drug use, Arch. Gen. Psychiatry 28:463, 1973.
Baldessarini, R.J., and Lipinski, J.F.: Risks vs benefits of antipsychotic drugs, N. Engl. J. Med. 289:427, 1973.
Coleman, J.H., and Hayes, P.E.: Drug induced extrapyramidal effects—a review, Dis. Nerv. Syst. 36:591, 1975.
Davis, J.M.: Overview: maintenance therapy in psychiatry. Part I. Schizophrenia, Am. J. Psychiatry 132:1237, 1975.
Denha, J., and Adamson, L.: Long-acting phenothiazines in the prevention of relapse of schizophrenic patients, Can. Psychiatr. Assoc. J. 18:235, 1973.
Hogarty, G.E., and Goldberg, S. C.: Drug and sociotherapy in the aftercare of schizophrenic patients, Arch. Gen. Psychiatry 28:54, 1973.
Hollister, L.E., and others: Specific indications for different classes of phenothiazines, Arch. Gen. Psychiatry 30:94, 1974.
Klawans, H.L., Jr.: The pharmacology of tardive dyskinesias, Am. J. Psychiatry 130:82, 1973.
Laska, E., and others: Patterns of psychotropic drug use for schizophrenia, Dis. Nerv. Syst. 34:294, 1973.
Van Putten, T.: Why do schizophrenic patients refuse to take their drugs? Arch. Gen. Psychiatry 31:67, 1974.

MANIC-DEPRESSIVE DISORDERS

Almy, G.L., and Taylor, M.A.: Lithium retention in mania, Arch. Gen. Psychiatry 29:232, 1973.
American Psychiatric Association Task Force on Lithium Therapy: The current status of lithium therapy: report of the APA Task Force, Am. J. Psychiatry 132:997, 1975.
Baldessarini, R.J., and Lipinski, J.F.: Lithium salts: 1970-1975, Ann. Intern. Med. 83:527, 1975.
Cade, J.F.J.: Lithium—when, why, and how? Med. J. Aust. 1:684, 1975.
Goldfield, M.D., and Weinstein, M.R.: Lithium carbonate in obstetrics: guidelines for clinical use, Am. J. Obstet. Gynecol. 116:15, 1973.
Goodwin, F.K., editor: Lithium ion: impact on treatment and research, Arch. Gen. Psychiatry 36:833, 1979.
Prien, R.F., and others: Factors associated with treatment success in lithium carbonate prophylaxis, Arch. Gen. Psychiatry 31:189, 1974.

Singer, I., and others: Mechanisms of lithium action, N. Engl. J. Med. **289**:254, 1973.

Tucker, W.I., and others: Effectiveness of lithium in the prevention of manic and depressive episodes, Med. Clin. North Am. **56**:681, 1972.

ANTIANXIETY DRUGS

Balter, M.B., and others: Cross-national study of the extent of antianxiety/sedation drug use, N. Engl. J. Med. **290**:769, 1974.

Blackwell, B.: Psychotropic drugs in use today: the role of diazepam in medical practice, J.A.M.A. **225**:1637, 1973.

Costa, E., and Greengard, P., editors: mechanisms of action of benzodiazepines, New York, 1975, Raven Press.

Glick, S.D., and Goldfarb, J., editors: Behavioral pharmacology, St. Louis, 1976, The C.V. Mosby Co.

Goodman, L.S., and Gilman, A., editors: The pharmacological basis of therapeutics, ed. 6, New York, 1980, The Macmillan Co.

Goth, A.: Medical pharmacology, ed. 10, St. Louis, 1980, The C.V. Mosby Co.

Greenblatt, D.J., and Shader, R.I.: Benzodiazepines, N. Engl. J. Med. **291**:1011, 1239, 1974.

Greenblatt, D.J., and Shader, R.I.: Benzodiazepines in clinical practice, New York, 1974, Raven Press.

Hitchens, E.A.: Helping psychiatric outpatients accept drug therapy, Am. J. Nurs. **77**:464, 1977.

Hollister, L.E.: Clinical use of psychotherapeutic drugs, Springfield, Ill., 1973, Charles C Thomas, Publisher.

Hollister, L.E.: Drugs for mental disorders of old age, J.A.M.A. **234**:195, 1975.

Hollister, L.E.: Clinical pharmacology of psychotherapeutic drugs, New York, 1978, Churchill Livingstone.

Hopper, J.J.: Effective therapy with anti-psychotic medications, Nurse Pract. **2**(1):32, 1976.

Hoyumpa, A.M., Jr.: Disposition and elimination of minor tranquilizers in the aged and in patients with liver disease, South. Med. J. **71**(suppl. 2):23, Aug. 1978.

Johnson, D.A.W.: The psychiatric side-effects of drugs, Practitioner **209**:320, 1972.

Lader, M.: Anxiolytic drugs, Practitioner **215**:468, 1975.

Lader, M., and others: Clinical comparison of anxiolytic drug therapy, Psychol. Med. **4**:381, 1974.

Lewis, A.J., editor: Modern drug encyclopedia, New York, 1977, Dun-Donnelley Publishing Corp.

Meyers, F.H., Jawetz, E., and Goldfien, A.: Review of medical pharmacology, ed. 4, Los Altos, Calif., 1974, Lange Medical Publications.

Modell, W., editor: Drugs of choice 1980-1981, St. Louis, 1980, The C.V. Mosby Co.

Osol, A., and Pratt, R.: The United States Dispensatory, ed. 27, Philadelphia, 1973, J.B. Lippincott Co.

Petit, J.M. Jr., and others: Tricyclic antidepressant plasma levels and adverse effects on overdosage, Clin. Pharmacol. Ther. **21**(1):47, 1977.

Prein, R.F.: Chemotherapy in chronic organic brain syndrome: a review of the literature, Psychopharmacol. Bull. **9**:5, 1973.

Rosenbaum, A.H., and others: Drugs that alter mood. I. Tricyclic agents and monoamine oxidase inhibitors. II. Lithium, Mayo Clin. Proc. **54**:335, 401, 1979.

Rosenbaum, J.F.: Psychotropic drugs and the cardiac patient, Drug Ther. (Hosp.), p. 80-88, March 1980.

Sellers, E.M.: Clinical pharmacology and therapeutics of benzodiazepines, Can. Med. Assoc. J. **115**:1533-1538, 1978.

DEPRESSION

Akiskal, H.S., and McKinney, W.T., Jr.: Overview of recent research in depression, Arch. Gen. Psychiatry **32**:285, 1975.

Alkalay, D., and others: Bioavailability and kinetics of maprotiline, Clin. Pharmacol. Ther. **27**(5):679-703, 1980.

Ashcroft, G.W.: Management of depression, Br. Med. J. **2**:372, 1975.

Ayd, F.J.: Single daily dose of antidepressants, J.A.M.A. **230**:263, 1974.

Davies, B.: Diagnosis and treatment of anxiety and depression, Drugs **6**:389, 1973.

Flemenbaum, A.: Methylphenidate: a catalyst for the tricyclic antidepressants, Am. J. Psychiatry **128**:649, 1973.

Glassman, A.H., and others: The clinical pharmacology of imipramine, Arch. Gen. Psychiatry **28**:649, 1973.

Johnson, D.A.W.: A study of the use of antidepressant medication in general practice. Br. J. Psychiatry **125**:186, 1974.

Kline, N.S.: Antidepressant medications: a more effective use by general practitioners, family physicians, internists, and others, J.A.M.A. **227**:1158, 1974.

Pinder, R.M., and others: Maprotiline: a review of its pharmacological properties and therapeutic efficacy in mental depressive states, Drugs **13**:321-352, 1977.

Riess, W., and others: The pharmokinetic properties of maprotiline (Ludiomil) in man, J. Intern. Med. Res. **3**(2):16-41, 1975.

Schildkraut, J.J.: Neuropharmacology of the affective disorders, Annu. Rev. Pharmacol. **13**:427, 1973.

ADDITIONAL REFERENCES

A.M.A. drug evaluations, ed. 4, New York, 1980, John Wiley & Son.

Avery, G.S., editor: Drug treatment, ed. 2, New York, 1980, ADIS Press.

Biggs, J.T., and others: Tricyclic antidepressant overdosage, J.A.M.A. **238**:135, 1977.

Collis, M.G., and Shepherd, J.T.: Antidepressant drug action on presynaptic receptors, Mayo Clin. Proc., **53**:567, 1980.

Council on Child Health: Medication for hyperkinetic children, Pediatrics **55**:560, 1975.

Garver, D.L.: Biogenic amine hypothesis of affective disorders, Life Sci. **24**:383, 1979.

Sabelli, H.C., and others: The methylphenidate test to differentiate between desipramine-responsive (type I) and nortriptyline-responsive (type II) depressions, Annual convention of American Psychiatric Association, San Francisco, Calif., May 3-9, 1980.

Sabelli, H.C., and others: Further evidence for a role of 2-phenylethylamine in the mode of action of delta 9-tetrahydrocannabinol, Life Sc. **14**:149, 1974.

Sprague, R., and Sleator, E.: What is the proper dose of stimulant drugs in children? Int. J. Ment. Health **4**:75, 1975.

CHAPTER 12

Substance and drug abuse

Although most drugs are prescribed and administered with a high degree of discrimination, all drugs potentially can be misused or abused. The prescription of drugs without adequate exploration of the patient's presenting complaint, for example, is representative of drug misuse by a physician. Prolonged and unsupervised administration of drugs for symptomatic relief is another such example. In general, drug misuse refers to nonspecific or indiscriminate use of drugs. Drug abuse, on the other hand, refers to self-medication or self-administration of a drug in chronically excessive quantities, resulting in psychologic and/or physical dependence, functional impairment, and deviation from approved social norms. Statistics from the National Institute of Drug Abuse on drugs abused in the United States are given in Table 12-1.

Drug abuse is neither a new nor a recent phenomenon. It has been known throughout history as one expression of an individual's search for relief of physical, psychologic, social, and economic problems. Indeed, investigations suggests that epidemics of drug abuse have occurred throughout human history. Currently over 43 million Americans have tried marijuana, and almost half that number may be regular users. The epidemic is now even reaching the preteenage group of our society.

Contemporary drug abuse has attained prominence as an issue with moral, legal, social, intrapsychic, and medical implications and is difficult to examine objectively. To fulfill their professional responsibility to society in relation to this pressing social issue, nurses need current knowledge about drugs most frequently abused, reasons for drug abuse, crisis intervention in relation to drug abuse, and regional treatment facilities to which they can refer patients either for emergency care or for long-term treatment.

It is beyond the scope of this chapter to explore all aspects of drug abuse in depth.

T A B L E 1 2 - 1 Drug abuse in the United States: percentage who have tried the drug at least once

Drug(s)	Age group		
	12 to 17 years old (%)	18 to 25 years old (%)	26 years old or older (%)
Marijuana, hashish	Over 20	Over 60	Over 15
Cocaine	Over 4	Over 19	Over 3
Heroin	Less than 2	About 4	About 1
Prescription stimulants with nonmedical use	About 6	About 22	About 5

Instead this chapter focuses on the actions and treatment of drug abuse. However, the nurse is urged to investigate other aspects of the complex phenomenon of drug abuse independently to achieve a more holistic frame of reference.

Etiologic factors of drug abuse

A characteristic common to most drugs which cause dependence is that they initially are taken because the individual believes that a desirable pharmacologic effect will result. To cause dependence, then, a drug must produce favorable, pleasant, unusual, or desirable effects. The person who is dependent on a drug has found something that provides relief from problems, and the drug generally is used as an adjustive, coping mechanism. Since very few drugs or substances without central nervous system effects are abused, one of the predominant factors contributing to drug abuse appears to be intrapsychic, that is, a desire to alter one's state of mind. This desire may arise from a number of factors, such as curiosity, boredom, peer pressure, multiple and diverse alienation, hedonism, mass media, and affluence. All or any combination may lead to misuse of drugs and substances. More individual or subjective reasons are personal inadequacy or failure, conflicts terminating in tension, shame, and depression as a personality trait predisposing one to emotional and behavior problems.

Pleasure-seeking behavior (hedonism) often seems to be a factor in drug abuse and, among other goals, may represent escape from inner tensions, a search for euphoria, an attempt to explore unknown aspects of cognitive function, or an attempt to discover one's self. More specifically, some psychologic hypotheses have been advanced in relation to persons prone to use drugs as escape mechanisms. Descriptions of potentially drug-dependent personalities have included characteristics of strong psychologic dependence, low threshold of frustration, fear of failure, and feelings of inadequacy. Other authorities dispute the "addiction-prone" personality hypothesis, maintaining that everyone has the potential to become dependent on something; however, the unstable immature person with a self-image of inadequacy and an inability to tolerate frustrations frequently seems to be a distraught, anxious, tense, and unhappy person and a candidate for drug or substance abuse. This person may self-administer "therapy" for his or her affective disorder to give relief from relationships that are unable to be endured and negotiated effectively.

Types of drugs and substances abused

All drugs have some abuse potential, and some sources indicate that drug abuse may be more related to the personality of the user than to the drug itself. Perhaps among the more frequently abused chemically active substances are the xanthines, which are contained in beverages such as coffee, tea, chocolate, and colas. Although these substances rarely are perceived as drugs by the lay public, they do produce mild stimulant and euphoric effects, and their use may lead to psychic dependence. Nicotine and ethyl alcohol are the most frequently misused and abused, with consequent physical and psychic dependence. Reserpine, anticholinergics, steroids, phencyclidine (PCP, angel dust), phenethylamines (for example, amphetamines, epinephrine), pentazocine, and cardiac glycosides, L-dopa, are examples of other drugs that may induce altered states of perception, thought, and feelings and drug-induced psychoses as a result of prolonged and concentrated therapeutic use or abuse.

However, as previously indicated, few drugs without CNS effects are misused or abused. Therefore the major categories of commonly abused drugs are narcotics and related compounds, barbiturates, alcohol and other sedative-hypnotics, amphetamines, cocaine, other CNS stimulants, cannabis drugs, and other mind-altering drugs that have been variably classified as mood modifiers and include the psychotomimetic agents (hallucinogens). When used for prolonged periods, depressant drugs like the opiates, barbiturates, and alcohol generally produce both physical and psychic dependence. Stimulant drugs like the amphetamines and cocaine appear to produce psychologic dependence and tolerance and may be associated with some physical dependence in increased dosages. The other mind-altering drugs have variable and, at this time, questionable dependence-producing qualities, but it seems generally agreed that they all produce psychic dependence and have a rapid onset of action for immediate satisfaction.

Before proceeding it is necessary to differentiate between the terms "hallucinogenic," "psychotomimetic," and "psychedelic." Although all three terms have been used interchangeably, they have some distinct differences. *Hallucinogenic* refers to the tendency of a drug to produce auditory and/or visual hallucinations. Hallucinogenic effects, however, are neither a uniform nor a primary property of all consciousness-altering drugs, and the term should be used with discrimination. *Psychotomimetic* refers to the ability of a drug to chemically induce a psychotic state that mimics a "natural" psychosis. Again, this term must be used with discrimination when referring to mind-altering drugs, since not all induce psychosis. The term *psychedelic* originally was intended to be a non-judgmental adjective referring to the "mind-manifesting" properties of a drug, that is, to a drug's ability to effect states of consciousness an individual would not usually experience. However, it has become more ambiguous in definition and has acquired some valuational connotations. It may be used to refer to self-administered mind-altering drugs for their subjective effects of inducing states of altered perception, thought, and feeling and also for their social-recreational purposes.

Drug abuse may take several forms. It may be experimental abuse, in which the individual uses drugs in an exploratory way after which he or she may accept or reject continuing use of the drugs. Drug abuse may occur only in social contexts; drugs that are frequently abused only in social situations include alcohol, marijuana, nicotine, and caffeine. Episodic drug abuse refers to the periodic abuse of excessive amounts of a drug, as frequently occurs with ethyl alcohol. Compulsive drug abuse is characterized by irrational, irresistible, or compelling abuse of a drug. Ritualistic drug abuse, on the other hand, may be related to religious or philosophic rites.

Polydrug or multiple drug abuse is a common condition that is emerging. Marijuana, alcohol, and other depressants frequently are used together. CNS stimulants are used in conjunction with depressants. Heroin may be used in conjunction with pentazocine and tripelennamine (known as T's and blues), alcohol, or other depressants. Patterns in use also develop regionally, for example, on the west and east coasts of the United States, and then are seen more inland toward the midwestern states. The common use of LSD in the 1960s led to the use of speed (amphetamines) in the middle to late 1960s; in the early 1970s the use of downers (CNS depressants) emerged heavily, and about the same time PCP usage became common and held a strong position into the late 1970s. Now in the early 1980s cocaine has become popular again, and its abuse is seen more frequently but is somewhat curtailed by its high cost. The bizarre, unpredictable reactions to PCP have encouraged the return to LSD and more frequent use of depressants. Throughout these changes in which substances are popular for abuse, marijuana and alcohol and other depressants have remained prominent.

Drug dependence

In the past drug abuse was defined in terms of habituation and addiction. These terms, however, have been used in so many ways that there is no longer any consensus regarding their definitions. Moreover, the terms "habituation" and "addiction" are nonspecific in that they do not describe the nature of the problem. Characteristics of drug abuse vary according to the particular agent abused, and different drugs have entirely different patterns of dependence and different characteristics of withdrawal. In an attempt to reduce the conceptual ambiguity of habituation and addiction, in 1964 the World Health Organization suggested that the use of these terms be replaced by the concepts of *psychic* and *physical dependence*. Its statement regarding this issue reads as follows:

Drug dependence is a state of psychic or physical dependence or both on a drug arising in a person following administration of that drug on a periodic or continuous basis. The characteristics of such a state will vary with the agent involved and these characteristics must always be made clear by designating the particular type of drug dependence in each specific case—e.g., drug dependence of the barbiturate type, of the morphine type . . .

Physical dependence on a drug (physiologic drug dependence) refers to an adaptive physiologic state that occurs after prolonged exposure to and administration of that drug which manifests itself by intense physical disturbances (objective withdrawal symptoms) when the drug's administration is discontinued. That is, physical dependence on a drug can be demonstrated only by production of an objective withdrawal syndrome. This syndrome can be relieved by readministering the drug or by administering a pharmacologically related drug. (Drugs are cross dependent when they are mutually capable of relieving withdrawal symptoms that result from the withdrawal of either drug.) Closely related to physical dependence is the production of drug tolerance with a tendency to increase the drug dosage.

Psychic, or psychologic, dependence, by contrast, is a subjective state of emotional reliance on a drug to maintain a drug-induced state that, to the involved individual, is preferable to a drug-free state of being. The manifestations of psychologic dependence range from a mild desire for a drug to craving to repeated compulsive use for subjectively satisfying or pleasurable effects. Either type of dependence can exist independently of the other, or both can exist simultaneously. Both types of dependence potentially can lead to compulsive patterns of drug use in which the user's life-style is focused in administration and procurement of the drug.

Pharmacologic basis of physical drug dependence and tolerance

Several hypotheses attempt to explain that pharmacologic basis of the physiologic adaptation that occurs in tolerance and physical drug dependence.

According to Martin's pharmacologic redundancy theory,* there are two or more pathways mediating the physiologic functions influenced by the opiates. Martin assumes that morphine sulfate interrupts one of the redundant pathways but does not interrupt the other. This results in hypertrophy of the uninterrupted pathway (pathway A), which then assumes the functions mediated by the interrupted pathway (pathway B). Therefore tolerance to morphine is the result of hypertrophy of pathway A. When the drug is withdrawn, pathway B resumes its normal level of excitability, but because pathway A is still overfunctioning, the total system then functions at a level that is higher than the predrug state of function. This exaggerated function, Martin states, is the hyperexcitability that is characteristic of the abstinence syndrome.

Collier,* on the other hand, hypothesizes that tissue may contain two types of receptors for particular drugs. One of these types, the *pharmacologic receptors*, produces a pharmacologic response when contact is made with the

*In Phillipson, R.V., editor: Modern trends in drug dependence and alcoholism, London, 1970, Butterworth & Co. (Publishers) Ltd.

drug. The other receptors are *silent receptors* that elicit no response. The development of drug tolerance results from a change in the number and production of these receptor types, the pharmacologic receptors decreasing in number and the silent receptors increasing in number.

From a third frame of reference, Crossland* states that physical adaptation to depressant drugs simply involves an increase in the amount of excitatory transmitter that is adequate to overcome the drug-depressed condition of the nerve cells. When the drug is withdrawn, hyperexcitability (abstinence symptoms) occurs if the nerve cells return to normal condition more rapidly than the transmitter supply.

As stated previously, the term "addiction syndrome" as used here refers to physiologic dependence on a substance that generally is found after extended exposure to the substance, and the period of exposure necessary to develop addiction varies with the substance. When the substance is discontinued abruptly, an objective withdrawal syndrome of physiologic changes occurs, and dependence is evident.

Although these and other theories of physical drug dependence are in hypothetical stages and still are being researched, they generally seem to agree that, in a state of dependence, a condition of latent hyperexcitability develops in the cells of the central nervous system following frequent and prolonged administration of depressant drugs.

Tolerance may exist with dependence or habituation. Tolerance may be viewed in two manners. First, receptor site tolerance, or tissue tolerance, is a form of adaptation in that the length of exposure of the CNS receptor site to a given drug concentration produces different effects, depending on the length of time and the concentration of the drug on the exposed receptor. This tolerance type has a reduced clinical effect as the duration of the substance exposure continues.

An example of receptor site tolerance is seen in the acute intoxicant effect of ethanol. The concentration of ethanol in the blood (and at

*Crossland, J.: Lewis's pharmacology, ed. 4, Baltimore, 1970, The Williams & Wilkins Co.

the receptor site in the brain) that follows the acute ingestion of ethanol may be higher in recovery from acute intoxication than earlier, when subjective manifestations of the intoxication are at a maximum.

The second type of tolerance is metabolic or pharmacokinetic tolerance, an aspect of drug disposition. This tolerance is the effect of prolonged exposure of the substance on the substance's own pharmacokinetic properties. This is described as the increase in drug clearance that is associated with repeated ingestion. An example of this tolerance type is seen with prolonged barbiturate exposure; the steady state blood concentrations of the substance administered chronically will fall progressively with continued administration of the same dose. This may be an attribute of the barbiturate drugs' effect on hepatic microsomal enzymes to stimulate their own metabolism.

Altered states of consciousness produced by drugs

The effects of various mind-altering drugs are unpredictable and highly variable. The same drug in the same dose may produce quite disparate effects in two different individuals. The primary factors influencing the effects of any drug are generally defined as (1) the pharmacologic properties of the drug itself, (2) the personality of the user, (3) the environment of the user, (4) the experience of the user, and (5) the interaction of these four components. The effects of mind-altering drugs, specifically, also are thought to be related to the purity of the drug used (drugs transferred illegally are frequently adulterated, or *cut*, with other substances), the underlying psychopathology of the user, and the age of the user. For example, many drug users are adolescents who are dealing with the intrapsychic problems accompanying this stage of maturation. The tenuous emotional equilibrium of this stage may particularly predispose the individual to negative reactions to mind-altering drugs. The effects of mind-altering drugs also appear to be particularly subject to the user's mood, expectations, and social environment. Most adverse reactions to marijuana, for example, are said to occur in

364 Drugs affecting mood and behavior

novice users, since they may enter the experience with a mental set of fear.

Adequate preparation for the drug experience, therefore, is a significant factor influencing the nature of that experience. In addition, the presence or lack of a supportive environment (particularly the presence and guidance of a trusted and knowledgeable person) and the presence or lack of an opportunity to understand and to reintegrate the experience following recovery from the drug are variables that may influence a drug experience either positively or negatively.

In describing the phenomenon of the psychedelic experience Houston* identifies some general effects that are commonly observed and experienced after the administration of mind-altering drugs. Among the most common and repeated effects, she identifies the following: changes in auditory, visual, olfactory, tactile, gustatory, and kinesthetic perception; changes in body image; changes in experiencing time and space; changes in rate and content of thought; abrupt and frequent changes in mood and affect; heightened suggestibility; possible occurence of depersonalization and ego dissolution; possible activation of repressed materials; awareness of internal organs and body processes; multiple and fragmentized consciousness; concern with philosophic, cosmologic, and religious questions; perception of a world released from its normal ordering; a sense of capacity to communicate better through nonverbal means; and feelings of empathy.

Houston states that these are not the only effects of psychedelic drugs but that this description should serve to convey some idea of their mind-altering effects. She goes on to categorize the effects of these drugs into four major levels of consciousness, as follows:

1 Sensory level. The drug user may experience a great variety of sensory awareness, including heightened awareness of visual phenomena, such as colors, lines, textures, and spatial relationships. This sensory awareness also may be focused on internal processes of the body. It may be a pleasant heightened awareness or a frightening one.

*Houston, J.: Phenomenology of the psychedelic experience. In Hicks, R.E., and Fink, P.J.: Psychedelic drugs, Hahnemann symposium, New York, 1969, Grune & Stratton, Inc., pp. 1-7.

Often it is the only alteration in consciousness the drug user experiences.

2 Recollective-analytic level. In this level of altered consciousness the drug user is described as experiencing psychologic involution and introspection and engaging in self-analysis of personal problems, values, and potentialities. Emergence of unconscious material may occur, and the drug user may experience regression. In an unsupportive context or in a context of latent psychosis this experience may result in an acute panic psychosis. With an appropriate, predetermined mental set and knowledgeable guidance the experience may be therapeutic.

3 Symbolic level. At this level of consciousness the drug user is described as experiencing rich symbolism in which life expands beyond the particular-personal orientation to a personal-universal orientation, and the individual may see life in terms of a guiding pattern or goal.

4 Integral level. The experience of this level of consciousness is described as extremely rare and is characterized as being similar to religious and mystic experiences in which profound and fundamental value and behavior changes occur or in which self-actualization occurs.

Houston's categorization provides a conceptual tool for comprehending experiences with mind-altering drugs, although it is by no means the only frame of reference to apply to the drug experience. Again, it must be emphasized that (1) expanding and continuing research is necessary to validate information regarding drug abuse, and (2) at this time the illicit drug experience appears to have as much (if not more) potential for being frightening and negative as it has for being pleasant and constructive.

Pathophysiologic changes characteristic of drug abuse

Physical and psychic dependence on drugs frequently is associated with debilitated physical states caused by the user's extensive involvement in procuring and using the drug. Malnutrition, dehydration, and hypovitaminosis often are evident. Respiratory complications such as pneumonia, pulmonary emboli, and abscesses frequently are associated with neglect, debilitation, and the respiratory depression produced by CNS depressants. The intravenous administration of illicit drugs often leads to a high incidence of sepsis and hepatitis

T A B L E 1 2 - 2 Illicit drug adulterants

Illicit drug(s)	Adulterants	Diluents
Cocaine	Lidocaine, procaine, antipyrine, boric acid, ethyl aminobenzoate (Benzocaine), ephedrine, tetracaine, phenylpropanolamine, barbiturates, amphetamines, CNS stimulants, caffeine, A.S.A., methapyrilene, PCP	Dextrose, quinine, inositol, mannitol, lactose
Heroin	Strychnine, tripelennamine, procaine, caffeine, barbiturates, PCP, methapyriline, cocaine, scopolamine, pentazocine, propoxyphene, antihistamines, quinine, dyes, amphetamines, phenylpropanolamine, hashish, those adulterants listed under cocaine	Similar to those of cocaine
Marijuana	PCP, hashish oil, organic solvents	
LSD	PCP, MDA, ethyl aminobenzoate, benzodiazepines, antihistamines	
Amphetamines and their derivatives	Caffeine, phenylpropanolamine	

T A B L E 1 2 - 3 Signs and symptoms of acute drug intoxication

Drug(s) abused	Signs and symptoms
Cannabis drugs	Tachycardia and postural hypotension, conjunctival vascular congestion, clear sensorium, distortions of perception, dryness of mouth and throat, possible panic
Opiates	Depressed blood pressure and respirations, fixed, pinpoint pupils, depressed sensorium, coma, pulmonary edema
Barbiturates and other general CNS depressants	Depressed blood pressure and respirations, ataxia, slurred speech, confusion, depressed tendon reflexes, coma, shock
Amphetamines	Elevated blood pressure, tachycardia, other cardia arrhythmias, hyperactive tendon reflexes, pupils dilated and reactive to light, hyperpyrexia, perspiration, shallow respirations, circulatory collapse, clear or confused sensorium, possible hallucinations, paranoid feelings
Hallucinogenic agents	Elevated blood pressure, hyperactive tendon reflexes, piloerection, perspiration, pupils dilated and reactive to light, anxiety, distortion of body image and perception, delusions, hallucinations

as a result of the use of contaminated equipment. In addition, cellulitis, sclerosis of the veins, phlebitis, and skin abscesses may occur. Last but not least, death from accidental overdose is not uncommon. Overdosage is a particularly significant potential danger because illegal drugs are notoriously unreliable in regard to the potency of their active ingredient. The drugs are frequently well adulterated with various substances by the time they reach the user (Table 12-2). If an individual who has been using cut drugs unknowingly receives pure or stronger drugs, there is the risk of toxicity and even death. Overdosage also may occur when an individual who has been withdrawn from drugs for some time (thereby having lost accumulated tolerance) injects the previous usual dose, which now is in excess of his or her tolerance level.

Parenthetically it must be said that the dose unreliability of most mind-altering drugs also affects research findings. Because dosage is difficult to control, and because most drug abuse research is ex post facto, research results frequently may be skewed.

As a consequence of all these factors, the life expectancy of persons who are physically dependent on drugs is generally lower than that of nondependent individuals.

Table 12-3 presents common drug groups that are abused with signs and symptoms of acute intoxication. The following are possible clinical signs and symptoms of a person who has been abusing drugs and which drug groups may be responsible for the toxicity; this list can be used for diagnostic purposes.*

Central nervous system

Coma: amphetamines, antihistamines, atropine, barbiturates, chloral hydrate, diazepam, ethanol, glutethimide, meprobamate, methaqualone, narcotics, PCP, pentazocine, propoxyphene, quinine, scopolamine, sedative-hypnotics, toluene, tricyclic antidepressants

Ataxia, or incoordination: atropine, barbiturates, cocaine, ethanol, glutethimide, hallucinogens, opiates, PCP, phenothiazines, propoxyphene, toluene, tricyclic antidepressants

Tetanic rigidity: caffeine, methaqualone, morphine, PCP, phenothiazines, scopolamine

Convulsions: amphetamines, antihistamines, atropine, barbiturates, benzodiazepines, caffeine, cocaine, ethanol, ethchlorvynol, glutethimide, meprobamate, methaqualone, methyprylone, opiates, PCP, propoxyphene, tricyclic antidepressants

Muscle weakness or paralysis: alcohol, hallucinogens, morphine, PCP, quinine

Muscle spasm: atropine, cocaine, methaqualone, phenothiazines

Anesthesia: barbiturates, benzene, cocaine, ethanol, ketamine, PCP

Paresthesia: barbiturates, benzene, cocaine, hallucinogens, morphine, psilocybin, quinine

Muscle fasciculations (twitchings): atropine, ethanol

Hallucinations: amphetamines, atropine, barbiturates, caffeine, cocaine, ethanol, ketamine, LSD, morphine, PCP, psilocybin

Headaches: atropine, barbiturates, benzene, caffeine, cocaine, ephedrine, ethanol, morphine, scopolamine, toluene, tricyclic antidepressants

Cardiovascular system

Circulatory collapse or shock: amphetamines, antihistamines, barbiturates, benzodiazepines, boric acid, caffeine, chloral hydrate, cocaine, ephedrine, ethanol, methaqualone, opiate withdrawal, procaine, procaine amide, propoxyphene, quinine

Bradycardia: codeine, ethchlorvynol, lidocaine, narcotics, quinine, sedative-hypnotics

Tachycardia: amphetamines, antihistamines, atropine, caffeine, cocaine, codeine, ephedrine, ethanol, glutethimide, methaqualone, methyprylon, PCP, quinine

Hypertension: amphetamines, ephedrine, glutethimide, PCP, methaqualone

Hypotension: barbiturates, benzodiazepines, caffeine, chloral hydrate, glutethimide, lidocaine, LSD, meprobamate, methyprylon, narcotics, propoxyphene, quinine

Arrhythmias: amphetamines, meprobamate, propoxyphene, quinine, toluene, tricyclic antidepressants

Vasoconstriction: amphetamines, cocaine, ephedrine

Hemorrhage, petechiae, purpura: barbiturates, benzene, quinine

Respiratory system

Rapid or deep breathing: amphetamines, atropine, barbiturates, boric acid, caffeine, chloral hydrate, cocaine, ethanol, LSD, quinine

Slow or labored breathing: atropine, barbiturates, benzene, benzodiazepines, chloral hydrate, cocaine, ethanol, ethchlorvynol, glutethimide, heroin, methaqualone, methyprylon, morphine, narcotics, propoxyphene, quinine, tricyclic antidepressants

Respiratory paralysis: barbiturates, ethanol, hypnotics, lidocaine, opiates, PCP, procaine, toluene

Cough: benzene, ethanol

Digestive system

Anorexia: amphetamines, cocaine, codeine, ethanol, morphine

Dysphagia: atropine, cocaine, ephedrine, tricyclic antidepressants

Thirst: atropine, chloral hydrate, morphine

Salivation: cocaine, morphine, quinine

Dry oral mucosa: amphetamines, antihistamines, atropine, benzene, glutethimide, morphine, scopolamine, tricyclic antidepressants

Nausea and vomiting: antihistamines, atropine, benzene, benzodiazepines, boric acid, caffeine, cocaine, codeine, ephedrine, ethanol, lidocaine, LSD, marijuana, opiates, propoxyphene, quinine, toluene

Colic: morphine

Diarrhea: boric acid, chloral hydrate, cocaine, quinine

Bloody stools: morphine

Constipation: anticholinergics, barbiturates, codeine, ephedrine, glutethimide, morphine, tricyclic antidepressants

Abdominal pain: benzene, chloral hydrate, cocaine, codeine, morphine, procaine, quinine, tricyclic antidepressants

Gastroenteritis: atropine, benzene, chloral hydrate, codeine, ethanol, nonbarbiturates, sedative-hypnotics

Skin and mucous membranes

Pruritus: atropine, boric acid, opiates, scopolamine

Rash, urticaria: barbiturates, glutethimide, halogens, LSD, meprobamate, methaqualone, non-

*From the Bio-Science Handbook of Clinical and Industrial Toxicology, ed. 1, Van Nuys, Calif., 1979, Bio-Science Laboratories Main Laboratory.

barbiturates, procaine, quinine, sedative-hypnotics

Dryness: atropine, benzene, boric acid, ephedrine, ethanol, heroin, morphine, scopolamine

Perspiration: ethanol, tricyclic antidepressants

Flush: amphetamines, antihistamines, atropine, codeine, ephedrine, ethanol, morphine, scopolamine

Pallor: barbiturates, benzene, cocaine, ephedrine, heroin

Discoloration of skin
    Cyanosis: barbiturates, ethanol
    Jaundice yellow: benzene, chloral hydrate, nitrobenzene
    Red: atropine, boric acid, scopolamine

Bullae: barbiturates, glutethimide

Burns, irritation, corrosion, ulcers: boric acid, cocaine, glutethimide, pentazocine

Dermatitis inflammation: amphetamines, atropine, barbiturates, benzene, boric acid, chloral hydrate, cocaine, codeine, ephedrine, morphine, quinine, toluene

Alopecia: boric acid, chloral hydrate, morphine

Hirsutism: antidepressants, barbiturates

Exfoliation, or desquamation: boric acid

Needle marks: (referred to as *tracks*) amphetamines, barbiturates, cocaine, narcotics, pentazocine, propoxyphene

Urine and breath

Glycosuria: atropine, caffeine, morphine

Hematuria: benzene

Oliguria: atropine, morphine, quinine

Polyuria: atropine, benzene, caffeine, cocaine, ethanol, scopolamine

Porphyrinuria: benzene

Proteinuria: benzene, caffeine, ethanol, methaqualone, morphine, quinine, toluene

Urobilinogenuria: benzene, chloral hydrate, cocaine, quinine

Breath odor: ethanol, fetid or pearlike with chloral hydrate, pungent with ethchlorvynol

Hematologic disorders

Anemia: barbiturates, benzene, ethanol, meprobamate, morphine, quinine

Hemolysis: benzene, quinine

Leukopenia: benzene, meprobamate

Polycythemia: benzene

Auditory, personality, and visual disturbances

Auditory disturbances
    Hearing impairment: atropine, benzene, cocaine, quinine
    Tinnitus: benzene, codeine, morphine, quinine

Personality alteration (such as irritability, confusion, delirium, psychosis): amphetamines (psychosis), antihistamines, atropine, barbiturates, benzene, benzodiazepines, caffeine, cocaine, codeine, ephedrine, ethanol, ethchlorvynol, hallucinogens, LSD, marijuana, morphine, pentazocine, PCP, procaine, scopolamine, toluene

Visual disturbances
    Blindness (partial or complete): ethanol, phenothiazines, quinine
    Blurred vision: alcohol, atropine, barbiturates, benzodiazepines, CNS depressants, ephedrine, hallucinogens, lidocaine, morphine, quinine, scopolamine
    Color distortions: ethanol, hallucinogens, LSD, quinine
    Miosis (pinpoint pupil): barbiturates, benzodiazepines, caffeine, chloral hydrate, codeine, heroin, morphine, pentazocine, propoxyphene
    Blank stare: PCP
    Mydriasis: amphetamines, cocaine, glutethimide, hallucinogens

Narcotics and related compounds
Opiates and opiate derivatives

The opium derivatives are the most abused narcotics, although some other narcotics also are abused. The pharmacologic types of drugs that cause opiate-like dependence include the opium alkaloids (heroin, morphine), the semisynthetic group (hydromorphone, oxymorphone), and the synthetic group, (meperidine, levorphanol, methadone). Of the opiates, heroin, codeine, and morphine are the most often abused, heroin (diacetylmorphine) being the most potent of the three.

Mode of administration. The opium derivatives generally can be administered through the percutaneous route (absorption through the mucous membranes), by sniffing, in the form of subcutaneous injections (known in street language as *skin popping*), or directly intravenously *(mainlining)*. The rate of absorption is correspondingly increased, with mainlining producing almost immediate drug effects.

Mechanism of action and effects. The opium derivatives, being narcotics, act as CNS depressants, probably acting on the sensory cortex, psychic or higher centers, and thalami. Because these drugs elevate mood, relieve tension, fear, and anxiety, and produce feelings of peace, euphoria, and tranquility, they are particularly likely to lead to physical and psychologic dependence. Rapid intravenous injection of these drugs produces warm, flushing sensations described as being similar to sexual orgasm. This is followed by a soothing state that seems to be best characterized as a state of complete drive satiation. The individual "high" on opiates feels no need to satisfy drives for basic biologic needs and is often described as being "on the nod"—drowsy, content, and euphoric. The drugs do not produce hallucinogenic or psychotomimetic effects.

Acute overdosage. Acute overdosage of opiate-type substances may result in coma, pulmonary edema, and cessation of respiration. These outcomes are dose dependent and are related to the degree of individual tolerance. Symptoms occur rapidly in most patients, and since tolerance occurs in dependent patients, a lethal dose is patient dependent.

Opiate toxicity manifests itself in various ways. Pupils are generally found to be pinpoint (miotic), but they may be dilated in mixed overdose conditions or severe acidosis. Thrombophlebitis, scarred veins, puckered scars from subcutaneous injections, conditions of severe acidosis, bradycardia, itching caused by histamine release, hypotension, hypoxia, muscle spasm, respiratory depression, and urinary retention may be seen also. There is rapid absorption of the opiates from the oral route as well as the intravenous route. These drugs tend to delay motility and gastric emptying time, so the revival of the patient may increase peristalsis and thus further increase absorption of the drug, producing a coma cycle. An overdose with methadone may produce prolonged toxicity of 24 to 48 hours, including respiration depression. Frequently, chronic abusers may present with abscesses, myelitis, anaphylaxis, arrhythmias, cellulitis, endocarditis, fecal impaction, glomerulonephritis, hyperglycemia or hypoglycemia, myoglobinuria, osteomyelitis, encephalopathy, tetanus, and thrombphlebitis. These are caused by a spectrum of factors ranging from injection technique to adulterants in the substance of abuse.

The treatment of choice after acute overdosage is administration of an antagonist and methods of respiratory support. Attention is focused on the opiate toxic reaction for shock and problems of apnea. The opiates depress brainstem sensitivity to carbon dioxide, and heavy dependence on a hypoxic respiratory drive device is paramount. When the triad of miotic pupils, coma or stupor, and bradypnea (slowed or periodic respirations such as four to six per minute) appear, the administration of a pure narcotic antagonist (naloxone [Narcan]) may differentiate the diagnosis of narcotic poisoning from that of other conditions. Naloxone is a pure narcotic antagonist and reverses the toxic effects of abused opiates and derivatives such as heroin, morphine, methadone, pentazocine, and propoxyphene. The usual adult dose is 0.4 to 0.8 mg intravenously. If a site for intravenous injection is not found because of abuse injections sites, the intramuscular (producing a longer lasting effect), subcutaneous, or sublingual route may be used.

Larger doses may be required to reverse acute overdoses of codeine, propoxyphene, and pentazocine; if a single dose fails, a dose of 2 to 4 mg may be used intravenously. A failure to respond to high doses may indicate a mixed substance overdose or that there is no opiate-type substance involved. Children should have a minimum of 0.1 mg intravenous push. Children with a known or suspected narcotic overdose may receive 0.01 mg/kg as the first dose. Naloxone may be diluted with Sterile Water for Injection.

Naloxone has prompt onset within minutes to reverse apnea and coma. The naloxone must be titrated to the patient's arousal with a respiratory rate in a range of 10 to 20 breaths per minute. Administration may be repeated to reverse narcotic respiratory depression in 2- to 3-minute intervals. Repeated dosages may be required within 1- to 2-hour intervals, depending on the amount, type (that is, short or long acting), and interval since the last administration of the narcotic. A positive response to naloxone may be characterized by dilation of the pupils and an increase in respiratory function, blood pressure, and cardiac rate. Blood and urine samples should be examined for a multiple drug screen to aid in diagnosis. Heroin itself may not be detected in the urine because it appears as a derivative of morphine and may be detected from 12 to 24 hours after administration. It is necessary to provide support of blood pressure and maintenance of respiration. Pupils may be dilated if hypoxia is severe or if the overdose is from meperidine, whereas miosis is observed in barbiturate, ethanol, and phenothiazine overdoses.

After satisfactory response is attained, the patient is kept under observation and naloxone doses repeated as necessary, since the duration of action of some narcotics (morphine, heroin, methadone) exceeds that of naloxone (1½ to 2 hours).

Physical dependence and withdrawal. In a patient physically dependent on opiates an abrupt and complete reversal of narcotic effects may precipitate an acute abstinence syndrome. Although the opiate abstinence syndrome may be reversible by opiate administration, the administration of narcotics to maintain an addict as a drug-dependent patient is prohibited by law except if the patient is an inpatient who was admitted for an emergency procedure or is being detoxified or maintained in an approved federal drug-treatment program. Methadone usually is considered the drug of choice in the treatment of this clinical condition.

Opiate physical dependence usually is described in terms of the opium derivative heroin, since the other derivatives manifest similar symptoms. Physical dependence on heroin is evident in the withdrawal syndrome that develops if the drug is withheld and in the marked tolerance that develops with continued use of the drug. Also, because persons dependent on heroin so frequently feel satiated, physical, emotional, and social deterioration often occur. The individuals may feel little need for food and become grossly malnourished and weak. Preoccupation with obtaining the drug makes participation in the usual social and vocational aspects of life difficult, if not impossible. While the drug craving grows, tolerance to the drug also increases, and eventually the motivation for using the drug becomes oriented more to the avoidance of withdrawal symptoms and less to the achievement of euphoria.

Common street names for heroin include bag, big H, big Harry, blanco, boy, caca, chip, crap, dirt, dogie, dope, H, Harry, heavy stuff, horse, junk, muzzle, pack, poison, salt, scag, shit, skid, smack, stuff, thing, TNT, and white junk.

Withdrawal symptoms. The initial withdrawal symptoms are related to the half-life of the narcotic being used. Symptoms of withdrawal from heroin are autonomic in origin and appear within 8 hours after the last dose in individuals who are physically dependent; these symptoms are less life threatening than with other substances of abuse. They may originally be manifested as restlessness, chills and hot flashes, piloerection on the skin (which gives rise to the term "cold turkey"), rhinorrhea, drowsiness, lacrimation, mydriasis, sneezing, yawning, generalized anxiety, abdominal cramps, lower back pain, lower extremity cramps (which probably resulted in the phrase "kick the habit"), vomiting and diarrhea, anorexia, diaphoresis, muscular twitching, elevated pulse, blood pressure, and temperature, and a craving for the drug. Such symptoms usually are followed by a restless sleep known as *yen* from which the patient may awaken irritable, weak, and depressed. Depending on the drug used, the abstinence syndrome develops within 2 to 48 hours and peaks at 72 hours.

Occasionally withdrawal symptoms are severe enough to result in cardiovascular collapse. If withdrawal is untreated, it may continue for up to 7 to 10 days, after which the physical dependence of the body on the presence of opiates is eventually lost. Psychic dependence continues for a longer period; some authorities claim it continues forever.

Treatment of opiate dependence

WITHDRAWAL PROGRAMS. Generally, opiate withdrawal is a difficult task, and repeated relapses to drug abuse can be expected. Abrupt and complete withdrawal *(cold turkey)* can be accomplished but is generally avoided as a dangerous and inhumane approach. Therapeutic withdrawal from an opiate may be somewhat more comfortably achieved by successively tapering the drug's dosage over a period of several days.

The choice of withdrawal program is partly influenced by the following factors: the patient's physical condition, the duration of drug dependence, the type of drug being taken and its daily dose, motivation for drug abuse, motivation for withdrawal, and whether the patient is also dependent on other drugs. In some instances, depending on these factors, opiate withdrawal may need to be accomplished within a hospital and with close medical supervision.

In identifying criteria for evaluating opiate withdrawal the Council on Mental Health emphasizes that recovery from dependence of the morphine type is not to be equated with cure. Regardless of repeated relapses to drug abuse, therapeutic programs should continue. Progress in withdrawal may be indicated by progressively longer periods of abstinence from opiates without resort to the use of other psychoactive drugs and by the patient's growing confidence in his or her ability to function effectively without drugs.

METHADONE TREATMENT AND MAINTENANCE. A currently preferred method of withdrawal is immediate withdrawal with concurrent substitution of methadone hydrochloride, a program pioneered by Drs. Vincent Dole and Marie Nyswander. Methadone hydrochloride is a synthetic opiate analgesic that, by virtue of cross-tolerance, permits effective substitution of methadone dependence for heroin dependence. Its effectiveness against heroin dependence results from its ability to forestall the euphoriant effects of heroin and the craving for the drug without producing heroin's deleterious physical and mental effects. When properly administered, methadone allows the individual to function adequately, without intellectual or emotional impairment. Methadone is taken orally, generally in daily doses of 15 to 20 mg and ranging up to 120 mg in a carrier of cherry syrup, orange juice, or the like. It is initiated usually in a 20-mg dose and titrated in 5- to 10-mg increments until there is symptom suppression. Detoxification may be made by decreasing the dosage by 5 mg/day (to 25 mg), and then decreasing it by 2.5 mg/day. Methadone therapy is initiated empirically based on patient symptoms, and as a general guide, 1 mg methadone may be used to substitute for 20 mg meperidine, 4 mg morphine, and 2 mg heroin.

Regular administration results in the development of tolerance to methadone and cross-tolerance to heroin. The opiate addict will not experience the opiate induced "rush" and euphoria unless higher doses than usual are used. When the addict is being treated with methadone, supportive psychologic or psychiatric counseling may relieve some of the burdens that motivate addiction. During this phase the methadone may be gradually withdrawn; however, this is controversial, since this program is not always successful. Previous opiate abusers who are unable to negotiate life in a drug-free state may revert to their former addiction or alternative substance abuse or may return to the methadone therapy detoxification.

In its eighteenth report the WHO Expert Committee on Drug Dependence defined methadone maintenance as follows: "Methadone maintenance is the continuing daily oral administration of methadone under adequate medical supervision, the dose being adjusted to (a) prevent the occurrence of abstinence phenomena (b) suppress partially or completely any continuous preoccupation with the taking of drugs of the morphine-type and (c) establish a sufficient degree of tolerance and cross tolerance to blunt or suppress the acute effects of such agents."* Because the procedure of injecting heroin *(fixing)* itself may be one factor in producing dependence, the oral administration of methadone discourages dependence on injections. Methadone also is available in tablet, dispersible tablet (for detoxification and maintenance only), and syrup form (Dolophine).

Methadone dependence does occur, but it is less serious than heroin dependence, and withdrawal symptoms are less severe but last for a longer period. Methadone withdrawal programs generally include supplemental rehabilitation techniques such as vocational and social rehabilitation. After the individual has functioned free from heroin for a sufficient period, secured steady employment, and readjusted his or her life-style, theoretically he or she can be withdrawn from methadone maintenance. Some treatment centers report having accom-

*Council on Mental Health: Narcotics and medical practice, J.A.M.A. **218**(4): 578, 1971.

plished withdrawal from methadone through the use of chlorpromazine, whereas others maintain that methadone may need to be taken indefinitely. Whether the latter can be avoided still is being researched.

Buprenorphine, a partial opiate agonist-antagonist, has proved useful in significantly suppressing the self-administration of heroin in control studies. The effects are dose dependent, and no withdrawal symptoms are reported after use of buprenorphine has been discontinued.

Clonidine (Catapres), a sympatholytic antihypertensive (central alpha adrenergic stimulator) drug approved for treatment of hypertension, is being investigated for relieving symptoms of acute withdrawal in addiction to opiates, such as heroin and methadone. Opiate withdrawal symptoms theoretically are thought to be a function of the hyperactivity of the locus ceruleus, a major noradrenergic nucleus of the brain. Inhibitory receptors in the locus ceruleus are thought to be stimulated by opiates through opiate reception and by stimulation with clonidine through the alpha-2 adrenergic receptors. The use of clonidine for this purpose is also a means of self-initiated treatment by an opiate abuser.

THERAPEUTIC COMMUNITY PROGRAMS. The ultimate goal of using any substance to treat addiction is to provide relief from the compulsive craving for the drug of abuse. To achieve rehabilitation, it has been found that the addict needs more than another substance to turn to. The addict also needs human dignity, sincerity, compassion, warmth, self-respect, and hope with positive reinforcement. To achieve independence and become a self-sustaining, productive member of the community, the addict must be provided with support, both emotionally and socially. These human resources have not been effectively addressed by many programs of methadone maintenance, and failures have resulted. However, there have been therapeutic community programs that have sprung up to help the addict. These programs include group psychotherapy, self-help approaches such as Phoenix House, and halfway houses. Because persons withdrawing from drugs frequently cannot make the transition easily, groups of persons who have decided to abstain from drug use can meet or live together in an attempt to support and guide one another through this transition. Ultimately an individual should emerge from such a program with sufficient personal growth and appropriate support systems so that he or she will be able to manage life satisfactorily without resorting to drug abuse.

NARCOTIC MAINTENANCE. In a number of countries, notably Great Britain, physicians have been permitted to prescribe opiates to persons who have a history of intractable dependence, thereby maintaining them and preventing withdrawal symptoms. Prescriptions currently are issued only through designated hospitals and only through the National Health Service. When such a system is implemented appropriately, it appears that the drug user can feel normal, function normally, and will seldom seek supplemental or illicit sources of drugs. There are, however, several reasons why such programs sometimes do not operate effectively and may be abused. Allowing patients to determine their own dose of the drug and supplying the drug in a form and quantity such that it can be easily resold or misused are examples of the ways in which such systems can be abused.

Nonnarcotic analgesics
Pentazocine (Talwin)

Sharp increases in the incidence of drug abuse and diversion involving pentazocine have led the Drug Enforcement Administration to place this drug in the controlled status (Class IV) under the Controlled Substances Act. Pentazocine is an analgesic for the relief of moderate to severe pain and is available in tablet and parenteral form. The recent rise in diversion, illicit marketing, and abuse of this drug may be reflections of the reductions in the quantity and quality of heroin available.

The shortages of heroin in large metropolitan areas have led to the use of pentazocine and tripelennamine, known as *T's and blues.* The *T* is for Talwin, and the *blue* is for the generic tablet color of tripelennamine. The use of this combination or pentazocine alone began to develop in 1969. In the past when heroin supply was low and prices were high, pentazocine was a viable choice. When tightened federal controls on pentazoncine placed it in the scheduled controlled substance classification, the price of pentazocine and tripelennamine had almost reached that of the heroin. T's and blues are tablets that are mixed together in solution and injected either through a cotton filter intravenously, like heroin or subcutaneously, techniques, possibly resulting in abscess and necrotic tissues (many users require hospitalization and grafting). Drug abusers have indicated that tripelennamine is used to increase the onset of action and prolong the duration of the euphoria produced by pentazocine.

Pentazocine is taken for the abuse-related motives of psychic effect and physical dependence. Pentazocine can cause psychotomimetic reactions such as visual hallucinations, feelings of depersonalization, and nightmares. This is a legitimate drug with illegitimate reasons for abuse, and the complex chemical synthesis deters illicit manufacturers. A dose of 20 mg injected intravenously produces analgesia after 15 to 45 minutes and has a duration of 1 hour.

The pattern of CNS effects is similar to that of the opiates, with analgesia, sedation, and respiratory depression. It may be lethal to combine it with other CNS depressants such as barbiturates and alcohol. Respiratory depression may be reversed by the opiate antagonist naloxone (not nalorphine). In high doses pentazocine causes an increase in blood pressure and heart rate. The repeated use of pentazocine may produce psychologic and/or physical dependence of the narcotic classification, which has been shown by a naloxone challenge in patients who have been administered pentazocine at the recommended medical dosage on a daily basis for several weeks.

Pentazocine's potential for producing psychologic and physical dependence is significant even in low doses, and infants born to pentazocine-dependent women experience withdrawal immediately postpartum.

Clinical effects of pentazocine abuse include death, lung problems caused by the talc binders and other particulate matter of crushed tablets accumulating in the lung, seizures, psychoto-

mimetic reactions (psychosis, hallucinations, delusions, etc.), and the ulceration and severe sclerosis of the skin and subcutaneous tissue and muscles, caused by subcutaneous or intramuscular injections of pentazocine. These ulcerated areas may measure 8 × 5 cm, and extensive cellulitis is observable. Such areas often require debridement and grafting.

The literature is replete with reports of dosages of 600 mg daily in 15 to 20 different administrations.

The treatment of pentazocine dependence is gradual reduction of the drug itself in a controlled environment. The psychotomimetic effects should be observed professionally and closely and may persist for 5 to 7 days.

Propoxyphene

The nurse should be acquainted with the warnings concerning use of propoxyphene products in excessive doses, either alone or in combination with other CNS depressants, including alcohol, which are a significant cause of drug-related deaths. Fatalities within the first hour of overdose are not uncommon. In a survey of deaths from overdosage conducted in 1975, in approximately 20% of the fatal cases death occurred within the first hour (5% occurred within 15 minutes). Propoxyphene should not be taken in doses higher than those recommended by the physician, and patients should be so warned. The judicious prescribing of propoxyphene is essential for safe use of this drug. With patients who are depressed or suicidal consideration should be given to the use of nonnarcotic analgesics.

Because of its added depressant effects, propoxyphene should be prescribed with caution for those patients whose medical condition requires the concomitant administration of sedatives, tranquilizers, muscle relaxants, antidepressants, or other CNS depressant drugs. Patients should be cautioned against the concomitant use of propoxyphene products and alcohol because of potentially serious CNS additive effects of these agents. Many of the propoxyphene-related deaths have occurred in patients with previous histories of emotional disturbances or suicidal ideation or attempts as well as histories of misuse of tranquilizers, alcohol, and other CNS active drugs. Some deaths have occurred as a consequence of the accidental ingestion of excessive quantities of propoxyphene alone or in combination with other drugs.

The clinical effects of overdose are an onset of symptoms within ½ hour and symptoms of coma and stupor (preceded by nausea, vomiting, and drowsiness). Within ½ to 1 hour of an oral overdose respiratory arrest, hypotension, and grand mal seizures are often seen. Miotic pupils are frequently seen in addition to diabetes insipidus, pulmonary edema, cardiac arrythmias (needing cardiopulmonary resuscitation measures) and bundle branch block, nonspecific ST and T wave alterations and prolongation of the QRS complexes, and hypoglycemia.

There is a high incidence of toxic psychosis, convulsions, and coma. The peak plasma level is 2 to 25 hours after a therapeutic dose, with a therapeutic half-life of 6 to 12 hours; however, the norpropoxyphene attains peak plasma concentration in 4 hours, and the half-life of the active metabolite is 30 to 36 hours.

The drug also may be abused by parenteral administration of the oral form. The tablet or capsule is dissolved in ethyl alcohol (vodka), placed in a syringe with a cotton filter or cigarette filter, and injected intravenously.

The severe and sometimes unpredictable course of propoxyphene intoxication has stimulated an interest in its clinical kinetics. It is primarily metabolized in the hepatic microsomal enzyme system through the major metabolic pathway of demethylation to norpropoxyphene and is primarily eliminated by renal excretion. The most severely intoxicated patients with the highest plasma levels also had metabolites with the longest half-life, which may indicate dose-dependent kinetics. Total urinary excretion of all metabolites is about 7 days. The systemic availability was reduced corresponding to extensive first pass metabolism of 30% to 70%, and the half-life was 8 to 24 hours for propoxyphene and 18 to 29 hours for the metabolite norpropoxyphene. The ranges indicate pronounced intraindividual dose-independent variations in oral clearance, and transient changes in hepatic blood flow at the time the drug passes through the liver may influence kinetics of high-clearance drugs such as propoxyphene. This is further influenced by a high-affinity binding site in some tissues, and this binding kinetics is also seen with tricyclic antidepressants.

Norpropoxyphene has less CNS depressant effect than propoxyphene but a greater local anesthetic effect, similar to that of amitriptyline and antiarrhythmic drugs (lidocaine and quinidine). Electrocardiographic monitoring is essential in management of overdosage.

Propoxyphene is pharmacologically related to the opiates; however, it may not elicit the narcotic response when naloxone is administered, and the patient will need more protracted respiratory support measures. The overdose may be accompanied by seizures (requiring anticonvulsants), and emergence from a coma may require restraints before administration of the naloxone antagonist because of the disorientation, agitation, and confusion encountered.

The FDA Drug Bulletin has carried the warning that propoxyphene should not be taken during pregnancy. The warning against use during pregnancy is based on demonstrations of withdrawal symptoms in newborn infants from mothers taking the drug during pregnancy. The symptoms include tremors, irritability, high-pitched cry, diarrhea and weight loss with ravenous appetite, and, infrequently, seizures.

Some street names for this drug are dummies, red and grays, and darvos.

Sedative-hypnotics
Barbiturates

Although it is not generally known by the lay public, the barbiturates and some nonbarbiturate sedative-hypnotics can cause physical as well as psychic dependence. It appears that short-acting barbiturates, in addition to drugs like glutethimide (Doriden), methaqualone, chloral hydrate, methyprylon (Noludar), and ethchlorvynol (Placidyl) are most likely to produce physical dependence, possibly because they produce sudden and forceful desired effects (rapid onset of action), which offer no

TABLE 12-4 Therapeutic and toxic reference values for some sedative-hypnotics

Substance of abuse	Levels	
	Therapeutic	Toxic
Barbiturates		
Short acting (blood, serum, plasma)	1 to 5 μg/ml	>5 μg/ml
Intermediate acting (blood, serum, plasma)	5 to 14 μg/ml	>30 μg/ml
Long acting (blood, serum, plasma)	15 to 35 μg/ml	>40 μg/ml
Amobarbital (blood)	5 to 8 μg/ml	>30 μg/ml
Secobarbital (blood)	3 to 5 μg/ml	>5 μg/ml
Pentobarbital (blood)	1 to 4 μg/ml	>5 μg/ml
Nonbarbiturates		
Methaqualone (blood)	0.9 to 8 μg/ml	>5 μg/ml
Methyprylon (blood)	<10 μg/ml	>30 μg/ml
Chloral hydrate (trichloriethanol—TCE—and trichloroacetic acid)	2 to 6 μg/ml (urine), 2 to 3 hours after ingestion 0.8 to 1.2 mg TCE/100 ml blood, 30 to 60 minutes after 1 g chloral hydrate	
Ethchlorvynol (blood)	0.5 to 6.5 μg/ml	>20 μg/ml
Glutethimide (blood, serum)	2 to 6 μg/ml	>10 μg/ml

delay to the abuser's gratification. The lipid solubility enables the drug to rapidly enter the central nervous system, with immediate appearance of effects.

Because these drugs are more extensively described in previous chapters, mechanisms of action and effects are not explored. Rather, this section focuses on acute intoxication and withdrawal syndromes resulting from dependence on these drugs. Table 12-4 presents the therapeutic and toxic serum reference values for some of these agents.

Both the acute and the chronic effects of barbiturate intoxication resemble those of alcohol intoxication. Manifestations may include emotional lability, muscular incoordination, difficulty in cognitive processes, and sedation. Toxic doses lead to stupor and respiratory depression. The reasons for barbiturate abuse are similar to those for ethyl alcohol abuse: both drugs produce disinhibition and mild euphoria.

The withdrawal syndrome accompanying cessation of barbiturate and previously identified nonbarbiturate hypnotic administration has been termed one of the most dangerous in the field of drug abuse. It may begin with weakness, tremulousness, restlessness, anxiety, insomnia, gastrointestinal disturbances, and orthostatic hypotension that may last 3 to 14 days but starts in the first 24 hours, possibly leaving the patient too weak to get out of bed. Symptoms of psychoses may progress to confusion, delirium, and hallucinations. In addition, major convulsive seizures are more common in barbiturate withdrawal than in alcohol withdrawal. Agitation and hyperthermia may lead to exhaustion, cardiovascular collapse, and death.

Coma and apnea from single high doses of mixed depressants may lead to high morbidity and mortality. If the withdrawal syndrome is untreated, it generally ends by the fourteenth day of drug abstinence, and its end generally is preceded by prolonged sleep. It is recommended that patients experiencing barbiturate withdrawal be hospitalized because even when, 24 hours after the last dose, the syndrome appears mild, it may herald impending convulsions and cardiovascular collapse, which may appear on the second or third day and last up to 2 weeks.

Treatment of barbiturate withdrawal generally consists of substitution of the drug with a longer-acting barbiturate such as phenobarbital, the dosage of which is then slowly tapered over a period of several weeks until it is completely withdrawn.

Some investigators prefer pentobarbital to phenobarbital as a withdrawal agent, and there is some controversy concerning the dose equivalents. Some clinicians use 30 mg phenobarbital for 100 mg pentobarbital, and others use a milligram per milligram equivalency. Phenobarbital intoxication may produce disinhibition and euphoria and may result in fewer patient management problems than with pentobarbital. Phenobarbital permits safer withdrawal with fewer blood level fluctuations and less risk of overdose fatality in the sedative-hypnotic–dependent patient.

Some abusers inject the tablet or capsule oral forms of the barbiturates and sedative-hypnotics intravenously, which could result in serum hepatitis, septicemia, pulmonary emboli, papilloma, bacterial endocarditis, abscesses, tetanus, and various skin rashes. Because of the highly alkaline sclerosing of veins, phlebitis and extravascular abscesses occur with intravenous injection abuse of barbiturates. The intoxication from barbiturates must be differentiated from other intoxication causes. The patient's breath odor is a factor with alcohol, inhalants, and chloral hydrate but not with the barbiturates. Specific and efficient antidotes to offset barbiturate/depressant drug overdoses are not available as with the naloxone for opiate overdose patients. Patients dependent on the sedative-hypnotics should never be abruptly withdrawn but should use the phenobarbital reduction regimen.

Long-acting barbiturates (phenobarbital, mephobarbital, metharbital, primidone [15% converted to phenobarbital]) are not generally the substances of abuse. Doses over 8 mg/kg have produced some toxic manifestations depending on the patient's exposure or addiction to the drug. Because of enzyme induction, long-term barbiturate use increases the metabolism of the barbiturate. Hepatic enzymes degrading barbiturates increase rapidly, metabolize the barbiturates, and reduce the barbiturate effect. Addicts have been known to abuse 1 barbiturate daily. Doses in therapeutic ranges may achieve levels as high as 5 mg/100 ml; however, patients on long-term therapy or those who abuse the drug have sustained levels of 10 to 25 mg/100 ml without clinical symptoms. Generally, a patient having a level of over 8 mg/100 ml in an acute overdosage may enter a comatose state.

Some clinical effects observed in the acute overdosage situation are depression, coma, hypotension, hypoxia, hypothermia, depressed kidney function caused by cardiovascular depression, respiratory or cardiac arrest, and aspiration pneumonia. Addiction has been observed in chronic ingestion of 300 to 700 mg daily for about 2 months. Withdrawal (lasting up to 14 days) presents as tremors, anorexia, insomnia, nausea, vomiting, muscular weakness, and hypotension. Convulsions (clonic-tonic, isolated, or status epilepticus) may ensue 16 to 24 hours after the last dose of the drug. The nurse should be aware that withdrawal may be seen in neonates of mothers who are abusing the drug and may be delayed up to 2 weeks or seen soon after delivery. Hyperirritability and seizures may be seen for several months following neonatal withdrawal. Treatment of the adult patient with phenobarbital poisoning should include forced alkaline diuresis. Withdrawal may be treated with phenobarbital by a gradual reduction regimen over a 3-week period.

Short-acting barbiturates possess clinical effects similar to those of the longer acting derivatives. Unlike with longer acting barbiturates, forced diuresis is of no value here. Hemodialysis is ineffective also; however, this may be used in patients with severe acid base or fluid and electrolyte problems even though the drug is not dialyzable. The seizure from barbiturate withdrawal may be treated with diazepam in the intravenous route. (See Chapter 8.) Withdrawal after the last dose may be treated with phenobarbital in a dosage of 30 mg for each 100 mg short-acting barbiturate used, administered every 6 hours daily for a gradual decrease. If withdrawal symptoms continue, the dosage should be increased until the patient is comfortable; then once stabilized, the patient is gradually withdrawn over a period of 3 weeks. Neonatal withdrawal occurs just as with the long-acting barbiturates. Fatalities from the synergistic combination of alcohol and barbiturates are well documented.

Nonbarbiturates

Ethchlorvynol (Placidyl)

Prolonged use of ethchlorvynol may result in tolerance, physical dependence, and psychologic dependence. Intoxication has been observed in patients taking 1-g dosages over prolonged periods (4 to 5 months). Some signs and symptoms of chronic intoxication are incoordination, tremors, ataxia, confusion, slurred speech, hyperreflexia, diplopia, and generalized muscle weakness. Some reversible symptoms seen are toxic amblyopia, nystagmus, and peripheral neuropathy. The liquid within the capsule form may be used by the intravenous route, which can result in pulmonary edema. Severe withdrawal symptoms, similar to barbiturate and alcohol withdrawal, have been seen as late as 9 days following abrupt cessation after prolonged use of this drug. Signs and symptoms of ethchlorvynol withdrawal are convulsions, delirium, schizoid reactions, perceptual distortions, retrograde amnesia, ataxia, insomnia, slurred speech, anxiety, irritability, agitation, tremors, anorexia, dizziness, nausea, vomiting, weakness, sweating, muscle twitching, and weight loss. Coma has been reported to last 12 days before recovery; a flat electroencephalogram during coma should not initiate cessation of supportive care. Hypotension responds to fluids and vasopressor agents, and hypothermia often is seen in the overdose patient. The respiratory depression necessitates artificial ventilation. Close nursing monitoring should include observations for bradycardia, pulmonary edema, peripheral neuropathy, cardiac arrest, and respiratory arrest. The half-life in an overdose may be over four times

that of the therapeutic half-life (25 hours). Just as with barbiturates, neonatal withdrawal has been observed. The nurse should be alert for mixed ingestion, as in other cases of substance abuse. Alcohol may be ingested with this drug, resulting in lower levels of ethchlorvynol leading to a coma.

The patient who manifests withdrawal symptoms is either reinstituted with ethchlorvynol or phenobarbital (30 mg phenobarbital for each 350 mg ethchlorvynol abused) and tapered gradually over a period of a day or weeks. The addition of a phenothiazine may be necessary for the patient exhibiting psychotic withdrawal symptoms. Hospitalization in the withdrawal stage is absolutely necessary. There is a narrow margin between the toxic and therapeutic dose ranges for this drug, and habituation is produced with lower doses. The overdose symptoms usually disappear in 1 to 2 weeks. The nurse should remember that since ethchlorvynol is very lipid soluble, 9 days may elapse after the last dose before the appearance of withdrawal symptoms. Since this is a tertiary alcohol, a characteristic pungent odor of the breath is frequently seen.

Some street names of ethchlorvynol are dyls, plastic red, K-H, and K-N.

Glutethimide (Doriden)

Glutethimide is widely abused. Signs and symptoms of chronic intoxication include impairment of memory and ability to concentrate, impaired gait, ataxia, tremors, hyporeflexia, and slurring of speech. Withdrawal reactions are seen after abrupt cessation of the drug when the patient has been on prolonged usage; reactions range from nervousness and anxiety to grand mal seizures, including abdominal cramps, chills, numbness of extremities, and dysphagia.

Acute overdosage is a life-threatening situation. The nurse should be alert for mixed drug ingestion (such as hypnotics, sedatives, alcohol, and illicit drugs) and suicide attempts. Signs and symptoms of acute intoxication vary in severity with the ingested dose and are difficult to distinguish from barbiturate intoxication. Mild intoxication produces drowsiness and lethargy, and moderate to severe intoxication produces different degrees of coma, which may last as long as 4 or more days. Glutethimide produces significant anticholinergic effects, which are seen in the adynamic ileus (diminished or absent peristalsis), urinary retention (atonic urinary bladder), dryness of the mouth, mydriasis, irritability, and convulsions. These are all potentiated by a mixed drug ingestion involving, among other substances, alcohol. There is also depressed or absent response to painful stimuli, hypotension, inadequate ventilation, sometimes with cyanosis, and sudden apnea (often with manipulation such as gastric lavage or endotracheal intubation). Cyclic coma (coma to wakefulness), a distinguishing feature from barbiturate overdosage, occurs because of the continued absorption of the glutethimide from the gastrointestinal tract. This may be interrupted by increasing the gastrointestinal tract emptying time with a cathartic and charcoal to adsorb and lavage or emesis. Prolonged coma may be caused by the accumulation in brain and plasma of the toxic active liver metabolite 4HG (4 hydroxy-2 ethyl-2-phenylglutarimide). As previously stated, the anticholinergic effects (cholinergic blockade) of glutethimide lower the motility of the gastrointestinal tract until the drug is metabolized, after which motility is resumed; following this, more glutethimide is absorbed, and the coma begins again. This circular pattern justifies the use of emesis, cathartics, and adsorbents. This anticholinergic effect and cyclic coma necessitate a period of observation to determine the toxicity of the ingestion. Death has been the outcome of ingestion of 5 g (10 tablets of 500 mg), and survival has been reported with 35 g. The lethal dose, then, is in a range of 10 to 20 g, and the mortality with the 10-g dose is reported to be 45%. Mild intoxication produces blood levels of 0.5 to 5.5 mg/100 ml, and severe intoxication is in a range of 1.8 to 12 mg/100 ml. A plasma level of 3 mg/100 ml is seen in severe poisoning. The half-life in acute massive overdose is unknown but is less than 7 hours after a 500-mg dose with a range of 6 to 45 g. Some street names that have been associated with this drug are cibas, D's, gluts, 354s, and USV's.

A phenobarbital equivalent dose of 30 mg is recommended for each 250 mg glutethimide

abused in cases of withdrawal. Overdose is a potential problem, since there is a narrow therapeutic-lethal range and the presence of active metabolites. Glutethimide remains in the gastrointestinal tract longer than the barbiturates, since absorption stops when a certain blood level is reached. As this level drops, gastric reabsorption occurs, leading to coma after the patient shows signs of recovery.

Methaqualone (Mequin, Parest, Quaalude, Sopor)

Illicit use of methaqualone for nontherapeutic ends can produce severe psychologic or physical dependence. Acute overdose may result in delirium and coma, with restlessness, irritability, and hypertonia, progressing to convulsions. Spontaneous vomiting and increased secretions are frequently seen and may lead to aspiration pneumonitis or respiratory obstruction. Large overdosages may result in edema (cutaneous and pulmonary), hepatic damage, renal insufficiency, bleeding, shock, and respiratory arrest. Coma has been reported with doses of 2.4 g and death with a dose of 8 g; patients have survived doses of 22 g. The nurses should be alert for multiple drug ingestion, and the concomitant abuse of alcohol may worsen the patient's prognosis. Hyperexcitability and hyperreflexia are seen frequently in addition to myoclonic jerking, tetany, and tachycardia. Myocardial damage may result from use of this drug. Addiction withdrawal symptoms are similar to those of barbiturates, and there may be hallucinations, jitteriness, irritability, agitation, depression, and gastrointestinal problems (abdominal pain) within 16 to 24 hours, with 20% to 40% of patients experiencing convulsions. The drug is rapidly absorbed from the gastrointestinal tract, so the use of emesis or lavage is necessary in addition to carthartics and charcoal. Convulsions may be controlled with intravenous diazepam. Pulmonary edema contraindicates the use of forced diuresis. Hemodialysis is reserved for the patient who is severely intoxicated with levels over 11 mg/100 ml. Withdrawal is initiated either with methaqualone or phenobarbital (30 mg phenobarbital for each 250 to 300 mg methaqualone abused). Methaqualone is used in decreasing dosages, and phenobarbital is usually initiated with 100 mg every 6 hours in the adult, titrated to patient comfort when symptoms of withdrawal subside for 1 or 2 days, and then gradually reduced. Continued absorption of the drug remaining in the gastrointestinal tract produces erratic peak plasma levels. Further, in abuse circumstances the continued exposure may be accounted for by differential metabolisms. It is estimated that levels exceeding 2.5 mg/100 ml are intoxicating in most patients.

Abusers describe the state as sensual, euphoric, and similar to opiate experiences. The convulsions produced with this drug make it more of a threat than overdose with other sedative-hypnotics that have dependence potential.

There is diversion of this drug from outside the borders of the United States, and it is suspected of being manufactured in clandestine laboratories in the United States either alone or in combination with other substances (such as benzodiazepines, PCP, and antihistamines). These tablets are manufactured to be identical in appearance to the legitimate drug tablet form.

Some street names used to describe this drug are 714s, ludes, sopors, west coast, lemmons, Mandrax, Parest, and Q's.

Methyprylon (Noludar)

Symptoms reported in methyprylon intoxication are coma (lasting up to 30 hours), hypotension, respiratory depression, tachycardia, hypothermia, hyperthermia, and paradoxic excitability. The most dangerous complication is the hypotension. Methyprylon can cause dependence similar to that of barbiturates and alcohol in high doses over extended periods. The symptoms of withdrawal are restlessness, auditory and visual hallucinations, diaphoresis, polyuria, excitement, confusion, and convulsions on the abrupt cessation of the drug. Methyprylon is water and lipid soluble, and 60% of the dose is excreted as a metabolite in the urine with a therapeutic half-life of up to 6 hours. Toxic blood levels are 3 to 5 mg/100 ml, and 10 mg/100 ml is potentially lethal, whereas therapeutic blood levels are less than 10 μg/ml (1 mg/100 ml).

Some symptoms of overdosage are somnolence, confusion, and constricted pupils in addition to the aforementioned coma, respiratory depression, and hypotension. The nurse should be alert for mixed substance ingestion in the overdosage situation. Some street names given to the drug are Roche 300s, nols, and purple and whites.

The dose of phenobarbital used in the withdrawal of this drug is 30 mg, equivalent to 300 mg methyprylon.

Ethyl alcohol

Ethyl alcohol is one of the most abused drugs in the world and, contrary to popular opinion, is not a stimulant. Rather, it is a primary and continuous depressant of the central nervous system. Alcohol is the most widely abused psychoactive substance of the sedative/depressant class, and that, being highly addictive, it produces the four characteristics of drug dependence: psychologic and physiologic dependence, tolerance, and the characteristic abstinence (withdrawal) syndrome.

Representatives of alcohol (ethanol) that are abused are wines, beer, whiskeys and other distillates, and drugs or foods with ethanol as the vehicle. By volume of alcohol beer has 3% to 6%, table wine has 8% to 14%, dessert wine has 15% to 20%, and distilled spirits have 40% to 50%. The *proof* of alcohol is double the ethanol concentration in volume percent (for example, 50 proof = 25% ethanol).

Alcoholics may misuse or abuse all drugs in the same manner as alcohol. They may increase the dosage regimen and refill prescription medication without the physician's knowledge or approval. The chronic alcoholic induces an enzyme system, the microsomal ethanol oxidizing system, which is associated with a nonspecific enhancement of a wide variety of microsomal enzymes, leading to metabolic alterations of prescribed drug regimens (sedative-hypnotics, tranquilizers, etc.). Half-lives are shortened in the absence of alcohol and are prolonged when the same medication is taken in combination with alcohol. Close nursing supervision of the alcoholic person should be maintained when other psychoactive medications

T A B L E 1 2 - 5 Effects of alcohol after ingestion in the nonhabituated individual*

Fluidounces of 90 proof whiskey (45% alcohol)	Blood level (mg/100 ml)	Effects
3	30 to 50	State of relaxation and sense of well-being, increased talkativeness, reduced reflexes, impaired driving skills
6	100	Slightly slurred speech, movement incoordination, impairment of judgment, reduced inhibitions, less emotional control, six-fold increase in driving fatalities and accidents
9	200	Gross intoxication with markedly impaired gait, gross effects on thinking and memory, distorted judgment, emotional lability, depression
18	300 to 700	Possible coma and death from respiratory depression

*One milliliter per kilogram of absolute (100%) ethanol results in blood levels of 100 mg/100 ml 2 hours after ingestion.

such as tranquilizers, sedatives, or hypnotics are used.

The classic manifestations of alcoholism—red face, bloodshot eyes, unsteady hands, enlarged liver, and malnutrition—are the last signs to look for in alcoholic individual. Many psychologic and physical manifestations of alcoholism provide evidence for early detection. Some of the more commonly observed early indications of alcohol abuse are the following:

Physical guides

Cardiovascular: tachycardia
Gastrointestinal: vague abdominal complaints, diarrhea, dysphagia, nausea, vomiting (prior to breakfast)
Neurologic: blackouts, headaches, insomnia
Traumatic: frequent accidents, cigarette burns on hands and chest, falls or injuries of vague origin
Laboratory guides: anemia, blood alcohol of 0.15%, hyperlipemia, abnormal kidney and/or liver function

Psychologic guides

Behavioral: excessive absenteeism, financial problems, improper use of drugs, marital disharmony, marital instability, poor performance on the job
Emotional: anxiety, depression, hallucinations, panic attacks, suicidal tendencies or expressions

With prolonged alcohol drinking sprees there is an accumulation of congeners (such as methanol, ethyl acetate, higher straight and branched chain alcohols, and fusil oil derivatives), which may contribute to the toxicity and hangover. Charcoal filtering in the bottling process reduces many of these congeners. The alcohol is efficiently and rapidly absorbed from the large mucosal surface, which aids diffusion in the small intestine. Food and high concentrations of consumed alcohol delay absorption from the stomach.

Mode of administration and pharmacodynamics. Ethyl alcohol is ingested orally and is well absorbed from the stomach and intestines. Peak blood levels are achieved 30 minutes to 3 hours after ingestion. Distribution to all tissues, including the brain, is rapid. The drug is metabolized in the liver to acetaldehyde by alcohol dehydrogenase at the rate of 10 to 20 ml/hour. Ninety percent is metabolized; 5% is excreted through the lungs and 5% through the kidneys. A physiologic role of microsomal ethanol oxidizing system has been described.

Mechanism of action. Ethyl alcohol acts by depressing the reticular activating system, which is thought to be largely responsible for integration of central nervous system activity.

Effects. The drug can foster a pseudostimulant effect that is a consequence of hyperactivity of various parts of the brain which have been suddenly released from the inhibitory control of the cortex. Some of the first mental processes affected are those that depend on this control. Further effects of alcohol on the central nervous system are proportionately related to blood concentrations of alcohol in the nonhabituated individual (Table 12-5). Memory, concentration, and finer discrimination abilities are successively lost with higher drug concentrations. Emotional lability may result, with sensory-motor disturbances following. Incoordination may be accompanied by slurred speech and followed by stupor as the drug continues to cause irregular descending depression of the central nervous system. Large doses of alcohol will produce anesthesia, which may be followed by medullary paralysis. Alcohol has also been implicated as a causative factor in cardiac arrhythmias and cardiomyopathies. These conditions may result from individual sensitization.

Physiologically, ethyl alcohol causes diuresis because of depressed secretion of antidiuretic hormone and vasodilation as a result of depression of the vasomotor center.

Repeated and prolonged use of large doses of ethyl alcohol results in the development of marked tolerance and physical and psychic dependence. Malnutrition may result, because although alcohol contains calories, it contains no vitamins. Cirrhosis of the liver, gastritis, peripheral polyneuropathy, portal hypertension, and lowered resistance to disease are also common adverse effects of dependence on ethyl alcohol.

Another significant and potentially adverse effect of alcohol lies in the fact that it potentiates the actions of many drugs and may, therefore, be instrumental in many drug fatalities.

Acute intoxication. If alcohol has been ingested in large quantities and within the past hour, emesis is indicated in a noncomatose and conscious patient. If a mixed drug ingestion is suspected, then gastric lavage is useful. An intravenous injection of 5% or 10% or dextrose in water may be started, and if blood glucose is below 60 mg/100 ml, then 50% intravenous glucose is necessary. If there are seizures induced by the ethanol withdrawal, the use of phenytoin may provide protection. Thiamine is used to treat possible Wernicke's encephalopathy.

Withdrawal symptoms. The intensity of the ethyl alcohol withdrawal syndrome depends on the duration of dependence on the drug and the degree of intoxication. Generally, within a few hours after the last dose of alcohol the physically dependent person begins to experience weakness, tremulousness, anxiety, gastrointestinal disturbances, and hyperreflexia. Within 24 hours acute alcoholic hallucinosis results, fol-

lowed by disorientation, confusion, and delusional thinking. Convulsive seizures may occur, and death from cardiovascular collapse is possible at the height of the withdrawal syndrome. If the person lives, recovery from the syndrome is complete by the fifth to seventh day of abstinence.

Treatment of the abrupt withdrawal syndrome may include the administration of longer acting depressant drugs, such as chlordiazepoxide, diazepam, clorazepate dipotassium mesoridazine, or paraldehyde, if the patient is seen in early stages of delirium tremens when withdrawal is severe. Once the withdrawal symptoms are controlled, the drug dosage can be safely and progressively reduced at a rate that prevents the development of further symptoms.

Long-term treatment of alcohol dependence includes methods similar to treatment of dependence of the opiate type, such as halfway houses, therapeutic organizations like Alcoholics Anonymous, patient/family clinics, counseling, and reinforcements for sobriety.

Aversion therapy is also used in treatment of alcohol dependence and involves the administration of drugs to prevent complete metabolism of alcohol, thereby causing unpleasant physical symptoms. Drugs such as emetine, apomorphine, and disulfiram (Antabuse) have been used as adjuncts in the treatment of chronic alcoholism. If ethyl alcohol is administered after treatment with disulfiram, the *aldehyde syndrome* (disulfiram reaction) is produced, with resulting body vasodilation, hypotension, pulsating headache, nausea, vomiting, diaphoresis, thirst, chest pain, vertigo, weakness, and blurred vision. If the patient wishes to avoid the experience of this syndrome, he or she must not ingest alcohol for at least 2 to 3 weeks after taking disulfiram. A blood alcohol level of 5 to 10 mg/100 ml may cause this reaction, but the full disulfiram reaction is seen with 50 mg/100 ml blood alcohol level.

The nurse should be aware of drugs other than disulfiram that produce similar ethanol reaction. This syndrome is also seen with two oral hypoglycemics, chlorpropamide (Diabinese) and tolbutamide (Orinase), which are aldehyde dehydrogenase inhibitors, and metronidazole (Flagyl), which is an alcohol dehydrogenase inhibitor.

Alcohol and pregnancy. Excessive use of alcoholic beverages by women during pregnancy may result in a pattern of congenital abnormalities labeled the fetal alcohol syndrome, characterized by prenatal onset and postnatal developmental and performance deficiencies. The syndrome consists of behavioral, craniofacial, limb, and neurologic anomalies and in about half the cases cardiac septal defects, genital abnormalities, and hemangiomas. Primary anomalies of the head and face include microcephaly, short fissures of the eyelids, midfacial defects, and a flattened, elongated vertical groove in the upper lip; those of the hands include abnormal palmar creases and joined deviated or permanently flexed fingers and toes. The IQ scores of those affected individuals who have been tested averaged 35 to 40 points below the normal scores. These observations demonstrate that ethanol is a potent teratogen, increasing also the incidence of stillbirths, resorptions, and spontaneous abortions. These risks and the extent of the abnormalities are a function of doses, since both have an incidence of increase in correlation with maternal ethanol consumption. The nurse must reinforce the concept of alcohol abstinence for patients with chronic and severe drinking problems and discourage pregnancy for patients who present with ethanol abuse until the problem is controlled and medically supervised.

When the pregnant patient is presented for care, the nurse should counsel her in definitive terms to refrain from any spree or binge drinking of ethanol. The nurse should inform the patient that high blood levels of ethanol may produce malformations during the first trimester and retard growth during the third trimester. About one third of the infants born to heavy drinkers demonstrated congenital anomalies, compared with about 10% in abstinent women and about 15% in moderate drinkers, and microcephaly was observed frequently.

Alcohol during pregnancy is the unequivocal factor when the full pattern of fetal alcohol syndrome is present. When all the characteristics are not present, the correlation between ethanol use and its adverse effects is more intricate in factors such as nutrition, smoking, caffeine, and other drugs and environmental agents.

The pregnant patient should be particularly aware of the ethanol impact on the fetus, since totally safe ethanol consumption levels are unknown. The risk is pronounced with six drinks daily that contain the equivalent of 3 fluidounces of absolute alcohol. The nurse should caution the patient that the peak blood alcohol concentration is the most critical factor of teratogenesis and that the patient must not exceed two alcoholic beverages daily. Further, the nurse should inform all women patients who have ethanol drinking habits of the risks involved if they are of childbearing age.

Tranquilizers (antianxiety and antipsychotic agents)

The fact that the use of tranquilizers can lead to psychic dependence is well known. Less well known is the fact that the use of these drugs may also produce physical dependence similar to dependence of the barbiturate type.

Phenothiazine-type tranquilizers, although not known to produce physical dependence, will result in anxiety, insomnia, and gastrointestinal disturbances if abruptly withdrawn. Drugs such as meprobamate, diazepam, and chlordiazepoxide may produce withdrawal symptoms such as hallucinations, confusion, and seizures; it is recommended to slowly withdraw the patient over several months to avoid these effects.

If the daily ingested dose of a benzodiazepine is subjected to nonmedical abuse over months as, for example, with 80 to 120 mg diazepam or 300 to 600 mg chlordiazepoxide, then withdrawal may occur. Initial management should include the use of the phenobarbital equivalent of 30 mg (equivalent to 5 mg diazepam and 25 mg chlordiazepoxide), or tapering the benzodiazepine by 10% daily for 10 to 14 days or more until the patient is comfortable.

Benzodiazepines are similar to the barbiturate-hypnotics in most actions but have relaxant qualities on skeletal muscles, are more selective in the relief of anxiety, are less sedative or hypnotic, and produce less incoordination and judgment impairment. Ingestion of only 500 to 1500 mg benzodiazepine have been reported with minor toxicity. The symptoms of the patient with benzodiazepine overdosage may be merely sleepiness and minor extrapyramidal signs with some excitement. Because of the high probability of a mixed ingestion, possible deep coma, marked hypotension, and respiratory depression should be watched for. The anticholinergic effects may be dry mouth, tachycardia, dilated pupils, and absent bowel sounds. It is important to recall that abrupt cessation of a benzodiazepine may result in withdrawal symptoms when the drug was taken for several months or years on a daily basis; hallucinations, confusion, and seizures often are reported. This may be overcome when the drug is gradually withdrawn, since there is a long half-life.

Phenothiazine overdosage most often produces a stiff neck, ataxia, protruding tongue, reduced activity and attentiveness, and psychomotor slowing; an initial period of agitation, hyperactivity, and seizures may precede emotional quieting stages. The disturbance of the temperature-regulating processes by phenothiazines creates hyperthermia or hypothermia. The alpha blocking and anticholinergic effects of phenothiazines frequently produce tachycardia, lethargy, and somnolence. The quinidine-like effect of the phenothiazines may produce a widening of the QRS complexes and ventricular tachycardia. The nurse should remember not to administer other sedatives, barbiturates, narcotics, or anesthetics, since these depressive drugs are potentiated by the phenothiazines and may create respiratory depression and increased CNS effects.

CNS sympathomimetics
Amphetamines

Persons who are amphetamine abusers may begin the cycle of abuse inadvertently. Amphetamine dependence may begin as infrequent use of the drug to stay awake (such as by students studying for examinations, night-shift work-

ers, double-shift workers, or overambitious, achievement-oriented persons) or use of the drug for appetite control. Although the use of amphetamines often begins for legitimate purposes and with legitimate prescriptions it seems that its exhilarating effects become so attractive that there are high rates of dependence.

Weight reduction currently accounts for 80% to 90% of amphetamine prescriptions, which totaled 3.3 million in 1978. The federal government currently is contemplating banning the use of amphetamines for exogenous obesity because of their wide-spread abuse. This would leave the treatment of narcolepsy and minimal brain dysfunction in children among the limited approved claims for the use of amphetamines, and some states already have enacted laws to only permit a prescription written for amphetamines for indications of narcolepsy, hyperkinesis in children, and possibly neurotic fatigue. Alternative drugs are available for obesity management (benzphetamine, chlorphentermine, clortermine, diethylpropion, fenfluramine, mazindol, phenmetrazine, and phentermine).

Some common amphetamine street names are A's, AMT's, bombitas (when with cocaine), bennies, black beauties (Biphetamine), black birds, copilots, crossroads, DES (methamphetamine [Desoxyn]), diet pills, footballs (SKF capsule), goofballs (when with barbiturates), grads (Abbott sustained action tablet), hearts (from the tablet shape of orange dextroamphetamines and purple amphetamines), jolly beans, pep pills, reducing pills, speed, truck drivers, uppers, and white crosses.

Preparations. Chemically, there are three types of amphetamines: salts of racemic amphetamines, dextroamphetamines, and methamphetamines, all of which vary in degree of potency and peripheral effects. Dextroamphetamine is said to have fewest peripheral effects, such as hypertension and tachycardia.

Other agents that have been called *psychotomimetic amphetamines* include 3,4-methylene-dioxyamphetamine (MDA), dimethyltryptamine (DMT), dimethoxy methylamphetamine (DOM), and diethyltryptamine (DET). These drugs seem to span the gap between amphetamines and LSD in producing their effects. DMT and DET produce short (1 to 2 hours) psychotomimetic reactions that are characterized by more pronounced autonomic nervous system effects than those produced by LSD. DOM (also called STP for Timothy Leary's slogan "serenity, tranquility, and peace" and for the brand name of a motor oil additive that promises added power) appears to produce longer psychotomimetic reactions (16 to 72 hours) with much more intense physiologic effects than the other two drugs.

Mechanism of action. The amphetamines are synthetic indirect sympathomimetic amines that are chemically and pharmacologically related to epinephrine and norepinephrine. The exact mechanism by which amphetamines act is unknown, but they result in CNS stimulation, probably by releasing catecholamines (norepinephrine and dopamine) from sympathetic nerve terminals. They are orally absorbed and concentrated in the kidneys, lungs, and brain. Peak effects are seen 15 minutes after intravenous administration. Approximately half the administered dose is excreted unchanged, with the balance being metabolized as deaminated metabolites. The half-life of the metabolites in the urine varies with changes in urine pH. Amphetamine (a basic drug with a pK_a level of 9.9, which is the point at which half the amount in the body is ionized and half is in an unionized form) half-life in patients with an acidic urine (pH less than 6.6) ranges from 7 to 14 hours. In patients with alkaline urine (pH over 6.7, as from use of sodium bicarbonate) the half-life range is prolonged to 18 to 34 hours. Deaths have occurred with doses of 5 mg/kg or more. Tolerance develops, and response is variable, since chronic abusers use from 5 to 8000 mg/day, as the desired effects occur within 1 hour after ingestion. The amphetamines and related derivatives possess a high pK_a, and therefore acid diuresis will enhance amphetamine excreton. Acidification is achieved with a goal of urine pH between 4.5 and 5.5.

Effects. The amphetamines usually are abused because they produce an elevation of mood, a reduction of fatigue, a sense of increased alertness, and "invigorating aggressiveness." Amphetamines do not create extra physical or mental energy; rather, they promote expenditure of present resources, sometimes to the hazardous point of fatigue that is often unrecognized. Intravenous injection results in marked euphoria, an orgasmic feeling known as the *flash* or *rush*, a sense of great physical strength and capacity, and a sense of crystal-clear thinking. The user feels little or no need for rest, sleep, or food and may continually engage in vigorous activity that may be perceived as exhilarating and creative. To an objective observer, inefficient, stereotyped, and repetitive behavior is common during an amphetamine high, and the drug user may engage in perseverating behavior such as repeatedly reconstructing mechanical devices. Depending on the dosage of the drug taken (as much as 1.5 g is known to have been injected in one dose by long-term users), the individual may experience a "run" of variable length, perhaps for several days. Some amphetamine users force themselves to lie down and close their eyes for a few hours during such a run and also will force-feed themselves in an attempt to prolong the run. Termination of the drug's use may result from a variety of factors, such as exhaustion, fright, or inability to obtain more of the drug. Withdrawal of the drug is followed by long periods of sleep. On awakening, the individual often feels hungry, extremely lethargic, and profoundly depressed, a phenomenon known as *crashing*. This phenomenon may be very severe, and the risk of suicide must be considered.

The stimulant properties of amphetamines can cause dramatic cardiorespiratory effects, such as tachycardia, dyspnea, and chest pain. Users of amphetamines may panic because of association of these signs and symptoms with those of a myocardial infarction. To deal with these disturbing symptoms, amphetamine users often use depressants, or *downers*. Some drugs (such as dextroamphetamine sulfate and amobarbital) combine CNS stimulant with a CNS depressant in an attempt to minimize the overstimulation produced by the amphetamine ingredient.

Amphetamines are also said to be psychotomimetic. Although there is some conflicting evidence regarding the etiology of amphetamine psychosis, it is claimed that heavy users may develop psychosis characterized by aggression, delusions of persecution depression, paranoia, euphoria, and fully formed visual and auditory hallucinations. Some authorities suggest that these phenomena may be related to the insomnia produced by prolonged amphetamine abuse because sleep deprivation, in and of itself leads to psychologic disturbance such as deterioration in performance, misperceptions, and hallucinations.

In addition, marked tolerance to amphetamines occurs.

If the intravenous route was employed, the nurse should be aware that the oral tablet form may have been the source of amphetamine. Although the intravenous amphetamine alone is not associated with pulmonary microemboli, tablet fillers such as magnesium silicate (talc) and cornstarch may be the foreign body that produces pulmonary emboli, resulting in granuloma formation within the lung. Pulmonary emboli have also been observed in methylphenidate table injectons. Talc also may appear in the cornea of the eye after chronic oral tablet parenteral administration of methylphenidate, (and probably does so with any oral tablet or capsule when injected). The lungs act as filters for these large talc particles; therefore the abuser of intravenous tablets complaining of nonspecific pulmonary symptoms should be considered a candidate for talc-containing microemboli, and an eye examination may reveal the same source of talc.

Withdrawal symptoms. Although amphetamines do not appear to lead to physical dependence, as identified by the criteria of a characteristic and reproducible withdrawal syndrome, some authorities maintain that the signs and symptoms characteristic of crashing may constitute just such a syndrome.

Treatment of amphetamine toxicity. Diazepam is the drug of choice for the treatment of hyperactivity caused by amphetamines. It may be given orally or intravenously. The nurse must remember the possibility of a mixed ingestion of other drugs such as barbiturates. The effect may be complete within 24 to 36 hours. Chlorpromazine may be employed only if the ingested substance is a pure amphet-

amine or is combined with a barbiturate. However, if the ingested drug is purported to be MDA, DMT, DOM, or similar agents, the chlorpromazine is contraindicated because of the synergistic hypotension; it also is contraindicated in patients with a seizure disorder because of the potentiation of seizures. If hypertension does not respond to chlorpromazine, or in an emergency that is refractory to chlorpromazine, the choice is phenoxybenzamine, phentolamine, diazoxide, or sodium nitroprusside. The intravenous route of chlorpromazine is effective with a slow infusion, since a rapid infusion will result in a rapid fall in blood pressure.

The nurse should remember that marked suicidal depression often follows an amphetamine overdose and chronic abuse by 24 to 72 hours; withdrawal results in sleepiness and apathy.

Cocaine

A potent CNS stimulant, cocaine is used therapeutically mostly as a local anesthetic, since it is likely to cause toxic side effects when administered by other routes. When it is used for its stimulant effects, it produces euphoria and increased expenditure of energy similar to that produced by amphetamines and may lead to a similiar psychotic state with strong elements of paranoia.

Cocaine as a social-recreational drug of abuse is achieving great popularity for its euphoric effect. Cocaine is classified as a narcotic but is a tropine, related to the belladonna alkaloids. When referred to illicitly, the female gender is generally applied to cocaine products, whereas the male gender is generally applied to heroin products. Some common street names for cocaine are Bernice, Bernies, C, Cadillac, Charley, coke, flake, gold dust, happy dust, ice, lady (her, she), nose candy, nose snuff, nose stuff, paradise, snow, and witch.

The purity of the illicitly produced drug varies greatly. This short-lived CNS stimulant is often adulterated; it is diluted or cut with agents such as amphetamines, boric acid, quinine, mannitol, procaine, or lidocaine. The vasoconstricting effect of cocaine may be responsible for limiting its own absorption. Abusers of this drug also are known to mix it with alcohol and term it a "liquid lady." The motivation for abuse is a search for euphoria.

Cocaine may be administered by sniffing (snorting) the white, fluffy crystalline powder (which resembles snow, hence the name), by direct intravenous injection, or by smoking the converted base form. Sometimes it is mixed with heroin for heightened effects, this combination being known as a *speedball*. Cocaine is rapidly metabolized, and the abuser of cocaine may use the drug every half hour or less to attain the high. Cocaine is metabolized rapidly in the liver by hepatic esterases, and plasma hydrolysis is the result of serum cholinesterase. It is absorbed from all mucous membranes. The serum levels are not proportional to the toxicity, and the elimination half-lives by oral, intranasal, and intravenous routes are similar (50, 80, and 60 minutes, respectively).

At this time there is no absolute level known to be lethal (20 mg to 10 or more per day), but with its growing abuse these data may become evident. The relatively rapid increase in blood level may be as important in determining fatal reactions as the peak blood concentration. Factors other than blood concentration of cocaine must be examined, such as tolerance, reverse tolerance, previous history of cocaine abuse, individual susceptibility, and presence of other drugs.

Side and toxic effects. Initial symptoms of cocaine use include restlessness, mydriasis, hyperreflexia, vasoconstriction, tachycardia, hallucinations, nausea, vomiting, and muscle spasms, which may be followed by respiratory failure, convulsions, coma, and circulatory collapse. In chronic abusers a toxic psychosis characterized by hallucinations and paranoid delusions as well as skin eruptions caused by self-inflicted skin irritation is frequently observed. The energetic patient may be prone to outbursts of violent behavior. Frequently blood in the nose and a perforated nasal septum are seen in those who chronically snort cocaine. Nasal inhalation may be achieved by a small spoon, rolled dollar bills, or inhalation device misused to accommodate cocaine (a spinhaler device for cromolyn sodium). A large dose of cocaine has direct cardiotoxicity, but death from overdose may result from respiratory failure.

Physical dependence does not seem to be characteristic of cocaine abuse, but strong psychologic dependence is evident.

Cannabis drugs (marijuana)

The cannabis drugs are derived from the leaves, stems, fruiting tops, and resin of both female and male hemp plants, *Cannabis sativa*. The potency of the active ingredient, tetrahydrocannabinol (Δ^9-THC), is greatest in the flowering tops of the plant and seems to vary according to the climatic conditions under which the plant was grown. In the United States the plant may grow wild or is illegally cultivated and thus generally varies in potency. The only legal cultivation is that by the federal government for research purposes.

More potent types (differentiating between species and varieties) of marijuana and alarmingly greater use among young teenagers require a new attitude of concern toward the substance. Imported marijuana and that which is grown scientifically in controlled conditions is often 10 times as potent as the domestic variety smoked in the past. Some of the marijuana from sources outside U.S. borders (Central and South America) have 4% to 6% THC. Many of the users are employing it more frequently, and the average age at which use begins is nearing 12 to 14 years.

The nurse should become familiar with the following street names to assist in identifying use of marijuana: Acapulco gold, ace, Aunt Mary, baby, bhang, blond, blue saze, bobo, bo, brown weed, burnie, bush cannabix, Chicago green, Columbian, dagga, ding, doobies, dope, drag weed, fu, gage, ganga, gange, gold, goof butts, grass, griffo, hemp, herb, Indian hemp, J, jive sticks, joint, juanita, lid, Maggie, Mary, Mary Jane, Mary Warner, Mexican green, MJ, mu, number, Panama gold, Panama red, pot, reefer, rick sticks, roach rope, sativa, sprue, sticks, tea, Texas tea, TJ, weed, wheat, and yerba.

Research protocols. THC, the most active ingredient derived from marijuana, is currently being investigated for use in the treatment of nausea and vomiting induced by cancer agents refractory to other commonly used antiemetics and in the treatment of glaucoma refractory to standard forms of treatment. Studies are still in process, and no conclusive data have been presented. It appears, however, that THC may have useful therapeutic uses and may not always be considered a drug of abuse with no benefit to mankind.

Preparations. Marijuana (average grown in U.S.A. 0.2% to 4% THC) and hashish (5% to 12% THC) are the most common forms of cannabis drugs used in the United States. Hashish refers to the powdered form of the plant's resin, which is five to eight or ten times as potent as some varieties of marijuana. Other forms of cannabis drugs used in different parts of the world (such as Jamaica, Mexico, Africa, and the Middle East) include *bhang*, *ganja*, and *charas*, which are commonly used in India and correspond, respectively, to American marijuana, hashish, and unadulterated resin. In Morocco *kif* is used, whereas in South America a cannabis drug often used is called *dagga*.

Mode of administration. Cannabis drugs may be absorbed when administered by oral, subcutaneous, or pulmonary routes but are most potent when inhaled. Either the pure resin or the dried leaves of the cannabis plant may be smoked in pipes or cigarettes. Because the smoke is acrid and irritating, some users prefer to smoke marijuana through a water pipe. The smoke is deeply inhaled and retained in the lungs as long as possible to achieve maximum saturation of the absorbing surface. Powdered hashish and marijuana may also be mixed with foods, a mode of administration that delays the drug's absorption. The sedative-hypnotic effects of smoking are rapid and generally last 2 to 3 hours, whereas the effects of the orally ingested drugs may not begin for several hours. Hashish oil has been used by the intravenous route, with a high incidence of mortality.

THC is the major active constituent of marijuana, and biologic activity may be caused by the 11-hydroxy metabolite. Marijuana cigarettes (joints) illicitly used in the United States generally have 1% to 2% THC and weigh approximately 500 mg, yielding THC from 5 to 10 mg. The effective dose may be reduced by one half when the dose is smoked, yielding from 2.5 to 5 mg THC per 500-mg weight.

Since the potency varies with plant strain and cultivation, marijuana cigarettes will produce moderate to intense psychopharmacologic effects, reaching a peak in 15 minutes and lasting 1 to 4 hours.

The nurse must keep in mind that the marijuana cigarette may be *dusted* (treated) or saturated with PCP (known as *super grass*), which may present a need to treat PCP overdosage. Such adulteration is also seen with hashish oil being used on the marijuana cigarette.

Mechanism of action. All the cannabis drugs seem to act as CNS depressants, their high resulting from depression of higher brain centers and consequent release of lower centers from inhibitory influence. Although there is some controversy regarding their classification, the cannabis drugs are not narcotic derivatives but are legally classified as controlled substances; they are more frequently classified as sedative-hypnotic-anesthetics or psychedelic drugs. Like the sedative-hypnotics, they appear to depress the ascending reticular activating system, and as their dosage increases, their effects proceed from relief of anxiety, disinhibition, and excitement to anesthesia. If dosage is high enough, respiratory and vasomotor depression and collapse may occur.

Research has yielded some marijuana homologs and analogs (such as synhexyl, which is one third as potent as marijuana); these should permit standardization of dosage and yield more information regarding structure-activity relationships of the cannabis drugs.

Pharmacokinetics. Peak plasma levels of THC after smoking one marijuana cigarette are reported to be from 0.020 to 0.050 µg/ml. Within a few hours these values decrease to between 0.005 and 0.010 µg/ml, and only trace amounts of the unmetabolized THC are detected in the urine.

The liver is the primary site of metabolism, and the major route of elimination of THC is the bile and feces. Prolonged enterohepatic circulation is reported with this lipophilic drug, and it is highly protein bound in the serum. Reports of death or overdose are rare. For several days both THC and its metabolites may be detected in plasma and urine. Marijuana may alter barbiturate and ethanol metabolism.

Effects. The drugs have intoxicating, mind-altering properties and induce an anxiety-free state of relaxation characterized by a feeling of extreme well-being. Perceptions of time and space are distorted; ideas flow freely and disconnectedly; there may be interruptions in thought that are blanks or gaps similar to *epileptic absence*; and there may be states of inwardness and/or occasional excitement in the form of hilarity. Hallucinations can occur with high doses of the drug but are generally reported to be pleasant, and dissociative phenomena also are reported. There has been some controlled research with these drugs, and some experiments suggest that impaired decision making and psychometric performance are related to the use of these drugs. The drug experience is highly subjective, and the presence of an altered state of consciousness may not be perceived by the novice until he or she is sensitized to it by colleagues. Some of the factors that influence the psychologic and behavioral effects of marijuana are drug dose, user's personality, user's drug expectations, environment, social influences, and life experiences.

The incidence of adverse reactions to marijuana appears to be low. Minor side effects include immediate tachycardia and delayed bradycardia, delayed hypotension, conjunctival vascular congestion (red eyes), dryness of the mouth and throat, hyperphagia, delayed gastrointestinal disturbances, possible vasovagal syncope, and enhanced appetite and flavor appreciation. More serious side effects that may occur are psychologic and include fear, panic (especially among first-time or naive users), feelings of paranoia, disorientation, memory loss, confusion, and a variety of perceptual alterations. Moreover, marijuana has been known to precipitate acute psychotic reactions and toxic psychoses in poorly organized personalities. The incidence of adverse effects appears to be highest in novice users of the drug. However, these adverse effects generally appear to be short lived and self-limiting.

Apparently psychological dependence and tolerance to marijuana develop but not physiologic dependence. Experimentally, however, marijuana withdrawal has been demonstrated. Subjects who had been given large daily dosages of synhexyl for 1 month, for example, demonstrated hyperexcitability when the drug was abruptly withdrawn, this excitability was relieved by readministration of the drug.

The effects of prolonged abuse of marijuana have not yet been scientifically proved. However, there seems to be some indication that amotivational states, apathy, memory problems, and some loss of mental acuity may occur. Physiologically, the possibility of chronic, long-term use of marijuana cigarettes leading to chronic bronchitis (bronchodilation and reduced airway resistance) and emphysema cannot be discounted.

There has also been some question regarding the use of marijuana leading to the use of opiates, a progression termed the "stepping-stone" theory. This theory, however, is somewhat controversial, and some authorities state that any progression in drug use stems from personality and environmental factors rather than from the pharmacologic properties of marijuana. The multiple drug use theory lends support to this hypothesis, stating that a person predisposed to abuse one drug is also likely to abuse other, and perhaps stronger, drugs.

Treatment of the rare acute overdose is directed at the symptoms, using support of respiration, blood pressure, and other functions as needed. Treatment of the depressive, hallucinatory, or psychotic reactions to this drug is to provide a quiet, nonthreatening area with positive verbal reassurance; the effects are short lived, in a range from a few minutes to about 4 hours. If the patient shows signs of excessive agitation, panic, or disorientation, then an oral dose of 5 to 10 mg diazepam may be useful.

Withdrawal symptoms. Physiologic withdrawal symptoms after discontinuation of marijuana use have been produced experimentally. Whether marijuana produces physical dependence outside of experimental situations is still being explored. Some restlessness, anxiety, irritability, and insomnia may be associated with withdrawal of the drug, but these symptoms are generally mild and of short duration.

Psychedelic drugs (hallucinogens, psychotomimetics, and psychotogens)
LSD and related compounds

Classifications of the most common hallucinogenic agents include (1) those drugs containing the indole nucleus, such as lysergic acid diethylamide (LSD) and its variants, dimethyltryptamine (DMT) and its analogs, and psilocybin, and (2) those drugs containing the phenyl ring, such as mescaline, DOM, and the anticholinergic hallucinogens. The phenylethylamine derivatives (such as mescaline) are structurally related to catecholamine, whereas LSD and DMT have structural relationships to serotonin that may involve the action of these agents as hallucinogens.

LSD

LSD is a colorless, odorless, and tasteless substance that is a synthetic derivative of lysergic acid, a compound that naturally occurs in ergot and some varieties of morning glory seeds and is structurally related to ergonovine, an ergotalkaloid.

The use of LSD has been revived recently, possibly because of the unpleasant effects of PCP. The users of LSD are more informed about the effects and are not experiencing the high incidence of bizarre or adverse effects to the substance such as loss of control and intense hallucinations, which were reported in the earlier days of its use at 150 μg levels in the 1960s. The strengths used today are lower on the average (approximately 85 μg), which may be the reason for the lesser degree of adverse effects. The doses used today produce speedy effects such as visual trails of color or light, laughing, facial grimacing, and bruxism. Forms of street LSD are microdots (tablets 2.5 × 5 cm or smaller) and blotter acid (a 6 × 6 cm square blotter paper with figures drawn on it or plain). The strengths may increase as the abusers are able to handle the doses required to produce their desired individual effects. Some of the common street names of LSD are acid, animal, beast, black star, blotter acid, blue acid, blue cheer, brown dots, California sunshine, cube, dots, flash flats, heavenly blue, instant Zen, Owsley's blue dot/acid, pearly gates, purple haze, purple barrel, sacrament, star, strawberries, sugar lump, twenty-five, windowpane, yellow sunshine, and zen.

Therapeutic uses. A number of potentially therapeutic uses of LSD have been proposed, all of which merit more investigation. These include the drug's use in the treatment of chronic alcoholism and in the reduction of intractable pain as is found in malignant disease and in phantom limb sensations. For a time some psychiatrists also used the drug to induce psychosis, thereby helping the patient revive repressed memories, the influence of which could then be dealt with by the patient and therapist. The psychotomimetic effects of the drug have also generated the theory that some chemical imbalance may be involved in the etiology of schizophrenia. However, such preliminary data regarding the therapeutic uses of LSD require much more research.

Mode of administration. LSD is usually distributed as a soluble powder and can be ingested in capsule, liquid, or tablet form. A frequent but now obsolete mode of ingestion was from an aqueous solution on sugar, although the drug can be licked off any object impregnated with it, such as a cookie, a stamp, or blotting paper. The drug may also be administered subcutaneously, intramuscularly, or intravenously. It is readily absorbed from the intestinal tract and mucous membranes as well as from body fluids.

Dosage. Pharmacologically on a weight-for-weight basis, LSD is more active than almost any other drug and can be detected in the body at concentrations of 1 part per billion. The human body reacts to relatively minute doses of the drug, and 100 to 250 μg administered orally can produce a potent experience of intense depersonalization for up to 12 hours in the majority of subjects.

Mechanism of action. LSD acts pharmacologically as a sympathomimetic agent. These effects, however, are secondary to the profound psychologic changes that it also produces. The drug is believed to be a serotonin antagonist and inactivates monoamine oxidase and acetyl-cholinesterase. Cross-tolerance to mescaline and psilocybin has been demonstrated. The exact biochemical mechanism of action, however, is not currently known.

Pharmacokinetics. After oral ingestion LSD is absorbed rapidly, strongly plasma protein bound, with high concentrations in the liver, kidneys, and lungs. Less than 1% of the orally administered dose will penetrate the central nervous system, but intense psychic alterations occur at levels of less than 3 ng LSD per gram of brain tissue. The concentrations of LSD in the brain are thought to be in the pituitary and pineal glands, the hypothalamus and limbic system, and the auditory and visual reflex areas. In humans the half-life of LSD is almost 3½ hours, and this is close to the duration of the peak psychosensory effect, which decreases over an 8- to 12-hour period. The substance is metabolized to inactive metabolites in the liver and excreted in the urine.

Effects. The effects of LSD usually begin within 20 to 50 minutes after administration and, like effects of other mind-altering drugs, cannot be reliably predicted. Autonomic nervous system changes are relatively mild and may include tachycardia, hypertension, nausea, vertigo, and perspiration. Effects vary widely among individuals and are in part related to the dosage, the mental set of the individual, and the environment of the individual. The drug experience may also vary for the same individual from time to time; he or she may have a pleasant experience, or a "good trip," one time, and the next may be an unpleasant or "bad trip."

The initial reaction to the drug may be one of vague anxiety and sometimes nausea. Later there are general changes of perception involving sound, sight, touch, body image, and time. The brightness of colors may be intensified, for example, and there is generally heightened awareness of the environment, creating a flood of sensations and impressions. There may be synesthesia, that is, the translation of one type of sensory experience into another sensory modality, such as "hearing a color." Every perception assumes an increased sense of significance and meaning. Changes in cognitive func-

tioning and value judgment formation may occur (good and bad may become equal). There may be blurring of boundaries between the self and the environment, and an ineffable state of transcendence may be achieved.

However, unpleasant experiences with LSD are also rather frequent. Clinically, evidence of impaired judgment in the toxic state is frequent, and examples of such behavior are well known, as demonstrated, for example, by LSD users attempting to stop traffic with their bodies. Some authorities state that if the previously described altered state of consciousness develops in the context of fear and disorganization, psychosis may occur. Moreover, one of the chief dangers of the drug is that it will precipitate a latent psychosis into activity. With the release of repressed material with which the individual cannot cope, an acute panic psychosis may result. Feelings of acute panic and paranoia during a toxic LSD psychosis can result in homicidal thoughts and actions. Toxic delirium, with altering and alternating levels of consciousness, follows toxic psychosis, and the experience generally resolves in a stage of exhaustion in which the user feels empty, unable to coordinate thoughts, and depressed. During this time suicide is a definite risk.

The chemical effects of LSD might be antidoted by administration of a tranquilizer, a barbiturate, or nicotinic acid. It is specifically recommended that the administration of chlorpromazine be avoided in LSD toxicity because it may accentuate anticholinergic-like drug effects and may, in high doses, lead to severe hypotension or confusion, further compounding the situation. However, the administration of medication is recommended only as an adjunct to psychotherapy of a crisis intervention nature. The latter is directed primarily toward the restoration of a positive mental set under the guidance of a stable and consistent human point of reference whom the patient trusts. A "talk-down" approach in a quiet environment is often used and consists of directing the patient's attention away from perceptions that produce panic and providing reassurance that the experience will dissipate and that he has not permanently harmed himself. Hospital practices of administering massive doses of tranquilizers, applying restraints, and isolating such patients are to be avoided. The patient's dramatically heightened awareness of the environment and distorted perceptions may render these measures traumatic rather than therapeutic.

Markedly unfavorable reactions induced by LSD include prolonged, delayed, and recurrent reactions such as depression and long-term schizophrenic or psychotic reactions. The recurrent reactions have been described as *flashback phenomena*, referring to the transient, spontaneous repetition of a previous LSD-induced experience that is unrelated to renewed administration of the drug. Moreover, a bad trip (anxiety or panic reaction) on LSD is likely to be a paranoid experience, and tendencies toward violence can be characteristic of LSD intoxication. Research reports of chromosomal damage related to LSD ingestion are increasing, although there appears to be some variation in susceptibility to chromosomal breaks that is of unknown origin. The drug does not seem to cause physical dependence, but tolerance to the drug occurs rapidly, and psychic dependence is frequent.

Pregnant women should be especially cautioned against taking LSD. Because lysergic acid is the base of all ergot alkaloids, it has uterine stimulant properties that can adversely affect a pregnancy and may have adverse cytogenetic effects.

Withdrawal symptoms. Insofar as is known, LSD does not produce physical dependence, and there are no withdrawal symptoms following discontinuation of long-term use. Tolerance develops in 3 to 7 days but disappears within 7 days of abstinence.

Mescaline

Mescaline is the chief alkaloid extracted from mescal buttons (flowering heads) of the peyote cactus, and it produces subjective hallucinogenic effects similar to those produced by LSD. Like the amphetamines, mescaline belongs to the phenylethylamine group, and its chemical structure distantly resembles that of norepinephrine. It is usually ingested in the form of a soluble crystalline powder that is either dissolved into teas or capsulated. The

usual dose of mescaline is about 500 mg. Each button contains about 45 mg mescaline.

The effects of mescaline from a dose of 5 mg/kg (6 to 12 buttons) appear within 2 or 3 hours and may last 4 to 12 hours or longer. Effects of doses of up to 500 mg are characterized by prodromal abdominal pain, nausea, vomiting, and diarrhea, which are followed by vivid and colorful visual hallucinations. Peyote cactus is used internally by Southwestern Plains Indians in religious practices.

Mescaline is not a very potent psychotomimetic, and the oral dose of 5 mg/kg in adults is 4000 times larger than the equivalent milligram dose of LSD. After oral ingestion a syndrome of sympathomimetic effects of anxiety, hyperreflexia, static tremors, and psychic perturbations with vivid visual hallucinations is encountered. The half-life of mescaline is about 6 hours, and it is excreted in the urine. Some street names for this substance are bad acid, bad seed, big chief, button, half moons, mesc, mescal button, and P.

Psilocybin

Psilocybin is a drug derived from Mexican mushrooms *(Psilocye mexicana)* that produces subjective hallucinogenic effects similar to those produced by mescaline but of shorter duration.

Psilocybin, a phosphate ester of DMT, occurs in the Mexican mushroom at a concentration of about 0.3%. In vivo dephosphorylation by alkaline phosphatase converts psilocybin to psilocin. Since the molecule is less polar because of the loss of the phosphoric acid radical, psilocin is able to more efficiently penetrate the blood brain barrier and therefore produce relatively greater hallucinogenic potency compared with psilocybin. Psilocin is not as potent as LSD (about 0.01% as active on a milligram for milligram basis) and creates a lesser psychedelic state, but when equivalent does are employed, the acquainted user may be unable to differentiate between the two drugs. Psilocin is 4 hydroxy-DMT and is the most active psychotogen of the N-alkylated tryptamines, and the 5 hydroxy-DMT (bufotenine from the skin and parotid glands of the toad *Bufo marinus*) and the cahobe bean has less psychotomimetic activity. Thus the position of the hydroxyl substitution on the indole nucleus is critical. Within ½ to 1 hour after ingestion of 5 to 15 mg psilocybin a hallucinogenic dysphoric state begins. A dose of 20 to 60 mg may produce effects lasting 5 or 6 hours. The mood is pleasant to some users, and others experience apprehension. The user has poor critical judgmental capacities and impaired performance ability. Also seen are hyperkinetic compulsive movements, laughter, mydriasis, vertigo, ataxia, paresthesias, muscle weakness, drowsiness, and sleep lasting only about 5 or 6 hours.

Phencyclidine (PCP)

Phencyclidine was developed in the late 1950s as an anesthetic for dissociative anesthesia, that is, production of a cataleptic state in which the patient appears to be awake but is detached from the surroundings and unresponsive to pain. It is related chemically to ketamine (Ketaject, Ketalar), an anesthetic used primarily for children, and the analgesic meperidine (Demerol). It is now restricted to veterinary use, since it was found to produce postanesthetic excitement, visual disturbances, delirium, and hallucinations.

Abuse of this anesthetic agent (ketamine) has begun to develop.

An increased frequency of emergency room visits for PCP-induced problems of intoxication, psychosis, and overdosage has been recorded. Chemically, PCP is 1-(1-phenylcyclohexyl)piperidine hydrochloride. Its illicit manufacture for less than $100 can bring thousands of dollars in sales. The ingredients to manufacture PCP are now under government regulation (regarding the piperidines). This has prompted clandestine laboratories to seek new chemical derivations for their sale of PCP analogs. It is frequently misrepresented and distributed as THC, mescaline, or LSD to the naive user or buyer of abuse substances. The most current application of the drug is soaking a dark wrapper cigarette in PCP, referred to as "Shermans" or "longs." In addition, the use of marijuana soaked with PCP is seen frequently. Smoking is the preferred route, since it permits titration by the user to the stage desired. Some of the common street names of PCP are angel dust, ele-

phant, kristal jointhog, mist, monkey, peace pill, pits, rocket fuel, TAX, THC, and TIC.

Pharmacodynamics. PCP is rapidly metabolized in the liver to inactive metabolites, and large ingestions have resulted in high concentrations of the unmetabolized drug in urine. PCP is lipophilic and has a half life of ½ to 1 hour in small doses and from 1 to 4 days in larger doses; the pK^a of the drug is 8.5. The "ion trapping" of the drug into extravascular areas (which are more acidic than the serum) is thought to be a major influence on prolonged toxicity, and the recirculation of the drug secretion to the acidic gastric fluid and reabsorption in the small intestine may also account for the prolonged toxicity and offer a key to the management of the toxicity of overdosage. These observations have led to treatment using urine acidification with diuresis and continuous gastric drainage in severe intoxication to enhance elimination. Urinary excretion is enhanced when the urine is acidified to 5.5 pH or less with ascorbic acid. The fact that PCP may be found in the adipose tissue may indicate that the long-term effects and sequelae are related to its lipophilic nature, and possibly during a nutritional fast the emergence of PCP is seen and interpreted as a flashback.

Effects. In humans common peripheral signs include flushing, profuse sweating, nystagmus, diplopia, ptosis of the eyelids, analgesia, and sedation. Other effects of PCP are:

1. A state similar to alcohol intoxication with ataxia and generalized numbness of extremities is produced.
2. Subanesthetic doses cause psychologic effects usually proceed in three stages.
   a. Change in body image and feelings of depersonalization
   b. Perceptual distortions—visual or auditory
   c. Discomforting feelings of apathy, estrangement, or alienation
3. Disorganization of thought and derealization is greater than with LSD.
4. Attention span, motor skills, and sense of body boundaries, movement, and position are impaired.
5. Hallucinations can recur unpredictably for days, weeks, or months after taking the drug.

PCP is similar to ketamine in producing stages of anesthesia. In addition, excitation, paranoid behavior, self-destructive acts (no sensation or feeling of pain because of anesthesia), horizontal and vertical nystagmus, tachycardia, hypertension, seizures, increased reflexes, muscle rigidity, respiratory depression, and coma (with open eyes) may ensue. PCP is a strong sympathomimetic and hallucinogenic dissociative anesthetic agent. Since the drug is now classified as a controlled substance (Class II), penalties for illegal manufacture have been enacted and enforced.

Effects of PCP are claimed by some investigators to mimic schizophrenia more accurately than those of other psychotomimetics or hallucinogenics (for example, LSD). Like the symptoms of schizophrenia, the effects of PCP are reduced by sensory deprivation. Currently no chemical antidote exists for inhibiting the effects of PCP. Keeping the user quiet and away from sensory stimuli may decrease the intensity of some of the effects.

Toxic effects. The pressor effects of PCP may cause hypertensive crisis, intracerebral hemorrhage, convulsions, coma, and death.

Intoxication and treatment. The clinical symptoms and signs of PCP intoxication are dose related, and the waxing and waning of the intoxicative signs may have a relationship to the pharmacokinetics of enteric reabsorption for the alkalized (nonionized) PCP with the recirculation and redistribution of the agent, as described earlier.

Low overdosages. With low overdosages the patient is conscious, disoriented, and may exhibit self-destructive acts of violence. This low dose is about 2 to 5 mg ingested by smoking or intranasal route, with serum levels in a range of 25 μ/ml.

In the low-overdose patient the treatment should include rest, minimal sensory situmlation in a quiet, lowly lit room, positive verbal reassurance, and psychologic support. This is useful because the patient is oblivious to the environment, so the environment should be nonthreatening. The patient should be protected from self-inflicted injury. The nurse should not talk down the anxious patient to the extent that anxiety is intensified or agitation produced. If treatment with an antipsychotic drug is necessary, the butyrophenone haloperi-

dol is preferred. Use of phenothiazine has resulted in hypotension with PCP patients, and other drugs with anticholinergic properties also should be avoided. The patient with low-dose toxicity of PCP often has a characteristic blank, open-eyed stare.

Intravenous diazepam may be used for convulsions (myoclonic and seizures) and calming the patient. The dosage is usually 2.5 mg at 1- to 15-minute intervals for adults. Oral administration is used for cooperative, low-dose patients. Diazepam also will assist in relief of muscle spasm, altering somatosensory dissociation, managing behavioral problems (as does haloperidol), and placing the patient in a position to accept treatment.

Moderate overdosage. The moderate dose of 5 to 25 mg with a serum level of 90 to 300 μg/ml is nonthreatening, since the patient is unconscious, in no immediate danger of death, responsive to noxious or painful stimulus, and unable to respond to verbal command.

For the moderately overdosed patient considerable caution must be used when attempting instrumentation to avoid deep oropharyngeal suctioning or intubation except when absolutely imperative. The somatosensory system is deadened, so pain and the stimulation of the autonomic relfex system of the airway should be avoided. The patient will not respond to verbal commands. The treatment is initially begun with the use of forced acid diuresis with a dosage of furosemide from 1 to 40 mg/kg/hour every 6 hours (to produce urine flow of 3 to 6 ml/kg/hour) along with urinary acidification with ascorbic acid (0.5 to 1.5 g slowly over 5 to 10 minutes) to a urinary pH of 4.5 to 5.5). The use of ammonium chloride is avoided, since ammonia-breakdown products place a burden on the damaged hepatocellular complex.

High overdosage. A high overdosage is generally 25 mg or more, perhaps by the oral route, with a serum level of 300 μg/ml or more; such patients may have underlying suicidal tendencies. This dose produces an adrenergic crisis and status epilepticus, possibly with fatal results, and respiratory failure is very late and frequently seen. The patient is comatose and unresponsive to deep or surgical pain stimulus.

This patient must be hospitalized and vital life processes maintained.

The high-overdosage management is as for a moderate overdose. Periodic respiration is seen, apnea is a terminal sign, and the protective airway reflexes that begin to obtund in moderate overdoses now are lost. The increased respiration with orotracheal secretions and sustained vomiting often initiates aspiration pneumonitis. At this stage, if the tachycardia and hypertension continue, congestive heart failure and a cerebro vascular accident may result. Board-like stiffness and myoclonus increase with opisthotonos and tonic-clonic seizure activity to status epilepticus, and the airway is lost. All the medical efforts are directed to management of the airway and control of the status epilepticus. The fixed dilated pupils are a sign of the patient's deep intoxication. An expert should perform orotracheal intubation, possibly in the operating room. A large-bore nasogastric tube is used for flushing gastric contents, since it is suggested that ion trapping of PCP occurs in an acid gastric content. Periodic lavage with a solution of 0.1 N hydrochloric acid to maintain a gastric pH of 2 is recommended. Since PCP has a high pK_a level and is ionized in an acid medium, PCP is not absorbed so long as it remains in the highly acidic gastric juice. When PCP passes to the small intestine where the pH is alkaline, it becomes non-ionized and unable to pass through the semipermeable membrane of the stomach to be absorbed into the blood. This is the key to the ion trapping and the reason for maintaining a highly acid pH in the stomach and urine.

The treatment of overdosage with high amounts of PCP should further include keeping the patient cool with sponging, the use of 1 mg propanolol intravenously over 1 minute to a maximum of 10 mg to titrate the hypertensive spikes and arrhythmia, a standing order for diazoxide for hypertensive crisis (150 to 300 mg over ½ minute by intravenous push), protection of the pulmonary system for edema (aspiration pneumonitis), and symptomatic control of the status epilepticus by intravenous anticonvulsant therapy, as indicated.

When the patients are recovering from moderate to high overdosages, the phenomena of anxiety or depression and confusion and (prior to this) an overlapping severe life-threatening dopaminergic storm may occur. The anxiety/depression state is different in each patient, but the use of diazepam or haloperidol may provide the proper modality to control such emergence reactions. The dopaminergic storm may be controlled with propranolol, since propranolol may cross the blood-brain barrier and act on the dopaminergic receptor sites of the limbic to achieve a central calmative effect.

The use of PCP causes a wide range of subjective effects, requiring careful observations of the overdosed patient. The prolonged and severe behavioral disturbances may change to respiratory and cardiovascular emergencies as emergence from different dosage levels ensues.

Inhalants

Volatile hydrocarbons and aerosols are other substances of abuse. Representatives of this group are toluene, xylene, benzene, gasoline, paint thinner, lighter fluid, and airplane glue. When sniffed (inhaled), these agents may produce a rapid generaly CNS depression with marked inebriaton, dizziness, floating sensations, exhilaration, and intense feelings of well-being that are at times seen as reckless abandonment, disinhibition, and feelings of increased power and aggressiveness similar to those seen with alcohol. Inhalation may result in bronchial and laryngeal irritation, transient euphoria, headache, giddiness, vertigo, ataxia, and renal tubular acidosis, especially with the glue sniffers. At high doses confusion and coma occur with blood syncrasia. After these early excitatory effects disappear, depression may follow. Chronic toluene abuse will lead to hepatic and renal toxicity, and death from cardiac arrhythmia and respiratory failure has been reported. Recovery from lower doses may be seen in 15 minutes to a few hours. These agents are used mainly by young children and preteens (6- to 15-year-olds), and use of the volatile hydrocarbons as propellants in aerosol products is seen frequently.

Butyl nitrite is a clear, yellow liquid sold as a room deodorizer under trade names such as

Rush, Bolt, and Bullet. The substance is sold in drug paraphernalia shops, adult book stores, and by mail order. The opened container is placed under the nose, and the individual inhales in deep, nasal breaths and becomes dizzy, feels faint, and possibly loses consciousness. This rush lasts less than 1 minute and may include a headache, perspiration, and flushing, all caused by rapid vasodilation. It strongly resembles the effects achieved from amyl nitrite (a prescription smooth muscle relaxant and vasodilator). The FDA may change the status of butyl nitrate from a room odorizer or deodorizer because of its potential for abuse and for harmful effects. Amyl nitrite also is abused and is known as poppers, snappers, stew-sticks, and by other names. It is abused sometimes to heighten a sexual orgasm in both partners. Both of these substances lower blood pressure and reduce the heart's oxygen consumption.

The abuse of phenylpropanolamine in the form of the over-the-counter anorexiants is frequently seen today. The drug is used for its central nervous system stimulation, since as a sympathomimetic amine it possesses in high doses many of the amphetamine effects. Many of the over-the-counter "nighttime" cough and cold remedies are also abused because of their considerable sedative potential, since they contain 25% alcohol with antihistamines.

Legal aspects of drug abuse

In May 1971 the Controlled Substances Act became effective, replacing the former Narcotics Acts and Drug Abuse Control Amendments. In July 1973 the Drug Enforcement Agency (DEA) become the sole law enforcement agency for combating drug abuse. The DEA is charged with the responsibility of controlling narcotics and dangerous drug abuse through enforcement and prevention by working cooperatively with other federal agencies and with state and local governments. The DEA also registers physicians and those authorized to administer, dispense, and prescribe controlled substances.

The possession and distribution of hallucinogens, opium poppy and straw, coca leaves, and certain opiates and opium derivatives are, of course, illegal. Since 1937 it has been illegal in the United States to possess or sell marijuana. Nevertheless controversy exists about the classification of marijuana as a narcotic in the same category as the opiates and cocaine. Although the sale and traffic of marijuana are felonies, some state statutes make the possession and use of marijuana a misdemeanor.

Nursing implications related to drug abuse

The nurse may be called on to function in any aspect of health care related to drug abuse: in prevention, in case-finding, in treatment of acute intoxication, and in long-term rehabilitation. To function with optimal effectiveness, the nurse needs current knowledge not only of drugs most frequently abused but also of other aspects of the nursing process, such as patient teaching, crisis intervention, administration of acute emergency care, and support of therapeutic and rehabilitative regiments. Because drug abuse is such a complex, multifaceted behavioral phenomenon, the nurse must relate to and treat the whole patient. Therefore the nurse must take into account the patient's reality and environment and must evolve an understanding of what mind-altering drugs realistically can and cannot do.

In their preventive role nurses may function either inside or outside the hospital environment. Within the hospital they will be required to make decisions regarding a patient's need for a narcotic or any other drug that may produce dependence. Many nurses are reluctant to administer narcotics to a patient in pain, for example, for fear of producing dependence. The tendency to avoid the use of narcotics should not be carried to such extremes, but it behooves nurses to exercise their repertoire of skills in a therapeutic attempt before administering a narcotic. A large component of pain is one's subjective response to pain. Many patients experiencing pain are also anxious or depressed. It has been found that if these conditions are relieved, the physical pain will also be alleviated. When medication is indicated, if a nonnarcotic analgesic will relieve the pain, it should be administered in place of a narcotic analgesic. Or, when narcotic analgesics are indicated, return to drugs that do not produce dependence should be accomplished as soon as possible. It must be emphasized that when other nursing interventions fail, prescribed drugs should never be withheld from patients who are experiencing physical or psychologic pain.

Preventive nursing roles both inside and outside the hospital environment also include education regarding drugs of all types but particularly those prone to producing dependence. The promotion of the use of functional coping mechanisms rather than the use of drugs is another crucial aspect of the nurse's preventive role in drug abuse. Persons who abuse drugs because of psychologic problems frequently have lost sight of their strength to deal with their problems in other ways. In such situations the nurse can apply knowledge of crisis intervention and of supportive psychotherapy.

As a health professional, the nurse also has a responsibility in identifying persons who are dependent on drugs in order to refer them to appropriate resources. The diagnosis of drug dependence usually is not difficult, and often the individual will admit a need for drugs. Observation for physical signs of drug abuse will frequently yield substantial evidence. Needle marks and scars of abscesses along intravenous routes and pupillary dilation are some overt signs that are often indicative of chronic drug abuse. Signs of acute intoxication differ according to the drug abused and may manifest themselves variably, as indicated in Table 12-3 and on p. 365. Striking changes in personality, interest patterns, and social relationships also may be indicative of drug abuse. A medical history of hepatitis, abscesses, or bacterial endocarditis may further substantiate an assumption, and diagnostic tests are available to detect the presence of some drugs in the bloodstream and in urine. Conclusive evidence of chronic drug dependence is the appearance of a withdrawal syndrome.

The nurse's role in acute drug intoxication, or in treatment of overdoses, can be twofold:

support of medical therapy and/or interviewing the patient or companions in an attempt to discover the specific agent that precipitated intoxication. With drugs increasingly being mixed, it is often difficult to identify the drug used and to provide an antidote. In such cases persistent, patient, nonjudgmental, and painstaking probing of the patient's history may be necessary.

The nurse also may be called on to care for a patient undergoing withdrawal, a most difficult physiologic phenomenon that requires astute observation of the patient's physical condition as well as a firm but supportive and reassuring interpersonal approach.

When withdrawal from the drug is completed, however, the role of the nurse does not end. Indeed physiologic withdrawal may be defined as the starting point for meeting the problem of the patient's drug dependence. Continuing help and contact are necessary and must be maintained for a long period. If such help is not available, relapse to the abuse of drugs is almost inevitable.

A person cannot be restructured in the manner of thinking, feeling and acting until a new image is achieved of how that person is seen by himself or herself. Many abusers suffer from a deprivation of basic biologic needs such as physical closeness and emotional openness, which may in part be caused by the dissolution of the basic family unit relationships, affecting individual needs and the expectations of what one is entitled to in these meaningful relationships. The unfulfillment of these needs leads to a pronounced disequilibrium that must be dealt with.

There are the five basic emotions: pleasure, pain, fear, anger, and love. Emotions are not logical and must be expressed rather than hidden or continually repressed; expression is therapeutic. The sharing of emotional pain, depression, guilt, tension, and anxiety brings the individual an experience of tremendous relief, strength, and a sense of self that may not have been felt in a long time. The individual is entitled to feel happiness, to feel pleasure, to have a good self-image, and to make relationships meaningful. The success of many group therapeutic communities for drug, alcohol, and substance abusers lies in their use of these concepts of human caring and their enabling individuals to express their happiness or unhappiness.

Summary of nursing considerations

Historically, people have turned to drugs in search of relief from physical and psychosocial problems. Drug abuse refers to self-medication or self-administration of a drug in chronically excessive quantities, resulting in psychologic and/or physical dependence, functional impairment, and deviation from approved social norms. Drug abuse may be experimental, social, episodic, compulsive, or ritualistic.

The major categories of commonly abused agents are narcotics and related compounds, sedatives and hypnotics, tranquilizers, central nervous sytem sympathomimetics, cannabis drugs (marijuana), psychedelic agents, and inhalants.

In the abuse of consciousness-altering drugs there are two types of drug dependence: physical and psychologic. Physical dependence on a drug can be demonstrated only by production of a withdrawal syndrome. This syndrome can be relieved by readministering the drug or by administering a pharmacologically related drug. Closely related to physical dependence is the development of drug tolerance with a tendency to increase the drug dose.

Psychological dependence, ranging from mild desire to craving to compulsive use, is an emotional reliance on a drug to maintain a drug-induced state. The psychologically dependent individual prefers a drug-induced state to a drug-free state of being.

A drug must produce favorable, pleasant, unusual, or desirable effects to cause dependence. Since very few drugs without central nervous system effects are abused, one of the predominant factors contributing to drug abuse appears to be intrapsychic, a desire to alter one's state of mind, for example, to search for euphoria or to escape from inner or societal tensions.

Although still in the research stages, theories of physical drug dependence agree that in a state of dependence a condition of latent hyperexcitability develops in the cells of the central nervous system after frequent and prolonged administration of depressant drugs.

The effects of various mind-altering drugs are unpredictable and highly variable. The primary factors influencing the effects of any drug are (1) the pharmacologic properties of the drug itself, (2) the personality of the user, (3) the environment of the user, (4) the experience of the user, and (5) the interaction of these four components. The effects of mind-altering drugs, specifically, are also thought to be related to the purity of the drug used, the underlying psychopathology of the user, and the age of the user. Houston describes the phenomenon of the psychedelic experience, identifies some general effects, and categorizes the effects into four major levels of consciousness: sensory, recollective-analytic, symbolic, and integral.

Cannabis drugs (marijuana and hashish), opiates (heroin), ethyl alcohol, barbiturates, anxiolytics, and neuroleptics act as CNS depressants. All are likely to lead to physical and/or psychologic dependence. All, with the exception of cannabis, whose effects of prolonged use are as yet scientifically unproved, cause withdrawal symptoms on cessation.

On the other hand, amphetamines, cocaine, and hallucinogenic agents such as LSD, mescaline, PCP, and psilocybin act as CNS stimulants. Insofar as is known none produces physical dependence, and none causes withdrawal symptoms following discontinuation of long-term use. However, strong psychologic dependence is often evident.

Inhalants such as toluene, benzene, lighter fluid, and airplane glue provide transient euphoria. This is usually followed by mental depression and adverse physiologic effects. These agents are used mainly by children from 6 to 15 years of age.

Physical and psychologic dependence on drugs is frequently associated with debilitated physical states caused by the user's extensive involvement in procuring and using the drug. The life expectancy of persons who are physically dependent on drugs is generally lower than that of nondependent individuals.

Although controversy exists about the penalties, it is still illegal to possess and distribute all the drugs discussed in this chapter (with the exception of butyl nitrite, which may be banned in the future) and which federal and state laws prohibit without a prescription.

The nurse may be called on to function in any aspect of health care related to drug abuse: in prevention, case-finding, treatment of acute intoxication, and long-term rehabilitation.

QUESTIONS

FOR STUDY AND REVIEW

1 Differentiate between drug misuse and drug abuse.
2 Define physical and psychologic drug dependence.
3 Identify the major categories of drugs that are commonly abused.
4 Identify four factors that are significant in influencing the nature of an individual's experience after administration of a mind-altering drug.
5 Describe some factors that are believed to be causative in the development of drug abuse.
6 Differentiate among the following terms: hallucinogenic, psychotomimetic, and psychedelic.
7 Compare and contrast the primary forms of the cannabis drugs used in the United States.
8 Identify the active ingredient of the cannabis drugs.
9 Describe the effects and adverse effects produced by the cannabis drugs.
10 Identify some therapeutic goals for which the use of marijuana has been proposed.
11 Describe the pharmacologic effects of the opium derivatives. Explain why these drugs can lead to dependence.
12 If heroin is withheld from an individual dependent on the drug, what physiologic effect might the nurse expect the patient to experience?
13 Explain the rationale for the use of methadone hydrochloride, itself a dependency-producing drug, for accomplishing heroin withdrawal.
14 List the narcotic antagonists that may be used safely in the treatment of dependence of the opiate type.
15 Describe the physical changes that occur in fetal alcohol syndrome. What information can the nurse provide the mother about alcohol abuse?
16 Explain why pregnant women should be especially cautioned against excessive alcohol use.
17 Identify the effects for which the amphetamines are most frequently abused and describe the experience of an amphetamine high.
18 Identify the three most commonly used amphetamines.

19 Explain why high doses of amphetamines may be dangerous to persons with cardiac problems.
20 Explain why individuals who abuse amphetamines often use depressants in conjunction with these drugs.
21 Describe the psychologic effects produced by LSD.
22 Identify the currently known major adverse effects of LSD.
23 Explain why pregnant women should be especially cautioned against taking LSD.
24 Describe how LSD intoxication or a bad trip might be treated.
25 List the most common pathophysiologic complications that result from physical drug dependence and explain why they occur.
26 Explain the significance of dosage control in relation to frquently abused drugs.
27 Describe the dose-related overdose symptoms of PCP.

BIBLIOGRAPHY

GENERAL

Abel, E.L.: Drugs and behavior, New York, 1974, John Wiley & Sons, Inc.

Avery, G.S.: Drug treatment, ed. 2, New York, 1980, ADIS Press.

Confidentiality of alcohol and drug abuse patient records, Federal Register **40**:27802, 1975.

Council on Mental Health: Narcotics and medical practice, J.A.M.A. **218**(4):578, 1971.

Detzer, E., and others: Detoxifying barbiturate addicts: hints for psychiatric staff, Am. J. Nurs. **76**:1306, 1976.

Distasio, C., and Nawrot, M.: Methaqualone, Am. J. Nurs. **73**:1922, 1973.

Ellinwood, E., and Kilbey, M., editors: Cocaine and other stimulants, New York, 1977, Plenum Press.

Fultz, J.M., and Senay, E.C.: Guidelines for the management of hospitalized narcotic addicts, Ann. Intern. Med. **82**:815, 1975.

Glauser, F.L., et al.: Ethchlozvynol (Placidyl)—induced pulmonary edema, Ann. Intern. Med. **84**:46, 1976.

Goodman, L.S. and Gilman, A.: The pharmacological basis of therapeutics, ed. 6, New York, 1980, Macmillan Publishing Co., Inc.

Goth, A.: Medical pharmacology, ed. 9, St. Louis, 1978, The C.V. Mosby Co.

Greene, M.H., and others: Evolving patterns of drug abuse, Ann. Intern. Med. **83**:402, 1975.

Hansen, A.R., and others: Glutethimide poisoning: a metabolite contributed to morbidity and mortality, N. Engl. J. Med. **292**:250, 1975.

Hunt, L.G.: Recent spread of heroin use in the United States, Am. J. Public Health **64**(Suppl.):16, 1974.

Martin, W.R., and others: Naltexone, an antagonist for the treatment of heroin dependence, Arch. Gen. Psychiatry **28**:784, 1973.

Methadone maintenance, Med. Letter Drugs Ther. **16**(26), Dec. 20, 1974.

Morgan, A.J., and Moreno, J.W.: Attitudes toward addiction, Am. J. Nurs. **73**:497, 1973.

Nightingale, S.L., and others: emergency services and drug abuse, Ann. Intern. Med. **83**:569, 1975.

Petersen, D.M., and Chambers, C.D.: Demographic characteristics of emergency room admissions for acute drug reactions, Int. J. Addict. **10**(6):963, 1975.

Pillari, G., and Narus, J.: Physical effects of heroin addiction, Am. J. Nurs. **73**:2105, 1973.

Pradhan, S.N., and Dutta, S.N., editors: Drug abuse: clinical and basic aspects, St. Louis, 1977, The C.V. Mosby Co.

Ray, O.S: Drugs, society, and human behavior, ed. 2, St. Louis, 1978, The C.V. Mosby Co.

Rumack, B., and Temple, A. editors: Management of the poisoned patient, Princeton, N.J., 1977, Science Press.

Seixas, F.A., Cadoret, R., and Egglestone, S., editors: The person with alcoholism, Ann. N.Y. Acad. Sci. **233**, Apr. 15, 1974.

Sellars and Kalanti: Alcohol intoxication and withdrawal, N. Engl. J. Med. **294**:757, 1976.

Teehan, B.P., and others: Acute ethchlorvynol (Placidyl) intoxication, Ann. Intern. Med. **72**:875, 1970.

Wiley, L., editor: Managing a hospitalized drug addict, Nursing '77, **7**(6):46, 1977.

Yowell, S., and Brose, C.: Working with drug abuse patients in the ER, Am. J. Nurs. **77**:82, 1977.

MARIJUANA

Abruzzi, V.: 5,000 bad trips, Contemp. Drug Prob. **3**:345, 1974.

Annis, H.M., and Smart, R.G.: Adverse reactions and recurrences from marijuana use, Br. J. Addict. **68**:315, 1973.

Butler, J.R., and Regelson, W.: Treatment effects of delta-9-THC in an advanced cancer population. In Cohen, S., and Stillman, R.C., editors: The therapeutic potential of marihuana, New York, 1976, Plenum Press.

Coggins, W.J., and others: The health status of chronic heavy cannabis users, Ann. N.Y. Acad. Sci. **282**:148, 1976.

Cohen, S.: The 94-day cannabis study, Ann. N.Y. Acad. Sci. **282**:211, 1976.

Dell, D.D., and Snyder, J.A.: Marijuana: pro and con, Am. J. Nurs. **77**:630, 1977.

Hollister, L.E., and others: Marijuana and setting, Arch. Gen. Psychiatry **32**:798, 1975.

Jones, R.T., and others: Clinical studies of cannabis tolerance and dependence, Ann. N.Y. Acad. Sci. **282**:221, 1976.

Klonoff, H., and others: Neuropsychological effects of marijuana, Can. Med. Assoc. J. **108**:150, 1973.

Lemberger, I., and Rubin, A.: The physiologic disposition of marihuana in man, Life Sci. **17**:1637, 1975.

Low, M.D., and others: The neurophysiological basis of the marijuana experience, Can. Med. Assoc. J. **108**:157, 1973.

Paton, W.D.M.: Pharmacology of marijuana, Annu. Rev. Pharmacol. **15**:191, 1975.

Regelson, W., and others: Delta-9-tetrahydrocannabinol as an effective antidepressant and appetite-stimulatory agent in advanced cancer patients. In Braude, M.C., and Szara, S., editors: Pharmacology of marijuana, New York, 1976, Raven Press.

Sallan, S.E., Zinberg, N.E., and Frei, E.: Anti-emetic effect of delta-9-tetrahydrocannabinol in patients receiving cancer chemotherapy, N. Engl. J. Med. **293**:795, 1975.

Stefanis, C., and others: Clinical and psychophysiological effects of cannabis in long-term users. In Braude, M.C., and Szara, S., editors: Pharmacology of marijuana, New York, 1976, Raven Press.

Tennant, F.S., and Groesbeack, C.J.: Psychiatric effects of hashish, Arch. Gen. Psychiatry **27**:133, 1972.

Volavka, J., and others: EEG, heart rate and mood change ("high") after cannabis, Psychopharmacologia **32**:11, 1973.

NARCOTICS

Clouet, D.H., and Iwatsubo, K.: Mechanisms of tolerance to and dependence on narcotic analgesic drugs, Annu. Rev. Pharmacol. **15**:49, 1975.

Dole, V.P., and Nyswander, M.C.: Methadone maintenance treatment: a 10 year-perspective, J.A.M.A. **235**(19):2119, 1976.

Fultz, J.M., and Senay, E.C.: Guidelines for the management of hospitalized narcotic addicts, Ann. Intern. Med. **82**:815, 1975.

Gold, M.S., and others: Opiate withdrawal using clonidine, J.A.M.A. **243**(4):343, 1980.

Gram, L., and others: D-propoxyphene kinetics after single oral and intravenous doses in men, Clin. Pharmacol. Ther. **26**(4):473, 1979.

Kay, D.C., and others: Morphine effects on human REM state, waking state, and NREM sleep, Psychopharmacologia **14**:404, 1969.

Kelleher, R.T., and Goldberg, S.R.: General introduction: control of drug-taking behavior by schedules of reinforcement, Pharmacol. Rev. **27**:291, 1975.

Martin, W.R., and others: Methadone—a reevaluation, Arch. Gen. Psychiatry **28**:286, 1973.

Martin, W.R., and others: Comparison of graded single intramuscular doses of morphine and pentobarbital in man, Clin. Pharmacol. Ther. **15**:623, 1974.

O'Brien, C.P.: Experimental analysis of conditioning factors in human narcotic addiction, Pharmacol. Rev. **27**:533, 1975.

Pert, C.B., and Snyder, S.H.: Opiate receptors: its demonstration in nervous tissue, Science **179**:1011, 1973.

Showalter, C.V.: T's and blues, J.A.M.A. **244**:(11):1224, 1980.

Showalter, C.V., and Moore, L.: Abuse of pentazocine and tripelennamine, J.A.M.A. **239**:1510, 1978.

Takemori, A.E.: Biochemistry of drug dependence, Annu. Rev. Biochem. **43**:15, 1974.

Tennant, F.S., Jr.: Complications of propoxyphene abuse, Arch. Intern. Med. **132**:191, 1973.

Warren and others: Fatal overdose of propoxyphene, napsylate and aspirin, J.A.M.A. **230**:259, 1979.

Wesson, D.R., and others: Managing narcotic and sedative withdrawal, Hosp. Physician **8**:52, 1972.

Young, D.J.: Propoxyphene suicides, Arch. Intern. Med. **129**:62, 1972.

STIMULANTS

Angrist, B., and others: Amphetamine psychosis: behavioral and biochemical aspects, J. Psychiatr. Res. **11**:13, 1974.

Angrist, B., and others: The antagonism of amphetamine-induced symptomatology by a neuroleptic, Am. J. Psychiatry **131**:817, 1974.

Barton, W.I.: Drug-related mortality in the United States, Drug Forum **4**:79, 1974.

Caldwell: Amphetamines, cocaine and LSD, Clin. Pharmacol. Ther. **16**:265, 1974.

Gay, G.R., and others: An old girl: flying low, dyin' slow, blinded by snow: cocaine in perspective, Int. J. Addict. **8**:1027, 1973.

Pittel, S.M., and Hofer, R.: The transition to amphetamine abuse, J. Psychedelic Drugs **5**:105, 1972.

Post, R.M.: Cocaine psychosis: a continuum model, Am. J. Psychiatry **132**:225, 1975.

Post, R.M., and others: The effect of orally administered cocaine on the sleep of depressed patients, Psychopharmacologia **37**:59, 1974.

Rabins, P., and others: A comparison of two methods of determining drug use among university students, J. Louisiana St. Med. Soc. **126**:1, 1974.

Schick, J.F.E., and others: An analysis of amphetamine toxicity and patterns of use, J. Psychedelic Drugs **5**:113, 1972.

Winburn, G.M., and Hays, J.R.: Dropouts: a study of drug use, J. Drug Educ. **4**:249, 1974.

HALLUCINOGENS

Accord, L.D., and Barker, D.D.: Hallucinogenic drugs and cerebral deficit. J. Nerv. Ment. Dis. **156**:281, 1973.

Burns, R.S., and others: Phencyclidine states of acute intoxication and fatalities, West J. Med. **123**:345, 1975.

Dewhurst, K., and Hatrick, J.A.: Differential diagnosis and treatment of lysergic acid diethylamide induced psychosis, Practitioner **209**:327, 1972.

Done, A.K., and others: Pharmokinetic observations in treatment of phencyclidine poisoning in management of the poisoned patient, Princeton, N.J., 1977, Princeton Science Press.

Forrest, J.A.H., and Tarala, R.A.: Sixty hospital admissions due to reactions to lysergide (LSD), Lancet **2**:1310, 1973.

Glass, G.S.: Psychedelic drugs, stress and the ego, J. Nerv. Ment. Dis. **156**:232, 1973.

Harper, R.W., and Knothe, B.U.C.: Coloured Lilliputian hallucinations with amantadine, Med. J. Aust. **1**:444, 1973.

Klock, J.C., and others: Massive LSD overdosage: a report of 8 cases, Clin. Toxicol. **7**:213, 1974.

McGlothlin, W.H., and others: LSD revisited. 10 year follow-up of medical LSD users, Arch. Gen. Psychiatry **24**:35, 1971.

Meyer, J.S., and others: A new drug causing symptoms of sensory deprivation: neurological electroencephalographic and pharmacological effects of Sernyl, J. Nerv. Ment. Dis. **129**:54, 1959.

Rappolt, R.T., and others: Emergency management of acute phencyclidine intoxication, J. Am. Coll. Emerg. Physicians **8**(2):68, 1979.

Rumack, B.H., and others: Ornade and anticholinergic toxicity: hypertension, hallucinations and arrhythmias, Clin. Toxicol. **7**:573, 1974.

Savage, C., and McCabe, L.: Residential psychedelic (LSD) therapy for the narcotic addict, Arch. Gen. Psychiatry **28**:808, 1973.

Showalter, C.V., and thornton, W.E.: Clinical pharmacology of phencyclidine toxicity, Am. J. Psychiatry **134**(11):1234, 1977.

Tucker, G.J. and others: Chronic hallucinogenic drug use and thought disturbance, Arch. Gen. Psychiatry **27**:443, 1972.

Wesson, D.R., and others: Drug crisis intervention: conceptual and pragmatic considerations, J. Psychedelic Drugs **6**:135, 1974.

PHENCYCLIDINE

Aranow, R., and others: Phenycyclidine overdose: an emerging concept of management, J. Am. Coll. Emerg. Physicians **7**:56, 1978.

Burns, R.S., and others: Causes of phencyclidine-related deaths, Clin. Toxicol. **12**:463, 1978.

Rappolt, R.T., and others: Emergency management of acute phenycyclidine intoxication, J. Am. Coll. Emerg. Physicians **8**:68, 1979.

Richards, M.L., and others: Phencyclidine psychosis, Drug Intelligence Clin. Pharm. **13**:336, 1979.

Stillman, R., and others: The paradox of phencyclidine abuse, Ann. Med. **90**:428, 1979.

PROPOXYPHENE

Ballin, J.C.: Propoxyphene: is it a hazard to health? J.A.M.A. **241**:1618, 1979.

Fatalities due to propoxyphene, FDA Drug Bull. **9**:2, 1979.

Harris, B.: Psychosis after dextropropoxyphene, Lancet **2**:743, 1979.

Schuckit, M.A., and others: Propoxyphene and phencyclidine (PCP) use in adolescents, J. Clin. Psychiatry **39**:7, 1978.

Whittington, R.M.: Dextropropoxyphene addiction, Lancet **2**:743, 1979.

UNIT FIVE

DRUGS ACTING ON THE AUTONOMIC NERVOUS SYSTEM

CHAPTER 13

Neuropharmacology of the autonomic nervous system

Autonomic nervous system

Autonomic (from the Greek words *auto*, self; *nomos*, law) means a law unto itself, or self-governing. The autonomic nervous system has been known by other names. Winslow (1732) called it sympathetic because he thought it controlled the sympathies of the body; Bichat (1800) called it vegetative to designate its control over nutrition, as opposed to voluntary processes. Gaskell called it the involuntary nervous system, to contrast it with the voluntary system, which controls skeletal movement. Langley, who studied and described the structure and many of the functions and effects of the autonomic nervous system, provided much of the terminology used today to describe this system. He used the terms "sympathetic" and "parasympathetic" for the two divisions of the autonomic nervous system, and he introduced the concept of receptor.

The autonomic nervous system functions primarily as a regulatory system for maintaining the internal environment of the body at an optimal level. This system automatically controls the function of smooth muscle, cardiac muscle, and secreting glands, which through an interacting mechanism perform a multitude of physiologic tasks necessary for the preservation of a constant internal environment (homeostasis). Digestion of a meal, pressure of circulating blood, and many other processes are quietly supervised by a system of efficient control.

REFLEX CONTROL SYSTEM

The nervous system in general is the important control and communication system of the body. It collects information about its external surroundings and about what is going on inside the body. The simplest means by which the nervous system responds to environmental change is through the action of the reflex arc. As a functional unit of the nervous system, the reflex arc

T A B L E   1 3 - 1   **Schema of components of feedback control mechanisms**

	← Sensory input →			← Motor output →	
1 Reflex arc (anatomy)	Receptor ⟶	Afferent neuron ⟶	CNS ⟶	Efferent neuron ⟶	Effector
2 Reflex act (physiology)	Stimulus ⟶	Sensory nerve impulse ⟶	Integration ⟶	Motor nerve impulse ⟶	Motor response (motion)
3 Blood pressure regulation	Baroreceptor ⟶	Afferent neuron ⟶	Medulla ⟶	Efferent neuron ⟶	Arteriolar smooth muscle
↑ BP	Stimulus ⟶	Afferent impulse ⟶	VSMC ⟶	Decrease in sympathetic ⟶ nerve impulse	Vasodilation (↓ PR ⟶ ↓ BP)
4 Visceral nervous system	←	Visceral afferent system →		Visceral efferent system → (ANS)	

CNS = central nervous system
BP = blood pressure
PR = peripheral resistance
ANS = autonomic nervous system
VSMC = vasomotor center
↑ = Increase
↓ = Decrease

The *sensory input* carries sensory information concerning pain, temperature, or pressure to the central nervous system. The *motor output* conducts the altered impulse from the central nervous system to the effector and produces motor activity or motion such as muscle contraction or glandular secretion. NOTE: The visceral efferent system or autonomic nervous system performs motor activity.

is defined as the automatic motor response to sensory stimuli. The term *reflex arc* is essentially anatomic. The work it does is the *reflex act*, which identifies its physiologic usage. In any reflex a nerve fiber conducts a nerve impulse. These impulses form the basis by which communication of information is transmitted through the nervous system.

The reflex act consists of two major functional processes: the *sensory input* and the *motor output*. The first component of the reflex arc is the *receptor*, whose function is to detect environmental changes such as temperature, pressure in blood vessels, and distention in the viscera. These changes are responsible for producing a stimulus in the receptor. Information from the sensitized receptor is then transmitted as a nerve impulse along the *afferent neuron* to the *central nervous system*, the site of integration. Following this process, the results in instructions are sent out as an altered motor nerve impulse along the *efferent neuron* to the *effector*, which produces the appropriate movements of muscles and glands (see parts 1 and 2 of Table 13-1).

The information carried *to* the central ner-

vous system (sensory input) and instructions sent *from* the central nervous system (motor output) constitute a *feedback control mechanism*. That is, information fed back to the central nervous system from a receptor is modulated so that nerve impulses may vary in frequency and pattern according to the degree of activity required of the effector. Physiologically, the control of visceral function is involuntary, and this mechanism must include all the components of a control system essential for performing the reflex act. Therefore reflex action functions as a feedback mechanism, operating from a receptor to an effector, and its purpose is to prevent extreme changes in function that may create a disturbance in the internal environment.

The mechanism of feedback control can be exemplified by the blood pressure–regulating reflex. Again, the sequence of events follows the pattern of the reflex arc. The carotid sinus in the carotid artery and the aortic sinus in the aortic arch serve as pressure receptors *(baroreceptors)* that are highly sensitive to stretch; the degree of wall stretching is determined by the amount of pressure within these vessels. Thus any *increase in blood pressure* stimulates the baroreceptors, and this information is conveyed as nerve impulses along the *afferent neuron* to the *vasomotor center in the medulla,* the central nervous system site for integration of blood pressure. Following the appropriate neuronal connections, a *decrease in sympathetic discharge,* conducted along the *efferent neuron* to the *effectors,* produces dilation of smooth muscle, decrease in peripheral resistance, and a return of blood pressure to normal (see part 3 of Table 13-1). This explanation provides only a partial account of blood pressure regulation, since a decrease in arterial pressure produces the opposite response in the same neuronal pathway. In addition, this control mechanism operates in coordination with cardiac function.

DIFFERENCES BETWEEN THE PARASYMPATHETIC AND SYMPATHETIC SYSTEMS

Divisions of the nervous system. The nervous system of the body may be classified on the basis of the reflex arc (see part 4 of Table 13-1). The two main divisions include the central nervous system and the peripheral nervous system. The central nervous system, consisting of the brain and spinal cord, performs the important integrative functions from the peripheral sources. The peripheral system has two divisions: the somatic nervous system, which innervates voluntary or skeletal muscles, and the visceral nervous system, which influences the involuntary activities of smooth muscles, cardiac muscles, and glands. The afferent fibers of both systems represent the first link in the reflex arc by carrying sensory information to the central nervous system. Following integration at various levels in the brain, the motor outflow from the central nervous system is conducted along either the somatic efferent system or the visceral efferent system. Both of these systems constitute the final link in the reflex arc. Anatomically and physiologically, the visceral efferent system is identified as the autonomic nervous system, which is conventionally considered to be a *motor system.* (See box for divisions of the nervous system.)

A number of centers in the central nervous system are concerned with integration of all autonomic nervous system activities. There is

---

Divisions of the nervous system

 I. Central nervous system
II. Peripheral nervous system
  A. Somatic nervous system
    1. Somatic afferent system
    2. Somatic efferent system
  B. Visceral nervous system
    1. Visceral afferent system
    2. Visceral efferent system or autonomic nervous system
      a. Sympathetic nervous system
      b. Parasympathetic nervous system

---

evidence that the hypothalamus, in particular, is concerned with such integrating activities. It contains centers that function in the regulation of body temperature, water balance, and carbohydrate and fat metabolism. It also integrates mechanisms concerned with emotional behavior, the waking state, and sleep. The medulla oblongata integrates the control of blood pressure, respiration, and cardiac function. A series of "vital centers," including the vasomotor center, respiratory center, and cardiac center, respectively, coordinates these activities. In addition, the midbrain, limbic system, cerebellum, and cerebral cortex are involved in the control of and in physiologic functions regulated by the autonomic nervous system. It should be remembered that the autonomic nervous system is part of the central nervous system, not a distinct entity.

During the many years of experimental studies of the autonomic nervous system, a proliferation of terms has evolved and many have been used interchangeably. To clarify usage in pharmacology, the following sets of terms must be correlated:

Terminology	Divisions	
Anatomic	Craniosacral	Thoracolumbar
Physiologic	Parasympathetic	Sympathetic
Pharmacologic	Cholinergic	Adrenergic

Physiologic differences. The autonomic nervous system is organized into two subdivisions: the parasympathetic system and the sympathetic system. The basic arrangement of each system consists of two motor nerves, a preganglionic nerve and a postganglionic nerve, with a ganglion (group of nerve cell bodies) connecting the two neurons (see Fig. 13-1).

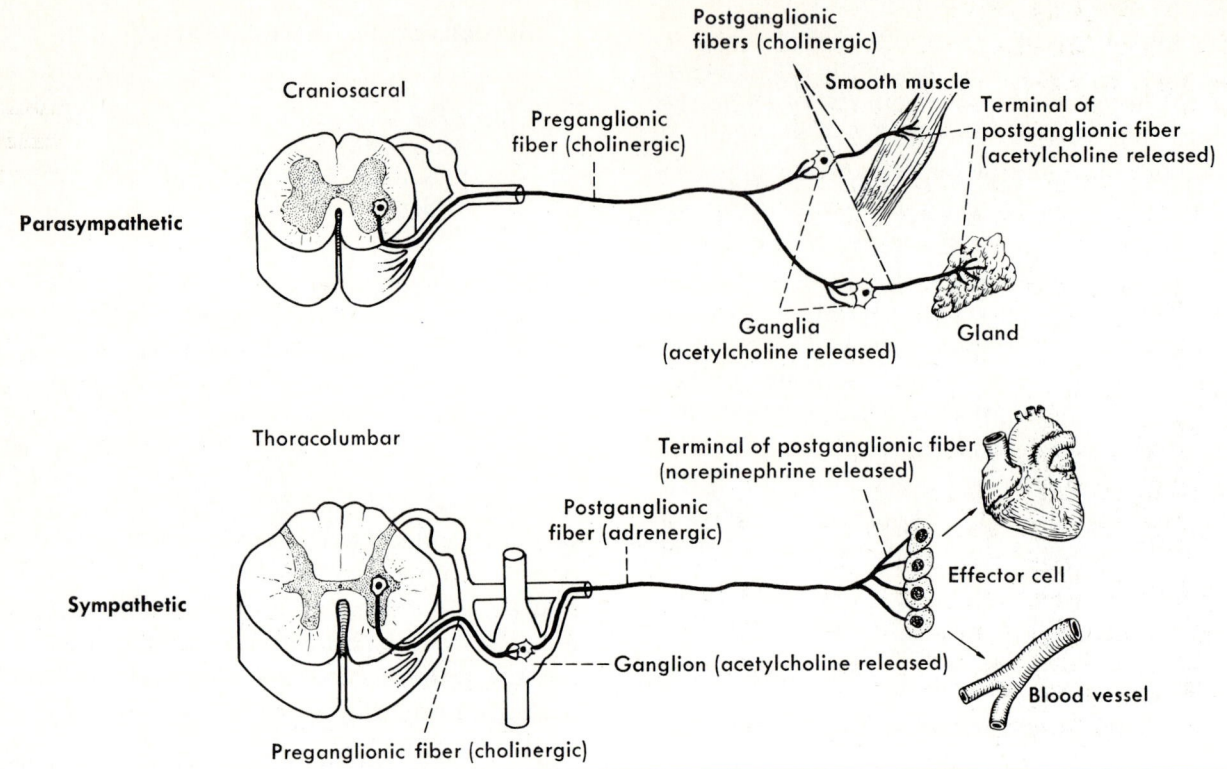

FIG. 13-1. Pre- and postganglionic fibers of the autonomic nervous system and neurohormonal transmitters.

Since the parasympathetic system and the sympathetic system simultaneously innervate many of the same organs, the actions of the two systems are opposed in a balanced antagonism. The functions stimulated by the parasympathetic system are mainly those concerned with conservation and restoration of body resources of the organism. These include cardiac deceleration, a rise in gastrointestinal activities associated with increased digestion and absorption, and an increase in excretion. In contrast, the functions stimulated by the sympathetic system are those that mobilize the organism during emergency and stress situations—the "fight or flight" responses. These involve expenditure of energy, such as emotional stress, and increases in the blood sugar concentration, heart activity, and blood pressure (see Table 13-2 for effector organ responses).

Anatomic and pharmacologic differences. The parasympathetic system is also called the craniosacral system because its preganglionic fibers emerge with the cranial nerves III, VII,

IX, and X and at the sacral spinal levels from about S3 through S4. The tenth cranial nerve or vagus nerve has extensive branches that supply fibers to the heart, lungs, and almost all the abdominal organs. The parasympathetic system is also known as the cholinergic system because the neurotransmitter released by its postganglionic fiber is acetylcholine (ACh).

The sympathetic system is aso called the thoracolumbar system because its preganglionic fibers originate in the spinal cord from the thoracic segment T1 to the lumbar segment L2 levels. Because the postganglionic fiber of this system releases the neurotransmitter norepinephrine or epinephrine from the adrenal medullary cells, this system is designated the adrenergic system (see Fig. 13-2 and Table 13-3).

NEUROHUMORAL TRANSMISSION

There is general agreement that transmission of information in the nervous system involves both electrical and chemical processes. This phenomenon is based on the fact that

T A B L E   1 3 - 2   Classification of the effector organ responses to autonomic nerve impulses

Effector organs	Response to parasympathetic (cholinergic) impulses	Sympathetic (adrenergic) impulses	
		Receptor	Response
Cardiovascular system			
Heart			
Sinoatrial node	Decreased heart rate	Beta$_1$	Increased heart rate
Atrioventricular node	Decreased conduction velocity	Beta$_1$	Increased automaticity and conduction velocity
Ventricles	No innervation	Beta$_1$	Increased force of contraction and conduction velocity
Arterioles			
(smooth muscle)			
Coronary*	Dilation	Alpha, beta$_2$	Constriction and dilation
Skin and mucosa	Dilation	Alpha	Constriction
Skeletal muscle	No innervation	Cholinergic	Dilation
Cerebral	Dilation	Alpha	Slight constriction
Abdominal viscera	—	Alpha, beta$_2$	Constriction and dilation
Renal	—	Alpha, beta$_2$	Constriction and dilation
Veins	—	Alpha, beta$_2$	Constriction and dilation
Lung			
Bronchial muscle	Bronchoconstriction	Beta$_2$	Relaxation (bronchodilation)
Bronchial glands	Stimulation		Inhibition
Gastrointestinal tract			
Motility	Increased motility	Alpha, beta$_2$	Relaxation (decreased motility)
Sphincters	Relaxation	Alpha	Contraction
Exocrine glands	Increased secretion	?	Decreased secretion
Salivary glands	Dilation: copious, watery secretion	Alpha	Constriction: thick, viscous secretion
Gallbladder and ducts	Contraction		Relaxation
Kidney	—	Beta$_2$	Renin secretion
Urinary bladder			
Detrusor muscle	Contraction	Beta$_2$	Relaxation
Sphincter	Relaxation	Alpha	Contraction
Eye			
Radial muscle	Contraction of sphincter	Alpha	Contraction (mydriasis)
Iris	Muscle (miosis, pupillary constriction)		
Ciliary muscle	Contraction		No innervation
Liver	Glycogen synthesis	Beta	Glycogenolysis, gluconeogenesis
Pancreas			
Acini	Secretion	Alpha	Decreased secretion
Islets (beta cells)	—	Alpha	Decreased secretion
	—	Beta$_2$	Increased secretion
Skin			
Sweat glands	No innervation	Cholinergic	Increased sweating
Pilomotor muscle	No innervation		Contraction (gooseflesh)
Lacrimal glands	Increased secretion		No innervation
Nasopharyngeal glands	Increased secretion		No innervation
Male sex glands	Erection		Ejaculation

*Receptors in coronary arteries are controversial; they are believed to have both alpha and beta$_2$ receptors.

nerve cells have two special characteristics: (1) They can conduct electrical signals. *The passage of a nerve impulse or an action potential along a nerve fiber or a muscle fiber is called conduction.* (2) They possess intercellular connections with other nerve cells and with innervated tissues such as muscles and glands. The presence of a specific chemical at these connections deter-mines the type of information a neuron can receive and the range of responses it can yield in return. *The passage of a nerve impulse across a synaptic or neuroeffector junction is called transmission.*

Although each nerve fiber may conduct an impulse along the neuron, it is solely the chemical substance called the *neurotransmitter* or

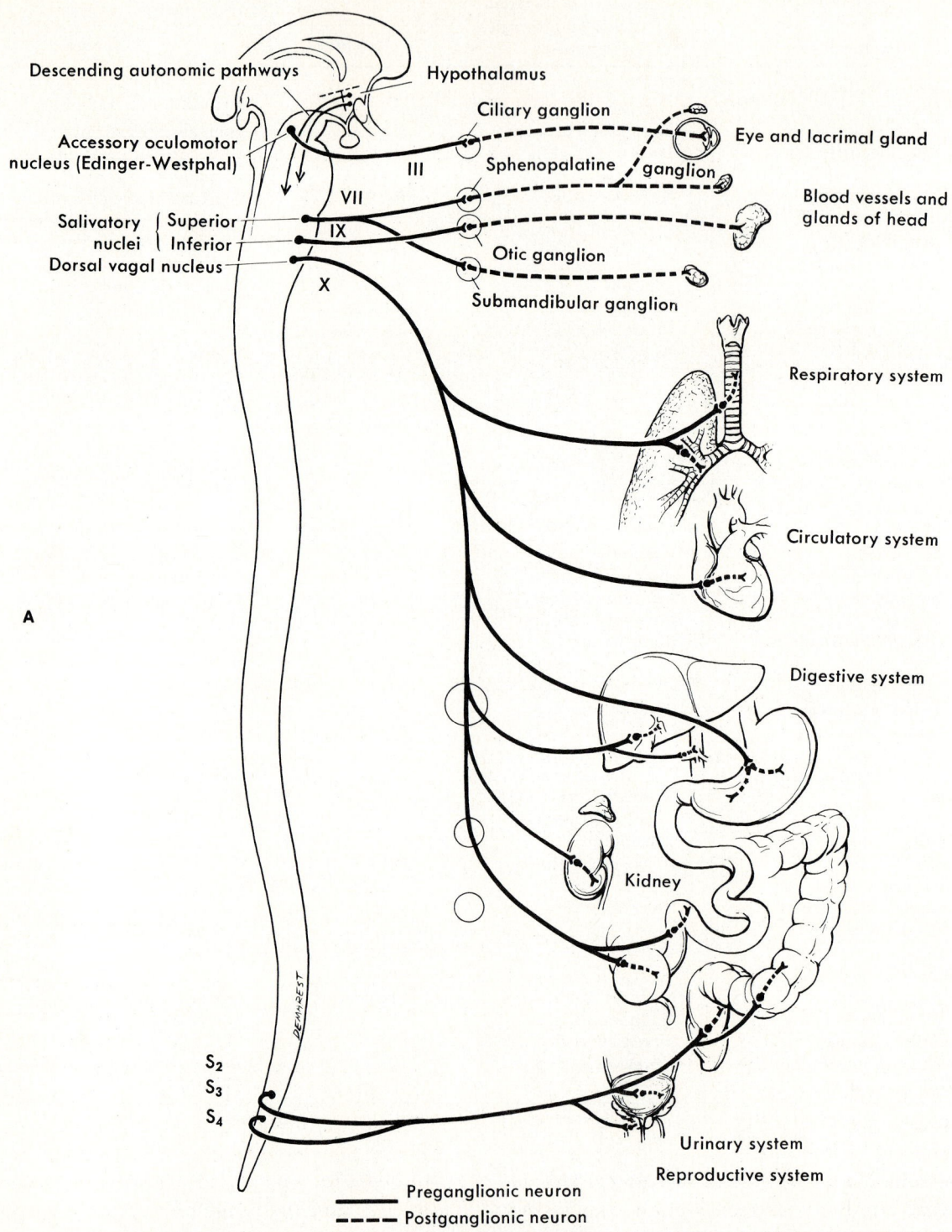

Descending autonomic pathways

Hypothalamus

Accessory oculomotor
nucleus (Edinger-Westphal)

Ciliary ganglion

Eye and lacrimal gland

III

Sphenopalatine ganglion

VII

Salivatory | Superior
nuclei | Inferior

Blood vessels and
glands of head

IX

Dorsal vagal nucleus

Otic ganglion

X

Submandibular ganglion

Respiratory system

Circulatory system

A

Digestive system

Kidney

DEMAREST

S₂
S₃
S₄

Urinary system

Reproductive system

———— Preganglionic neuron
- - - - Postganglionic neuron

FIG. 13-2. A, Diagram of the parasympathetic (craniosacral) division of the autonomic nervous
system. **B,** Diagram of the sympathetic (thoracolumbar) division of the autonomic nervous system. (From The nervous system, introduction and review by Noback, C., and Demarest, R. Copyright 1977, McGraw-Hill Book Co. Used with the permission of McGraw-Hill Book Co.)

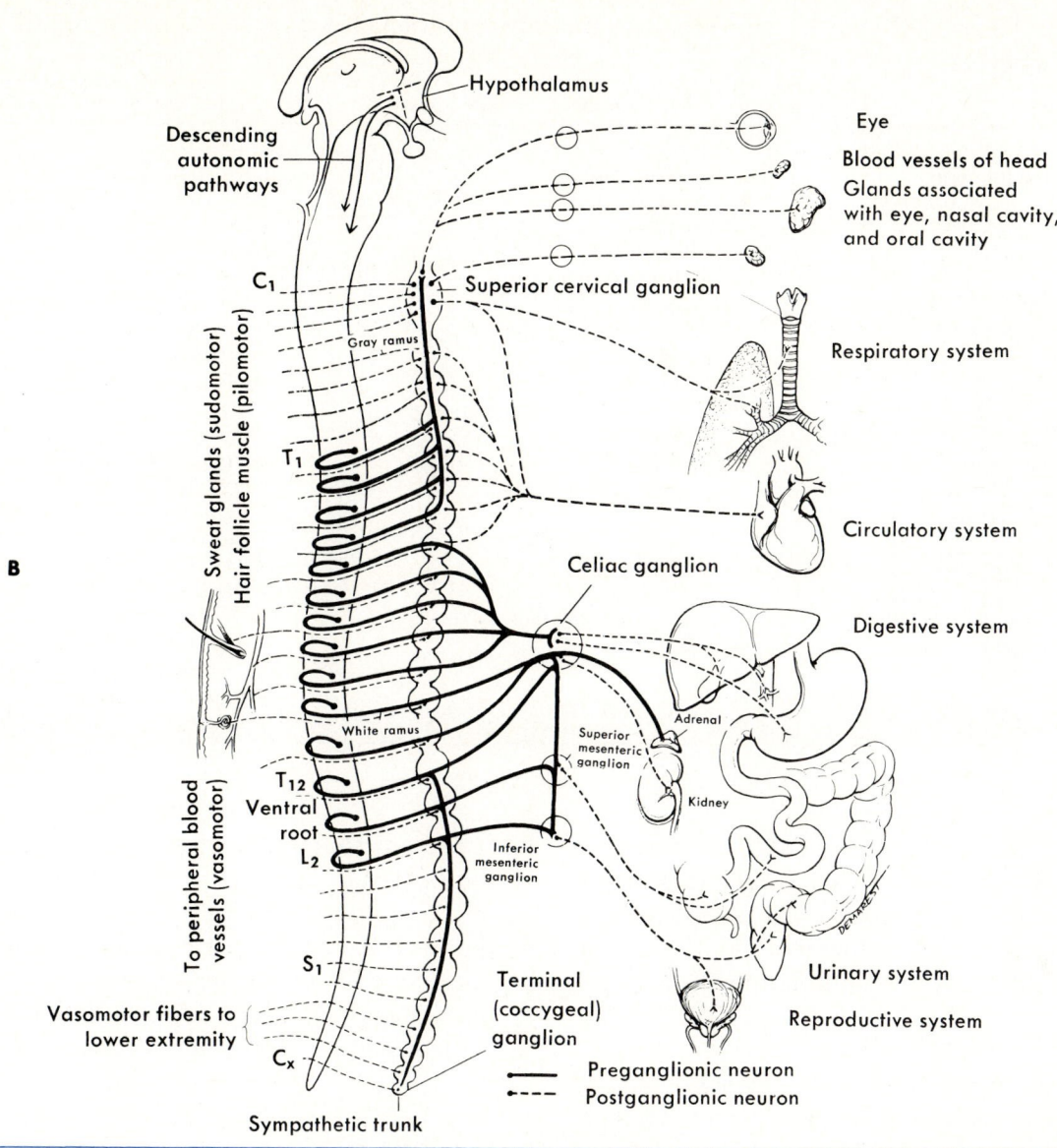

Fig. 13-2, cont'd. For legend see opposite page.

neurohormone that permits the action potential of a neuron to *cross* (1) the *synaptic junction* from one neuron to another neuron or (2) the *neuroeffector junction* from a neuron to an effector organ. In this mechanism the arrival of an action potential at a nerve terminal initiates the release of the neurotransmitters, and these hormones or mediators act as messengers by which nerve cells communicate information to the structures they innervate. It must be emphasized that the neurotransmitter exerts its influence primarily at the junctional space to facilitate the transmission of impulses to their final destination. Many drugs also act selectively at these junctions (see Fig. 13-3).

The compounds acetylcholine and norepinephrine are the neurohormones responsible for neurohumoral transmission. Neurons are classified according to the mediator released in them; nerves that contain acetylcholine are called *cholinergic neurons* and are involved in cholinergic transmission, and nerves that contain norepinephrine are known as *adrenergic neurons* and are associated with adrenergic transmission.

In neurohumoral transmission the sequence of events includes the following steps: (1) synthesis, (2) storage, (3) release, (4) action, and (5) inactivation of the mediator. Many autonomic drugs act by affecting one of these individual

T A B L E   1 3 - 3   **Differentiating characteristics between the parasympathetic and sympathetic nervous systems**

Characteristic	Parasympathetic nervous system	Sympathetic nervous system
Origin	Craniosacral	Thoracolumbar
Structure innervation	Cardiac muscle	Cardiac muscle
	Smooth muscle	Smooth muscle
	Glands	Glands
	Viscera	Viscera
Ganglia	Near the effector (vagus, atria of heart)	Near central nervous system
Length of fibers	Preganglionics (long)	Preganglionics (short)
	Postganglionics (short)	Postganglionics (long)
Ratio of preganglionics to postganglionics	Divergence is minimal (1:2), very discrete, fine responses	High degree of divergence (1:11, 1:17)
Response	Discrete	Diffuse
Ganglion transmitter	Acetylcholine	Acetylcholine
Transmitter substance (postganglionic nerve endings)	Acetylcholine	Norepinephrine (most cases); epinephrine and norepinephrine (adrenal medulla)
		Acetylcholine for sweat glands and blood vessels of skeletal muscles
Blocking drugs (postganglionic nerve endings)	Cholinergic blocking agents (atropine)	Adrenergic blocking agents Alpha-phenoxybenzamine (Dibenzyline) Beta-propranolol (Inderal)

events, and for this reason it is essential to understand the basic mechanisms involved in this complicated process. These drugs have been found useful in the treatment of many patients afflicated with autonomic disorders.

Cholinergic transmission

Synthesis and storage. Acetylcholine is synthesized in a reaction catalyzed by the enzyme choline acetylase (choline acetyltransferase) in the cytoplasm of the nerve terminal:

$$\text{Acetyl coenzyme A} + \text{Choline} \underset{\text{Acetylcholinesterase}}{\overset{\text{Choline acetylase}}{\rightleftarrows}}$$
$$\text{Acetylcholine} + \text{Coenzyme A}$$

Once synthesized, the acetylcholine is stored in packets called synaptic vesicles or granules, which are located in the nerve terminal.

Release and action. The arrival of an action potential at the nerve ending causes the vesicle to approach the membrane and release the acetylcholine molecules into the synaptic cleft or space. The presence of calcium ions is essential for an efficient release. Once free, the acetylcholine diffuses across the synaptic or junctional cleft and attaches itself to specialized receptors

called postjunctional sites on the membrane of the next neuron or neuroeffector. The binding of acetylcholine to the receptor increases the permeability of the membrane to sodium and potassium ions, a depolarizing action that finally results in excitation or inhibition of neural, muscular, or glandular activity (see Fig. 13-4).

Inactivation. Once acetylcholine has exerted its effect on the postjunctional sites, the excess amount is inactivated rapidly by the enzyme acetylcholinesterase (AChE). The metabolites formed in this reaction are chemically inactive and are the same compounds from which acetylcholine is formed. Inactivation of this neurohormone is shown as a reverse action in the preceding formula (see Fig. 13-4).

Adrenergic transmission

The term "catecholamine" refers to a group of chemically related compounds: norepinephrine (noradrenalin), epinephrine (adrenaline), and dopamine. They are all involved in some aspect of adrenergic transmission.

Synthesis and storage. The catecholamines produced by the sympathetic nervous system

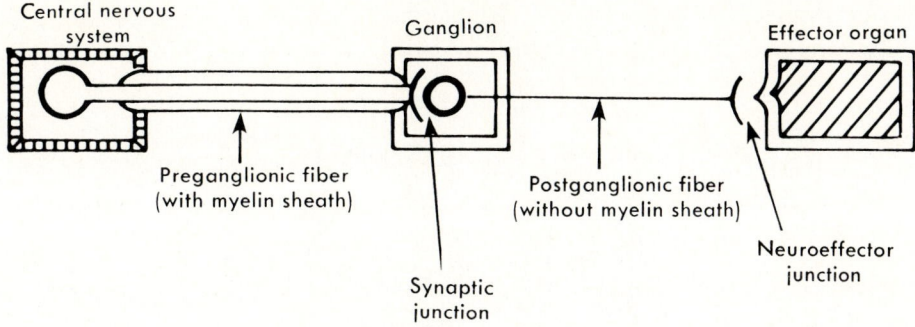

FIG. 13-3. Schematic representation to show the relationship between a neuron in the central nervous system, a neuron in a peripheral ganglion, and an effector organ. Note that the synaptic junction occurs as a space (cleft) or connection between the preganglionic fiber and the postganglionic fiber, and the neuroeffector junction occurs as a connection between the postganglionic fiber and the effector organs. These junctions act as important sites of neurohumoral transmission.

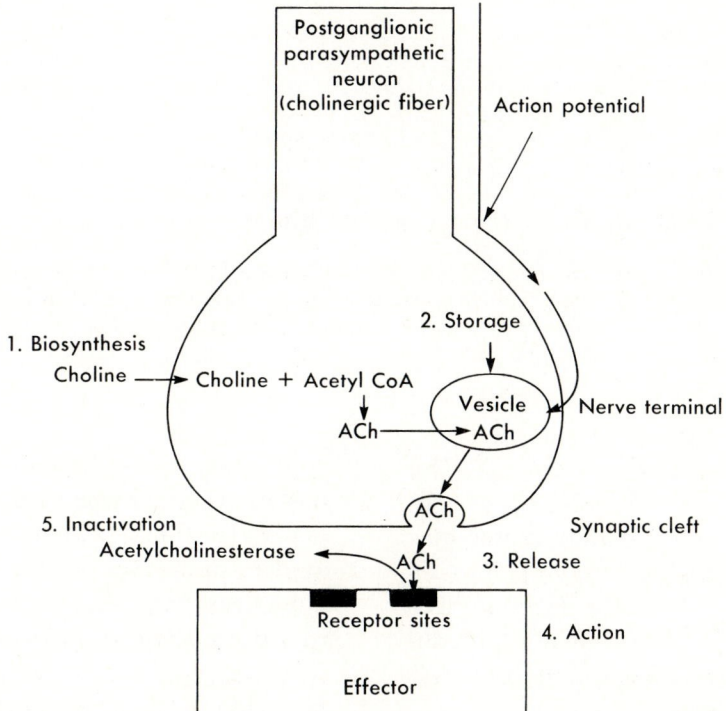

FIG. 13-4. Schematic diagram of parasympathetic postganglionic neuron showing steps in cholinergic transmission at the neuroeffector junction. *1. Biosynthesis* of acetylcholine (ACh): Choline is taken up by the nerve terminal and it interacts with acetyl CoA to synthesize ACh. *2. Storage:* Following synthesis, ACh is stored in the vesicle until the arrival of a nerve impulse. *3. Release:* An action potential at the nerve terminal causes the vesicle to attach itself to the membrane and release ACh. The neurohormone then diffuses across the synaptic cleft and combines with the receptors on the effector cell. *4. Action:* The interaction of ACh with the receptor sites results in a motor response. *5. Inactivation* of ACh: At the synaptic cleft, ACh is hydrolyzed by the enzyme acetylcholinesterase.

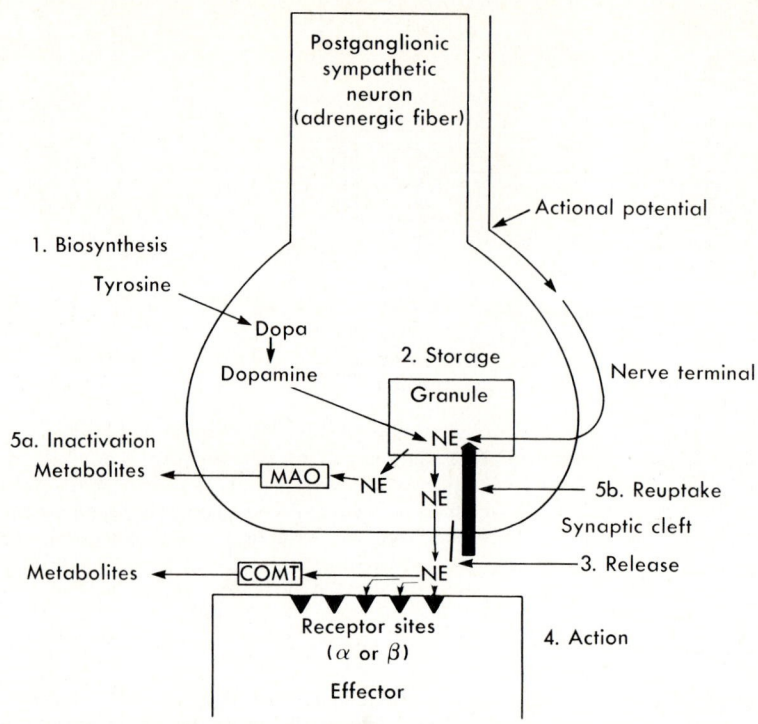

FIG. 13-5. Schematic diagram of sympathetic postganglionic neuron showing steps in adrenergic transmission at the neuroeffector junction. *1. Biosynthesis* of neropinephrine (NE): Tyrosine is taken up by the nerve terminal and converted to dopamine, which after transport into the storage granule is finally synthesized into NE. *2. Storage:* Following synthesis, NE is stored in the granule until the arrival of a nerve impulse. *3. Release:* Action potential along the neuron stimulates release of NE from the granule; NE then diffuses into the synaptic cleft to the receptor site of the effector cell. *4. Action:* The interaction of NE with the receptor sites (α or β) results in a motor response. *5a. Inactivation of NE:* Enzymatic metabolism of NE occurs within the neuron by action of the enzyme monamine exidase (MAO) or outside the neuron by the enzyme catechol-O-methyltransferase (COMT). *5b. Reuptake* of NE: reuptake into the nerve terminal and reentry into the storage granule (shown by heavy arrow) comprise another method of removal of NE.

include norepinephrine and epinephrine. The complex pathway for synthesis of these neurotransmitters is mediated by different enzymes located in the postganglionic nerve terminals and in the chromaffin cells of the adrenal medullary glands. The production of norepinephrine and epinephrine proceeds through the following biochemical steps:

$$\text{Tyrosine} \xrightarrow[\text{hydroxylase}]{\text{Tyrosine}} \text{Dopa} \xrightarrow[\text{decarboxylase}]{\text{Dopa}}$$

$$\text{Dopamine} \xrightarrow[\text{β-hydroxylase}]{\text{Dopamine}} \text{Norepinephrine} \xrightarrow[\text{transferase}]{\text{Methyl}}$$

$$\text{Epinephrine}$$

The formation of norepinephrine is initiated by the circulating tyrosine, an amino acid derived from proteins in the diet. When tyrosine enters the cytoplasm of the nerve terminal, it is converted by the enzyme tyrosine hydroxylase into dopa, which in turn is decarboxylated to dopamine by the cytoplasmic enzyme dopa decarboxylase. Dopamine is then taken up into the storage vesicles or granules where it is transformed into the neurotransmitter norepinephrine by the enzyme dopamine β-hydroxylase. Fig. 13-5 shows the steps of the synthetic process. In the adrenal medullary gland, the action of the enzyme methyl transferase carries chemical synthesis one step further by converting norepinephrine to epinephrine. On stimulation, both epinephrine and norepinephrine are released from the adrenal medulla and carried by the circulation to all parts of the body. The autonomic drugs may inhibit the actions of

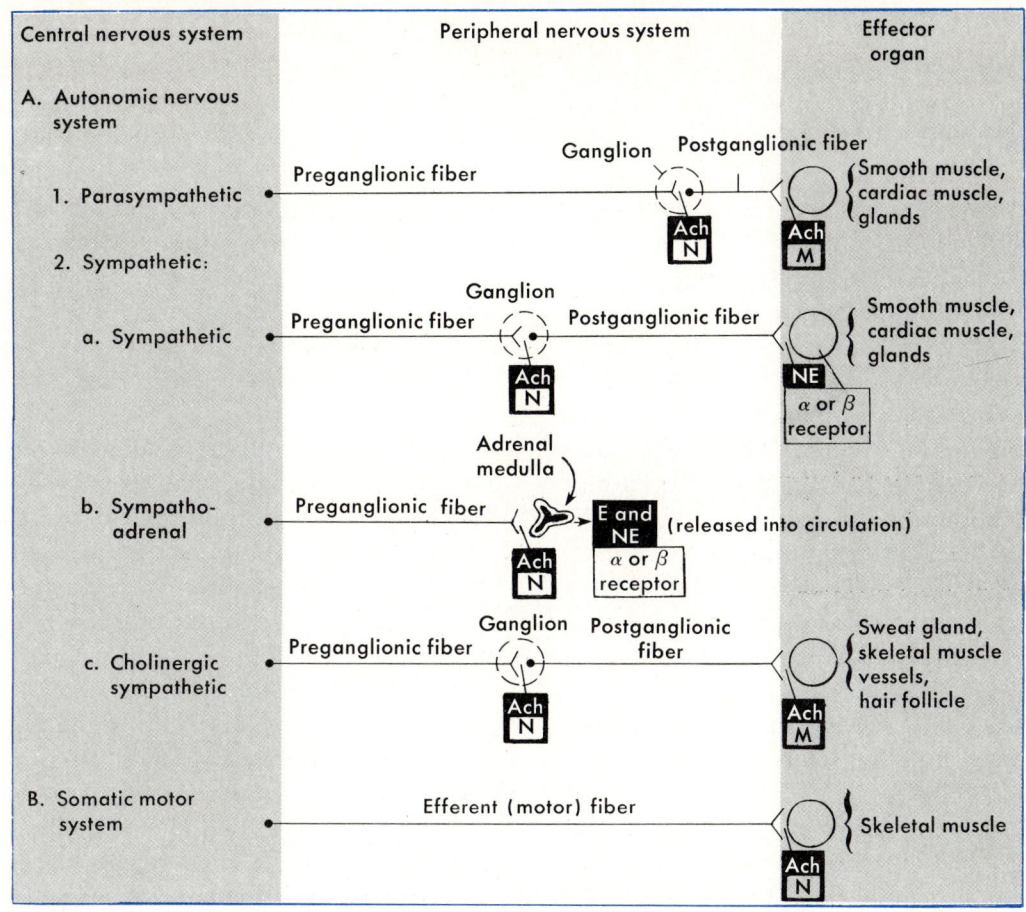

FIG. 13-6. Schema of sites of neurohumoral transmission. **A,** In the autonomic nervous system, the preganglionic fibers of both the parasympathetic and sympathetic divisions synapse in the ganglia of the postganglionic fibers and the adrenal medulla. The release of acetylcholine *(ACh)* by terminals of preganglionic fibers interact with nicotinic *(N)* receptors in the membrane of the postganglionic neurons or adrenal medullary cells. *1,* In the parasympathetic system, the terminals of the postganglionic fibers release acetylcholine and interact with muscarinic *(M)* sites in the membrane of smooth muscle, cardiac muscle, and glands. *2,* In the sympathetic system, there are three types of postganglionic fibers: *a.* The *sympathetic* neuron—releases norepinephrine *(NE)* and activates alpha (α) or beta (β) receptors in the membrane of smooth muscle, cardiac muscle, and glands. *b.* The *sympathoadrenal* neuron of the adrenal medulla—secretes norepinephrine and epinephrine *(E),* which are circulated in the blood to all parts of the body to activate alpha or beta receptors. *c.* The cholinergic *sympathetic* neuron—releases acetylcholine and interacts with muscarinic sites on sweat glands and skeletal muscle vessels. **B,** The somatic motor nervous system has a single fiber whose terminals release acetylcholine and activates nicotinic receptor sites on the skeletal muscle.

tyrosine hydroxylase and dopamine β-hydroxylase, causing a decrease in the rate of formation of norepinephrine.

Release. The arrival of an action potential at the nerve terminal of the postganglionic fibers causes the vesicles to fuse with the cell membrane and extrude the stored supply of norepinephrine into the junctional cleft. The presence of calcium ions is required to enhance the release of norepinephrine from the vesicles. The free form of norepinephrine then diffuses across the cleft to the receptor sites on the postjunctional membrane of neuroeffector cells (smooth muscle, cardiac muscle, or glands).

Action. Once the transmitter combines with either the alpha or beta receptor sites on the membrane of the neuroeffector cells, a series of chemical and electrical events is initiated to produce either an excitatory or an inhibitory effect. The alpha receptor activation is primarily responsible for excitatory response, although it results in intestinal relaxation. By contrast, beta receptor activation is usually inhibitory except in the myocardial cells, where norepinephrine produces an excitatory effect.

Inactivation. Once norepinephrine has performed its adrenergic function, its action must be rapidly terminated to prevent the prolongation of its effects, which could lead to a loss of regulatory control of visceral function. The inactivation of norepinephrine is accomplished by (1) enzymatic transformation, (2) reuptake into nerve terminals, and (3) diffusion.

Catecholamines are metabolized by two enzymes, monoamine oxidase (MAO) and catechol-O-methyltransferase (COMT). Free norepinephrine liberated endogenously *within* the cytoplasm of the nerve terminal is metabolized by MAO, which is stored in the mitochondria of sympathetic neurons. The second or alternate metabolic pathway involves the action of COMT, which is located *outside* the neuron or at the synaptic cleft. COMT participates in the inactivation or metabolism of *extraneural* norepinephrine.

The *reuptake* mechanism plays a more significant role than enzymatic transformation in catecholamine inactivation. In the reuptake process norepinephrine is removed by active transport ("amine pump") from the junctional sites (synaptic and neuroeffector junctions) and is returned to the sympathetic nerve terminal and storage vesicles. Thus this mechanism provides a means other than the synthetic process for maintaining an adequate supply of norepinephrine.

Finally, a small portion of norepinephrine released at the synaptic cleft may be picked up by the circulation and metabolized elsewhere in the body. This is known as the diffusion process. Fig. 13-5 portrays the steps in adrenergic transmission.

Sites of neurohumoral transmission

In 1933, Dale and his co-workers determined the chemical differences between fibers that release acetylcholine (cholinergic fibers) and those that release norepinephrine and epinephrine (adrenergic fibers). The distribution of these fibers in the autonomic and somatic nervous systems is summarized in Fig. 13-6. In the autonomic nervous system, all the preganglionic fibers originate in the central nervous system and synapse with the ganglia of the postganglionic fibers. The terminals of all the preganglionic fibers release acetylcholine and interact with nicotinic receptors in the membrane of the postganglionic fibers or the adrenal medulla.

In the parasympathetic system the terminals of the postganglionic fibers also release acetylcholine and interact with muscarinic receptors in the membrane of the smooth muscle, cardiac muscle, and glands.

In the sympathetic nervous system there are three different kinds of postganglionic neurons: (1) the sympathetic neuron, the major type, which releases norepinephrine and activates either alpha or beta receptors in the membrane of the smooth muscle, cardiac muscle, and glands; (2) the sympathoadrenal neuron, in which the preganglionic fiber synapses with a modified sympathetic ganglion, the adrenal medulla, and releases mostly epinephrine and a small amount of norepinephrine, which are secreted into the circulation and carried to all parts of the body; and (3) the cholinergic sympathetic neuron, which releases acetylcholine and stimulates muscarinic receptor sites on the sweat glands to produce sweating and on the blood vessels in skeletal muscle to increase vasodilation and enhance blood flow.

In the somatic nervous system a single neuron, the efferent (motor) fiber, releases acetylcholine and interacts with the nicotinic sites on the skeletal muscle membrane. The autonomic drugs play an important role by either enhancing or inhibiting physiologic activity at these sites of neurohumoral transmission (Fig. 13-6).

Autonomic drugs and related compounds

The autonomic drugs mimic, intensify, or block the effects of the sympathetic and parasympathetic divisions of the autonomic nervous system. As a class, they are divided into the following groups:

1 Cholinergic (parasympathomimetic) drugs, such as bethanechol, that act like mediators of the parasympathetic nervous system

TABLE 13-4   Muscarinic and nicotinic actions of acetylcholine

	Muscarinic action	Nicotinic action	
Cardiovascular			
Blood vessels	Dilation	Constriction	With large doses after atropine
Heart rate	Slowed	Increased	
Blood pressure	Decreased	Increased	
Gastrointestinal			
Tone	Increased	Increased	
Motility	Increased	Increased	
Sphincters	Relaxed	—	
Glandular secretions	Increased salivary, lacrimal, intestinal, and sweat secretion	Initial stimulation, then inhibition of salivary and bronchial secretions	
Skeletal muscle	—	Stimulated	
Autonomic ganglia	—	Stimulated	
Eye	Pupil constriction Decreased accommodation	—	
Blocking agent	Atropine	Tubocurarine	
Remarks	Effects increase as dosage increases	Increased dosage inhibits effects and causes receptor blockade	

2 Cholinergic blocking (parasympatholytic) drugs, such as atropine, that block the action of the parasympathetic nervous system
3 Adrenergic (sympathomimetic) drugs, such as norepinephrine and epinephrine, that act like mediators of the sympathetic nervous system or the adrenal medulla, respectively
4 Adrenergic blocking (sympatholytic) drugs, such as propranolol, that block the action of the sympathetic nervous system

Cholinergic (parasympathomimetic) drugs

As previously mentioned, acetylcholine plays an important role in transmission of nerve impulses in both the sympathetic and parasympathetic divisions of the autonomic nervous system.

Acetylcholine has two major actions on the nervous system: (1) it has stimulant effects on the ganglia, adrenal medulla, and skeletal muscle, and (2) it has stimulant effects at postganglionic nerve endings in cardiac muscle, smooth muscle, and glands. The first action resembles the effects of nicotine and therefore is referred to as the "nicotinic action" of acetylcholine. The effects of acetylcholine at the effector cell are like that of muscarine (an alkaloid obtained from the toadstool *Amanita muscaria*), and they are referred to as the "muscarinic action" of acetylcholine. These terms are used in describing acetylcholine effects because both

nicotine and muscarine and their effects on nerve impulses were studied long before acetylcholine was identified or synthesized. See Table 13-4 for these actions and Fig. 13-6 for nicotonic and muscarinic sites.

Drugs that bring about effects in the body similar to those produced by acetylcholine are called *cholinergic drugs*. These agents are also designated *parasympathomimetics* because they appear to mimic the action produced by stimulation of the parasympathetic nervous system.

Cholinergic fibers are widespread: they are present in heart, spleen, uterus, vas deferens, colon, and the vessels of the skin and muscles. It is quite likely that cholinergic fibers are present in many more tissues of the body. In the gastrointestinal tract parasympathetic innervation predominates: it stimulates both motor and secretory action.

Although acetylcholine itself is important physiologically, it has no therapeutic value because (1) its actions are very brief owing to rapid hydrolysis by acetylcholinesterase and (2) no selective purpose can be achieved through its use, since it has multiple sites of action.

Cholinergic drugs may be obtained from plant sources or synthesized. The synthetic drugs are more stable and have a more selective action on particular organs. There are two groups of cholinergic drugs available: *direct acting* and *indirect acting. Direct-acting drugs combine directly with the cholinergic receptors in*

TABLE 13-5   Prominent cholinergic agents including the anticholinesterase drugs*

Generic name	Trade name	Single adult dose	Usual route of administration
Ambenonium	Mytelase	5-25 mg	Oral
Benzpyrinium	Stigmonene	2 mg	Intramuscular
Bethanechol	Urecholine	10-30 mg	Oral
			Sublingual
		2.5-5 mg	Subcutaneous
Isoflurophate	Floropryl	1-3 gtt 0.1% solution	Topical (eye)
Neostigmine	Prostigmin		
Bromide	Bromide	15 mg	Oral
Methylsulfate	Methylsulfate	0.5 mg (1-2 mg)	Intramuscular
Physostigmine	Eserine	0.02%-1% solution	Topical (eye)
Pilocarpine		0.5%-4% solution (1 gtt)	Topical (eye)
Pyridostigmine	Mestinon	Highly variable	Oral

*Effects to be expected are similar to those that can be expected from stimulation of the parasympathetic nervous system (see Table 13-3). Drugs are listed in alphabetical order. The majority of drugs mentioned are administered in the form of their salts.

postsynaptic membranes innervated by parasympathetic neurons and evoke effects similar to those produced by acetylcholine. By contrast, instead of a direct effect on receptors, *indirect-acting drugs act primarily on the enzyme by inhibiting the action of cholinesterase (acetylcholinesterase)* that normally degrades acetylcholine. This results in an accumulation of acetylcholine at all the sites where it is liberated. By rendering the enzymatic action ineffective, the anticholinesterase drugs cause a prolonged and intensified cholinergic response at the various effector sites.

Cholinergic drugs are used:

1 To stimulate the intestines and bladder postoperatively
2 To lower intraocular pressure in glaucoma
3 To promote salivation and sweating
4 To dilate peripheral blood vessels in conditions of vasospasm
5 To terminate curarization
6 To treat myasthenia gravis symptomatically

The use of cholinergic agents to treat cardiac dysrhythmias has been almost abandoned, since newer and more effective antidysrhythmic agents have been developed. The therapeutic effectiveness of cholinergic drugs depends primarily on their muscarinic action; however, some of them also possess nicotinic action. This latter action usually requires doses much larger than those used therapeutically. However, some drugs may exhibit more nicotinic than muscarinic effects.

The ideal cholinergic or anticholinesterase drug would:

1 Mimic or inhibit the effect of acetylcholine on a particular structure or organ
2 Be effective when administered orally
3 Be more stable and less easily inactivated than the drugs now available
4 Produce a therapeutic effect with minimal side effects

Although these ideal drugs are not yet available, progress has been and is being made in this direction.

Cholinergic drugs used primarily to lower intraocular pressure will be discussed in Chapter 17; these include pilocarpine and carbachol. Table 13-5 lists the prominent cholinergic and anticholinesterase drugs.

DIRECT-ACTING CHOLINERGIC DRUGS (CHOLINE ESTERS)

Drugs that are chemically similar to the neurotransmitter acetylcholine include bethanechol, carbachol, and methacholine. All compounds in this group are quarternary amines and as a result are poorly absorbed orally. Their actions are comparable to those of the physiologic mediator acetylcholine, but they are longer acting. The side effects of these drugs are a consequence of parasympathetic stimulation. They include bradycardia, hypotension, sweating, salivation, vomiting, diarrhea, and intestinal cramps.

Bethanechol chloride (Urecholine, Myotonachol)

Bethanechol is a cholinergic agent that has rather selective effects on the smooth muscle of the gastrointestinal and urinary tracts, where it promotes motility of the intestines and contraction of the bladder. Its action is primarily muscarinic. It does not exhibit any ganglion-stimulating effect. Bethanechol is not destroyed by cholinesterase; therefore its action is comparatively long. It is less potent than some of the other choline derivatives but is also less toxic. Cardiovascular effects are minimal.

Uses. Bethanechol is useful in conditions in which stimulation of the parasympathetic nervous system is indicated. It is used to treat gastric retention after vagotomy or gastric surgery, for postoperative abdominal distension, and for nonobstructive urinary retention.

Preparation, dosage, and administration. Bethanechol chloride is available in 1-ml ampules containing 5 mg of the drug and also in 5-, 10-, and 25-mg tablets. Bethanechol chloride is administered orally, sublingually, or subcutaneously. It must not be given intramuscularly or intravenously.

Oral and sublingual doses of 10 to 30 mg three or four times daily will usually control symptoms. The effect of the drug can usually be observed in about 30 minutes. When given orally it should be administered with meals, since it increases the volume and acidity of gastric secretions. The usual subcutaneous dose is 2.5 to 5 mg three or four times daily.

For children and infants the dosage is 0.6 mg/kg body weight divided into three oral doses. For subcutaneous use the dose is one third to one fourth the oral dose.

Side effects and toxic effects. Side effects of bethanechol include headache, flushing, abdominal cramps, sweating, asthmatic atacks, and sometimes a drop in blood pressure. Parenteral administration of atropine promptly abolishes side effects. The major advantage of bethanechol over other choline derivatives is its greater margin of safety and low incidence of severe toxic effects.

Contraindications. Bethanechol should not be used after gastrointestinal anastomosis until healing has occurred; it should not be used when peritonitis is present or when there is inflammatory disease. Its use is also contraindicated during pregnancy or in patients with coronary disease, hyperthyroidism, asthma, and gastrointestinal or urinary obstruction.

Methacholine chloride (Mecholyl Chloride)

At the present time methacholine is not a popular drug. It has been used for many different conditions—to improve muscle tone of various organs, increase secretions, treat paroxysmal atrial tachycardia—and in the diagnosis of pheochromocytoma. For the latter, a positive test results when the patient responds to a subcutaneous injection of methacholine with a rise in blood pressure caused by catecholamine release from the tumor. It has primarily muscarinic action and little nicotinic action.

Pilocarpine

Pilocarpine is found in the leaves of the plant *Pilocarpus jaborandi*. It is employed in ophthalmology because it constricts the pupil. The drug also causes considerable salivation and sweating when given orally or by subcutaneous injection.

INDIRECT-ACTING CHOLINERGIC DRUGS (ANTICHOLINESTERASES)

The indirect-acting cholinergic drugs are called anticholinesterases because they inhibit the action of the enzyme cholinesterase, thereby prolonging the effect of acetylcholine. Anticholinesterase agents exert their influence on both muscarinic and nicotinic sites. They are used in the treatment of myasthenia gravis and glaucoma. (See Chapters 10 and 17.) Certain compounds in this group are considered to be potent agents for chemical warfare.

DRUGS USED FOR TREATMENT OF MYASTHENIA GRAVIS

Myasthenia gravis is a condition characterized clinically by weakness of the skeletal muscles innervated by the somatic efferent fibers. Since the disease affects cholinergic transmission, the anticholinesterase drugs are used because they elevate the concentration of acetylcholine at the myoneural junctions. The prolonged activity of the neurohormone at these sites results in a dramatic increase in muscle strength and function. A more extensive discussion of myasthenia gravis and its treatment can be found in Chapter 10.

Cholinergic blocking (parasympatholytic) drugs

The cholinergic blocking drugs, which act selectively on postganglionic sites and block the muscarinic effects of acetylcholine, have many important uses in medicine. These agents are also called anticholinergic or parasympatholytic drugs. They act as competitive inhibitors of acetylcholine by occupying receptor sites normally taken up by acetylcholine. When stimulation of the nerve fiber occurs, the acetylcholine liberated from the terminal is unable to bind to the receptor site and thus fails to produce a cholinergic effect.

ATROPINE-LIKE GROUP

Cholinergic blocking agents are also known as antimuscarinics, and their prototype is atropine, a belladonna alkaloid. They relax smooth muscle, inhibit secretions of duct glands, and dilate the pupils. In toxic doses these agents produce skeletal muscle paralysis. Anticholinergic agents may be obtained from natural sources, or they may be synthesized. The synthetic drugs tend to have fewer side effects than the natural products.

A number of plants belonging to the potato family (Solanaceae) contain similar alkaloids. Included are *Atropa belladonna* (deadly nightshade), *Hyoscyamus niger* (henbane),* *Datura stramonium* (jimsonweed or thorn apple),† and several species of *Scopolia*. The principal alkaloids of these plants are atropine, scopolamine (hyoscine), and hyoscyamine.

---

*Henbane is thought to be a corruption of hennebell, which suggests a musical instrument. In medieval Latin, henbane was referred to as *Symphoniaca herba*, symphoniaca being a rod with many bells on it. (Wootton.) Henbane is the bane of domestic fowl.
†Jimsonweed is a corruption of Jamestown weed, so called because it was early observed as a weed in Jamestown, Virginia. It is given its other name, thorn apple, because of its spiny capsule.

Atropa belladonna was the name conferred on one of these plants by Linnaeus in 1753. The first part of the name was selected because of the poisonous qualities of the plant and is called Atropa after Atropos, the eldest of the Greek Fates who supposedly cut the thread of life. The second part of the name, belladonna, means beautiful lady and was chosen because of the custom practiced by certain Roman women who placed belladonna preparations in their eyes to make them appear larger and more lustrous.

Atropine

Atropine is the chief alkaloid of the plant *Atropa belladonna*, which is grown for commercial purposes in Germany, England, Austria, and North America. It is also synthesized.

Atropine is the prototype of the anticholinergic drugs. It has been in use for over half a century and continues to be a popular drug because of its therapeutic effectiveness.

Action and result. Atropine may have a local, central, or peripheral action.

Local. There is a slight amount of absorption when atropine or belladonna is applied to the skin, especially if it is oily or alcoholic preparation or in the form of a plaster.

When an aqueous solution of atropine is dropped into the conjunctival sac of the eye, it quickly produces dilation of the pupil, diminished secretion of tears, and impaired ability to focus objects close to the eye. If the eye if normal, there is little change in intraocular tension, but it may increase in patients who have glaucoma.

Central. Atropine has prominent effects on the central nervous system and in large doses causes excitement and maniacal behavior. These behavioral effects suggest the existence of important cholinergic pathways and receptors within the central nervous system.

CEREBRUM. Small or moderate doses of atropine have little or no cerebral effect. Large or toxic doses cause the patient to become restless, wakeful, and talkative. This condition may develop into delirium and finally stupor and coma. The exalted, excited stage has sometimes been called a "belladonna jag." A rise in temperature is sometimes seen, especially in infants and young children. This is probably the result of suppression of sweating rather than action on the heat-regulating center.

Atropine has been used to diminish tremor in Parkinson's disease. It probably reduces cholinergic synaptic transmission.

MEDULLA. Therapeutic doses of atropine stimulate the respiratory center and make breathing faster and sometimes deeper. When respiration is seriously depressed, atropine is not always reliable as a stimulant; in fact, it may deepen the depression. Large doses stimulate respiration, but they can also cause respiratory failure and death.

Small doses stimulate the vagus center in the medulla, causing primary slowing of the heart. The vasoconstrictor center is stimulated briefly and then depressed. Because depression follows rather soon after stimulation, atropine has been called a borderline stimulant of the central nervous system.

Peripheral. The main therapeutic uses of atropine are the result of its peripheral action rather than its central action. The more important effect is on the smooth muscle, cardiac muscle, and gland cells, which are supplied by postganglionic cholinergic nerves. Atropine is a competitive antagonist of acetylcholine; by occupying receptor sites, atropine prevents or reduces the muscarinic action of acetylcholine. To some extent, atropine brings about effects similar to those produced by stimulation of postganglionic fibers in the sympathetic nervous system. The following results of peripheral action are seen.

EYE. The pupil is dilated (mydriasis) and the muscle of accommodation is paralyzed (cycloplegia). The sphincter muscle of the iris and the ciliary muscle are both innervated by cholinergic nerve fibers and therefore are affected by atropine. Since the spincter muscle is unable to contract normally, the radial muscle of the iris causes the pupil to dilate. Pupil dilation may reduce outflow of aqueous humor, causing a rise in intraocular pressure, a hazardous situation for patients with glaucoma. These effects in the eye are brought about by both local and systemic administration of atropine, although

the usual single therapeutic dose of atropine given orally or parenterally has little effect on the eye. After the pupil is dilated, photophobia occurs, and when the drug has reached its full effect, the usual reflexes to light and accommodation disappear.

RESPIRATORY TRACT. Secretions of the nose, pharynx, and bronchial tubes are decreased. The muscles of the bronchial tubes relax and the airway widens to ease breathing. Atropine and scopolamine are less effective than epinephrine as bronchodilators and are seldom used for asthma.

HEART AND BLOOD VESSELS. When the usual clinical doses are given, the cardiac rate is temporarily and slightly slowed because of the central action of the drug on the cardiac center in the medulla. Moderate-to-large doses accelerate the heart by interfering with the response of the heart muscle to vagal nerve impulses. The latter is a peripheral action. The ability of atropine to interfere with vagal stimuli explains its use in the treatment of sinus bradycardia and atrioventricular heart block. In therapeutic doses atropine has little or no effect on blood pressure, although large and sometimes ordinary doses cause vasodilation of vessels in the skin of the face and neck. This may result from a direct dilator action or from histamine release. Reddening of the face and neck is seen, especially after large or toxic doses.

GLANDS. Since the sweat glands of the skin are supplied by cholinergic nerves, atropine decreases or abolishes their activity. This causes the skin to become hot and dry. The flow of saline and mucus from glands lining the respiratory tract is reduced, and drying of the mucous membranes of the mouth, nose, pharynx, and bronchi occurs. Patients who have been given atropine, particularly for preoperative preparation, often complain of a dry mouth and thirst. Some of this discomfort may be relieved by frequent rinsing of the mouth.

Although some difference of opinion exists among authorities as to the effect of atropine on the activity of gastric glands, it appears that the amount and character of the gastric secretion are little affected by atropine given in ordinary therapeutic doses. The secretion of acid in the stomach is presumably less under vagal control than under hormonal or chemical control. The effect of atropine on the secretion of the pancreas and intestinal glands is not therapeutically significant.

SMOOTH MUSCLE. Atropine and other belladonna alkaloids decrease tone and peristalsis in the stomach and small and large intestine. Atropine does not affect the secretion of bile, but it exerts a mildly antispasmodic effect in the gallbladder and bile ducts. The drug exerts a relaxing effect on the ureter, especially when it has been in a state of spasm. Therapeutic doses decrease the tone of the fundus of the urinary bladder. When the detrusor muscle is hypertonic, it is relaxed by atropine.

The power of atropine to decrease the activity of uterine muscle is thought to be negligible. It is at best only mildly antispasmodic.

USES. Atropine is especially useful as a preliminary medication before surgical anesthesia. It decreases secretions of the mouth and respiratory passages and is effective in the prevention of laryngospasm.

Atropine and shorter-acting anticholinergics may be used as mydriatics and cycloplegics in examinations of the eye and in the treatment of certain eye conditions. Atropine is used especially for refraction of the eyes of children who need a potent drug to paralyze the muscle of accommodation. Homatropine, a shorter-acting cycloplegic and mydriatic, is usually satisfactory for adults.

Atropine is sometimes given with morphine to relieve biliary and renal colic. Atropine tends to relieve the muscular spasm induced by morphine.

Preparations of belladonna or its alkaloids are administered for their antispasmodic effects in conditions characterized by hypermotility of the stomach and bowel—pylorospasm, spastic colon, biliary and renal colic, and hypertonicity of the urinary bladder and ureters. These drugs are also found in certain cough remedies (antiasthmatic mixtures), in which case they are given to relieve mild conditions of bronchial spasm and excessive secretions. Atropine has a mild antihistaminic effect.

Symptoms in selected cases of Parkinson's disease are also relieved—the tremor, muscular rigidity, and cramps. However, other drugs are superior to atropine for this use.

Preparation, dosage, and administration. The following are the available preparations of atropine.

Atropine sulfate. Tablets containing 0.3, 0.4, and 0.6 mg of drug are available. These correspond to gr $\frac{1}{200}$, $\frac{1}{150}$, and $\frac{1}{100}$, respectively. The drug is also available in multiple-dose vials (gr $\frac{1}{150}$ per milliliter) for injection and in the form of atropine sulfate ophthalmic ointment. Atropine sulfate is usually administered subcutaneously, orally, or topically (in the eye). The usual subcutaneous or oral dose is 0.5 mg (gr $\frac{1}{120}$), although 0.4 mg (gr $\frac{1}{150}$) is frequently ordered. The ophthalmic solution and the ointment are usually used in a 0.5% or 1% concentration.

Belladonna extract. The extract is prepared from belladonna leaf and contains alkaloids of the leaf. It is given orally, usually in doses of 15 mg (gr $\frac{1}{4}$).

Belladonna tincture. The usual dose is 0.6 ml (10 minims), although the range of dosage may be from 0.3 to 2.4 ml. It is given orally.

Absorption, distribution, and excretion. Atropine (and also scopolamine) is readily absorbed after oral and parenteral administration. It is also absorbed from mucous membranes, as is noted when ophthalmic solutions escape through the lacrimal ducts to the mucous membrane of the nose. To a lesser extent, atropine is also absorbed from the skin. The drug is widely distributed in the fluids of the body and easily passes the placental barrier to the blood of the fetus. It is excreted chiefly by way of the kidney. Some is excreted through the bile. The remainder is apparently metabolized in the liver. Traces are found in other secretions, such as the milk.

Side effects and toxic effects. Atropine is a potent alkaloid, but is has a wide margin of safety. Poisoning occurs but is rarely fatal. The fatal dose is said to be about 100 mg for adults and 10 mg for children. Survival has occurred after much larger doses.

Symptoms develop rapidly after overdosage and consist of dry mouth, great thirst, and difficulty in swallowing and talking. Vision becomes blurred, pupils are dilated, and photophobia is present. A rash may develop, chiefly over the face, neck, and upper trunk. Rash is seen particularly in children, although it may occur in adults. The body temperature is elevated, and in young children and infants it may reach 107° F and more. The skin of the face and neck is flushed; the pulse becomes rapid and may be weak. Urinary urgency and difficulty in emptying the bladder may be noted. The patient becomes restless, excited, talkative, and confused. This may progress to delirium and mania and may be mistaken for an acute psychosis. The patient may also experience giddiness, staggering, stupor, coma, and respiratory and circulatory failure. (See Table 13-6.)

Young children who are given atropine or scopolamine as a preanesthetic medication often have a pronounced cutaneous flush after administration of the drug. Parents may be much disturbed about this and think that the child is ill with an acute disease. This is a side effect and is not seen as often in adults as in children.

Contraindications. Atropine and related alkaloids are usually contraindicated for patients with glaucoma because of the tendency to mydriatics to increase intraocular tension.

Treatment of overdosage. If the drug has been taken by mouth, the stomach should be lavaged promptly with tannic acid solution. Administration of syrup of ipecac or activated charcoal will help to inhibit further absorption of the drug. Neostigmine or pilocarpine is sometimes given subcutaneously in doses of 10 mg until the mouth is moist. Physostigmine has also been recommended and is becoming an important antidote in atropine poisoning. Artificial respiration, oxygen, or oxygen and carbon dioxide may be indicated. Short-acting barbiturates, chloral hydrate, or paraldehyde may be given to relieve excitement. Ice bags and alcohol sponge baths aid in reducing the fever.

Scopolamine (hyoscine)

Action. Scopolamine resembles atropine in its peripheral effects but differs in its central action, since doses of the drug given parenterally depress the central nervous system, producing drowsiness, euphoria, relief of fear, relaxation, sleep, and amnesia. Some "over-the-

TABLE 13-6 Side effects characteristic of cholinergic blocking agents

Dryness of mouth	Mental confusion
Dilation of pupils (mydriasis)*	Excitement
	Dizziness; headache
Blurred vision	Constipation
Heart palpitation	Urinary retention
Flushing and dryness of skin	

*A symptom such as mydriasis is not a side effect when this is the purpose for which a drug is given.

counter" sleeping pills (for example, Sleep-Eze) contain small amounts of scopolamine.

Uses. Scopolamine is used as a preanesthetic medication, usually along with morphine or one of the barbiturates, to check secretions and to prevent laryngospasm, as well as for its sedative (twilight sleep) and amnesic effects.

It is used for motion sickness because of its depressant action on vestibular function, but for this use it has largely been supplanted by newer drugs. It is employed as a sedative for certain maniacal and delirious patients and also for postencephalitic parkinsonism and paralysis agitans.

It is also used as a mydriatic and cycloplegic. Its effects appear more promptly and disappear more rapidly than those of atropine. Scopolamine is less likely to cause irritation in the eyes than atropine.

Preparation, dosage, and administration. The following are the available preparations of scopolamine.

Scopolamine hydrobromide; hyoscine hydrobromide. This drug is available in 0.6-mg (gr 1/200) tablets, which can be given orally or parenterally. The usual adult dose is 0.6 mg orally or subcutaneously; the range of dose is 0.3 to 0.8 mg. The dose for children is 0.006 mg/kg body weight orally or subcutaneously. Ophthalmic solutions are applied topically to the eye in 0.2% concentration.

Hyoscine eye ointment. The ointment contains 0.25% hyoscine hydrobromide.

Scopolamine hydrobromide injection; hyoscine injection. The injection is available in ampules containing 0.3, 0.4, and 0.6 mg in 1 ml and 0.4 mg in 0.5 ml. The dosage is 0.3 to 0.8 mg subcutaneously.

SYNTHETIC SUBSTITUTES FOR ATROPINE (ANTISPASMODICS)

The usefulness of atropine is limited by the fact that it is a complex drug and produces effects in a number of organs or tissues simultaneously. When it is administered for its antispasmodic effects, it also produces prolonged effects in the eye, causing dilated pupils and blurred vision, as well as dry mouth and possibly rapid heart rate. When the antispasmodic effect is the one desired, other effects become side effects, which may be distinctly undesirable.

A large number of drugs have been synthesized in an effort to capture the antispasmodic effect of atropine without its other effects. Drugs of this type are frequently used to relieve hypertonicity and hypersecretion in the stomach and to treat patients with gastric and duodenal ulcers.

The ideal drug for the management of peptic ulcer should block the mechanism of gastric secretion without producing blockage in the autonomic ganglia and without causing curariform effects (muscle weakness). It should be relatively nontoxic and palatable and should reduce both the volume and the acidity of the gastric secretion over long periods of time. It should be effective when given orally. It should not produce troublesome or adverse side effects. The ideal drug has not been found, which probably explains why so many different preparations are available. Seemingly no single preparation excels.

The synthesis of new anticholinergic drugs continues, and if the claims for longer action and greater effectiveness are substantiated after long trial, more useful therapeutic agents may become available.

Like most of the cholinergic blocking agents, the atropine substitutes are contraindicated for patients with glaucoma, pyloric obstruction, and prostatic hypertrophy.

Methscopolamine bromide (Pamine Bromide)

Action. Methscopolamine bromide is an anticholinergic drug that produces antispasmodic and antisecretory effects. It can suppress both volume and acidity of gastric secretion if large enough doses are given. It slows the emp-

tying of the stomach and reduces peristalsis in the bowel. It decreases secretion of salvia and sweat. Tolerance to the medication does not seem to develop.

Uses. Methscopolamine bromide is used as an antispasmodic in the treatment of patients with peptic ulcer and forms of gastritis associated with hypermotility and hyperacidity. It is also occasionally used to relieve excessive salivation and sweating.

Preparation, dosage, and administration. Methscopolamine bromide is available in 2.5-mg tablets and in solution for injection (1 mg/ml). The usual dosage for adults is 2.5 mg administered before meals and at bedtime. The usual parenteral dose is 0.5 mg intramuscularly or subcutaneously every 6 to 8 hours as needed to control symptoms. It is also available as a syrup and as an elixir containing phenobarbital.

Side effects of toxic effects. The side effects most frequently encountered include dry mouth, constipation, and blurred vision. Other effects encountered less frequently may include dizziness, palpitation, flushed dry skin, difficult urination, headache, and nausea.

Overdosage may bring about a ganglionic blocking action and a curare-like effect on skeletal muscle.

Methantheline bromide (Banthine Bromide)

Action. Methantheline bromide has an anticholinergic action similar to that of atropine. It has a ganglionic blocking action in the autonomic nervous system, as well as a curare-like effect on skeletal muscle. It inhibits motility of the stomach and delays emptying time, inhibits motility of the small intestine and genitourinary tract, and diminishes secretions.

Uses. It is used as an antispasmodic in the treatment of patients with pylorospasm, hypermotility of the intestine, spastic colon, and spasm of the ureter and urinary bladder. Some degree of pupillary dilation accompanies the antispasmodic effect.

Preparation, dosage, and administration. Methantheline bromide is available in 50-mg tablets for oral administration and in ampules, each containing 50 mg. The content of the ampule is dissolved in physiologic saline solution for the purpose of injection (intramuscularly or intravenously). Parenteral administration is not recommended if the patient can take the drug orally. The tablets should not be chewed because they have an unpleasant taste. Antacids with adsorbent action, such as aluminum hydroxide, should not be given with methantheline.

The usual initial dose for adults is 50 mg, although the usual effective dose is 100 mg four times a day, before meals and at bedtime. Some patients require more, some less, than this amount. The recommended dosage is the smallest amount that will effectively relieve the symptoms. Onset of action occurs within 30 to 45 minutes and persists for 4 to 6 hours. The dosage for children is 6 mg/kg body weight daily in four divided doses.

Side effects and toxic effects. Side effects may occur in the form of dryness of the mouth, dilated pupils, and inability to read fine print. Some patients may have constipation and require a laxative. Varying degrees of urinary retention have been observed in patients with prostatic hypertrophy. A small percentage of patients complain of general malaise and weakness and do not tolerate the drug well. The general side effects characteristic of cholinergic blocking agents are presented in Table 13-6.

Propantheline bromide (Pro-Banthine Bromide)

Action. Propantheline bromide is an analog of methantheline bromide and is said to be more effective than the latter drug in reducing the volume and acidity of gastric secretions. It is also said to produce less severe side effects. It has come to replace the older drug to a great extent.

Preparation, dosage, and administration. Propantheline is available in 7.5- and 15-mg tablets, 30-mg prolonged action tablets, and 30-mg vials as a powder for intramuscular or intravenous injection. The content of the vial is dissolved in not less than 10 ml of water for injection before intravenous administration. Parenteral administration is reserved for patients who cannot take the drug orally. Propantheline bromide is also available in tablets that contain phenobarbital.

The dosage of propantheline must be carefully adjusted to the needs of individual patients. The initial recommended dose is one tablet (15 mg) with meals and two tablets at bedtime, with subsequent adjustment depending on the patient's reaction and tolerance to the medication. The bitter taste of methantheline bromide has been controlled by sugar-coating the Pro-Banthine tablet. The dosage for children is 1.5 mg/kg body weight daily in four divided doses.

Side effects. Propantheline is thought to have less severe but not less frequent side effects than methantheline bromide.

Homatropine methylbromide (Novatrin, Mesopin)

Action. Homatropine methylbromide is one of the older cholinergic blocking agents used in the United States. Its effects are similar to those of atropine, but it is without the latter drug's effect on the central nervous system. Its anticholinergic potency is said to be considerably less than that of atropine, but it is also less toxic. Its effect on gastric secretion and motility and its duration of action are said to be much the same as those of atropine.

Uses. Homatropine methylbromide is used for the treatment of gastrointestinal spasm and as an adjunct in the treatment of patients with peptic ulcer.

Preparation, dosage, and administration. Homatropine methylbromide is available in 2.5-, 5-, and 10-mg tablets and as an elixir containing 5 mg in 5 ml. The usual oral dose is 2.5 to 5 mg three or four times daily. Solutions are also available for injection and for oral administration. The dosage for children is 3 to 6 mg, in chewable tablets four times daily. The dosage for infants with colic is 1 mg (elixir) four times daily.

Side effects. Side effects of homatropine methylbromide include dryness of the mouth and blurring of vision.

Pipenzolate bromide (Piptal)

Action and result. Pipenzolate bromide is a synthetic anticholinergic drug with effects comparable to those of atropine. It diminishes gastric acidity and gastric motility and relieves

TABLE 13-7 Summary of some of the anticholinergic agents*

Generic name	Trade name	Usual single adult dose	Usual route of administration
Atropine		0.5 mg	Oral or subcutaneous
		0.5%-1% ophthalmic solution	Topical
Scopolamine		0.6 mg	Oral or subcutaneous
Hyoscine		0.2% ophthalmic solution	Topical
Synthetic mydriatics and cycloplegics			
Homatropine hydrobromide		1%-2% ophthalmic solution	Topical
Synthetic antispasmodics			
Homatropine methylbromide	Novatrin, Mesopin	5-10 mg	Oral
Methscopolamine bromide	Pamine	2.5-5 mg	Oral
Methantheline bromide	Banthine	50 mg	Oral
Propantheline	Pro-Banthine	15 mg	Oral
Pipenzolate	Piptal	5 mg	Oral

*Drugs listed are usually administered in the form of their salts.

spasms. It is used to treat peptic ulcers. The ability of pipenzolate to relax spasms of the lower gastrointestinal tract of the sphincter of Oddi makes it useful in the treatment of ileitis, irritable colon, and biliary colic.

Preparation, dosage, and administration. Pipenzolate bromide is available in 5-mg tablets for oral administration. The average adult dose is 5 mg three times daily before meals and 5 to 10 mg at bedtime. The onset of action is about 1 hour; the duration of effect is 4 hours.

Side effects and toxic effects. Pipenzolate has a minimum of side effects, and those are chiefly atropine-like in nature. No serious toxic reactions have been reported to date.

Ganglionic stimulant
Nicotine

Nicotine is a liquid alkaloid, freely soluble in water. It turns brown on exposure to air. It is the chief alkaloid found in tobacco.

Nicotine has no therapeutic use but is of great pharmacologic interest and toxicologic importance. Its use in experiments performed on animals has helped to increase understanding of the autonomic nervous system.

Absorption. Nicotine is readily absorbed from the gastrointestinal tract, respiratory mucous membrane, and skin.

Action and result. Nicotine produces a temporary stimulation of all sympathetic and para-

sympathetic ganglia. This is followed by depression, which tends to last longer than the period of stimulation. Its effects on skeletal muscle is similar to its effects on the ganglia; that is, a depressant phase follows stimulation. During the depressant phase nicotine exerts a curare-like action on skeletal muscle.

In addition, nicotine stimulates the central nervous system, especially the medullary centers (respiratory, emetic, and vasomotor). Large doses may cause tremor and convulsions. Stimulation is followed by depression. Death is caused by respiratory failure, although it may be caused more by the curariform action of nicotine on nerve endings in the diaphragm, which prevents respiratory muscles from responding, than by action on the respiratory center.

The actions and effects of nicotine on the blood-vascular system are complex. The rate of the heart is frequently slowed at first, but later it may beat faster than usual. Various disturbances in rhythm have been observed. The small blood vessels in peripheral parts of the body constrict but may later dilate, and the blood pressure will fall. The latter condition is observed in nicotine poisoning. Nicotine also has an antidiuretic action.

Repeated administration of nicotine causes tolerance to develop to some of its effects.

Toxic effects. Nicotine can cause acute or chronic poisoning.

Acute poisoning. Nicotine is a rapid-acting,

extremely toxic drug. Cases of gardeners who were poisoned while handling the drug as an insecticide have been reported. Death occurred in a few minutes. Black Leaf 40 is a commercial preparation that contains nicotine and is used as a spray to kill various types of insects.

Symptoms of poisoning include increased flow of saliva, nausea, vomiting, abdominal cramps, diarrhea, cold sweat, confusion, fainting, drop in blood pressure, rapid pulse, prostration, and collapse. Convulsions sometimes occur. Death results from respiratory failure.

Treatment is directed toward keeping the patient breathing. Artificial respiration with oxygen is said to be more effective than central respiratory stimulants. If life can be prolonged to give the tissues an opportunity to detoxify the drug, the patient may recover.

If the poison has been swallowed, gastric lavage with a solution of potassium permanganate (1:10,000) is recommended. Other forms of treatment depend on the symptoms present.

Tobacco smoking and nicotine. The effect of tobacco in the individual who smokes is a subject about which there is considerable difference of opinion. The effects of excessive smoking seem to afford more agreement than the effects of mild or moderate use of tobacco. Excessive smoking is known to cause irritation of the respiratory tract, and it is now generally accepted that tobacco smoke exerts carcinogenic effects in the human lung. Chronic dyspepsia may develop in heavy smokers, and patients with gastric ulcer are usually advised to avoid overindulgence. Of considerable importance is the fact that smokers absorb sufficient nicotine to exert a variety of effects on the autonomic nervous system.

In patients with peripheral vascular disease such as thromboangiitis obliterans (Buerger's disease), nicotine is generally believed to be a contributing factor in the disease and may precipitate spasms of the peripheral blood vessels and thus reduce the blood flow through the affected vessels. Vasospasm in the retinal blood vessels of the eye, associated with smoking of tobacco, is thought to be the cause of a serious disturbance of vision.

Roth found that nicotine in cigarettes must be reduced more than 60% before vascular effects of smoking fail to appear or are only slight.

Some physicians recommend that patients with hypertension and peripheral vascular disease sharply limit their smoking habits or discontinue smoking entirely. The adverse effects of cigarette smoking on the cardiovascular system are increasingly emphasized as a contributing factor in pulmonary emphysema and bronchogenic carcinoma.

Adrenergic (sympathomimetic) drugs

DIRECT-ACTING ADRENERGIC DRUGS

The adrenergic drugs included in this group—the catecholamines—depend on their ability to interact *directly* with adrenergic receptors (alpha and beta) and are called *direct-acting* drugs. Thus the response of these agents is mediated by directly stimulating the adrenergic receptors.

CATECHOLAMINES

As previously discussed, the three naturally occurring catecholamines in the body—dopamine, norepinephrine, and epinephrine—are a part of the synthetic pathway.

In the past great interest was evoked by confusing and conflicting reports that the effects of sympathetic nerve stimulation and the effects of epinephrine injection did not always correspond. In the mid-1940s it was shown that epinephrine had a twin, norepinephrine. With the recognition that these were separate substances that occurred naturally in the body, the confusion began to resolve. With further research one more catecholamine has been positively identified—dopamine. Dopamine is a precursor of norepinephrine and epinephrine. However, dopamine has a transmitter role of its own in certain portions of the central nervous system. Epinephrine acts mainly as an emergency hormone, while norepinephrine is an important transmitter of nerve impulses. It is also an intermediary in epinephrine biosynthesis.

The term "catecholamine" originates from organic chemistry. Catechol is dihydroxybenzene, and a glance at Fig. 13-7 will show that dopamine, norepinephrine, and epinephrine are all catechols as well as amines.

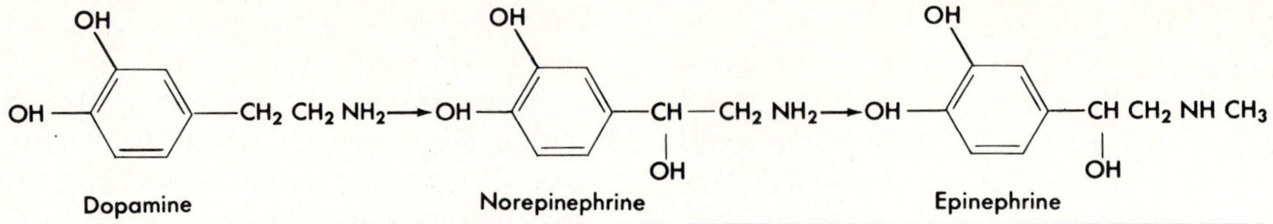

FIG. 13-7. Structural similarity of catecholamines.

T A B L E 1 3 - 8   Adrenergic receptor stimulation

Organ	Alpha receptor	Beta receptor
Heart	—	
Cardiac muscle		Increased contractility of atria and ventricles
Sinoatrial node		Increased heart rate
Atrioventricular node		Increased conduction velocity;
Conductive tissue		shortened refractory period
Arteries	Constriction	Relaxation
Veins	Constriction	Relaxation
Bronchial smooth muscle		Relaxation

In 1948 Ahlquist helped to clarify the varied actions of the catecholamines by showing that in the sympathetic nervous system the adrenergic effector cells contained two distinct receptors, the alpha (α) and beta (β) receptors. Norepinephrine acts mainly on alpha receptors and may cause pure vasoconstriction, whereas epinephrine acts on both alpha and beta receptors and produces a mixture of vasodilation and vasoconstriction. Isoproterenol, a synthetic catecholamine, acts only on beta receptors.

The most important alpha adrenergic activities in man are (1) vasoconstriction of arterioles in the skin and splanchnic area, resulting in a rise in blood pressure; (2) pupil dilation; and (3) relaxation of the gut. Beta adrenergic activity includes (1) cardiac acceleration and increased contractility; (2) vasodilation of arterioles supplying skeletal muscles; (3) bronchial relaxation; and (4) uterine relaxation. The effects of both alpha and beta stimulation will result from a summation of action where they are interrelated. That is, a change in blood pressure will depend on the degree of vasoconstriction in the skin and splanchnic area *and* the extent of vasodilation in skeletal muscles. Large arteries and veins contain both alpha and beta receptors; the heart contains only beta receptors (see Table 13-8).

While there are specific drugs that stimulate the alpha or beta receptors, there are also drugs that selectively block alpha or beta receptors. Most adrenergic blocking agents are alpha blockers; these drugs include ergot derivatives such as phenoxybenzamine. In the United States in 1968 a beta receptor blocking agent, propranolol, became available for clinical use. These agents effect blockade at peripheral autonomic sites, which distinguishes them from ganglionic blocking agents that act as the ganglia. The beta receptors may be subdivided on the basis of their responses to drugs into $beta_1$ and $beta_2$ receptors. The $beta_1$ receptors are located mainly in the heart, whereas the $beta_2$ receptors mediate the actions of catecholamines on bronchioles and arterial smooth muscles (dilator actions).

As catecholamines, norepinephrine and epinephrine are neurohormones that serve important functions in neural and endocrine integration. They are continuously present in arterial blood, although the amount varies widely during any one day. Certain physiologic stimuli such as stress and exercise significantly increase blood levels of catecholamine.

Studies indicate that the major source of circulating norepinephrine comes from stimulated sympathetic nerve endings. Organs that receive a large fraction of blood and contain large numbers of sympathetic nerve endings contain the greatest amount of catecholamines. (Examples of such organs are the heart and blood vessels.) Thus the number of sympathetic nerve endings or adrenergic nerves to various organs determines the magnitude of response of these organs to increased levels or injections of catecholamines.

Pharmacologic effects. Catacholamines produce a variety of physiologic responses as evidenced by the following effects.

Cardiac effects. Epinephrine and nonepinephrine produce almost the same cardiac responses when injected. These responses include the following.

MARKED INCREASE IN MYOCARDIAL CONTRACTION (POSITIVE INOTROPIC EFFECT). This increase is probably the result of an enhancement of influx of calcium into cardiac fibers. The strong myocardial contractions result in more complete emptying of the ventricles and an increase in cardiac work and oxygen consumption. The strong contractions brought about by isoproterenol and epinephrine also increase cardiac output, or minute volume. Norepinephrine, on the other hand, may not alter cardiac output and may even decrease it slightly. This effect of norepinephrine is believed to result from its potent vasoconstricting action, which increases resistance to ejection. The increased work of the heart to move the blood against increased pressure is "pressure work" rather than "volume work."

It has been shown experimentally and clinically that 0.5 mg of epinephrine injected into arterial or venous blood and circulated by cardiac compression or massage may stimulate spontaneous and vigorous cardiac contractions. Even though the heart is in ventricular fibrillation, epinephrine increases fibrillation vigor and frequently promotes successful electric defibrillation of the patient. In these situations the drug may be injected repeatedly. Use of other drugs is also necessary, such as sodium bicarbonate to overcome acidosis. However, epinephrine cannot be used repeatedly to improve the function of a failing heart (congestive heart failure), since it increases oxygen consumption by cardiac muscle. It can also cause anginal pain in patients with angina pectoris because it increases cardiac oxygen demand. Therefore, although it increases coro-

nary blood flow, its use is contraindicated for patients with angina.

The production of strong contractions provided the rationale for the use of epinephrine in cardiac arrest. Injection of epinephrine is made directly into heart muscle.

MARKED INCREASE IN CARDIAC RATE (POSITIVE CHRONOTROPIC EFFECT). Acceleration of heart rate by the catecholamines is the result of the increased rate of membrane depolarization in the pacemaker cells in the sinus node during diastole: action potential threshold is reached sooner, pacemaker cells fire more often, and heart rate increases.

Norepinephrine with its predominantly alpha adrenergic activity may not produce as severe a tachycardia as epinephrine. The increased vasoconstriction and increased blood pressure may produce a reflex bradycardia. Dosage and patient variables affect these responses. Isoproterenol usually produces a tachycardia, since its direct and reflex effects act in the same direction.

INCREASE IN ATRIOVENTRICULAR CONDUCTION (POSITIVE DROMOTROPIC EFFECT). Because epinephrine increases atrioventricular conduction, some cardiologists use it in the treatment of heart block.

PURKINJE FIBER EFFECTS. Catecholamines may produce spontaneous firing of Purkinje fibers, resulting in their exhibiting pacemaker activity. This effect may produce ventricular extrasystoles and increase the susceptibility of ventricular muscle to fibrillation. These effects are more likely to occur with epinephrine than norepinephrine.

Blood pressure and blood flow effects. Vascular effects of the catecholamines depend on the dose and the vascular bed affected. Low doses of epinephrine may produce a decrease in blood pressure due to a decrease in total peripheral vascular resistance. In large doses epinephrine activates alpha receptors in the greater peripheral vascular system, which leads to increased resistance and increased blood pressure. Norepinephrine elevates blood pressure by increasing peripheral resistance and decreasing blood flow through skeletal muscles.

Norepinephrine is a vasoconstrictor and it increases total peripheral resistance. Isoproterenol is not a vasoconstrictor but a pure vasodilator; epinephrine is both a vasoconstrictor and vasodilator, with vasodilation being greater in its overall net effects. For example, during great stress (fright, fight, flight phenomena) the release of epinephrine from the adrenal medulla constricts blood vessels in the skin and splanchnic areas but dilates those of muscles, thus shunting blood from noncritical to critical areas.

There is greater renal artery constriction and resistance with epinephrine than with norepinephrine. In large doses epinephrine may actually stop blood flow through some nephrons (up to 40%) and stimulate release of antidiuretic hormone (ADH), thereby reducing urinary excretion.

Central nervous system effects. Epinephrine and isoproterenol in sufficient amounts can lead to alertness, tremulousness, respiratory stimulation, and manifest anxiety. Norepinephrine is less likely to cause anxiety and tremulousness. Beneficial cerebral effects from epinephrine and norepinephrine in cases of hypotension are thought to be the result of increased systemic pressure with a resultant improvement in cerebral blood flow.

Smooth muscle effects. Generally, the catecholamines relax nonvascular smooth muscles. Smooth muscle of the gastrointestinal tract is relaxed, and amplitude and tone of intestinal peristalsis are reduced. This may retard propulsion of food and gastrointestinal emptying. However, this effect is rarely produced in humans with therapeutic doses.

The musculature of the splenic capsule is stimulated, thereby increasing contractions of that organ, which results in increasing the number of circulating red cells and blood viscosity. This effect is not of great significance in humans.

In some situations smooth muscle of some organs reacts like vascular smooth muscle and contracts. For example, radial and sphincter muscles of the iris contract and the smooth muscle that inserts into the lids may contract, giving rise to the widened, staring eyes seen in sympathetically stimulated individuals.

In the urinary bladder epinephrine causes trigone and sphincter contraction and detrusor relaxation with a delay in the desire to void.

Bronchodilator effects. Catecholamines dilate bronchial smooth muscle. Isoproterenol is a more active bronchodilator than epinephrine, which in turn is a stronger bronchodilator than norepinephrine. Epinephrine, in addition, constricts bronchial vessels and inhibits bronchial secretions, which accounts for its time-honored use in the treatment of acute bronchial asthma.

Effect on glands. Epinephrine may increase the amount of viscid saliva excreted, but as a rule sympathomimetics decrease secretion and produce a dry mouth. Catecholamines may produce local sweating on the palms of the hands and in the axillary and genital areas. The exact mechanism for these effects is not clear.

Metabolic effects. Epinephrine inhibits insulin secretion. Catecholamines have antagonistic effects on gluconeogenesis, and they decrease liver and skeletal muscle glycogen and increase lipolysis in adipose tissue. The result of these effects is a rise in blood sugar and an increase in free fatty acids. Thus in response to stress (fright, fight, flight response) there can be an abundant supply of fuel and energy.

Catecholamines also have a calorigenic effect (increased oxygen consumption) resulting from the sum of the preceding effects. Norepinephrine's action in relation to these effects is weaker than that of epinephrine or isoproterenol.

Other effects. Catecholamines cause a decrease in circulating eosinophils. The mechanism of this action is unknown.

Drug interactions. Among the various drug interactions that can occur between the catecholamines and other drugs are the following:

1 Digitalis and the catecholamines may have an additive effect and precipitate ectopic pacemaker activity.
2 Catecholamines given to patients receiving MAO inhibitors may cause a hypertensive crisis.
3 Certain anesthetics, such as chloroform, cyclopropane, halothane, and trichloroethylene, sensitize the heart to catecholamines, and injection of these drugs during surgery is hazardous because the risk of induced dysrhythmias is increased.
4 Tricyclic antidepressants, other sympathomimetic drugs, and reserpine and related drugs may potentiate the effects of the catecholamines.
5 Diuretics and some antihypertensive drugs antagonize the effects of the catecholamines.

6 Epinephrine and isoproterenol should not be administered concomitantly, since their combined effects may produce serious dysrhythmias. Their use may be alternated if at least 4 hours have elapsed.

Epinephrine (Adrenalin)

General characteristics. Epinephrine can be prepared synthetically or obtained from the adrenal glands of domestic animals. Most epinephrine used in medicine at the present time is a pure synthetic preparation. Chemically, epinephrine is an amine and reacts with acids to form salts. Epinephrine hydrochloride solutions are unstable; they react to light, heat, and air, turn pink and then brown when oxidized, and should be kept in the refrigerator. Discol-ored solutions should be discarded, since there will be loss of potency.

Epinephrine acts on both alpha and beta receptors. It is a more potent alpha receptor stimulator than norepinephrine at some sites. Beta receptors are also more sensitive to epinephrine than to norepinephrine. (See Table 13-9.)

Action and uses. The ability of epinephrine to constrict blood vessels makes it useful for topical application in stopping capillary bleeding from the nose, mouth, mucosal surfaces, and skin abrasions. It should not be used on fingers, toes, or ears, since the vasoconstriction may cause tissue necrosis and sloughing. It is often added to local anesthetic solutions to delay their absorption from the site of injection

TABLE 13-9 Direct adrenergic drug effects—catecholamine type

	Epinephrine	Norepinephrine	Isoproterenol
Trade names	Adrenalin	Noradrenalin Levarterenol	Isuprel
Mode of action			
Alpha receptors	Stimulates	Stimulates	N.S.*
Beta receptors	Stimulates	Stimulates the heart	Stimulates
Effects			
Cardiovascular			
Myocardium	Increases rate and strength of contractions Increases output	Slows rate reflexly	Like epinephrine
Pacemaker cells	Stimulates Increases irritability May cause dysrhythmias	Stimulates—like epinephrine	Like epinephrine
Coronary vessels	Dilates—increases blood flow	Dilates	Like epinephrine
Blood pressure	Increases (depending on dose)	Increases	Decreases diastolic Slightly increases systolic
Bronchi	Relaxes Improves airway	Relaxes less than epinephrine	Potent bronchodilator—more effective than epinephrine
Blood vessels			
Skeletal muscle	Dilates—increases blood flow	—	Dilates—increases blood flow
Kidney	Constricts—decreases blood flow	Constricts—decreases blood flow	N.S.
Gastrointestinal tract	Relaxes smooth muscle Inhibits peristalsis	Like epinephrine	N.S.
Metabolic	Increases oxygen consumption Mobilizes glycogen Causes hyperglycemia	Increases metabolic rate but less than epinephrine	N.S.
Remarks	Tolerance does not develop	Infiltration into tissues may cause necrosis and sloughing	
Uses	Widely used for allergic states, cardiac arrest; with local anesthetics Given by injection or inhalation	To elevate blood pressure, given by slow intravenous infusion	Heart failure Asthma

*N.S., Not significant.

by promoting local vasoconstriction, which in turn restricts the action of the anesthetic to that given area, prolongs the anesthetic action, and checks bleeding.

This same vasoconstrictor ability accounts for the use of epinephrine to relieve congestion and swelling of particular tissues—thus its use in treating allergic conditions such as urticaria and angioneurotic edema. When applied to the eye in a 2% solution, it dilates the pupil, decreases the blood flow, and reduces intraocular tension. This last effect makes it useful in treating chronic simple glaucoma.

Epinephrine may also be given by inhalation (in a 1:100 solution) to asthmatics to relieve bronchial spasm and swelling and to promote a patent airway. However, the usual treatment of an acute asthmatic attack is the subcutaneous injection of epinephrine, 0.2 to 0.5 ml of a 1:1000 solution. The dose may be repeated every 10 to 15 minutes or hourly if necessary. However, physiologic resistance to epinephrine may develop. Therefore its use should be restricted to acute asthmatic attacks. Asthmatics may also develop an emotional dependence on epinephrine.

Epinephrine has not proved an effective drug in the relief of nasal congestion because of its rebound or secondary vasodilator effect, which brings about a greater swelling of the nasal mucosa than was present initially.

Epinephrine has a significant effect on beta receptors; consequently, it can dilate some vessels, such as those of skeletal muscle. Because of this and its potent action on cardiac beta receptors, epinephrine is not the drug of choice in most cases of shock or hypotension. On the other hand, it is the drug of choice for treating anaphylactic shock. Epinephrine may also be used to treat cardiac arrest.

Absorption and excretion. Although epinephrine is readily absorbed from mucous membranes, it is destroyed by digestive enzymes and is therefore useless if given by mouth. Rapid effects may be noted when the drug is given hypodermically or intramuscularly, and almost immediate effects occur when it is given intravenously. The drug is rapidly inactivated in the body by enzymatic alteration and is taken up by adrenergic nerves.

Preparation, dosage, and administration. The following are available preparations of epinephrine.

Epinephrine nasal solution. The 1:1000 aqueous solution is for topical application only. This solution is not sterile.

Epinephrine injection; adrenaline injection. This 1:1000 solution is available in ampules and 30-ml vials. The dosage is 0.5 ml given subcutaneously or intramuscularly for treatment of shock in adults. This may be followed by 0.25 to 0.5 ml of a 1:10,000 solution given intravenously every 5 to 15 minutes.

For children, the initial dose is 0.3 ml of a 1:1000 solution given subcutaneously or intramuscularly; this dose may be repeated at 15-minute intervals for three or four doses. In emergencies the drug may be given intravenously. This preparation is sterile and contains 1 mg of drug in each milliliter of solution. Subcutaneous administration is most often used. Promptness of action can be facilitated by massaging the injection site. When the intravenous route is used, the drug must be given very slowly and in a very low concentration.

Epinephrine inhalation. This 1:100 (1%) epinephrine solution can be administered as a 1% solution or diluted to a 0.1% solution for administration with a special nebulizer to provide a fine mist for oral inhalation. Epinephrine is well absorbed from mucous membranes. The effectiveness of this preparation for the asthmatic patient is explained on the basis of achieving a relatively high concentration of the drug in the throat and respiratory passages rather than from a systemic action. *Special precautions should be taken to avoid confusing the 1:100 solution with the 1:1000 solution.*

Sterile epinephrine suspension (epinephrine in oil injection). Dosage for adults is 0.2 to 0.5 ml intramuscularly. It is available in 1-ml ampules (1:500). The duration of action is prolonged.

Epinephrine bitartrate. This preparation is available as a 2% ophthalmic solution.

Adrenaline injection. This is a 1:1000 solution of epinephrine tartrate for subcutaneous injection. It is a sterile solution.

Epinephrine suspension (aqueous). Available preparations are Sus-Phrine, 1:200 solution (5 mg/ml) in 0.5- and 5-ml containers, and Asmolin, 1:400 solution (2.5 mg/ml) in 10-ml vials.

The subcutaneous dose for treating asthma in adults is 0.1 to 0.3 ml of the aqueous 1:200 solution; for children the dosage is 0.005 ml/kg. Since this is a concentrated solution, the dose should not be repeated for 4 hours.

Medihaler-Epi is a suspension, 7 mg/ml in 15-ml vials with or without an oral adapter. Each measured dose contains 0.3 mg epinephrine bitartrate.

• • •

Unofficial preparations of epinephrine such as epinephrine suppositories (1:1000 with cocoa butter), are also available.

Solutions of epinephrine do not keep well; deterioration is evidenced by formation of sediment and brownish discoloration. These solutions should be discarded.

For children the recommended subcutaneous injection dose for asthma is 0.01 ml of 1:1000 aqueous solution per kilogram of body weight, with a maximum dose of 0.5 ml. This dosage may be repeated every 4 hours. When the intramuscular injection of epinephrine in oil (1:500) is used, the dose is 0.01 to 0.02 ml/kg body weight every 12 to 24 hours as needed. However, the intramuscular route is not recommended, since bioavailability is not uniform and fatal cases of gas gangrene have been reported.

Because epinephrine is such a potent drug, the nurse must be particularly careful to give the correct dose. If the preparation at hand is an ampule containing 1 ml of the drug, it does not follow that 1 ml is the usual dose. Very often, the dose is only a few minims. The minimal fatal dose of epinephrine subcutaneously seems to be about 10 ml of a 1:1000 solution.

Toxic effects. Toxic effects and death from epinephrine may result from overdosage caused by errors in preparation of solutions or the intravenous administration of a subcutaneous dose. Symptoms of toxicity include tachycardia, palpitations, dyspnea, pulmonary edema, severe headache, pallor, pupillary dilation, anxiety, high blood pressure, and rapid collapse. Toxic effects may be counteracted by injection of an alpha blocker and a beta blocker. Cardiac dysrhythmias that may be evoked by epinephrine include atrial fibrillation, atrioventricular nodal rhythm, ventricular extrasystoles, ventricular tachycardia, and ventricular fibrillation.

A nurse is expected to recognize an obvious error. The strength of solution, dosage ordered, and route of administration should be carefully checked.

Contraindications. Epinephrine should not be used for patients on a regimen of digitalis, since together these drugs have a synergistic action and predispose the heart to premature beats or dysrhythmias. Epinephrine should be avoided in patients with hyperthyroidism, hypertension, cerebral arteriosclerosis, and nervous instability. The drug should not be used in elderly or debilitated patients. Use of epinephrine preoperatively in patients with angle-closure glaucoma is contraindicated. Administration of epinephrine to patients with cerebral arteriosclerosis may result in cerebral hemorrhage.

Levarterenol bitartrate (Levophed Bitartrate, norepinephrine); noradrenaline acid tartrate

Levarterenol bitartrate is a grayish white, crystalline powder, freely soluble in water. It darkens on exposure to light and air. It can be synthesized or obtained from the medullary portion of the adrenal glands of animals. It has positive inotropic and chronotropic effects on the heart (beta$_1$-adrenergic activity) and a potent constrictor action on blood vessels (alpha-adrenergic activity). (See Table 13-9.)

Uses. Levarterenol bitartrate is used to maintain blood pressure in acute hypotensive conditions caused by vasomotor depression, trauma, and shock. It does not take the place of intravascular fluids if the fall in blood pressure is caused by diminished blood volume.

Levarterenol may be lifesaving in cardiogenic shock because of its direct stimulating effect on the myocardium and its vasoconstricting action. These effects restore the cardiac output and blood pressure to a more normal level.

Preparation, dosage, and administration. Levarterenol bitartrate is available in 4-ml ampules containing 0.2% solutions of the drug (1 mg/ml). Usually 4 ml is added to 1000 ml of

5% glucose in distilled water or to 5% glucose in physiologic saline solution. It is administered slowly by intravenous infusion with a control drip bulb, 2 to 3 ml/minute at first. The amount may be decreased to 0.5 to 1 ml/minute, depending on the response of the patient. Vessels in the hand and ankle should not be used because of the risk of inducing gangrene. Since the drug is quickly metabolized, its pressor effects disappear within 1 to 2 minutes after the infusion is stopped. Heparin is usually added to the infusion solution to inhibit venous thrombosis. The drug is also used for immediate intravenous or intracardiac administration in patients with cardiac arrest. It is ineffective when given orally.

During administration the blood pressure of the patient must be taken frequently (every 2 to 5 minutes), since the rate of infusion is determined by changes in the patient's heart rate and blood pressure. Direct arterial measurement with an intra-arterial catheter is the preferred method of taking the blood pressure. However, the indirect measurement of blood pressure using the sphygmomanometer may be used. It should be kept in mind that blood pressure measurement obtained indirectly is significantly lower than that obtained by direct measurement; the difference may be as much as 15 mm Hg.

Precautions. Overdosage can produce marked hypertension, severe headache, photophobia, chest pain, pallor, and vomiting. *Great care must be taken that the drug does not leak into subcutaneous tissue, since its marked local vasoconstricting effect may cause the tissues to slough.* If infiltration occurs, the area should be promptly infiltrated with 5 to 10 mg of phentolamine in 10 to 15 ml of normal saline solution using a hypodermic needle.

A solution that is brown or contains a precipitate should not be used.

Levarterenol should not be given to patients with mesenteric thrombosis, since the drug may increase ischemia and extend the area of infarction. Edema, hemorrhage, and necrosis of the intestine; hepatic and renal necrosis; focal myocarditis; subpericardial hemorrhage; and gangrene of the extremities have been reported following prolonged administration of levarterenol. Moreover, since splanchnic and renal blood flow are reduced by the drug, circulation to the kidneys and other vital organs may be compromised. Therefore, levarterenol is not recommended as a first choice vasopressor drug in the restoration of an adequate blood pressure.

Dobutamine hydrochloride (Dobutrex)

Dobutamine is a synthetic catecholamine that acts directly on the heart muscle to produce an increased force of myocardial contraction. This response is attributed to the direct stimulation of the $beta_1$ adrenergic receptors of the heart. At the same time dobutamine produces comparatively little increase in heart rate or peripheral vascular resistance. By enhancing stroke volume, this agent is an effective positive inotropic drug. Because of its minimal influence on heart rate and blood pressure (both major determinants of myocardial oxygen demand), it is of value in patients with the low cardiac output syndrome. In contrast to dopamine, which also is capable of increasing myocardial contractility, dobutamine does not produce renal vasodilation. In a comparative study of dobutamine and dopamine, the improvement in peripheral blood flow, urine flow, and sodium excretion noted with the use of dobutamine was probably caused by the elevation in cardiac output.

Uses. Dobutamine is administered intravenously in the *short-term* management of patients requiring inotropic support. It is employed to strengthen the decompensated heart in individuals with the low cardiac output syndrome. It is currently used in the short-term treatment of acute and chronic (low cardiac output) congestive heart failure. Its beneficial effect results in a progressive increase in cardiac output and a decrease in pulmonary capillary wedge pressure, thereby improving ventricular contraction. Dobutamine also is used to promote myocardial performance in patients following cardiac surgical procedures such as cardiopulmonary bypass. In patients with acute myocardial infarction, the drug has been recommended only when congestive heart failure is superimposed. If cardiogenic shock also is present, hypovolemia should be corrected by the administration of a suitable plasma volume expander before treatment with dobutamine is instituted.

Preparation, dosage and administration. Dobutamine hydrochloride is supplied in a 20-ml vial that contains 250 mg of the compound. This preparation is dissolved in sterile water or 5% dextrose in water, and the solution is further diluted to at least 50 ml for use. Because of its short half-life in plasma (about 2 minutes), dobutamine is administered by continuous intravenous infusion at a usual dose of 2.5 to 10 μg/kg/minute. Occasionally infusion rates up to 40 μg/kg/minute have been required to obtain the desired effect. During therapy, the electrocardiogram and blood pressure should be continuously monitored. If possible, the pulmonary capillary wedge pressure and cardiac output also should be monitored to ensure safe infusion of the drug. If the patient responds by an increase in heart rate (30 beats/minute or more) and an increase in systolic blood pressure (50 mm Hg or greater) during the course of treatment, a reduction of dosage usually reverses these adverse effects because the drug is rapidly metabolized.

Side effects. The adverse reactions include a marked increase in heart rate and blood pressure and ventricular ectopic activity. Since dobutamine enchances atrioventricular conduction, its use should be avoided in patients with atrial fibrillation. Other side effects include nausea, headache, dyspnea, palpitations, and anginal pain.

Contraindications. Dobutamine is contraindicated in patients with marked obstruction to cardiac ejection. Its positive inotropic effect prevents its use in idiopathic hypertrophic subaortic stenosis.

Precautions. Safety for use of dobutamine following myocardial infarction has not been established. There is concern that because dobutamine increases the force of myocardial contraction, it may increase the size of an infarction and thereby intensify the ischemia. The safety of dobutamine for use in children and pregnant women also has not been established.

Drug interactions. In a surgical procedure such as cardiopulmonary bypass, the concomitant use of sodium nitroprusside and dobutamine results in a higher cardiac output and a lower pulmonary capillary wedge pressure than when either drug is used alone. Because of the vasodilating effect of nitroprusside, the decrease in peripheral resistance lessens the workload on the heart.

The concurrent use of dobutamine with other drugs such as digitalis preparations, furosemide, spironolactone, lidocaine, glyceryl trinitrate, isosorbide dinitrate, morphine, atropine, heparin, protamine, potassium chloride, folic acid, and acetaminophen has shown no evidence of drug interaction.

Dobutamine is incompatible with alkaline solutions and should not be mixed with products such as 5% Sodium Bicarbonate Injection.

Dopamine

Dopamine (Intropin) is a naturally occurring catecholamine that has been introduced as a vasopressor agent for the treatment of certain forms of hypotension.

Dopamine, administered by intravenous infusion, causes an elevation of blood pressure by acting on alpha receptors. At the same time, it dilates the renal and mesenteric vessels, and these actions may be exerted on specific dopaminergic receptors that are blocked by the phenothiazine group of drugs. In addition, dopamine acts on $beta_1$ receptors of the heart, causing increased contractility and heart rate.

Uses. Dopamine infusions are used in some cases of shock. It should be administered only if the blood volume is adequate. The drug can cause adverse effects that include cardiac arrhythmias, nausea, vomiting, and occasionally hypotension. The cardiac effects of dopamine are antagonized by propranolol, its hypertensive effects are prevented by phentolamine, and its vasodilator actions are antagonized by the phenothiazines.

Preparation, dosage, and administration. Dopamine hydrochloride (Intropin) is available in 5-ml ampules containing 200 mg of dopamine. The drug should be diluted in a 250- or 500-ml sterile intravenous solution. Infusion rates should be adjusted so that 2 to 5 μg/kg/minute is administered.

Isoproterenol

Isoproterenol has predominant beta adrenergic action. It is a synthetic catecholamine with potent cardiovascular properties. Its chemical structure resembles that of epinephrine and norepinephrine.

The positive inotropic and chronotropic actions of isoproterenol are greater than those of epinephrine. These effects result in increased stroke volume, cardiac output and cardiac work, and coronary flow. Therefore it is a useful drug for patients with some types of heart disease, particularly heart block. (See Table 13-9.)

Uses. Isoproterenol's effects improve atrioventricular conduction and enhance the rhythmicity of the sinoatrial and ventricular pacemakers. This makes isoproterenol an important drug—and for many authorities the drug of choice—for the treatment of atrioventricular heart block and asystole. By accelerating the action of the basic pacemakers of the heart, the drug suppresses ectopic pacemaker activity and dysrhythmias. However, its effect on cardiac automaticity can enhance ventricular irritability. Thus some cardiologists recommend its use in atrioventricular block only for patients with slow ventricular responses who do not respond to atropine. Pacemaker implantation may be preferred.

In addition, isoproterenol relaxes arterial and bronchial smooth muscles. Isoproterenol produces both pulmonary and systemic arterial dilation, which decreases vascular resistance. It can be used to reverse pulmonary hypertension caused by pressor agents, pulmonary embolism, and incompatible blood transfusion.

Isoproterenol is a more active bronchodilator than epinephrine. It shrinks swollen mucous membrane and reduces mucus secretion. This makes it a useful drug in the treatment of bronchial asthma and pulmonary emphysema and for the prevention and treatment of bronchospasm and laryngospasm during anesthesia. It is also used for the patient who is no longer benefited by the use of epinephrine and for the patient in status asthmaticus.

Isoproterenol is used during cardiac catheterization to simulate exercise to help determine its effects on cardiovascular activity, particularly in evaluating congenital cardiac defects and acquired valvular disease. The use of isoproterenol for patients in shock is still experimental.

Preparation, dosage, and administration

Isoproterenol hydrochloride (Isuprel, Aludrine). Isoproterenol hydrochloride is available in 10- and 15-mg sublingual tablets. However, their absorption is variable, unreliable, and at times associated with pronounced side effects such as nausea, tachycardia, and palpitations. Extended-release tablets, 15 and 30 mg, are available. Isoproterenol is used as a solution for inhalation in concentrations of 1:100, 1:200, and 1:400 and as a solution for injection in 1:5000 concentration. Solutions of isoproterenol turn pink on exposure to air, and patients should be told that saliva and sputum may appear pink after oral inhalation of the drug.

Isoproterenol sulfate (Norisodrine Sulfate, Isonorin Sulfate); isoprenaline sulfate. This is available in the form of a powder for insufflation (10% and 25%), as a solution for inhalation (1:100), and in tablets (10 mg) for sublingual administration.

• • •

Isoproterenol is also available in metered dose inhalers for bronchodilation and treatment of asthmatic attacks.

Isoproterenol may be given intravenously. From 1 to 2 µg/minute may be given in a continuous drip. From 5 to 40 µg/minute has been used to arouse a pacemaker. It has been shown that isoproterenol is an effective drug in the treatment of Stokes-Adams syndrome when 1 mg is administered in 200 ml of 5% dextrose in water starting at 20 drops/minute. Thereafter, flow is regulated to maintain the ventricular rate at 35 to 50 beats/minute.

Side effects and toxic effects. Untoward effects of isoproterenol include precordial pain, heart palpitation, anginal pain, headache, nausea, tremor, and flushing of the skin. There may be a fall in arterial blood pressure. The drug is contraindicated for pateints who have insufficient coronary blood flow and those with a history of tachycardia. Toxic effects can be counteracted by administering propranolol.

Precautions. Isoproterenol must be used cautiously in patients with valvular stenosis. Caution should also be exercised when the patient has digitalis-induced heart block.

INDIRECT- AND MIXED-ACTING ADRENERGIC DRUGS

As was discussed previously, the *direct-acting adrenergic drugs*—the catecholamines—act *directly on alpha and beta receptors* to stimulate adrenergic response. On the other hand, the *indirect-acting adrenergic drugs* act *indirectly on receptors* by first triggering the release of catecholamines norepinephrine and epinephrine from their storage sites, which then activate the alpha and beta receptors. Finally, the *mixed-acting adrenergic drugs* have *both indirect and direct* effects. These drugs are used widely in medicine and will be discussed next.

Ephedrine

Ephedrine is the name given to an active principle isolated from an Asiatic herb, ma huang (*Ephedra vulgaris*, var. *helvetica)*, which has been used in the practice of medicine in China for more than 5000 years. In chemical composition it is an amine, closely allied to epinephrine, and an alkaloid. Presently, most of the ephedrine used is produced synthetically.

Action and result. Ephedrine has both a direct and an indirect sympathomimetic action. Its indirect action is caused by its release of norepinephrine or the impairment of norepinephrine uptake by storage granules. Ephedrine is both an alpha and beta adrenergic stimulant. Like epinephrine and norepinephrine, ephedrine has positive inotropic (myocardial stimulation) and chronotropic (increased heart rate) activity, but it is a less effective vasoconstrictor. However, it does raise the blood pressure and is used for this purpose during spinal anesthesia and to treat orthostatic hypotension. It is beneficial for the treatment of hypotension caused by shock from any cause.

Ephedrine resembles epinephrine but differs from it in a number of ways. Ephedrine is more stable than epinephrine, it is well absorbed from the gastrointestinal tract, and it is effective when given orally. Its action is slower, more prolonged, but less intense than that produced by epinephrine. In addition, ephedrine stimulates the central nervous system by acting on the cerebral cortex and medulla. This accounts for its use in the treatment of narcolepsy, a state in which the patient persistently falls asleep. However, for this use ephedrine has been largely replaced by the amphetamines.

Ephedrine's ability to stimulate the respiratory center in the medulla makes it a useful drug for the treatment of narcotic, barbiturate, and alcohol poisoning.

Ephedrine relaxes hypertonic muscle in the bronchioles and in the gastrointestinal tract. Emptying time of the stomach and intestine is delayed. Sphincter muscles in the urinary and gastrointestinal tracts are stimulated. The effect on metabolism is similar to that of epinephrine.

In the treatment of bronchial asthma, ephedrine is useful in preventing acute attacks. Epinephrine is preferable when attacks are acute because of its more rapid effect.

As a constituent of nasal drops, jellies, and sprays, ephedrine relieves acute congestion of hay fever, sinusitis, head colds, and vasomotor rhinitis. Shrinkage of mucous membranes begins immediately and lasts for several hours. Vasodilation does not ordinarily follow vasoconstriction, as may occur after administration of epinephrine.

Ephedrine exhibits a tendency to increase the tone of skeletal muscle. It is used in the treatment of muscle weakness associated with myasthenia gravis. It is most effective, however, when combined with prostigmine.

Ephedrine may be used in solution as a mydriatic when a cycloplegic action is not desired. It is not useful if inflammation is present. It acts as a mydriatic in the eye by acting on the radial muscles of the iris. This occurs with local application to the eye and with systemic administration of the drug. (See Table 13-10.)

A 3% to 4% solution is used for eyedrops, and the oral range of dosage is 20 to 50 mg (gr ⅓ to ¾) every 3 or 4 hours. The oral dose for children is 3 mg/kg body weight daily, divided into four or six portions. Children are more resistant

TABLE 13-10 Indirect- and mixed-acting adrenergic drug effects

	Ephedrine	Phenylephrine	Mephentermine	Metaraminol	Methoxamine
Trade names		Neo-Synephrine	Wyamine	Aramine Pressonex	Vasoxyl
Mode of action					
Alpha receptors	Stimulates	Stimulates	Stimulates	Stimulates	Stimulates
Beta receptors	Stimulates More prolonged but less intense action than epinephrine	N.S.*			
Effects					
Cardiovascular.					
Myocardium	Variable	N.S. Bradycardia may occur reflexly	Increases contractility and rate May cause bradycardia	Some increase in contractility Bradycardia may occur	— Reflex bradycardia may occur
Pacemaker cells	N.S.	N.S.	N.S.	—	—
Coronary vessels	Dilates—increases blood flow	Dilates—increases blood flow	Dilates—increases blood flow	—	—
Blood pressure	Increases	Increases	Increases	Increases	Increases
Bronchi	Dilates	Dilates but less than epinephrine	Dilates but less than epinephrine	N.S.	
Cerebral effects	Stimulating action	N.S.	N.S.	—	—
Blood vessels					
Skeletal muscle	N.S.	—†	N.S.	N.S.	—
Kidney	Constricts	Constricts	Constricts but less than ephedrine	Constricts—decreases blood flow	Decreases blood flow
Gastrointestinal tract	Decreases peristalsis	Decreases motility	Relaxes smooth muscle—inhibits	Some inhibition	Inhibits
Metabolic	Increases metabolic rate	Some increase in metabolic rate	N.S.	N.S.	N.S.
Remarks	Serious dysrhythmias may occur if used with digitalis Can be given orally			Prolonged duration of action, cumulative effects may occur—give drug slowly May cause tissue sloughing—do not give subcutaneously	
Uses	Vasopressor Allergic states Nasal decongestant Enuresis Myasthenia gravis	Nasal decongestant Vasopressor Paroxysmal atrial tachycardia Mydriatic	Vasopressor Nasal decongestant	Vasopressor Nasal decongestant	Vasopressor Paroxysmal atrial tachycardia Nasal decongestant

*N.S., Not significant.
†Effect is slight, nonexistent, or unknown in humans.

than adults to the stimulant effects of ephedrine.

Preparation, dosage, and administration. The following are the preparations and dosages of ephedrine.

Ephedrine sulfate capsules; ephedrine sulfate tablets. These are available in 25 to 50 mg for oral administration. The usual dose is 25 mg (gr ⅜) taken three or four times daily. Effects occur 30 minutes to 1 hour after oral administration.

Ephedrine sulfate injection. This is available in 1-ml ampules and 10-ml vials containing 25 or 50 mg (gr ⅜ to ¾) of drug per milliliter for injection. The usual dose is 25 mg (gr ⅜).

Ephedrine hydrochloride. This is available in capsule and tablet form, and the usual dose is 25 mg (gr ⅜).

Ephedrine sulfate nasal solution. This is available in 1% and 3% solutions of the drug in 0.36% sodium chloride solution, to be further diluted with an equal amount of isotonic saline before use.

Ephedrine sulfate syrup. The usual dose is 5 ml (20 mg ephedrine sulfate).

Ephedrine sulfate and phenobarbital capsules. Each capsule contains 25 or 50 mg of ephedrine sulfate and 15 or 30 mg of phenobarbital.

(The main difference between the hydrochloride and the sulfate salts of ephedrine is that the latter are more freely soluble in water.)

Side effects and toxic effects. Older men taking ephedrine may have difficulty voiding because of the drug's ability to relax bladder musculature. Anxiety, irritability, headache, tremor, anorexia, palpitation, and insomnia are common side effects. Nausea and vomiting may also occur. Ocassionally a patient exhibits symptoms of hypersensitivity. The same precautions are recommended for the use of ephedrine as for epinephrine. Barbiturates or some type of sedative is sometimes prescribed for the patient who is receiving the drug over a period of time. This is to counteract the central stimulating effect of ephedrine. Diminished response to the drug occurs with repeated administration. Although tolerance develops, ephedrine has not been known to cause addiction.

Phenylephrine hydrochloride (Neo-Synephrine Hydrochloride)

Phenylephrine hydrochloride is a synthetic adrenergic drug chemically related to epinephrine, norepinephrine, and ephedrine.

Action and uses. Phenylephrine hydrochloride is relatively nontoxic, exhibits fewer side effects than epinephrine, and has longer-lasting therapeutic effects. It has no effect on the central nervous system.

Phenylephrine hydrochloride is a powerful stimulator of alpha receptors and is therefore a potent vasoconstrictor. It elevates both the systolic and diastolic blood pressures. Its vasoconstricting action is more prolonged than that of epinephrine—it lasts 20 minutes after intravenous administration and 50 minutes after subcutaneous injection. For these reasons it is often used to treat hypotension caused by myocardial infarction, orthostatic hypotension, and hypotension resulting from loss of vasomotor tone from spinal anesthesia. It is not effective in shock caused by loss of blood volume.

Phenylephrine has little inotropic or chronotropic effect. It does cause a reflex bradycardia as a result of its ability to elevate the blood pressure, which stimulates the baroreceptors and vagal activity. It is therefore an effective drug in converting paroxysmal tachycardia to a normal rate.

When applied topically to mucous membranes, it reduces swelling and congestion by constricting the small blood vessels.

It is useful in the treatment of sinusitis, vasomotor rhinitis, and hay fever and is used alone or with other drugs for the relief of bronchial asthma. It is sometimes combined with local anesthetics to retard their systemic absorption and to prolong their action.

Phenylephrine hydrochloride is used as a mydriatic for certain conditions in which dilation of the pupil is desired without cycloplegia (paralysis of the ciliary muscle). (See Table 13-10.)

Preparation, dosage, and administration. Phenylephrine hydrochloride is marketed in 10- and 25-mg capsules for oral administration, as a solution for injection (10 mg/ml in 1- and 5-ml containers), and in a number of forms for topical application—solutions, an ophthalmic solution, a jelly, and an emulsion.

For topical application to the nasal mucous membrane, 0.25% solution is ordinarily used. As a mydriatic, 1 or 2 drops of the 1% solution or emulsion or the 2.5% ophthalmic solution is used.

The intramuscular or subcutaneous dose for adults ranges from 1 to 10 mg; the dose for children is 0.1 mg/kg body weight. The dose for hypotensive states is 10 mg of phenylephrine in 500 ml of 5% dextrose by slow intravenous infusion, or 0.25 to 0.5 mg diluted in sodium chloride injected slowly. For orthostatic hypotension the oral dose for adults is 20 mg three times daily; for children the dose is 1 mg/kg body weight in 24 hours divided into six doses.

Side effects and cautions. Oral doses may cause mild gastrointestinal symptoms, which may be avoided by giving the drug after meals. Phenylephrine may cause tremor, insomnia, and palpitations. Intravenous doses may induce ventricular extrasystoles, paroxysmal ventricular tachycardia, a feeling of fullness in the head, and paresthesias.

Phenylephrine should be used with great caution in elderly patients or patients with hyperthyroidism, bradycardia, partial heart block, myocardial disease, or severe arteriosclerosis.

Ophthalmic solutions are contraindicated in patients with narrow-angle glaucoma.

Mephentermine sulfate (Wyamine Sulfate)

Mephentermine sulfate is a white crystalline powder that is freely soluble in water.

Action. Mephentermine's effects are similar to those of ephedrine, but it brings about far less cerebral stimulation. Local application in the eye produces dilation of the pupil.

Mephentermine is an indirectly acting sympathomimetic. It releases catecholamines from storage sites in the heart and other tissues. Therefore it tends to bring about both alpha and beta stimulating effects and inotropic and chronotropic effects on the heart.

Its vasoconstrictor effect is used to treat hypotensive states not associated with hemorrhage. In these cases the drug is given intramuscularly or intravenously. The onset of action occurs within 5 to 15 minutes, and the effects last 1 to 2 hours. Since mephentermine improves cardiac contraction and mobilizes blood from venous pools, thereby increasing cardiac output, it is used in heart failure following a myocardial infarction. It also increases cardiac conduction and shortens the refractory period of the heart. This makes it useful in treating certain cardiac dysrythymias.

Like ephedrine, mephentermine constricts the small blood vessels of the nasal mucosa and can be used topically or by inhalation to relieve nasal congestion. It does not cause rebound congestion. (See Table 13-10.)

If catecholamine storage sites have been depleted, there may be no pressor response from mephentermine. In this case administration of norepinephrine resupplies these depots or storage sites, which restores the action of mephentermine.

Preparation, dosage, and administration. Mephentermine sulfate is administered topically for nasal congestion and orally, intramuscularly, and intravenously for systemic effects. It is available in injection form containing 15 to 30 mg/ml; as an elixir, 5 mg/ml; in tablets (12.5 and 25 mg) for oral administration; and as a solution (0.5%) for topical administration to nasal membranes (2 or 3 drops every 4 hours as needed). Dosage for systemic effect varies from 10 to 30 mg. Inhalers that contain 250 mg of the drug are also marketed. The dose for children is 0.4 mg/kg body weight.

When given by continuous intravenous drip, 600 to 1000 mg may be added to 1 liter of 5% glucose in water. Continuous blood pressure monitoring is required, since adverse blood pressure responses may occur.

Side effects and precautions are similar to those of previously discussed sympathomimetics.

Metaraminol bitartrate (Aramine Bitartrate, Pressonex Bitartrate)

Metaraminol is a vasopressor agent with both direct and indirect effects on the sympathetic system. It acts indirectly by releasing norepinephrine from tissues and storage sites and directly as a neurohormone. Metaraminol also has positive inotropic effects. Since it constricts blood vessels, increases peripheral resistance, elevates both systolic and diastolic blood pressure, and improves cardiac contractility and cerebral, coronary, and renal blood flow, it is a valuable drug for the treatment of shock. It is used to overcome hypotension associated with myocardial infarction, surgical procedures, barbiturate poisoning, and trauma.

Since metaraminol exhibits beta as well as alpha adrenergic activity, it is often effective in raising blood pressure when alpha adrenergic agents are ineffective. This may be because of its ability to bring about more effective venous flow. It does not appear to cause dysrhythmias.

Although the action of metaraminol is similar to that of norepinephrine, it is a less potent drug. Its onset of action is more gradual than that of norepinephrine, but it is longer acting. It exerts a smoother blood pressure response than some of the other vasopressor agents, which makes the rate of flow easier to determine when the drug is given intravenously. (See Table 13-10.)

Preparation, dosage, and administration. Metaraminol is available in 1- and 10-ml units containing 10 mg/ml. It may be given intramuscularly in a 2- to 10-mg dose, or by intravenous drip, 15 to 100 mg in 500 ml of 5% dextrose in physiologic saline. The intramuscular dose for children is 0.1 mg/kg body weight. Effects appear in 10 minutes after intramuscular injection, and within 1 or 2 minutes following intravenous administration. In emergency situations, 500 µg to 5 mg of metaraminol may be injected intravenously. The AMA does not recommend the subcutaneous route, since tissue sloughing may occur. Care should be taken to prevent tissue infiltration of intravenous infusions of metaraminol.

The same precautions should be employed when giving metaraminol as when giving other powerful vasoconstrictors.

Methoxamine hydrochloride (Vasoxyl)

Methoxamine is an alpha adrenergic stimulator that appears to be devoid of beta receptor activity. Therefore it is almost exclusively a

Principal uses of adrenergic drugs

Vasoconstrictor (pressor) action (treatment of hypotensive states)
  Epinephrine
  Isoproterenol
  Levarterenol (norepinephrine)
  Metaraminol
  Methoxamine
  Mephentermine
  Phenylephrine
  Phenylpropanolamine
Local vasoconstrictor action (hemostasis; prolong local anesthetic action)
  Epinephrine
  Methoxamine
Nasal decongestant action (in treatment of allergic rhinitis, common cold, hay fever)
  Ephedrine
  Mephentermine
  Methoxamine
  Phenylephrine
  Phenylpropanolamine
  Propylhexedrine
Bronchodilator action (in treatment of asthma)
  Ephedrine
  Epinephrine
  Isoproterenol
  Methoxyphenamine
  Phenylpropanolamine
  Protokylol
Vasodilator action (in treatment of peripheral vascular disease)
  Nylidrin
Mydriatic action (for ophthalmologic examination)
  Ephedrine
  Phenylephrine

vasoconstrictor. It is used in treating nasal congestion and hypotension; it may also be used to maintain blood pressure during anesthesia. Since it has no stimulating effect on the heart, the rise in blood pressure causes a reflex bradycardia. This effect makes it useful in treating paroxysmal supraventricular tachycardia. (See Table 13-10.)

Preparation, dosage, and administration. Methoxamine is supplied in solution form for intramuscular or intravenous injection. It is available in 1-ml ampules containing 20 mg, in 10-ml vials containing 10 mg/ml, and in 1-ml ampules containing 15 mg methoxamine and 10 mg procaine hydrochloride. It is also available in a 0.5% nasal solution. The intramuscular dose for adults ranges from 5 to 20 mg; for children the dose is 0.25 mg/kg body weight.

When methoxamine is given intravenously, its effects occur almost immediately and last for 1 hour; intramuscularly, effects occur within 15 minutes and persist for about 90 minutes. Slow intravenous infusions of the drug may also be used—35 to 40 mg methoxamine in 250 ml of 5% dextrose.

Side effects. Side effects include severe headache, urinary urgency, and vomiting.

Adrenergic blocking (sympatholytic) drugs
ALPHA BLOCKING AGENTS

Most alpha adrenergic blocking agents are competitive blockers; that is, they compete with the catecholamines at receptor sites and inhibit adrenergic sympathetic stimulation. They are more effective against the action of circulating catecholamines than against catecholamines released from storage sites. These drugs may be obtained from natural sources, such as ergot and its derivatives, or they may be synthesized.

Alpha blocking agents are used in the treatment of peripheral vascular disease; ergotamine is used to treat migraine headache. Phentolamine is used in the diagnosis and surgical management of pheochromocytoma (tumors of the medullary portion of the adrenal gland that secrete large amounts of epinephrine and norepinephrine). Most adrenergic blocking agents are not drugs of choice in the treatment of essential hypertension because their action is too unpredictable and side effects too troublesome.

Phenoxybenzamine hydrochloride (Dibenzyline)

Phenoxybenzamine abolishes or decreases the receptiveness of alpha receptors to adrenergic stimuli. Its effects are predominantly those of vasodilation and inhibition of vasospasm. This drug lowers peripheral resistance and increases the size of the vascular space. For these reasons it is a useful drug in the treatment

of peripheral vascular diseases such as Raynaud's disease.

Since phenoxybenzamine competes with the catecholamines, it is also useful in decreasing the blood pressure of patients with pheochromocytoma. It does not block sympathetic impulses on the heart and therefore does not impair cardiac output directly. It has mild antihistaminic activity and may cause nasal drying.

Preparation, dosage, and administration. Phenoxybenzamine is available in 10-mg capsules for oral use. The initial dose is usually 10 mg daily. The dosage may be increased by increments of 10 mg at 4-day intervals. The maintenance dosage is usually 20 to 60 mg daily. The onset of action occurs in about 2 hours, and the duration of action is 24 to 36 hours. Daily administration causes cumulative effects, intensifies side effects, and makes the patient susceptible to toxic effects.

Side effects and toxic effects. Common side effects from phenoxybenzamine include nasal congestion, miosis, reflex tachycardia, and postural hypotension. Sedation, drowsiness, and failing to ejaculate occur occasionally.

Toxic symptoms include severe postural hypotension, vomiting, lethargy, shock, and circulatory failure.

Phentolamine hydrochloride (Regitine Hydrochloride); phentolamine mesylate (Regitine Mesylate)

Phenotolamine is a direct vasodilator and an inhibitor of hypertension when there are excessive levels of epinephrine and norepinephrine. Its direct effect is more potent than its adrenergic blocking action.

Phentolamine is used in the diagnosis of pheochromocytoma. Since this tumor secretes large amounts of catecholamines, which produce elevated blood pressure, a marked fall in blood pressure following administration of phentolamine suggests the presence of pheochromocytoma. However, this test lacks precision. A false-positive test may occur if the patient recently received a sedative, narcotic, or antihypertensive drug.

This drug is also used to reverse the vasoconstrictive action of an overdose or excessive response to injected norepinephrine (levarterenol). The subcutaneous injection of phentolamine following extravasation of intravenous norepinephrine will prevent tissue necrosis if prompt action is taken.

Preparation, dosage, and administration. Phentolamine hydrochloride is available in 50-mg tablets for oral use. The usual adult dose is 50 mg four to six times daily; for children the dose is 5 mg/kg body weight daily divided into four or six doses.

Phentolamine mesylate is administered intramuscularly or intravenously. It is prepared in 5-mg vials to which 1 ml of diluent is added for injection. The amount used in the test for pheochromocytoma is 5 mg. A decrease in blood pressure of more than 35 mm Hg systolic and 25 mm Hg diastolic implies pheochromocytoma. The preoperative dose for removal of the adrenal tumor is 2 to 5 mg given 1 or 2 hours before surgery. For children the dose is usually 1 mg or 0.1 mg/kg.

Side effects. Side effects include tachycardia, orthostatic hypotension, nausea and vomiting, diarrhea, weakness, dizziness, and flushing. Phentolamine should be used with caution in patients with gastritis or peptic ulcer, since it has a stimulant action on the gastrointestinal tract, and in patients with coronary artery disease.

ERGOT ALKALOIDS

Alkaloids found in extracts of a fungous disease of rye called *ergot* are derivatives of lysergic acid; some of these alkaloids cause alpha receptor blockade. The ergot alkaloids have many other effects. They are powerful constrictors of vascular or uterine smooth muscle. This action has nothing to do with the slight adrenergic effect they possess.

Ergotamine tartrate

Ergotamine has marked vasoconstrictor activity. All ergot alkaloids stimulate uterine smooth muscle; both tone and amplitude of uterine contractions are increased. However, ergotamine is no longer used as an oxytocic. It is now used chiefly to treat migraine headache and is considered almost a specific for this condition. Its efficacy in migraine is thought to result from cerebral vasoconstriction, which decreases the amplitude of the pulsations of cranial arteries. The earlier the drug is taken, the smaller the dose needed and the more rapid the effect. Administration of the drug should be followed by bed rest in a quiet, darkened room for an hour or two.

This drug also has been used to relieve intense itching and hives associated with jaundice, cirrhosis of the liver, or Hodgkin's disease.

Since ergotamine has a cumulative action, it must be used with caution. It is capable of producing all the symptoms of ergotism: numbness and tingling of the fingers and toes, muscle pains and muscle weakness, gangrene, and blindness. Thus daily use is not advised. Its use is contraindicated in pregnant patients and those with diabetes mellitus, hepatic and renal disease, and peripheral vascular disease.

Preparation, dosage, and administration. The following are the ergotamine preparations available.

Ergotamine tartrate (Gynergen). The usual oral dose is 2 mg, and the usual intramuscular or subcutaneous dose is 0.25 mg. The oral dose for children over 5 years of age is 1 mg. Ergotamine tartrate is available in tablets for oral administration (1 mg), 2-mg sublingual tablets, in ampules of solution for parenteral administration (0.25 mg in 0.5 ml and 0.5 mg in 1 ml), as a solution for inhalation (9 mg/ml in 2.5-ml containers; a single inhalation contains 0.36 mg), and as suppositories for rectal administration.

Ergotamine with caffeine (Cafergot). Each tablet contains 1 mg ergotamine tartrate and 100 mg caffeine. The usual dose is one to two tablets for headache. The dose may be repeated if necessary every 30 minutes; no more than six tablets should be taken per attack. The caffeine presumably increases the effectiveness of ergotamine because of its own vasoconstrictor action.

Dihydroergotamine (D.H.E. 45). This compound is prepared by hydrogenating ergotamine. It is available in 1-ml ampules that contain 1 mg of the drug. Administration is intramuscular or intravenous. To relieve acute migraine, the dose is 1 mg at onset of the attack; this may be repeated in 1 hour. Dihydroergotamine is said to produce fewer side effects than ergotamine tartrate. However, its effects are less predictable.

Methysergide maleate (Sansert)

Methysergide maleate, a drug related structurally to the ergot alkaloids, is effective for the prophylactic treatment of vascular headaches. It is of no value for treating acute attacks or preventing tension headache. Each tablet contains 2 mg of methysergide maleate. The drug is a serotonin antagonist.

Retroperitoneal fibrosis has been noted in a small number of patients on methysergide therapy. Its signs and symptoms usually present themselves as urinary tract obstruction. Pleuropulmonary and cardiac fibroses have also been reported. If there are symptoms of peripheral vascular insufficiency, such as cold, numb, or painful extremities and diminished pulse, the drug should be discontinued to prevent severe tissue ischemia. Because of these serious complications and numerous side effects, the approved package insert should be consulted before the drug is used. The usual dose is two to four tablets, preferably one tablet with each meal. Because of the potential dangers of prolonged therapy, a rest period of 3 to 4 weeks should follow 6 months of treatment with methysergide. The dosage should be gradually reduced to avoid rebound headaches. In addition, patients should be instructed to report promptly any dysuria, back pain, dyspnea, or chest pain.

Dihydroergocornine dihydroergocristine dihydroergokryptine mesylate (Hydergine)

Sublingual tablets of Hydergine are sometimes administered to elderly patients, and some improvement in self-care, sociability, and alertness in patients with hypertensive brain disease may be subsequently observed. The drug is controversial, and the pharmacologic mode of action in elderly patients is not understood. Hydergine does not cause vasoconstriction. Sublingual tablets may produce buccal irritation and nausea.

BETA BLOCKING AGENT

In the United States the most widely used beta blocking agent is propranolol (Inderal). This drug is chemically related to isoproterenol. Metoprolol (Lopressor) has recently been approved for treating hypertension.

Beta blockers inhibit the beta receptors by competing with the catecholamines at the effector site. These agents *block* beta receptors in myocardial, bronchial, and vascular smooth muscle.

Propranolol hydrochloride (Inderal)

Propranolol inhibits the inotropic and chronotropic actions caused by beta adrenergic stimulation and has a quinidine-like effect and local anesthetic effect. Propranolol inhibits pacemaker activity (normal as well as ectopic), decreases atrioventricular conduction, and prolongs cardiac diastole. It also decreases heart rate and myocardial activity, suppresses myocardial automaticity, increases systolic ejection time, and increases cardiac volume. These actions account for its clinical effectiveness in controlling various ventricular arrhythmias including digitalis-induced arrhythmia when hypokalemia is not present. It may be used in the preparation of patients for cardioversion when digitalis must be withheld before cardioversion.

Propranolol has been found effective in the treatment of some cases of angina, probably owing to its ability to prevent an increase in cardiac rate during exercise. There is evidence that patients treated with propranolol can undertake a greater amount of exercise before experiencing anginal pain.

In addition, propranolol increases airway resistance, inhibits glucogenolysis in skeletal and cardiac muscles, and blocks adrenergic release of free fatty acids and insulin. It also has a hypotensive effect when taken orally for a prolonged period. Propranolol may cause electrocardiographic changes such as higher voltage T waves and an increase in the Q-T interval. Propranolol is also used in antihypertensive therapy either alone or with another hypotensive agent.

Dosage and administration. Propranolol may be administered orally or intravenously. It may be used alone or in conjunction with other antidysrhythmic agents. When given orally, it is most readily absorbed if the patient is in the fasting state and therefore should be given before meals. It is effective within 30 minutes, peak action occurs in 60 to 90 minutes, and the effect lasts about 6 hours. The usual oral dose is from 30 to 120 mg daily. The drug is available in 10- and 40-mg tablets. Propranolol is metabolized by hepatic enzymes. The optimal dosage for children has not been determined.

When propranolol is administered intravenously, the maximal effect occurs within 3 to 5 minutes; the duration of effect is 2 to 4 hours. The range of dose for intravenous administration is usually 1 to 5 mg. The drug is available in 1-ml ampules containing 1 mg of drug per milliliter. This drug *must* be given slowly with careful monitoring of vital signs with the electrocardiogram. Administration should be discontinued when a desirable change in heart rate or rhythm is noted.

Side effects. Side effects include nausea and vomiting, light-headedness, lethargy, mental depression, and mild paresthesia.

Toxic effects. Toxic effects include hypotension, bradycardia, heart block, congestive heart failure in patients with limited cardiac reserve, and intensified hypoglycemia in diabetic patients receiving insulin or oral hypoglycemic drugs. The last effect occurs because beta-receptor activity is necessary for a rise in blood sugar and free fatty acids. Special precautions should be taken when propranolol is used along with other adrenergic blocking agents, since the effects are additive, or when used with MAO inhibitors, since the enhanced alpha effect may lead to hypertension.

Contraindications. Propranolol is contraindicated in patients with congestive heart failure, hypotension, asthma, and atrioventricular heart block.

• • •

Additional therapeutically useful autonomic drugs are described in greater detail elsewhere in the text where their actions are more specifically relevant to the systems discussed.

Summary of nursing considerations

The primary function of the autonomic nervous system is to modulate and integrate a multitude of physiologic tasks necessary to preserve internal homeostasis, emergency mechanisms, and repair. Its activities are integrated by a number of centers within the central nervous system: the hypothalamus, medulla oblongata, midbrain, limbic system, cerebellum, and cerebral cortex. The autonomic nervous system innervates the smooth muscles, cardiac muscles, and glands. It is composed of two divisions, the parasympathetic and the sympathetic; their actions are opposed in a balanced antagonism.

Functions stimulated by the parasympathetic system are chiefly those concerned with digestion, excretion, near vision, cardiac deceleration, and anabolism. Functions stimulated by the sympathetic system are primarily those concerned with the expenditure of energy and are called into play by physical or emotional stress.

Nerve impulse transmission is caused by the activity of chemical substances called *mediators*, acetylcholine and the catecholamines. Nerve fibers that synthesize and liberate acetylcholine are known as *cholinergic* fibers; those that synthesize and secrete norepinephrine and epinephrine are called *adrenergic* fibers.

Drugs that cause physiologic effects similar to those of acetylcholine are called *cholinergic drugs* (formerly known as parasympathomimetics). Drugs that produce effects such as those caused by the adrenergic mediators are called *adrenergic drugs* (formerly called sympathomimetics).

Three principal catecholamines have been positively identified: dopamine, epinephrine, and norepinephrine. Dopamine is a precursor of the other two but like norepinephrine is an important transmitter of nerve impulses. Epinephrine acts mainly as an emergency hormone.

Within the sympathetic nervous system, the adrenergic effector cells contain two distinct receptors, the alpha and beta receptors. The beta receptors are further divided into beta$_1$ and beta$_2$ receptors. Norepinephrine acts mainly on alpha receptors, whereas epinephrine acts on both alpha and beta receptors. Principal alpha adrenergic activities are vasoconstriction of arterioles in the skin and splanchnic areas, elevation of blood pressure, pupil dilation, and relaxation of the gut. Beta$_1$ adrenergic activity includes cardiac acceleration and increased contractility; beta$_2$ adrenergic activity includes bronchial and uterine relaxation. Norepinephrine and epinephrine are continuously present in arterial blood, although the amount varies widely during any one day and is increased by stress and exercise.

Drugs chemically related to acetylcholine that produce similar effects are cholinergic drugs. Acetylcholine has two major actions on the nervous system: (1) *Nicotinic*—stimulates ganglia, adrenal medulla, and skeletal muscles, and (2) *Muscarinic*—stimulates postganglionic nerve endings in cardiac muscle, smooth muscles, and glands. Cholinergic drugs are used to stimulate intestines and bladder postoperatively, lower intraocular pressure in glaucoma, promote salivation and sweating, and dilate peripheral blood vessels in vasospasm.

Some drugs act as cholinergic agents by inactivating or inhibiting the enzyme cholinesterase that normally degrades acetylcholine thus prolonging the activity of acetylcholine. These agents are called *anticholinesterase drugs.* Nicotine has no therapeutic use but is of great pharmacologic interest because its use in animal experiments has helped increase understanding of the autonomic nervous system. Its effect resembles the "nicotine" effect of acetylcholine.

Cholinergic blocking drugs (anticholinergic drugs) that act selectively to block the muscarinic effects of acetylcholine relax smooth muscles, inhibit secretions of duct glands, and dilate the pupils. Their prototype is atropine, a belladonna alkaloid, which may produce local, central, or peripheral action. Atropine is readily absorbed and potent, but it has a wide margin of safety. It is contraindicated for patients with glaucoma because of the risk of increased intraocular tension. Scopolamine resembles atropine in structure and peripheral effects but differs in its central action. Given parenterally, scopolamine depresses the central nervous system, producing drowsiness, euphoria, and amnesia. Its primary use is as a preanesthetic medication.

Atropine is limited in its usefulness because of the simultaneous effects produced in multiple organs and tissues. Many drugs have been synthesized to capture the antispasmodic effect of atropine without its other effects, but these efforts have been less than totally successful. Among the synthetic substitutes are methscopolamine bromide, methantheline bromide, propantheline bromide, homatropine methylbromide, and pipenzolate bromide. Like most of the cholinergic blocking agents, they are contraindicated for patients with glaucoma, pyloric obstruction, and prostatic hypertrophy.

Catecholamines have a high potential for drug interaction when given with other drugs, particularly with digitalis, MAO inhibitors, certain anesthetics, tricyclic antidepressants, diuretics, and antihypertensive drugs.

Many drugs, structurally related to the catecholamines, affect alpha and beta receptors *indirectly* by releasing catecholamines from adrenergic nerves. Others act *directly* on the receptors, and some have both *indirect and direct* effects. These widely used drugs include ephedrine, phenylephrine hydrochloride, mephentermine sulfate, metaraminol bitartrate, and methoxamine hydrochloride.

Most alpha adrenergic blocking agents compete with the catecholamines at receptor sites and inhibit adrenergic sympathetic stimulation. They are used to treat peripheral vascular disease, migraine headache, and certain adrenal tumors. Because their action is too unpredictable and their side effects too troublesome, these are not drugs of choice for hypertension. These drugs include phenoxybenzamine hydrochloride, phentolamine hydrochloride, the ergot alkaloids, and methysergide maleate.

The beta blocking agent that has a variety of clinical uses is propranolol hydrochloride (Inderal). Its exact mode of action is unknown, but it blocks beta receptors in the myocardium and bronchial and vascular smooth muscles. Propranolol is used to control various ventricular arrhythmias including digitalis-induced dysrythymia when hypokalemia is not present. It has also been found effective in the treatment of angina, and the drug is now used in antihypertensive therapy. Propranolol is contraindicated in patients with congestive heart failure, hypotension, asthma, and atrioventricular heart block.

QUESTIONS

FOR STUDY AND REVIEW

1 Explain what is meant by the muscarinic action of a drug; by the nicotinic action of a drug.
2 What is the difference between cholinergic fibers and adrenergic fibers? Between cholinergic drugs and adrenergic drugs?
3 Explain the pharmacologic actions of nicotine.
4 Why is atropine often given as a preoperative medication?
5 Are there differences between the effects of scopolamine and atropine? Explain.
6 What side effects can be expected from antispasmodics?
7 What nursing action should be taken if these side effects occur?
8 What are the actions of epinephrine that make it a useful drug in the following situations:
  a treatment of an acute asthmatic attack
  b injection along with a local anesthetic
  c treatment of glaucoma
9 Which drugs potentiate the action of the catecholamines; antagonize the action of catecholamines?
10 Discuss the therapeutic effects resulting from stimulation of alpha receptors; $beta_1$ and $beta_2$ receptors.
11 Discuss the desired therapeutic effects of alpha blocking agents; beta blocking agents.
12 What treatment should be given if levarterenol infiltrates subcutaneous tissues?
13 Which autonomic drugs are used in the treatment of severe hypotension? Explain.
14 Explain why after prolonged use of a pressor drug the drug may no longer have a vasoconstrictor effect.
15 Discuss the use of ergot preparations in the treatment of migraine headache.

BIBLIOGRAPHY

BOOKS

A.M.A. drug evaluations, ed. 3, Acton, Mass., 1977, Publishing Sciences Group, Inc.

Avery, G.S., editor: Drug treatment, Acton, Mass., ed. 2, 1980, Publishing Sciences Group, Inc.

Bhagat, B.D.: Mode of action of autonomic drugs, Flushing, N.Y., 1979, Graceway Publishing Co.

Bowman, W.C., and Rand, M.J.: Textbook of pharmacology, ed. 2, London, 1980, Blackwell Scientific Publications.

Bowsher, D.: Introduction to the anatomy and physiology of the nervous system, ed. 4, London, 1979, Blackwell Scientific Publications.

Burn, J.: The autonomic nervous system: for students of physiology and pharmacology, ed. 5, London, 1975, Blackwell Scientific Publications.

Cooper, J., Bloom, F., and Roth, R.: The biochemical basis of neuropharmacology, New York, 1974, Oxford University Press.

Goodman, L.S., and Gilman, A., editors: The pharmacological basis of therapeutics, ed. 6, New York, 1980, Macmillan, Inc.

Goth, A.: Medical pharmacology, ed. 10, St. Louis, 1981, The C.V. Mosby Co.

Levine, R.R.: Pharmacology: drug actions and reactions, ed. 2, Boston, 1978, Little, Brown & Co.

Lewis, A.J., editor: Modern drug encyclopedia, ed. 15, New York, 1979, Dun-Donnelley Publishing Corp.

Meyers, F.H., Jawetz, E., and Goldfien, A.: Review of medical pharmacology, ed. 5, Los Altos, Calif., 1980, Lange Medical Publications.

Modell, W., editor: Drugs of choice 1980-1981, St. Louis, 1980, the C.V. Mosby Co.

Noback, C., and Demarest, R.: The nervous system: introduction and review, ed. 2, New York, 1977, McGraw-Hill Book Co.

Turner, P., and Richens, A.: Clinical pharmacology, Edinburgh, 1973, Churchill Livingstone.

PERIODICALS

Axelrod, J.: Noradrenaline: fate and control of its biosynthesis, Science **173:**598, 1971.

Axelrod, J.: Neurotransmitters, Sci. Am. **230:**58, 1974.

Axelsson, J.: Catecholamine functions, Annu. Rev. Physiol. **33:**1, 1971.

Beta blockade in cardiovascular therapeutics, Drugs **7:**1, 426, 1974.

Catecholamines, Br. Med. Bull. **29:**91, 1973.

DiPalma, J.R.: Cholinergic and anticholinergic drugs, R.N. **37:**83, May, 1974.

Geffen, L.B., and Livett, B.G.: Synaptic vesicles in sympathetic neurons, Physiol. Rev. **51:**98, 1971.

Gravenstein, J.S., and others: Atropine on the electrocardiogram, Clin. Pharmacol. Ther. **10:**660, 1969.

Greenblatt, D.J., and Shader, R.I.: Anticholinergics, N. Engl. J. Med. **288:**1215, 1973.

Huss, P., and others: The new inotropic drug, dobutamine, Heart Lung **10:**121,1981.

Koelle, G.B.: Acetylcholine—current status in physiology, pharmacology and medicine, N. Engl. J. Med. **286:**1086, 1972.

Kosman, M.E.: Current status of propranolol hydrochloride (Inderal), J.A.M.A. **225:**1380, 1973.

Lawrence, T., and others: Beta adrenergic receptor blocking drugs, Med. Clin. North Am. **57:**944, 1973.

Littman, A., and Pine B.H.: Antacids and anticholinergic drugs, Ann. Intern. Med. **82:**544, 1975.

Moreli, H.F.: Propranolol, Ann. Intern. Med. **78:**913, 1973.

Patil, P.N., and others: Molecular geometry and adrenergic drug activity, Pharmacol. Rev. **26:**323, 1974.

Piper, D.W.: Antacid and anticholinergic drug therapy, Clin. Gastroenterol. **2:**361, 1973.

Pohorecky, L.A., and Wurtman, R.J.: Adrenocortical control of epinephrine synthesis, Pharmacol. Rev. **23:**1, 1971.

Reid, P., and Thompson, W.: The clinical use of dopamine in the treatment of shock, Johns Hopkins Med. J. **13:**276, 1975.

Rosenberg, J.: Anticholinergics: where additive side effects matter, Curr. Prescribing, July 1976, p. 36.

UNIT SIX

DRUGS ACTING ON SYSTEMS OF THE INTERNAL ENVIRONMENT

CHAPTER 14

Respiratory system drugs

The respiratory system

The respiratory system includes all that is involved in the exchange of oxygen and carbon dioxide—such as all airway passages, the lungs, nasal cavities, pharynx, larynx, trachea, bronchi, bronchioles, pulmonary lobules with their alveoli, the diaphragm, and the muscles concerned with respiration itself.

Although a large number of specific substances must be supplied to maintain life, the most urgent and critical need is a continued, uninterrupted supply of oxygen. This specific need for oxygen is supplied through the process of respiration. Respiration is a term loosely used to describe three distinct but interrelated processes. These include:

1 Pulmonary ventilation, which involves the movement of air into and out of the lungs
2 Gas transport, which involves the exchange of gas-

es between the air in the lungs, the blood, and the cell
3 Cellular respiration, which involves the utilization of oxygen in the catabolism of energy-yielding substances for the production of energy

The process of respiration is one of the regulating systems that helps to maintain physiologic dynamic equilibrium. It also functions as a compensatory mechanism for rapid adjustment to changes in metabolic states.

The air passages serve the dual purpose of permitting air to flow from the external environment to pulmonary blood and of modifying the air taken in by warming and moistening it and removing noxious substances. Airway efficiency is determined by the following factors:

1 Shape and size of each portion of the respiratory tract (nasal cavity, pharynx, larynx, trachea, bronchi, bronchioles, alveolar sacs)

2 Presence of a ciliated, mucus-secreting, epithelial lining throughout most of the respiratory tract
3 Character and thickness of respiratory tract secretions
4 Compliance of the cartilaginous and bony supports
5 Pressure gradients
6 Traction on airway walls
7 Absence of foreign substances in the lumen of the respiratory tract

An alteration from normal of any of these factors will affect the ease with which air flows through the air passages. Congenital anomalies, injuries, allergies, or disease will cause air flow resistance if the preceding factors are abnormally affected. Resistance occurs, for example, if there is stenosis or narrowing of any portion of the respiratory tract, loss of cilia that ordinarily sweep out foreign substances, presence of thick or tenacious secretions, loss of elasticity, or presence of foreign objects.

RESPIRATORY TRACT SECRETIONS

Secretory glands. The tracheobronchial tree, made up of repeated branching tubes, is a tubular airway that serves as a conduit for passage of air from the external environment to the alveolar-capillary exchange unit. The inner surface of the tracheobronchial tree is lined with ciliated columnar epithelium that is interspersed with *goblet cells*. The gelatinous mucus (gel layer) produced by these goblet cells is normally discharged into the tubular lumen. During respiratory disease, goblet cells multiply in great numbers and the viscosity of the mucus also increases, thus making it difficult for the cilia to transport the secretions along the airway (Fig. 14-1).

The second source of respiratory secretions is located in the submucosa of the tracheobronchial tree. These are the *bronchial glands*, which secrete a relatively watery fluid (sol layer) through ducts that lead to the surface of the ciliated epithelium. Under vagal (parasympathetic) control, the glands can be stimulated by irritant agents or aerosol drugs to release or discharge their contents into the lumen of the airway (Fig. 14-1, *B*).

The products of these two sources—goblet cells and bronchial glands—form the *sol-gel film* that constitutes the *mucociliary blanket*.

This protective blanket of fluid bathes the ciliated epithelium of the tracheobronchial tree. Moreover, the cilia keep the secretions in constant motion by continuously propelling the sol-gel film in an upward direction toward the larynx along the respiratory tree. The normal adult produces approximately 100 ml of respiratory secretions a day, and this material is swallowed without the individual being aware of it. The process of moving mucus along the tracheobronchial tree is called *mucokinesis*. The mucociliary blanket is a fundamental concern associated with most chronic obstructive pulmonary disease. The cilia must sustain appropriate function; a dry atmosphere causes the respiratory secretions to become thick and tenacious, which tends to interfere with ciliary movements. Thus, adequate humidity of the atmosphere should be maintained to prevent the change in the normal consistency of the respiratory secretions (see Fig. 14-1, *B*, for mucociliary blanket).

BRONCHIAL SMOOTH MUSCLE

Smooth muscle arrangement. An important structural component of the tracheobronchial tree is the smooth muscle. The mass of muscle fibers along the bronchi progressively increases as it extends down toward the distal bronchioles. Isolated muscle fibers may be found even as far down as the alveolar ducts. The arrangement of the smooth muscle fibers along the length of the tubular tree appears in a double helical or spiral pattern, and this formation has a profound regulatory influence on the diameter or the lumen of the airways. As a consequence of this structural feature, the effect of muscle contraction reduces both the caliber and length of the bronchus (Fig. 14-1, *A*).

Nerve supply. The airway or tracheobronchial tree is innervated by the automatic nervous system. In the healthy subject the bronchial smooth muscle tone is influenced by the balance maintained between parasympathetic and sympathetic stimuli during rest. Activation of the parasympathetic fiber (vagus nerve) releases acetylcholine, and this results in bronchoconstriction and narrowing of the airway. By contrast, the stimulation of the sympathetic fiber and also the sympathoadrenal system,

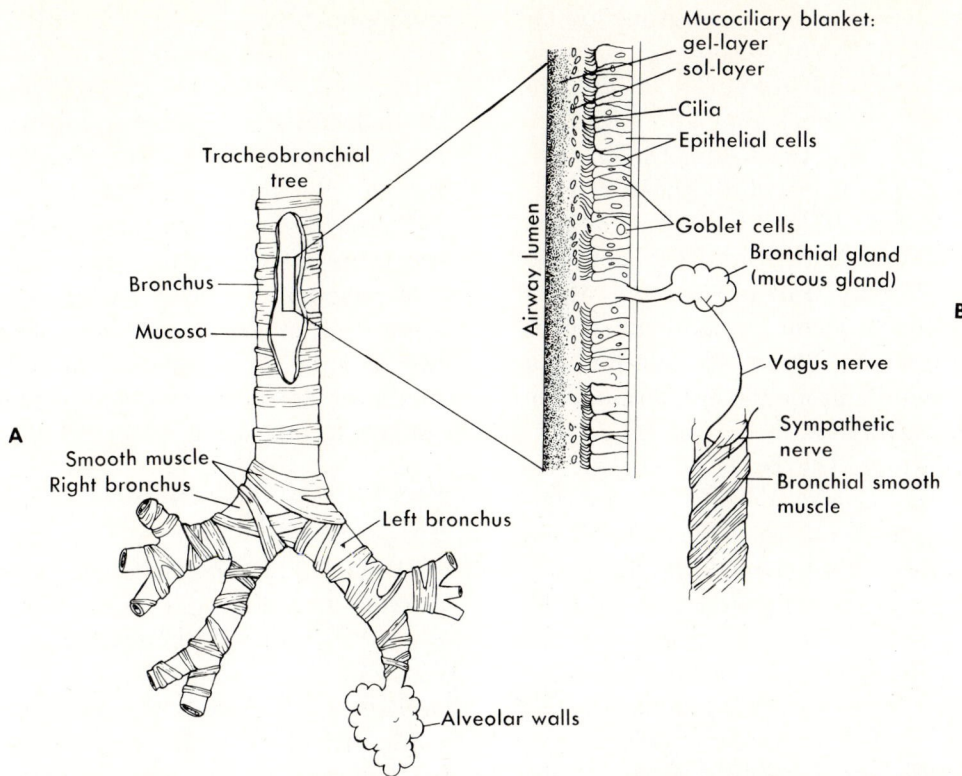

FIG. 14-1. Tracheobronchial tree and bronchial smooth muscle. **A,** Diagram of the tracheobronchial tree illustrates the double helical or spiral arrangement of the bronchial smooth muscle along the bronchi. Cut-out section shows the inner lining or the mucosa of the bronchus. **B,** The elements of the mucosal lining are enlarged to show details of structures that contribute to the mucociliary blanket. Note that the cilia move in an upward direction toward the larynx. The goblet cells interspersed between the columnar epithelium produce a gelatinous mucus, called the gel-layer, whereas the bronchial gland has a tubular duct to the lumen of the tracheobronchial tree through which it secretes a watery fluid, the sol layer. Thus, the sol-gel layer forms the mucociliary blanket, a protective fluid film that bathes the ciliated epithelium of the tracheobronchial tree. The normal adult produces approximately 100 ml of respiratory secretions a day. Furthermore, the bronchial gland is under vagal control and on stimulation by foreign substances increases production of watery secretion. The sol-gel fluid is kept in constant motion by cilia. When a foreign particle from inspired air becomes trapped in the fluid layer, cilia move it in an upward direction toward the mouth for excretion. By this process, the accumulation of bacteria and foreign material in the lung is prevented.

The innervation of the bronchial smooth muscle is also shown. Activation of the vagus nerve results in bronchoconstriction whereas the sympathetic nerve produces bronchodilation.

release epinephrine and norepinephrine from the adrenal medulla into the circulation. Their action on the beta$_2$ receptor sites in the bronchial smooth muscle is particularly effective in producing bronchodilation during smooth muscle relaxation (see Fig. 14-1, *B*, for nerve supply).

Receptors. Several kinds of receptors are found along the bronchial airway. The release of acetylcholine results in activation of muscarinic receptors during stimulation of the para-

sympathetic system. On the other hand, the sympathetic system affects adrenergic receptors. Most of the adrenergic receptors present in the bronchial smooth muscle belong to the beta$_2$ classification; these receptors are stimulated mainly by epinephrine released from the adrenal medulla. However, beta$_1$ receptors are also found. The ratio of beta$_2$ to beta$_1$ receptors is approximately 3:1; thus it can be concluded that the bronchial smooth muscle is supplied primarily by beta$_2$ receptors. The sympathomimetic drugs used principally as bronchodilators stimulate the beta$_2$ receptors. Because many of these agents are not purely selective in their pharmacologic effect, they also stimulate the beta$_1$ receptors in the heart. Under such circumstances, the effects on the heart constitute unwanted side effects such as increased cardiac output, tachycardia, and a tendency to dysrhythmia. Finally, the presence of alpha receptors on the bronchial smooth muscle is relatively scarce, and their stimulation can result in only mild bronchoconstriction. (See Fig. 13-6 for receptors.)

Bronchodilation. The beta$_2$ adrenergic receptors mediate bronchodilation. This mechanism presumably is initiated by epinephrine released from the adrenal medulla. This hormone then reaches the lung via the circulation and interacts with the beta$_2$ adrenergic receptor in the cell membrane of the bronchial smooth muscle cell. Also located in the cell membrane is an enzyme system known as adenylcyclase. In the presence of magnesium ions, adenylcyclase catalyzes the action of adenosine triphosphate (ATP) in the cytoplasm of the cell to produce cyclic 3'5' adenosine-monophosphate (cyclic 3'5'AMP or c3'5'AMP). Cyclic AMP then performs its important function, that is, inducing relaxation of bronchial smooth muscle or bronchodilation. The hormone epinephrine is designated as the "first messenger" and cyclic 3'5'AMP as the "second messenger." As a final action, cyclic 3'5'AMP is inactivated by an enzyme, phosphodiesterase, which catalyzes it to the inactive 5'AMP. This results in a fall in the cyclic 3'5'AMP level. The action of phosphodiesterase may be inhibited by a xanthine drug such as theophylline. As a consequence, the cyclic 3'5'AMP level increases, thereby effecting smooth muscle dilation (Fig. 14-2).

Bronchoconstriction. The bronchial smooth muscle is innervated by the parasympathetic fibers from the vagus nerve. Acetylcholine released from the terminal interacts with the muscarinic receptors on the membrane of the cell. Stimulation of the muscarinic receptor increases the activity of the enzyme guanyl cyclase in the membrane, thereby promoting the rate of formation of cyclic 3'5' guanosine monophosphate (cyclic 3'5'GMP) from guanosine triphosphate (GTP). The cyclic GMP level affects the bronchial muscle by producing bronchoconstriction. In addition, there are alpha receptors found on the bronchial smooth muscle that have a similar involvement with this mechanism. On activation, the alpha receptors also increase the cyclic GMP level. Furthermore, cyclic 3'5'GMP stimulates the release of chemical mediators from the mast cell during an asthmatic attack, and these mediators are responsible for causing bronchoconstriction (see Fig. 14-2).

REGULATORY CONTROL OF RESPIRATION

Breathing is primarily controlled and coordinated involuntarily by the medullary rhythmicity area located beneath the lower part of the floor of the fourth ventricle in the medial half of the medulla. In this area inspiratory and expiratory neurons intermingle and discharge or fire impulses alternately. Thus it is in this area that the basic rhythm for respiration is initiated and maintained. However, signals from the spinal cord, the cerebral cortex and midbrain, the apneustic area of the pons, and the pneumotaxic area of the upper pons can enter the medullary rhythmicity area and modify the rhythm of respiration as well as contribute to the normal pattern of respiration.

Normally, the human organism is unaware of the respiratory process. However, voluntary influence and control of breathing are possible. This becomes of paramount importance in a situation in which a patient must learn to voluntarily control breathing patterns.

The medullary rhythmicity area is also influenced by various forms of sensory and peripheral stimuli, the vasomotor center, reflex mechanisms (such as the Hering-Breuer reflex), the chemoreceptors in the carotid and aortic bodies, and the baroreceptors in the carotid sinus and aortic arch. Fear, pain, stress, blood pressure, body temperature, and blood levels of oxygen and carbon dioxide can all modify the activity of the respiratory centers.

Humoral regulation of respiration is primarily achieved through changes in the concen-

BRONCHIAL SMOOTH MUSCLE FIBER CELL

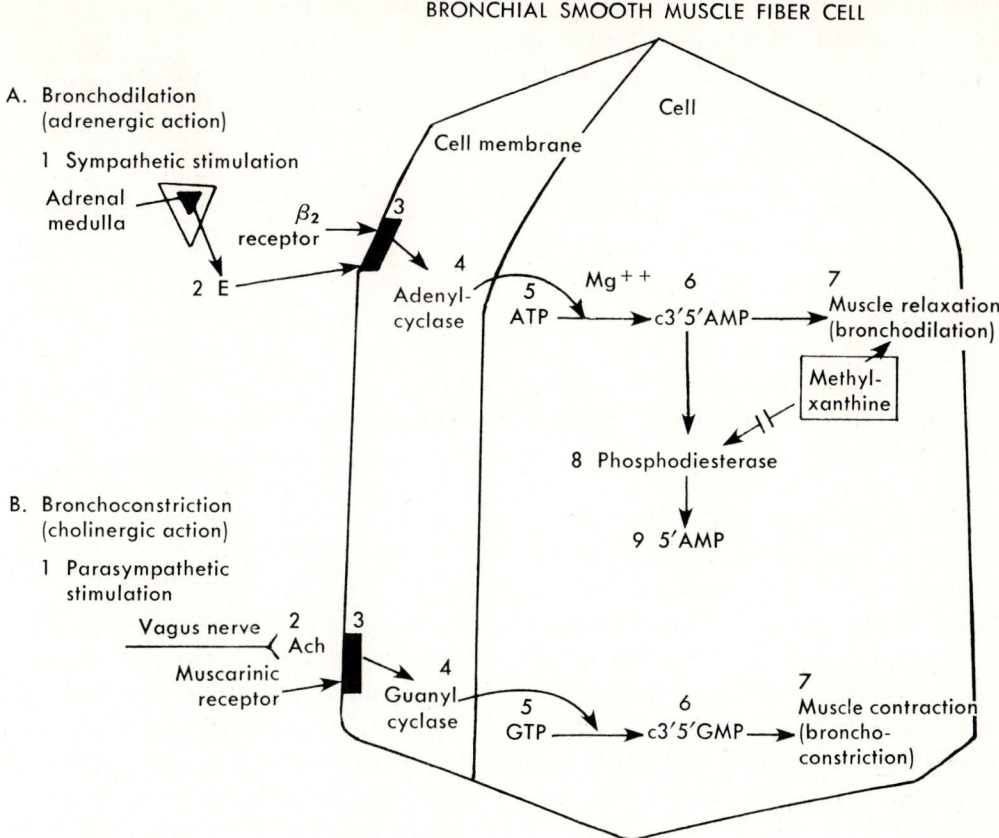

FIG. 14-2. Mechanism of bronchial smooth muscle action: **A,** Bronchodilation involves the adrenergic action. The sequence is numbered from *1* through *9.* Sympathetic stimulation releases epinephrine *(E)* and norepinephrine *(NE),* the "first messengers," from the adrenal medulla. The interaction of mainly epinephrine with the beta₂ receptor in the cell membrane activates adenylcyclase, an enzyme also in the cell membrane. Adenylcyclase catalyzes the conversion of adenosine triphosphate (ATP) to cyclic 3'5'AMP (c3'5'AMP), the "second messenger" that in some way induces muscle relaxation or bronchodilation. Magnesium (Mg++) is required to promote the reaction. Normally, c3'5'AMP undergoes fairly rapid hydrolysis to inactive 5'AMP by the intracellular enzyme *phosphodiesterase.* Methylxanthine is capable of inhibiting the action of the enzyme *phosphodiesterase* so that the level of c3'5'AMP is increased and bronchodilation is prolonged. **B,** Bronchoconstriction involves cholinergic action. The sequence is numbered from *1* to *7.* The steps in this mechanism include the release of acetylcholine *(Ach)* following vagal nerve stimulation. Interaction of Ach with the muscarinic receptor in the cell membrane activates the enzyme guanyl cyclase, also found in the membrane. Guanyl cyclase catalyzes the reaction that converts guanosine triphosphate (GTP) to cyclic 3'5' guanosine monophosphate (c3'5'GMP). The production of c3'5'GMP causes muscle contraction or bronchoconstriction.

trations of oxygen, carbon dioxide, or hydrogen ions in body fluids. In the normal well individual carbon dioxide is the chief respiratory stimulant. An increase in the carbon dioxide tension of the blood directly stimulates the inspiratory and expiratory centers, which increases both the rate and depth of breathing. This results in a blowing off of carbon dioxide to keep the carbon dioxide tension of the blood constant. The pH of the blood is determined by the ratio of bicarbonate ion (HCO₃) to carbon dioxide. When the carbon dioxide content of the blood is increased, there is a subsequent increase in the formation of carbonic acid in the blood. This alters the bicarbonate/carbonic acid ratio from the normal value of 20:1 and results in acidosis. Conversely, a decrease in the carbon dioxide content of the blood results in alkalosis. There-

TABLE 14-1   Pharmacologic actions of the main drug groups
used in the management of respiratory diseases

Drug groups	Respiratory structure	Pharmacologic action
Mucokinetic drugs	Goblet cells, bronchial glands, and ciliated epithelium	Alters character of respiratory secretions
Bronchodilator drugs	Bronchial smooth muscle	Maintains airway caliber by bronchodilation
Mucosal constrictor drugs	Alpha receptors in blood vessels	Relieves nasal congestion

fore, respiration is important for regulating the pH of the blood by controlling the carbon dioxide tension of the blood.

Basically, changes in arterial oxygen concentration have little, if any, direct effect on the respiratory center. However, if the arterial oxygen concentration falls below normal, the chemoreceptors in the carotid and aortic bodies are stimulated and in turn stimulate the respiratory center to increase alveolar ventilation. This mechanism operates primarily under abnormal conditions, such as chronic obstructive pulmonary disease.

• • •

In the management of respiratory diseases the main groups of drugs used to maintain and restore the integrity of lung structure may be classified according to their sites of tissue action. Thus the pharmacologic aspects associated with these drugs include the factors shown in Table 14-1.

Aerosol therapy

Aerosol therapy is a form of topical pulmonary treatment administered mainly by aerosols. An aerosol is a suspension of fine liquid or solid particles dispersed in a gas. Liquid or solid particles range in size from about 0.005 to 50 μm in diameter. Nebulizers are designed to deliver a maximum number of particles of a desired size. Thus aerosol therapy is delivered through nebulization. The terms "aerosol therapy" and "nebulization therapy" are often used interchangeably.

In aerosol therapy the medication is inhaled as a fine mist that is deposited on the respiratory tract. This form of therapy is used to promote:

1 Bronchodilation and pulmonary decongestion
2 Loosening of secretions
3 Topical application of antibiotics, steroids, and antifoaming agents
4 Moistening, cooling, or heating of inspired air

The effectiveness of nebulization therapy depends on the number of droplets that can be suspended in an inhaled aerosol. The number of droplets that can be suspended is directly related to the size of the droplets. Small droplets can be suspended in greater numbers than large droplets. Smaller droplets (about 2μm in diameter) are more likely to reach the periphery of the lungs—the alveolar ducts and sacs. Currently, in many institutions, ultrasonic nebulizers are utilized in the treatment of bronchial constriction and pulmonary congestion. Larger droplets (8 to 15 μm in size) will be deposited primarily in the bronchioles and bronchi. Droplets of more than 40 μm will be deposited primarily in the upper airway (mouth, pharynx, trachea, and main bronchi).

Rate and depth of breathing are other important factors. Rapid or shallow breathing decreases the number of droplets reaching the periphery of the lungs as well as their retention. Rapid breathing permits escape of significant amounts of fine droplets during expirations. Few droplets will escape if the breath is held long enough after deep inspiration to permit droplet deposit in the lung periphery. Small droplets are more effective for absorption of antibiotics and bronchodilators.

Almost all large droplets will be retained somewhere in the air passage. Large droplets are used for keeping large airways moist (nose, trachea) and for loosening secretions. Slow and deep breathing is required for proper lung aeration and penetration of the mist into peripheral lung areas. The breath should be held for a few seconds after a full inspiration. Nebulizers commonly used in hospitals all produce similar mists. Droplet size can be controlled by the amount of pressure used to force oxygen or room air through the solution to produce a mist. The tubing used, its length, and number of bends affect turbulent flow and mist temperature. With most nebulizers maximum density of the inhaled mist is achieved by making the flow of mist as smooth and direct as possible. *A note of precaution:* drug reconcentration can occur with both jet and ultrasonic nebulizers if a humidity deficit occurs. Evaporation of water molecules causes a gradual increase in drug concentration in the droplets being returned to the fluid reservoir, thus increasing the risk of drug toxicity. Control of temperature and humidity can prevent this.

The main groups of drugs that are conventionally administered for their pulmonary action include mucokinetic agents, which loosen and liquefy the mucus, and the bronchodilator agents, which relieve bronchospasm. However, other drugs such as antimicrobial and steroid agents also are given for their effect on the respiratory mucosa.

One major consideration to bear in mind is that the lung is an *absorptive organ*, and therefore, it provides a route of access for drugs to enter the systemic circulation. For example, after inhalation anesthetic agents enter the blood and exert their main effect on the central nervous system. Aerosol therapy, when used as a method of administering drugs, is supposed to minimize their side effects. Yet certain bronchodilator aerosols do produce cardiovascular effects simply because the drug may possess a property that adversely influences cardiac action after it is absorbed into the bloodstream.

Systemic antibiotics are often the drugs of choice to combat pulmonary infection. Certain antibiotics that can be given in limited doses only when administered systemically because of their toxicity can often be given in large doses by nebulization. These antibiotics include polymyxin, colistin, neomycin, and bacitracin. Since these antibiotics are irritating and may cause *broncospasm,* bronchodilators are usually given prior to, or along with, the antibiotic.

Antifoaming agents (ethyl alcohol or octyl alcohol) have been used to supplement therapy to reverse severe fulminating pulmonary edema. Alcohol reduces the surface tension of pulmonary edema bubbles and causes them to break, and it produces some bronchodilation. The result is better ventilation. This form of aerosol therapy must not be administered rapidly since it will cause irritation and coughing. It should be used with intermittent positive pressure breathing (IPPB) for effective oxygenation. Aerosol alcohol should be discontinued as soon as the lungs are dry to prevent ciliary damage.

Mucokinetic drugs

A mucokinetic drug is an agent that thins hyperviscous secretions or sputum and removes it from the respiratory tract. *Sputum (or phlegm) may be defined as an abnormal, viscous secretion that is an excretory product of the lower respiratory tree.* It consists mainly of mucus, a proteinaceous material that is identified chemically as having a mucopolysaccharide as its major component. In addition, it contains molecules of deoxyribonucleic acid (DNA) that are derived from the breakdown of mucosal cells, leukocytes, and bacteria, and these products are responsible for the characteristic heavy quality and yellow color of the sputum. The terms "sputum" and "mucus" should not be used interchangeably. Sputum is a secretion that originates in the *lower respiratory tract,* whereas mucus is produced by the *surface cells* in the mucous membrane.

Patients with respiratory disorders such as chronic bronchitis develop disturbances of the mucociliary system, and this results in a significant impairment of the mucus clearance process. As a consequence, mucous plugging and pathogenic colonization of microorganisms occur in the lower respiratory tract. These changes then lead to overproduction of thick, tenacious sputum. Thus the advantage provided by the mucokinetic drugs is that they alter the consistency of the sputum, thereby promoting the eventual expulsion of these secretions.

Diluents

Water

The most commonly used diluent of the respiratory secretion is water. Patients with chronic obstructive pulmonary disease frequently suffer from dehydration. This clinical finding causes retention of respiratory secretions, which then become highly viscous in consistency and lead to widespread plug formation in the respiratory tree.

Water may be administered by ultrasonic nebulizer. Small amounts of water deposited on the gel layer of the respiratory tree appear to reduce the adhesive characteristics and general viscosity of the gelatinous substances found in this layer. Care is needed with patients on restricted fluid intake, since water can be absorbed through the inhalation route. (If fluid intake is being measured, water absorbed through the inhalation route must be added to the patient's intake record.) If a patient's fluid intake is not restricted, large amounts of water are usually encouraged to liquefy the respiratory secretions.

Saline solutions

Normal saline (0.9% sodium chloride) is physiologic salt solution or isotonic solution that exerts the same osmotic pressure as plasma fluids. Therapy by nebulization is well tolerated, resulting in hydration of respiratory secretions. Hypotonic solution (0.45% sodium chloride) is thought to provide deeper penetration into the more distal airways or in the alveoli via the inhalation route, whereas inhalation of hypertonic solution (1.8% sodium chloride) stimulates a productive cough since the particles deposited on the respiratory mucosa are irritating. Hypertonic solution osmotically attracts fluid out of the mucosa and into the respiratory secretions, thereby promoting their excretion.

Surface-active drugs

Hygroscopic drugs

Hygroscopic drugs are detergents that facilitate hydration and emulsification of tenacious secretions by readily absorbing and retaining water. Additionally, these agents provide a soothing effect in the respiratory tree. Tyloxapol (Alevaire) had been used for this purpose. However, there is reason to suspect that it is no more effective than water. Although the FDA has attempted to remove this preparation from the market, tyloxapol is still available but is now seldom used.

Propylene glycol

Propylene glycol is usually administered by nebulization. It absorbs moisture and decreases the viscosity of the gel component of respiratory secretions. It is administered in concentrations of 2% to 10% in volumes of 1 to 5 ml as needed.

Ethanol

Ethanol or ethyl alcohol decreases surface tension of respiratory secretions. In pulmonary edema, airway obstruction is caused by increased production of very stable foam that fills the air spaces. Thus ethanol may be administered by nebulization. It can also be given by bubbling oxygen through diluted ethanol; this produces a vapor that is inhaled through a face mask. The drug acts by dispersing the bubbles in the airway and thereby relieving the obstruction. Ethanol is an effective antifoaming agent in pulmonary edema, but because of its irritating effect on airway tissue, it is not recommended for use in routine mucokinetic therapy.

Mucolytic drugs

Mucolytic agents reduce the thickness and stickiness of purulent and nonpurulent pulmonary secretions by breaking up the linkages or bonds of mucoprotein molecules of the respiratory secretions into smaller, more soluble, and less viscous strands. In addition to altering the molecular composition of the mucopolysaccharides, this type of agent also effects similar changes in the DNA molecule and cellular debris. These drugs are usually administered by aerosol inhalation to facilitate the removal of secretions and permit more adequate pulmonary ventilation. These drugs are used in the management of individuals with chronic bronchitis, emphysema, bronchiectasis, cystic fibrosis, pneumonia, and as an adjunct for tracheostomy care. When used appropriately, few adverse effects are seen. Some patients may develop nausea and vomiting, but this is probably due to the odor and quantity of respiratory secretions eliminated. With the aid of these agents and postural drainage most individuals can expectorate pulmonary secretions without further assistance; however, in the elderly or debilitated, suctioning may be indicated.

Acetylcysteine (Mucomyst, Respaire)

Acetylcysteine is an amino acid derivative that is administered by nebulization as a 10% or 20% solution. The 20% solution may be converted to a 10% solution by dilution with isotonic sodium chloride or sterile water.

Preparation, dosage, and administration. Range of dosage is from 1 to 10 ml of the 20% solution, or 2 to 20 ml of the 10% solution for about 15 minutes, three or four times daily. Since the solution tends to concentrate, it should be diluted with sterile water when three fourths of the original volume has been used. It may also be administered for a single continuous treatment by means of a closed tent or croupette. This may require up to 300 ml of a 20% solution. It is effective within 1 minute; however, it takes 5 to 10 minutes for maximum effect to occur.

Side effects. Acetylcysteine may cause stomatitis, nausea, and rhinorrhea. Bronchospasm may occur in patients with bronchial asthma. This drug has a wide margin of safety. Currently, in some institutions a 2% to 5% saline solution is being used instead of acetylcysteine to avoid side effects.

Because of release of hydrogen sulfide, solutions of acetylcysteine will harden rubber and become discolored on contact with certain metals. Acetylcysteine solutions should be used with equipment made of glass, plastic, or stainless steel. If the vacuum seal has been broken on the bottle, the solution should be refrigerated to retard oxidation and then used within 48 hours.

Following nebulization, the face should be washed with water to remove the sticky coating left by the drug. Acetylcysteine has an unpleasant rotten-egg odor caused by the disruption of the disulfide linkages (hydrogen sulfide). This factor along with the excess volume of liquefied bronchial secretions may cause nausea and vomiting. However, with continued inhalation, the odor becomes less noticeable; the patient should be advised of this fact so that therapy may be continued.

Deoxyribonuclease (Dornavac)

Deoxyribonuclease is an enzyme obtained from beef pancreas that degrades DNA. It reduces the tenacity or thickness of pulmonary secretions. Deoxyribonuclease is available in powder form, 100,000 units per vial. The powder is dissolved in 1 to 2 ml of sterile saline. The average dose is 50,000 to 100,000 units three times a day by aerosol inhalation for 2 to 6 days. It is relatively free of side effects; however, individual sensitivity to the drug should be watched for. The drug is expensive, which is one disadvantage to be considered.

Bronchomucotropic drugs

The bronchomucotropic drugs previously have been classified as expectorants, a term sometimes used in pharmacology. These agents act on bronchial glands to increase the volume and reduce the viscosity of secretions, thereby facilitating their expulsion from the airway. They are used to enhance bronchial drainage and cough in chronic bronchitis, emphysema, and other respiratory disorders.

The exact mode of action of these drugs is not clearly understood. Since bronchial glands are innervated by the vagus (parasympathetic) nerve, it is thought that the oral intake of bronchomucotropic drug causes gastric irritation. This stimulus then reflexly activates the afferent (vagal) nerve to the gastric mucosa, and after the information is relayed to the medullary center, the impulse is carried by the efferent (vagal) nerve to the bronchial glands, causing the increased volume of secretions. This mechanism is referred to as the gastropulmonary reflex action.

Sodium iodide; potassium iodide

Iodides increase bronchial secretions reflexly by causing gastric irritation. These preparations are too irritating to be used in acute inflammatory conditions of the respiratory tract. They are given to liquefy the secretions or loosen the cough when sputum becomes particularly tenacious. The average expectorant dose for adults is 300 mg every 4 to 6 hours; dosage for children is 0.25 to 1 ml in two to four doses daily. The salts may be administered in a saturated solution or in a cough mixture. With long-term use these drugs frequently produce symptoms of iodism. These are caused by irritation of the nasal passage, bronchi, and skin and include coryza and pain in the region of the frontal sinus and various skin eruptions, generally of a papular character. When such toxic symptoms occur, the drug should be discontinued, but it may be resumed in smaller doses after the disappearance of the symptoms.

Ammonium chloride; ammonium carbonate

Ammonium chloride is frequently administered in some vehicle such as wild cherry syrup, citric acid syrup, or orange syrup. The ammonium ions produce local gastric irritation, which acts reflexly to stimulate respiratory tract secretory activity. Used as an expectorant, ammonium chloride is given in doses of 250 to 500 mg four times a day in some suitable medium. It should be accompanied by a full glass of water because increased fluid intake also plays a part in the formation of increased mucus, thus decreasing viscosity of secretions.

Ammonium carbonate acts like ammonium chloride except that it causes gastric distress more easily. It is given in much the same manner and dosage as ammonium chloride. It is an alkaline salt and cannot be given in acid syrups. The usual dose is 250 to 500 mg.

Ipecac syrup

Ipecac syrup is prescribed in doses of 1 to 8 ml with a glass of water for adults and 5 min-

ims for infants 1 year of age. A small increase of dosage is made for each additional year. In children, it is used to increase secretions and relieve bronchitis associated with croup. Ipecac syrup is also used as an emetic, particularly in children.

Terpin hydrate

Terpin hydrate occurs as colorless, lustrous crystals, nearly odorless, having a slightly aromatic odor and somewhat bitter taste. Terpin hydrate is antiseptic, diaphoretic, and diuretic in action, but it is used chiefly as a vehicle for other drugs. The usual dose of terpin hydrate elixir and terpin hydrate and codeine elixir is 4 to 5 ml (1 fluidram) every 4 to 6 hours. When terpin hydrate is combined with codeine, it is the high alcohol content of the elixir that produces its expectorant action. The amount of terpin hydrate in the combined preparation is usually too small to exert a significant effect and therefore it acts only as a vehicle for the codeine.

Agents that antagonize bronchial secretions

Atropine, although not used as an expectorant, may be given cautiously to check secretions and excessive expectoration in certain forms of bronchitis.

Many remedies used to treat colds contain atropine. Morphine, codeine, and papaverine not only act as sedatives but also tend to dry the mucous membranes. In many cases the best treatment of a cold or inflammation of the respiratory mucous membranes consists of prescribing extra rest, forcing fluids, and simple but nutritious food.

Bronchodilator drugs

The principal agents used in the treatment of airway obstruction include sympathomimetic drugs and methylxanthine drugs. Prophylactic antiasthmatic agents are also effective in the prevention of airway obstruction in patients with certain types of asthma. Most of these drugs enhance the production of cyclic AMP to effect bronchodilation.

In the management of constricted airways the use of bronchodilator drugs includes the following therapeutic goals:

1 Maximal bronchial smooth muscle relaxation
2 Prolonged activity of the drug
3 Minimal adverse adrenergic effects not associated with bronchodilation

Sympathomimetic drugs

Based on their receptor action, three groups of sympathomimetic drugs are recognized: (1) nonselective adrenergic drugs that have alpha, $beta_1$, and $beta_2$ activities (for example, epinephrine); (2) nonselective beta drugs with both $beta_1$ and $beta_2$ effects (for example, isoproterenol); and (3) selective $beta_2$ receptor drugs that act solely on $beta_2$ receptors and produce minimal adrenergic side effects.

NONSELECTIVE ADRENERGIC DRUGS

The drugs in this category possess both alpha and beta receptor stimulating properties. Alpha activity appears to mediate vasoconstriction to reduce mucosal edema. $Beta_2$ stimulation increases the level of cyclic AMP, producing bronchodilation and vasodilation. In contrast, $beta_1$ receptor action causes unwanted side effects such as an increase in heart rate and in the force of cardiac contraction (Table 14-2).

Epinephrine

Epinephrine stimulates $beta_2$ as well as alpha and $beta_1$ receptors. The main effect of epinephrine on respiration is to increase cyclic 3'5'AMP, which induces bronchial smooth muscle relaxation ($beta_2$ activity).

Uses. Epinephrine is particularly useful in the treatment of asthma because of its powerful bronchodilator action. It also increases vital capacity by relieving congestion of the bronchial mucosa. When epinephrine is administered as an aerosol, it aids in the relief of congestion by constricting bronchial vessels (alpha activity). In normal subjects, epinephrine increases respiratory rate and tidal volume and results in a reduction in alveolar carbon dioxide.

Preparation, dosage, and administration. Epinephrine is administered parenterally and by aerosol because it is destroyed by enzymes present in the gastrointestinal tract. The subcutaneous and intramuscular dose for an adult is 0.1 to 1 ml of a 1:1000 aqueous solution; the intravenous dose is 0.05 to 0.1 ml of a 1:1000 solution injected very slowly and with caution. Epinephrine hydrochloride is available for oral inhalation as a 0.1% to 1% solution or suspension; epinephrine bitartrate is marketed in a 15-ml aerosol package (Medihaler) containing 7 mg/ml. The pediatric dose for asthma is 0.01 mg/kg body weight of the 1:1000 aqueous solution given subcutaneously.

During acute allergic emergencies such as anaphylactic shock and angioedema of the larynx, parenteral epinephrine, 1:1000, is the most effective drug. Its alpha receptor action will constrict blood vessels and raise the blood pressure.

Racemic epinephrine is a synthetic mixture of d- and l-epinephrine. It is favored for aerosal therapy in place of l-epinephrine. It is available as Vaponephrin in a 2.25% solution. It is believed that this preparation offers the advantage of a more potent $beta_2$ activity.

Side effects. Nervousness, insomnia, fear, tremors, headache, palpitations, tachycardia, and dyspnea may occur as distressing side effects.

Precautions. The drug is not recommended for individuals with coronary artery disease, hypertension, and hyperthyroidism. Anginal

T A B L E 1 4 - 2 **Adrenergic receptor activity**

Tissue	Alpha	Beta₁	Beta₂
Heart		Increased rate and force of contraction	
Lungs			
Bronchial smooth muscle			Relaxation
Bronchial glands			? Inhibition of secretions
Blood vessels	Vasoconstriction		Vasodilation

pain may be induced in patients with coronary insufficiency.

Drug interactions. Concurrent use with monamine oxidase inhibitors that increase the catecholamine levels will precipitate severe hypertension.

NONSELECTIVE BETA ADRENERGIC DRUGS

The nonselective beta adrenergic drugs exhibit both beta$_2$ and beta$_1$ activities. Their main action is on the bronchial smooth muscle as well as the heart.

Isoproterenol hydrochloride (Isuprel Hydrochloride)

Isoproterenol is an adrenergic drug frequently used for its bronchodilator effect. This drug and its various preparations are discussed in more detail in Chapter 13.

Isoproterenol relaxes bronchial smooth muscle because of its beta$_2$ effect. It is known as one of the most powerful bronchodilators. In additon, it exerts strong beta$_1$ effects, producing tachycardia and palpitations of the heart, which are disturbing side effects that could limit its use for certain patients. Isoproterenol is rapidly metabolized by the enzyme catechol-O-methyltransferase (COMT), and therefore it is a relatively short-acting agent. Another concern about this drug is that the more it is used, the less effective it might become as a bronchodilator.

SELECTIVE BETA$_2$ RECEPTOR DRUGS

The high incidence of undesirable cardiotoxic effects caused by the beta$_1$ property of sympathomimetic agents has led investigators to search for a more specific beta$_2$ receptor agonist. There are two types: (1) the catecholamine beta$_2$ receptor agonist (for example, isoetharine) and (2) the noncatecholamine beta$_2$ receptor agonist (for example, metaproterenol and terbutaline).

The structural arrangement of the catechol nucleus in the basic catecholamine molecule plays a major role in determining alpha and beta adrenergic activity. In the catecholamine group of drugs, the presence of hydroxyl groups in the 3,4 ring positions of the nucleus mediates both alpha and beta activity. By contrast, in the noncatecholamine group of drugs, modification of the ring structure enhances beta$_2$ activity. This involves placement of phenolic hydroxyl groups in the 3,5 positions, which results in the formation of a resorcinol nuclear arrangement. The drug presenting this resorcinol nuclear arrangement not only *provides a more selective beta$_2$ activity* but also *prolongs its duration of action* because the molecule resists degradation by COMT. Figs. 14-3 and 14-4 show structural arrangements of these drugs.

CATECHOLAMINE BETA$_2$ RECEPTOR DRUGS
Isoetharine hydrochloride (Bronkosol)

Isoetharine was the first of the sympathomimetic agents to exhibit predominant beta$_2$ activity. It has relatively little beta$_1$ activity, and as a bronchodilator it is less potent than isoproterenol. This drug increases cyclic AMP and thus provides rapid symptomatic relief of bronchospasm and significantly increases vital capacity. Because it is a catecholamine, it is susceptible to metabolism by COMT, which shortens its duration of action.

Uses. Isoetharine is administered as a bronchodilator to patients with bronchial asthma and to relieve bronchospasm in patients with bronchitis and emphysema.

Preparation, dosage, and administration. Isoetharine hydrochloride (Bronkosol) was originally marketed as a product containing phenylephrine. It was initially thought that the addition of phenylephrine would improve the caliber of the airway by acting as a topical vasoconstrictive decongestant. Because of doubt that the compound provides such a benefit, the ingredient has been removed.

In many hospitals, isoetharine enjoys considerable popularity and is the bronchodilator of choice.

When the drug is administered as isoetharine solution by a hand nebulizer, three to seven inhalations are recommended. It is diluted (0.25 to 1 ml in three parts saline solution) when the preparation is delivered by intermittent positive pressure breathing (IPPB). Isoetharine mesylate (Bronkometer) is administered as an oral nebulized drug that provides a metered dose of 340 μg per puff—the dosage is one to four puffs every 3 to 6 hours.

Side effects. Frequent use of isoetharine

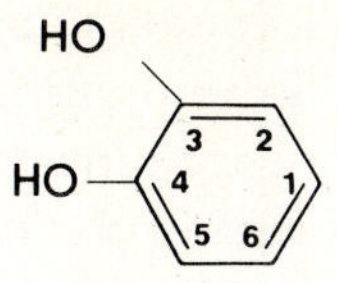

Catechol:
Dihydroxybenzene

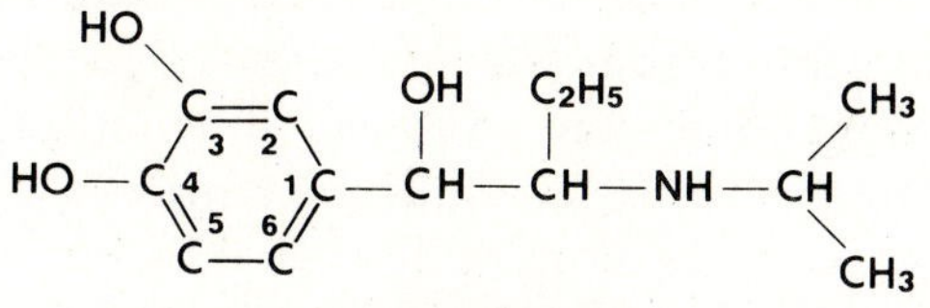

A Catecholamine:
Isoetharine

Fig. 14-3. Note the catechol nucleus with phenolic hydroxyl groups at positions 3 and 4. Isoetharine is a derivative of this structure.

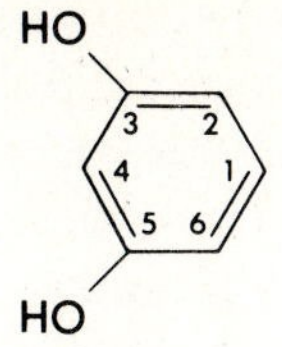

Resorcinol

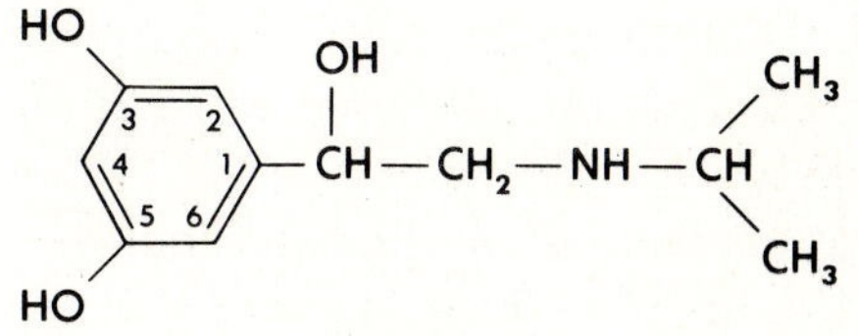

Metaproterenol

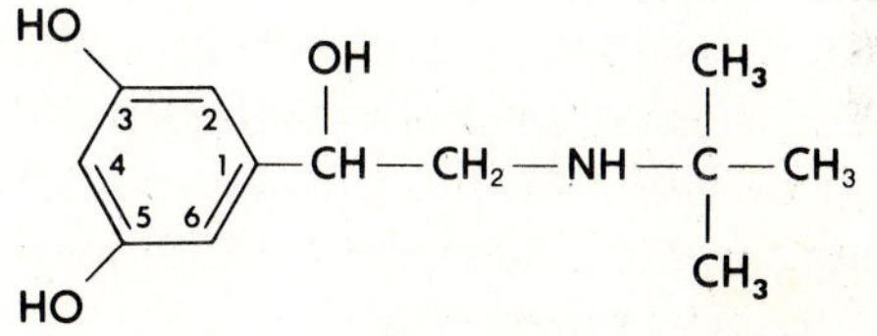

Terbutaline

Fig. 14-4. The noncatcholamine beta$_2$ receptor agonist shows the resorcinal nucleus with phenolic hydroxyl groups at positions 3 and 5. Metaproterenol and terbutaline are the derivatives of the resorcinol structure.

may cause tachycardia, palpitations, nausea, headache, dizziness, weakness, and excitement.

Excessive use of the aerosol can lead to loss of effectiveness. Occasionally, patients have developed paradoxic airway resistance.* In this case, alternative therapy should be instituted. The dosage of isoetharine must be carefully adjusted in patients with hyperthyroidism, hypertension, and coronary disease to prevent tachycardia, palpitations, nausea, and other epinephrine-like side effects.

Isoetharine should not be given to individuals who are hypersensitive to any of its ingredients.

NONCATECHOLAMINE BETA$_2$ RECEPTOR DRUGS
Metaproterenol sulfate (Alupent, Metaprel, Orciprenaline Sulfate)

Metaproterenol is a synthetic compound quite similar to isoproterenol except that the hydroxyl groups are attached at the 3,5 positions on the benzene ring or catechol nucleus (Fig. 14-4). As a consequence, the drug is resistant to degradation by COMT. When administered orally, this property provides a longer duration of action than does isoproterenol.

Metaproterenol has a greater stimulating

*In paradoxic response, some patients with asthma develop resistance to a bronchodilator. In this condition the drug actually causes bronchospasm.

effect on the beta$_2$ receptors of the bronchial and vascular smooth muscles and a lesser effect on the beta$_1$ receptors of the heart than does isoproterenol.

Uses. Metaproterenol is used as a bronchodilator in the symptomatic treatment of asthma and bronchospasm. It has a longer duration of action, has a lower incidence and severity of cardiac side effects, and is more effective after oral administration than isoproterenol. Onset of action occurs 1 minute after oral inhalation and 15 minutes after oral administration. Peak effect occurs in about 1 hour with a duration of effect of about 4 hours with either route of administration. Duration of action may shorten with long-term use, but metaproterenol retains its efficacy to a greater extent than isoproterenol.

Preparation and dosage. Metaproterenol is available in 20-mg capsules and tablets for oral administration and as a powder, 225 mg in metered dose vials of 15 ml, with mouthpiece. Each metered dose delivers approximately 0.65 mg metaproterenol; range of dose is one to three inhalations with 2 minutes between inhalations. Inhalations may be repeated every 3 to 4 hours but should not exceed 12 inhalations in 24 hours. For oral inhalation the patient should be instructed to shake the container, exhale through the nose as completely as possible, then administer the aerosol while breathing deeply through the mouth; the patient should hold his breath for a few seconds before exhaling slowly.

Oral dosage of metaproterenol is 20 mg three to four times daily. A syrup preparation of 10 mg/5 ml is available for children; the dose may be 10 mg three or four times daily. This drug should be protected from light and air.

Side effects and toxic effects. Adverse effects are usually dose related and occur with high doses. The most common side effects include tachycardia, nervousness, palpitations, tremor, hypertension, headache, dizziness, nausea and vomiting, and bad taste.

Metaproterenol should be used cautiously in patients with hypertension, coronary artery disease, hyperthyroidism, congestive heart failure, or diabetes mellitus and in those sensitive to sympathomimetic drugs. It is contraindicated in patients with a history of tachycardia.

Metaproterenol should not be used concurrently with other sympathomimetic drugs (such as epinephrine), since the additive effects may induce serious dysrhythmias and toxic reactions. It is not recommended for pregnant women.

Terbutaline sulfate (Brethine, Bricanyl)

Terbutaline is a synthetic compound similar to metaproterenol in chemical structure and pharmacologic action. It is a beta$_2$ stimulant. Its main effect is relaxation of smooth muscles of the bronchial tree and the peripheral vasculature; thus the drug is a beta$_2$ agonist.

Terbutaline is used as a bronchodilator in the treatment of bronchial asthma and bronchospasm. Compared to ephedrine, its bronchodilator activity is about equal, but onset and duration of action are longer. Compared to metaproterenol, terbutaline has equal or slightly greater effectiveness, a slower onset of action, and a longer duration of action.

After oral administration, onset of action occurs in 30 minutes and peak action in 2 to 3 hours, with a duration of action ranging from 4 to 8 hours. After subcutaneous injection, onset of action occurs in 15 minutes, and duration of action ranges from 1½ to 4 hours.

Preparation and dosage. Terbutaline is available in isotonic solution for injection containing 1 mg of drug/ml and in 2.5- and 5-mg tablets for oral administration. The subcutaneous dose for adults is 0.25 mg injected into the lateral deltoid area; for children the subcutaneous dose is 3.5 to 5 μg/kg body weight. The use of the drug in children under 12 is still being investigated.

Oral dosage for adults is 2.5 or 5 mg three times daily at 6-hour intervals; dosage should not exceed 15 mg daily. For children 12 to 15 years of age, dosage is 2.5 mg three times daily; daily dosage should not exceed 7.5 mg.

Side effects and toxic effects. Since terbutaline is a potent beta$_2$ stimulator, it also produces peripheral vasodilation, which in a larger dose can result in a fall in blood pressure. The lowering of pressure stimulates a reflex hemodynamic response so that tachycardia may occur. In this situation the rapid heart rate is not a direct result of stimulation of beta$_1$ receptors of the heart muscle. The marked muscle tremors are caused by stimulation of the neuromuscular receptors. With continued drug administration, the tremors usually disappear. Other commonly observed side effects include nervousness, palpitations, and dizziness. These effects usually occur when the subcutaneous dosage is in excess of 0.25 mg. Headache, nausea and vomiting, anxiety, restlessness, lethargy, drowsiness, sweating, and tinnitus have also been reported.

Precautions. Terbutaline should be used with caution in patients with diabetes, hypertension, hyperthyroidism, or cardiac disorders associated with dysrhythmias. Terbutaline should not be given concurrently with other sympathomimetic agents because of the possibility of additive cardiovascular side effects. However, it can be used with an adrenergic aerosol bronchodilator to relieve acute bronchospasm.

OTHER BETA₂ SELECTIVE DRUGS

Salbutamol has a greater specificity for the beta₂ receptors of the bronchial muscle than metaproterenol. As a consequence, less adverse reactions are encountered with this drug. Salbutamol is a slightly more powerful bronchodilator than terbutaline. In addition, there is evidence that this agent is the safest of the bronchodilators for intravenous management of bronchospasm. As a bronchodilator, it is effective orally as well as by inhalation. Despite these advantages, the drug has been approved only recently in the United States market because of the development of neoplastic toxicities in experimental rats.

Carbuterol and fenoterol are agents that are also available in Europe but not in the United States.

Albuterol (Ventolin Inhaler)

Albuterol is one of the most recently introduced sympathomimetic bronchodilators now in clinical use in the United States. The international generic name of this drug is salbutamol.

Albuterol possesses a useful degree of selectivity for beta₂ adrenergic receptors and therefore is less likely to give rise to unwanted cardiac effects. Its interaction with the beta₂ receptor in the cell membrane of the bronchial smooth muscle stimulates the enzyme adenyl cyclase, which is also located in the membrane, to produce cyclic 3'5'-adenosine monophosphate (cyclic AMP). The cyclic AMP thus formed mediates a response that is capable of relaxing smooth muscle of the bronchi (see Fig. 14-2, *A*). This mechanism also causes relaxation of the smooth muscle of the uterus and blood vessels of skeletal muscle. However, it has been reported that high doses of the drug administered intravenously would be required to inhibit uterine contractions to delay premature labor.

Because albuterol has a greater specificity for the beta₂ adrenergic receptors of the bronchial smooth muscle, it produces fewer cardiovascular side effects and more prolonged bron-

chodilation than does isoproterenol. Yet when this drug is taken in excessive doses, even by aerosol, long-lasting cardiac effects may be observed. This is the result of a systemic accumulation of albuterol, whose prolonged effects are caused by its gradual absorption from the bronchi along with its slow rate of metabolism and excretion.

Since it is resistant to metabolic degradation, the therapeutic effect of albuterol may be active for up to 5 hours. Studies of urinary excretion have shown that its elimination half-life is 3.8 hours. Approximately 72% of the inhaled dose is excreted in the urine within 24 hours and consists of 28% unchanged drug and 44% metabolites.

Uses. When used as Ventolin Inhaler, this drug relieves bronchospasm in patients with reversible obstructive airway disease. In individuals with asthma, clinical experience indicates that a therapeutic response may be sustained generally for 3 to 4 hours.

The use of Ventolin Inhaler is contraindicated in patients with a history of hypersensitivity to the drug. Because it is an adrenergic aerosol, it has a potential for producing paradoxic bronchospasm. The drug should be discontinued immediately if this occurs. Also, since this agent is a sympathomimetic amine, excessive inhalation doses should be avoided. Some fatalities have been reported and it is suspected that cardiac arrest has been implicated. Therefore, Ventolin Inhaler should be used with caution in patients with cardiovascular disorders including coronary insufficiency and hypertension, as well as in individuals with hyperthyroidism and diabetes mellitus.

Preparation, dosage, and administration. Ventolin Inhaler is a metered-dose aerosol unit prepared for oral inhalation. It contains a microcrystalline suspension of albuterol in propellants along with oleic acid. Ventolin Inhaler is marketed in a 17-g canister in a box and is supplied with an oral adapter and patient's instructions. The metered product delivers from the mouthpiece 90 μg albuterol per puff. Each canister contains at least 200 inhalations.

The usual dosage for adults and children 12 years or older is two inhalations repeated every

4 to 6 hours. In some patients one inhalation every 4 hours may be sufficient. A larger number of inhalations or more frequent administration is not recommended. If symptoms get worse, medical consultation should be sought promptly. The loss of effectiveness of a previous dosage regimen is a sign of increasing severity of asthma which is a serious condition that requires immediate reassessment of therapy.

Since the contents of Ventolin Inhaler are under pressure, the container should not be punctured. Also, it should not be stored near heat or an open flame, for exposure to temperatures above 120° F may cause it to burst. This means that a container should never be thrown into fire or incinerator.

Side effects and toxic effects. Because of the greater specificity of albuterol for the beta$_2$ receptors of the bronchial smooth muscle, cardiovascular toxicity is significantly less than with the older bronchodilator aerosol currently in use, such as isoproterenol. The results of a study have shown that the incidence of tachycardia, increased blood pressure, tremor, dizziness, or nausea is decreased with the administration of this agent. However, like other sympathomimetic agents, adverse reactions such as hypertension, angina, vomiting, vertigo, insomnia, unusual taste, and drying or irritation of the oropharynx may occur in some patients.

Drug interactions. Other sympathomimetic aerosol bronchodilators or epinephrine should not be used when albuterol is administered. In addition, the drug should be used with special caution in patients being treated with monoamine oxidase inhibitors or tricyclic antidepressants for the action of albuterol on the vascular system may be potentiated. Also, beta receptor blocking agents used concomitantly with albuterol negate the effect of each other.

During a study, albuterol caused a significant dose-related increase in incidence of mesovarian leiomyomas in rats. The relevance of this finding is not known in the human. Additionally, there are no adequate and well-controlled studies of the drug in pregnant women. However, albuterol has been shown to be teratogenic in mice. Also, the importance of the drug in nursing mothers must be carefully assessed because of its potential for tumorigenicity seen in animal studies.

Methylxanthine drugs

The methylxanthine group of drugs includes caffeine, theophylline, and theobromine. Beverages from aqueous extracts of plants containing these alkaloids have been used by humans since ancient times. Methylxanthines relax smooth muscle, particularly bronchial muscle, stimulate cardiac muscle, stimulate the central nervous system, and also produce diuresis probably through a combined action of increased renal perfusion and increased sodium and chloride ion excretion.

The drugs in this category are methylated forms of xanthines, hence the name methylxanthines. The effectiveness of these preparations as bronchodilators depends on their conversion to *theophylline*, which is the active constituent. The mode of action of methylxanthines is to inhibit the enzyme phosphodiesterase, a compound that catalyzes the hydrolysis of cyclic 3′5′AMP to the inactive form 5′AMP. The increased levels of cyclic 3′5′AMP then mediates a beta adrenergic effect that results in relaxation of bronchial smooth muscle and pulmonary blood vessels. In addition, it inhibits mast cell degranulation and the release of histamine and other mediators that are responsible for bronchoconstriction. Because they impede enzymatic action, the methylxanthines are also called phosphodiesterase inhibitors (see Fig. 14-2).

Uses. The methylxanthines relieve acute bronchial asthma and reversible bronchospasms associated with chronic bronchitis. They also are of value in maintenance and prophylactic therapy in patients with chronic bronchospasm.

Precautions. The half-life of methylxanthines in smokers is shorter than in nonsmokers; therefore smokers may require larger doses. Methylxanthines must also be used with great care in patients with bleeding peptic ulcer, liver disease, hypertension and hyperthyroidism, and in the elderly.

Contraindications. Methylxanthines should not be administered to patients with glaucoma. The safe use in pregnant women has not been established. Hypersensitivity to xanthines is another contraindication.

Drug interactions. Toxic synergism with high doses of ephedrine may occur as well as some other sympathomimetic bronchodilator when combination therapy is used.

The prototype agent of the methylxanthines is theophylline.

Aminophylline (Theophylline Ethylenediamine)

Aminophylline, a theophylline derivative, provides a prototype for most of the other theophylline compounds. It is a conjugate of 78% anhydrous theophylline and 12% ethylenediamine. The latter is added to render theophylline water soluble. Aminophylline plays an important role in the management of asthma and other disorders resulting in bronchial constriction and spasm. It is also used in the treatment of pulmonary edema.

Preparation, dosage, and administration. Aminophylline is available for oral administration in 100- and 200-mg tablets and is usually given three times a day. For intravenous administration, ampules containing 250 mg/10 ml and 500 mg/20 ml are available. Rectal suppositories come in 100-, 250-, and 500-mg strengths.

When given intravenously, aminophylline should always be well diluted (25 mg/ml) and the flow rate should not exceed 25 mg/minute. If a loading dose is required, 6 mg/kg body weight of aminophylline is infused intravenously over a 20- to 30-minute period. The maintenance infusion dosage is 0.9 mg/kg/hour. *The therapeutic serum theophylline concentration level is 10 to 20 μg/ml.* When the serum drug level exceeds 20 μg/ml, toxic effects begin to appear, and the dosage should be lowered.

The drug is metabolized in the liver and excreted in the urine. Smokers tend to metabolize the drug more rapidly than nonsmokers and usually require a larger dose of the drug.

Side effects. Given orally, aminophylline may cause gastric irritation, nausea, and vomiting. However, this is more likely produced by stimulation of the vomiting center than by gastric irritation. Nevertheless, this constitutes a generally accepted drawback to its use in individuals with gastrointestinal conditions. The central nervous system effects include headache, nervousness, insomnia, and convulsions. These symptoms occur in a more severe form in children. The cardiovascular effects are usually mild and they include tachycardia and palpitations. The drug may also produce urinary frequency. If administered intravenously too rapidly, cardiovascular distress may occur. Intramuscular injection produces local pain at the injection site; therefore it is the least desirable route and is not recommended.

Nursing considerations. Nursing interventions important in the administration of theophylline include the following:

1 Vital signs, especially the quality and rate of the pulse and respirations, should be carefully monitored.
2 When administered intravenously, it should be given slowly to avoid cardiovascular distress.
3 Oral preparations should be given with food to minimize gastric irritation.
4 Rectal preparations should be administered when the rectum is free of feces, since this will enhance the absorption of the drug.
5 Any form of this drug given over a long period of time may have cumulative effects or may become ineffective.
6 If side effects occur, the drug should be discontinued and the physician should be notified.
7 Ephedrine given in conjunction with theophylline has a combined central stimulant action and may necessitate the administration of a barbiturate.

OTHER THEOPHYLLINE DERIVATIVES

Various other theophylline derivatives and other preparations used for their bronchodilating effects are choline theophylline (Choledyl) and theophylline (Aqualin, Elixophyllin). These oral preparations cause less gastric irritation and have a more rapid rate of absorption than aminophylline.

Theophylline and ephedrine combination therapy

Some physicians advocate the combined use of theophylline and ephedrine, which appears to produce a *synergistic effect* on cyclic AMP levels. Theophylline effects bronchodilation and also dislodges thick tenacious sputum by increasing mucus secretion. At the same time it also causes cerebral vasoconstriction, thereby reducing the oxygen content of the brain. Ephedrine, by contrast, effects cerebral vasodilation and increases oxygen content of the brain. Since theophylline produces mental sluggishness in certain patients, this condition can be controlled by the combined effect of ephedrine and theophylline. The advantage of the mixture is that the synergistic effects allow smaller doses of each agent to be given, thereby lowering the risk of untoward reactions. On the other hand, other physicians contend that this mixture of drugs has no value because ephedrine provides no enhancement of bronchodilation, rather they believe that it contributes to the production of disturbing adverse effects.

Prophylactic asthmatic drugs

Cromolyn sodium (Aarane, Intal)

Cromolyn is a bronchial asthmatic prophylactic agent. It is not a bronchodilator, antihistaminic, or antiinflammatory drug. Cromolyn appears to act primarily through a local effect on lung mucosa. It inhibits the release of histamine and the slow-reacting substance of anaphylaxis (SRS-A) from sensitized mast cells following exposure to various allergens. It inhibits late allergic reactions to a lesser extent.

Cromolyn has no role in the treatment of an acute attack of asthma or in status asthmaticus. Its approved use is as an adjunct to the overall management of patients with severe, perennial, bronchial asthma. A satisfactory response to cromolyn therapy is indicated by a reduction in the number of attacks, reduced cough, decreased sputum production, and/or a decreased need for other antiasthma drugs. Some patients show improvement in pulmonary function. These responses usually occur in the first 2 to 4 weeks of treatment. Only those patients showing improvement should continue to receive cromolyn (see full description of cromolyn sodium in Chapter 15).

CORTICOSTEROID DRUGS

Corticosteroid drugs are used in chronic asthma to lessen airway obstruction. As antiinflammatory agents, they stabilize the membranes of lysosomes, thus preventing the release of hydrolytic enzymes that produce the inflammatory process in the tissues. The exact mechanism in asthma is still poorly understood, but it does involve suppression of antibody formation that is responsible for provoking the asthmatic attack. In addition, corticosteroids potentiate an increase in cyclic AMP, a

compound needed to promote bronchodilation. At the same time it is thought that they prevent the formation of cyclic GMP, which induces smooth muscle constriction.

Corticosteroids are used in asthmatic patients to treat *status asthmaticus*, which is a life-threatening exacerbation of asthma associated with bronchospasm. The patients with this condition are usually unresponsive to nonsteroid bronchodilators. These drugs are also indicated for patients with severe chronic asthma when relief is difficult to obtain from other bronchodilating agents.

Steroids should not be used when other measures are available. Although maintenance programs of steroid therapy decrease the frequency of severe asthmatic attacks, they do not prevent all asthmatic episodes. Furthermore, it is not known whether all episodes of asthma could be prevented by continuous administration of large doses of these drugs. Actually, prolonged administration of large doses are associated with severe adverse effects that are permanent—osteoporosis, subcapsular cataracts, and stunting of growth in children. There are other adverse effects caused by this group of drugs, but fortunately they are reversible.

Daily administration of systemic corticosteroid therapy provides great therapeutic benefits, but the high incidence of adverse effects has led to the use of the alternate-day schedule of treatment. This regimen provides the best benefit/risk ratio for prolonged therapy because it minimizes the likelihood of unwanted side effects. The corticosteroids that generally are used have relatively short durations of action, and they include prednisone, prednisolone, and methylprednisone (see Chapter 27 for details of these drugs).

Recently, the use of steroid aerosols has become increasingly popular. Topical corticosteroid therapy offers the possibility of limiting action at the site of application and thereby *avoiding systemic effects*. By chemically modifying the structural arrangement of the steroid molecule, several compounds have been developed in an effort to diminish systemic absorption from the respiratory tract. One such topical agent is beclomethasone dipropionate (Vanceril), and it does offer the advantage of producing few systemic adverse effects including that of limited or no adrenal suppression.

Beclomethasone dipropionate (Vanceril Inhaler, Beclovent)

Beclomethasone is a synthetic corticosteroid chemically related to prednisolone and having high antiinflammatory activity. Because it is an inhalational agent, only a limited amount of systemic absorption occurs from respiratory and gastrointestinal tissues with excretion in the feces and urine (less than 10%).

Uses. It is indicated only for patients who require chronic treatment with corticosteroids for control of bronchial asthma in conjunction with other therapy. It may be used after bronchodilator or cromolyn failure when long-term steroid control is considered or when oral steroids are producing undesirable side effects.

Beclomethasone is used in patients not receiving systemic steroids (withheld because of concern of potential adverse reactions) whose disease is inadequately controlled with nonsteroid measures; improvement in pulmonary function appears in 1 to 4 weeks.

Stable asthmatic patients who are dependent on receiving systemic steroids and are to be transferred to beclomethasone have a more difficult subsequent management because of the slow (resumption of adrenal function) recovery from impaired adrenal function. Suppression of adrenal function may last up to 1 year. Beclomethasone may be effective in managing these patients and may permit significant reduction in the oral corticosteroid dosage. The slow rate of withdrawal is emphasized. During withdrawal from systemic steroids some patients exhibit symptoms of systemically active steroid withdrawal (for example, joint and muscle pain, lassitude, and depression).

Beclomethasone may also be used in treatment of nonasthmatic bronchitis.

Preparation, dosage, and administration. This metered dose oral inhaler has 200 doses per inhaler (10 mg); each activation of the inhaler releases about 50 μg into the adapter. The usual adult dosage is two inhalations (100 μg) three or four times daily. Patients with severe asthma may initially administer 12 to 16 inhalations three or four times daily and adjust

the dosage downward to correspond with response but not exeeding 20 inhalations daily. Children (6 to 12 years old) receive one or two inhalations three to four times daily based on response but not exceeding 10 inhalations daily. The nurse should instruct the patient who is also using a bronchodilator by inhalation (for example, isoproterenol) in addition to the beclomethasone to use the bronchodilator first because this enhances penetration of the steroid into the bronchial tree. Several minutes should elapse before using the steroid inhaler to reduce the potential toxicity of the fluorocarbon propellants.

Side effects and toxic effects. Patients may complain of hoarseness or dry mouth; additionally, localized infections with *Candida albicans* or *Aspergillus* have occurred frequently in the mouth and pharynx and occasionally in the larynx.

Deaths caused by adrenal insufficiency have occurred during and after transfer from systemic corticosteroids to aerosol beclomethasone, and suppression of hypothalamic-pituitary-adrenal (HPA) function (reduction of early morning plasma cortisol levels) has been reported in adults receiving 1600 μg daily for 1 month. During periods of stress (trauma, surgery, infections) or severe asthmatic attacks, a patient transferred from systemic (oral tablets) steroids will require supplementary treatment with additional systemic (oral tablets) steroids for a short course, with gradual tapering as symptoms subside. The nurse should warn the patient that the steroid inhaler is not useful in aborting an acute attack but that the catecholamine inhalation product is useful for this purpose. The patient should be told also that the steroid inhaler may take weeks before the full benefit is realized.

Contraindications. The steroid inhaler is contraindicated in the treatment of status asthmaticus or other acute asthmatic episodes needing intensive measures.

Precautions. The nurse should encourage the patient to carry a warning card indicating the need for supplementary systemic steroids during stressful periods or a severe asthma attack. After withdrawal from systemic corticosteroids, a number of months are required for

HPA function recovery, and during this HPA suppression the patient exhibits signs and symptoms (hypotension, weight loss, particularly gastroenteritis) of adrenal insufficiency when exposed to stress. The beclomethasone inhaler does not provide the systemic steroid necessary for coping with these emergencies. Before the patient is discharged the nurse should encourage the patient to see the physician to have routine tests of adrenal cortical function done to assess the risks of adrenal insufficiency in emergency situations. This can include measurement of early morning resting cortisol levels.

Patients transferred from systemic steroid therapy should be told by the nurse that they may experience unmasked allergic conditions previously suppressed (such as rhinitis, conjunctivitis, and eczema).

Dexamethasone sodium phosphate (Decadron Phosphate, Turbinaire)

Dexamethasone is used for allergic or inflammatory nasal conditions and nasal polyps (excluding polyps originating within the sinuses).

Adults should receive two sprays in each nostril two or three times a day; children should receive one or two sprays in each nostril two times a day, depending on age.

The nurse should review the instructions for use of the Decadron Turbinaire for nasal use with the patient. The patient should be reminded to blow accumulated mucus and secretions from the nose immediately before use and, while holding his breath, to press the cartridge to release one measured dose of medication. The patient should not inhale, but the breath should be held (to avoid systemic absorption by the lungs) for several seconds after applying the medication for its full nasal topical effectiveness. The patient should be told not to blow the nose immediately after applying the medication. Each cartridge delivers 170 metered nasal sprays; 12 sprays deliver about 1 mg of dexamethasone. The maximum daily dosage for adults is 12 sprays, and for children it is 8 sprays.

Side effects and toxic effects. The most common side effects are nasal irritation and dry-ness. Headache, light-headedness, urticaria, nausea, epistaxis, rebound congestion, bronchial asthma, perforation of the nasal septum, and anosmia have occured. Signs of adrenal hypercorticism may occur, especially with overdosage.

Dexamethasone sodium phosphate (Decadron Phosphate, Respihaler)

The Decadron Respihaler is for oral inhalation; with each metered dose approximately 84 μg dexamethasone is delivered. Adult dosage is three inhalations (oral) three or four times daily to a maximum of 12 inhalations daily. The dosage for children is two inhalations three or four times daily with a maximum of eight inhalations daily.

Drugs that affect the respiratory center
Therapeutic gases
Oxygen

Oxygen was discovered by Priestley in 1772. Later, Lavoisier described the role of oxygen in the respiratory process. Beddoes introduced the utilization of oxygen as a therapeutic modality in England in the eighteenth century.

Oxygen is a gas that constitutes 20.93% of inspired air and is essential for maintaining life. Oxygen is a colorless, odorless, and tasteless gas. It is not flammable, but it supports combustion much more vigorously than does air.

Oxygen is compressed and marketed in steel cylinders that are fitted with reducing valves for the delivery of the gas. The cylinders are usually color coded; green is used in the United States. Since the gas is under considerable pressure, the tanks must be handled carefully to prevent their falling or bumping into each other or into anything that may cause undue jarring.

Oxygen must be continuously supplied to tissue cells, since no fiber or cell can remain hypoxic for very long and survive. The adult human brain consumes from 40 to 50 ml oxygen/minute. The cortex consumes more than the centers in the medulla or spinal cord. Cerebral oxygen consumption proceeds without respite, and the replenishment of oxygen by the blood must be maintained continuously. Whenever any circulatory stress exists, cerebral blood flow tends to be preserved at the expense of other less vital organs. Of all the tissues affected by hypoxia, the brain is most susceptible to disruption of normal function and irreversible damage. An acute reduction of the Po_2 to 50 mm Hg decreases mental functioning, emotional stability, and finer muscular coordination. Further reduction of the Po_2 to 40 mm Hg produces impaired judgment, decreased pain perception, and impairment of muscular coordination. When the Po_2 is reduced to 32 mm Hg or less, unconsciousness and a progressive descending depression of the central nervous system ensue.

The kidneys constitute other vital organs in which there must be considerable constancy of blood flow and oxygen supply. Oxygen consumption is greater in the renal cortex; renal medullary tissue has an oxygen consumption that is 15% less than that of the renal cortex. This difference is related to the variation in pressure gradient and the fact that cortical flow is rapid while the medullary flow is slower. The renal cortex is highly dependent on oxygen, whereas the renal medulla can function relatively independently of the oxygen supply.

The rate of oxygen consumption by the kidneys is approximately 0.06 ml/g/minute. They consume more oxygen than most other tissues. For each 100 ml of blood entering the kidney, 1.4 ml of oxygen is consumed. The oxygen consumed by the kidneys is primarily used for sodium reabsorption. When the arterial content falls to less than 55% of normal, renal vasoconstriction occurs. It is currently believed that this response is mediated by the chemoreceptors, which stimulate the vasomotor center to produce renal vasoconstriction. Renal vasoconstriction also occurs as a result of the action of ether, barbiturates, and other anesthetics. Renal blood flow is also decreased during periods of exercise. In relation to the preceding, it is important to note that autoregulation of renal perfusion does occur.

In skeletal muscles oxygen consumption is related to blood flow. Oxygen consumption and blood flow are decreased when muscle is at rest and significantly increased during exercise.

Reduction of oxygen supply to the intestinal tract is regarded by some investigators as a key factor for inadequate splanchnic vascular compensation (splanchnic vasoconstriction) during hypotension.

Inadequate oxygen supply impairs myocardial metabolism and function. Recent research seems to indicate that ethyl alcohol decreases myocardial oxygen consumption.

Arterial blood pressure determinations, when used alone, are unreliable indicators of the adequacy of tissue perfusion. Therefore arterial blood gas determinations should be obtained, since these results provide a more accurate and reliable indication of shifts in the partial pressures of oxygen and carbon dioxide. Severe hypoxia may produce changes in the ST segment and T wave of the ECG, dysrhythmias, ectopic beats, and myocardial infarction.

Indications for use. Oxygen is used in medicine chiefly to treat hypoxia (oxygen lack) and hypoxemia (diminished oxygen tension in the blood). There are basically four types of hypoxia described in the literature. These include the following:

1 Hypoxic hypoxia—produced by any condition causing a decrease in Po_2
2 Ischemic hypoxia—inadequate blood flow to an organ or tissue in the presence of a normal Po_2 and hemoglobin content
3 Anemic hypoxia—inadequate hemoglobin to carry O_2 in the presence of a normal Po_2
4 Histotoxic hypoxia—adequate Po_2 and hemoglobin, but inability of tissues to utilize oxygen delivered because of a toxic agent

Clinically, hypoxic hypoxia is the most common form of hypoxia seen. There is a variety of pathologic conditions that result in hypoxic hypoxia necessitating the utilization of oxygen as a treatment modality. Some of these include hypoventilation, increased airway resistance, pneumothorax, respiratory center depression, abnormal ventilation/perfusion ratio, congenital cyanotic heart disease, decreased pulmonary compliance, and breathing oxygen-poor air. The use of oxygen is also indicated in the following: (1) cardiac failure or decompensation and coronary occlusion, (2) anesthesia, to increase the safety of general anesthetics, and (3) treatment of certain types of headache.

Administration of oxygen. Oxygen is administered in a number of ways, including oxygen tent, nasal catheter or cannula, face mask, hood, and oxygen chamber. Each of these methods of administering oxygen has advantages and disadvantages.

When a *nasal catheter* is used it should be lubricated with a water-soluble jelly and passed through the nose until the tip is just above the epiglottis. This distance is usually the same as the distance from the patient's external nares to the tragus of the ear, minus 1 cm. The catheter should not be inserted so far that the patient swallows oxygen, since this will cause stomach distention and abdominal discomfort. The catheter is fastened with tape to the forehead and/or nose. Flow rate varies according to patient need, but 3 to 4 liters oxygen/minute is commonly used. Since this form of therapy is very drying to the mucous membrane, the oxygen should be humidified. In addition, nasal and oral hygiene is important to maintain cleanliness and intact mucous membrane and to prevent infection and discomfort. Most patients receiving oxygen therapy are mouth breathers, and frequent mouth care is required to prevent sores. Nasal catheters become obstructed with encrusted secretions and must be removed and cleaned or replaced several times a day.

Nasal cannulas are much more comfortable for patients than catheters. They are less likely to become obstructed with secretions. Nasal and oral mucosa still require frequent attention. A flow of 3 liters of oxygen is adequate for many patients.

Oxygen masks are the most effective means of delivering needed oxygen. Oxygen concentrations of 90% to 100% can be administered by mask. To be effective the mask must fit well over the nose and mouth; high flow rates can compensate to some extent for a poor fit. Masks are better tolerated when used intermittently or when disposable plastic masks are used. Only absolutely clean and uncontaminated rubber masks should be used, since they can be a source of nosocomial infection.

Oxygen tents and hoods have the advantage of temperature and humidity regulation. Disadvantages include oxygen loss, carbon dioxide accumulation, and claustrophobic effect. Oxygen concentration in a tent rarely reaches 50%; in a hood the concentration may reach 90% to 100%. The tent and hood should be periodically tested with an oxygen analyzer for oxygen concentrations. Oxygen should be flowing into the tent *before* it is secured over the patient. The usual rate of flow is 15 liters/minute for the first 15 to 30 minutes after the patient is in the tent, and 10 to 12 liters/minute thereafter. Tent leakage should be prevented by careful planning of care so that the tent is removed or opened as seldom as possible. The tent should also be securely tucked under the mattress and around the patient. The mattress should be covered with plastic or a rubber sheet to prevent oxygen saturation of the mattress and undue loss of oxygen. Oxygen tents and hoods are less popular today than formerly since the advent of plastic face masks and face tents.

For a child with a respiratory infection adequate oxygen concentration can be maintained in a croup tent with an open top. When indicated, the top may be covered to increase the mist.

Face tents are the most convenient, comfortable way to administer high concentrations of oxygen. A flow of 15 liters/minute can provide an oxygen concentration of 70%.

Since oxygen supports combustion and combustible material burns with greater ease and intensity, and since the patient is surrounded with combustible materials (linens, wooden furniture), smoking and the use of matches or electric equipment that may cause sparks are strictly forbidden in rooms where oxygen is being administered.

The effectiveness of oxygen administration will depend on the carbon dioxide content of the blood. Patients with chronic obstructive pulmonary disease have difficulty with carbon dioxide and oxygen exchange and are subject to hypercapnia (high carbon dioxide content in the blood). Because of the long-term presence of hypercapnia, the medullary center of these patients is relatively insensitive to stimulation of carbon dioxide; rather a low Pao_2 serves as a stimulant to respiration. Therefore oxygen must be administered to these individuals with caution in an attempt to prevent the further accumulation of carbon dioxide, with the subsequent development of toxic and narcotic levels resulting in further depression of respiration and respiratory acidosis. The nurse should be alert to the development of neurologic symptoms indicative of accumulation of carbon dioxide. Symptoms may include drowsiness, mental confusion, paresthesias, and visual disturbances. The occurrence of carbon dioxide narcosis may be prevented by gradually increasing the concentration of oxygen administered or, according to some investigators, by using intermittent positive pressure breathing. When there is no danger of accumulation of carbon dioxide, the medullary center retains its sensitivity to carbon dioxide stimulation and high concentrations of oxygen can be administered.

Oxygen administration in the premature infant. Nurses who care for premature babies in incubators must be constantly aware of the potential danger of the development of retrolental fibroplasia. This is a vascular proliferative disease of the retina that occurs in some premature infants who have been subjected to high concentrations of oxygen at birth.* The oxygen concentrations should be kept between 30% and 40%; however, higher concentrations can be administered to cyanotic infants without increasing the danger of retrolental fibroplasia because it is the Pa_{O_2}, not inspired P_{O_2}, that is implicated in the development of this disease. Therefore careful monitoring of arterial blood gases is essential. Some models of incubators are equipped with a safety valve that automatically releases any excess oxygen outside the chamber.

When orders for an infant include oxygen p.r.n. as required, the nurse must make certain that it is administered only as needed and at low concentrations, rather than continuously. Frequently, the removal of a very small plug of mucus can clear the baby's airway, thus enabling him to breathe oxygen without assistance.

Oxygen administration in tumor therapy. Hy-

___
*Excessive oxygen constricts the developing retinal vessels of the eye. Consequently, normal vascularization is suppressed, and since the endothelial cells become disorganized, they cause destruction of the immature retina. This results in blindness.

poxic cells are resistant to radiation damage. Therefore, if a tumor outgrows its blood supply, hyperoxygenation of the blood may increase oxygen supply to these cells and make them more sensitive to radiation. This particular therapy is still under investigation, and it will be several years before its efficacy can be accurately evaluated.

Use of hyperbaric oxygen. In recent years, hyperbaric oxygen has been used in the treatment of various conditions. In the treatment of infections caused by *Clostridium welchii*, the anaerobic bacillus producing gas gangrene, hyperbaric oxygen used intermittently has been of some value. It is believed that an increased oxygen pressure in the tissue may exert an inhibitory effect on enzyme systems of these bacteria. This same inhibitory effect may be implicated in the use of hyperbaric oxygen on other anaerobic microorganisms. Hyperbaric oxygen has been used in the treatment of tetanus, but the results are less satisfactory than those obtained in the treatment of gas gangrene.

Hyperbaric oxygen has also been used in certain circulatory disturbances. In shock, in which there is a generalized circulatory deficit, hyperbaric oxygen may be of some value. It has also been used in certain local circulatory disturbances such as various peripheral vascular diseases.

Helium-oxygen mixtures. Helium-oxygen mixtures have been used for some time to treat obstructive types of dyspnea. Helium is an inert gas and so light that a mixture of 80% helium and 20% oxygen is only one third as heavy as air. Helium is only slightly soluble in body fluids and has a high rate of diffusion. Its low specific gravity makes it possible for mixtures of this gas with oxygen to be breathed with less effort than either oxygen or air alone when there is obstruction in the air passages.

These mixtures are recommended for status asthmaticus, bronchiectasis, and emphysema, and during anesthesia for a patient with respiratory tract obstruction.

Carbon dioxide

Carbon dioxide is a colorless, odorless gas that is heavier than air. It was discovered by Priestley in the eighteenth century; Lavoisier elucidated its role in the respiratory process. Its use as a pharmacologic agent has implications for respiration, circulation, and the central nervous system. Whether it affects the respiratory center directly or by increasing the hydrogen ion concentration is still a matter of debate. However, inhalation of carbon dioxide for a short period of time increases both the rate and the depth of respiration unless the respiratory center is depressed by narcotics or disease.

Carbon dioxide has two opposing effects in the human body:

1 It stimulates cells of the sympathetic nervous system, the respiratory center, and the peripheral chemoreceptors.
2 It depresses the cerebral cortex, myocardium, and smooth muscle of the peripheral blood vessels.

Carbon dioxide may also interfere with nerve conduction and transmission. When carbon dioxide increases the rate and force of respiration, venous return to the heart is usually enhanced as a result of decreased peripheral resistance; there is improved rate and force of myocardial contraction and less likelihood of myocardial irritability and dysrhythmias.

Too much carbon dioxide has a depressant effect and results in acidosis as well as unresponsiveness of the respiratory center to carbon dioxide. Therefore, it is important that carbon dioxide be administered with caution.

Indications for use. The following are indications for use of carbon dioxide.

Carbon monoxide poisoning. A 5% to 7% concentration of carbon dioxide in oxygen is sometimes used in the treatment of carbon monoxide poisoning. Physiologically, carbon dioxide increases the rate of dissociation of carbon monoxide from carboxyhemoglobin as well as gas exchange.

General anesthesia. Most general anesthetics cause a reduction in response to carbon dioxide, which reflects central nervous system depression. The degree of depression is directly related to the depth of anesthesia. The more deeply the patient is anesthetized, the greater the depression of the central nervous system. In the beginning carbon dioxide speeds up anesthesia by increasing pulmonary ventilation. By lessening the sense of asphyxiation, it reduces

struggling. After anesthesia, it hastens the elimination of many anesthetics. Inhalation of 5% to 7% carbon dioxide increases cerebral blood flow by approximately 75%, primarily by dilation of cerebral vessels.

Respiratory depression. The use of carbon dioxide as a respiratory stimulant in the presence of depressed respiration is limited. When used, close monitoring of Pao_2 is important; if desired results are not obtained, it should be discontinued. In cases of respiratory depression, mechanical assistance to respiration plus oxygen administration is the usual treatment.

Postoperative use. Occasionally, carbon dioxide is used postoperatively in an effort to increase ventilation and prevent atelectasis. Most investigators think that the use of deep breathing exercises, coughing, frequent turning, tracheal suction, and intermittent positive pressure breathing produces better results. Carbon dioxide administration has also been used in the treatment of postoperative singultus (hiccups). Relief of singultus is apparently accomplished by stimulating the respiratory center, causing large excursions of the diaphragm that submerge spasmodic contractions of that muscle, thereby promoting regular contractions.

Administration. Carbon dioxide is kept in metal cylinders and vaporizes as it is delivered from the cylinder. When carbon dioxide is used for medical purposes, it is administered in combination with oxygen. A 5% to 10% concentration of carbon dioxide delivered through a tight-fitting face mask is inhaled by the patient until the depth of respiration is definitely increased, which usually occurs within 3 minutes. For the postoperative individual, the procedure should be repeated every hour or two for the first 48 hours, and then several times a day for several days.

Another way of administering carbon dioxide is to allow the patient to hyperventilate with a paper bag held over his face. He reinhales his expired air in which the carbon dioxide content is continually increased.

Signs of carbon dioxide overdosage are dyspnea, breath-holding, markedly increased chest and abdominal movements, nausea, and increased systolic blood pressure. Administration of the gas should be discontinued when these symptoms appear. The administration should, in fact, be stopped as soon as the desired effects on respiration have been obtained.

Direct respiratory stimulants

Direct respiratory stimulants come under a broader classification of central nervous system stimulants and are often referred to as *analeptics*. These drugs act directly on the medullary center to increase rate and tidal exchange. Although drugs from this category are available for stimulating depth of respiration and concomitantly, but to a lesser degree, rate of respiration, airway management and support of ventilation are more effective in the treatment of respiratory depression. Indeed, the latter is often superior to the use of drugs, since respiratory stimulants in large doses are convulsants.

Respiratory stimulants (analeptics) have in the past been advocated in the treatment of drug-induced respiratory depression, but since these drugs are not specific antagonists to sedatives or narcotics, their use in drug-induced respiratory depression is now considered obsolete. Indeed, repeated doses of an analeptic may potentiate the depressant effects of central nervous system depressants.

Analeptics have also been used to counteract respiratory depression caused by anesthetics or to shorten postanesthetic recovery time. However, these methods of therapy are not recommended, since decreasing the concentration of the anesthetic agent in the blood is accomplished more effectively with mechanical ventilatory measures.

Doxapram hydrochloride (Dopram)

Doxapram is a centrally acting respiratory stimulant. It is particularly useful for treatment of postanesthetic respiratory depression and to hasten return of protective pharyngeal and laryngeal reflexes after anesthesia. The depth of respiration is significantly increased by doxapram, and the rate of respiration may also increase. The action of doxapram is thought to be primarily caused by stimulation of the respiratory center. It may also have some effect on chemoreceptors. Mild vasopressor activity is noted with the use of doxapram, resulting in elevation of blood pressure and heart rate. In addition, doxapram produces an increase in salivation, body temperature, gastric secretions, and tone and motility of the gastrointestinal tract and urinary bladder.

Preparation, dosage, and administration. Doxapram is available in solution form for intravenous injection, 20 mg/ml in 20-ml, vials. When administered postoperatively, a single dose of 0.5 to 1.5 mg/kg body weight may be given over a period of 30 to 90 seconds. Repeated doses may be necessary, but maximum dosage, even when multiple injections are used, should not exceed 2 mg/kg. Intravenous infusion may also be used. With this method of administration the dose is usually 5 mg/minute initially; this is reduced to 1 to 3 mg/minute when the desired response has been obtained. Doxapram is metabolized rapidly and has a brief duration of action. During administration, the patient's blood pressure, heart rate, and other vital signs should be carefully monitored to prevent overdosage and toxic reactions.

Side effects. Doxapram can cause a wide variety of side effects as a result of its central stimulating effect. Minor side effects include singultus, nausea, vomiting, sneezing, headache, fever, spontaneous urination, confusion, dyspnea, and cough. The most serious side effects are hypertension, tachycardia, muscle rigidity, and cardiac dysrhythmias.

Precautions. The adverse cardiovascular effects of doxapram may be greatly increased in individuals receiving sympathomimetic drugs or monoamine oxide inhibitors. Doxapram is contraindicated for patients with hypertension, convulsive disorders, cardiac dysrhythmias, cerebral edema, or hyperthyroidism. It is not recommended for use in patients with chronic pulmonary disease.

Nursing considerations. Nursing interventions in the administration of doxapram include:

1 Maintenance of a patent airway
2 Monitoring of vital signs continuously during administration and for 30 to 60 minutes following discontinuation of the drug
3 Availability of oxygen and equipment for mechanical ventilation

4 Periodic determination of arterial blood gases to ascertain degree of effective ventilation

Nikethamide (Coramine)

Nikethamide is a synthetic compound chemically related to nicotinamide, the vitamin that prevents pellagra. Apparently, nikethamide has its most pronounced effect on the respiratory center when the center is in a state of depression. Respiratory stimulation is a result of increasing the sensitivity of the respiratory center to carbon dioxide, or possibly to action on the chemoreceptors. When used on experimental animals, the medullary centers give evidence of stimulation, resulting in increased rate and depth of respiration and inconsistent peripheral vasoconstriction.

Nikethamide may be used to treat acute respiratory depression caused by hypnotics, anesthetics, or alcohol. It has low toxicity and is considered to be a relatively safe stimulant, since it is less likely to cause convulsions than other centrally acting stimulants; however, it is seldom used today.

Nikethamide is available in solution form for parenteral injection. It is usually given intravenously. The dose varies according to the degree of respiratory depression and may range from 1 to 10 ml of a 25% solution (250 mg to 2.5 g). Anxiety, nausea, and vomiting may occur, but side effects are usually mild.

Reflex respiratory stimulants

Camphor, ammonia, and carminatives act as mild respiratory stimulants when taken orally. Ammonia, however, is the only drug given by inhalation for its action as a reflex respiratory stimulant. In cases of fainting aromatic spirits of ammonia is administered by inhaling the vapor. When given orally, 2 ml of aromatic ammonia spirits is diluted with at least 1 fluidounce of water. Reflex stimulation of the medullary center occurs through peripheral irritation of sensory nerve receptors in the pharynx, esophagus, and stomach. The rate and depth of respiration are then increased through afferent messages to the control centers. Reflex stimulation of the vasomotor center results in a rise in blood pressure.

Respiratory depressants

The most important respiratory depressants are the central depressants of the opium group and those of the barbiturate group of drugs. These drugs depress the respiratory center, thereby making breathing slower and more shallow and lessening the irritability of the respiratory center. Respiratory depression, however, is seldom desirable or necessary, although it is sometimes unavoidable. It is frequently a side effect in otherwise very useful drugs. Occasionally, a cough is so painful or harmful that an opiate, such as codeine, is administered to inhibit the rate and depth of respiration. A greater value, however, lies in its action to depress the cough reflex. Too-high concentrations of carbon dioxide in inhalation mixtures may paradoxically act to depress respiration.

Cough suppressants

Coughing is a protective reflex for clearing the respiratory tract of environmental irritants, foreign bodies, or accumulated secretions and thus should not be depressed indiscriminately. The afferent impulses that arise from irritated pharyngeal and laryngeal tissues initiate the cough reflex. Drugs act either by suppressing the cough center in the medulla oblongata or peripherally by lessening irritation of the respiratory tract. A cough is *productive* when irritants or secretions are removed from the respiratory tract; it is *nonproductive* when it is dry and irritating. The severity of frequent and prolonged coughing should be diminished since it can be exhausting, painful, and taxing to the circulatory system and the elastic tissue of the respiratory system, particularly in the elderly and in young children. Most coughs can be suppressed without danger to the patient and thereby foster comfort and rest. Some coughs occur primarily at night or when the patient is recumbent because of the accumulation of secretions, and some coughs occur in the morning on arising as a result of the gravitational movement of secretions. Coughing is to some extent under voluntary control; an individual can cough at will and at times can suppress coughing. However, coughing is usually initiated by respiratory tract reflexes responding to irritations by sending impulses to the cough center. The value of adequate hydration of the patient, by oral intake of fluids as well as by inhalation of fully water-saturated vapors (steam), should be stressed as one of the most important means of producing increased amounts of mucus as well as thinning such secretions.

Treatment of the cough is secondary to treatment of the underlying disorder. Antitussives should not be given in situations in which retention of respiratory secretions or exudates may be harmful. The therapeutic objective is to decrease the intensity and frequency of the cough yet permit adequate elimination of tracheobronchial secretions and exudates. Medications that may be used to relieve the cough include narcotic and nonnarcotic antitussive agents.

Narcotic antitussive agents

Narcotics such as morphine, dihydromorphinone, and levorphanol are potent suppressants of the cough reflex, but their clinical usefulness is limited by their side effects. They inhibit the ciliary activity of the respiratory mucous membrane, depress respiration, and may cause bronchial constriction in allergic or asthmatic patients. In addition, they can cause drug dependence.

Codeine and dihydrocodeinone exhibit less pronounced antitussive effects but they also have fewer side effects. They have been widely used. Dihydrocodeinone is more active than codeine, but its drug dependence liability is also greater. The usual dose is 5 to 10 mg three to four times a day.

Methadone is not an opiate, but it resembles morphine in a number of respects. Its ability to suppress the cough reflex is similar to that of morphine. A dose of 1.5 to 2 mg will effectively relieve a cough. Its main disadvantage as an antitussive agent lies in its drug dependence qualities.

Nonnarcotic antitussive agents

The instillation of a local anesthetic agent prior to various diagnostic techniques such as bronchoscopy has proved effective in suppressing the cough reflex. This has led to the investigation of other agents that exert a similar action. The clinical effectiveness of these drugs against pathologic cough still remains to be established. Newer nonnarcotic drugs in this group have fewer gastrointestinal side effects than do codeine and related compounds.

Benzonatate (Tessalon)

Benzonatate is chemically related to the local anesthetic tetracaine. It is *effective* for symptomatic treatment of cough. It relieves cough without suppressing respiration. Benzonatate relieves cough through two mechanisms, one of which is a peripheral action involving selective anesthesia of stretch receptors in the lungs. The second mechanism involves a direct action on the sites of medullary transmission.

Preparation of dosage. Benzonatate is marketed in 100-mg capsules, and the dosage is 100 mg three times a day for adults and children over 10 years of age. For younger children the dose is 8 mg/kg body weight in three to six divided doses. It is also available in intravenous and intramuscular preparations. However, oral administration is the route of choice. After oral administration its effects are noticed within 15 to 20 minutes, and they last for 3 to 8 hours. Benzonatate produces temporary local anesthesia of the oral mucosa, so the patient should be told to swallow the capsule immediately.

Side effects. Side effects do not seem to be serious but may include drowsiness, nausea, tightness in the chest, skin eruptions, chilling, and nasal congestion. On occasion, benzonatate may produce constipation. Side effects like those associated with the narcotic antitussives have not been reported.

Carbetapentane citrate (Toclase)

Carbetapentane is a synthetic preparation said to exhibit properties similar to atropine and certain local anesthetics. Its antitussive potency seems to be similar to that of codeine phosphate. It is marketed in 25-mg tablets and as a syrup (1.45 mg/ml) for oral administration. The proposed dosage for adults is 15 to 30 mg three to four times a day.

Noscapine (Tusscapine, Actol)

Noscapine is one of the isoquinoline alkaloids of opium, formerly known as narcotine. It is structurally related to papaverine and resembles it in its effects on smooth muscle, but its present use is based on its ability to depress the cough reflex. Noscapine resembles codeine in potency but does not produce opiate effects such as constipation, respiratory depression, constriction of the pupils, analgesia, and psychologic or physical dependence.

Preparation and dosage. Noscapine is marketed for oral administration. The usual adult dose is 15 to 30 mg three or four times a day. Side effects after therapeutic dosage are minimal and include drowsiness, headache, nausea, rhinitis and conjunctivitis.

Dextromethorphan hydrobromide (Romilar Hydrobromide)

Dextromethorphan is a synthetic derivative of morphine but is employed only as an agent to relieve cough. However, it possesses no significant analgesic properties, does not depress respiration, and does not cause dependence. It is the only agent in this group whose antitussive effects have been well documented through extensive experimental and clinical studies.

Preparation and dosage. Dextromethorphan hydrobromide is available in a variety of mixtures with other drugs and in a syrup (3 mg/ml). The usual adult dose is 15 to 30 mg, three or four times daily. The dose for children is 1 mg/kg body weight daily in divided doses. It acts within 20 to 30 minutes and is effective for 3 to 5 hours. Adverse reactions are mild and infrequent; they include slight drowsiness, nausea, and dizziness. Dextromethorphan may be purchased without a prescription.

Levopropoxyphene napsylate (Novrad)

Levopropoxyphene has no analgesic properties, but it does have antitussive effects and is effective for the symptomatic treatment of cough. Adverse reactions include nausea and vomiting, epigastric distress, headache, dizziness, tremors, urticaria, rash, dry mouth, and drowsiness.

Preparation and dosage. Levopropoxyphene is available in 50- and 100-mg capsules and as a suspension containing 50 mg/5 ml. Dosage for adults is 50 to 100 mg every 4 hours as needed. Dosage for children is 6 mg/kg body weight daily.

Chlophedianol hydrochloride (Ulo)

Chlophedianol has been cited as having cough suppressant potency comparable to that of the narcotics but with a slower onset of peak effect and a longer duration of action. It has mild anticholinergic properties. Dependence has not been reported.

Adverse reactions include nausea and vomiting, urticaria, dry mouth, vertigo, visual disturbances, excitability, nightmares, and hallucinations. Chlophedianol should be used with caution in patients taking drugs that stimulate or depress the central nervous system and in debilitated patients.

Preparation and dosage. Chlophedianol is available as a syrup containing 25 mg/5 ml. Usual dosage for adults is 25 mg three to four times daily; for children over 6 years of age, 2 mg/kg body weight in four divided doses; for children 2 to 6 years of age, 1 mg/kg in divided doses.

NURSING IMPLICATIONS

Nursing interventions that apply to this entire group of agents should include the following:

1 Accurate reporting of the frequency and quality of coughing and sputum production
2 Deep breathing exercises, postural drainage, frequent change of position, limitation or cessation of smoking, maintenance of adequate humidity in the environment, and adequate hydration
3 Observing for and reporting to the physician any untoward side effects of the drug
4 Proper administration of liquid antitussives (A liquid nonnarcotic antitussive agent should be administered undiluted, and the individual should be instructed not to drink water for approximately 30 to 35 minutes.)

Mucosal constrictor drugs (nasal decongestants)

Perhaps the attribute for which vasoconstricting drugs are most commonly used is their capacity to shrink the engorged nasal mucous membranes in mild upper respiratory infections. Many drugs are used exclusively as nasal vasoconstrictors. Because of their wide popular use and lack of serious hazard (when used topically), a confusingly large number of preparations have been provided by the pharmaceutical industry for direct sale to the public. Some of the more widely used agents in this group are phenylephrine hydrochloride (Neo-Synephrine), ephedrine sulfate, mephentermine sulfate (Wyamine Sulfate), propylhexadrine (Benzedrex), tuaminoheptane (Tuamine), xylometazoline hydrochloride (Otrivin Hydrochloride), phenylpropylmethylamine hydrochloride (Vonedrine), and naphazoline hydrochloride (Privine). Students will recognize these drugs as adrenergic agents. They act on alpha receptors of blood vessels in the nasal mucosa to produce mucosal constriction. However, many nasal decongestant agents also possess a beta property that causes an adverse effect of vasodilation following vasoconstriction.

Nasal decongestant drugs are used to shrink engorged mucous membranes of the nose and to relieve nasal stuffiness. However, there is a tendency on the part of patients to misuse them by using them in too large an amount and too frequently. This may result in "rebound" engorgement or swelling of the mucous membranes. Preservatives, antihistaminics, detergents, and antibiotics are sometimes added to the preparation of the decongestant. In some cases untoward reactions are believed to be caused by the additive rather than by the decongestant. Too-frequent interference with the vasomotor mechanism in the nose may do more harm than good, and there is always the possibility of spreading the infection deeper into the sinuses or to the middle ear. Sprays and nose drops are of benefit when used judiciously under the advice of a physician.

Antihistaminic agents for colds

Considerable difference of opinion exists at the present time as to the usefulness of the antihistaminic drugs for the prevention or treatment of the common cold. These drugs include diphenhydramine hydrochloride (Benadryl) and tripelennamine hydrochloride (Pyribenzamine) as well as a number of others. They are discussed in Chapter 15. Some investigators are of the opinion that if these drugs are taken early during the onset of a cold, the allergic manifestations of the disease are relieved. The patient experiences relief from the tickling sensation in the nose, sneezing, and the continuous irritating discharge from the nasal mucous membrane. The Council on Drugs warns that their indiscriminate use is not without harmful effects—people may become excessively drowsy and fall asleep while driving a car or operating machinery. It is also possible that profound effects may occur in the central nervous system and the blood-forming tissues after prolonged use of these drugs.

Summary of nursing considerations

The most critical requirement for maintaining life is an uninterrupted supply of oxygen. This need is met through the process of respiration, a process that includes pulmonary ventilation, gas transport, and cellular respiration.

Respiration is regulated by the medulla, but signals from other parts of the brain and spinal cord can modify the rhythm and pattern of respiration. Fear, pain, stress, blood pressure, body temperature, and blood levels of oxygen and carbon dioxide can all alter the activity of the respiratory center.

Aerosol therapy deposits medication in the respiratory tract in the form of droplets suspended in air. Drugs used for aerosol therapy include mucokinetic agents, mucolytic agents, bronchodilators, antibiotics, steroids, and antifoaming agents.

Mucokinetic agents thin hyperviscous secretions or sputum, and their removal prevents mucous plugging and pathogenic colonization in the lower respiratory tract. The most commonly used diluent of respiratory secretions is water. This may be administered by ultrasonic nebulizer. If patients are not on restricted fluid intake, they are usually encouraged to drink large amounts of water to liquefy the respiratory secretions.

Mucolytic agents reduce the viscosity of pulmonary secretions by breaking up the bonds of mucoprotein molecules of the secretion into smaller, more soluble strands. This facilitates removal of secretions and promotes more adequate pulmonary ventilation; an example is acetylcysteine.

Bronchodilators are used to relieve intermittent and recurring bronchial constriction, which, if prolonged and untreated, disrupts normal exchange of gases at the alveolar-capillary membrane. These drugs relax the smooth muscle of the tracheobronchial tree and decrease congestion in the respiratory tract through vasoconstriction and a decrease in mucous membrane swelling. Among these agents are the sympathomimetic drugs and the methylxanthines.

Cromolyn sodium is not a bronchodilator, antihistaminic, or an antiinflammatory drug but is effective as a prophylactic adjunct to the overall management of patients with severe, perennial bronchial asthma. It is administered as a prophylactic agent to prevent bronchoconstriction, thereby protecting the individual against asthmatic attacks.

Corticosteroids are also used as prophylactic agents in chronic asthma. They lessen airway obstruction by increasing the cyclic 3'5'AMP, thereby promoting bronchodilation. The two types of corticosteroids are systemic and nonsystemic. The latter type of agent is administered as a steroid aerosol, and because of its topical application, adverse systemic effects are avoided. Corticosteroids are given in conjunction with bronchodilator therapy. They are used only when simpler and less dangerous forms of therapy have failed.

Nasal decongestants are primarily adrenergic agents used as nasal vasoconstrictors to relieve nasal stuffiness. Because of their wide popular use and lack of serious hazard, many are available without prescription. Patients may take too large a dose too frequently, thereby experiencing rebound swelling of the mucous membrane and other untoward reactions.

Oxygen must be continuously supplied to tissue cells; without it, cells die. Of all the tissues affected by hypoxia, the brain is the most susceptible to disruption of normal function and irreversible damage. The kidneys also demand considerable constancy of blood flow and oxygen supply for normal function. Arterial

blood gas determinations are necessary to indicate the adequacy of tissue perfusion.

Oxygen is administered to treat hypoxic hypoxia, ischemic hypoxia, anemic hypoxia, histotoxic hypoxia, and hypoxemia (diminished oxygen tension in the blood). It is also indicated in cardiac failure or decompensation, coronary occlusion, anesthesia, and treatment of certain types of headache. It may be administered by oxygen tent, nasal catheter or cannula, face mask, hood, and oxygen chamber.

Effectiveness of oxygen administration depends on the carbon dioxide content of the blood. Nurses should be alert for the possible development of hypercapnia and subsequent development of toxic and narcotic levels of carbon dioxide.

Oxygen concentrations above 40% can cause retrolental fibroplasia in premature infants; therefore careful monitoring of blood gases is essential.

Hyperbaric oxygen has been used with some success in the treatment of gas gangrene, tetanus, and in certain circulatory disturbances. Helium-oxygen mixtures are used for treatment of obstructive types of dyspnea—status asthmaticus, bronchiectasis, and emphysema.

Carbon dioxide has two opposing effects in the human body: (1) it stimulates cells of the sympathetic nervous system, the respiratory center, and the peripheral chemoreceptors, and (2) it depresses the cerebral cortex, myocardium, and smooth muscle of the peripheral blood vessels.

Inhalation of carbon dioxide for a short time increases both the rate and the depth of respiration unless the respiratory center is depressed by narcotics or disease; excessive carbon dioxide has a depressant effect and results in acidosis.

Carbon dioxide is used in the treatment of carbon monoxide poisoning and in anesthesia; it initially speeds anesthesia by increasing pulmonary ventilation and later speeds the elimination of anesthetics.

Carbon dioxide overdosage is signaled by dyspnea, breath-holding, markedly increased chest and abdominal movements, nausea, and increased systolic blood pressue.

Direct respiratory stimulants are often

referred to as analeptics. They act directly on the medullary center to increase respiratory rate and tidal volume. However, airway management and support of ventilation are preferred in the treatment of respiratory depression, since respiratory stimulants may potentiate the effect of CNS depressants or may cause convulsions. When an analeptic is used, the drug of choice is doxapram.

Medications used to relieve coughing include narcotic and nonnarcotic antitussives, demulcents, antiseptics, expectorants, and others. Narcotics such as morphine, dihydromorphinone, levorphanol, codeine, and methadone are potent suppressants of the cough reflex, but these drugs are limited in their usefulness by their side effects, which include drug dependence.

Nonnarcotic antitussive agents have fewer gastrointestinal side effects than do codeine and related compounds. These drugs include benzonatate, carbetapentane citrate, noscapine, dextromethorphan, levopropoxyphene, and chlophedianol hydrochloride.

QUESTIONS

FOR STUDY AND REVIEW

1 Explain the effects of mucokinetic agents. Name two such agents and what therapeutic advantages each has.
2 Describe the mechanism of action of an adrenergic bronchodilator agent. What adverse effect is caused by nonselective adrenergic bronchodilator?
3 What are the advantages of aerosol therapy?
4 When is it advantageous to use large droplets for aerosol therapy? To use small droplets?
5 Discuss the use and pharmacokinetic properties of theophylline.
6 Which bronchodilator also has a diuretic effect?
7 Explain the pharmacologic action of cromolyn sodium.
8 What is beclomethasone? What therapeutic advantage does it have when used in status asthmaticus?
9 What is the nurse's role in caring for patients undergoing steroid therapy?
10 Discuss the therapy and nursing care for a patient with an acute asthmatic attack.
11 Explain the therapeutic uses of carbon dioxide and state what precautions should be taken when carbon dioxide is administered.

12 What precautions must be taken when oxygen is administered to patients with severe respiratory disease?
13 Discuss the beneficial and harmful effects of coughing.
14 Discuss the advantages and disadvantages of "over-the-counter" preparations for coughs and nasal congestion.
15 How do drugs act to produce relief from coughing?

BIBLIOGRAPHY

Avery, G.S., editor,: Drug treatment, ed. 2, Acton, Mass., 1980, Publishing Sciences Group, Inc.

Bowman, W.C., and Rand, M.J.: Textbook of pharmacology, ed. 2, London, 1980, Blackwell Scientific Publications, Ltd.

Brogden, R.N., and others: Sodium cromoglycate: a review of its mode of action, pharmacology, therapeutic efficacy and use, Drugs 7:164, 1974.

Brooks, S.M., and others: Adverse effects of phenobarbital on corticosteroid metabolism in patients with bronchial asthma, N. Engl. J. Med. 286:1125, 1972.

Caplin, I.: Choosing the right drugs for bronchial asthma, Mod. Med. 47:70, 1979.

Collins, J.V., and others: The use of corticosteroids in the treatment of acute asthma, Q.J. Med. 44:259, 1975.

Editorial: Analgesics and asthma, Br. Med. J. 3:419, 1973.

Goodman, L., and Gilman, A., editors: The pharmacologic basis of therapeutics, ed. 6, New York, 1980, Macmillan, Inc.

Goth, A.: Medical pharmacology: principles and concepts, ed. 10, St. Louis, 1981, The C.V. Mosby Co.

Greene, J.: Bronchial asthma: a chronic disease, Today's Clin. Oct. 1978, p. 33.

Griffith E.W.: Nursing process: a patient with respiratory difficulty, Nurs. Clin. North Am. 6:145, 1971.

Harvey, L.L., and others: Beclomethasone dipropionate aerosol in the treatment of steroid-dependent asthma, Chest 70:345, 1976.

Hyde, J.S., and others: Metaproterenol in children with chronic asthma, Clin, Pharmacol. Ther. 20:207, 1976.

Jacobs, M.Y., and others: Clinical experience with theophylline, J.A.M.A 235:1983, 1976.

Jenne, J.S., and others: Pharmacokinetics of theophylline, Clin. Pharmacol. Ther. 13:349, 1972.

John, J.: The clinical pharmacology of bronchodilators, Basics Resp. Dis. 6:1, 1977.

Klock, L.E., and others: A comparative study of atropine sulfate and isoproterenol hydrochloride in chronic bronchitis, Am. Rev. Respir. Dis. 112:371, 1975.

Lehnert, B., and Schachter, E.: The pharmacology of respiratory care, St. Louis, 1980, The C.V. Mosby Co.

McFadden, E.R., and others: Acute bronchial asthma: relations between clinical and physiological manifestations, N. Engl. J. Med. 288:221, 1973.

Mitchell, R.: Synopsis of clinical pulmonary disease, ed. 2, St. Louis, 1978, The C.V. Mosby Co.

Mitenko, P.A., and Ogilvie, R.I.: Bioavailability and efficacy of a sustained-release theophylline tablet, Clin. Pharmacol. Ther. 16:720, 1974.

Mitenko, P.A., and others: Rational intravenous doses of theophylline, N. Engl. J. Med. 289:600, 1973.

Modell, W., editor: Drugs of choice 1980-1981, St. Louis, 1980, The C.V. Mosby Co.

Morris, H.: Benefits vs. risks of corticosteroid therapy in patients with asthma, Adv. Asthma Allergy **5:**19, 1978.

Morrison, R.J., and Boyd, R.N.: Organic chemistry, ed. 3, Boston, 1973, Allyn & Bacon, Inc.

Nalepka, C.: The oxygen hood for newborns in respiratory distress, Am. J. Nurs. **75:**2185, 1975.

Nicholson, D.P., and others: A re-evaluation of parenteral aminophylline, Am. Rev. Respir. Dis. **108:**241, 1973.

Niewoehner, D., and others: Mechanisms of airway smooth muscle response to isoproterenol and theophylline, J. Appl. Physiol. **47:**2, 1979.

Rebuck, A.S.: Antiasthmatic drugs. I. Pathophysiological and clinical pharmacological aspects, Drugs **7:**344, 1974.

Rebuck, A.S.: Antiasthmatic drugs. II. Therapeutic aspects, Drugs **7:**370, 1974.

Sackner, M.A., and others: Bronchodilator effects of terbutaline and epinephrine in obstructive lung disease, Clin. Pharmacol. Ther. **16:**499, 1974.

Sedlock, S.A.: Detection of chronic pulmonary disease, Am. J. Nurs. **72:**1407, 1972.

Silverglade, A.: Cardiac toxicity of aerosol propellants, J.A.M.A. **222:**827, 1972.

Steen, S.N., and others: Evaluation of a new mucolytic drug, Clin. Pharmacol. Ther. **16:**58, 1974.

Szidon, J.P., Pietra, G.G., and Fishman, A.P.: The alveolar-capillary membrane and pulmonary edema, N. Engl. J. Med. **286:**1200, 1972.

Toogood, J.: Steroids in asthma, Lancet, **2:**1185, 1979.

Townley, R.: Pharmacologic blocks to mediator release: clinical application, Adv. Asthma Allergy **2:**7, 1975.

Webb-Johnson, D., and Andrews, J.: Drug therapy. I. Bronchodilator therapy, N. Engl. J. Med. **297:**476, 1977.

Webb-Johnson, D., and Andrews, J.: Bronchodilator therapy, II, N. Engl. Med. **297:**758, 1977.

Weinberger, M.M., and Bronsky, E.A.: Evaluation of oral bronchodilator therapy in asthmatic children, J. Pediatr. **84:**421, 1974.

Weinberger, M.M., and others: Rational use of theophylline, N. Engl. J. Med. **291:**151, 1974.

West, J.: Pulmonary pathophysiology, Baltimore, 1977, The Williams & Wilkins Co.

Williams, M.H.: Corticosteroid aerosols for the treatment of asthma, J.A.M.A. **231:**406, 1975.

Ziment, I.: Respiratory pharmacology and therapeutics, Philadelphia, 1978, W.B. Saunders Co.

CHAPTER 15

Histamine and antihistamines

Histamine

Storage and release
Pharmacologic actions
Pathologic effects
Clinical uses

Antihistamines

H_1 receptor antagonists
    Agents used in allergic conditions
    Drugs used for motion sickness
    Inhibitor of histamine release
    Nursing implications
H_2 receptor antagonists

Summary of nursing considerations

Histamine

Histamine is a chemical mediator that occurs naturally in almost all tissues of the body. It is present in highest concentration in the skin, lung, and gastrointestinal tract. These structures are frequently exposed to environmental assaults and require protection against damage. When liberated from their cells, the free form of histamine plays an early transient role in the inflammatory process that defends the exposed tissues against injury. Histamine is derived from the Greek words, *histos*, meaning tissue, and *amine*, meaning a nitrogen-containing compound, hence the name "tissue amine" or histamine. It was isolated from extracts of ergot in 1910 and firmly established as a natural body substance in 1927.

Since it is an amine, this compound possesses the basic group NH_2. Histamine is formed by enzymatic decarboxylation of histidine, a common amino acid derived from protein. The reaction proceeds as follows:

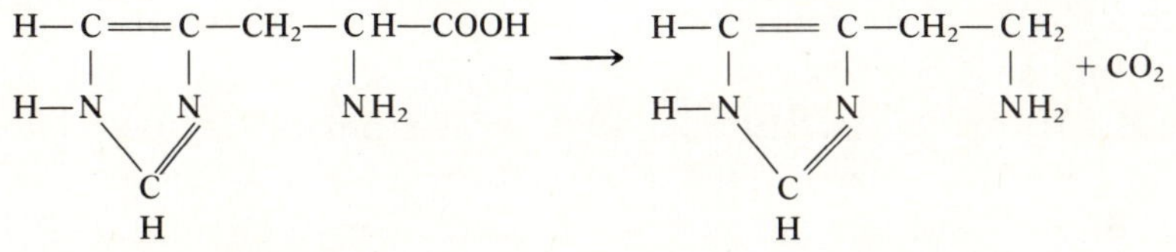

Storage and release

In many tissues the chief site of production and storage of histamine occurs in the cytoplasmic granules of the mast cell or, in the case of circulation, of the basophil, which closely resembles the mast cell in function. The mast cells are small, ovoid-shaped structures widely distributed in the loose connective tissue. They are especially abundant along small blood vessels and along the bronchial smooth muscle cell, which appears to have the highest concentration of mast cells of any organ in the body. Both the mast cells and basophils make up the *mast-cell histamine pool*. A second major site of histamine production is known as the *nonmast pool*, where the amine is stored in the cells of the epidermis, gastrointestinal mucosa, and the central nervous system. Although histamine is present in various foods and is synthesized by intestinal flora, the amount absorbed does not contribute to the body's stores of this amine.

In the storage sites, histamine is pharmaco-

H—C═C—CH₂—CH—COOH   →   H—C═C—CH₂—CH₂
    | | | | | | $+ CO_2$
H—N   N NH_2 H—N   N NH_2

Histidine   **Histamine**

TABLE 15-1   Receptor-mediating effects of histamine

Structure	Histamine receptors	Pharmacologic effects
Vascular system		
Capillary	H_1 and H_2	Dilation
(Microcirculation)		Increased permeability
Arteriole	H_1 and H_2	Dilation
(Smooth muscle)		
Smooth muscle		
Bronchial	H_1	Contraction
Gastrointestinal	H_1	Contraction
Exocrine glands		
Gastric	H_2	Gastric acid secretion
Epidermis	H_1	Triple response (flush, flare, wheal)
Adrenal medulla	—	Epinephrine and norepinephrine release
Central nervous system	H_1	Motion sickness

logically inactive. Stimulation of the mast cell membrane by certain agents such as antigen-antibody reactions, enzymes (trypsin), and other surface-active compounds activates the release of the amine from its granular binding sites into the extracellular environment of the smooth muscle, epidermis, and other involved tissues. It is solely the free form of histamine when in contact with the invading tissues that elicits the many untoward reactions that may range in intensity from mild itching to fatal anaphylactic shock.

Pharmacologic actions

The reactions mediated by histamine are attributed to receptor activity, which involves two distinct populations of receptors called H_1 and H_2 receptors.

The principal actions of histamine include (1) vascular effects mediated by H_1 and H_2 receptors of both arterioles and capillaries, (2) smooth muscle effects of the bronchi and the gastrointestinal tract as a result of activation of the H_1 receptors, and (3) secretory glandular effects caused by H_2-receptor stimulation of the gastric mucosa.

Vascular effects. In the mircocirculatory component of the cardiovascular system (constitutes arterioles, capillaries, and venules) the liberation of histamine has been shown to involve both the H_1 and H_2 receptors. Stimulation of these receptors exerts a twofold effect: (1) it dilates the capillaries and venules, producing an increased localized blood flow, and

(2) it promotes capillary permeability, allowing the escape of plasma protein and fluids through the capillary wall into the interstitial space. These are localized responses that result in erythema and swelling of the tissues. By activating the H_1 and H_2 receptors on the smooth muscles of the arterioles, histamine is also capable of eliciting a systemic response. In certain conditions it causes massive vasodilation of the arterioles that can bring about a profound fall in blood pressure.

Smooth muscle effects. Although histamine exerts a powerful relaxing effect on the smooth muscles of the arterioles, it produces a contractile action on smooth muscles of many nonvascular organs such as the bronchi and gastrointestinal tract. In sensitized individuals activation of the H_1 receptors of the lungs can cause marked bronchial muscle contraction that often progresses to dyspnea and leads to airway obstruction.

Secretory glandular effects. Histamine stimulates the gastric, salivary, pancreatic, and lacrimal glands. The chief effect on humans, however, is seen in the gastric glands. Stimulation of H_2 receptors in the exocrine glands of the stomach increases production of gastric acid secretions. Its high H^+ concentration is attributed to the activity of the parietal cells of the stomach and is implicated in the development of peptic ulcers.

Histamine is also known to be present throughout the tissues of the brain. Its effects seem to involve both H_1 and H_2-receptor mediation. The activation of H_1 receptors of the semicircular canals is associated with motion sickness (see Table 15-1 for receptor-mediating sites).

An intradermal injection of histamine causes a series of reactions called the "triple response." This is characterized as a local action resulting from stimulation of H_1 receptors in the skin. Blood vessels (capillaries) immediately affected by the histamine dilate and produce a *flush* or redness. Surrounding blood vessels then dilate to produce a *flare* or diffuse redness. This reaction is probably the result of a neural mechanism—axon reflexes stimulate sensory nerves and their branches to produce dilation of blood vessels. Widely dilated blood vessels have increased permeability. There is an increase in tissue fluid or local edema, which is termed a *wheal*. Any chemical or mechanical injury to the skin can cause this triple response of flush, flare, and wheal. Therefore it is believed that histamine is released from injured skin. The triple response is believed to be one of the body's protective mechanisms, since increased permeability of blood vessels permits the passage of plasma proteins and white cells into the tissues.

Pathologic effects

Histamine as a chemical mediator is implicated in many pathologic disorders. An important class of conditions for which drugs are used to counteract this compound is concerned with the hypersensitivity response known as the allergic reaction. Although there are four different types of hypersensitivity responses to immunologic injury, the type I–anaphylactic reaction is the one associated with the disorders caused by histamine release.

Individuals with type I–mediated hypersensitivity develop allergies as a result of sensitization to a foreign agent that may be ingested, inhaled, or injected. An incalculable number of these agents acting as antigens exist. They vary widely in that seasonal exposure to pollens, grasses, and weeds or nonseasonal agents such as housedust, feathers, molds, and other similar substances can develop different forms of allergic reactivity. Hypersensitivity to a variety of foods such as shellfish or strawberries requires ingestion of the antigen. Insects such as bees or wasps and even drugs, particularly penicillin, also possess allergic properties that may induce a severe response in hypersensitive individuals. Thus type I–anaphylactic hypersensitivity accounts for a substantial number of allergic diseases, and it involves a complex series of anomalies that range in severity from mild urticaria to a fatal condition known as anaphylactic shock.

The mechanism of type I–anaphylactic reaction involves the attachment of an antigen (Ag) to an antibody (Ab), specifically the IgE, which in turn becomes fixed to the mast cell. The pathologic manifestations of Ag-IgE interaction are caused by mast cell degranulation resulting in the release of histamine and other mediators responsible for producing the allergic symptoms. The type I–anaphylactic reaction causes various disorders such as urticaria, atopy (allergic rhinitis, hay fever), bronchial asthma, food allergies, and systemic anaphylaxis.

Urticaria. Urticaria is a vascular reaction of the skin characterized by immediate formation of a wheal and flare accompanied by severe itching. Contact with an external irritant such as drugs or foods produces the Ag–IgE mediated response with resultant release of histamine from the mast cell into the skin. The local vasodilation produces the red flare, and the increased permeability of the capillaries leads to tissue swelling. These swellings are called "hives," and when giant hives occur they are known as *angioneurotic edema*. Antihistaminic drugs administered prior to exposure to the antigen will prevent this response.

Atopy. Atopy occurs in genetically susceptible individuals and is usually due to seasonal pollen. This condition is manifested as an upper respiratory tract disorder known as allergic rhinitis (hay fever). Following the interaction of Ag-IgE antibody on the surface of the bronchial mast cells, histamine is released, producing local vascular dilation and increased capillary permeability. This change causes a rapid fluid leakage into the tissues of the nose resulting in swelling of the nasal linings. In certain individuals antihistaminic therapy can prevent the edematous reaction if the drug is administered before antigenic exposure.

Bronchial asthma. When the inhaled antigen combines with the IgE antibody, stimulation of the mast cells triggers the release of mediators in the lower respiratory tract, usually in the bronchi and bronchioles. Histamine plays a minor role in this response because the slow-reacting substance of anaphylaxis (SRS-A) is a more potent mediator causing a long-term contraction of the bronchiolar smooth muscle. The difficulty in breathing may be relieved by a bronchodilator such as epinephrine. The administration of antihistaminic drugs actually has no value in relieving this condition, since more potent chemical mediators than histamine are responsible for causing the reaction.

Food allergies. Food allergies involve intestinal IgE–mast cell responses to ingested antigens. If the upper gastrointestinal tract is affected, vomiting results; if the lower gastrointestinal tract is invaded, cramps and diarrhea occur. This condition also has been known to produce systemic anaphylaxis following ingestion of a large amount of antigen.

Systemic anaphylaxis. Systemic anaphylaxis is a generalized reaction manifested as a life-threatening systemic condition. The Ag–IgE mediator response involves the basophils of the blood and the mast cells in the connective tissue. The most common precipitating causes of this response are drugs, particularly penicillin; insect stings (wasps and bees); and occasionally certain foods. The massive release of histamine into the circulation causes widespread vasodilation, resulting in a profound fall in blood pressure. The excessive dilation also allows plasma to leave the capillaries so that a loss of circulatory volume ensues. When the reaction is fatal, death is usually caused not only by shock but also by laryngeal edema. The symptoms of the latter condition include smooth muscle contraction of the bronchi and pharyngeal edema, which usually leads to asphyxiation. Since the mediator, SRS-A, is also released from the cells, spasm of the smooth muscle of the bronchioles elicit the asthmalike attack.

Antihistaminic drugs are less effective against true anaphylaxis because these agents do not antagonize the SRS-A mediator that causes the severe bronchoconstriction. Therefore a drug such as epinephrine, a bronchodilator, is indicated for this life-threatening situation. The relief produced by this drug is due to the beta$_2$-receptor action that relaxes bronchial smooth muscles.

Drug allergies frequently develop in susceptible individuals who show no adverse effects following the first dose of drug administration. However, a second or subsequent reexposure to even a minute amount of this same antigen may elicit an exaggerated IgE response either locally or systemically. Individuals who exhibit such reactions are said to be allergic to the drug. The IgE-mediated response, particularly with penicillin, may occur either in the skin, producing severe urticaria, or in the respiratory tract, causing bronchial asthma. On the other hand, even limited contact in certain sensitized individuals can produce a fatal systemic anaphylaxis. Allergic reactions to penicillin account for nearly 100 deaths per year in the United States. Therefore, if an individual exhibits even the mildest sign of an allergic response such as a slight skin rash, this symptom should be reported immediately to the physician. In all probability the drug will be discontinued to avoid the possibility of an exaggerated IgE reaction (see Table 15-2 for symptoms of drug allergies involving various organ systems).

Clinical uses

Histamine is rarely used therapeutically but occasionally has been employed for diagnostic purposes. One diagnostic use of histamine is to determine the ability of the stomach to produce gastric acid. Histamine is a potent stimulus to the secretion of gastric hydrochloric acid, and there is evidence that it may be the natural trigger that starts the secretion of hydrochloric acid. Accordingly, it can be used to reveal the absence of gastric acid (achlorhydria), a diagnostic aid for pernicious anemia or cancer of the stomach. If a patient does not respond with a significant secretion of gastric acid to the challenge of a small dose of histamine, it is likely that he cannot make gastric acid. This is believed to be caused by a degenerative change in the gastric mucosa.

T A B L E 1 5 - 2   Common manifestations of allergic reactions in the human

Tissue or organ	Symptom	Hapten commonly involved
Skin	Hives (urticaria) and generalized itching	Penicillin, aspirin
	Rashes	Barbiturates, sulfonamides, streptomycin
	Exfoliative dermatitis (loss of superficial skin layers)	Tetracycline, streptomycin, phenobarbital
Mucous membranes (particularly of nose and eye)	Inflammation, swelling, and excessive secretions	Sulfonamides, barbiturates
Respiratory tract	Difficulty in breathing	Penicillin, local anesthetics, aspirin, heroin
Vascular system	Fall in blood pressure	Penicillin, aspirin
Blood and blood-forming tissues*	Reduction in the number of one or more types of circulating blood cells	Aminopyrine (Pyramidon) Quinidine

From Levine, R.: Pharmacology: drug actions and reactions, ed. 2. Copyright © 1978 by Little, Brown & Co. Used with the permission of Little, Brown & Co.

*The presence of an antibody that reacts specifically with the sensitizing drug has been demonstrated in the case of each of the drugs cited as well as for a number of other drugs. Such demonstrations provide proof that drug allergy can account for some disorders of blood and the blood-forming tissues.

Another use is in the diagnosis of pheochromocytoma. Tumors of the medullary portion of the adrenal gland that secrete epinephrine and norepinephrine are uncommon, but their discovery is important since they represent one type of hypertension that can be permanently cured by surgery. Small doses of histamine stimulate the secretion of the adrenal medulla; in the normal individual the pressor amines secreted by the adrenal gland are insufficient to produce a marked rise in blood pressure, but in the patient with pheochromocytoma histamine may lead to a very prominent secretion of medullary amines with a resultant striking rise in blood pressure. The histamine test is one of several "pharmacologic" provocative tests for pheochromocytoma.

Histamine may also be used to test the capacity of capillaries to dilate in certain peripheral vascular diseases.

The administration of histamine is also of diagnostic value in determining whether asthma is an underlying cause of respiratory tract symptoms. Asthma is a disease characterized by widespread narrowing of the airway. In such instances when the specific diagnosis of this disease is in doubt, it is helpful to evaluate a patient's reaction to a drug that will stimulate or "provoke" a bronchospastic response in susceptible airways. This is known as provocative testing, and under carefully controlled conditions, histamine inhalation produces a response that resembles an asthmatic attack. Following

administration of the drug, it reacts at specific receptor sites (H_1 receptors) on the membrane of the smooth muscle cells, causing bronchoconstriction. In addition, the histamine increases bronchial secretions and vascular permeability. This results in edema formation in the submucosa. In normal individuals inhalation of histamine produces only slight bronchospasm, wheras in asthmatic patients a markedly hyperreactive bronchial response occurs. Thus inhalation testing will reliably produce a significant bronchospasm in asthmatic patients. With the patient's safety and welfare always the uppermost consideration, only those pulmonary function laboratories with experienced, qualified personnel and adequate testing equipment should conduct pulmonary provocative studies.

Preparation, dosage, and administration. Before the test for gastric acid production the patient should have fasted and rested for 12 hours. A gastric tube is inserted and the gastric contents are aspirated. The patient may then be given 300 ml water. The histamine is injected subcutaneously; the dose is usually 0.5 to 0.75 mg histamine in the form of a 1:1000 solution. Pulse and blood pressure should be taken immediately after injection; the usual response is increased pulse rate and slightly decreased blood pressure. Observations for side effects should be continued during the test. Epinephrine hydrochloride 1:1000 (0.5 to 1 ml) should be readily available to treat severe reactions if they occur. After injection of histamine, gastric contents are aspirated every 10 to 15 minutes for 1 hour and tested for volume, total acidity, blood, bile, and mucus. Maximum secretory response to histamine usually occurs in 30 minutes; the effect lasts about 1½ hours. Gastric achlorhydria after histamine injection is usually pathologic and often indicates pernicious anemia or stomach cancer.

In the test for pheochromocytoma the first dose is 0.01 mg histamine injected intravenously. The patient should be at rest and his basal blood pressure level should have been determined. Following a decrease in blood pressure within 30 seconds, if a marked rise in blood pressure occurs (60 mm Hg systolic, 30 mm Hg diastolic) in 1 to 4 minutes associated with symptoms of pallor, fear, sweating, and so on, the test is positive for the presence of the tumor. Blood pressure usually returns to preinjection levels within 5 to 15 minutes. If no response occurs within 5 minutes, a dose of 0.05 mg is given. Pulse rate and blood pressure must be frequently determined both during and following the test. This test is contraindicated for elderly persons or for those with marked hypertension (blood pressure in excess of 150 mm Hg systolic and 100 mm Hg diastolic).

For the pulmonary provocative test for asthma, histamine phosphate comes in a solution and is aerosolized in concentrations of 0.02 to 10 mg/ml. The concentrations recommended vary—0.03, 0.06, 0.12, 0.25, 0.5, 1, 2.5, 5, and 10 mg/ml. Some experts recommend 10 breaths of the lowest selected concentration, followed by a 2-hour wait before trying a higher concentration.

All these procedures should be carried out by the physician.

Side effects and toxic effects. Symptoms of overdosage include rapid drop in blood pressure, intense headache, dyspnea, flushing of the skin, vomiting, diarrhea, shock, and collapse. The toxic symptoms are rarely dangerous, although they may be alarming. If the patient goes into shock, the blood volume may need to be restored. Epinephrine is a specific physiologic antagonist and will prevent or counteract symptoms if administered promptly.

Contraindications. Histamine should not be administered to the elderly or to those with cardiovascular disease such as angina. Histamines cause hypotension, and this should be avoided in patients with angina. It is also contraindicated in individuals with bronchial asthma, since histamine can precipitate bronchospasm. In addition, individuals with a history of hypersensitivity to histamine should not be given this drug.

Betazole hydrochloride (Histalog)

Betazole is an analog of histamine with similar pharmacologic actions. It is also used in diagnostic tests of gastric secretion. It stimulates gastric secretion equal to that of histamine, particularly during the first hour of gastric analysis; however, the amount of acid secreted during the second hour and later is usually greater with betazole. Betazole produces fewer side effects than histamine. The dosage is 50 mg for adults or 0.5 mg/kg body weight given intramuscularly or subcutaneously.

Side effects. Flushing, sweating, and a feeling of warmth occur in about 20% of the patients tested with betazole. Headache occurs in about 3% of the patients, and urticaria and syncope occur rarely.

Precautions. Betazole should be used with caution in patients with bronchial asthma, recent gastrointestinal bleeding, or heart disease.

Antihistamines

Antihistamines are drugs that compete with histamine for its receptor sites. With the discovery of two histamine receptors, known as H_1 and H_2, the antihistamines should be divided into the H_1-receptor antagonists and the H_2-receptor antagonists. The generally available antihistamines are H_1-receptor antagonists. The newer compounds, such as cimetidine (an H_2-receptor antagonist), are of great recent interest because they can block gastric secretion and are of value in the treatment of peptic ulcers.

Antihistamines are believed to act not by

opposing but by preventing the physiologic action of histamine. It is postulated that the antihistamines act by preventing histamine from reaching its site of action, that is, by competition for the receptors. The first antihistamine was found in 1933 as a result of a conscious attempt to discover a compound with this activity. Although the initial compounds were quite toxic and therefore not very useful, hundreds of antihistamines have been synthesized and tested. Many of these compounds have similar chemical features.

A common structural feature is a short straight chain terminating in a tertiary amine

$$-C-C-N\begin{array}{c}\diagup R' \\ \diagdown R''\end{array}$$

and it has been suggested that this portion of the antihistamines is an analog of the $-C-C-NH_2$ chain of histamine.

Pharmacologically, it is known that antihistamines block histamine action somewhat selectively. They tend to prevent the muscular (circulatory and bronchiolar) action of histamine but are not as effective against the secretory actions of histamine.

H₁-receptor antagonists

During the past few years histamine antagonists of various types have been tried for histamine shock, anaphylactic reactions, and allergy. The antihistamines of the H₁ type have the greatest therapeutic effect on nasal allergies, particularly on seasonal hay fever. They relieve symptoms better at the beginning of the hay fever season than during its height but fail to relieve the asthma that frequently accompanies hay fever. These preparations are palliative and do not immunize the patient or protect him over a period of time against allergic reactions. Their benefits are therefore comparatively short lived and provide only symptomatic relief. They must be regarded only as adjuncts to more specific methods of treatment. They do not begin to replace such remedies as epinephrine, ephedrine, and aminophylline. In acute asthmatic reactions, the antihistamine drugs serve only as supplements to these older remedies. Furthermore, relief of various symptoms

of allergy is obtained only while the drug is being taken. Antihistamines do not appear to have a cumulative action and can therefore be taken over a period of time.

Different antihistamines are either more or less effective in different individuals. If one drug provides an unsatisfactory clinical response, a different antihistamine may provide a favorable effect. Although the use of antihistamines for treatment of the common cold is controversial, many over-the-counter cold remedies contain an antihistamine.

One peculiar and unanticipated action of many of the antihistamines of the H₁ type is their ability to relieve or abolish the symptoms of motion sickness, both in animals and in humans. Thus a number of antimotion sickness agents are also potent antihistamines. The commonly used compound dimenhydrinate (Dramamine), for example, is simply diphenhydramine with a different acid neutralizing the basic nitrogens of the antihistamine itself.

The most common untoward effect of these preparations is drowsiness, which may become so marked that deep sleep may result. Other untoward symptoms include dizziness, dryness of the mouth and throat, nausea, disturbed coordination, lassitude, muscular weakness, and gastrointestinal disturbances. Sedation may disappear after 2 or 3 days of treatment. However, in some patients symptoms of excitation occur, such as insomnia, nervousness, and even convulsions.

Patients receiving these preparations for continuous treatment should have the benefit of periodic medical examinations since blood dyscrasias can occur.

AGENTS USED IN ALLERGIC CONDITIONS
Brompheniramine maleate (Dimetane)

Brompheniramine is an effective antihistaminic for treatment of allergic reactions and as an adjunct for anaphylactic reactions after the acute manifestations have been controlled. Principal side effects are drowsiness and rash. Usual oral adult dosage is 4 to 8 mg three or four times daily, or one timed-release tablet every 8 to 12 hours; parenteral dosage is 5 to 20 mg twice daily. The dosage for children is 0.5 mg/kg body weight divided into three or four doses. *Dimetapp* is brompheniramine with phenylephrine.

Chlorcyclizine hydrochloride (Di-Paralene)

Advantages claimed for chlorcyclizine are a prolonged action and low incidence of side effects. It is effective in 30 minutes; action may last for 12 hours. A dosage of 50 mg or more is given orally up to four times a day. For children the dosage is 1.5 mg/kg body weight divided into two doses. Chlorcyclizine tablets are available in 25 and 50 mg each. It is contraindicated in pregnancy because of potential harm to the fetus.

Chlorpheniramine maleate (Chlor-Trimeton, Histaspan, Teldrin)

Chlorpheniramine produces a low incidence of side effects but compares favorably with other antihistamines in therapeutic usefulness and does so after comparatively low dosage. The drug may be given to alleviate acute urticaria as a result of eating shellfish or after a penicillin injection to which an individual is allergic. The effect of the drug is prolonged by the use of a special tablet form that contains twice the average single dose, half of which is contained in an enteric-coated core that delays absorption. The drug is available in dosage forms suited for parenteral as well as oral administration. Its action tends to be slow. The usual adult oral dosage is 2 to 4 mg three or four times daily. Tablets of 4 mg are available. The repeat-action tablet and sustained-release capsules are available in 8 and 12 mg; the syrup contains 2 mg/5 ml; the injection solution contains 10 and 100 mg/ml. The usual parenteral dose is 5 to 40 mg. For children the dosage is 0.35 mg/kg body weight divided into four doses.

Diphenhydramine hydrochloride (Benadryl)

Diphenhydramine is similar to other members of the group. In addition to its antihistaminic activity it has a moderate antispasmodic action for control of spasmodic bronchial cough. This is sometimes significant in cases of bronchial asthma. When given in full therapeutic doses, it causes a high incidence of sedation, which makes it more suitable for use at night than during the day. The average oral dosage for adults is 25 to 50 mg given three or four times daily. For children under 12, the dosage is 5 mg/kg body weight in four divided doses over a 24-hour period. It is available in a number of dosage forms suited for topical, oral, and parenteral administration. The usual intravenous dose is 10 to 50 mg.

It is the antihistamine of choice for treatment of anaphylactic and other allergic reactions, but it is not a substitute for epinephrine. For anaphylactic reactions it is given intravenously or by deep intramuscular injection.

Diphenhydramine is also an effective antiemetic and antiparkinsonism drug.

Promethazine hydrochloride (Phenergan)

Promethazine exhibits a number of pharmacologic effects although its pronounced sedative effect limits its use. It is a potent antihistamine, it can be used for the relief of motion sickness, and it relieves apprehension. It potentiates the action of drugs that depress the central nervous system, making possible a reduction of their dosage. It has a relatively prolonged action, lasting up to 18 to 24 hours. Its sedative action is utilized clinically for surgical and obstetric patients. Promethazine is administered orally, parenterally, and rectally. The usual oral dose is 25 mg, although the range of dosage may be 6 to 75 mg. Parenterally, the dosage is up to 1 mg/kg body weight. The dosage for children is 0.13 mg/kg body weight taken when necessary. It is available in 12.5-, 25-, and 50-mg tablets, as a syrup, and as a sterile solution for injection (25 mg/ml). Promethazine suppositories are available (25 and 50 mg). Since it is a phenothiazine, precautions applicable to phenothiazines should be observed.

Pyrilamine maleate (Neo-Antergan, Histalon); mepyramine maleate (Anthisan)

Pyrilamine is available in 25- and 50-mg tablets and as a syrup, 2.5 mg/ml, for oral administration, after which effects last 4 to 6 hours. The usual adult dosage is 25 to 50 mg three or four times daily. The incidence of sedation is low, but it may cause gastrointestinal irritation. It is used for allergic rhinitis and mild urticaria.

Tripelennamine hydrochloride (Pyribenzamine)

Tripelennamine hydrochloride is therapeutically effective, and the incidence of untoward reactions is low. Stimulation of the nervous system does occur as well as gastrointestinal irritation, but the latter is not severe. Sedation is moderate. This agent is available in a number of dosage forms for topical, oral, and parenteral (subcutaneous, intramuscular, and intravenous) administration. The usual oral adult dosage is 25 to 75 mg three or four times a day, although doses of 100 to 150 mg are tolerated by most patients. It is used to ameliorate allergic symptoms and reactions to blood and plasma.

Tripelennamine citrate (Pyribenzamine)

Tripelennamine citrate is more palatable than the hydrochloride when administered in a liquid form. It provides the same therapeutic action as does the hydrochloride. The dosage is greater for the citrate than for the hydrochloride preparation of the drug because of the difference in the molecular weights of the compounds. The usual adult dosage is 50 mg three or four times a day.

Other antihistamines

A tremendous number of H_1-blocking drugs are available, but little distinction can be made between them on the basis of efficacy as antagonists. Some of these include bromodiphenhydramine (Ambodryl), carbinoxamine maleate (Clistin), methapyrilene hydrochloride (Dozar, Histadyl), cyproheptadine (Periactin), dimethindene (Forhistal, Triten), and pyrrobutamine phosphate (Pyronil).

DRUGS USED FOR MOTION SICKNESS

Motion sickness is a reaction to certain kinds of movement, sometimes any kind if it is sufficiently severe. Most persons are well adjusted to horizontal movements, but some are unable to tolerate continuous vertical movements. Such persons are likely to become ill when traveling in cars, trains, airplanes, or ships. Disturbance of the cells in the labyrinth of the ear is believed to be the cause of motion sickness. The person usually becomes pale, perspires, feels chilly or warm, and salivates freely. If he continues to be subjected to the motion, symptoms usually progress to nausea and vomiting.

A number of drugs have been used for motion sickness, including sedatives such as barbiturates, autonomic drugs such as scopolamine, and a number of the tranquilizing agents. Promethazine, mentioned previously, has been widely tested and found effective. The following agents have also been found useful for prevention of motion sickness and vestibular dysfunction (disturbance of functions of the inner ear). The exact mechanism of their action is unclear, but most of them appear to depress the central nervous system and decrease sensitivity of the labyrinth of the ear. Like other antihistamines they should be used with caution by persons who are responsible for the operation of power machines.

Cyclizine hydrochloride (Marezine)

Cyclizine is an antihistaminic drug that has been found effective in a high percentage of cases in the prevention of nausea and vomiting associated with motion sickness.

Although dry mouth, drowsiness, and blurred vision can be observed after large doses, these symptoms seldom appear after ordinary therapeutic doses. Cyclizine is teratogenic in the rat. This fact should be taken into consideration before its use in pregnancy is contemplated.

Cyclizine is administered orally and rectally. The usual adult dosage is 50 mg 30 minutes before departure and 50 mg three times daily before meals. Reduction of dosage may be indicated after the initial dose, depending on the duration of the trip, type of travel, and reaction of the individual. For the relief of dizziness and associated symptoms of vestibular disorder (in conditions other than motion sickness) the usual dosage is 50 mg three times a day.

Cyclizine hydrochloride is available in 50-mg tablets and 50- and 100-mg suppositories. Cyclizine lactate has the same effects as cyclizine hydrochloride but is suited for intramuscular injection. The dosage is the same as that for cyclizine hydrochloride.

Dimenhydrinate (Dramamine)

As mentioned previously, dimenhydrinate is chemically related to diphenhydramine (Benadryl). It produces mild sedation. It is effective for a high percentage of persons who suffer from motion sickness. It is also used to control nausea, vomiting, and dizziness associated with a number of conditions such as stapedectomy operations, radiation sickness, and Meniere's disease. It has also been employed for the relief of postoperative nausea and vomiting. Its status as an antiemetic for this purpose is not well established because of the variety of factors that contribute to the illness.

Dimenhydrinate is available in a number of dosage forms for oral, rectal, or intramuscular administration. The usual oral dose is 50 mg 30 minutes before departure to prevent motion sickness. Dosage up to 100 mg every 4 hours may be prescribed not only for motion sickness but also for the control of nausea and vomiting associated with other conditions. The usual intramuscular dose is 50 mg.

Meclizine hydrochloride (Bonine)

Meclizine exerts a mild but prolonged antihistaminic action and is effective in the prevention of motion sickness. The duration of its effects may be as long as 24 hours. Like other members of this group of drugs, it appears to affect the central nervous system and the inner ear.

The incidence of its side effects seems to be low, although like most other antihistaminic drugs it can cause drowsiness, blurred vision, dryness of the mouth, and fatigue. Meclizine is teratogenic in the rat and thus should not be taken during pregnancy.

It is administered orally. The usual adult dosage is 25 to 50 mg once a day for the prevention of motion sickness (1 hour before departure). For the relief of nausea and vomiting from other causes the dosage is 25 to 100 mg daily. The drug is available in tablets of 25 mg, as well as in chewable tablets of 25 mg.

INHIBITOR OF HISTAMINE RELEASE
Cromolyn sodium (Disodium Cromglycate, Aarane, Intal)

Cromolyn sodium is the first successful antiasthma prophylactic drug that has been developed as a result of knowledge of the mechanisms of allergic reactions. Cromolyn sodium exerts a local protective effect in the mucosal airways by inhibiting the granulation of pulmonary mast cells and thereby preventing the release of histamine and SRS-A. Although the drug permits the union of antigen and specific IgE on the surface of mast cells, its membrane stabilizing activity suppresses the release of chemical mediators responsible for causing the asthmatic symptoms. Thus the mode of action of cromolyn sodium is fundamentally prophylactic. It also lessens the need for steroids in asthmatic patients who are dependent on corticosteroid drugs. Since this agent possesses no direct bronchodilator or antiinflammatory properties, it has no value in terminating an allergic attack that is already in progress.

Pharmacokinetics. Cromolyn sodium should be given only by inhalation. Since it is a lipid-soluble agent, the oral dosage is poorly absorbed through the gastrointestinal tract. About 8% of the inhaled dose reaches the lung and enters the systemic circulation. The remainder is either exhaled or deposited at the back of the throat. The peak plasma concentrations occur within 15 minutes, and the drug has a half-life of about 80 minutes. Cromolyn sodium is eliminated in the unchanged form in the feces and also in the urine.

Clinical uses. In the management of patients with severe bronchial asthma, cromolyn sodium is used prophylactically to prevent attacks. It is also indicated in certain other patients to prevent exercise-induced bronchospasm.

Preparation, dosage, and administration. Cromolyn sodium is a powdered inhalant that is available in 20-mg capsules containing lactose powder to enhance the flow properties of the drug.

The initial dose for adults and children 5 years of age and over, is 20 mg or the contents of one capsule. This should be repeated four times daily at *regular* intervals to obtain beneficial effects. Therapeutic response will usually occur within the first 4 weeks of use; otherwise the drug should be discontinued.

Since cromolyn sodium is administered by inhalation only, the patient should be taught how to use the spinhaler correctly. The enclosed instructions with the particular device used must be followed carefully. The drug is administered only when the acute asthmatic episode has been brought under control. In addition, the airway must be cleared so the patient is able to inhale adequately. Mild throat irritation, hoarseness, and cough can be minimized by swallowing a little water following administration of the drug.

Side effects and toxic effects. Following inhalation therapy, cromolyn sodium causes mild throat irritation, cough, and hoarseness. This discomfort can be remedied by drinking water or sucking a lozenge. On occasion, inhalation of the finely powdered drug may produce bronchospasm. Esophageal irritation as indicated by sensations of substernal burning can be relieved by an antacid or drinking a glass of milk before each cromolyn dose to protect the gastrointestinal mucosa from direct contact with the drug.

Cromolyn sodium demonstrates a low order of toxicity. However, various forms of hypersensitivity have occurred in certain patients. Allergy to cromolyn sodium has appeared in the form of skin rashes and eosinophilic pneumonia. Thus the eosinophil count should be monitored because progressive eosinophilia is a reliable indicator of developing allergy, even though clinical symptoms may be absent. The clinical signs of dermatologic or respiratory discomfort together with eosinophilia indicate the need for discontinuation of drug therapy.

Precautions. Cromolyn sodium should be used with caution in patients with hepatic and renal disorders undergoing prolonged treatment. The renal and biliary routes of excretion of this drug may require a decrease in dosage or discontinuation of its administration in certain individuals.

Contraindications. Cromolyn sodium is contraindicated in pregnant women and in individuals with previous hypersensitivity. Because of

the difficulty in using the inhaler device by which the drug is administered, cromolyn sodium should not be given to children under 5 years of age.

NURSING IMPLICATIONS

1 Many antihistamines that antagonize the H_1 receptors produce sedation, which causes drowsiness and even some slowing of reflexes. Patients should be cautioned about driving cars or motor bikes if drowsiness occurs and to be careful when around hazardous machinery or tools.
2 Patients should be informed that antihistamines can potentiate the effects of other sedatives, hypnotics, tranquilizers, and alcohol.
3 The drying effect of some antihistamines may produce a dry cough and even hoarseness. If this occurs, dosage may need to be decreased, the antihistamine stopped for a few days, or a different antihistamine prescribed.
4 Some antihistamines can cause an increase in blood pressure, particularly if overdosage occurs.
5 Patients with hypertension or cardiovascular disease should be advised not to use over-the-counter cold remedies except with the permission of their physician. The vasoconstrictor effects may be detrimental to their condition.

H_2-receptor antagonists
Cimetidine (Tagamet)

Among the first H_2-receptor antagonists, metiamide received some clinical testing, but the drug was abandoned because a few cases of agranulocytosis were attributed to it. A chemical modification of metiamide resulted in the drug cimetidine, which has been approved for clinical use in the United Kingdom and the United States.

Cimetidine (Tagamet) is an antihistamine that selectively and competitively inhibits the action of histamine by occupying the H_2 receptors of the parietal cells of the stomach. The drug inhibits both daytime and nocturnal basal gastric acid secretion. When given orally or intravenously, cimetidine inhibits gastric acid secretion stimulated by food, pentagastrin, histamine, caffeine, and insulin. Both the volume of secretion and H^+ concentration are reduced by the drug. The output of pepsin, which appears in the secretion, is also reduced. Now widely used to reduce the production of gastric acid, cimetidine provides prompt relief from ulcer pain and accelerates healing.

Pharmacokinetics. Cimetidine is readily absorbed after oral administration with peak levels occurring in 45 to 90 minutes. The plasma half-life is approximately 2 hours. Most of an oral or intravenous dose of cimetidine is eliminated in the urine within 24 hours of administration. About 40% to 70% of a usual dose is excreted as unchanged drug. In patients with impaired renal function, excretion is delayed; therefore the frequency of the dose may need to be increased to every 8 hours or even more.

Clinical uses. Cimetidine is effective in the treatment of duodenal ulcer and gastric ulcers. In addition, it is used to control pathologic hypersecretory conditions such as Zollinger-Ellison syndrome, systemic mastocytosis, and multiple endocrine adenomas. The effect of prophylaxis on stress ulceration in patients who are ulcer prone or those who are receiving steroids that may produce ulcers still needs to be evaluated. For uncomplicated duodenal ulcers, therapy should normally not exceed 8 weeks.

Preparation, dosage, and administration. Cimetidine (Tagamet) is available in 300-mg tablets and in 2-ml vials containing 300 mg of the drug. The adult dose for the treatment of duodenal ulcer is 300 mg four times a day to be given with meals and at bedtime. It is essential to administer antacids concurrently with cimetidine as needed for relief of pain and to promote effectiveness of the drug. Cimetidine also can be used intramuscularly at a dosage of 300 mg every 6 hours or by intravenous unfusion at a dosage of 300 mg every 6 hours (diluted in 100 ml of 5% dextrose) to be given over a 15- to 20-minute period.

Treatment should be continued for 4 to 6 weeks although healing of the ulcer may occur within 1 to 2 weeks after therapy is started. Complete ulcer healing should be verified by endoscopy. When given on a long-term basis, the role of cimetidine in delaying ulcer recurrence has not been established.

Side effects and toxic effects. Important side effects caused by cimetidine include mild transient diarrhea, muscular pain, dizziness, and rash. A few cases of reversible confusional states have been reported in the elderly and in those individuals with impaired renal function or organic brain syndrome. This effect may have been the result of an overdosage. In a few patients treated for 1 month or longer, mild gynecomastia also has been observed. Cimetidine does not cause drowsiness like the H_1-blocking drugs.

Cimetidine is relatively nontoxic, but in patients with impaired renal function and in the elderly the dosage needs to be reduced. There are some individuals in whom slight elevations of plasma creatinine have occurred, but this disappears at the end of therapy.

Precautions. To avoid relapses, patients with ulcers should be cautioned to maintain therapy at the prescribed dose without interruption. For patients with impaired renal function, dosage adjustment must be made to avoid toxicity.

Contraindications. Safety of cimetidine during pregnancy has not been established; therefore it should not be used in pregnant women or women of childbearing potential. Because of insufficient clinical information, cimetidine is not recommended for children under 16 years of age.

Drug interactions. Information concerning drug interaction with cimetidine is limited. This drug may be prescribed to patients receiving tetracycline, which produces gastrointestinal upset, nausea, vomiting, diarrhea, and mucous membrane lesions. These symptoms generally occur when administration of tetracycline is prolonged and the dosage is high. In a recent study it was found that the use of cimetidine does not interfere with tetracycline absorption as it was originally thought. The investigation also revealed that this antibiotic is poorly absorbed, particularly when administered with an antacid. Therefore cimetidine may be used in place of antacids if control of gastric acid suppression is needed in patients taking tetracycline.

Cimetidine does potentiate warfarin-type anticoagulants. For this reason, close monitoring of prothrombin time is recommended, and the adjustment of the dose of the anticoagulant should be made accordingly during concomitant administration of cimetidine.

Summary of nursing considerations

When released, histamine, the enigma of pharmacology, can provoke allergic responses and troublesome side effects that range in intensity from mild itching to angioneurotic edema, shock, and death. Histamine occurs naturally in the body. It is an amine possessing the basic group NH_2. The principal actions of histamine are contraction of bronchial and intestinal smooth muscle, dilation of capillaries, and promotion of gastric acid secretion. In humans a noticeable dilation of the arterioles also occurs.

The reactions mediated by histamine are attributed to receptor activity. This involves two distinct populations of receptors, H_1 and H_2 receptors. The response of the H_1 receptor is generally associated with type I–mediated hypersensitivity caused by sensitization of an individual to a foreign agent, which may be ingested, inhaled, or injected. The mechanism of type I–anaphylactic reaction involves attachment of an antigen (Ag) to an antibody (IgE), which in turn becomes fixed to the mast cell. The interaction of the complex (Ag/IgE/mast cell) triggers degranulation of the mast cell, resulting in release of histamine and other mediators responsible for causing the allergic symptoms. The disorders of type I–anaphylactic reaction include urticaria, atopy (allergic rhinitis, hayfever), bronchial asthma, food allergies, and systemic anaphylaxis. Certain compounds that prevent the pharmacologic action of histamine (histamine antagonists and antihistamines) have very useful effects, including the prevention of relief of allergic symptoms and motion sickness. Cromolyn sodium is now used as a prophylactic agent in bronchial asthma to prevent the degranulation of bronchial mast cells, thereby inhibiting the release of histamine.

The presence of endogenous histamine in the gastric secretion has led to the discovery of H_2 receptors in the gastric mucosa. The introduction of the H_2 blocking agent cimetidine has provided a new and effective therapeutic approach to the treatment of peptic ulcers and Zollinger-Ellison syndrome.

QUESTIONS

FOR STUDY AND REVIEW

1 Explain the rationale for linking histamine with allergic reactions.
2 Explain the difference between the H_1 and H_2 receptors.
3 Do a comparative study of diphenhydramine (Benadryl) and one other antihistamine. Include range of dosage, possible side effects, use in children, and efficacy.
4 Explain how histamine may be used for diagnosing achlorhydria; for diagnosing pheochromocytoma.
5 Describe the mechanism of action of cimetidine and give some of its side effects.
6 Explain how drug allergy occurs. Why is it important to obtain a history of allergies from the patient before administering certain medications?

BIBLIOGRAPHY

Aas, K.: Biochemical and immunologic basis of bronchial asthma, Triangle **17**:97, 1978.
A.M.A. drug evaluations, ed. 3, Littleton, Mass., 1977, PSG Publishing Co., Inc.
Anderson, W.A., and Scotti, T.M.: Synopsis of pathology, ed. 10, St. Louis, 1980, The C.V. Mosby Co.
Beaven, M.: Histamine, N. Engl. J. Med. **294**:30, 320, 1976.
Bellanti, J.: Immunology II, Philadelphia, 1978, W.B. Saunders Co.
Black, J.W., and others. Definitions and antagonism of histamine H_2-receptors, Nature **236**:385, 1972.
Dix, M.R.: Vertigo, Practitioner **211**:295, 1973.
Editorial: Hayfever, Lancet **1**:786, 1975.
Fiedenberg, H., Stites, D., and Caldwell, J.: Basic and clinical immunology, ed. 2, Los Altos, 1978, Lange Medical Publications.
Garty, M., and Hurivitz, A.: Effect of cimetidine and antacids on gastrointestinal absorption of tetracycline, Clin. Pharmacol. Ther. **28**:203, 1980.
Goth, A., and Johnson, A.R.: Current concepts on the secretory function of mast cells, Life Sci. **16**:1201, 1975.
Grollman, A.: How cimetidine works, Consultant **19**:170, 1979.
Johnson, L.R., editor: Gastrointestinal physiology, St. Louis, 1977, The C.V. Mosby Co.
Kumagai, A., and Tomioka, H.: Pharmacological models for characterizing new anti-asthmatics, Triangle **17**:135, 1978.

Lehnert, B., and Schachter, E.N.: The pharmacology of respiratory care, St. Louis, 1980, The C.V. Mosby Co.

Levine, R.: Pharmacology: drug actions and reactions, ed. 2, Boston, 1978, Little, Brown and Co.

Lewis, A.J., editor: Modern drug encyclopedia, ed. 14, New York, 1977, Dun-Donnelley Publishing Corp.

Parker, P.: Food allergies, Am. J. Nurs. **80:**236, 1980.

Pearlman, D.S.: Rationale for therapy of allergic disorders, Pediatr. Clin. North Am. **22:**101, 1975.

Townley, R.: Pharmacologic blocks to mediator release: clinical applications, Adv. Asthma Allergy **2:**7, 1975.

Weissman, G.: The pain mediators, Hosp. Prac. Suppl. p. 17, Jan. 1977.

West, S., and others. A review of antihistamines and the common cold, Pediatrics **56:**100, 1975.

Ziment, I.: Respiratory pharmacology and therapeutics, Philadelphia, 1978, W.B. Saunders Co.

CHAPTER 16

Drugs acting on the gastrointestinal tract

Gastrointestinal disorders vary in nature, and they are the most common of human problems. Since the cause of many gastrointestinal diseases remains obscure, pharmacologic management often may be directed at alleviating symptoms rather than at control or cure.

The major purpose of the gastrointestinal system is to provide nutrients to the cells of the body. The normal activity of this system is concerned with four physiologic processes: muscular movements, secretion, digestion, and absorption. Following ingestion of food, nutritive material is propelled by muscular contractions through the different regions of the gastrointestinal system. Located along the route are exocrine glands that secrete a number of digestive juices. The enzymes in these secretions require

an appropriate pH to hydrolyze the complex food materials to smaller molecules. This biochemical activity, otherwise known as digestion, is a process that is essential for facilitating absorption. The simple molecules of nutritive material can then be readily transported from the intestinal lumen across the wall of the small intestine into the blood and lymph, which ultimately distribute them to the cells of the body. Meanwhile, the remaining unabsorbed residues of food and waste products are moved to the end of the tract and eliminated from the body.

The secretory and muscular activities of the gastrointestinal system are regulated by neural mechanisms. An interconnecting network of neurons is located within the smooth muscle and secretory cells. This network is referred to as the *internal nerve plexus*. This system is self-regulating because it is capable of controlling exocrine gland secretions and muscular contractions without any external influence. By contrast, the *external innervation* of the gastrointestinal system is supplied by the two divisions of the autonomic nervous system. Their major function is to correlate activities between different regions of the gastrointestinal system and also between this system and other parts of the body. The influence of the parasympathetic system is mediated by two branches of the vagal nerve. This division predominates in the gastrointestinal system by exerting an excitatory action, which increases digestive secretions and muscular activity. By contrast, the splanchanic nerves of the sympathetic division are primarily inhibitory, depressing digestive secretions and muscular activity. Under normal conditions, the two divisions of the autonomic nervous system maintain a delicate balance of control of functions.

Drugs affecting the gastrointestinal tract exert their action mainly on muscular and glandular tissues. The action may be directly on the smooth muscle and gland cells or indirectly on the autonomic nervous system. Drugs also may bring about increased or decreased function, tone, emptying time, or peristaltic action of the stomach or bowel. In addition, they may be used to relieve enzyme deficiency, to counteract excess acidity or gas formation, to produce or prevent vomiting, or as diagnostic aids.

Drugs that affect the mouth

On the whole, drugs have little effect on the mouth. Good oral hygiene that includes adequate measures for mechanically cleansing the mouth and teeth has more influence than most medicines.

Flavoring agents

Oral medications that have an unpleasant taste are usually encapsulated, but occasionally it is necessary to give a drug in liquid or powder form. Licorice syrup is particularly effective in disguising the taste of a saline substance because of its colloidal properties and because the taste lingers in the mouth. Other popular syrup flavors are raspberry and cherry.

Unpleasant-tasting drugs that are disguised in a suitable flavoring agent are further improved (psychologically, at least) by the addition of a coloring agent. A chocolate-colored medicine is often thought to have the taste of chocolate even when the flavoring agent added is something entirely different. Since the oral route of drug administration is most acceptable, consultation with the pharmacist is useful when taste problems arise.

Mouthwashes and gargles

The efficacy of a mouthwash or gargle depends largely on the length of time it is allowed to remain in contact with the tissues of the mouth and throat. Ordinarily, these preparations cannot be used in sufficient concentration or over a period of time sufficient to ensure germicidal effects.

A 1% solution of sodium bicarbonate (½ teaspoon in a glass of water) is useful to remove mucus from the mouth and throat. A 0.9% sodium chloride solution is probably as good a gargle as most mixtures used.

Chloraseptic mouthwash and *Cēpacol mouthwash* are used in some institutions. Chloraseptic mouthwash provides surface anesthesia when this is indicated for oropharyngeal discomfort, and it maintains oral hygiene. It is to be diluted with equal parts of water or sprayed full strength.

Cēpacol is also available commercially. It is to be used full strength and is also produced in lozenge form.

Sodium perborate is a white, odorless, salty tasting powder that contains not less than 9% available oxygen. It is used in 2% solution as a mouthwash and local disinfectant. Its action results from the liberation of oxygen. It may be obtained in flavored preparations that disguise the salty taste. It is a popular ingredient of tooth powder and is said to be particularly effective against Vincent's infection and pyor-rhea. *Potassium permanganate* (0.1%), *potassium chlorate* (1%), or *hydrogen peroxide* (25%) may also be used; they are oxidizing agents.

Other substances used in the treatment of stomatitis include boric acid, formalin, gentian violet, and zinc chloride.

Many hospital pharmacies prepare the mouthwash used in that particular institution. Nurses should inquire regarding the content of the preparation and whether or not the mouth-wash should be diluted before use.

Dentifrices

The ordinary dentifrice contains one or more mild abrasives, a foaming agent, and fla-voring materials made into a powder or paste to be used as an aid to the toothbrush in the mechanical cleansing of accessible parts of the teeth.

The following ingredients, alone or mixed, are found in a number of dentifrices:

Glycerin
Alcohol
Sweetening agents
Propylene glycol
Precipitated calcium
  carbonate
Pumice (flour)
Stannous fluoride
Soap
Sodium borate
Milk of magnesia

The essential requirement of a tooth powder or cleaner is that it must not injure the teeth or surrounding tissues. In the absence of tooth-paste the nurse may feel justified in having the patient use only a toothbrush and proper tooth-pick techniques, since thorough mechanical cleansing of bacterial plaques and food debris is the primary objective.

Therapeutic dentifrices. Accepted Dental Therapeutics (ADT) claims that the incidence of dental caries is low in communities with fluo-rine-bearing water. Approximately 1 part of flu-oride to a million parts of water will help to control dental caries. In those communities without fluorinated water, dentists can pre-scribe individualized doses of sodium fluoride to children from infancy to adolescence.

The Council of Dental Therapeutics of the American Dental Association has accepted the toothpastes Crest and Colgate MFP as being effective in reducing the incidence of dental caries. Crest contains 0.4% stannous flouride; Colgate MFP contains 0.76% sodium mono-fluorophosphate.

Drugs that affect the stomach

Conditions of the stomach requiring drug therapy include hyperchlorhydria, hypochlo-rhydria, peptic ulcer, nausea and emesis, and hypermotility. Drugs are also used for diagnos-tic test purposes. Some of the drugs utilized for these conditions are not unique in their treat-ment of gastric dysfunction but are members of other major groups of drugs, such as anticholin-ergic preparations and sedatives.

Antacids

Antacids are indicated for the relief of symp-toms associated with hyperacidity related to the diagnosis of peptic ulcer, gastritis, peptic esophagitis, gastric hyperacidity, heartburn, or hiatal hernia. The nurse should remember that since all antacids (except Oxaine-M because of the anesthetic oxethazaine) require no prescrip-tion and there is no medically supervised restriction, patients may abuse or misuse ant-acids through self-medication.

The weakly basic metal alkali compounds of antacids combine with the existing hydrochlo-ric acid of the stomach to form neutral salts or weak acids and therefore reduce the acidity or neutralize the stomach contents. The major acid-neutralizing capacity (this is one of the sig-nificant factors in antacid therapy selection) is seen with calcium carbonate; it is slightly less with magnesium hydroxide, and aluminum hydroxide has the least neutralizing capacity (Table 16-1). There is a similar duration of action for these three antacid compounds. A dose in a fasting patient shows neutralizing effects in approximately 30 minutes, but when a patient has food in the stomach, the duration of action is prolonged to 2 or 4 hours. The slightly longer duration of action with magne-sium hydroxide is due to the molecules remain-

TABLE 16-1 **Acid-neutralizing capacity of liquid antacids**

Antacid	Ingredients	mEq/30 ml	ml/140 mEq dose*
ALternaGEL	Aluminum hydroxide gel	72	58
Aludrox	Aluminum hydroxide gel, magnesium hydroxide	84	50
Amphojel	Aluminum hydroxide gel	39	107
Basaljel	Aluminum carbonate	84	50
Camalox	Aluminum and magnesium hydroxides, calcium carbonate	108	39
Delcid	Aluminum and magnesium hydroxides	262	16
Di-Gel	Aluminum and magnesium hydroxides, simethicone	74	56
Gelusil	Magnesium hydroxide, aluminum hydroxide gel, simethicone	40	61
Gelusil-M	Simethicone hydroxide, aluminum and magnesium hydroxides	68	64
Gelusil-II	Magnesium and aluminum hydroxides, simethicone	144	30
Kolantyl Gel	Aluminum and magnesium hydroxides	63	66
Maalox	Magnesium and aluminum hydroxide gels	81	54
Maalox Plus	Magnesium and aluminum hydroxide gels, simethicone	81	54
Maalox Therapeutic Concentrate	Magnesium and aluminum hydroxides	170	25
Mylanta	Magnesium and aluminum hydroxides, simethicone	72	58
Mylanta-II	Magnesium and aluminum hydroxides, simethicone	124	28
Phosphaljel	Aluminum phosphate gel	12	350
Riopan	Magnesium and aluminum hydroxides (magaldrate)	66	64
Riopan Plus	Magnesium and aluminum hydroxides (magaldrate), simethicone	66	64
Titralac	Glycine, calcium carbonate	114	36
WinGel	Aluminum and magnesium hydroxides, hexitol stabilized	69	61

Data modified from Fordtran, J.S., and others: N. Engl. J. Med. **288**:923, 1973.
*Volume (in milliliters) of each antacid necessary to provide 140 mEq of neutralizing capability.

ing in the stomach reacting with further secreted acid. Raising the gastric pH above 4 will inhibit the proteolytic activity (pH 1.5 to 2.5 necessary) of pepsin.

Traditionally, the antacids have been termed nonsystemic or systemic. Nonsystemic indicates the almost negligible (nonabsorbable) degree of absorption reaching the circulation, with only local activity within the gastrointestinal tract. The nonsystemic metal ion, however, is absorbed to some degree. The aluminum ion is absorbed the most and magnesium the least, and calcium is absorbed slightly more than magnesium. The circumstances in which increased adverse effects are seen with metal ion absorption are in impaired renal function and long-term excessive use of calcium carbonate and magnesium hydroxide.

Sodium bicarbonate is a systemically active antacid that is highly soluble and absorbed readily through the gastrointestinal tract, fast acting and that possesses the best neutralizing capacity. Its use as an antacid is not by the physician's orders but by the patient's self-medication and initiative. Since sodium and the bicarbonate ions are released into the circulation in such excessive amounts, potential serious disturbances in electrolytes may occur. The product is seldom prescribed and has fallen into disuse as an antacid. Sodium bicarbonate is also contained in many over-the-counter drugs that are effervescent, such as Alka Seltzer and Instant Metamucil.

Preparation, dosage, and administration. Antacid doses are calculated from the milliequivalents (mEq) of neutralizing activity and then converted to volume. In gastric ulcer disease the antacid dose is about 40 mEq, in duodenal ulcer disease the antacid dose is about 80 mEq, and for the relief of occasional indigestion a dose of 20 to 40 mEq is adequate.

The neutralizing activity or buffering capacity is the volume (expressed in milliliters) of O.1 N hydrochloric acid at 120 minutes titrated to a pH of 3 with 1 ml of the antacid. Table 16-1 shows the variation in neutralizing capacity, which is dependent on the amount of antacid and formulation differences. Magnesium hydroxide has a greater capacity than mixtures of magnesium and aluminum hydroxide mixtures.

The patient who is not hospitalized may be placed either on an intensive or an "as needed" dosage regimen. The "as needed" regimen involves taking one or two doses (that is, 15 to 30 ml) seven times daily at 1 and 3 hours after each meal and at bedtime. As stated earlier, the antacid effect is prolonged to 2 to 4 hours when there is food in the stomach. The intensive regimen is used to maintain a gastric pH of 5 or more in a patient with acute pain. This consists of a scheduled 15- to 30-ml antacid dose administered every hour or two through the day. The healing of the ulcer is only achieved with the antacid when the dose is close to 1000 mEq/day neutralizing capacity (seven doses daily of 140 mEq/dose neutralizing capacity).

The hospitalized patient is able to receive continuous antacid benefit through administration by continuous feeding through a nasogastric tube for over 12 hours daily. This is given to the patient who is having a severe ulcerative attack or to a patient following surgery to reduce acid secretion. This method allows for changes in doses after hourly gastric analysis.

The antacids are available in liquid suspensions, chewable tablets, swallow tablets, capsules, and powders. The liquid preparations are the dosage forms of choice, since the dispersion, surface area covered, and onset of action are all superior to the tablet forms. The liquid forms are not very palatable and decrease the patient's compliance. The nurse may consider refrigeration of the antacid to improve the taste. Because of its frequent administration and taste, the liquid antacid may reduce the patient's desire for food or drink. For this reason, the thoroughly chewable tablets followed by adequate water may offer some value and convenience. Table 16-2 lists the most common antacids used and dosages at which they are normally given.

All the liquid preparations (suspensions) must be shaken vigorously before administration to achieve a uniform dispersion.

Side effects. Two inconvenient side effects are constipation and diarrhea. Aluminum and calcium products form insoluble salts that precipitate in the intestine and on accumulation lead to constipation. Magnesium antacids form compounds that attract and retain water, creating an osmotic effect, and are unabsorbed, which leads to diarrhea. Many products often contain both magnesium and aluminum compounds to create a balance and minimize constipation and diarrhea. While increasing the neutralizing effect, magnesium hydroxide also increases the laxative effect.

Magnesium trisilicate has some potential to form silicate salts, which may precipitate as renal calculi stones.

Aluminum ions may decrease smooth muscle contraction, which decreases gastric emptying time; the nurse should exercise caution with this antacid ingredient in patients with obstructions of gastric outlets. The aluminum antacids may cause white speckled feces.

The diarrhea produced by the magnesium-containing antacids has the risk of potassium depletion and acidosis.

Calcium-containing antacids produce acid rebound because the calcium carbonate neutralizes gastric acid initially but subsequently stimulates greater gastric acid production and release of gastrin than before the calcium carbonate administration. This is seen particularly during sleep when the antacid is not taken at close intervals as it is during the day. Table 16-3 summarizes some of the side effects seen with antacid preparations.

Precautions and contraindications. In patients who have normal renal function and are using antacids for short-term therapy, only infrequent toxic effects are seen. If renal function is impaired, the metal ions accumulate in the compromised kidney, producing additional kidney impairment, systemic alkalosis, and fluid and electrolyte disturbances. This is seen with long-term excessive use of the calcium and magnesium antacid products. The excess magnesium absorption may create neurologic, cardiovascular, and neuromuscular dysfunctions. The excess calcium absorption is seen with

TABLE 16-2 **Common antacid preparations**

Preparation*	Dosage
Aluminum carbonate gel, basic (Basaljel)	As antacid: two capsules or tablets, or 10 ml regular suspension (diluted in juice or water), or 5 ml of extra strength suspension as needed every 2 hours; not more than 12 doses daily
	To prevent phosphate stones (urinary phosphate stones are reduced by binding; the phosphate is decreased in the urine): two to six capsules or tablets, 10 to 30 ml suspension, or 5 to 15 ml extra-strength suspension taken 1 hour after meals and at bedtime; both suspensions diluted in juice or water
Aluminum hydroxide gel (ALternaGEL, Alu-Cap, Alu-Tab, Amphogel, Dialume)	600 mg three or four times daily between meals and at bedtime
Aluminum phosphate gel (Phosphaljel)	15 to 30 ml undiluted every 2 hours between meals and at bedtime
Calcium carbonate (Alka-2, Amitone, Chooz, Dicarbosil, Tums, others); chewable tablets range from 330- to 650-mg strengths	0.5 to 2 g as needed
Dihydroxyaluminum aminoacetate (Robalate)	Two to four tablets chewed well with water four times daily between meals and at bedtime
Dihydroxyaluminum sodium carbonate (DASC) (Rolaids)	One or two tablets chewed as needed; repeat hourly if symptoms return
Magaldrate (Riopan); available in tablets (chewable and swallow) and suspension (This is a distinct chemical entity, hydroxymagnesium aluminate, equivalent to approximately an average of 33% magnesium oxide and 21% aluminum oxide.)	400 to 800 mg between meals and at bedtime
Magnesium carbonate powder	0.5 to 2 g between meals with a half glass of water
Magnesium hydroxide (Milk of Magnesia—MOM, various manufacturers); available in tablets and liquid	As antacid: adults, 5 to 15 ml four times daily; children, 2.5 to 5 ml with water
	As laxative: adults, 30 to 60 ml with water once daily; children, 7.5 to 30 ml
Magnesium oxide (various); available in tablets, capsules, and powder	250 to 1500 mg administered with water or milk four times daily
Magnesium trisilicate (various); available in tablets and power	1 to 4 g four times daily with water
Sodium bicarbonate (Soda mint, Bell-ans, various); available as tablets and powders ranging from 325 to 650 mg	0.3 to 2 g one to four times daily

*Other ingredients found as single entities and in combination are: bismuth aluminate, bismuth subcarbonate, defatted skim milk, glycine, ipecac, mineral oil, simethicone bismuth subnitrate, sorbitol, and others. Effervescent tablets and powders contain acetaminophn, citric acid, flavoring, potassium bicarbonate, sodium bicarbonate, sodium citrate, and tartaric acid. Simethicone is a gastric defoaming additive breaking or coalescing gas bubbles. Several antacid combinations have added this agent for acute gas-related symptoms.

impaired renal function and intake of foods high in calcium and vitamin D content (the milk-alkali syndrome). Vitamin D increases the absorption of calcium ions and the antacid. The result is renal damage, systemic alkalosis, hypercalcemia, and other manifestations such as weakness and mental confusion.

Antacid products vary in their sodium content. Some patients require a low-sodium antacid (for example, in cases of hypertension and congestive heart failure). Table 16-4 presents the sodium content of some antacids. Many manufacturers are making modifications in their antacid products to reduce the sodium content.

Altered drug solubility, stability, and absorption. Many drugs are either weak acids or weak bases, and the pH of the stomach is an important factor in the absorption of these drugs. Drugs that are weak acids are un-ionized in the acidic environment of the stomach. These are lipid soluble and are absorbed by simple diffusion across the gastric mucosal cells. The administration of an antacid either with a weak acidic drug or shortly before or after its administration will raise the pH of the stomach contents, causing the formation of a more ionized drug that will not be absorbed to the degree the un-ionized lipid-soluble form was absorbed. A weakly basic drug is absorbed in a more alka-

T A B L E 1 6 - 3 Side effects of antacids

Ion involved	Side effects
Aluminum	Constipation, phosphate depletion via feces (including weakness, apnea, hemolytic anemia, and tetany), delay in gastric emptying, concretions, encephalopathy from aluminum intoxication, impairment of drug absorption, bone demineralization
Bicarbonate	Systemic alkalosis (elevates plasma pH, carbon dioxide, anorexia, mental confusion, and so forth); enhanced effects of amphetamines, quinidine, and quinine
Calcium	Milk-alkali syndrome, nephrocalcinosis, rebound hyperacidity, antagonism of digitalis preparations, stimulation of gastric secretions, hypercalcemia, kidney failure, constipation
Magnesium	Diarrhea, hypokalemia, hypermagnesemia, iron deficiency
Sodium	Salt and water retention exacerbating edema, ascites, effusion, and hypertension
Antacids collectively elevate pH of gastrointestinal tract	Cause a release of enteric-coated tablets in the stomach instead of the duodenum; enhancement of absorption of drugs such as dicumarol and L-dopa (all weak bases); reduction of absorption of phenothiazines, INH, and nalidixic acid (all weak acids)

T A B L E 1 6 - 4 Sodium content of antacids (liquid and solid dosage forms)

Antacid	Sodium content
Aludrox suspension	0.10 mEq Na/5 ml
Aludrox tablets	0.70 mEq Na/tablet
Alutabs	0.066 mEq Na/tablet
Amphogel suspension	0.3 mEq Na/5 ml
Basaljel suspension	0.104 mEq Na/5 ml
Basaljel tablets	0.091 mEq Na/tablet
Gelusil liquid	0.039 mEq Na/5 ml
Gelusil tablets	0.069 mEq Na/tablet
Gelusil-II liquid	0.057 mEq Na/5 ml
Gelusil-II tablets	0.117 mEq Na/tablet
Gelusil-M liquid	0.044 mEq Na/5 ml
Gelusil-M tablets	0.131 mEq Na/tablet
Maalox suspension	0.109 mEq Na/5 ml
Maalox Plus suspension	0.109 mEq Na/5 ml
Maalox Plus tablets	0.061 mEq Na/tablet
Maalox No. 1 tablets	0.037 mEq Na/tablet
Maalox No. 2 tablets	0.078 mEq Na/tablet
Mylanta liquid	0.030 mEq Na/5 ml
Mylanta tablets	0.0218 mEq Na/tablet
Mylanta-II liquid	0.061 mEq Na/5 ml
Mylanta-II tablets	0.044 mEq Na/tablet
Riopan suspension	0.013 mEq Na/5 ml
	0.013 mEq Na/tablet

*1 mg of sodium (Na) = 0.0435 mEq.; 1 mEq of sodium = 23 mg sodium.

line medium. Changes in pH will modify drug solubility and stability, which also affects absorption.

As the pH of the gastric contents increases, alterations of absorption of weak acids and bases occur as a result of altering the degree of ionization in the following manner: for basic drugs absorption increases because as the pH increases there is an increase in the un-ionized concentration of basic drugs; for acidic drugs absorption decreases because as the pH increases there is a decrease in the un-ionized concentration of acidic drugs.

Examples of drugs that are weak bases are morphine sulfate, quinine, pseudoephedrine, antihistamines, amphetamines, theophylline, tricyclic antidepressants, and quinidine. Examples of weak acids are isoniazid, barbiturates, nalidixic acid, nonsteroidal antiinflammatory agents, sulfonamides, salicylates, nitrofurantoin, and coumarins.

In summary, the antacids given with weak acidic drugs will increase the gastric pH and increase their ionization, therefore delaying or decreasing the drug's absorption. When antacids are administered with weak basic drugs, the increase in gastric pH and increase in the unionized form of the drug will cause an increase in the drug's absorption.

Drug interactions. The mechanisms of drug interactions involve adsorption, renal elimination, alteration of the gastric pH, formation of complexes, and absorption. Alterations in the pH of the gastrointestinal tract and its effect on drug absorption will be discussed.

Aluminum antacids (hydroxides and carbonate gel) cause phosphate depletion because the aluminum ion binds to the phosphate in the gastrointestinal tract (this is beneficial in patients with hyperphosphatemia in chronic renal failure). Phosphate deficiency and hypophosphatemia, if severe, may lead to weakness, tetany, hemolytic anemia and respiratory arrest, and congestive cardiomyopathy.

Digitalis preparations are potentiated by hypercalcemia or potassium depletion and when administered with calcium or magnesium antacids there is a risk of digitalis intoxication. Antacids also adsorb the digitalis preparations and thus impair digitalis absorption.

The antacid will remove the acid-resistant enteric coating on tablets, changing the pH of the stomach and causing release of the medication under the enteric coating into the stomach instead of the alkaline duodenum.

If aluminum-containing antacids are administered with an ion-exchange resin (for example, sodium polystyrene sulfonate used to remove serum potassium), a calculus-like mass forms within the stomach. The resin may also bind calcium and magnesium, producing anion absorption (as bicarbonate) and creating systemic alkalosis. This may be avoided by rectal administration of the resin.

The aluminum, calcium, and magnesium antacids complex, chelate, and impair dissolution of the tetracycline drugs when given together. This clinically significant interaction occurs with many drugs; therefore the nurse should not administer any oral drug within 1 to 2 hours before or after an antacid dose. Magnesium antacids inhibit the absorption of iron alone or in vitamin-mineral preparations.

Magnesium trisilicate, aluminum hydroxide, and magnesium hydroxide gel antacids decrease plasma chlorpromazine (phenothiazines) levels by decreasing absorption of phenothiazines. Indomethacin is adsorbed by antacids and kaolin, delaying the concentration peak and reducing bioavailability when administered simultaneously with antacids.

The nurse should remember that raising the pH with an antacid may alter the dissolution, disintegration, solubility, ionization, and gastric emptying time of a drug administered concomitantly with the antacid, creating either an increase or decrease in the drug's absorption. Antacids also modify the urinary pH, which alters drug elimination.

The absorption of levodopa is increased threefold when the antacid is given with the antiparkinsonian drug because raising the pH

increases the gastric emptying, placing more levodopa in the duodenum where it is absorbed readily. Therefore, relapse or toxicity may occur if the patient begins to use antacids while being treated with levodopa.

Aluminum antacids interfere with the absorption of isoniazid. By separating the administration of isoniazid and aluminum antacids over 1 hour or by administering a nonaluminum-containing antacid, this interaction will not occur.

Propranolol is significantly decreased in absorption when administered with antacid gels. The nurse may prevent this by administering these drugs several hours apart.

ANTACID COMBINATIONS

There are many antacid combinations as alluded to in Table 16-2; however, the antacid combination Gaviscon deserves particular attention because of its uniqueness and widespread use.

Gaviscon

Gaviscon forms a viscous cohesive foam that floats on the surface of the stomach contents, providing neutralization of refluxed stomach acid. This helps protect the sensitive mucosa from irritation because the foam contains antacid that precedes the stomach contents into the lower esophagus when reflux occurs. The foam is the result of the alginic acid contained in the product. The other ingredients are aluminum hydroxide, magnesium trisilicate, and sodium bicarbonate; it is available in two tablet strengths and a liquid suspension.

NURSING IMPLICATIONS

1 Patients who self-medicate with antacids for recurring gastrointestinal symptoms should be advised to seek medical care, since they are treating symptoms and not the cause of the symptoms. They may be treating themselves in vain. Nurses should thoroughly question patients who routinely self-medicate with antacids.
2 Helping a patient identify the source of his gastric discomfort, such as overeating, eating a wide variety of foods at one time, or tension, anxiety, or other emotional stress, may enable him to avoid the causes of his discomfort and eliminate the need for antacid therapy.
3 The nurse should be alert to drugs that may cause

or exacerbate ulcers. Some of these drugs are aspirin, ibuprofen, indomethacin, phenylbutazone, prednisone, potassium chloride supplements, reserpine, sulindac, tetracycline, and tolmetin.

4 Patients on a low-sodium diet and patients with hypertensive, cardiac, or renal disease should be instructed to avoid antacids containing sodium, particularly if antacids are used frequently.

5 Patients taking antacid tablets that should be chewed should be instructed to thoroughly chew or pulverize the tablet. These tablets are usually hydrophobic and do not mix readily with water. The wettability of an antacid is related to its ability to provide prompt and complete action. Thus liquids are better than tablets. Chewing the tablets slowly and thoroughly helps to obtain small particle size like that present in liquid antacids and helps to more thoroughly wet those particles for more prompt action.

6 Antacid suspensions should be shaken well before being taken.

7 There are a few foods the patient should avoid (caffeine, alcohol, and highly spiced foods) that increase acid secretion or irritate the ulcer. Diets high in milk and cream increase gastric acid production. Smoking impairs the normal neutralization of acid in the duodenum and is to be avoided. These facts should be communicated to the patient before discharge and reinforced with each visit.

8 Patients receiving medical antacid therapy should be encouraged to strictly adhere to their antacid schedule and should be given responsibility for taking their own antacids while still hospitalized.

9 Outpatients take only one-third to one-half of the prescribed dosage regimen. The compliance decreases proportionally with time as the patient only takes the dose when the symptoms arise and thus antagonizes healing. The nurse must educate the patient to comply with this regimen and life-style adjustment.

10 Patients should be cautioned about side effects and instructed to consult their physician if these occur.

11 Evaluation of antacid therapy is important. The patient's subjective response to antacid therapy and the nurse's objective observations (for example, frequency with which the patient takes his antacid) can help determine the effectiveness of antacid therapy.

12 The age of an antacid is important. For example, aluminum hydroxide gel becomes less reactive as it ages. Also, there is wide variation in aluminum hydroxide batches to neutralize acid, one batch being more or less effective than another. A patient not responding well to aluminum hydroxide therapy may need a different supply of aluminum hydroxide.

Antiflatulents
Simethicone

Simethicone acts in the stomach and intestines to alter the surface tension of gas bubbles, causing them to coalesce and free the gas that is eliminated by belching or passing flatus. The mechanism of action of this defoaming agent relieves flatulence by dispersing and preventing the formation of mucus-surrounded gas pockets in the gastrointestinal tract.

The approved clinical use is for relief of painful symptoms of gas in the gastrointestinal tract. Gas retention is a problem in conditions such as air swallowing, diverticulitis, functional dyspepsia, peptic ulcer, postoperative gaseous distention, and spastic or irritable colon.

The tablets are chewed thoroughly four times daily, after meals and at bedtime, and as needed for flatulence. They are available in 40- and 80-mg tablets (Mylicon, Silain) and in drops (40 mg/0.6 ml) to be shaken before administration. Several antacid combination products contain simethicone.

H_2-receptor antagonist

Continued research to develop drugs that will selectively inhibit gastric secretion or increase mucous secretion has finally resulted in the advent of drugs with just such actions. These drugs represent a significant pharmacologic revolution.

Cimetidine (Tagamet)

Cimetidine is a specific histamine H_2 receptor antagonist. Histamine stimulates gastric acid secretion in the stomach's parietal cells. Cimetidine substantially reduces stomach acid secretion by blocking the H_2 receptors, which also reduces the intrinsic factor output of the parietal cells. There is a negligible effect on gastrin secretion or stomach emptying time. As a consequence of decreased gastric juice volume, the pepsin output from the chief cell is decreased.

It is highly protein bound (85%), widely distributed, and rapidly absorbed (70% bioavailable) orally. Following oral administration, peak levels are achieved in 45 to 90 minutes. About half the oral dose is excreted substantially unchanged in the urine. The serum half-life is about 2 to 3 hours in normal renal function. Following parenteral administration, most of the drug is secreted unchanged. Metabolism occurs in the liver. The onset of gastric acid secretion inhibition occurs within 15 to 60 minutes. When administered with meals, a 300-mg oral dose has up to a 7-hour duration of action. No gastric acid secretion is seen for 2 hours after a 300-mg dose, and a 90% reduction in secretion is seen for up to 4 hours. Peak blood levels are reached within 75 minutes. Blood levels of 0.5 mg/ml inhibit about 80% of basal acid secretion and 50% of stimulated (by gastrin, insulin, food) acid secretion for 4 to 5 hours. The nurse may readily see the advantage of administering antacids between doses of cimetidine for the relief of duodenal ulcer pain. Cimetidine increases gastric mucosal cyclic AMP content. Serum prolactin levels are unaffected. A short-lived decrease in creatinine clearance occurs. Administration of cimetidine to patients with renal failure requires a decrease in total dose and prolonged intervals between doses because of the blood level accumulation and prolonged half-life. (The dosage for renal failure is 300 mg every 12 hours by any route, up to every 8 hours, based upon response.) It may be excreted in breast milk and should be used cautiously by breast-feeding mothers. The peripheral antagonism of androgens by cimetidine may be responsible for male gynecomastia and impotence, since the circulating hormone level is not altered.

Preparation, dosage and administration. Cimetidine is available in tablets of 200 and 300 mg; liquid containing 300 mg/5 ml; and injection of 300 mg/2 ml. The 200-mg tablet is a reduced-dose form for patients with renal impairment.

For duodenal ulcer, 300 mg is given four times orally daily with (not before) or immediately following meals and at bedtime. The bedtime dose increases blood levels of the drug since there is no added buffering capacity from food to inhibit acid secretion. The dose in Zollinger-Ellison syndrome is up to 2400 mg/day divided into four doses. Pediatric doses may be 20 to 40 mg/kg/day orally or parenterally in divided doses, but there has been limited experience with such use.

With parenteral administration the intravenous dose is 300 mg every 6 hours diluted in normal saline or 5% dextrose in water to a total volume of 20 ml and slowly injected over a 2-minute period. When given by intravenous infusion, the cimetidine dose is diluted in 100 ml of 5% dextrose in water or normal saline. It is infused at a rate of 1 to 4 mg/kg/hour over a 20- to 30-minute period. This slow injection or infusion avoids the possible risk of cardiac arrhythmias and arrest resulting from rapid injection. The drug is given orally when there are no signs of ulcer bleeding for 48 hours once the gastric pH is maintained at 5 or more. Cimetidine is physically incompatible with aminophylline or barbiturates in an intravenous infusion. The intramuscular route has a pharmacokinetics profile similar to the intravenous route, but some patients have some transient pain at the injection site.

Uses. Approved uses are to hasten healing of duodenal ulcer (hypersecretion of stomach acid), Zollinger-Ellison syndrome (a triad of gastrin-secreting non-beta-cell pancreatic tumors, extreme gastric hyperacidity, and intractable atypical peptic ulcer), patients unable to undergo gastrectomy, or pathologic hypersecretory conditions. Many investigations for unapproved uses have been made with cystic fibrosis, gastrointestinal hemorrhage, chronic urticaria, stress ulcer prophylaxis, psoriasis, and gastric ulcer, to name a few.

Precautions. Abrupt discontinuation of cimetidine produces a rebound or relapse perforation of the ulcer (duodenal and esophageal). Use during pregnancy subjects the fetus to potential hazards. Patients who are elderly or who have diminished renal or hepatic function may experience mental confusion (effect ceases 48 hours after discontinuation of cimetidine) associated with elevated serum concentrations due to decreased clearance.

Side effects and toxic effects. Adverse reactions include mild diarrhea, muscular pain, dizziness, rash, and neutropenia. Less frequently seen are galactorrhea, bradycardia, impotence, alopecia, hallucinations, and delirium.

Drug interactions. Cimetidine potentiates warfarin's anticoagulant effect by increasing prothrombin time. Cimetidine inhibits drugs degraded by hepatic microsomal oxidative enzyme systems. This results in an increase in plasma levels of drugs such as benzodiazepines (only those metabolized in the liver to desmethyldiazepam, therefore not by glucuronidation), phenytoin, propranolol, and theophylline. The resulting exaggerated response in the patient's therapy requires careful nursing observation. For example, elderly persons and those with liver disease *then* may have increased sedation from the benzodiazepines.

Nursing considerations. The nurse will notice the patient has more relief of abdominal pain and discomfort. The patient should be told to take cimetidine on a scheduled basis with or immediately after a meal. Antacids may be used between doses to relieve pain. The patient must report to the physician any medications that are or will be concurrently used. Ulcer healing should take place within 6 to 8 weeks.

Digestants

Digestants are drugs that promote the process of digestion in the gastrointestinal tract. Some of these agents previously used for replacement therapy are no longer considered to be effective or their use justifiable. Included in this category are dilute hydrochloric acid and glutamic acid hydrochloride (Acidulin). However, since nurses may still encounter their use, these agents are included in the text.

Diluted hydrochloric acid; dilute hydrochloric acid

Diluted hydrochloric acid contains 10% hydrochloric acid, which should be further diluted in at least one-half glass of water and should be administered through a tube to avoid injury to the enamel of the teeth. The usual dose is 5 ml, although some physicians recommend doses up to 10 ml. The acid may be sipped with the meal or taken just after the meal. Even though the acid is diluted well, the taste is very sour. Food should be eaten after the last swallow of the acid or the mouth rinsed with an alkaline mouthwash.

Glutamic acid hydrochloride (Acidulin, Fibertone)

Glutamic acid hydrochloride is a combination of glutamic acid and hydrochloric acid (1.8 mEq) and is available in capsules, which avoids exposure of dental enamel to the acid. The hydrochloric acid is released when the preparation comes in contact with water. The dose is 1 to 3 capsules or tablets three times daily before meals.

Pancreatin (Panteric)

Pancreatin is a powdered substance obtained from the pancreas of the hog or ox. It principally contains pancreatic amylase, trypsin, and pancreatic lipase. Acid chyme entering the duodenum and vagal stimulation regulate pancreatic secretion, so replacement therapy may be necessary for patients who have had vagal fibers surgically severed or surgical procedures that cause food to bypass the duodenum. Pancreatin and pancrelipase aid in the digestion and absorption of fats, carbohydrates, and triglycerides. In addition, replacement therapy is usually necessary in exocrine pancreatic enzyme deficiency states, chronic pancreatitis, cystic fibrosis, pancreatic tumors, pancreatic obstruction, and pancreatectomy. The drug is available in enteric-coated capsules to avoid destruction in the stomach.

Pancreatin is available in 300-, 325-, and 1000-mg tablets, capsules, and powder. The dosage for adults is 325 mg to 1 g daily in divided doses before meals, during meals, or within 1 hour after meals, with an extra dose taken with any food eaten between meals. In high doses this drug may cause nausea, diarrhea, hyperuricosuria, and hyperuricemia. To avoid temporary indigestion the patient must maintain a dietary balance of fat, protein, and starch.

Viokase (VioBin)

Viokase is obtained from the pancreas of cattle. It is available in 325-mg tablets or in powder form.

Pancrelipase (Cotazym, Pancrease, Isozyme)

Pancrelipase is similar to other pancreatic enzyme preparations, but its lipase activity is greater and it can be given in lower doses to control steatorrhea. It is a concentrate of pancreatic enzymes from hogs. It is available in capsules, tablets, and packets. The dosage for adults is one to three capsules or tablets or one to two packets before or with each meal or snack. In extreme deficiency the dosage interval may be changed to hourly if no nausea or diarrhea develops. Because of its enteric-coated microsphere formulation, Pancrease resists gastric inactivation, so enzymes reach the duodenum to hydrolyze fats into glycerol and fatty acids, proteins into proteases, and starch into dextrins and sugars.

Chenodeoxycholic acid (bile acid)

Chenodeoxycholic acid is a primary bile acid under clinical investigation for the nonsurgical treatment of cholesterol gallstones. Cholesterol gallstones occur when bile contains an excess of cholesterol relative to the bile salts and phospholipid content. Since chenodeoxycholic acid is a common bile acid in humans, it alters this ratio in favor of bile salts and the phospholipid content and presumably prevents the precipitation of cholesterol. It is under investigation to determine its ability to dissolve or reduce the size of cholesterol gallstones. Dosage varies from 0.75 to 4.5 g. The drug has been administered for 6 to 22 months.

Side effects and toxic effects. Diarrhea has been reported as an adverse reaction to chenodeoxycholic acid. Some concern has been expressed about its chronic use, since it is dehydroxylated in the intestines to lithocholic acid, a known hepatotoxin in some animal species.

Antiemetics

Antiemetics are drugs given to produce symptomatic relief of nausea and vomiting. Control of vomiting is important and often difficult. Numerous preparations have been used, but effective treatment usually depends on treating the cause of vomiting. Vomiting may result from such diverse phenomena as strong emotion, severe pain, increased intracranial pressure, and labyrinthine disturbances. Other factors include motion sickness, endocrine disturbances, toxic reaction to drugs, gastrointestinal pathology, reaction to roentgenographic treatments, and chemotherapy.

In mild cases of nausea and vomiting, a cup of plain hot tea will often relieve a patient's nausea. Carbonated drinks are popular remedies when medication is unavailable and seem to be more effective when administered at room temperature. In patients who cannot eructate, however, they will only increase gastric distention and discomfort.

The following drugs are used as antiemetics:

1 Sedatives and hypnotics (for example, phenobarbital) centrally depress the cerebral cortex and the vomiting center.
2 Anticholinergics, such as scopolamine, reduce the excitability of labyrinth receptors, depress conduction in the vestibular cerebellar pathways, or prevent impulses from stimulating the chemoreceptor trigger zone.
3 Antihistamines affect neural labyrinth pathways, for example, cyclizine (Marezine) and dimenhydrinate (Dramamine).
4 Phenothiazines act on the chemoreceptor trigger zone and on the vomiting center. These are the most effective antiemetics and often the drugs of choice, for example, chlorpromazine (Thorazine) and promethazine (Phenergan).
5 Antacids relieve gastric irritation, for example, Gelusil.
6 Miscellaneous drugs include diphenidol (Vontrol), which acts on the aural vestibular apparatus, and benzquinamide (Emete-Con), which acts on the chemoreceptor trigger zone.

Most of these drugs have been discussed elsewhere in the text (see Index). Antiemetics exert their effects on the vomiting center, the cerebral cortex, the chemoreceptor trigger zone, or the aural vestibular apparatus.

Precautions should be taken when administering antiemetics, since antiemetics may mask signs of overdosage of toxic drugs, such as sedatives or hypnotics, and may obscure diagnosis of complications such as paralytic ileus. They also may have additive effects when used with narcotic analgesics or when given to patients with unexcreted levels of anesthetic agents.

Diphenidol hydrochloride (Vontrol)

Diphenidol is recommended for the prevention and control of nausea and vomiting, the vertigo of Meniere's disease, labyrinthitis following middle or inner ear surgery, and motion sickness. It is used to control postoperative vomiting, drug-induced vomiting, and vomiting resulting from radiation therapy. It is not recommended for control of nausea and vomiting of pregnancy, since its safety during pregnancy has not been determined. Its use to control vertigo in children has not been investigated.

Diphenidol controls nausea and vomiting by inhibiting the medullary chemoreceptor trigger zone; it controls vertigo by a specific antivertigo effect on the vestibular apparatus.

Side effects and toxic effects. Diphenidol should be restricted to hospitalized or carefully supervised patients because of untoward effects that may occur, which include hallucinations, disorientation, and confusion. These usually occur within 3 days after initiation of therapy and subside within 3 days after discontinuing the drug. Other side effects include drowsiness, depression, sleep disturbances, and dry mouth. Dizziness, rash, malaise, headache, and mild transient hypotension occur rarely.

Since diphenidol has a weak peripheral anticholinergic effect, it should be used cautiously in patients with glaucoma or gastrointestinal or urinary obstructions.

Preparation, dosage, and administration. Recommended oral dosage for adults is 25 to 50 mg four times a day; for children the dosage is 5 mg/kg body weight daily divided into four doses. Intravenous or intramuscular dose for adults is 20 mg; 20 to 40 mg may be given four times daily. Diphenidol is not recommended for infants under 6 months of age or for those weighing less than 25 pounds. Intravenous administration is not recommended for children of any age.

Diphenidol is available in 25-mg tablets and in 2-ml ampules containing 20 mg diphenidol/ml.

Trimethobenzamide hydrochloride (Tigan)

Trimethobenzamide exhibits an antiemetic action similar to the phenothiazine derivatives but has a weak antihistaminic action. It is believed to depress the chemoreceptor trigger zone in the medulla rather than the vomiting center directly. It has the advantage of long duration of action and little or no sedative effect. It is recommended for the prevention or relief of nausea and vomiting caused by radiation sickness, infection, and operative procedures. It has also been used to relieve nausea and vomiting caused by a number of other conditions. It is not particularly effective for the treatment of motion sickness.

Trimethobenzamide is marketed in 100- and 250-mg capsules for oral administration, in vials and ampules for intramuscular injection containing 100 mg/ml, and in 100- and 200-mg rectal suppositories. The usual adult oral dose is 100 to 250 mg. The usual adult parenteral dose is 200 mg. After oral or parenteral administration the drug is effective in 20 to 40 minutes, and action persists 4 to 6 hours. Dosage for children is 15 mg/kg body weight divided into three or four doses during a 24-hour period.

Side effects. Incidence of adverse effects is low. Dizziness, drowsiness, diarrhea, irritation after rectal administration, and pain at the site of injection have been noted. Occasionally, the patient's nausea is intensified.

Thiethylperazine maleate (Torecan)

Thiethylperazine is a phenothiazine derivative with pronounced antiemetic and antinauseant activity. Studies indicate that this drug is a more effective antiemetic than other phenothiazines. It effectively controls vertigo caused by pathology in the inner ear and nausea and vomiting caused by anesthetics, radiation therapy, and chemotherapy. It is not useful for preventing motion sickness.

Preparation, dosage, and administration. Thiethylperazine is available in 10-mg oral tablets and in 10-mg ampules and suppositories. The dosage for adults is 10 to 30 mg daily.

Side effects and toxic effects. Side effects occur infrequently and are usually mild and transitory. Drowsiness, dry mouth, tachycardia, and anorexia may occur. Like other phenothiazines, thiethylperazine may cause extrapyramidal symptoms. Moderate orthostatic hypotension has also been reported.

Contraindications. Thiethylperazine is contraindicated during pregnancy, for children under 12 years of age, and for use in patients with severe central nervous system depression.

Benzquinamide hydrochloride (Emete-Con)

Benzquinamide is an antiemetic agent chemically unrelated to the phenothiazines or other antiemetic drugs. Studies in animals indicate the drug has antiemetic, antihistaminic, anticholinergic, antiserotonin, and sedative effects. Its antiemetic action is probably due to a depressant effect on the vomiting center.

After parenteral administration, the antiemetic effect occurs in 15 minutes; the duration of effect is 3 to 4 hours. Benzquinamide is used for the prevention and treatment of nausea and vomiting associated with anesthetics and surgery in those patients in whom emesis would endanger the results of surgery or harm the patient.

Preparation, dosage, and administration. Benzquinamide is available for injection in 2-ml vials, containing 50 mg of base, which is reconstituted with 2.2 ml of sterile water to produce a solution containing 25 mg/ml. It is usually given by *deep* intramuscular injection. The initial dose is 50 mg, which may be repeated in 1 hour with subsequent doses every 3 to 4 hours as necessary. When used prophylactically for nausea and vomiting associated with anesthetics, the drug should be given 15 minutes prior to emergence from anesthesia.

Benzquinamide may be given intravenously in a single dose of 25 mg. It should be administered slowly (1 ml over 30 seconds to 1 minute.) Subsequent doses should be given intramuscularly.

Side effects. The most common reaction to benzquinamide is drowsiness. Other side effects include insomnia, restlessness, headache, dry mouth, shivering, sweating, hiccups, flushing, salivation, and blurred vision. Intravenous administration has been associated with sudden increase in blood pressure and transient cardiac arrhythmias.

Contraindications. Benzquinamide should not be given intravenously to patients with cardiovascular disease. It should not be given to patients who demonstrate hypersensitivity to the drug (pyrexia, urticaria). Its safe use during pregnancy has not been established.

Drugs that affect the intestines

Constipation is a symptom of an underlying condition manifesting itelf by abnormally infrequent and difficult fecal evacuation. This physical body malfunctioning is an objective aspect of constipation. A subjective aspect of constipation is the individual patient's feeling or attitude of dissatisfaction regarding his bowel function. The nurse will be confronted with both of these aspects in the daily routines of the patient. There are patients who may be described as "stool gazers" who often relate their daily life to the inadequacy or subjective dissatisfaction with their bowel function.

Chronic constipation is sometimes caused by organic disease, such as benign or malignant tumors, which produces obstruction in the bowel; megacolon; hypothyroidism; anal and rectal disorders; and diseases of the liver and gallbladder. Patients who suffer from disorders of the gastrointestinal tract frequently complain of constipation. On the other hand, many persons complain of constipation when no organic disease or lesion can be found. A number of factors may operate to cause constipation in such persons.

1 Faulty diet and faulty eating habits (A diet that provides inadequate bulk and residue will contribute to the development of constipation. The gastrointestinal tract should function normally if fluids and residue are supplied in sufficient quantities to keep the stool formed but soft.)
2 Failure to respond to the normal defecation impulses and insufficient time to permit the bowel to produce an evacuation
3 Sedentary habits and insufficient exercise (Bedridden patients may be constipated because of inactivity or unnatural position for defecation.) Constipation, when not a result of organic causes, is generally attributable to the above three factors.
4 The effect of drugs (The use of morphine, tricyclic antidepressants, codeine, aluminum hydroxide, ganglionic blocking agents, anticholanergic activity, and so forth often leads to constipation as a side effect.)
5 Febrile states, psychosomatic disorders, anemias, and sick headaches (Constipation can be a symptom of both functional and organic disorders.)
6 Atonic and hypertonic conditions of the musculature of the colon (These may result from habitual use of cathartics.)

Laxatives

Laxatives are oral drugs administered to induce defecation. They may be administered for the following purposes:

1 In preparation of abdominal viscera prior to roentgenographic examination or surgery
2 Postoperatively
3 In cases of food and drug poisoning to promote the elimination of the offending substance from the gastrointestinal tract; saline cathartics are considered useful for this purpose
4 To keep the stool soft when it is essential to avoid the irritation or straining that accompanies the passage of a hardened stool (a rectal disorder, irritated polyps in the bowel, or cases in which straining should be avoided, as after the repair of a hernia or after a cerebrovascular accident)
5 To expel parasites and toxic anthelmintics; cathartics are routinely prescribed after certain anthelmintics for the purpose of expelling the parasites as well as the anthelmintic, which may be toxic
6 To secure a stool specimen to be examined for parasites; a saline cathartic is often preferred
7 To relieve constipation during pregnancy or the postnatal period
8 In geriatric patients
9 In children with megacolon
10 To overcome decreased intestinal motility caused by drugs
11 For gastrointestinal tract roentgenogram preparation

The laity, however, frequently misuses laxatives, and misconceptions about the function of the bowel have long been harbored by mankind.

CLASSIFICATION

Laxatives may be classified according to their source, site of action, degree of action, or method of action. The latter two classifications will be described.

Degree of action
1 Laxatives—stimulate few bowel movements, which are formed and usually unaccompanied by cramping
2 Purgatives—produce more frequent bowel movements, which are soft or liquid in nature and are frequently accompanied by cramping

Method of action
1 Saline laxatives—retain and increase water content of feces by virtue of osmotic qualities; may also be considered as bulk laxatives
2 Stimulant laxatives—increase peristalsis in the

colon by irritating sensory nerve endings in the mucosa
3 Bulk laxatives—increase the volume of nonabsorbable intestinal contents, thereby distending the bowel and initiating reflex bowel activity
4 Intestinal lubricants—mechanically lubricate feces to facilitate defecation
5 Fecal softening agents—act as dispersing wetting agents, facilitating mixture of water and fatty substances within the fecal mass; when a homogeneous mixture is produced, the feces become soft

Table 16-5 summarizes the traditional laxatives that can be bought without a prescription. Their differences and advantages and disadvantages are presented.

CONDITIONS FOR WHICH LAXATIVES MAY BE CONTRAINDICATED

There are a number of conditions for which laxatives should be given with caution, if at all.

1 Inflammatory disorders of the alimentary tract, such as appendicitis, typhoid fever, and chronic ulcerative colitis
2 Cases of undiagnosed abdominal pain; should the pain be caused by an inflamed appendix, a laxative may bring about a rupture of the appendix by increasing intestinal peristalsis
3 After some operations such as repair of the perineum or rectum (for a time, at least)
4 Pregnancy and severe anemia; debilitated patients
5 Chronic constipation and spastic constipation
6 Bowel obstruction, hemorrhage, or intussusception

A number of ill effects may follow the use or overuse of irritant laxatives in particular; one of these is a disturbance of electrolyte balance. The small intestine contains an abundance of sodium, potassium, chloride, and bicarbonate ions that will be lost when the bowel is emptied vigorously. This can result in alkalosis or acidosis, dehydration, and potassium deficiency. Young and healthy adults may recover from the purgation without noticeable ill effect, but the same may not be true in the elderly or the debilitated patient or the patient with renal impairment.

The different groups of laxatives will be presented according to their method of action and the way they are used. Lactulose, mentioned in Table 16-5, is in a classification all its own. It is a disaccharide that is broken down in the colon

TABLE 16-5 Traditional laxatives

	No prescription required					Prescription required
	Irritant/ stimulant type	Osmotic/ saline type	Stool softener/ surfactant or wetting agent type	High-fiber and bulk-forming type	Lubricant/ emollient type	Lactulase syrup
Disadvantages with repeated frequent (long-term) administration	Watery stools, griping	Watery stools, cramps	Unreliable results, may contribute to liver toxicity	Obstruction of narrowed lumen, some difficulty in chewing and swallowing	Anal leakage, lipid pneumonia	Early, transient flatulence and cramps; nausea has been reported
Increases rate of transit in small bowel	Yes	Yes	Yes	Yes	Unknown	Possibly
Causes net secretion of water and electrolytes in small bowel	Yes	Yes	Yes	Yes	No	No
Inhibits absorption in small bowel	Yes	Yes	Yes	Yes	Yes	Not reported
Increases mucosal permeability in small bowel	Yes	Not studied	Yes	Not reported	Not reported	No
Causes mucosal damage in small bowel	Yes	Not studied	Yes	Not reported	Not reported	No
Acts only in colon (not small bowel)	No	No	No	No	Yes	Yes
Indicated for long-term treatment	No	No	No	Probably	No	Yes
Examples of type	Anthraquinone and isatin derivatives, phenolphthalein, castor oil	Magnesium salts, MOM, sodium phosphate, magnesium citrate	DSS, DCS	Methylcellulose, sodium CMC, psyllium seed, agar, plantago	Mineral oil	Chronulac
Physical or chemical property responsible for action	Mucosal surface irritation to stimulate or increase intestinal motor function or activity	Hyperosmolar ingredients trap water in intestinal lumen; hypertonicity of colon increases liquid in colon	Changes surface tension of fecal mass, provides increased penetration of colonic water; penetrates and softens fecal mass by wetting agents	Absorbs water on surface, increases soft fecal mass, adds bulk and moisture to feces causing distention and elimination	Coats over fecal mass, passes with ease, lubricates gastrointestinal tract and softens feces	Colon-specific increase in stool water content and stool softening by increase in osmotic pressure and colon acidification

by bacteria to lactic acid, formic acid, acetic acid, and carbon dioxide. These products cause an increase in osmotic pressure and slightly acidify the colonic contents, which results in an increase in stool water content and stool softening.

SALINE LAXATIVES

The saline laxatives are soluble salts that are only slightly absorbed from the alimentary canal. Because of their osmotic effect, these salts retain and increase the water content of feces. An isotonic saline solution will inhibit absorption of water from the bowel and will therefore increase the total fluid bulk. Peristalsis will be increased and several liquid or semi-liquid stools will result. A hypertonic saline solution will cause diffusion of fluid from the blood in the wall (semipermeable membrane) of the bowel and into the lumen of the organ until the solution has been made isotonic. This type of fluid is especially effective in relieving edema, although the action may prove exhausting to the patient. Laxation results in 30 minutes to 3 hours.

The intestinal membrane is not entirely impermeable to the passage of saline laxatives. Electrolyte disturbances have been reported with their long-term daily use. Some find their way into the general circulation only to be excreted by the kidney, in which case they act as saline diuretics. Hypertonic saline solutions in the bowel may result in so much loss of fluid that little or no diuretic effect will be possible. Some ions may have a toxic effect in impaired renal function if they accumulate in the blood in sufficient quantity. This may occur with magnesium ions if a solution is retained in the intestine for a long time or if the patient suffers from renal impairment. It may also occur when large doses of the salt are given intravenously. Magnesium acts as a depressant of the central nervous system and neuromuscular activity.

Uses. The saline laxatives are the laxative of choice for the relief of edema (cerebral, cardiac), for securing a stool specimen for examination, and for fecal impactions, as well as for use with certain anthelmintics and in some cases of food and drug poisoning. Phosphate enemas are useful as preparations for a barium enema.

When the object is merely to empty the intestine, magnesium citrate, magnesium sulfate, sodium phosphate, or milk of magnesia is effective. Milk of magnesia (magnesium hydroxide) is the mildest of the salines and is often the cathartic of choice for children. As a rule, heavy magnesium oxide is better for adults. Magnesium sulfate is probably the best to relieve edema, although it has a disagreeable taste. Sodium sulfate is the most disagreeable and is seldom prescribed, except in veterinary practice. The effervescent preparations are the most agreeable to take.

The sodium salts are contraindicated in cardiac patients or those on a low sodium diet. The magnesium and potassium salts are contraindicated in patients with renal disease.

Preparation, dosage, and administration. The following salts, when given for their laxative effect, are usually given orally. Certain of them may be given rectally as an enema. The salts tend to have a rapid action, especially if administered in the morning before breakfast. Patients sometimes complain of gaseous distention after taking saline laxatives. All preparations should be accompanied by a liberal (8-ounce) intake of water, since the salts do not readily leave the stomach and may cause vomiting unless well diluted. On the other hand, if the saline is given to reduce edema, the patient's total daily intake of fluids will probably be restricted.

When a salt such as magnesium sulfate is administered to a patient, it should not only be dissolved in an adequate amount of water but it should also be disguised in fruit juice. Grape juice is excellent unless the patient is nauseated, in which case it is better to give it in plain water (chilled) or on chipped ice, since the grape juice, if vomited, will stain bedclothing.

Sodium sulfate (Glauber's salt). Sodium sulfate occurs as a white powder that is readily soluble in water. It has a strong disagreeable saline taste that may be improved with lemon juice. It is one of the least expensive of saline laxatives and is the basis of many proprietary saline laxatives such as Sal Hepatica. The usual dose is 15 g.

Magnesium sulfate (Epsom salt). Magnesium sulfate occurs as glassy, needlelike crystals or as a white powder and is readily soluble in water. It has a bitter saline taste. The usual dose for laxative effect is 15 g (½ ounce), although the range of dosage may be from 10 to 30 g.

Milk of magnesia; magnesium hydroxide mixture. Milk of magnesia (mom) is also used as an antacid. In the stomach the magnesium hydroxide reacts with the hydrochloric acid to form magnesium chloride, which is responsible for the laxative effect. The usual dose for adults is 15 ml (½ fluidounce), although the range of dosage is 5 to 30 ml. *Magnesium hydroxide tab-*

lets contain 0.3 g of the drug. Results occur in 30 minutes to 3 hours.

Magnesium oxide. Magnesium oxide depends on the conversion of the oxide into soluble salts of magnesium, which are responsible for the laxative effect. The usual laxative dose is 1 to 4 g.

Heavy magnesium carbonate; light magnesium carbonate. Magnesium carbonate is a bulky white powder that is practically insoluble in water. It is used as an antacid as well as a laxative. The laxative effect depends on the formation of a soluble salt of magnesium. The usual dose is 2 to 8 g.

Magnesium citrate solution. Magnesium citrate solution is not very soluble, hence the need for a relatively large dose. It is not unpleasant to take because it is carbonated and flavored. The usual dose is 200 ml, and results occur in 30 minutes to 3 hours.

Sodium phosphate. Sodium phosphate is a white crystalline substance readily soluble in water. Its taste is less disagreeable than that of either sodium sulfate or magnesium sulfate. The usual dose is 4 g.

Effervescent sodium phosphate. Effervescent sodium phosphate is made effervescent by the addition of sodium bicarbonate and citric and tartaric acids. The usual dose is 10 g.

A concentrated aqueous solution of sodium biphosphate and sodium phosphate is available under the name of Fleet Phospho-Soda. The usual dose as a laxative is 4 to 15 ml. It is also marketed in a disposable enema unit and should be used cautiously in patients on low-sodium diets.

Potassium sodium tartrate (Rochelle salt). The usual dose is 5 to 10 g orally. Potassium sodium tartrate occurs as crystals or white powder, is very soluble, and does not have an unpleasant taste.

Mineral waters. Mineral waters are usually artificially prepared solutions made in a factory and contain magnesium sulfate or sodium sulfate or both. Their use in the treatment of constipation is thought inadvisable.

Lactulose syrup (Chronulac)

Lactulose syrup is used in the treatment of constipation in patients with a history of chronic constipation to increase the number of bowel movements daily and the number of days on which bowel movements occur. Lactulose syrup (15 ml) contains lactulose (10 g), galactose (2.2 g), lactose (1.2 g), and other sugars (less than 1.2 g); 97% of the oral dose of lactulose is unabsorbed and reaches the colon unchanged. The normal colonic bacteria (*Lactobacillus* and *Bacteroides*) metabolize it to organic acids, primarily lactic acid, plus small amounts of carbon dioxide, acetic acid, and formic acid, thus producing a drop in pH (7 to 5) of the contents of the ascending colon and softening of the feces. There is also an increase in the number of osmotically active molecules as a result of the formation of low molecular weight acids.

Acidification of the colon results in the transformation of free ammonia to ammonium ions, which are not absorbed from the colon, to the general circulation by a principle of nonionic diffusion. The acidic colonic contents cause a retention of the ammonia as the ammonium ion. Since the colon contents are now more acidic than the blood, the ammonia molecule can migrate from the blood into the colon to form the ammonium ion. The acid colonic contents convert the ammonia (NH_3) to the ammonium ion (NH_4^+), trapping it and preventing its absorption. The laxative action of the metabolites of lactulose expel the trapped ammonium ion from the colon.

The drop in pH and the increased osmotic action combine to stimulate the colon's own propulsive activity. A stool of increased weight, volume, and moisture content results. This unique colon-specific laxative does not cause net secretion of water and electrolytes in the small intestine and does not inhibit absorption in the small bowel. Effectiveness is seen from a few hours to 24 or 48 hours, producing normal bowel movements. There are no signs of tolerance. There are 60 calories in a 15-ml dose; however, less than 18 calories are in the absorbable sugars, with the remainder of the calories not available. This same dose contains from 0.4 to 0.7 mg sodium.

Dosage and administration. The usual dose is 1 to 2 tablespoons (15 to 30 ml) daily, and the dose may be increased in 5- and 10-ml increments to 60 ml daily following breakfast. A patient with a history of severe constipation and treatment with other laxatives plus enemas and suppositories may require an initial dose of 30 ml. The dose may be taken in juice, water, or milk for acceptance of the sweet taste.

If the patient has a recent onset of constipation caused by postsurgical or postpartum complications or other special circumstance (posthemorrhoidectomy pain), a 15-ml dose may be suitable. This product is available only by a prescription (physician's order), which keeps the condition under medical supervision and decreases the propensity to laxative abuse and misuse and the harmful effects that result.

Lactulose is also used to reduce blood ammonia levels in portal systemic encephalopathy. An initial dose of 30 to 50 ml, three times daily, is given and adjusted to produce a fecal pH of 5 to 5.5 and two to three soft, formed stools daily. Lactulose has been used successfully as a retention enema to produce a decrease in the fasting blood ammonia level.

Another application of lactulose is in the treatment of constipation in the geriatric population. An initial dose of 15 ml at bedtime is given for 3 or 4 days followed by a maintenance dose of 7.5 ml to 30 ml daily. This gives the nurse more assurance that the invasive and time-consuming enemas or suppositories will not have to be administered. A dose of 5 to 10 ml administered two to three times daily is effective in bowel emptying and preventing retention of barium in the elderly patient undergoing the gastrointestinal series. There is a greater margin of safety with lactulose in the elderly than the conventional laxatives because of less side effects and adverse reactions and the "prescription only" status.

Side effects and toxic effects. Initially, dose-related flatulence and intestinal cramps, gas, belching, and extension (transient) are seen, and excessive doses may produce some diarrhea (hypokalemic) and nausea (caused by the sweet taste). No irritation or damage to the colon or to normal or diseased rectal or perianal tissue has been reported. Lactulose has no effect on absorption or secretion in the small intestine, and the dose does not need to be increased in long-term therapy.

Precautions, contraindications, and drug

interactions. The effectiveness of lactulose may be reduced if used concomitantly with an antibiotic that has activity in the colon by reducing the normal colonic bacteria. A nonabsorbed antibiotic such as neomycin destroys enough luminal colonic bacteria to interfere with the effective action of lactulose. Most systemic, highly absorbable antibiotics do not affect the colonic bacteria in the lumen. No laxative should be given when an acute surgical condition in the abdomen might be suspected. Since lactulose contains galactose (less than 2.2 g/15 ml), it is contraindicated in low-galactose diets. Studies during pregnancy of the effect on the mother and fetus have not been evaluated. The galactose and lactose contained in the syrup require caution in diabetic patients monitoring for blood glucose increases, which may rarely occur. Elderly and debilitated patients receiving lactulose for 6 months or more should have serum electrolytes (potassium, chloride, and carbon dioxide) periodically measured.

STIMULANT LAXATIVES

The principal members of the stimulant group of laxatives are botanical glycoside drugs obtained from the bark, seed pods, leaves, and roots of a number of plants. Cascara, senna, rhubarb, and aloe yield anthraquinones in the alkaline portion of the small intestine; these are absorbed and later secreted to produce irritation in the large intestine. These compounds are partially absorbed from the intestine and may cause discoloration (yellow-brown in acid urine, alkaline urine pink to red) of the urine. They have also been found to impart a purgative effect to the milk of nursing women. The anthracene laxatives act in 6 to 24 hours and exert their main action on the small and large intestines, which explains their tendency to produce cramping. Aloe and rhubarb are almost obsolete because of their irritating properties.

Stimulant laxatives are used in preparation for barium enemas, in some cases of acute constipation, and before a proctologic examination. The nurse is cautioned that the stimulant laxative may lead to mucous secretion and fluid evacuation.

Side effects and toxic effects. The side

TABLE 16-6   **Oral stimulant laxatives**

Generic name	Trade name	Therapeutic effect (hours)	Stool consistency	Remarks
Bisacodyl	Dulcolax	6	Soft	Not to be taken within 1 hour after ingestion of milk or antacids to prevent premature dissolving of enteric coating and gastrointestinal irritation
Castor oil	Neoloid emulsion, Castor Oil	2-6	Watery	Chilling, mixing with fruit juice or carbonated drinks increases palatability
Cascara sagrada	Cascara sagrada	6-8	Soft, formed	Gives a yellowish brown color to acid urine; reddish color to alkaline urine
Danthron	Dorbane, Modane	6-8	Soft, semifluid	Gives a pink color to alkaline urine; do not give to nursing mother; drug is excreted in milk
Phenolphthalein	Ex-Lax Feen-A-Mint Phenolax	4-8	Semifluid	Gives pink color to alkaline urine or feces; action may persist for 3 to 4 days; may cause skin eruptions as dermatitis
Senna	X-prep, Senokot	6-12	Soft	Crude senna may cause urine discoloration like cascara

effects and toxic effects of stimulant laxatives include hypokalemia, enteric loss of protein, and malabsorption. Senna, cascara sagrada, danthron, and aloe are passed through the breast milk, initiating laxation in the nursing infant. Their occasional use should be restricted to 1 week, since long-term abuse may lead to a poorly functioning large intestine. Table 16-6 presents a comparison of the stimulant laxatives in use in medicine today.

Cascara sagrada

Cascara sagrada is obtained from the bark of the *Rhamnus purshiana*, a shrub or small tree, and is one of the most extensively used laxatives. Its action is mainly on the small and large bowel and, although its effects are comparatively mild, it does act by irritation. It is less likely to cause griping than some of the other laxatives belonging to this group of compounds. The active ingredients reach the large bowel by way of the bloodstream, after absorption in the small bowel, as well as by passage along the alimentary tract. Bowel evacuation occurs in about 8 hours. Prolonged use leads to melanotic pigmentation in rectal mucosa, which is reversible 4 to 12 months after discontinuation of the drug.

Preparation, dosage, and administration. Cascara is used in one of three preparations obtained by extracting the crude drug with hot water.

Cascara sagrada extract. Cascara sagrada extract is a powder obtained by evaporating the water extract to dryness and adding starch; each gram represents 3 g cascara sagrada. The usual dose is 300 mg; range of dose is 120 to 500 mg.

Cascara sagrada fluidextract; cascara liquid extract. Each milliliter of cascara sagrada fluidextract represents the activity of 1 g of crude drug. Alcohol is added as a preservative. The usual dose is 0.5 to 2 ml. This preparation has a very bitter taste.

Aromatic cascara fluidextract. Aromatic cascara fluidextract is prepared using magnesium oxide as a debitterizing agent to make it more palatable. Flavoring agents, sweeteners, and alcohol are also added. Each milliliter represents 1 g cascara sagrada. The presence of magnesium oxide decreases some bitter irritating substances and the laxative action requiring a higher dosage than the other preparations. The usual dose is 5 ml; range of dose is 5 to 15 ml. For infants the dose is 1 to 2 ml; for children, 2 to 8 ml.

Cascara tablets. Cascara tablets are available in 120-, 200-, and 300-mg tablets. The average dose is 300 mg (gr 5) for adults. The dose of cascara tablets is 120 to 250 mg.

Senna

Senna is obtained from the dried leaves of the *Cassia acutifolia* plant and may cause hemorrhagic gastritis and nephritis. The dried leaves have been used to make a homemade infusion of the drug, which is decidedly potent. It produces a thorough bowel evacuation in 6 to 12 hours and is likely to be accompanied by abdominal pain or gripping. It resembles cascara but is more powerful. It is found in the proprietary remedies Castoria and Syrup of Figs.

Senna tea is an infusion of senna leaves made from a teaspoonful of leaves to a cup of hot water.

A powdered concentrate of senna, obtained from the pod of the plant, is said to contain the desirable laxative components but to be free of the impurities that in previous preparations have been the cause of griping. This compound is sold under the name of Senokot (tablets, syrup, and granules), and the usual adult dose is two tablets or 1 teaspoon of the granules.

Preparation, dosage, and administration

Senna syrup. The usual dose is 8 ml orally for adults.

Senna fluidextract. The usual dose is 2 ml orally for adults.

OTHER STIMULANTS
Castor oil (oleum ricini)

Castor oil is obtained from the seeds of the castor bean, *Ricinus communis,* a plant that grows in India but that is also cultivated in a number of places where the climate is warm. Castor oil is a bland, colorless, emollient glyceride that passes through the stomach unchanged, but, like other fatty substances, it retards the emptying of the stomach and for this reason is usually given when the stomach is empty. In the small intestine the oil is hydrolyzed by pancreatic lipase to glycerol and a fatty acid, ricinoleic acid. This fatty acid is responsible for the irritation of the bowel, especially the small intestine. It rarely reaches the large intestine before causing irritation. Its irritating effect causes a rapid propulsion of contents from the small intestine, including any of the oil that may have escaped hydrolysis. A therapeutic dose will produce several copious semiliquid stools in 2 to 6 hours; it should not be given at bedtime. Some persons have little or no gripping or coliclike distress, whereas others may experience considerable abdominal cramping and exhaustion. Patients who have an irritable bowel or lesions in the bowel may be made very ill.

The fluid nature of the stool is caused by the rapid passage of the fecal content rather than by a diffusion of fluid into the bowel. Castor oil tends to empty the bowel completely; hence, no evacuation is likely to occur for a day or so after its administration. The drug is excreted into the milk of nursing mothers.

Uses. Castor oil is used much less often today than formerly. It continues to be used in the preparation of certain patients who are to have a roentgenographic examination of abdominal viscera. Because of its irritant action, it is contraindicated for patients with ulcerative lesions of the bowel, pregnant women, or nursing mothers.

Preparation, dosage, and administration. The usual adult dose of castor oil is 15 to 60 ml, and it is given orally. Dose for children is 5 to 15 ml.

The natural oil may be unpleasant and nauseating. This may be overcome by the use of fruit juices or pharmaceutical mixtures (neoloid) to emulsify and disguise the oil.

Phenolphthalein tablets

Phenolphthalein, a phenol derivative, is a synthetic substance, the laxative action of which is similar to that of the anthracene group. It is a white powder insoluble in water but soluble in the juice of the intestine, where it exerts its relatively mild irritant action. Evacuation is produced in 6 to 8 hours, unaccompanied by gripping. It acts on both the small and the large bowels, particularly the latter. When given orally, part (15%) of the drug is absorbed and resecreted into the bile (enterohepatic), and thus a prolonged laxative action may be obtained for 3 to 4 days. If the urine and feces are alkaline, they will be pink-red in color from this drug.

Repeated large doses may cause cardiac and respiratory distress, nausea, and in some susceptible individuals an allergic skin rash (pink-purple color) may appear. In other cases a prolonged and excessive purgative effect may indicate individual idiosyncrasy. The drug is odorless and tasteless and relatively pleasant to take; it is found in a number of proprietary preparations and is sold in a candylike form (Ex-Lax) and in a chewing gum (Feen-A-Mint). Children should not be allowed free access to these preparations, since they are likely to regard them as ordinary candy or gum and may get an overdose of the drug. Deaths have been reported from such accidents, although the dose causing toxicity is large.

Preparation, dosage, and administration. Tablets are available in 60- and 120-mg amounts. The usual dose is 60 mg orally.

Phenolphthalein is found in some proprietary preparations with other laxatives such as agar and liquid petrolatum, as well as with other irritant laxatives.

Bisacodyl (Dulcolax, others)

Bisacodyl is a relatively nontoxic laxative agent that reflexly stimulates peristalsis on contact with the mucosa of the colon. Bisacodyl has been successful in the treatment of various types of constipation. In larger doses, it is also widely used for cleansing the bowel before some surgeries and proctoscopic and roentgenographic examinations. Bisacodyl is insoluble in neutral or alkaline solution and should not be taken within 1 hour after antacids have been administered. It may cause abdominal cramps.

Preparation, dosage, and administration. Bisacodyl is available in 5-mg tablets for oral administration, 10-mg suppositories for rectal administration, and an enema (10 mg/30 ml). The suppositories act within 15 to 60 minutes, while the tablets produce evacuation of the bowel in 6 to 10 hours. The suppositories may cause a burning sensation and proctitis. The tablets are enteric coated and should not be

chewed or administered chipped. (To avoid release of the drug in the stomach and the possibility of emesis, therefore, the tablets should not be administered with milk, dairy products, or antacids.) They should be administered with water only.

BULK-FORMING LAXATIVES

Hydrophilic colloids stimulate peristalsis by increasing bulk and therefore modifying the consistency of the stool. This mechanism of laxative action is a normal stimulus and is one of the least harmful. These drugs do not interfere with absorption of food, but they can cause fecal impaction and obstruction, so it is important to give them with adequate fluids (8 ounces). The effect of these laxatives may not be apparent for 12 to 24 hours, and their full effect may not be achieved until the second or third day after administration. Some physicians maintain that bran and dried fruits (such as prunes and figs) exert the same effect, and they prefer to advise these foods rather than the bulk-forming laxatives.

The bulk-forming or bulk-producing laxatives are often the first choice for constipation. They are also used in irritable bowel syndrome, diverticular disease, postpartum constipation, and the elderly.

The laxatives comprising this group are polycarbophil and other natural or semisynthetic cellulose derivatives made from agar, plantago seed, kelp, and plant gums. Often these products are combined with fecal softeners (Dialose) or stimulant laxatives (Dialose Plus). They may also be emulsified with liquid petrolatum (Petrogalar, Agoral), cascara, phenolphthalein, or milk of magnesia.

The mineral oil and agar emulsions are widely advertised but are of little value because the agar content is so small (2% to 6%). The laxative effect of these emulsions is usually caused by the addition of some other ingredient.

Side effects and toxic effects. Flatulence and bulky stools may occur with the use of the bulk-forming laxatives. Because of the possibility of impaction or obstruction if fluid intake is not substantial, these laxatives should be avoided in patients with stenosis, adhesions, or dyspha-

Drugs acting on the gastrointestinal tract **517**

gia. The effervescent type of bulk-producing laxatives has sodium carbonate as an ingredient in the amount of about 250 mg per dose (Metamucil Instant Mix), and this is to be avoided by a patient on sodium restriction. The bulk-forming laxatives interact with salicylates, digitalis drugs, and other drugs by inhibiting their absorption from the gastrointestinal tract. When moistened, they swell, forming a mass of material that passes through the intestine without being affected by the digestive juices, and by their blandness and bulk they make the stool large and soft so that it is easily moved along the colon and into the rectum.

Polycarbophil calcium (Mitrolan)

Polycarbophil is used to normalize stools both in diarrhea and in constipation by restoring the normal moisture level and providing bulk in the intestinal tract. In diarrheal conditions the intestinal mucosa is unable to absorb the excess fecal water. This agent absorbs the water by forming a gel in the intestinal lumen, thus creating formed stools. In constipation the agent retains water in the lumen; each dose for constipation is followed by at least 8 ounces of water or other suitable liquid. Nonsystemic effects have been reported. Each tablet has a sodium content of about 0.02 mEq (0.46 mg). As with all hydrophilic agents, polycarbophil is not to be used in patients with intestinal obstruction. The even spacing of small doses overcomes abdominal fullness. Tablets (citrus/vanilla flavor and contains calcium) should be chewed thoroughly before swallowing. Adults may use up to 12 tablets in 24 hours. Children ages 6 to 12 use no more than 6 tablets in 24 hours, and children ages 3 to 6 may use up to 3 tablets in 24 hours.

Methylcellulose (Cologel, Hydrolose)

Methylcellulose is a synthetic hydrophilic colloid. It is a grayish white, fibrous powder that, in the presence of water, swells and produces a viscous, colloidal solution in the upper part of the alimentary tract. In the colon this solution loses water and forms a gel that increases the bulk and softness of the stool.

Preparation, dosage, and administration. Methylcellulose is available in 500-mg tablets or as a syrup (200 mg/ml). It is administered orally two to four times daily in doses of 1 to 1.5 g. It should be accompanied by one or two glasses of water. The dosage is gradually reduced as normal defecation reflexes establish a normal pattern for the behavior of the bowel. Tablets should not be chewed to avoid risk of esophageal obstruction. Results occur within 12 to 72 hours.

Plantago seed (psyllium seed)

Plantago seed is the dried ripe seed of the *Plantago psyllium, Plantago indica,* or *Plantago ovata.* The small, brown or blond seeds contain a mucilaginous material that swells in the presence of moisture to form a jellylike indigestible mass. The main disadvantage lies in the fact that although the seeds swell, their ends remain sharp and may be the cause of irritation in the alimentary tract. At present, only the preparations of the extracted gums are available, and these have the advantage of causing less mechanical irritation.

Preparation, dosage, and administration. The following are preparations of plantago.

Psyllium hydrophilic mucilloid (Metamucil). Psyllium hydrophilic mucilloid is a white- to cream-colored powder containing about 50% powdered mucilaginous portion (outer epidermis) of blond psyllium seeds and about 50% dextrose. This mixture is used in the treatment of constipation because it promotes the formation of a soft, water-retaining gelatinous residue in the lower bowel within 12 to 72 hours. In addition, it has a demulcent effect on inflamed mucosa. The dosage is 4 to 7 g one to three times daily. It should be stirred into an 8-ounce glass of cool water or other fluid, drunk while in suspension, followed by an additional 8-ounce glass of cool fluid to avoid an obstruction of the esophagus.

Plantago ovata coating (Konsyl). *Plantago ovata* coating is a cream- to brown-colored granular powder obtained from the *Plantago ovata* (blond psyllium, mucilaginous portion). The dosage is 5 to 10 g three times daily before meals in a glass of water or milk. It should be swallowed before it thickens. Results occur within 12 to 72 hours.

LUBRICANT OR EMOLLIENT LAXATIVES
Mineral oil; liquid paraffin

Mineral oil (liquid petrolatum, mo) is a mixture of liquid hydrocarbons obtained from petroleum. The oil is not digested and absorption is minimal. It softens the fecal mass and prevents excessive absorption of water. It is especially useful when it is desirable to keep feces soft and when straining at stool must be reduced, as after abdominal surgery, rectal operations, prevention of hemorrhoidal tearing, repair of hernias, cerebrovascular or spinal cord accidents, aneurysm, or myocardial infarction. It may be useful for patients who have a chronic type of constipation because of prolonged inactivity, as in the case of patients with orthopedic conditions.

Some physicians object to the use of mineral oil on the basis that it dissolves (acts as a lipid solvent) certain of the fat-soluble vitamins (A, D, E, and K), food, and bile salts and inhibits their absorption. Others maintain that only the precursor to vitamin A (carotene) is so affected and that natural vitamin A is quantitatively absorbed from the intestine in the presence of mineral oil. Another objection to its use is that in large doses it tends to leak or seep from the rectum, which may interfere with healing of postoperative wounds in the region of the anus and perineum. Although absorption of mineral oil is limited, it is said to give rise to a chronic inflammatory reaction in tissues where it is found after absorption. Indiscriminate use by the elderly and weak should not be encouraged. Mineral oil may also produce a lipid pneumonia if drops coating the pharynx gain access to the trachea. It should not be used routinely by pregnant women, since it decreases vitamin K availability to the fetus. The vitamin K deficiency is important in patients receiving oral anticoagulant therapy. Concurrent use with fecal moistening agents should be avoided, since they increase absorption of mineral oil.

Preparation, dosage, and administration. Mineral oil is administered in doses that range from 15 to 45 ml for adults to 10 to 15 ml for children over 6 years of age. It is best given on an empty stomach or at bedtime. The onset is 6 to 8 hours. It should not be given immediately after meals, since it may delay the passage of food from the stomach. Most patients may have a slice of orange or glass of orange juice to relieve the oily taste in the mouth. Mineral oil is also to be found as the major ingredient of some oil retention enemas (such as, Fleet mineral oil enema).

Olive oil; corn oil; cottonseed oil

Olive oil and cottonseed oil are digestible oils, but if given in sufficient quantity, they may act as emollient laxatives, since part of the oil will escape hydrolysis.

When administered in doses of 30 ml, these oils act as laxatives. They may be given orally or rectally. The dose for infants is 4 to 8 ml.

FECAL MOISTENING AGENTS (STOOL SOFTENERS, SURFACTANTS, OR WETTING SOLUTIONS)

With the introduction of fecal moistening agents and other less toxic synthetic drugs, there seems to be more restricted use of stimulant laxatives. Fecal moistening agents are constantly being improved and have achieved a level of popular therapy.

Sodium docusate (dioctyl sodium sulfosuccinate)

Sodium docusate acts in a manner similar to that of detergents and permits water and fatty substance to penetrate and to be well mixed with the fecal material. Thus this agent promotes the formation of soft formed stools (occasionally diarrhea) and is a useful aid in the treatment of constipation. One or 2 days may be required for full effects.

It is said to have a wide margin of safety and negligible toxicity. There is some question about the advisability of giving it concurrently with mineral oil, since there is a possibility that it may promote absorption of the oil.

Uses. Sodium docusate is indicated for patients with rectal impaction, hemorrhoids, chronic constipation, postpartum constipation, and painful conditions of the rectum and anus and for those who should avoid straining (such as with rectal surgery or myocardial infarction) at the time of defecation. It is particularly useful for bedridden patients, especially children. When used with aspirin, an increased incidence of mucosal damage occurs. It may interfere with the absorption of nutrients and some vitamins.

Preparation, dosage, and administration. The following are available preparations of dioctyl sodium sulfosuccinate.

Sodium docusate (Colace DSS, Doxinate, Comfolax). Sodium docusate is available in 50-, 60-, 100-, and 240-mg capsules; in solution, 10 and 50 mg/ml; and as a syrup, 4 mg/ml. The usual dosage for adults and children over 12 is 50 to 360 mg daily and 10 to 50 mg for infants and young children. Solutions of the drug are best given in fruit juice or milk.

Peri-Colace. Peri-Colace includes casanthranol, which provides gentle peristaltic stimulation. Either dioctyl sodium sulfosuccinate or casanthranol produces a bowel movement in 8 to 12 hours.

Calcium docusate (dioctyl calcium sulfosuccinate) (Surfak, DCS). Calcium docusate is claimed to provide superior surfactant activity to the older chemical, dioctyl sodium. It is indicated in conditions in which cathartic therapy is undesirable but in which prevention of constipation is necessary. A wide margin of safety is claimed. The drug is administered in 240-mg capsules; the usual dose is one capsule daily.

Dialose. Dialose is a combination of dioctyl sodium sulfosuccinate and sodium carboxymethylcellulose. It combines the advantages of both drugs—fecal-moistening and bulk-producing agents. Dialose Plus also includes oxyphenisatin acetate, which is a peristaltic stimulant. Recommended dosages are one capsule two or three times a day, taken with a glass of water.

Hyperosmotic suppository

Glycerin suppositories are available in adult, child, and infant sizes. They promote peristalsis through local irritation of the mucous membrane of the rectum. The adult dose is 3 g; for children under 6 years of age the dose is 1.15 g. The effects are achieved in 15 minutes to 1 hour.

NURSING IMPLICATIONS

As is true for all medications, the nurse must exercise caution in giving advice about laxatives. Persons who seek help because they are becoming increasingly dependent on laxatives should be encouraged to seek the advice of a physician. Frequently, powerful, self-prescribed laxatives empty the whole colon, which then requires time to collect material. In the meantime, the patient may again be distressed because there has been no daily bowel movement and take another laxative, thereby initiating a vicious cycle that may lead to dependency. Whatever the case, the patient should be helped to overcome his dependency.

Nurses should direct their efforts toward teaching the patient practices that promote normal bowel habits. In doing so, they must bear in mind that teaching in this area may be met with some resistance, so they should attempt to achieve a nonthreatening atmosphere. The patient's bowel complaints should be listened to and his habits explored to determine the possible cause of the bowel disorder. Appropriate teaching can then be directed to the problem in relation to the patient's intellectual level, his socioeconomic background (which influences the type of food he eats), and his receptivity. Frequently, entire families have similar bowel habits and sometimes the mother is an excellent intermediary for change. Individuals may have anywhere from three bowel movements each day to three bowel movements each week. Alterations in the diet to provide more fiber and bulk, such as whole grain breads and cereals, more fruit, less refined foods, vegetables, and bran sprinkled on selected foods, may relieve some of the constipation. The consumption of at least eight glasses of liquid daily is recommended. If the patient is able to incorporate more exercise into the daily routine such as walking, bicycling, or using stairs instead of an elevator, this aids in decreasing the constipation.

Elderly persons who have some degree of constipation cannot be treated in the same way as younger patients. They cannot be expected to change the habit patterns of a lifetime or to subject themselves to tiresome diets that disturb the peace required by the elderly person. It may be decidedly unwise to urge an elderly person to increase the roughage of his diet. He may not have the teeth or the type of bowel to make such an adjustment happily. After an examination, the physician frequently prescribes a laxative for more or less regular use, and if it produces satisfactory results (no gripping or gaseous distention), there is probably little need to worry about the laxative habit.

The nurse should be familiar with the following drugs that have been implicated in constipation: antacids containing aluminum, anticholinergics, calcium carbonate, ganglionic blocking agents, iron, opiates, phenothiazines, sedatives, tricyclic antidepressants, and multivitamins containing iron; the abuse of laxatives will also cause constipation. If the patient intends to nurse an infant, stimulant laxatives should not be used, since they may be passed into the breast milk. Chronic constipation may be linked to hemorrhoids, diverticulosis, and cancer of the colon, and laxatives may mask the underlying symptoms of these and other conditions (such as a drug's side effect of constipation). There may also be aspects of the patient's life-style that cause constipation.

Antidiarrheals

The term "diarrhea" is descriptive of a symptom of an underlying disease, which describes the abnormal passage of stools with increased frequency, increased fluidity, or increased weight. Diarrhea is acute when it is of a sudden onset in a previously healthy individual, lasting about 3 days to a few (3) weeks, is self-limiting, and resolves without sequelae. Morbid and mortal consequences are seen in the following: underdeveloped and malnourished populations, the elderly, infants, and debilitated persons. Chronic diarrhea lasts for over 3 to 4 weeks, with the recurring passage of diarrheal stools, anorexia, weight reduction, and chronic weakness; it is the result of multiple etiologic factors, necessitating definitive treatment directed to the organic cause(s).

Some causes of both acute and chronic diarrhea are outlined on p. 521. The causes are variable and exist in a spectrum of psychogenic to neoplastic origins.

The objectives of treatment are to (1) replenish fluid and electrolyte loss, (2) ascertain, if possible, the cause(s) of diarrhea, (3) reduce the frequency of evacuation, (4) adsorb toxins, (5) restore the intestinal flora, and (6) direct treatment at underlying cause(s).

Nonspecific treatment is directed at the increased stool frequency, which burdens daily life-style; the alleviation of abdominal cramps; the prevention of dehydration and metabolic acidosis from fluid and electrolyte loss; and the minimization of weight loss and nutritional deficits resulting from malabsorption. Specific treatment is directed at the cause or condition creating the diarrhea.

Ideally, the nursing process lends itself to ascertaining the type or cause of diarrhea to be treated through careful individual patient evaluation. Such evaluative questions for discovering the cause(s) may be used in assessing the following criteria:

Age of the patient
Occupation
Duration of diarrhea (precipitating factors tantamount to onset)
Stool description (frequency of evacuation, rectal bleeding or black stool appearance, foul-smelling odor, light color, or greasy consistency)
Medication profile (prescribed and self-administered as over-the-counter drugs)
Presence or absence of anorexia, weight reduction (involuntary), fever
Ingestion of foods, toxic substances, milk intake, alcohol use
Travel abroad or bordering countries
Symptom description (location)
Relief obtained, if any, and treatment modality
Chronic diseases, presence of acute or concurrent illness, emotional or behavioral problems

The extent of fluid and electrolyte loss may be seen by tachycardia, postural hypotension, elevated hematocrit or blood urea nitrogen, and poor skin turgor. The stool specimen may reveal occult blood (gastrointestinal bleeding), fecal leukocytes, parasites, or fat. Endocrine diseases such as diabetes mellitus and hyperthyroidism should not be overlooked. Hospitalization is needed for dehydration that would

---

Causes of acute and chronic diarrhea

Causes of acute diarrhea

A. Bacterial
  1. Invasive organisms
     a. *Campylobacter fetus (jejuni)*
     b. *Escherichia coli* (enteropathogenic)
     c. *Salmonella*
     d. *Shigella*
     e. Staphylococci
  2. Noninvasive toxigenic organisms
     a. Cholera *(Vibrio cholerae)* endotoxin
     b. *Escherichia coli* (enterotoxigenic) toxin
  3. Food poisoning as toxin mediated
     a. *Bacillus cereus*
     b. *Clostridium perfringens*
     c. *Salmonella*
     d. *Staphylococcus aureus*
B. Viral
  1. Adenoviruses
  2. Coxsackievirus
  3. Coronaviruses
  4. Echoviruses
  5. Norwalk agent
  6. Rotavirus
C. Protozoal
  1. Amebic dysentery *(Entamoeba histolytica)* amebiasis
  2. Giardiasis *(Giardia lamblia)*
D. Drug induced
  1. Antacids (magnesium containing)
  2. Antiadrenergic antihypertensives
     a. Guanethidine
     b. Methyldopa
     c. Reserpine
  3. Antibiotics
     a. Ampicillin
     b. Cephalexin
     c. Clindamycin (clindamycin colitis associated with toxin-producing *Clostridium difficile*)
     d. Chloramphenicol
     e. Erythromycin
     f. Lincomycin
     g. Neomycin
     h. Penicillin G
     i. Tetracyclines
     j. Trimethoprim-sulfamethoxazole
  4. Antineoplastics
  5. Antitubercular agents
  6. Chenodeoxycholic acid
  7. Colchicine
  8. Digitalis
  9. Ferrous sulfate
  10. Laxatives
  11. Nitrofurantoin
  12. Parasympathomimetic (alpha agonist) drugs
  13. Quinidine
  14. Sorbitol
E. Nutritional
  1. Allergy
  2. Ingestion without discretion (spicy, fatty, roughage, seeds, preformed toxin)
F. Other
  1. Carcinoma
  2. Diverticulitis
  3. Neurogenic
  4. Psychogenic
  5. Radiation therapy
  6. Regional and ulcerative colitis
  7. Stress

Causes of chronic diarrhea

A. Addison's disease
B. Diabetic enteropathy/neuropathy
C. Iatrogenic
  1. Bacterial overgrowth
  2. Postsurgical
D. Inflammatory bowel disease
  1. Chronic ulcerative and granulomatous colitis
  2. Chron's enteritis
E. Irritable bowel syndrome
F. Malabsorption syndrome
G. Pancreatic adenoma—nongastrin secreting, such as watery diarrhea-hypokalemia-achlorhydria (WDHA)
H. Pancreatic insufficiency
I. Thyroid—hyperthyroidism
J. Tumors
  1. Carcinoma of colon and rectum
  2. Intestinal
  3. Lymphoma
  4. Polyposis
  5. Villous adenoma
K. Other
  1. Blind loops
  2. Carcinoid syndrome
  3. Enteritis
  4. Gastrointestinal hormones
  5. Gluten enteropathy
  6. Lactose deficiency
  7. Medullary carcinoma of thyroid
  8. Scleroderma
  9. Strictures
  10. Tuberculosis
  11. Uremia
  12. Whipple's disease
  13. Zollinger-Ellison syndrome

---

compromise a patient with congestive heart failure or chronic renal disease, since this complicates fluid replacement efforts. If any child or infant is unable to consume oral replacement fluid, hospitalization is needed to replace fluids and maintain urine flow. Bed rest alone may reduce stool frequency. In addition to the child or infant, the elderly patient with a poor medical history, a patient with chronic illness, and pregnant women are at risk from acute or chronic diarrhea.

Maintenance of fluid and electrolyte balance

is the most important goal of supportive therapy in acute diarrhea; if left untreated, a loss of anions (bicarbonate, organic anions as short-chain fatty acids) will create a gain of hydrogen ion resulting in metabolic acidosis, which will be exacerbated by the often concomitant ketoacidosis of starvation and acidosis of prerenal azotemia. As volume increases in diarrhea, a rise in sodium and chloride develops with a decrease in potassium concentration. The decreased contact time of the luminal contents with the mucosal surface decreases the passive secretion of potassium. The electrolyte composition of stool water will then be close to that of plasma. The electrolyte loss of sodium, potassium, chloride, and bicarbonate is the basis of the therapy.

It is recommended that clear liquids (noncarbonated soft drinks, fruit juice, diluted and flavored gelatin, and apple juice) and a bland diet are continued for 1 to 2 days. According to the cause of the diarrhea, several different medications can be given along with bed rest and nutritional support. These are listed below:

Activated attapulgite
Activated charcoal
Adsorbents
Aluminum hydroxide
Antibiotics, some
Anticholinergic activity drugs
Antiemetics
Aspirin
Belladonna alkaloids
Bismuth salts
Bulk-forming products
Cholestyramine
Colestipol
Digestive enzymes
Kaolin and pectin
Lactobacillus cultures
Metronidazole
Narcotic derivations
Quinacrine
Sedatives
Smooth muscle relaxants
Steroids
Sulfasalazine
Tranquilizers
Zinc phenolsulfocarbolate
Zinc phenolsulfonate

This section will focus on the drugs with a direct pharmacologic effect on the gastrointes-

tinal tract. The drugs providing symptomatic therapy do not alter the pathophysiology of diarrhea and do not provide electrolyte and fluid loss prevention. Although these drugs decrease the number, consistency, and fluidity of the stool, there is no absolute clinical evidence that an effective antidiarrheal therapeutic benefit accrues to the patient, but there is a relief of the bothersome symptoms that interrupt daily life routines.

ADSORBENTS

Adsorbents act by coating the walls of the gastrointestinal tract, adsorbing the bacteria or toxins causing the diarrhea, and passing them out with the stools. Examples of drugs in this class *not requiring* a prescription are activated charcoal, aluminum hydroxide, bismuth salts, kaolin, pectin, and activated attapulgite. Colestipol and cholestyramine are anion exchange resins *requiring a prescription.*

Kaolin is a natural hydrated aluminum silicate that is relatively inert but carries the danger of obstruction; stools appear to be more formed with this agent. The adsorbents kaolin, pectin, activated charcoal, and attapulgite are recognized as safe in therapeutic doses. Pectin causes a decrease in the intestinal pH, which destroys bacterial growth due to the unfavorable acid medium. The anion exchange resins (colestipol and cholestyramine) have adsorbent affinity directed at acidic materials (bile acids and so forth). The bismuth salts are used as adsorbents, astringents, and protectives.

Generally the adsorbent preparations are taken after each loose bowel movement until the diarrhea has been controlled. Constipation may develop because of the large amounts of the adsorbent products that must be used.

Drug interactions. A caution with all the adsorbents is the interference with absorption of medications given concurrently (such as, digoxin, clindamycin, lincomycin, and quinidine). The interactions are a function of their adsorbent properties. The drugs and nutrients adsorbed include a wide range of ingested substances. These may be decreased by administering the adsorbent 2 or more hours before or after a drug (except when used to inactivate a drug or desired poison for overdose therapy).

Kaolin with pectin (Kaopectate, others)

Kaolin with pectin is a suspension with 6 g kaolin and 130 mg pectin/30 ml; the dosage is 60 to 120 ml after each loose bowel movement.

Preparations, dosage, and administration

Kaopectate concentrate. Kaopectate concentrate is a mint-flavored liquid with 8.78 g kaolin and 195 mg pectin/30 ml; the dosage is 45 to 90 ml after each loose bowel movement.

Pectocel. Pectocel is a suspension of kaolin, pectin, and zinc phenolsulfonate; the dosage is 30 to 60 ml every 1 or 2 hours for 3 or 4 doses.

Quintess

Quintess suspension contains activated attapulgite, colloidal activated attapulgite, and 0.9% alcohol. The dosage is 30 ml immediately, then 15 ml after each loose bowel movement. Polymagma Plain Tablets contain activated attapulgite, pectin, and hydrated alumina powder. The dosage is four tablets immediately, followed by two tablets after each loose bowel movement.

Bismuth subsalicylate (Pepto-Bismol)

Bismuth subsalicylate is available in suspension and chewable tablets. The adult dosage is 30 ml or two tablets chewed or dissolved every 30 minutes to 1 hour up to eight doses. In a dose of 2 ounces every 6 hours it can be used prophylactically against pathogens by preventing them from attaching themselves to the intestinal wall and impeding their replication in the gut.

Since bismuth subsalicylate is a salicylate, it may be contraindicated in those with an allergy to aspirin (such as, asthmatic patients with nasal polyps and allergy to Tartrazine dye) and should be used with caution when the patient is taking a coumarin anticoagulant. A dose of 2 ounces of bismuth subsalicylate produces the same blood level as an aspirin tablet. It can be used to prevent traveler's diarrhea

as an alternative to antibiotic (doxycycline) therapy.

Activated charcoal (Charcocaps, charcoal)

Activated charcoal is indicated for the prevention and relief of intestinal gas and diarrhea and gastrointestinal distress associated with indigestion by acting as an adsorbent and detoxicant of irritants. It may also adsorb medication, nutrients, and enzymes.

The activated vegetable charcoal is administered as two capsules repeated every 30 minutes to 1 hour as needed up to eight doses (16 Charcocaps) for treatment of diarrhea symptoms. Tablets may be chewed or dissolved in mouth followed by water.

Cholestyramine (Questran)

Cholestyramine has a direct adsorbent affinity for acidic materials (bile acids and so forth). It must be diluted with suitable liquid (fruit juice) or added to applesauce and administered not less than 2 hours before meals or drugs to lessen the chances of binding with fat-soluble vitamins and other materials.

ANTICHOLINERGICS

The belladonna alkaloids—atropine, hyoscyamine and hyoscine, and homatropine methylbromide—are found in antidiarrheal products often with the adsorbents and other antidiarrheal agents as opium extracts. These are effective agents in treating diarrhea, but the recommended doses found in nonprescription products are somewhat ineffective. The higher effective doses have a narrow margin of safety in both children and adults.

The belladonna alkaloids, however, offer effectiveness in the treatment of diarrhea by causing an intestinal tone increase and peristalsis at doses of 0.6 to 1 mg of atropine sulfate, thus decreasing intestinal cramps and pain. The "cotton mouth" or "dry mouth" effect usually indicates therapeutic effective drug levels when these doses are administered. This dose of atropine, however, requires a prescription.

The following warnings on these products should be heeded by the nurse: not to be used by persons having glaucoma or excessive pressure within the eye; not to be used by children under 6 years of age; discontinue use if blurring of vision, rapid pulse, or dizziness occurs; a dry mouth may occur, necessitating a lower dosage. These anticholinergics are also contraindicated in urinary retention; they may precipitate ileus and the toxic megacolon of ulcerative colitis.

The following toxic effects of belladonna alkaloids are dose related: an increase in viscosity of bronchial mucus; bradycardia and tachycardia; obstructive uropathy. They are contraindicated in patients with heart disease, hypertension, hyperthyroidism, and prostatic hypertrophy.

Donnagel

Donnagel is a suspension of kaolin and pectin, with 0.137 mg hyoscyamine sulfate, 0.019 mg atropine sulfate, and 0.0065 mg hyoscine hydrobromide in each 30 ml. The dosage is 30 ml immediately, then 15 to 30 ml after each loose bowel movement.

OPIATES

The opiates (codeine and paregoric) act by virtue of their constipative and sedative action; they lower the propulsive motility of the bowel, reduce pain, and relieve tenesmus. The delay in transit time of food permits contact time of intestinal contents with the absorptive surface of the bowel, which permits an increase in the reabsorptive capacity of water and electrolytes and reduces stool frequency and net volume.

The anticholinergics and opium derivatives decrease the motility of the bowel. They should not be used when the cause of diarrhea is an invading organism (as toxigenic bacteria or pseudomembranous enterocolitis) because these drugs permit epithelial penetration and multiplication of the organism by decreasing the intestinal motility with the subsequent lowered excretion of the organisms and their toxins.

Codeine and paregoric cause CNS depression and sedation, and this is a factor to consider if the patient is taking other CNS depressant drugs because of the additive effects. The opiates are short acting; frequent administration (4- to 6-hour intervals) is needed to control the gastrointestinal smooth muscle function.

Parepectolin suspension contains 15 mg opium, equivalent to 3.7 ml paregoric/30 ml, with kaolin and pectin and 0.69% alcohol; the dosage is 15 to 39 ml after each loose bowel movement. This Class V drug may not require a prescription. Parelixer is a liquid containing 0.2 ml tincture of opium/30 ml with pectin in an 18% alcoholic elixir with fruit flavor; the dosage is 15 to 30 ml three to four times daily. This Class V drug may not require a prescription. Dia-Quel liquid has 0.03 ml tincture of opium (0.75 ml paregoric) per 5 ml and homatropine and pectin in a 10% alcoholic base; the dosage is 15 to 30 ml three to four times daily. This Class V drug may not require a prescription.

Opium tincture deodorized

Tincture of opium, a hydroalcoholic (19% alcohol) solution, contains 10% opium with an average dose of 0.6 ml to 1.5 ml (which contains 6 to 15 mg morphine, respectively) four times daily. This is a Class II prescription under the Controlled Substances Act.

Paregoric

Paregoric (camphorated opium tincture) requires a prescription. It is a Class III drug and contains 20 mg of powdered opium/5 ml, which is equivalent to 2 mg of morphine. It is important that the nurse not confuse opium tincture deodorized (10 mg morphine equivalent/1 ml) and camphorated opium tincture (0.4 mg morphine equivalent/1 ml) because opium tincture deodorized has 25 times more of the morphine equivalent than camphorated opium tincture. Addiction liability has been reported with these preparations. When paregoric is in combination with another product, the schedule of the Controlled Substance Act permits it to become a Class V product when the product contains no more than 100 mg of opium or 25 ml of paregoric/100 ml of the mixture.

Codeine

Codeine, when administered at a dosage of 15 mg four times daily, has shown effective antidiarrheal properties, although a range of up to 240 mg daily is suggested. Donnagel-PG suspension contains 24 mg powdered opium/30 ml with kaolin, pectin, hyoscyamine, atropine, hyoscine, and a 5% alcohol base. The dosage is 30 ml immediately then 15 ml every 3 hours as needed for loose stools. The adult dose is 5 to 10 ml (2 to 4 mg morphine) four times daily and for children 0.25 to 0.5 ml/kg body weight.

INTESTINAL FLORA MODIFIERS

Intestinal flora modifiers are bacterial cultures that consist of viable *Lactobacillus* organisms to suppress the growth of diarrhea-causing pathogens and to reestablish the normal intestinal flora. They may be useful in the treatment of uncomplicated diarrhea (including that caused by antibiotic therapy) and acute fever blisters and canker sores. The nurse may consider the use of a diet rich in milk or buttermilk and yogurt and high in lactose or dextrose, since this is equally effective in colonizing the intestine.

Lactinex

Lactinex (*Lactobacillus acidophilus* and *bulgaricus*) is available in tablets and granules; they need to be refrigerated. The dosage for gastrointestinal disturbances is one packet of granules (or four tablets) added to or taken with cereal, food, milk, fruit juice, or water three or four times daily.

Bacid

Bacid capsules are *Lactobacillus acidophilus* in sodium carboxymethylcellulose. They should be administered with milk. The dosage is two capsules two to four times daily. A fruity odor may be apparent in the stools from these drugs.

OTHER ANTIDIARRHEALS
ANTIDIARRHEA AGENTS
Diphenoxylate hydrochloride (with added atropine sulfate) (Lomotil)

Diphenoxylate, a narcotic chemical analog of meperidine, inhibits intestinal propulsive motility by acting directly on intestinal smooth muscles and thus decreases transit time.

The half-life is about 2.5 hours (range 1.9 to 3.1 hours). Because of its short duration of action, it is administered four times or more daily. About half the total daily dose is excreted in the urine within 96 hours as metabolites.

This is indicative of an enterohepatic recycling through biliary elimination. Trace amounts are found in the breast milk.

An active free metabolite, difenoxine, is five times more potent in antidiarrheal effects.

The CNS depressant effects are potentiated by alcohol and other CNS depressant drugs. Long-term use with chronic toxicity has resulted in physical dependence and intestinal obstruction.

The patient with an overdose initially has an anticholinergic symptom followed by a delayed opiate effect. Subtherapeutic amounts of atropine are added to discourage or deter deliberate, intentional abuse by causing undesirable side effects. This contributes to the initial overdose picture of dry mucous membranes and skin, flushing, and urinary retention, which may render the gastrointestinal tract atonic, requiring lavage for up to 24 hours after ingestion. Abuse is directed at the morphine-like euphoria from diphenoxylate. The overdose of diphenoxylate is similar to that of morphine, including respiratory and cardiac arrest necessitating hospitalization and treatment with naloxone for respiratory depression. Habituation is reported even with the atropine added to deter abuse.

A dose of one tablet or 5 ml (2.5 mg diphenoxylate and 0.025 mg atropine sulfate) of the liquid is similar in antidiarrheal effect to 4 ml paregoric.

Preparation, dosage, and administration. One tablet is equivalent to 5 ml liquid. For adults, one to two tablets (5 to 10 ml) is given three or four times a day until symptomatic control is achieved, then the dosage is reduced. Liquid dosage form only, with a calibrated dropper, for children. For children from 2 to 5 years (13 to 20 kg), 4 ml (2 mg) is given three times a day; for those 5 to 8 years (20 to 27 kg), 4 ml (2 mg) is given four times a day; for children 8 to 12 years (27 to 36 kg), 4 ml (2 mg) is given five times a day.

Contraindications. Diphenoxylate is not recommended in children under 2 years of age. The therapeutic-to-toxic ratio range is narrow. The 0.025 mg/5 ml of atropine (or one tablet) can produce acute atropine toxicity in young children. Because of its enterohepatic recycling, it is contraindicated in jaundiced patients or those with advanced hepatic disease. Intestinal bowel obstruction may occur in patients with ulcerative colitis.

Side effects. Drowsiness, dizziness, and dry mouth are frequently reported. Because of the potential for serious intoxication in children (with only six tablets), parents must keep this medication in secure storage to prevent a child's access.

Methscopolamine bromide (Pamine)

Methscopolamine bromide is a parasympatholytic drug that inhibits gastric secretion and also decreases gastrointestinal motility. The recommended dosage is 2.5 mg before meals and at bedtime.

Aspirin and other prostaglandin inhibitors

Aspirin and other prostaglandin inhibitors (such as, indomethacin and bismuth subsalicylate) may be used in diarrhea by preventing the activation of adenylcyclase; prostaglandins may affect the fluid production created by the microorganisms or the enterotoxin produced. Aspirin has also been used for the diarrhea produced by abdominal radiation (972 mg four times daily before meals).

Loperamide hydrochloride (Imodium)

Loperamide is a synthetic oral antidiarrheal with a chemical structure related to haloperidol and similar to diphenoxylate. It inhibits peristalsis in the intestinal wall, improving both stool frequency and consistency. The slowing of intestinal motility is a direct effect on the modulating cholinergic and noncholinergic neuronal pathways of the intestinal wall. This may be related to loperamide's binding affinity to opiate receptors in the ileum.

Uses. Indications include symptomatic control of acute and chronic diarrhea (as in inflammatory bowel disease) and in ileostomy patients to decrease the volume of intestinal discharge due to the intestinal resection. The results are prolonged intestinal transit time, increase in density and viscosity of discharge, and normalization of diarrheal-induced loss of fluid and electrolytes. It may be used in diarrhea secondary to radiation therapy or diarrhea

following gastrointestinal surgery. Investigational uses indicate that peak plasma levels are highest within 5 hours after administration of a dose. Plasma half-life ranges from 7 to 15 hours, with elimination half-life up to 15 hours (11-hour average). One hour following an oral dose, 85% of loperamide is found in the gastrointestinal tract; 25% of a 4-mg dose is excreted in the feces within 3 days, while 1.3% is found in the urine.

Antidiarrheal agents (like diphenoxylate, loperamide, or narcotics) should not be administered for acute diarrhea or traveler's diarrhea that are caused by bacteria (enterotoxin-producing strains of *Escherichia coli*, *Salmonella* or *Shigella*), parasites *(Giardia lamblia)*, and viruses (parvovirus or reovirus) because these penetrate the intestinal wall if retained in the intestine and must be eliminated in the feces. These agents must not be used with antibiotic-induced pseudomembranous colitis. If after 48 to 72 hours of therapy the symptoms of acute diarrhea have not clinically improved, if fever persists, or if blood and/or mucus appear in the stool, these agents should be discontinued.

Dosage and administration. For acute diarrhea, 4 mg is given orally, then 2 mg after each loose stool, usually not exceeding eight capsules (16 mg) daily. The long duration of action lends itself to twice daily dosage. Safety and effectiveness in children under 12 years have not been assessed. Paralytic ileus and prolonged stool retention occur in young children. For chronic diarrhea, the dose begins as in acute diarrhea and is then titrated to individual patient needs. The dosage may be administered in single dose (because of the long duration of action) or divided doses.

Side effects and toxic effects. Central nervous system fatigue and dizziness are seen only when therapeutic doses are greatly exceeded. This may be related to the structural similarity to haloperidol. Drug-induced gastrointestinal side effects are difficult to separate from those of diarrhea itself (epigastric pain, abdominal cramps, nausea, dry mouth, vomiting, anorexia). Skin rash hypersensitivity has been reported. Overdose symptoms include CNS depression, constipation, gastrointestinal irritation, nausea, and vomiting. Naloxone may reverse the CNS depression but the long duration of action of loperamide requires the nurse to monitor the vital signs for at least 24 hours and to repeat naloxone (because of naloxone's short duration of action) when necessary for recurring symptoms. Fluid and electrolyte levels must also be carefully watched.

NURSING IMPLICATIONS

The nurse is often required to provide information to persons traveling outside the United States. The following advice is critical in the prevention of "traveler's diarrhea." Where it is thought that sanitation is less than optimal, the traveler should avoid tap water, salads, cold sandwiches, uncooked vegetables, and ice. The water used in oral hygiene for brushing the teeth from the tap is also to be avoided. The traveler should only eat cooked food that is hot when served, and fruit should be peeled by the traveler. Only the following should be recommended to drink: water that is boiled or disinfected with chlorine or iodine compounds, carbonated water bottled with the cap closed from the manufacturer, soft drinks, beer, or wine. Milk products whether pasteurized or not are to be avoided.

The nurse may provide a simple formula to the traveler to be used conveniently as a glucose-electrolyte replacement solution that may be prepared in advance or obtained with ease.

The traveler may prepare and refrigerate a formula of glucose (from honey or corn syrup) and salts (sodium and potassium chloride) for the voluminous cholera-like losses of water and electrolytes. The combination can be placed in small waterproof plastic vials. The formula is as follows: glucose, 20 g; sodium chloride (table salt), 3.5 g; sodium bicarbonate (baking soda), 2.5 g; and potassium chloride (salt substitutes), 1.5 g. This combination is placed into 1 liter of boiled or bottled water and refrigerated to retard bacterial growth. The addition of these ingredients to the water should be made at time of use.

The glucose absorption stimulates the absorption of water and sodium since the small intestine's absorptive capacity is not radically altered during acute secretory diarrhea. This oral glucose and electrolyte solution will con- serve the net fluid and electrolytes; however, the stool volume will increase initially.

There are commercial solutions available such as Pedialyte, Lytren, or Gatorade that have electrolytes and contain high glucose concentrations. A preparation high in sodium may cause hypernatremia in children under 2 years of age. Gatorade has 23 mEq sodium/liter and 2.5 mEq potassium/liter. Pedialyte has 30 mEq sodium/liter and 20 mEq potassium/liter. Lytren provides 25 mEq/liter of potassium and 30 mEq/liter sodium.

Diagnostic agents
Agents used to determine gastric acidity
Histamine phosphate

Histamine phosphate is also known as histamine diphosphate or histamine acid phosphate. When given during an augmented histamine test, it is accompanied by simultaneous administration of an antidote (usually epinephrine) so that all effects of histamine, except those on gastric secretions, are antagonized. It is given subcutaneously in doses of 0.04 mg/kg body weight, and the patient is to have had nothing by mouth since midnight. It has been rated *effective* for testing gastric secretions.

Betazole hydrochloride (Histalog)

Betazole hydrochloride, an analog of histamine, is used more frequently than histamine phosphate because of its lower incidence of side effects. The routine administration of an antihistaminic compound is unnecessary, and augmentation of gastric secretion is equally effective. Betazole hydrochloride is to be used cautiously in patients with allergies. It is administered subcutaneously or intramuscularly in doses of 0.5 mg/kg body weight. Oral administration is under investigation. It has been rated *effective* for clinical testing of gastric secretion.

• • •

Both of these agents are discussed in more depth in Chapter 15.

Gastrointestinal stimulator

Metoclopramide (Reglan)

Metoclopramide is structurally similar to procaine and procainamide but without significant anesthetic or cardiac effects. The precise mechanism of action is not defined. As a central dopaminergic antagonist, it increases the release of acetylcholine and may increase the sensitivity of muscarinic receptors to acetylcholine. Effects of metoclopramide are directed at both the gastrointestinal tract and the central nervous system. The cholinergic-like contractions produced are altered by anticholinergic drugs and potentiated by cholinergic agonists. Metoclopramide inhibits gastric relaxation induced by dopamine. Levodopa blocks the effects of metoclopramide.

Metoclopramide increases the resting gastroesophageal sphincter tone pressures (reducing reflex esophagitis), increasing both the force of esophageal peristalsis and the rate of antral gastric emptying time, without an effect on the acid secretion rate. The increase in pyloric activity and duodenal bulb peristalsis increases transit time through the duodenum, jejunum, and ileum. Minimal motility effects are produced in the large intestine.

Blocking dopamine receptors results in the central nervous system effect, which is a central antiemetic effect mediated by inhibition of the chemoreceptor trigger zone. Stimulation of prolactin secretion is also seen by another mechanism.

In prolonged administration, extrapyramidal symptoms (similar to the antipsychotic drug–induced dyskinesias) are seen in children and young adults. Characteristic hypertonia of muscles is seen. This may result from the blocking of central dopaminergic receptors. Examples of these symptoms include restlessness (akathisia), involuntary limb twitching, facial spasms, buccal-lingual-facial movements (opisthotonos, torticollis), dystonias, dysphagia, and oculogyric crises. Sedation is also seen. These reactions occur within 36 hours of therapy and subside when the drug is discontinued.

The onset of action is ½ to 1 hour after oral dose, 10 to 15 minutes after an intramuscular dose, and within 3 minutes after an intravenous dose. Effects last up to 3 hours after an intravenous dose and 2 to 3 hours by the oral route. Significant metabolic first pass effects are seen (50% bioavailability). The half-life is up to 4 hours. Renal impairment requires dose adjustments (since 70% to 85% is excreted within 72 hours in the urine unchanged), because plasma levels are increased once the half-life is extended to 24 hours. The drug is moderately (25%) bound to protein.

Uses. The oral dosage form is used in diabetic gastroparesis both improving peristalsis and decreasing vomiting. Metoclopramide in the injectable form is used to facilitate transit of small bowel biopsy tubes in persons where the tube does not pass the pyloric sphincter with conventional maneuvers. It is also useful in stimulating gastric emptying and intestinal transit of barium in cases where delayed emptying interferes with radiologic examination of the stomach and small intestine. Because the drug speeds gastric emptying, it is effective for symptomatic relief of reflux esophagitis, a condition that results from reflux of the acid and peptic gastric contents into the esophagus.

Investigational uses include the following: antiemetic in drug-induced vomiting and nausea (cancer chemotherapy, radiation therapy, opiate analgesics, antitubercular drugs), persistent hiccups, postoperative vomiting, ulcer, migraine, reflux esophagitis (heartburn), and defective lactation (elevating prolactin levels). It has also been used investigationally to increase ureteral peristalsis.

Preparation, dosage, and administration. Metoclopramide is available as monohydrochloride monohydrate in 2-ml ampules for intravenous use. For diabetic gastroparesis 10 mg is given orally 30 minutes before each meal and at bedtime for 2 to 8 weeks, based on response to beneficial results. A dosage of 10 mg is given intravenously to adults to facilitate small bowel intubation if the biopsy tube has not passed the pylorus in 10 minutes. In patients where delayed gastric emptying of barium interferes with radiologic examination of the stomach or small intestine, a single dose of 10 mg for adults is administered *slowly* by the intravenous route over a 1 to 2 minute period. The dosage for children 6 to 14 years of age is

2.5 to 5 mg. Rapid intravenous administration of the drug should be avoided since a transient but intense feeling of anxiety and restlessness, followed by drowsiness, may occur.

Contraindications. Contraindications include states where stimulation of gastrointestinal motility is hazardous (such as gastrointestinal hemorrhage or mechanical obstruction), patients with pheochromocytoma (catecholamine release from tumor producing a hypertensive crisis), and concurrent therapy with drugs having extrapyramidal side effects (phenothiazines, butyrophenones, anticonvulsants). No controlled study has been done on use in pregnancy. Metoclopramide crosses the brain barrier and placental barrier.

Drug interactions. Motility effects are antagonized by anticholinergic drugs, narcotic analgesics, and drugs with CNS sedative effects. Ethanol, acetaminophen, ampicillin, tetracyclines, and L-dopa substantially decrease drug absorption from the stomach, while small bowel drug absorption is accelerated.

Side effects and toxic effects. Adverse reactions include dizziness, lassitude, restlessness, drowsiness, fatigue, insomnia, bowel disturbances, and extrapyramidal effects (dystonia is seen with dosages exceeding 0.5 mg/kg/day).

Agents used for roentgenographic studies

Barium sulfate

Barium sulfate is a fine, white, colorless, tasteless, and bulky powder free from grittiness. It is more impermeable to roentgen rays than are tissues and is therefore employed as an opaque contrast medium for roentgenographic examination of the hypopharynx, esophagus, upper gastrointestinal tract, small intestines, or colon. Its property of insolubility renders it safe to use; all soluble barium salts are exceedingly poisonous. The patient is usually first examined by means of a fluoroscope, and flat plate views are later taken to determine the rate of barium passage through the digestive tract and to locate sites of abnormality.

Preparation, dosage, and administration. For examination of the stomach, the patient is to have had nothing by mouth since midnight and is given barium orally in doses of 300 g (usually in 400 ml water). Suitable colors, flavors, and fluidizing agents may be added to improve the palatability of this mixture. If the large bowel is to be examined, the patient should have nothing by mouth after midnight in addition to laxatives and/or cleansing enemas. The barium is then given in enema form. The patient should be instructed to attempt to retain the barium during the roentgenographic examination, a feat that sometimes proves difficult. After the examination, either cleansing enemas or laxatives should be administered, so that the remaining barium does not contribute to bowel obstruction. In both cases the patient should be informed that his stool will be very light in color after the examination.

Organic iodine compounds in radiographic contrast media, with specific emphasis on cholecystography

Numerous organic iodine compounds are used as diagnostic aids in examination of the liver, gallbladder, and bile ducts. These compounds are excreted by the liver into the bile and concentrated in the gallbladder. Since they cast a shadow on the roentgenogram, they are used to visualize the gallbladder outline and the presence of stones and to determine whether the organ fills and empties normally. If the gallbladder is not functioning, it does not absorb the dye and is not visualized on the film. Because an empty stomach and a clear intestinal tract are necessary for visualization of the gallbladder, patients are prepared with fat-free suppers and laxatives and may have nothing by mouth after midnight. Occasionally, after films are taken, the patient is given a fat-containing meal and additional films are taken to determine the ability of the organ to contract.

It is recommended that iodinated compounds be used cautiously, if at all, for patients with severe renal disease, diabetic nephropathy, hepatic disease, iodine allergy, bronchial asthma, allergy suggesting histamine sensitivity, or prior reaction (such as urticaria, sneezing, chest tightness, wheezing, and laryngeal spasm) to other contrast media. The compounds are contraindicated for patients sensitive to iodine, because the iodine content ranges from 5% to 66%. Their use will interfere with diagnostic radioactive isotope uptake studies, such as ^{131}I thyroid. Injectable radiopaque agents may exacerbate pheochromocytoma and sickle cell anemia. Metrizamide may lower seizure threshold and precipitate seizures when patients receiving drugs such as butyrophenones, CNS stimulants, monoamine oxidase inhibitors, phenothiazines, and tricyclic antidepressants.

Some other agents used as radiographic contrast media and their uses are as follows:

Tests	Radiographic contrast media
Angiography	Diatrizoate and iothalamate as meglumine and sodium
Cholangiography (intravenous)	Iodipamide meglumine
Cholecystography (oral)	Iopanoic and iocetamic acids
	Ipodate sodium and calcium
	Tyropenate sodium
Cystourethrography	Diatrizoate and iothalamate as meglumine
Gastrointestinal radiography	Diatrizoate as meglumine or sodium
Urography (intravenous and retrograde)	Diatrizoate and iothalamate as meglumine and sodium
	Iodamine meglumine
	Methiodal sodium
	Metrizoic acid

Iopanoic acid (Telepaque)

Iopanoic acid is a radiopaque medium used in cholecystography. It is claimed that undesirable side effects seldom occur and that it produces greater opacification of the gallbladder. When side effects do occur, they include nausea, diarrhea, and dysuria. The usual dose of 3 to 6 g is given orally 14 to 17 hours before the roentgenogram is to be made. The drug is available in 500-mg tablets.

Iodipamide meglumine (Cholografin Meglumine)

Iodipamide is a water-soluble organic iodine compound that is administered intravenously for cholecystography when patients are unable to ingest or absorb oral agents or when rapid visualization of the gallbladder is essential for diagnosis in emergencies and before sur-

gery. It is the agent of choice for cholangiography. After injection, cholangiography can be performed in 25 minutes and cholecystography in 2 to 2½ hours. Sensitivity reactions are more common with this agent than with the oral iodides.

Summary of nursing considerations

Drugs affecting the gastrointestinal tract exert their action mainly on muscular and glandular tissues. The action may be directly on the smooth muscle and gland cells or indirectly on the autonomic nervous system. Drugs may bring about increased or decreased function, tone, emptying time, or peristaltic action of the stomach or gut. In addition, drugs may be used to relieve enzyme deficiency, to counteract excess acidity or gas formation, to produce or prevent vomiting, or as diagnostic aids. Mouthwashes, gargles, and dentifrices can be used to maintain good oral hygiene.

Conditions of the stomach requiring drug therapy include hyperchlorhydria, hypochlorhydria, peptic ulcer, nausea and emesis, and hypermotility. Systemic and nonsystemic antacids, anticholinergics, antispasmodics, and histamine H$_2$-receptor inhibitors are chemical substances used to treat hyperchlorhydria and peptic or gastric ulcers. Drugs are also used as diagnostic acids, for example, in determining gastric acidity and conducting roentgenographic studies.

Drugs that affect the intestine are laxatives, antidiarrheals, and carminatives. Laxatives are oral drugs administered to induce defecation. Carminatives are mild, irritant drugs that increase gastrointestinal motility and aid in expulsion of gas from the stomach and intestine.

QUESTIONS

FOR STUDY AND REVIEW

1 Differentiate between systemic and nonsystemic antacid characteristics.
2 Why is betazole hydrochloride (Histalog) preferred over histamine phosphate in diagnostic stimulation of hydrochloric acid secretion?

3 Differentiate between systemic and nonsystemic antacids.

4 What effect do calcium or magnesium antacids have on digitalis? Name two other drugs that interact with antacids and explain the adverse effects produced by each.

5 Discuss the use of syrup of ipecac.

6 Name several preparations that are useful to check vomiting.

7 What are several popular misconceptions about constipation?

8 Name several conditions in which laxatives are contraindicated.

9 If a patient is scheduled to have a cholecystogram and a T_3 uptake on the same day, what nursing judgment would be exercised?

10 Identify and define the major modes of laxative action, giving a drug example of each.

11 In case of food poisoning, why would castor oil be a more suitable laxative than cascara?

12 What suggestions would you give to a person who asked you what could be done to overcome habitual constipation?

13 Evaluate the claims made for laxatives on present-day television and radio programs.

14 Identify two major objections to the use of mineral oil.

15 Discuss the use of pancreatic enzymes.

16 How do opiate preparations relieve diarrhea? Name a preparation.

MULTIPLE CHOICE

Circle the answer of your choice.

17 Which of the following is a good example of a systemic antacid?
  a. calcium carbonate
  b. sodium bicarbonate
  c. lime water
  d. rhubarb and soda

18 Which of the following is a good example of a nonsystemic antacid?
  a. aluminum hydroxide
  b. calcium chloride
  c. sodium biacarbonate
  d. sodium carbonate

19 The physiologically least harmful of the following laxatives is:
  a. cascara sagrada
  b. milk of magnesia
  c. Dulcolax
  d. Metamucil

20 Indicate whether each of the following antacids is constipating or diarrheal.
  a. aluminum hydroxide gel
  b. magnesium trisilicate
  c. calcium carbonate
  d. milk of magnesia

21 The active proteolytic enzyme in gastric juice is:
  a. pepsin
  b. pepsinogen
  c. trypsin
  d. amylase

22 The pharmacologic action of cascara sagrada primarily results from:
  a. central nervous system stimulation
  b. hydrophilic action
  c. antispasmodic effect
  d. mild irritating effect on the intestine

BIBLIOGRAPHY

A.M.A. drug evaluations, ed. 4, New York, 1980, John Wiley & Sons, Inc.

Ambre, J., and others: Effect of coadministration of aluminum and magnesium hydroxides on absorption of anticoagulants in man, Clin. Pharmacol. Ther. **14:**231, 1973.

Avery, G.S., editor: Drug treatment, ed. 2, New York, 1980, ADIS Press.

Bank, S., and Marks, I.N.: Evaluation of new drugs for peptic ulcer, Clin. Gastroenterol. **2:**379, 1973.

Berry, L.H.: Gastrointestinal pan-endoscopy, Springfield, Ill., 1974, Charles C Thomas, Publisher.

Bodemarg, G., and Wallana, A.: Cimetidine in the treatment of active duodenal and prepyloric ulcers, Lancet **2:**161, 1976.

Brooks, F.P., editor: Gastrointestinal pathophysiology, ed. 2, New York, 1978, Oxford University Press, Inc.

Brown, M.S.: Over-the-counter gastrointestinal drugs. I. Antacids, Nurse Practitioner **1**(5):15, 1976.

Brown, M.S.: Over-the-counter gastrointestinal drugs. III. Antidiarrheal drugs, Nurse Practitioner **2**(1):23, 1976.

Code, C.F.: New antagonist excites an old histamine prospector, N. Engl. J. Med. **290:**738, 1974.

Davenport, H.W.: Physiology of the digestive tract, ed. 4, Chicago, 1977, Year Book Medical Publishers, Inc.

Donaldson, R.M.: Breakdown of barriers in gastric ulcers, N. Engl. J. Med. **288:**316, 1973.

Editorial: Burimamide, metiamide, cimetidine, Lancet **2:**802, 1975.

Farrell, R.L., and others: Cholinergic therapy of chronic heartburn, a controlled trial, Ann. Intern. Med. **80:**573, 1974.

Fordtran, J.S., and others: In vivo and in vitro evaluation of liquid antacids, N. Engl. J. Med. **288:**923, 1973.

Goodman, L.S., and Gilman, A., editors: The pharmacological basis of therapeutics, ed. 6, New York, 1980, Macmillan, Inc.

Goth, A.: Medical pharmacology, ed. 10, St. Louis, 1980, The C.V. Mosby Co.

Goulston, K.: Diagnosis and treatment of the irritable bowel syndrome, Drugs **6:**237, 1973.

Greenblatt, D.J., and others: Anticholinergics, N. Engl. J. Med. **288:**1215, 1973.

Griffinhagen, G.B., and Hawkins, L.L., editors: Handbook of non-prescription drugs, Washington, D.C., 1980, American Pharmaceutical Association.

Hill, R.B., and Kern, F., Jr.: The gastrointestinal tract: structure and function in disease, Baltimore, 1977, The Williams & Wilkins Co.

Hollander, D., and Harlan, J.: Antacids vs placebos in peptic ulcer therapy, J.A.M.A. **226:**1181, 1973.

Isenberg, J.I.: Therapy of peptic ulcer, J.A.M.A. **233:**540.

Knoben, J.E., Anderson, P.O., and Watanabe, A.S.: Handbook of clinical drug data, ed. 4, Hamilton, Ill., 1978, Drug Intelligence Publications, Inc.

Lennard-Jones, J.E., and Ritchie, J.K.: The diagnosis and management of colitis, Br. J. Hosp. Med. **11:**180, 1974.

Littman, A., and Pine, B.H.: Antacids and anticholinergic drugs, Ann. Intern. Med. **82:**544, 1975.

Modell, W., editor: Drugs of choice 1980-1981, St. Louis, 1980, The C.V. Mosby Co.

Morrissey, J., and Barreras, R.F.: Antacid therapy, N. Engl. J. Med. **290:**550, 1974.

Peterson, W.L., and others: Healing of duodenal ulcer with antacid regimen, N. Engl. J. Med., **297:**341, 1977.

Pietrusko, R.G.: Pharmacology of diarrhea, Am. J. Hosp. Pharm. **36:**757, 1979.

Sparberg, M.: The therapy of peptic ulcer disease, Ration. Drug Ther. **7:**1, 1973.

Spiro, H.M.: Clinical gastroenterology, ed. 2, New York, 1977, Macmillan, Inc.

Tompkins, R.K.: Comments on chemotherapy of cholesterol cholelithiasis, Am. J. Surg. **127:**501, 1974.

Trowbridge, J.E., and Carl, W.: Oral care of the patient having head and neck irradiation, Am. J. Nurs. **75:**2146, 1975.

Wilkins, R.W., and Levinsky, N.G., editors: Medicine: essentials of clinical practice, ed. 2, Boston, 1978, Little, Brown & Co.

CHAPTER 17

Drugs that affect the eye

The eye and ophthalmic agents

The eye is the receptor organ for one of the most delicate and valuable senses—vision; it demands only the most thoughtful and expert care. The eyeball has three layers or coats: the protective external (corneoscleral) coat, the nutritive middle vascular (uveal) coat, and the light-sensitive inner neural receptor (retinal) layer. Fig. 17-1 shows these parts of the eye.

The eyeball is protected in a deep depression of the skull, the orbit, and is moved in the orbit by six small extraocular muscles. The retina is connected to the brain by the optic nerve, which leaves the orbit through a bony canal in the posterior wall.

The cornea is normally transparent, allowing light to enter the eye. This transparency depends on normal intraocular pressure; increased intraocular pressure results in loss of transparency. The cornea has no blood vessels and receives its nutrition from the aqueous humor and its oxygen supply by diffusion from the air and surrounding structures. In order to act as a lens, the cornea must have air in front of it. The corneal surface consists of a thin layer of epithelial cells, which are quite resistant to infection. However, an abraded cornea is very susceptible to infection. The cornea is also supplied with 60 to 80 sensory fibers which elicit pain whenever the corneal epithelium is damaged. Seriously injured corneal tissue is replaced by scar tissue, which is usually not transparent. The sclera, which is continuous with the cornea, is nontransparent; it is the white fibrous envelope of the eye.

The iris gives the eye its brown, blue, gray, green, or hazel color. It surrounds the pupil; the sphincter and dilator muscles in the iris alter pupil size. The sphincter muscle, which encircles the pupil, is parasympathetically inner-

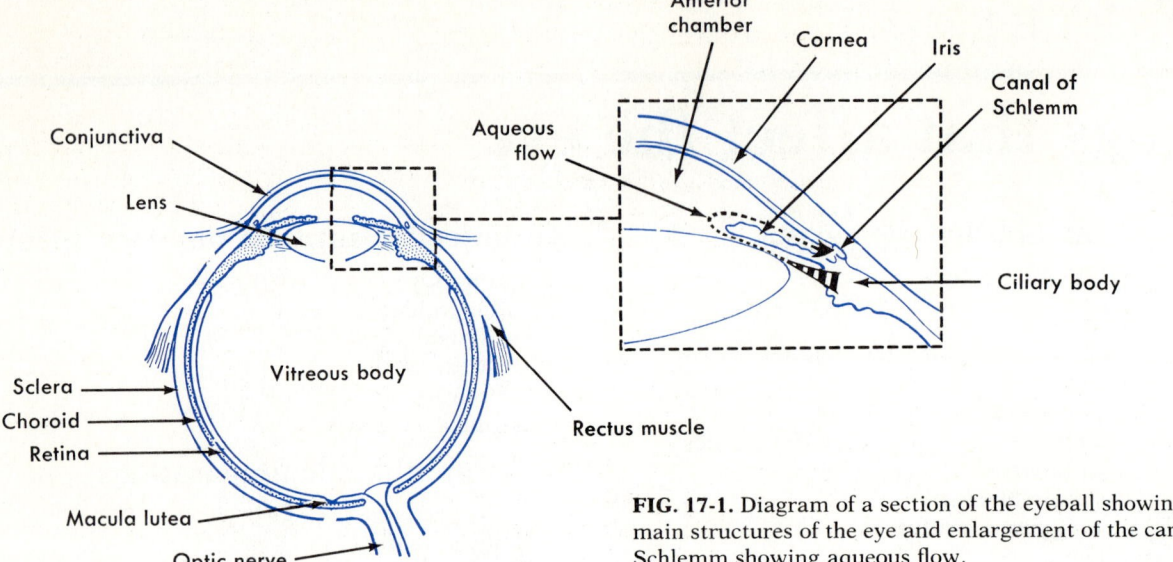

FIG. 17-1. Diagram of a section of the eyeball showing the main structures of the eye and enlargement of the canal of Schlemm showing aqueous flow.

vated; the dilator muscle, which runs radially from the pupil to the iris periphery, is sympathetically innervated. Contraction of the sphincter muscle, either alone or in association with relaxation of the dilator muscle, causes constriction of the pupil, or *miosis*. Contraction of the dilator muscle and relaxation of the sphincter muscle causes dilation of the pupil, or *mydriasis*.

Drugs producing miosis (miotics) act by (1) interfering with cholinesterase activity or (2) acting like acetylcholine at receptor sites in the sphincter muscle. Drugs producing mydriasis (mydriatics) act by (1) interfering with the action of acetylcholine or (2) stimulating sympathetic or adrenergic receptors. Pupil constriction normally occurs with light and when the eye is focusing on nearby objects. Pupil dilation normally occurs in dim light and when the eye is focusing on distant objects.

The lens is situated behind the iris. It is a transparent gelatinous mass of fibers uniformly arranged in a complex architectural pattern and encased in a thin elastic capsule. Its protein concentration is higher than that of any other tissue of the body.

The function of the lens is to ensure that the image on the retina is in sharp focus. The lens does this by changing shape (accommodation). This occurs readily in young persons, but with age the lens becomes more rigid, the ability to focus close objects is lost, and the *near point*

(the closest point that can be seen clearly) recedes. With age the lens may also lose its transparency and become opaque. This is known as a cataract. Unless it can be treated or removed surgically, blindness can occur. However, if the opaque (cataract) portion is located peripherally in the lens, vision is not compromised.

The lens has suspensory ligaments called zonular fibers around its edge, which connect with the ciliary body. Their tension helps to change the shape of the lens. In the unaccommodated eye, the ciliary muscle is relaxed and the zonular fibers are taut. For near vision the ciliary muscle fibers contract, and this relaxes the pull of the ligaments. Accommodation depends on two factors: (1) ciliary muscle contraction, and (2) the ability of the lens to assume a more biconvex shape when tension on the ligaments is relaxed. The ciliary muscle is innervated by parasympathetic fibers. Paralysis of the ciliary muscle is termed *cycloplegia*.

Aqueous humor is formed by the ciliary body, and it bathes and feeds the lens, iris, and posterior surface of the cornea. After it is formed, it flows forward between the lens and the iris into the anterior chamber. It drains out of the eye through drainage channels located near the junction of the cornea and sclera. A trabecular meshwork leads into the canal of Schlemm through which the aqueous drains into the venous system of the eye.

Protective mechanisms. Eyelashes, eyelids, blinking, and tears all serve to protect the eye. There are about 200 eyelashes for each eye. The eyelashes evoke a blink reflex whenever a foreign body touches them, momentarily closing the lids to prevent the foreign substance from entering the eye. Blinking, which is bilateral, occurs every few seconds during waking hours and serves to keep the corneal surface free of mucus and spreads the lacrimal fluid evenly over the cornea. Tears are secreted by lacrimal glands and contain lysozyme, a mucolytic enzyme with bactericidal action. Tears provide lubrication for lid movements. They wash away noxious agents, and by forming a thin film over the cornea they provide it with a good optical surface. Tear fluid is lost by evaporation and by draining into two small ducts (the lacrimal canaliculi) at the inner corners of the upper and lower eyelids.

Ophthalmic agents. Drugs used in the treatment of eye disorders can be divided into three major groups: the antiglaucoma agents, the mydriatics and cycloplegics, and the antiinfective/antiinflammatory agents. The ophthalmic drug groups most likely to be encountered by the nurse in clinical practice are outlined in the box. There are many other eye preparations, including ophthalmic diagnostic products, enzymes, irrigating solutions, eyewashes, and hyperosmolar preparations. This chapter will discuss the major groups and these other eye preparations, along with their major dosage and administration and other nursing considerations.

Antiglaucoma agents

Glaucoma is an eye disease characterized chiefly by abnormally elevated intraocular pressure that may result from excessive production of aqueous humor or from diminished ocular fluid outflow. Increased pressure, if sufficiently high and persistent, may lead to irreversible blindness. There are three major types of glaucoma—primary, secondary, and congenital. Primary glaucoma includes narrow-angle (acute congestive) glaucoma and wide-angle (chronic simple) glaucoma. These are determined by the angle of the anterior chamber

Ophthalmic drug groups

Antiglaucoma agents
  Miotics, direct acting
  Miotics, indirect acting
  Epinephrine
  Beta blockers
  Carbonic anhydrase inhibitors
  Osmotic agents
Mydriatics and cycloplegics
Antiinfective/antiinflammatory agents
  Antibacterial
    Antibiotics
    Sulfonamides
  Antifungal
  Antiviral
  Antiseptic
  Corticosteroids
Anesthetics
Artificial tears
Contact lens products
  Cleaning
  Cushioning
  Disinfecting
  Soaking
  Wetting
  Rinsing
  Storage
Decongestants

where aqueous humor reabsorption takes place. Wide-angle glaucoma has a gradual insidious onset, and its control depends on permanent drug therapy. Drugs are also necessary for controlling the acute attack associated with narrow-angle glaucoma, followed usually by surgery (such as iridectomy or laser surgery). Secondary glaucoma may result from previous eye disease or may follow cataract extraction; therapy for secondary glaucoma is usually with drugs for an indefinite period. Congenital glaucoma requires surgical treatment. Cholinergic and anticholinesterase drugs are used to treat glaucoma; selection of a drug is determined largely by the requirements of the individual patient.

Miotics

These miotics are topically applied agents useful in treating glaucoma and accommodative esotropia. The parasympathomimetic miotic agents are cholinergic (mimicking the effects of acetylcholine at autonomic synapses or the neuroeffector junction of the parasympathetic nervous system) or anticholinesterase (inactivating the enzyme cholinesterase by preventing hydrolysis of acetylcholine and thus prolonging the effect of acetylcholine).

CHOLINERGIC (PARASYMPATHOMIMETIC) MIOTICS

Cholinergic drugs are chemically related to acetylcholine, the neurohormone that mediates nerve impulse transmission at all cholinergic or parasympathetic nerve sites. Applied topically to the eye, cholinergic drugs (1) cause contraction of the sphincter muscle of the iris, resulting in pupil constriction (miosis), (2) cause spasms of the ciliary muscle and deepening of the anterior chamber, and (3) cause vasodilation of intraocular vessels (such as those in the iris) or where intraocular fluids leave the eye. The ciliary muscle effect leaves the eye in accommodation for near vision.

The cholinergic agents have a duration of miotic action of approximately 2 to 4 hours (pilocarpine drops) or 2 to 8 hours (carbachol). These agents are very effective in many cases of chronic glaucoma. Their side effects are less severe and occur less frequently than those caused by anticholinesterase agents.

The cholinergic drugs are used to lower intraocular pressure in glaucoma. Unless the elevated pressure is lowered, the result is an impaired blood supply to the optic nerve, with eventual atrophy of the nerve and visual field loss. Contraction of the ciliary muscles and constriction of the pupil may widen the filtration angle and permit increased outflow of aqueous humor. Increased outflow may also result from dilation of collector channels and veins peripheral to the canal of Schlemm.

Clinical toxicity from overdosage or unusual sensitivity to these drugs is manifested by headache, salivation, sweating, abdominal discomfort, diarrhea, asthmatic attacks, and a fall in blood pressure.

Acetylcholine chloride (Miochol Intraocular Ophthalmic)

Although not useful as an antiglaucoma agent, acetylcholine chloride is a common parasympathomimetic drug. A 1:100 solution (2 ml) of acetylcholine chloride (0.5 to 2 ml) is instilled into the anterior chamber or on the iris for rapid, intense miosis (pupil constriction) during surgery on the anterior chamber of the eye or for cataract removal, keratoplasty, peripheral iridectomy, or cyclodialysis. The miosis, occurring within seconds, protects the vitreous face and facilitates placement of corneal sutures by reducing the danger of imprisoning iris tissue during wound closure. Acetylcholine is promptly destroyed by cholinesterase; thus miosis may last only 10 minutes. This fact plus acetylcholine's poor corneal penetration makes it of no value in the treatment of glaucoma. Because of its instability, it is prepared immediately before use.

Carbachol (Miostat, Isopto Carbachol)

The only dosage form of carbachol officially approved in the United States is the solution for ophthalmic use, 0.75%, 1.5%, 2.25%, or 3%. It is used to treat open-angle or narrow-angle glaucoma and to produce miosis during or after cataract surgery (0.01% Miostat Intraocular).

Carbachol must be combined with a wetting agent, such as benzalkonium chloride, for increased corneal penetration. Carbachol produces intense and prolonged miosis, since it is resistant to destruction by cholinesterase. Its miotic action lasts 4 to 8 hours, and it is usually prescribed as 1 drop in each eye up to four times daily. After intracameral injection, miosis, occurring within 2 to 5 minutes, may persist for 15 hours. Carbachol may produce a slight conjunctival hyperemia, altered distance vision, decreased night vision, aching of the eyes, and headache during the first few days of treatment. These symptoms subside as therapy continues. The absorption of carbachol is enhanced by massaging the cornea lightly through the eyelid (on the lacrimal sac) for 1 minute.

Pilocarpine nitrate ophthalmic solution, pilocarpine hydrochloride

Pilocarpine is the drug of choice for primary glaucoma. It is used in 0.25% to 10% solution. One drop in the eye will cause miosis and spasm of accommodation in 15 minutes, reaching a maximum in 30 to 60 minutes. The pupillary effect lasts as long as 20 hours, but the fixation of the lens for near vision disappears in about 2 to 3 hours. At first intraocular pressure is increased, but this is followed by a persistent fall in pressure.

The dosage of pilocarpine for wide-angle glaucoma is usually 1 to 2 drops of a 1% or 2% solution every 6 to 8 hours. One drop of a 2% pilocarpine solution contains 1000 μg pilocarpine. For acute glaucoma pilocarpine in a 2% solution may be instilled every 10 minutes for an hour, then every 1 to 2 hours three or more times. Excess solution must be wiped away promptly to prevent its flow into the lacrimal system and the production of systemic symptoms. Pilocarpine is also used to neutralize mydriatics used during eye examinations. Pilocarpine is widely used for the treatment of early stages of wide-angle glaucoma; it is less beneficial in advanced stages. It may be used alternately with mydriatics to break adhesions between the iris and the lens. Patients may become resistant or intolerant to this drug. It is the safest and most widely used miotic.

Pilocarpine is also available in Ocuserts: Ocusert Pilo-20 and Ocusert Pilo-40. This preparation is used to treat patients with chronic open-angle glaucoma. These units deliver the drug at a rate of 20 to 40 μg/hour for 1 week (±20% rate variation) following an initial 6-hour period of more rapid release. Patients controlled with 0.5% to 1% pilocarpine may require a Pilo-20 unit; those controlled with 2% to 4% solution may require a Pilo-40 unit.

This dosage form has advantages and disadvantages. One advantage is a constant rate of released drug (zero-order kinetics), in contrast to the variation of medication available at the ocular receptor site that occurs with an eyedrop delivery system. The total active drug released is greatly reduced, and therefore the potential for systemic toxicity is decreased. The side effects of miosis and spasm of accommodation are decreased, and patient compliance is increased because drop instillation is eliminated. The disadvantages include difficulty of insertion and removal, increased expense, occasional rupture of the device, initial conjunctival irritation, and manual dexterity required for insertion.

The Ocusert units are elliptical devices

designed for continuous release of drug following placement in the cul-de-sac of the eye. Since pilocarpine-induced myopia occurs during the first few hours of therapy, the patient begins the therapy at bedtime and by morning the myopia is stable. For best retention in the evening, the unit is manipulated from the lower lid to the upper conjunctival cul-de-sac with gentle digital massage through the lid. If the unit slips out during sleep, the ocular hypotensive effect following the loss will continue for a period of time similar to that of pilocarpine eyedrops. However, the patient should continue to check the placement of the unit before sleeping and on awakening.

ANTICHOLINESTERASE MIOTICS

Anticholinesterase drugs inhibit the enzymatic destruction of acetylcholine by inactivating cholinesterase. This leaves acetylcholine free to act on the effector cells of the iris sphincter and ciliary muscles causing pupil constriction and spasm of accommodation.

The anticholinesterases are either reversible (physostigmine) and possess a miotic action lasting 12 to 36 hours or are irreversible (isoflurophate, demecarium bromide, echothiopate iodide) and possess a prolonged miotic action of days to weeks. These drugs are often effective in treating chronic glaucoma when other agents have been ineffective. Instillations may be less frequent with these drugs because of their prolonged action. Another advantage is better control over the intraocular pressure and less fluctuation in pressure.

After combination with the enzyme physostigmine is gradually dissociated and inactivated. Neostigmine is not as readily absorbed as physostigmine, and higher concentrations must be used for topical treatment of glaucoma.

The irreversible anticholinesterase drugs form stable complexes with cholinesterase and thus irreversibly impair the destructive function of the enzyme. Destruction of acetylcholine then depends on synthesis of new enzymes. These drugs are used primarily in the management of glaucoma in patients who have failed to respond to weaker miotics, carbonic anhydrase inhibitors, or direct-acting cholinergics.

Physostigmine salicylate (Eserine salicylate [solution], Eserine sulfate [ointment])

Physostigmine is used in solutions of 0.25%, 1 or 2 drops one to four times daily. The aqueous solutions of this compound tend to oxidize on exposure to light and air and turn pink or brown. Such colored solutions should never be used. The maximal effect of topical application is reached in 30 minutes and may last 12 to 36 hours. Physostigmine is used in the treatment of wide-angle glaucoma. It may be applied alternately with atropine to break adhesions between the iris and lens, and it may be used after instillation of a mydriatic to shorten the period of pupil dilation and minimize the dangers of increased ocular pressure.

Physostigmine is often irritating to the eye and is rarely tolerated for prolonged periods of treatment. Conjunctivitis and allergic reactions occur frequently with this drug; therefore, it is not a popular drug.

Physostigmine ointment (0.25%) may be prescribed for bedtime use to prevent nocturnal rise in ocular tension.

Demecarium bromide (Humorsol)

Demecarium bromide is prepared as a 0.125% and 0.25% ophthalmic solution. It is an extremely powerful and toxic agent, and 1 drop will produce miosis within 1 hour and ciliary muscle contraction for as long as 5 to 12 days. Care must be taken to prevent general systemic absorption. One drop is instilled every 12 to 48 hours.

It is effective for the same conditions as those listed for isoflurophate.

Echothiophate iodide (Echodide, Phospholine Iodide); ecotiopate iodide

Echothiophate is used as a 0.03%, 0.06%, 0.125% and 0.25% solution. It is very potent agent with prolonged effects similar to those of demecarium bromide. It is extremely effective in the control of chronic wide-angle glaucoma, aphakic glaucoma, and congenital glaucoma.

Miosis occurs within 10 to 45 minutes and may persist from several days to 4 weeks. Solutions of echothiophate are relatively unstable and gradually lose their potency at room temperature; refrigeration prolongs potency. In the treatment of glaucoma, 1 drop of the 0.03% solution is usually instilled into the eye on retiring (to avoid inconvenience of miosis) and in the morning. Frequency of administration and strength of dosage must be individually adjusted for each patient. Finger pressure should be applied at the inner canthus after instillation to minimize drainage into the nose and throat. This drug may induce cataract formation.

It is effective in the management of accommodative esotropia and wide-angle and congenital glaucoma.

Isoflurophate (diisopropyl fluorophosphate, Floropryl)

Isoflurophate is available only as an ophthalmic ointment, 0.025%. It produces miosis within 20 minutes, and the effect may last 2 or more weeks. It is topically applied (¼ inch per dose) into the conjunctival sac. The tip of the tube must not come in contact with moisture, since it will form hydrofluoric acid. Therefore, the tube must be kept closed, dry, and away from tears or the cornea. To minimize effects of blurred vision, the application should take place at bedtime. The dose is repeated every 8 to 72 hours, and the intraocular pressure decreases within a few hours of the initial dose. This dose is for glaucoma and differs from the dose used in the diagnosis and treatment of accommodative esotropia.

The effects of isoflurophate are similar to those of physostigmine, but it is more powerful. Isoflurophate has been rated *effective* in the management of accommodative esotropia, wide-angle glaucoma, and conditions obstructing aqueous outflow.

SIDE EFFECTS AND TOXIC EFFECTS OF THE MIOTICS

The disadvantages to instillation of cholinergic and anticholinesterase drugs into the eye include the following.

1 Visual blurring and headache result from stimulation of accommodation.
2 Miosis makes it difficult to adjust quickly to changes in illumination. This may be serious in elderly persons, since their light adaptation and visual acuity are often reduced. Nighttime is particularly hazardous for these patients.

3 These drugs may cause irritation, conjunctivitis, blepharitis, dermatitis, and so on.

4 Cysts of the iris, synechiae, retinal detachments, obstruction of tear drainage, and even cataracts may develop.

5 Tolerance and resistance may develop; this can occur with any of the miotics.

6 Instillation must be frequent.

7 Systemic side effects include salivation, vomiting, diarrhea, precipitation of asthmatic attack, nausea, fall in blood pressure, and other symptoms of parasympathetic stimulation (see Chapter 9).

8 Anticholinesterase drugs may cause spasm of the wink reflex, which is annoying to the patient.

9 Anticholinesterase agents lower plasma pseudocholinesterase activity, and if an adjunctive skeletal muscle relaxant such as succinylcholine (a neuromuscular blocking agent) is used during surgery, respiratory and cardiovascular collapse will result. Because of their long duration of effects, the eyedrops must be discontinued several weeks before surgery or electroshock therapy. Another depolarizing neuromuscular blocking agent is decamethonium bromide; some nondepolarizing agents are metocurine iodide, tubocurarine, gallamine, and pancuronium bromide.

10 Cholinesterase inhibitors also interact with organophosphate-type insecticides and pesticides, causing additive systemic effects from absorption through the respiratory tract or skin. Nursing intervention includes advising patients of the need for a respiratory mask and frequent bathing and changes of clothing if these substances are encountered.

Two antidotes are available for overcoming effects caused by cholinergic stimulation—atropine and pralidoxime. Pralidoxime chloride (Protopam) is effective only against anticholinesterases that phosphorylate the enzyme. Given early enough, it reactivates the enzyme.

Sympathomimetics
Epinephrine hydrochloride (adrenaline)

Preparation, dosage, and administration. Epinephrine is available in 0.25%, 0.5%, 1%, and 2% solutions, as the bitartrate, borate, or hydrochloride salt. Dilute solutions are used at times to treat local allergies and superficial hyperemia. It is sometimes added in dilute solutions (for example, 1:50,000) to local anesthetics, since its vasoconstricting effect prevents too rapid absorption of the anesthetic. In the initial treatment of primary open-angle glaucoma it is usually combined with pilocarpine or another miotic for greater effectiveness in lowering intraocular pressure and overcoming miosis. It may also be used during cataract surgery.

Instillation of 1 drop of a 2% solution of epinephrine causes immediate vasoconstriction that lasts 2 to 3 hours; mydriasis occurs within a few minutes and lasts for several hours; fall in intraocular pressure occurs within 1 hour, reaches a maximum in 4 hours, and persists for 24 hours or longer. Frequency of instillation should be individualized and may vary from every 2 or 3 days to two times a day in each eye.

Side effects and toxic effects. Systemic effects such as tachycardia and elevated blood pressure may occur with its use. Other possible side effects include eye pain, ocular irritation, and tearing. There have also been reports of epinephrine causing macular edema. Tricyclic antidepressants potentiate the pressor response of epinephrine. Exaggerated sympathomimetic effects occur with monoamine oxidase inhibitors.

Dipivefrin hydrochloride (Propine)

Action and result. Dipivefrin is a prodrug of epinephrine formed by the diesterification of epinephrine and pivalic acid. The enzymatic activity (hydrolysis) occurring within the eye converts dipivefrin (the prodrug of the parent drug) to epinephrine (the therapeutic active drug form). Prodrugs undergo biotransformation to produce pharmacologic effects. The chemical modification creates a more lipophilic compound that facilitates absorption and penetration through the cornea into the anterior chamber of the eye. The penetration and absorption of dipivefrin are greater than those of epinephrine. Dipivefrin is reported to have a lower intensity of side effects (hyperemia, stinging) than epinephrine. Dipivefrin produces less miosis than pilocarpine.

The epinephrine liberated from dipivefrin acts as an adrenergic agonist and decreases the intraocular pressure by reducing aqueous humor production and enhancing aqueous outflow. A dose of 1 drop of dipivefrin every 12 hours produces the same therapeutic response as 1 drop of 2% epinephrine four times daily. This 12-hour regimen can increase patient compliance by decreasing the number of instillations the patient must administer.

The onset of action occurs in 30 minutes, and the maximal effect is seen within 1 hour.

Uses. Dipivefrin is indicated as initial therapy to control intraocular pressure in chronic open-angle glaucoma. It is contraindicated in patients with narrow-angle glaucoma because pupil dilation may exacerbate the condition. In aphakic patients (those devoid of a crystalline lens), dipivefrin or epinephrine may cause macular edema. There are no controlled studies of the use of dipivefrin in pregnant women. It is unknown if this drug is excreted in breast milk of nursing mothers.

A special procedure is needed when changing from other antiglaucoma agents to dipivefrin. On the first day, the patient continues the previous medication and adds 1 drop of dipivefrin to the eye(s) every 12 hours. He discontinues the former agent on the second day while continuing with the dipivefrin therapy.

Side effects and toxic effects. The cardiovascular effects reported with epinephrine are also seen with dipivefrin: tachycardia, arrhythmias, and hypertension. Burning and stinging are also reported. Both dipivefrin and epinephrine may lead to adrenochroma deposits in the conjunctiva and cornea.

Beta adrenergic blocker
Timolol maleate (Timoptic)

Action and result. Timolol maleate is a nonselective or general beta adrenergic blocker that, when applied topically to the eye, reduces elevated and normal intraocular pressure. Elevated intraocular pressure may lead to visual field loss in glaucoma as a result of optic nerve damage. The drug's onset of action in lowering intraocular pressure occurs within 30 minutes, with maximal effects occurring in 1 or 2 hours. The lowered intraocular pressure is maintained for up to 24 hours. Although the precise mechanism is not understood, the action may be related to the reduction of aqueous humor formation.

Uses. The reduction of elevated intraocular

pressure is necessary for patients with chronic open-angle glaucoma, aphakic glaucoma, and secondary glaucoma and for those who have inadequate response to epinephrine or pilocarpine and other miotics. Small pupil size and occasional reduced visual acuity are common side effects; the latter results from the increased accommodation. The effects of dim and blurred vision and night blindness are not seen with timolol. Patients with glaucoma who wear hard contact lenses (PMMA) may use timolol.

Preparation, dosage, and administration. Timolol is available in 0.25% and 0.5% concentrations, with 5 ml and 10 ml units having 2.5 mg and 5 mg timolol in each milliliter. The initial dose is 1 drop of 0.25% solution in each eye twice daily. If the clinical response is inadequate, the patient can be given 1 drop of 0.5% solution in each eye twice daily. The dose is lowered to 1 drop daily in each eye when a satisfactory intraocular pressure is maintained. Higher doses do not further reduce the intraocular pressure. If the intraocular pressure cannot be lowered to the anticipated satisfactory level with timolol, concomitant therapy with pilocarpine and other miotics, epinephrine, or systemically administered carbonic anhydrase inhibitors such as acetazolamide may be useful.

If timolol is to replace a single antiglaucoma agent, the patient should continue the previous agent and add 1 drop of 0.25% timolol in each eye twice on the first day. On the second day the patient discontinues the previous therapeutic agent completely and continues with timolol. The same procedure is used for the 0.5% solution.

If timolol therapy is to replace several antiglaucoma agents used concomitantly, one agent a week should be withdrawn in the manner just described.

Side effects and toxic effects. Usually timolol is well tolerated with occasional signs of mild ocular irritation. Local hypersensitivity (rash) occurs rarely. A slight reduction of resting heart rate may occur, and acute bronchospasm in patients with bronchospastic disease has been reported.

Precautions. There is sufficient absorption

from the conjunctiva and nasopharynx to produce systemic effects such as cardiopulmonary complications and exacerbation of asthma. Caution must be exercised administering timolol to patients who have bronchial asthma, heart disease, sinus bradycardia or greater than first-degree heart block, cardiogenic shock, right ventricular failure caused by pulmonary hypertension, or congestive heart failure (CHF). Concomitant administration of timolol and adrenergic augmenting psychotropic drugs, including monoamine oxidase inhibitors, should be done cautiously. Pulse rates of patients with cardiac disease must be checked for bradycardia and other abnormalities. If the patient is receiving a systemic beta adrenergic blocker there is a potential for additive effects on intraocular pressure or systemic beta blockage; nursing observation is needed. Tolerance associated with other antiglaucoma drugs and diminished responsiveness do not occur with timolol.

Timolol is contraindicated in patients with hypersensitivity reactions. No studies of use in pregnant women are available, and the benefits should be weighed against the risks.

Carbonic anhydrase inhibitors

The intraocular pressure is maintained by the production of an aqueous humor inside the eye. It has been found that one substance necessary for the production of this fluid is the enzyme carbonic anhydrase. In glaucoma, where the intraocular pressure is abnormally high, it is desirable to slow the production of this fluid and thus decrease the pressure. The specific drugs used to inhibit carbonic anhydrase are quite effective when taken orally. Side reactions are usually not severe and consist of lethargy, anorexia, numbness, and tingling of the face and extremities. Diuresis is produced, and potassium depletion can occur.

Commonly used carbonic anhydrase inhibitors include the following.

1 Acetazolamide (Diamox)—125-mg and 250-mg tablets, 500-mg sustained release capsules, and injection. Tablets have an onset within 1½ hours and a duration of action of up to 14 hours. The

capsule onset is 2 hours and duration of up to 24 hours.
2 Ethoxzolamide (Cardrase, Ethamide)—125-mg tablets. Onset is 1 to 2 hours and duration up to 14 hours.
3 Methazolamide (Neptazane)—50-mg tablets. Onset is 2 to 4 hours and duration is up to 18 hours.
4 Dichlorphenamide (Daranide, Oratrol)—50-mg tablets. Onset is within 1 hour and duration is up to 12 hours.

Teratogenic effects from acetazolamide, ethoxzolamide, and methazolamide have been reported in animals. These agents should not be used in the first trimester of pregnancy.

Osmotic agents

Osmotic agents are administered intravenously or orally to reduce the intraocular pressure of glaucoma. These agents generally do not cross the blood-aqueous barrier into the anterior chamber of the eye and are rarely found in ocular humor.

The osmotherapeutic agents (glycerin and mannitol) create ocular hypotension by producing an osmotic gradient (making the blood hypertonic relative to the intraocular fluids). This gradient forces the water from the aqueous and vitreous humors into the bloodstream. The effect on the eye is reduction of volume of intraocular fluid, producing a decrease in intraocular pressure.

Glycerin (Glycerol, Glyrol, Osmoglyn), glycerol

Preparation, dosage, and administration. Glycerin is available as 50% or 75% oral solutions and as a 0.5% ophthalmic solution. Topical application of 1 or 2 drops is used for edema of the superficial layers of the cornea; it reduces edema, clears the cornea, and improves visualization for ophthalmoscopic examination.

Oral administration of glycerin is used to reduce intraocular pressure before iridectomy in patients with acute narrow-angle glaucoma. It is used preoperatively and postoperatively in conditions such as congenital glaucoma, retinal detachment, cataract extraction, and keratoplasty (corneal transplant). It may also be used in some secondary glaucomas.

The oral dose as an osmotic agent is 1 to 1.5 g/kg body weight 60 to 90 minutes before surgery for adults and children; it may be administered at 5-hour intervals. Following oral administration, intraocular pressure begins to decrease within 10 minutes and reaches a minimum in 30 minutes to 2 hours; the effect may persist 4 to 6 hours. Glycerin may be used with carbonic anhydrase inhibitors and miotics; these drugs may prolong the effects of glycerin.

Side effects. Glycerin has a slower onset of action and fewer side effects than mannitol or urea. Side effects include headache, backache, nausea and vomiting, dizziness, thirst, and diarrhea. Headache is the result of cerebral dehydration and may be relieved by having the patient lie down during and after oral administration of glycerin. Flavoring glycerin with lemon or lime juice, pouring it over cracked ice, and having the patient sip it through a straw may decrease the incidence of nausea and vomiting.

Precautions. Glycerin should be used cautiously in patients with cardiac, renal, or hepatic disease; the shift in body water may cause pulmonary edema or congestive heart failure. Elderly patients may be subject to dehydration because of a mild diuretic action. Diabetic patients receiving the drug should be carefully observed for symptoms of acidosis, since the metabolism of glycerin may cause transient hyperglycemia and glycosuria (glycerin is metabolized to carbohydrates).

Isosorbide (Ismotic)

Isosorbide (adihydric alcohol) is an oral osmotic agent used for emergency treatment of acute angle-closure glaucoma and conditions in which rapid reduction in intraocular pressure is indicated. It is available as a 45% solution. The dosage is 1 to 2 g/kg body weight. The drug's onset is within 30 minutes and duration of action is up to 90 minutes. Side effects are similar to those seen when using glycerin except that isosorbide is not metabolized and does not adversely affect blood glucose levels (an advantage in diabetic patients). The nurse must use isosorbide cautiously in patients placed on sodium restriction, since the 220 ml of isosorbide contains 105 mEq sodium and 34 mEq potassium.

Mannitol (Osmitrol)

Mannitol is a sugar alcohol with osmotic and diuretic properties. It is administered intravenously to reduce intraocular pressure. It is available in 5% to 25% solutions. The usual dosage is 0.5 to 2 g/kg (as a 25% solution; this is 2 to 8 ml/kg) body weight for adults and children. The solution should be infused slowly over 30 to 60 minutes. Maximal decrease in intraocular pressure occurs 30 to 60 minutes after administration and lasts about 6 to 8 hours.

Mannitol is used for the same conditions as glycerin. It should be used cautiously in patients with cardiovascular or pulmonary disease, in severely ill patients, and elderly persons.

Side effects. Side effects are similar to those for glycerin. In addition, the drug has caused agitation, disorientation, and convulsions. Fatalities have been reported after administration of large doses. Patients receiving mannitol should be carefully monitored for fluid and electrolyte balance, urinary output, and vital signs, since it produces more diuresis than urea. At cooler temperatures solutions crystallize; warming returns crystals to solution.

Urea (Ureaphil)

Urea is administered intravenously to reduce intraocular pressure. It is available as a powder; 40 g/150 ml of diluent makes a 30% solution with 10% invert sugar. The usual dosage for adults is 1 to 1.5 g/kg body weight of a 30% solution administered at a slow rate (not exceeding 4 ml/minute), because this hypertonic solution may produce hemolysis and a direct effect on cerebral vasomotor centers, producing an increase in capillary bleeding. The dosage for children is 0.5 to 1.5 g/kg of a 30% solution administered over 30 minutes. Maximal decrease in intraocular pressure occurs within 1 hour after injection and may last 8 to 12 hours. Urea is used for the same conditions as glycerin. It is unstable in solution and must be freshly prepared for administration.

Side effects. Headache, nausea and vomiting, dehydration, electrolyte imbalance, and massive diuresis are common side effects of urea. Dizziness, disorientation, syncope, and agitation may also occur. Pulmonary edema, convulsions, and death have occasionally been reported.

Urea is irritating to the tissues and causes pain at the site of injection. Extravasation should be prevented, since tissue necrosis can occur. Patients should be carefully monitored for vital signs and side effects. Urea should not be used in patients with severely impaired renal function, active intracranial bleeding, marked dehydration, or liver failure.

Mydriatic and cycloplegic agents

These topically applied autonomic drugs can cause pupillary dilation (mydriasis) and paralysis of accommodation (cycloplegia). The autonomic drugs cause mydriasis by a sympathomimetic or parasympatholytic mechanism of action. The effects of these agents depend on the patient's age, race, and color of iris. Mydriatic agents evoke a lesser response in persons with heavily pigmented irides than in persons with lighter pigmented irides. Thus blacks tend to respond less to these agents than whites. The maximal mydriatic effect occurs within 10 to 40 minutes, with a duration of 2 hours to 2 weeks. The maximal cycloplegic effect is 15 minutes to several hours, with a duration of 6 hours to 1 week.

The mydriatics and cycloplegics are also used to treat inflammations such as uveitis and keratitis. These drugs relieve ocular pain by relaxing inflamed intraocular muscles and by putting the eye at rest.

The pharmacologic actions of these drugs allow for accurate measurement of refractive errors, which permits proper lens determination for eyeglasses. They are also used preoperatively and postoperatively in intraocular surgery.

The parasympatholytic (anticholinergic) drugs cause mydriasis and cycloplegia by making the pupillary sphincter and the ciliary muscles insensitive to acetylcholine. The sympathomimetic (adrenergic) drugs either mimic (direct acting) or potentiate (indirect acting) the action of epinephrine in affecting the dilator muscle of the iris. Except for cocaine, they do not induce cycloplegia. Table 17-1 presents these parasympatholytic and sympathomimetic agents and their mydriatic and cycloplegic effects on the eye.

Anticholinergic (parasympatholytic) drugs

The circular smooth muscles of the iris, which constrict the pupil, are innervated by parasympathetic fibers from the oculomotor

TABLE 17-1 Mydriatics and cycloplegics: approximate maximum range of effects

	Maximal mydriasis	Duration of mydriasis	Maximal cycloplegia	Duration of cycloplegia
Parasympatholytic (anticholinergic) agents				
Atropine	30 to 40 minutes	12 days	Several hours	14 days
Cyclopentolate	15 to 30 minutes	24 hours	15 to 45 minutes	24 hours
Homatropine	10 to 30 minutes	6 hours to 4 days	30 to 90 minutes	10 to 48 hours
Scopolamine	15 to 30 minutes	Several days	30 to 45 minutes	5 to 7 days
Tropicamide	20 to 35 minutes	4 hours	20 to 25 minutes	6 hours
Sympathomimetic (adrenergic) agents				
Direct acting				
Epinephrine	Minimal		—	—
Phenylephrine	20 minutes	3 hours	—	—
Indirect acting				
Cocaine	20 minutes	2 hours	—	—
Ephedrine	30 minutes	3 hours	—	—
Hydroxyamphetamine	40 minutes	6 hours	—	—

(third cranial) nerve. Anticholinergics (parasympatholytics) block the neurohormonal mediator, acetylcholine. This leaves the pupil (radial fibers of the iris) under the unopposed influence of its sympathetic, or adrenergic, nerve supply, and pupil dilation occurs. The oculomotor nerve also supplies the ciliary muscle. Contraction of this muscle slackens the suspensory ligament of the lens and allows the lens to become more convex. Accommodation for near vision depends on the ciliary muscle's ability to contract.

The anticholinergic drugs used topically in the eye include atropine, scopolamine, homatropine, cyclopentolate, and tropicamide.

Homatropine, cyclopentolate, and tropicamide are short-acting cycloplegics. They are used for refraction in older children and adults. Instillation of a 1% pilocarpine solution may be used to counteract the mydriasis and cycloplegia of short-acting cycloplegics. Pilocarpine is not useful in counteracting the effects of atropine or scopolamine because of its short duration of action. All cycloplegics may produce flushing of the face and may induce fever.

Systemic absorption of these drugs can result in serious side effects, such as dryness of the mouth, inhibition of sweating, flushing, tachycardia, psychiatric and behavioral problems, fever, delirium, and coma. Pupillary dilation from either local or systemic administration can precipitate acute glaucoma in predisposed persons, which, if unrecognized or untreated, can result in blindness.

Atropine sulfate

Atropine is the most potent of all cyloplegic drugs and has a long duration of action. It is available in 0.125% to 3% aqueous solutions and in ointments containing 0.5% or 1% of atropine. Atropine produces mydriasis within 30 to 40 minutes; cycloplegia however, takes several hours and several applications over 1 or 2 hours may be required. Residual cycloplegia may persist for 5 to up to 14 days; the mydriatic effect lasts for 10 to 12 days and in some individuals 2 to 3 weeks.

Atropine is the drug of choice for refraction of children with accommodative esotropia. It is often preferred for refraction of children under 6 years of age. It is commonly used for the initial examination of patients with convergent strabismus. It is not a desirable drug for refraction in adults because of its long duration of effect.

Atropine in a 1% solution or ointment is also used to treat inflammations of the eye such as iritis, uveitis, and keratitis. In severe cases the drug may be instilled three times a day; in mild cases administration is usually once daily. Patients should be instructed that the next instillation should be omitted if side effects (dryness of mouth, tachycardia) are present. The patient must be aware that during therapy he may be unable to focus on nearby objects and will be unusually sensitive to light. Dark glasses should be worn to decrease photophobia. The eye will be accommodated for distant vision.

Atropine is contraindicated in patients with glaucoma. Dilation of the pupil causes a narrowing of the iridocorneal angle where the canal of Schlemm is located. This restricts drainage of intraocular fluids, although secretion continues and intraocular pressure rises. This may precipitate an attack of acute glaucoma.

Since atropine is highly toxic, it should be stored in a safe place out of the reach of children.

Scopolamine hydrobromide, hyoscine hydrobromide

Scopolamine in aqueous solutions of 0.25% and 0.3% and a 0.2% ophthalmic ointment has actions and side effects similar to those of atropine. Scopolamine is a more rapidly acting mydriatic and cycloplegic than atropine, but its effects are of shorter duration. Instillation of scopolamine solution causes mydriasis in 15 to 30 minutes; cycloplegia occurs in 30 to 45 minutes and effects may persist for 5 to 7 days. It is used in patients sensitive to atropine and for uveitis and refraction.

Homatropine hydrobromide

Of the short-acting cycloplegics, homatropine has the slowest onset and most prolonged action. Mydriasis occurs in 10 to 30 minutes and cycloplegia in 30 to 90 minutes. These effects may last from 24 to 48 hours. For mydriasis or ophthalmoscopic examination the 1% solution is usually adequate; for cycloplegia instillation of several drops of a 2% or stronger (up to 5%) solution at intervals of 10 to 15 minutes may be required. It is contraindicated in patients with glaucoma and those with narrow angle or shallow anterior chambers because of their susceptibility to glaucoma. It must be used cautiously in older patients.

Cyclopentolate hydrochloride (Cyclogyl)

Cyclopentolate is more potent than homatropine and has a shorter duration of action. Mydriasis and cycloplegia occur within 15 to 45 minutes; effects may last up to 24 hours. It is used solely as a mydriatic and cycloplegic. Dosage is usually 1 drop of a 1% solution or 2 drops of 0.5% solution 5 minutes apart. In children, 3 drops 10 minutes apart may be used.

Cyclopentolate has proved to be effective for mydriasis and cycloplegia for diagnostic purposes.

Tropicamide (Mydriacyl)

Tropicamide is a rapid-acting cycloplegic and mydriatic agent with a short duration of action. Two drops of a 1% solution of tropicamide 5 minutes apart has a mydriatic effect within 20 to 35 minutes. The cycloplegic effect begins to reach a maximum in 20 to 25 minutes and appears to wear off in 30 to 40 minutes, with complete recovery in 2 to 6 hours. Examination must be performed within 35 minutes after instillation, or an additional drop must be applied.

It is effective for diagnostic use for refraction but ineffective in inflammatory conditions.

Adrenergic (sympathomimetic) drugs

Mydriasis and decreased congestion of conjunctival blood vessels are produced when adrenergic, or sympathomimetic, drugs are applied topically to the eye. Five adrenergic drugs are used in ophthalmology—epinephrine (see previous section on Antiglaucoma agents—sympathomimetics), phenylephrine, hydroxy-amphetamine, naphazoline, and tetrahydrozoline.

Adrenergic drugs applied topically to the eye elicit the following sympathetic responses:

1 Mydriasis brought about by contraction of the radial or dilator muscle of the eye
2 Constriction of conjunctival blood vessels
3 Slight relaxation of the ciliary muscle
4 Decreased formation of aqueous humor and increased outflow with a resultant drop in intraocular pressure

Exactly how these effects are produced remains uncertain, but there is some evidence that alphadrenergic receptors are present in the outflow mechanism of the eye and, when stimulated, they increase outflow of aqueous humor. It has also been shown experimentally that vasoconstriction decreases the rate of aqueous humor formation.

Adrenergic drugs are used to treat wide-angle glaucoma and glaucoma secondary to uveitis, to produce mydriasis for ocular examination, and to relieve congestion and hyperemia. Adrenergic drugs are contraindicated in the treatment of narrow-angle glaucoma since dilation of the pupil will further restrict ocular fluid outflow and this may cause an acute attack of glaucoma. Serious systemic side effects from these drugs are unusual, but care must be taken in patients with cardiovascular disease, since tachycardia and elevated blood pressure can occur with these agents.

As with other sympathomimetic amines, the potential exists for drug interactions between these adrenergic drugs and monoamine oxidase inhibitors, creating exaggerated adrenergic effects. The potientation of adrenergic pressor effects is increased with the use of the tricyclic antidepressants.

Phenylephrine hydrochloride ophthalmic solution (Neo-Synephrine)

Phenylephrine is commonly used in 0.08%, 0.12%, and 0.15% solution as a decongestant in over-the-counter products. In the 2.5% and 10% solution it is used as a mydriatic for ocular examination and requires a prescription. The 2.5% solution is used in conjunction with cycloplegics to decrease the amount of cycloplegic needed for refraction and to aid in rapid satisfactory cycloplegia. The 10% solution is used in intraocular surgery, as a decongestant and vasoconstrictor, and for uveitis, pupil dilation, and wide-angle glaucoma. The 10% solution should be used with special caution in persons taking monoamine oxidase inhibitors and in patients with advanced arteriosclerosis or hypertension. Care must be taken to prevent systemic absorption, since 1 drop (0.05 ml) of a 10% (100 mg/ml) solution contains about 5 mg of drug. This is equal to the usual subcutaneous dose (in mild to moderate hypotension), and it can produce a substantial rise in blood pressure. Phenylephrine's effects are produced within 20 minutes. It should not be used if the solution is brown or has a precipitate. Prolonged exposure to light or air causes oxidation and discoloration.

Hydroxyamphetamine hydrobromide (Paredrine)

Hydroxyamphetamine is available in a 1% solution. It is extensively used as a mydriatic; 1 or 2 drops are usually instilled into the conjunctival sac. It produces mydriasis in 45 to 60 minutes; recovery occurs in about 6 hours. Its major use is in diagnosing the pupil abnormality of Horner's syndrome.

Naphazoline hydrochloride

Common brand-name solutions with naphazoline include Albalon, Naphcon Forte, and Vasocon Ophthalmic (0.1% naphazoline) sold by prescription, and Clera (0.05%), Vaso Clear (0.02%), and Clear Eyes and Naphcon Eyedrops (0.012%), sold without a prescription. Used for topical ocular vasoconstriction, these solutions are usually administered as 1 or 2 drops into the conjunctival sac every 3 to 4 hours.

Tetrahydrozoline hydrochloride (Murine Plus, Visine)

This 0.05% ophthalmic solution is sold without a prescription for relief from minor eye irritation and after contact lens removal as a topical eye decongestant. One or 2 drops are instilled in each eye every 3 to 4 hours.

Ophthalmic surgery aids
Sodium hyaluronate (Healon)

Sodium hyaluronate is used during anterior segment and vitreous procedures in cataract surgery (intracapsular and extracapsular). During intraocular lens implantation it is used to coat the instruments and the lens before insertion. A dose of 0.5 ml in the anterior chamber before insertion of the new lens delivery protects the corneal endothelium from damage when a cataractous lens is being removed. Other indications include glaucoma filtration surgery and corneal transplant surgery. Sodium hyaluronate is also used as a vitreous replacement after retinal detachment surgery and vitrectomy. The 1% solution protects corneal endothelial tissues and ocular structures by decreasing the chances for formation of adhesions and synechiae. Additionally the drug maintains a deep anterior chamber during surgery, thus permitting easier manipulation and causing less trauma to the corneal endothelium. This product is an extract from avian tissue and has the risk of any foreign biological (protein) material when injected.

Antiinfective/ antiinflammatory agents

The basic principles guiding the use of chemotherapy for ocular infections are the same in all branches of medicine. The drug of choice and the dose required should be established by adequate laboratory isolation of the offending organism; the initial culture from the infected area should be obtained before any antiinfective/antiinflammatory agent is applied. However, treatment should not be withheld if the time required to make these determinations may result in increased severity of infection and if the type of infection (for example, most cases of conjunctivitis) does not warrant the expense of laboratory analysis; the latter tend to be self-limiting. Prophylactic use of antiinfective/antiinflammatory agents in general is useless as well as wasteful and potentially dangerous. A large proportion of the inflammatory diseases seen in ophthalmology are caused by viruses or other agents that are not susceptible to any currently available antiinfective agents; obviously, the use of these agents in such situations is unwarranted.

Most antiinfective agents do not readily penetrate the eye when applied. However, some drugs will penetrate the inflamed eye when the blood-aqueous barrier is decreased by injury or inflammation. Topically applied antiinfective agents can cause sensitivity reactions (stinging, itching, angioneurotic edema, urticaria, dermatitis) and patients sensitized to one drug may show cross reactions to chemically related drugs. In addition, topical application of antiinfective agents interferes with the normal flora of the eye, which may encourage growth of other organisms. Eye infections require prompt treatment to help prevent spread of infection. Severe infections may damage the eye and impair vision. Solutions are preferred for treatment of eye infections, since ointment bases often tend to interfere with healing.

Antibiotics

All known systemically administered antibiotics are available and used at indicated times to treat ocular infections. Care must be taken to use an antibiotic that will not cause local or general sensitivity and to use drugs that are unlikely to ever be used systemically, in order to avoid possible sensitization to common systemic antiinfective drugs and to discourage development of resistant strains of offending organisms.

Selection of an antibiotic for ocular infection is based on (1) clinical experience, (2) nature and sensitivity of the organisms most commonly causing the condition, (3) the disease itself, and (4) sensitivity and response of the patient.

Some of the common ocular infections treated with antibiotics include the following.

conjunctivitis—Acute inflammation of the conjunctiva (the mucous membrane lining the back of the lids and the front of the eye, except for the cornea) resulting from bacterial invasion. "Pink eye" is the acute contagious epidemic form of conjunctivitis usually caused by pneumococci. Symptoms include redness and burning of the eye, lacrimation, itching, and at times photophobia. Conjunctivitis is usually self-limiting. The eye should be protected from light.

hordeolum (sty)—An acute localized infection of the eyelash follicles and the glands of the anterior lid margin resulting in the formation of a small abscess or cyst.

chalazion—Infection of the meibomian (sebaceous) glands of the eyelids. A hard cyst may form from blockage of the ducts.

blepharitis—Inflammation of the margins of the eyelid resulting from bacterial infection or allergy. Symptoms are crusting, irritation of the eye, and red and edematous lid margins.

keratitis—Corneal inflammation caused by bacterial infection; herpes simplex keratitis is caused by viral infection.

uveitis—Infection of the uveal tract, or the vascular layer of the eye, which includes the iris, ciliary body, and choroid.

Bacitracin ophthalmic ointment (Baciguent); bacitracin zinc

Bacitracin is rarely used systemically because of its nephrotoxic effects. Ophthalmic bacitracin is available as an ointment containing 500 units/g of suitable base and as a powder containing 10,000 and 50,000 units for making solutions for topical use. It is particularly useful in treating superficial infections caused by gram-positive bacteria. Ointment is instilled into the lower conjunctival sac of the affected eye one to three times daily or more often.

A broader spectrum of antimicrobial activity is produced when bacitracin is used in combination with gramicidin, neomycin, and polymyxin (Neosporin, Neo-polycin) than when it is used alone. Bacitracin does not penetrate the cornea in therapeutic amounts, is nonirritating to the eye, and causes no systemic effects. Ointment preparations are stable for about 1 year at room temperature. Bacitracin is preferable to neomycin for topical use, since fewer organisms are resistant to it, allergic reactions occur less frequently, and sensitization is avoided.

Chloramphenicol (Chloromycetin, Chloroptic, Econochlor, Opthochlor)

Chloramphenicol's effectiveness against a wide variety of gram-positive and gram-negative organisms makes it an extremely useful drug for intraocular infections. It penetrates the eye much more readily than many other antibiotics. Chloramphenicol is applied topically as a 1% ointment or a 0.16% to 0.5% solution. Drops may be instilled two to four times a day or every 3, 4, or 6 hours, and the ointment may be applied at bedtime. With severe infection, 1 drop may be instilled every 30 minutes until improvement occurs. Prolonged or frequent use should be avoided. A case of bone marrow hypoplasia has been reported following prolonged (23 months) use of the eyedrops.

Erythromycin (Ilotycin)

Erythromycin is applied one or more times daily in a 0.5% ointment. It is effective against all gram-positive and many gram-negative organisms and for treating superficial eye infections.

Neomycin sulfate (Myciguent)

Neomycin is available as an ointment containing 3.5 mg/g of base. It has a broad antibacterial spectrum and a low index of allergenicity. Because of auditory and renal toxicity, it is generally not used parenterally and thus is often preferred for local use. However, it is an active topical sensitizer and can cause cross-sensitivity reactions to systemically used antibiotics that are chemically related. It is effective for treating superficial ocular infections involving the conjunctiva and cornea.

Polymyxin B sulfate (Aerosporin)

Polymyxin B is used largely for its activity against gram-negative bacteria. Hypersensitivity reaction to the topical solution is practically unknown. For topical application 1 drop of a solution containing 20,000 units/ml is instilled; frequency of the dosage depends on the severity and type of infection. An intact corneal epithelium prevents penetration of polymyxin B into the eye, but epithelial damage from abrasion or ulceration permits effective penetration.

It is available in combination with neomycin (Polyspectrin, Statrol), bacitracin (Polysporin), gramicidin, and oxytetracycline.

Tetracyclines

The tetracyclines are used topically to treat superficial infections of the eye. Generally, they are bacteriostatic rather than bactericidal; they have a broad antimicrobial spectrum. Organisms resistant to one tetracycline are usually resistant to the others. Trachoma may be treated with both topical and oral tetracycline therapy. The tetracyclines have been recommended for prophylaxis of gonorrheal ophthalmia neonatorum, since they produce a lower incidence of conjunctivitis and less irritation of the eye than does silver nitrate. Topical tetracyclines rarely cause adverse reactions.

Tetracycline hydrochloride (Achromycin) is applied topically as 1% ointment or 1% suspension in oil.

Chlortetracycline hydrochloride (Aureomycin) is applied as a 1% ointment; a sterile powder is also available for making a 0.5% solution.

Oxytetracycline hydrochloride (Terramycin) is applied as a 0.5% ointment in combination with polymixin B.

Gentamicin sulfate (Garamycin, Genoptic)

Gentamicin is effective against a wide variety of gram-negative and gram-positive organisms. It is particularly useful against *Pseudomonas*, *Proteus*, and *Klebsiella* organisms and *Escherichia coli*, as well as staphylococci and streptococci that have developed resistance to other antibiotics. It is applied as an ointment two or three times daily or 1 drop of solution (3 to 10 mg/ml) is applied every 1 to 4 hours.

Tobramycin (Tobrex)

This water-soluble aminoglycoside is for topical use on a wide variety of gram-positive and gram-negative external ophthalmic pathogens. It is of particular value in gentamicin-resistant infections. Among the pathogens affected by the aminoglycoside are the staphylococci, streptococci, *Pseudomonas*, *Escherichia coli*, *Klebsiella*, *Enterobacter*, *Proteus*, *Haemophilus influenzae*, *Moxaxella*, *Acinetobacter*, and some *Neisseria*. Adverse reactions include ocular toxicity, hypersensitivity including lid itching, swelling, and conjunctival erythema. When topical aminoglycosides are used concurrently with systemic aminoglycosides, the total serum concentration will be affected and should be monitored. The dose for mild to moderate infection is 2 drops in the affected eye every 4 hours. For severe infections 2 drops are instilled hourly in the eye until improvement is seen, and then the dose is reduced before the drops are discontinued. The solution is incompatible with tetracycline because it contains tyloxacol. It is available in 5-ml containers (3 mg/ml) as a 0.3% solution.

Sulfonamides
Sulfacetamide sodium (Isopto Cetamide, Bleph-10 Liquifilm, Sodium Sulamyd)

Used in a 10% ointment or a 10% to 30% solution, sulfacetamide provides high local concentrations that are relatively nonirritating. The presence of purulent drainage or exudate interferes with the action of the sulfonamides, since the purulent matter contains para-aminobenzoic acid. Sulfacetamide is available only for topical use and thus is preferred over other sulfa drugs used systemically. It may cause local irritation.

Sulfisoxazole diethanolamine (Gantrisin)

Sulfisoxazole is available in 4% ophthalmic solution and a 4% ophthalmic ointment. It is applied topically to the conjunctiva three or more times daily.

Antifungal agent
Natamycin (Natamycin Ophthalmic Suspension)

Natamycin is derived from *Streptomyces natalenis* and is active against certain yeast and filamentous fungi. The apparent mechanism of action involves binding of the agent to the fungal cell membrane, which alters the permeability and causes depletion of the essential cellular constituents. Antifungal activity is dose-related but without gram-positive or gram-negative activity. The effective concentration is found within the corneal stroma but not in intraocular fluid. There is little systemic absorption measured.

This is the drug of choice in *Fusarium solanae* keratitis and is used in treating fungal blepharitis and conjunctivitis or keratitis caused by fungal organisms that is confirmed by clinical and laboratory diagnosis (smear and culture or corneal scrapings).

Adherence of the suspension to epithelial ulceration or retention in the fornices occurs with regularity, and possible tolerance must be checked at least twice weekly.

Initial doses are 1 drop every 1 or 2 hours, then 1 drop six or eight times daily for 3 to 4 days, with gradual weekly reduction over 2 to 3 weeks.

Antiviral agents
Idoxuridine (Herplex, Dendrid, Stoxil)

Idoxuridine (IDU) inhibits the replication of certain viruses when applied directly to the eye. The drug is too toxic for systemic use. When applied locally in the eye in a 0.1% solution, the drug is effective in the treatment of keratitis caused by the herpes simplex virus and the vaccinia virus. One drop of the drug may be applied to the conjunctiva every 1 to 2 hours (day and night) for several days and continued for 3 to 5 days after healing is complete. The solution should be kept refrigerated and the expiration date observed.

Idoxuridine is also available as a 0.5% ointment; it is usually applied five times a day. Its effectiveness is reported to be equal to that of the drops.

Vidarabine (Vira-A Ophthalmic)

Action and result. The antiviral mechanism of action is not established for this agent, but it appears to interfere with early steps of viral DNA synthesis. Activity is directed against herpes simplex (types 1 and 2), varicella-zoster, and vaccinia viruses. The deaminated metabolite arabinosylhypoxanthine (Ara-Hx) has less antiviral activity than the parent compound. An epithelial defect in the cornea permits trace amounts of the parent and metabolite to be found in the aqueous humor. Systemic absorption is not expected after ocular administration or by swallowing lacrimal secretions.

Uses. Vidarabine is used for ocular herpes simplex. A slit-lamp eye examination will reveal herpes simplex by establishing the presence of typical dendritic or geographic lesions (the clinical diagnosis).

Preparation, dosage, and administration. The ointment (3%) is the only form available for ophthalmic use. About ½ inch of ointment into the lower conjunctival sac five times daily every 3 hours is the recommended dose. Although some cases need longer treatment, improvement after 1 week or reepithelialization after 3 weeks must occur before other therapy is considered. To prevent recurrence, a dose twice daily for 1 week is recommended.

Side effects and toxic effects. Patients taking Vidarabine may experience lacrimation, foreign body sensation, burning, irritation, pain, photophobia, conjunctival injection, and keratitis. Ophthalmic ointments usually produce a temporary visual haze; the patient should be forewarned by the nurse. The possibility of viral resistance may exist but is not well established. Since the ophthalmic dose is small, the drug is relatively insoluble and ocular penetration is low. The possibility of embryonic or fetal damage in pregnant women is remote but to be overlooked. Contraindications center on hypersensitivity to the drug.

Drug interactions. Topical antibiotics (chloramphenicol, erythromycin, gentamicin sulfate) may be administered concurrently without interaction. The topical steroid (dexamethasone or prednisolone) administered concurrently may induce corticosteroid-induced ocular side effects such as glaucoma or posterior subcapsular cataract formation and progression of bacterial or viral infections.

Trifluridine (Viroptic)

Action and result. Trifluridine is a fluorinated pyrimidine nucleoside with activity against herpes simplex virus (types 1 and 2), vaccinia virus, and some strains of adenovirus. The mechanism of action is not completely understood, but it does interfere with DNA synthesis in cultured mammalian cells. Animal studies indicate that there is penetration of the intact cornea, since both the parent form (trifluridine) and the major metabolite (5-carboxy 2'-deoxyuridine) were recovered on the endothelial side of the cornea. In the absence of corneal epithelium, the penetration is enhanced twofold. Intraocular penetration occurs for the parent but not for the metabolite. A decrease in corneal integrity or presence of uveal inflammation enhances the penetration of the parent compound into the aqueous humor, yet there appears to be negligible systemic absorption of both the parent compound and the metabolite. It is well diluted in body fluids and has a half-life of 12 minutes.

Uses. Trifluridine is used for treatment of primary keratoconjunctivitis and recurrent epithelial keratitis caused by herpes simplex virus, types 1 and 2; epithelial keratitis unresponsive to idoxuridine or when ocular toxicity or hypersensitivity occurs as a result of idoxuridine therapy; and the small number of patients resistant to topical vidarabine. Trifluridine is not effective against bacterial, chlamydial, fungal, or nonviral trophic lesions of the cornea.

Preparation, dosage, and administration. Trifluridine is supplied as a 1% solution. One drop is instilled into the cornea every 2 hours while the patient is awake for a daily maximum number of 9 drops until the corneal ulcer has reepithelialized, then 1 drop every 4 hours for 7 more days for a minimum daily dosage of 5 drops. If after 1 week there is no sign of improvement or if complete reepithelialization has not occurred after 2 weeks, other forms of therapy should be considered. Continuous therapy for over 3 weeks is not recommended because of potential ocular toxicity.

Side effects. Mild transient burning or stinging and palpebral edema have been seen. Other reported adverse reactions in less than 3% of cases, in decreasing order, include superficial punctate and epithelial keratopathy, hypersensitivity, stromal edema, irritation, keratitis sicca, hyperemia, and increased intraocular pressure.

Precautions. Trifluridine is used only when clinical diagnosis is positive for herpetic keratitis. The possibility of viral resistance may follow multiple exposure. There is also the possibility that mutagenic agents may cause genetic damage. The oncogenic potential is unknown at this time. It is not prescribed for pregnant women or nursing mothers unless the potential benefits outweigh the potential risks. Trifluridine is contraindicated in persons who are sensitive or intolerant to it.

Drug interactions. The following drugs have been used topically and concurrently *without evidence of adverse interaction:* antibiotics (bacitracin, chloramphenicol, erythromycin, gentamicin sulfate, neomycin sulfate, polymyxin B sulfate, sulfacetamide, sodium, tetracycline hydrochloride), steroids (dexamethasone, fluorometholone, hydrocortisone, prednisolone), and other drugs (atropine sulfate, cyclopentolate, hydrochloride, homatropine, hydrobromide, ephedrine hydrochloride, naphazoline hydrochloride, pilocarpine, scopolamine hydrobromide, sodium chloride).

Antiseptics

Many of the antiseptics that were used to treat surface infections of the eye prior to the advent of antibiotics are now obsolete. Not only were many of these drugs relatively ineffective, they also delayed healing and in some cases caused permanent damage to the eye. Antiseptic solutions are employed in ophthalmology for irrigation, dissolution of secretions, and precipitation of mucus and in certain instances in which specific antimicrobial agents cannot be used. A 2.2% boric acid solution is used as an irrigant; this concentration is thought to be isotonic with tear fluid.

Inorganic mercuric salts such as yellow mercuric oxide ophthalmic ointment, thimerosal (Merthiolate), and ammoniated mercury formerly served as bacteriostatic agents. Today they are seldom used, since they do not completely sterilize, spores are resistant to them, and they are irritating to the eye.

Silver nitrate

A solution of 1% or 2% silver nitrate is routinely employed immediately after birth as a prophylaxis against ophthalmia neonatorum. In many states this is required by law. The gonococci are particularly susceptible to silver salts. Silver nitrate is preferred to effective antibiotic agents, since these may sensitize the patient and silver nitrate has stood the test of time. Silver nitrate ophthalmic solution is

available in collapsible capsules containing about 5 drops of a 1% solution. The solution should be in contact with the conjunctival sac for not less than 30 seconds to produce a mild chemical conjunctivitis. Irrigation following use is not recommended.

Benzalkonium chloride

Benzalkonium chloride is a cationic surface-active wetting agent that has several applications in ophthalmology. Its antiseptic properties make it useful in the preservation of other solutions and the sterilization of small instruments. It is also used in balanced salt solutions (B.S.S.) to aid in the cleansing and application of contact lenses. For topical application to the conjunctiva a 1:10,000 solution is used (1 ml of a 0.01% solution).

Zinc sulfate (Eye-Sed, Op-Thal-Zin, Zinc Sulfate Bufopto)

An aqueous solution of 0.2% to 0.25% zinc sulfate is used as an astringent and a mildly antiseptic eyewash in conjunctivitis caused by the Morax-Axenfeld bacillus.

Iodine tincture

Iodine tincture contains 2% iodine and 2% sodium iodide in dilute alcohol. Its only ophthalmic use is for chemical cautery of corneal lesions produced by herpes simplex virus.

Steroids

Corticosteroid therapy is indicated for all allergic reactions of the eye, nonpyogenic inflammations, and severe injury. Allergic reactions of the eye may be caused by drugs applied to the eye or by contact with substances such as weed pollen to which the individual is hypersensitive.

Ophthalmic corticosteroid therapy is not used for pyogenic (pus-producing) inflammations of the eye, since corticosteroids decrease defense mechanisms and reduce resistance to pathogenic organisms.

Eye structures are relatively delicate, and inflammation can cause functional damage, scarring, and impaired vision. Inflammation increases capillary permeability. In the eye, this results in the escape of proteins and cells from the blood vessels into the aqueous humor; this in turn may cause a rise in intraocular pressure.

The glucocorticoids used in ophthalmology may be applied topically, injected into the conjunctiva, or given systemically.

Corticosteroid therapy is not recommended for minor corneal abrasions. Steroids may actually increase ocular susceptibility to fungous infection. When steroids are used for various eye conditions, they should be used for a limited time only and the eye should be checked for increase in ocular pressure. Clinical evidence indicates that prolonged ocular steroid therapy can cause systemic side effects, glaucoma, and cataracts.

The following corticosteroids are available for topical use as solutions, suspensions, or ointments. They are available in varying strengths and in combinations with various antibiotics.

> Cortisone acetate
> Dexamethasone
> Fludrocortisone acetate
> Fluorometholone
> Hydrocortisone
> Medrysone
> Methylprednisolone
> Prednisolone

Other ophthalmic preparations
Topical anesthetics

Local anesthetics are used to prevent pain (deep anesthesia) during surgical procedures (removal of sutures and foreign bodies), tonometry, and examinations. Unfortunately, all of the topical anesthetic drugs interfere with healing of epithelial tissue, particularly of the cornea. The practice of repeatedly applying such an anesthetic to an eye after removal of a foreign body is to be condemned. Besides delaying wound healing, this can produce sensitivity, permanent corneal opacification, visual loss, or perforation of the cornea. These agents are used only under close medical supervision and are rarely self-administered by the patient.

Cocaine hydrochloride

Cocaine was the first drug to be used for anesthesia of the eye (1884). One drop of cocaine produces anesthesia of the cornea in 5 to 10 minutes. Complete anesthesia lasts for approximately 10 minutes; less anesthetic effect persists for 1 or 2 hours. In addition to its anesthetic effects, cocaine produces mydriasis and constriction of conjunctival vessels. Since the surface of the eye becomes dry, this may cause damage to the corneal surface. It may precipitate an acute attack of glaucoma. For these reasons, cocaine has largely been replaced by newer anesthetics.

Solutions of 0.5% to 4% are used for deep topical anesthesia of the eye. The drug has both anesthetizing and adrenergic effects. Local administration may produce acute cocaine poisoning with sudden severe confusion, delirium, and convulsions. Short-acting barbiturates must be given at once to prevent fatality.

Tetracaine hydrochloride (Pontocaine, Anacel)

Tetracaine is used topically in a 0.5% to 2% solution for rapid, brief, superficial anesthesia. It is a widely used local ocular anesthetic. One drop of a 0.5% solution of tetracaine will produce anesthesia within 30 seconds; the patient may feel a burning sensation. The anesthetic effect lasts for 10 to 25 minutes. Tetracaine can cause epithelial damage; therefore, it is not recommended for prolonged home use by patients. It is physically incompatible with the mercury (such as thimerosal [merthiolate]) or silver salts often found in ophthalmic products.

Proparacaine hydrochloride (Ophthaine, Ophthetic, Alcaine)

This drug is similar to tetracaine. A 0.5% solution is administered by topical instillation. Anesthesia is produced within 20 seconds and lasts for 15 minutes. It is relatively free from the burning and discomfort of other anesthetics and is highly toxic if it enters systemic circulation. Allergic contact dermatitis, softening and erosion of corneal epithelium, pupillary dilation, cycloplegia, conjunctival congestion and hemorrhage, and stromal edema have been reported.

Benoxinate hydrochloride (Dorsacaine)

Benoxinate is similar to proparacaine. Anesthesia occurs within 1 minute after instillation of 1 drop of a 0.4% solution and lasts about 10 to 15 minutes. A series of three instillations (2 drops in each eye at 90-second intervals) may extend the anesthesia to 20 minutes. The incidence of side effects is low.

Artificial tears

Lubricants, or "artificial tears," are used to provide moisture and lubrication in diseases in which tear production is deficient, to lubricate artificial eyes and moisten contact lenses, and to protect the cornea during procedures on the eye. These agents are also incorporated into ophthalmic preparations to prolong the contact time of topically applied drugs.

Methylcellulose (Methulose, Visculose, Isopto Tears, Lyteers, Tearisol)

Methycellulose is used as a 0.5% to 2.5% solution. For decreased tear production 1 or 2 drops of the 0.5% solution is applied to the eye as needed; to lubricate contact lenses and artificial eyes the solution is applied directly to the lens or artificial eye. Most preparations contain benzalkonium chloride or chlorobutanol as preservatives.

Methylcellulose is nonirritating to ocular tissue and can be used for prolonged periods without damaging the eye. However, if an excess is instilled into the eye and dries on the eyelids, it may cause discomfort similar to having sand in the eyes. If this occurs, an eyewash or sterile, nonirritating irrigating solution should be used.

Polyvinyl alcohol (Wetting Solution, Lens Mate, Liquifilm Tears)

Polyvinyl alcohol is a nontoxic agent that is less viscous than methylcellulose and therefore must be applied more frequently when used as a substitute for tears. As artificial tears, 1 or 2 drops are applied to the eyes as needed. To moisten contact lenses, the solution is applied to the lens before insertion. Preparations also contain a preservative such as benzalkonium chloride or chlorobutanol.

Prosthetic cleaning agent
Enuclene

Enuclene contains tyloxapol, benzalkonium chloride, and methylcellulose and is used for cleaning, wetting, and lubricating an artificial eye. One or 2 drops are applied onto the artificial eye three or four times daily.

Diagnostic aids
Fluorescein sodium

Fluorescein is a nontoxic water-soluble dye that is used as a diagnostic aid. When applied to the cornea, only areas denuded of epithelium (corneal lesions or ulcers) are stained a bright green color; foreign bodies appear surrounded by a green ring. These effects permit detection of corneal epithelial defects caused by injury or infection and location of foreign bodies in the eye. Loss of conjunctiva is indicated by a yellow hue. The dye is also used in fitting contact lenses. Areas that lack fluorescein-stained tears will appear black under ultraviolet light, indicating the contact lens is touching the cornea at those areas. Fluorescein is used in retinal photography to determine retinal vascular status and to identify defects in the retinal pigment epithelium. In addition, it may be used to test lacrimal patency; if after the dye is instilled into the eye it appears in the nasal secretions, the nasolacrimal drainage system is open.

Solutions of this dye are easily contaminated by *Pseudomonas aeruginosa*, which causes intense corneal ulceration. For this reason prepared solutions are never used, but strips of filter paper impregnated with the dry dye (Ful-Glo, Fluor-I-Strip) are moistened just before use. Staining of the eye disappears in 30 minutes. Hypersensitivity can occur in allergic and asthmatic patients.

Fluress is a combination of the dye fluorescein and the local anesthetic benoxinate hydrochloride. It is useful for removal of foreign bodies in the eye since it provides for simultaneous staining and anesthesia. One drop of a 0.25% solution is usually used.

Irrigating solutions

The sterile isotonic external irrigating solutions are used in tonometry, fluorescein procedures, removal of foreign material, gonioscopy and to cleanse and soothe eyes of patients wearing hard contact lenses. These external products do not require a prescription and are available in drops, irrigations, and eyewashes.

Enzyme
Alpha-chymotrypsin (Alpha Chymar, Zolyse, Catarase)

This proteolytic enzyme is used in selected cases to facilitate cataract extraction. It is injected behind the iris into the posterior chamber where it dissolves the filaments or zonules that hold the lens, thereby facilitating intracapsular lens extraction. This effect is usually obtained in 1 to 2 minutes with 0.2 to 0.5 ml of a freshly prepared 1:5000 solution. Chymotrypsin may cause a transient glaucoma lasting about 1 week, which can be relieved by the use of pilocarpine. The following products inactivate this enzyme: acids, alcohol, alkalies, antiseptics, blood, detergents, and serum. The enzyme is inhibited by chloramphenicol and isoflurophate. Epinephrine inactivates the enzyme in 1 hour. It is available in ampules containing 150, 300, or 750 units (proteolytic activity) of lyophilized enzyme dissolved in 2 to 10 ml of diluent.

Hyperosmolar preparation
Sodium chloride ointment (Muro) and Solution (Adsorbonac, Hypersal, Murocoll)

This 5% ointment and 2% or 5% solution are used to reduce the corneal edema that occurs in certain corneal dystrophies and to aid gonioscopy, funduscopy, and biomicroscopy. The dose is 1 to 2 drops in affected eye(s) every 3 to 4 hours as directed.

Summary of nursing considerations

Drugs used in the treatment of eye disorders are administered by topical application of a solution or ointment. They also are administered by packs, iontophoresis, subconjunctival injection, retrobulbar injection, injection directly into the chambers of the eye, and by a new method, an ocular insert with a centrally located reservoir of drug.

Glaucoma is an eye disease characterized chiefly by abnormally elevated intraocular pressure that may result from excessive production of aqueous humor or from diminished ocular fluid outflow. Increased pressure, if sufficiently high and persistent, may lead to irreversible blindness.

Drugs used in glaucoma therapy to decrease intraocular pressure are (1) the miotics (topical cholinergic and anticholinesterase agents), epinephrine (a sympathomimetic), and timolol maleate (a beta adrenergic blocker), which decrease resistance to aqueous humor outflow; (2) carbonic anhydrase inhibitors, which decrease aqueous production; and (3) osmotic agents, which reduce the volume of intraocular fluid.

Anticholinergic (parasympatholytic) drugs are applied topically to the eye primarily to produce mydriasis and cycloplegia to aid in refraction and eye examination for diagnostic purposes and to facilitate eye surgery. Adrenergic (sympathomimetic) drugs are used to produce mydriasis without cycloplegia.

Antiinfective/antiinflammatory agents used in treating ocular infection include antibiotics, sulfonamides, antifungal and antiviral agents, antiseptics, and steroids. Topical anesthetics, lubricants, and diagnostic aids are also used during ocular surgical procedures.

Ocular drug administration

In addition to developing a working knowledge of the ophthalmic agents available, the nurse must be especially aware of the special considerations in administering these drugs.

Ocular drugs are administered by topical application of a *solution* or *ointment*. Ocular solutions are sterile, have the advantage of being easily administered, and usually do not interfere physically with vision. Their main disadvantage is the short duration of time the drug is in contact with the eye. Ocular ointments have the advantages of being quite comfortable on instillation and keeping the drug in longer contact with the eye for more prolonged effects. However, ointments form a film over the eye that interferes with vision and cause a higher incidence of contact dermatitis than solutions. In addition, most ointments are not sterile.

Packs may also be used to apply drugs to the eye. These are cotton pledgets saturated with an ophthalmic solution and inserted into the inferior or superior cul-de-sac. Ocular drugs may also be administered by iontophoresis, subconjunctival (sub-tenon's) injection, retrobulbar injection, and injection directly into the vitreous or anterior chamber of the eye.

When the nurse instills topical preparations, the patient's head is placed on a suitable rest so that his face is directed upward. He is then instructed to fix his gaze on a point above his head. Gentle traction with clean fingertips is applied to the lid bases at the bony rim of the orbit; care is taken not to apply any pressure to the eyeball itself. The dropper or ointment tube approaches the eye from below, outside the patient's field of vision, with care to avoid contact with the eye. The drop is applied gently and is not allowed to fall more than 1 inch before it strikes the eye (Fig. 17-2). Following instillation of common ophthalmic drugs, ocular massage is not necessary because these drugs have solubility characteristics that permit adequate corneal penetration.

Many of the solutions employed in ophthalmology are extremely potent and care must be taken when indicated to prevent their systemic absorption. Gentle pressure can be applied for 2 minutes to the lacrimal canaliculi at the inner corner of the eyelids and is directed inward and downward against the bones of the nose. This will help (1) to prevent the solution from entering the nasal cavity and being absorbed through the highly vascular nasal and pharyngeal mucosa and (2) to maintain a higher drug concentration for a longer time.

OCUSERT

A new method of delivery for eye drugs has recently been developed. It consists of an ocular insert with a centrally located reservoir of drug. It is inserted into the upper or lower cul-de-sac. It has been successfully used in the management of glaucoma using pilocarpine-releasing devices. It is expected that other Ocuserts con-

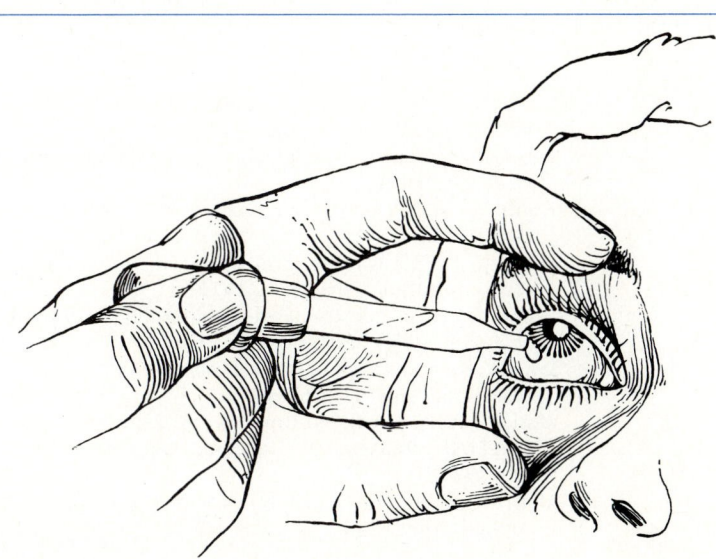

FIG. 17-2. Instillation of drops into the eye.

taining steroids, antivirals, and antibiotics will soon be available. Advantages of the Ocusert include the following.

1 The device delivers continuous, steady medication for 24 hours or more. Ocuserts containing pilocarpine are supposed to release the drug for 7 days; at the end of this period, an Ocusert replacement is necessary.
2 Less medication may be needed and toxicity may be reduced when this method rather than eyedrops is used. Eyedrops produce an initial high local concentration of drug. Some of the drug may escape from the ocular cul-de-sac, resulting in a lower concentration of drug, which may remain below optimal level until the next eyedrop application.
3 It is more convenient to use and may increase patient compliance, particularly in unreliable patients.
4 In younger patients with glaucoma, the miosis and spasm that occur with eyedrops are less prominent with Ocusert.
5 It may provide better daytime control of intraocular pressure.

Following are some limitations of the Ocusert.

1 The Ocusert is considerably more expensive than other methods of therapy.
2 Some patients require more therapy than can be delivered by the Ocusert; these patients need frequent administration of eyedrops.
3 Conjunctival irritation may occur during initial use.
4 There is variability in duration of action; some units proved to be effective for only 2 to 4 days.
5 Sudden leakage of the device has occurred.
6 Migration onto the cornea will obstruct vision and cause pain.
7 The Ocusert may not be retained; it may fall out of the cul-de-sac without the patient noticing the loss.
8 The unit may fall out at night; the patient should check that the unit is in place every morning.
9 Not all patients will be able to learn to insert them.

QUESTIONS

FOR STUDY AND REVIEW

1 Explain how the cholinergic and anticholinesterase miotics produce miosis.
2 How do the adrenergic (sympathomimetic) drugs lower intraocular pressure? How do osmotic agents reduce intraocular pressure?
3 What precaustions should be observed with the use of timolol maleate?
4 What are the therapeutic effects for which mydriatics are used?
5 What precautions should be used with ophthalmic antibiotics?
6 For what type of viral infection of the eye is vidarabine indicated? Explain how it acts.
7 State the legal purpose of the routine administration of silver nitrate in the eyes of newborn infants.
8 Compare the advantages and disadvantages of ophthalmic solutions and ointments.
9 Explain the ophthalmic use of chymotrypsin.
10 When are ophthalmic dyes (fluorescein, fluress) used?
11 Discuss the advantages and disadvantages of the Ocusert.
12 Select two over-the-counter eye preparations. Note the ingredients, instructions, and if there is an expiration date on the labels. Through library research determine the safety and effectiveness of the preparations.

BIBLIOGRAPHY

Abel, R., Jr.: Therapeutic indications for soft contact lenses, Del. Med. J. **47**:515, 1975.
Abrams, J.D.: The nature of glaucoma, Nurs. Times **68**;707, 1972.
Ahmad, S.: Cardiopulmonary effects of timolol eyedrops, Lancet **2**:1028, 1979.
Armaly, M.F., and Rao, K.R.: The effect of pilocarpine ocusert with different release rates on ocular pressure, Invest. Ophthalmol. **12**:491, 1973.
Benson, H.: Permeability of the cornea to topically applied drugs, Arch. Ophthalmol. **91**:313, 1974.
Ellis, P.P.: Ocular therapeutics and pharmacology, ed. 5, St. Louis, 1977, The C.V. Mosby Co.
Grant, M.: Toxicology of the eye, Springfield, Ill., 1973, Charles C Thomas, Publisher.
Havener, W.H.: Ocular pharmacology, ed. 4, St. Louis, 1978, The C.V. Mosby Co.
Jones, F.L.: Exacerbation of asthma by timolol, N. Engl. J. Med. **301**:270, 1979.
Kaufr....., r1.E.: Ocular virus disease, Ann. Clin. Res. **5**:189, 1973.
Leopold, I.H.: Advances in anaesthesia in opthalmic surgery, Opthalmic Surg. **5**:13, 1974.
Leopold, I.H., editor: Symposium on ocular therapy, vol. 7, St. Louis, 1974, The C.V. Mosby Co.
Levine, S., and Leopold, I.H.: Disorders of the eye, Med. Clin. North Am. **57**:1167, 1973.
Mandell, A.I., and others: Dipivalyl epinephrine: a new prodrug in the treatment of glaucoma, Ophthamology **85**(3):268, 1978.
Maurice, D.M.: Prolonged release systems and topically applied drugs. Sight Sav. Rev. **42**:42, 1972.

Modell, W., editor: Drugs of choice 1980-1981, St. Louis, 1979, The C.V. Mosby Co.

Newell, F.W.: Current trends in ophthalmic anaesthesia, Ophthalmic Surg. **6:**15, 1975.

Periera, P.: Screening for glaucoma, Nurs. Times **68:**771, 1972.

Podos, S.M., Becker, B., and Kass, M.A.: Prostaglandin synthesis, inhibition and intraocular pressure, Invest. Ophthalmol. **12:**426, 1973.

Smith, M.B.: Handbook of ocular pharmacology, Littleton, Mass., 1974, PSG Publishing Co., Inc.

Trevor-Rapor, P.D.: Lecture notes on opthamology, ed. 5., London, 1975, Blackwell Scientific Publications.

Cardiac drugs

The development of microelectrode techniques and recordings has resulted in new knowledge and greater understanding of cardiac activity. The resulting anatomic, electrophysiologic, and pharmacologic information has permitted greater precision in diagnosing and treating cardiac disease, particularly the dysrhythmias. Concomitant with these advances has been the increasing use of electrocardiographic monitoring of acutely ill patients and of those with known or suspected cardiovascular disorders. In addition, the nurse's clinical role has continued to expand and now includes responsibility for the care of patients on monitoring equipment. This in turn requires that the nurse be able to recognize and understand abnormal electrocardiographic patterns and in some cases to institute therapy, including pharmacologic therapy, to prevent serious complications and unnecessary deaths. Therefore it is necessary for nurses to understand the electrophysiology of the heart and drug effects on cardiac activity if they are to keep their knowledge current and their nursing care therapeutically effective.

The continuing sophistication of microelectrode techniques has provided a greater understanding of the electrophysiologic properties of cardiac fibers and of the mechanisms responsible for causing various cardiac disorders. Fortunately, these advances have led to the discovery of new drugs that are therapeutically useful in alleviating specific types of clinical cardiac conditions.

Cardiac drugs largely involve the action of three major tissues of the heart. The physiologic properties of these structures along with the various drug groups used therapeutically to produce a specific pharmacologic response are summarized in Table 18-1.

The heart

The heart is a hollow muscular organ that consists of two main pumping chambers: the right ventricle, which is linked with the pulmonary circulation, and the left ventricle, which is connected to the systemic circulation. The cardiac muscle or myocardium is the largest and most important structure of the heart. As a contractile muscle, it is capable of adapting its performance by adjusting the cardiac output according to the body's systemic needs. However, when the heart is incapable of adapting

TABLE 18-1   Effect of cardiac drug groups on physiologic properties of cardiac tissues

Cardiac tissue	Physiologic property	Drug group	Pharmacologic action
Cardiac muscle (Myocardium) Sarcomere (functional unit)	Force of myocardial contraction (Frank-Starling's law) Contractility and conductivity	Cardiac glycosides	Positive inotropic effect—increases cardiac output
Specialized conduction system	Automaticity (rhythm and rate) Conductivity	Antidysrhythmic drugs	Converts to normal sinus rhythm or abolishes dysrhythmia
Coronary arteries	Nutritional blood flow to myocardium and other cardiac structures	Antianginal drugs	Coronary vasodilation or lessens work of the heart

itself to a variable output, the therapeutic use of digitalis or cardiac glycosides exerts a powerful influence on defects in cardiac muscle performance, particularly in the management of congestive heart failure. Since cardiac glycosides, that is, the digitalis drugs, effect a change at the cellular level, a description of myocardial ultrastructure and the contractile process will help facilitate the understanding of the fundamental mechanisms involved in cardiac glycoside action.

CARDIAC MUSCLE
Ultrastructure

The pumping action of the heart depends on the contractile property of the cardiac muscle or myocardium. Structurally, the myocardium is composed of numerous interconnecting branching fibers or cells that form the walls of the two atria and two ventricles of the heart. The individual myocardial fiber contains a centrally located nucleus and a limiting plasma membrane (cell membrane), the sarcolemma (Fig. 18-1, A and B). By joining end to end, the cells form a long fiber, and each cell is separated from the other by a plasma membrane called the intercalated disk. It is thought that the intercalated disk provides sites of low electrical resistance to permit the spread of excitation throughout the cardiac muscle.

The individual muscle fiber (cell) is comprised of a group of multiple parallel myofibrils, and each myofibril is arranged longitudinally into a series of repeating units called the sarcomere. By using a light microscope, examination of the muscle fiber reveals its most characteristic feature, the cross-striations of alternating light and dark bands. These striations are due to the cross banding of the multiple parallel myofibrils, which are aligned in register with one another (Fig. 18-1, C).

At the level of the Z line, the sarcolemma of the muscle fiber invaginates at the end of each sarcomere to form the transverse sarcotubule or T system, which penetrates deeply into the cell. Furthermore, a system of internal membranes form an extensive network called the sarcoplasmic reticulum. The sarcoplasmic reticulum encircles groups of myofibrils and makes contact with the sarcotubules. Evidence of the tremendous energy requirements for cardiac muscle contraction is the presence of the great numbers of mitochondria that are lined up in long chains between the myofibrils (Fig. 18-1, C).

Fig. 18-1, D, shows the *sarcomere*, which is the fundamental unit of myocardial contraction. It is that portion of the myofibril that lies between two successive Z lines. The sarcomere consists of dark bands that are A bands and lighter bands called I bands.

The ultimate unit of the myofibril constitutes the myofilaments. The dark appearance of the A bands is attributed to the thicker *myosin* filaments, and the light appearance of the I bands is attributed to the thinner *actin* filaments. Cross-bridges, which are small projections that extend from the sides of the myosin filament, appear along the entire length of the thick filament. It is the interaction between these cross-bridges of the myosin and the active sites of the actin that finally produce contraction. In the sarcomere the H zone represents the middle, less dense portion of the A band, and the myosin filament is continuous through the length of this band. The I band, on the other

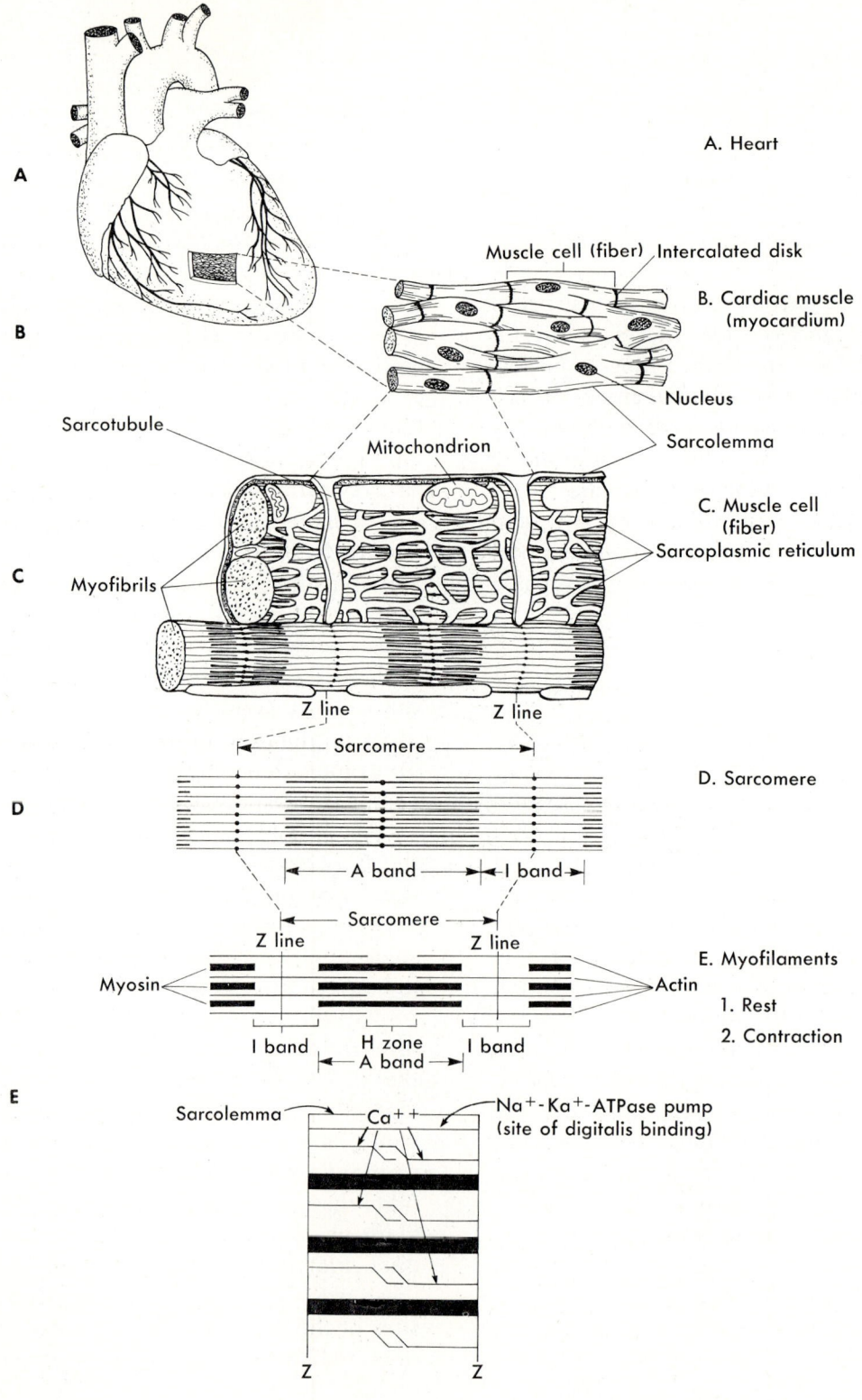

A. Heart

Muscle cell (fiber)   Intercalated disk

B. Cardiac muscle
(myocardium)

Nucleus

Sarcolemma

Sarcotubule

Mitochondrion

C. Muscle cell
(fiber)

Sarcoplasmic reticulum

Myofibrils

Z line   Z line

Sarcomere

D. Sarcomere

A band   I band

Sarcomere

Z line   Z line

E. Myofilaments

Myosin   Actin

1. Rest

2. Contraction

I band   H zone   I band

A band

Sarcolemma Ca^{++} Na^{+}-Ka^{+}-ATPase pump
(site of digitalis binding)

Z   Z

hand, is bisected by the Z line. The actin filament is continuous throughout the I band and terminates at the H zone. This arrangement is shown in Fig. 18-1, *E*.

Myocardial contraction: excitation-contraction coupling

During the last decade there has been a tremendous increase in our understanding of the fundamental mechanisms governing contraction of cardiac muscle in both normal and pathologic states. Yet there are some aspects of this complicated process that still are precisely unknown. The important steps involved in myocardial excitation-contraction coupling include (1) electrical excitation, (2) mechanical activation, and (3) contractile mechanism.

Electrical excitation. Initiation of cardiac muscle contraction begins with an electrical event that constitutes excitation or stimulus of the myocardial fiber. The source of electricity in the heart is found in the charges of ion concentration—mainly Na^+, K^+, and Ca^{++}—across the cardiac cell membrane or sarcolemma.

The action potential that produces the ion fluxes occurs in the myocardial cell. The *resting state* of an inactive ventricular muscle cell is created by the *difference* in electrical charge across the sarcolemma. In this case the inside of the cell is negative with respect to the cell's exterior, which is positively charged. Because the sarcolemma separates the opposite charges, the membrane in effect is *polarized*. At rest, the extracellular environment is rich in Na^+ and

the intracellular environment in K^+, with Ca^{++} concentration in the region of the sarcolemma and its invagination, the sarcotuble (Fig. 18-2, *B*).

The cardiac action potential is divided into two stages: depolarization and repolarization. These are subdivided into five stages of ionic changes. The resting potential of an inactive myocardial cell is called phase 4; in this phase the membrane is polarized with a charge of approximately -90 millivolts (mv). At this voltage the interior of the cell is negative with respect to the cell's exterior. During this time the membrane is impermeable to ions. However, any stimulus that changes the resting membrane potential to a critical value, called the *threshold*, can generate an action potential. (Follow Fig. 18-1, *A*, for steps of the action potential.) Threshold is attained when the voltage is decreased slightly to -60 or -70 mv and is referred to as a fall in membrane potential. Thus the potential difference of the membrane is quickly lost and in fact results from the influx of Na^+ and becomes positively charged to $+20$ mv. This sudden initial upstroke is depolarization and is designated as phase 0 of the action potential. Phase 0 in the ventricular muscle is the contraction phase and is represented by QRS on the surface electrocardiogram. Soon after, the repolarization period occurs, and this process has three phases. The beginning of phase 1 is the overshoot, and it makes a brief change toward repolarization. Phase 2 is a slow period that forms a plateau with slow influx of Ca^{++} and efflux of K^+. *Ca^{++} entry into the cell is*

FIG. 18-1. The heart and the ultrastructure of the cardiac muscle cell (fiber).

The heart *(A)* is mainly a muscular organ. The enlargement of the square illustrates a portion of the cardiac muscle (myocardium) *(B)* that is composed of myocardial cells. Each cell contains a centrally located nucleus and a limiting plasma membrane (sarcolemma), which forms the intercalated disk at the termination of each cell. An individual muscle cell (fiber) *(C)* consists of multiple parallel myofibrils. Each myofibril is arranged longitudinally in a series of light and dark repeating units, and the content of a unit is called a sarcomere. At the Z line, the sarcolemma invaginates to form the transverse sarcotubules or T system. An extensive network, called the sarcoplasmic reticulum, encircles groups of myofibrils and makes contact with the sarcotubules. The sarcoplasmic reticulum contains a high concentration of calcium ions. The mitochondria appear in long chains between the myofibrils. The sarcomere *(D)* is the unit of muscle contraction. It is composed of two types of bands, the A band and the I band. The latter is divided by the Z line. Myofilaments *(E)* of the sarcomere include the thin filament, actin, and the thicker filament, myosin. The dark appearance of the A bands is caused by the myosin and the lighter appearance of the I band by the actin. Here, the sarcomere is at rest, (1). On contraction (2) the thick filaments approach the Z line and the width of the H zone narrows between the thin filaments. Calcium ions are needed for systolic contraction.

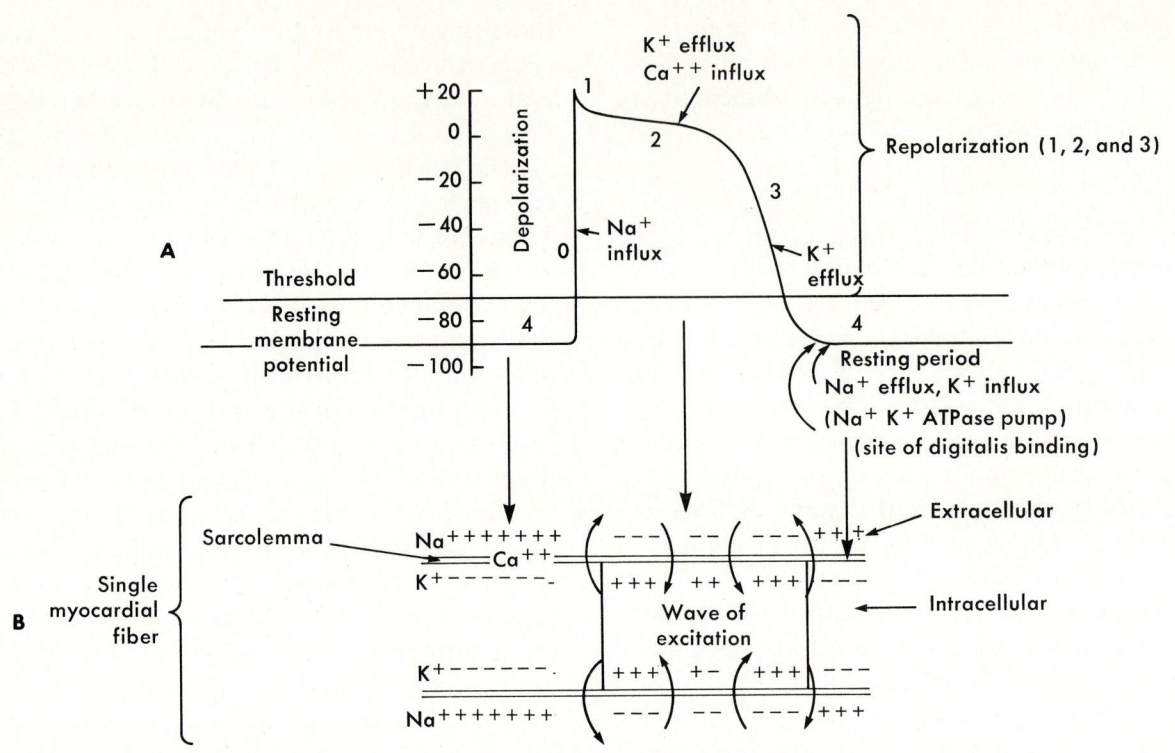

FIG. 18-2. A, Action potential of a single myocardial fiber (cell). **B,** Ionic exchanges that occur across the cell membrane of a single myocardial fiber during an action potential.

essential for the excitation-contraction coupling mechanism, which will be explained later. Phase 3 is accomplished by rapid K^+ efflux from the cell. Following repolarization, phase 4 recovery or resting period ensues, whereby the cell membrane *actively* transports Na^+ outside and K^+ inside, returning the cell membrane to a state of rest or polarization. These cation exchanges during recovery require the energy-utilizing transport mechanism of the Na^+-K^+-ATPase pump. The adenosine triphosphatase (ATPase) pump is an enzyme that is located in the cell membrane or sarcolemma; it furnishes the energy needed for active transport to return Na^+ and K^+ to their original resting positions at the membrane. Digitalis plays a key role at this site. By binding to the *sarcolemma Na^+-K^+-ATPase pump,* digitalis inhibits the return of Na^+ and K^+ to their resting positions. Consequently, digitalis allows more Na^+ and Ca^{++} to enter the cell to strengthen myocardial contraction. However, it is also thought that if an excessive amount of these ions appears intracellularly, digitalis toxicity may occur (see Fig. 18-2).

Mechanical activation. As previously stated, the unit of contraction is the sarcomere. It consists of two contractile proteins, actin and myosin. The thicker filament, myosin, contains the ATPase enzyme system that is needed to hydrolyze ATP. This process is required to provide the energy for contraction. The site of synthesis for ATP is the mitochondria, which are normally abundant in cardiac muscle. Actin, the thin filament, is involved with Ca^{++} activity, and this combination occupies a central role in effecting cardiac contraction.

The contractile process is initiated when the nerve impulse reaches the myocardial cell and travels along the sarcolemma of the muscle fiber. As the depolarization wave spreads along the sarcotubules, it arrives at the sarcoplasmic reticulum, causing the release of its large quantities of calcium ions. Ca^{++} then binds to special receptors on the actin filaments. Hence, the plateau, which is phase 2 of the action potential, is achieved by the slow inward calcium current flow. *Calcium ion movement is the chief component that links or couples electrical excitation of the sarcolemma with muscle activation of the myofilaments in the sarcomere.* Thus *mechanical activation* finally is accomplished when Ca^{++} binds to troponin, a regulator protein located on the actin filaments, and this, in turn, then mediates the interaction of actin and myosin.

Contractile mechanism. As soon as the actin filaments are activated by the calcium ions, the myosin filaments immediately become attracted to the active sites of the actin filament. This interaction pulls the actin filaments along the immobile myosin filaments toward the center of the A band, thus shortening the sarcomere and producing muscle contraction. In this process the lengths of individual filaments remain unchanged. The I band narrows as the thick filaments approach the Z line, and the width of the H zone narrows between the ends of the thin filaments when they meet at the center of the sarcomere (Fig. 18-1, *E*). It must be noted that the greater the quantity of Ca^{++} delivered to troponin, the faster will be the rate and numbers of interactions between actin and myosin. As a result of this response, the development of tension and contractility are increased.

In the presence of magnesium, ATP is cleaved by myosin ATPase. This reaction releases the energy needed to perform work. *The conversion of chemical energy to mechanical energy by ATP plays an essential role in energizing muscle shortening.* In other words, it provides the energy for movement of actin-myosin filaments to effect muscle contraction. Although this is a somewhat simplified explanation of the contractile mechanism, it serves to illustrate the important events that are pertinent to the understanding of cardiotonic drug action.

Finally, relaxation of the muscle depends on removal of Ca^{++} from the sarcomere. The *calcium pump ATPase* (located in the walls of the sarcoplasmic reticulum) actively returns Ca^{++} to the sarcoplasmic reticulum and the sarcolemma, thereby allowing the actin-myosin filaments of the sarcomere to again assume their original resting positions.

Myocardial failure

In heart failure the primary disorder appears to result from defective *excitation-contraction coupling*, and in some individuals dys-

function of *contractile proteins* may occur as an additional abnormality. It appears that ineffective calcium pumping by the sarcoplasmic reticulum alters the normal relaxation process. Furthermore, the mitochondria and *not* the sarcoplasmic reticulum may be the dominant calcium uptake storage site. If so, little calcium is available for release from the sarcoplasmic reticulum to activate contraction. Thus excitation-contraction coupling fails to occur, and as a consequence, depressed myocardial contractility results. Concerning dysfunction of contractile proteins in heart failure, attention has been focused on abnormal energy utilization. It has been demonstrated by some workers that the activity of myosin ATPase is decreased. With diminished activity of this enzyme in heart failure, the intensity of interaction between actin-myosin filaments is reduced, and thus the force of contractility is lowered.

In the normal heart the greater the numbers of interacting myosin-actin sites, the greater the force of myocardial contraction. This is *Frank-Starling's law of the heart*, which states that the longer the muscle fibers are at the end of diastole, the more forceful will be the contraction during systole. This law applies only when the muscle fiber is lengthened within physiologic limits. If a diseased heart is dilated and the fibers are stretched to a critical point beyond their limits of extensibility, the force of contraction and cardiac output are both diminished and ineffective. Thus the functional significance of Frank-Starling's law is that an effective cardiac output can be brought about only by adequate relaxation and refilling after each myocardial contraction.

CARDIAC CONDUCTION SYSTEM

The effective pumping action of the heart depends on the regularity of events that occurs in the cardiac cycle. Each cycle consists of a period of relaxation called *diastole* followed by a period of contraction known as *systole*. The *rhythm* and *rate* of the cardiac cycle are regulated by the conduction system, which has the ability to initiate and transmit electrical impulses needed to stimulate contraction of the cardiac muscle.

The conduction system is made up of the fol-

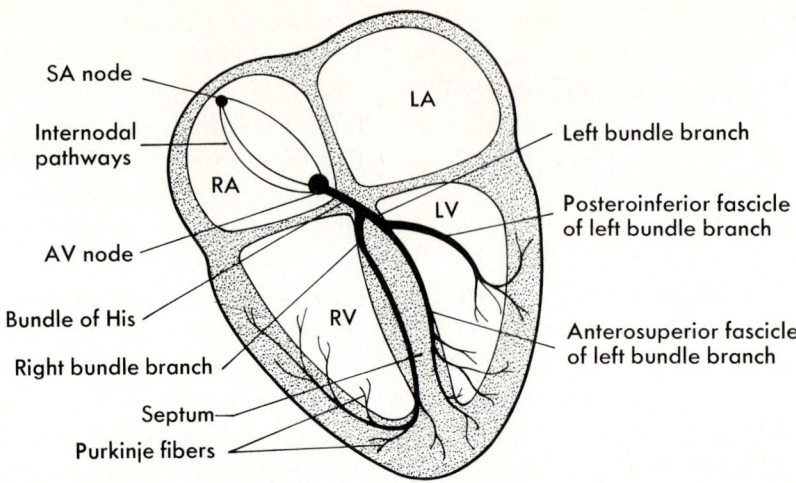

FIG. 18-3. Conduction system of the heart. The cardiac impulse is initiated at the S-A node and is transmitted through the internodal pathways to the two atria, resulting in atrial contraction. At the A-V node, the electrical impulse is delayed. Conduction then speeds up at the bundle of His, with the impulse traveling through the right bundle branch and the left bundle branch continuing through the posteroinferior fascicle and anterosuperior fascicle of the latter bundle branch. Finally, the arrival of impulses at the Purkinje fiber result in their distribution to all parts of both ventricles, whereupon excitation, ventricular contraction, is produced. *RA*, Right atrium; *RV*, right ventricle; *LA*, left atrium; *LV*, left ventricle. (Modified from Andreoli, K., and others. Comprehensive cardiac care, ed. 4, St. Louis, 1979, The C. V. Mosby Co.)

lowing structures: (1) SA node, (2) internodal pathways, (3) AV node, (4) bundle of His, (5) right and left bundle branches, and (6) Purkinje fibers. These latter fibers penetrate the endocardium and terminate in the myocardial cells. The AV node and the His area form the *AV junction*, which extends from the atrial fibers, through the AV node, to the bifurcation of the bundle of His. When referring to this region, the term *"AV junction"* is considered to be more accurate than *"AV node"* (Fig. 18-3).

In the normal heart the SA node initiates the heartbeat. The impulses generated here are then conducted through the internodal pathways to the "working" fibers of the atrial myocardium, producing atrial contraction. When the impulses move through the AV node, electrical conduction is delayed. However, at the bundle of His, conduction speeds up and the impulses travel through the right bundle branch and the left bundle branch continuing through the posteroinferior and anterosuperior fascicles of the latter bundle branch. The transmission of impulses at the Purkinje fibers, which consist of tiny fibrils that spread around

the ventricles and connect directly with the myocardial cells, is very rapid. Finally, the simultaneous depolarization of both ventricles produces ventricular contraction, whereupon blood is propelled through the pulmonary artery and aorta.

Electrophysiologic properties

The coordinated pumping action of the heart is initiated and regulated by the specialized fibers of the conduction system. The individual fibers of this system possess two basic electrophysiologic properties: (1) automaticity and (2) conductivity.

Automaticity. The specialized fibers of the conduction system have the inherent ability to *spontaneously initiate* an electrical impulse without any external stimuli. This is the most fundamental mechanism of impulse formation, and the cells that possess this property of automaticity or self-excitation are called pacemaker cells. They are found in specialized conducting tissues such as the SA node, the AV node, and the His-Purkinje system. Normally, the impulse of the heart is spontaneously and regularly initiated at the pacemaker cells of the SA node. During resting potential (phase 4), the membrane of the cell depolarizes itself—spontaneously and gradually—until it reaches threshold and an action potential occurs. The slow depolarization of the membrane in the resting state is called *spontaneous diastolic depolarization* or *phase 4 depolarization* and defines automaticity. Thus, the membrane of pacemaker cells is never at rest, and this property is attributed to the fact that there is a continuous influx of Na^+ ions into the interior of the cells, which readily drives the membrane to threshold. The resting potential of automatic pacemaker cells differs from that of the nonautomatic myocardial cells. After full repolarization, the membrane of myocardial cells maintains a steady resting potential until an external stimulus causes it to achieve threshold. To summarize, automaticity is a property of cardiac fibers normally controlling heart rhythm but not of "working" muscle—atria and ventricles. It is evident in the fibers that make up the conduction system. However, under pathologic conditions, myocardial cells do have the potential for exhibiting spontaneous depolarization.

The spontaneous excitation of pacemaker cells establishes the normal rhythm of the heart. The regularity of such pacemaking activity is termed *rhythmicity*. Under normal circumstances, there exists only one functional pacemaker, the SA node, which predominates because it has the highest frequency of depolarization. The normal rate of impulse formation is about 72 beats/minute. If the SA node decreases its rate of impulse formation to a level below the AV junction (40 to 60 beats/minute), then the AV junction becomes the primary pacemaker of the heart and will drive the heart at about 40 beats/minute.

Conductivity. The speed at which the electrical impulses set by the SA node are transmitted through the conduction system and the atrial and ventricular musculature is called conductivity. In other words, conductivity refers to the ability to transmit an action potential or nerve impulse from cell to cell. The property of conductivity therefore exists not only in the cells of the conduction system but also in the cardiac musculature. The speed of impulse conduction varies as it passes from one tissue to another in the heart. It is slowest in the AV node and fastest in the Purkinje fibers. The marked delay of conduction at the AV node allows more time for ventricular filling. On the other hand, the rapid depolarization of Purkinje fibers effects an instantaneous spread of impulses from the terminals to the ventricular muscles. Simultaneous activation of the musculature is essential for producing powerful ventricular contraction.

Velocity of conduction. The speed with which electrical activity is spread within the sinus node is quite slow, about 0.05 m/second. The impulse then spreads out rapidly over the atrial musculature at a rate of about 1.0 m/second. When the impulse reaches the AV node, a delay of about 0.05 m/second occurs and atrial systole takes place. The impulse then spreads rapidly, 2 to 4 m/second, along the right and left bundle branches and Purkinje fibers. Studies indicate that no more than 22 msec may elapse during this time. This rapid activation of contractile elements evokes a synchronous contraction of the ventricles.

The velocity of conduction is determined by the magnitude of the resting potential of the cell membrane and the rate of rise of phase 0 of the action potential. This defines membrane responsiveness. Antidysrhythmic drugs may affect conduction by lowering phase 0, thereby decreasing membrane responsiveness.

Refractoriness. Cardiac tissue is refractory to stimulation during the initial phase of systole (contraction). Throughout most of repolarization, the cell cannot respond to a stimulus. The *effective refractory period* represents that period in the cardiac cycle during which a stimulus, no matter how strong, fails to produce an action potential. Antidysrhythmic drugs can lengthen or shorten the refractory period of cardiac tissues by influencing the level of responsiveness of the cell membrane. Following the effective refractory period and as repolarization nears completion, *relative refractory period* occurs. This is defined as that period during which a propagated action potential can be elicited, provided the stimulus is of stronger intensity than normally required in diastole. When this happens, the fiber is stimulated to contract prematurely.

Autonomic nervous system control

Although the conduction system possesses the inherent ability for spontaneous, rhythmic initiation of the cardiac impulse, the autonomic nervous system has an important role in the regulation of the rate, rhythm, and force of myocardial contraction of the heart. The heart is innervated by both the parasympathetic and sympathetic nerves. Vagal nerve fibers of the parasympathetic branch are found primarily in the sinoatrial (SA) node, atrial muscles, and atrioventricular (AV) node, whereas the sympathetic fibers innervate the SA node, AV node, and the atrial and ventricular muscles.

Vagal stimulation to the heart is mediated by the release of the neurohormone acetylcholine, which acts on the muscarinic receptors to decrease heart rate and is also believed to decrease ventricular contraction. The main effect of acetylcholine on the AV node is to slow the rate of conduction and lengthen the refrac-

tory period. By contrast, stimulation of the sympathetic fiber is mediated by the release of norepinephrine, which acts specifically on the beta$_1$ receptors in the cardiac tissue. Circulating epinephrine from the adrenal medulla may also elicit cardiac responses. By acting on the beta adrenergic receptors, norepinephrine and epinephrine increase both heart rate and force of myocardial contraction. They also increase conduction velocity and shorten the refractory period of the AV node. Epinephrine has a very potent effect on the heart. In large doses its direct effect on the electrophysiologic properties of cardiac tissue can induce cardiac dysrhythmias. Normally, the heartbeat is under the continuous influence of both parasympathetic and sympathetic control, so that the resting heart rate is the result of their opposing influences.

Electrocardiogram

Electrocardiograms are graphic representations of the sequence of cardiac excitation. Nurses caring for patients on monitor equipment should be able to detect and interpret

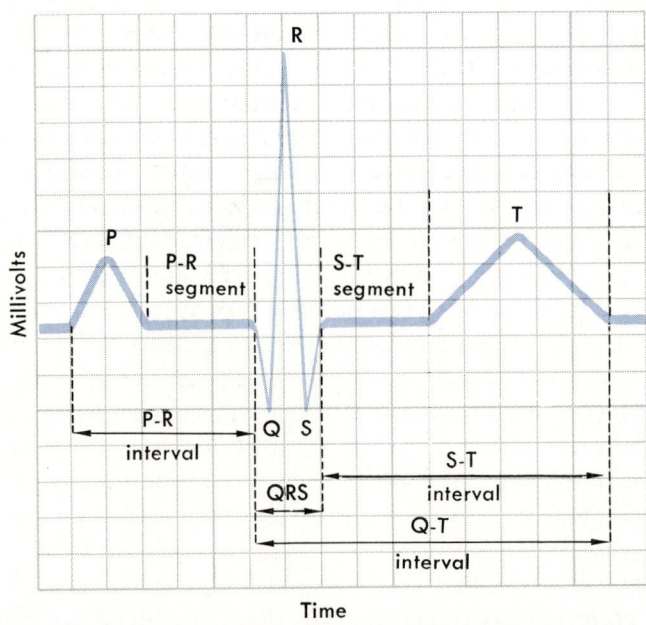

FIG. 18-4. Graphic representation of the normal electrocardiogram. Vertical lines represent time, each square represents 0.04 second, and every five squares (set off by heavy black lines) represents 0.20 second. The normal P-R interval is less than 0.20 second; the average is 0.16 second. The average duration of the P wave is 0.08 second; the QRS complex is 0.08 second; the S-T segment is 0.12 second; the T wave is 0.16 second; and the Q-T interval is 1.36 seconds. Each horizontal line represents voltage; every five squares equals 0.5 millivolt.

changes in the cardiac rate or rhythm or in the conduction of the wave of electric activity or excitation. The electrocardiogram (ECG) is a useful tool in determining the therapeutic effectiveness of certain drugs. Drugs used in the treatment of cardiovascular disease may alter the electric activity of the heart. The electrocardiogram may provide the earliest objective evidence of a drug's effectiveness or its toxic manifestations. A knowledgeable and observant nurse can use the information obtained from the electrocardiogram for assessing the effectiveness of drug therapy in the treatment of various cardiac dysrhythmias.

Electric activity always precedes mechanical contraction. Immediately after a wave of electric activity moves through atrial muscle, the muscle contracts and blood flows from the atria into the ventricles. (See Fig. 18-4 for the graphic illustration of the normal electrocardiogram.) The P wave is produced by a wave of excitation through the atria (atrial depolarization). The onset of the P wave follows the firing of the SA node. After the P wave, a short pause or interval (PR interval) occurs while the electric activity is transmitted to the AV node, conduction tissue, and ventricles. The electrocardiogram now records the QRS complex, or ventricular depolarization. This leads to contraction of the ventricles. Repolarization, or recovery, of the ventricles is indicated by the T wave. Atrial recovery or repolarization does not show on the ECG because of being hidden in the QRS complex. The ECG records receding activity as a negative potential, downward deflection; activity approaching an exploring electrode is recorded as a positive potential, an upward stroke on the graph paper or oscilloscope.

Drugs that affect the heart

Drugs may change the rate, force, and rhythm of the heart. Pharmacologic terms that have specific meaning for the actions of drugs on the cardiovascular system include the terms "inotropic," "chronotropic," "dromotropic," and "pressor effects."

Drugs with an *inotropic* (Gr. *inos*, fiber; *tropikos*, a turning or influence) effect influence myocardial contractility. If the drug has a positive inotropic effect, it strengthens or increases the force of myocardial contraction. A drug with a negative inotropic effect weakens or decreases the force of myocardial contraction.

Drugs with *chronotropic* (Gr. *chronos*, time) action affect the rate of the heart. If the drug increases the heart rate by increasing the rate of impulse formation in the SA node, it has a positive chronotropic effect. A negative chronotropic drug has the opposite effect and slows the heart rate by decreasing impulse formation.

When drugs have a *dromotropic* (Gr. *dromos*, a course) effect, they affect conduction velocity through the specialized conducting tissues. A drug having a positive dromotropic action speeds conduction. A drug with negative dromotropic action delays conduction.

Drugs with a *pressor* effect increase blood pressure by increasing peripheral arteriolar resistance through vasoconstriction.

Cardiac glycosides
DIGITALIS AND DIGITALIS-LIKE DRUGS

Drugs in the digitalis group are among the oldest and most effective therapeutic agents available to the physician for treatment of congestive heart failure. Cardiac glycosides act with specificity and rapidity and have unrivaled value in the treatment of congestive heart failure. Their use in medicine dates from the thirteenth century. However, it was not until 1785, when the English physician and botanist William Withering published his rigorous and systematic observations on the treatment of various ailments with digitalis, that cardiac glycosides became indispensable to a physician's drug armamentarium.

Chemically, all cardiac glycosides are closely related; each is composed of a sugar (glycoside), a steroid, and a lactone. The sugar portion of the molecule will vary in different glycosides. These sugars increase the substance's water solubility and cell penetrability, alter absorption, and modify toxicity. Removal of the sugar portion from the glycoside leaves a molecule known as an aglycone or genin in which pharmacologic activity resides. However, the lactone portion is essential to the characteristic cardiotonic properties of the molecule. The basic digitalis nucleus, the steroid portion, is similar to that of the sex hormones and corticosterones. This may cause gynecomastia in male patients.

Many substances, of which digitalis is the most important, are characterized by their action on the heart. These substances belong to many different botanical families. For ages they have been used empirically in therapeutics. The action of each is fundamentally the same, so that the description for digitalis, with minor differences, will apply to all.

The most important plants that contain digitaloid substances are as follows:

Digitalis purpurea—purple foxglove
Digitalis lanata—white foxglove
Strophanthus hispidus, S. kombé—an African arrow poison
Scilla maritima—squill or sea onion

While all cardiac glycosides have similar pharmacologic properties, they differ in absorption and rate of elimination, time of onset of action, and duration of action. The absorption of various cardiac glycosides varies from a minimal amount to almost 100% after oral administration. Digitoxin is almost completely absorbed, digoxin is 80% to 90% absorbed, less than 50% of lanatoside C is absorbed, while ouabain is even less completely absorbed. Oral preparations are readily absorbed from the intestinal tract. Distribution is widespread throughout body tissues. Selection of which cardiac glycoside to use is based on the needs of a particular individual and his reactions to the drug.

Digitalis

Digitalis is the dried leaves of *Digitalis purpurea*, or purple foxglove. This plant is cultivated for the drug market in England, North America, and Germany and grows wild in Europe, the United States, and Australia. Early investigators gave the plant the name *Digitalis purpurea* because the flower is purple and resembles a finger. Digitalis leaves contain a number

of glycosides; the most important are digitoxin, digoxin, and gitalin.

Action and results. Digitalis affects cardiac function through two important mechanisms:

1 Digitalis has *positive inotropic* action. It influences the mechanical performance of the heart by increasing the strength of myocardial contraction.
2 Digitalis has *negative chronotropic* and *negative dromotropic* actions. It involves alteration of *electrophysiologic* properties such as automaticity, conduction velocity, and refractory period.

Positive inotropic action. The main function of digitalis is the inotropic action. It results from direct action on the myocardium independent of extracardiac factors. Digitalis does not alter the amount of energy available for myocardial contraction; the increased contractility is associated with more efficient use of available energy. If the failing heart is enlarged and the positive inotropic action of digitalis increases cardiac output, heart size may be reduced with resultant decrease in oxygen utilization. This alteration in cardiac activity also produces a decrease in venous pressure and relief of edema.

The direct positive inotropic effect is attributed to the fact that digitalis *inhibits the membrane-bound Na^+-K^+-ATPase enzyme.* Normally, the hydrolysis of ATP by this enzyme provides the energy for the Na^+-K^+ pump, which actively extrudes Na^+ and transports K^+ across the membrane of the cardiac fiber during repolarization. By binding specifically to the Na^+-K^+-ATPase, digitalis inhibits the active transport of Na^+ and K^+. (See Fig. 18-2.) As a consequence, an accumulation of intracellular Na^+ results. This ionic action then brings about an exchange of intracellular Na^+ for extracellular Ca^{++} from the sarcolemma and T tubules. The resulting increased intracellular Ca^{++} carries a current along the T tubule, which in turn excites the sarcoplasmic reticulum causing a rapid release of its large quantities of Ca^{++}. This is free Ca^{++}, which is essential for linking the electrical excitation of the cell membrane to the mechanical contraction of the muscle fibers, a mechanism known as excitation-contraction coupling. Ultimately, the increase in free Ca^{++}

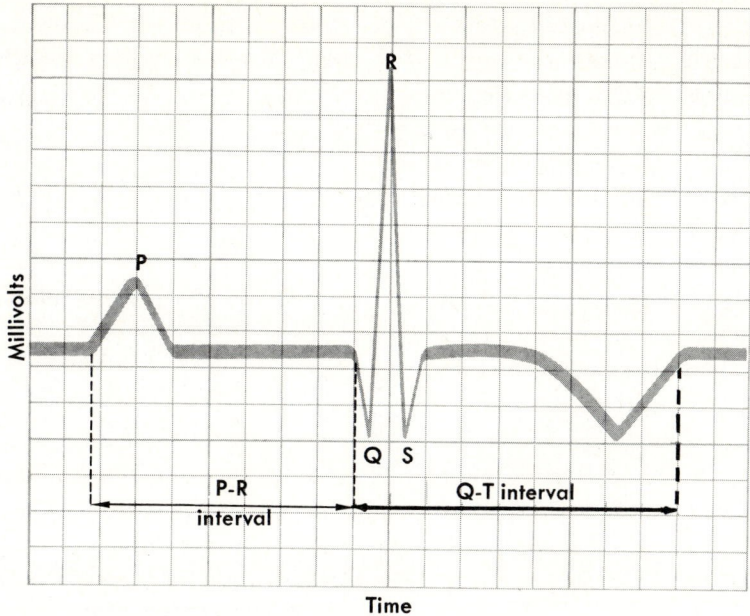

FIG. 18-5. Representation of typical effects of digitalization on the electric activity of the heart as shown on the electrocardiogram. Note the prolonged P-R interval, the shortened Q-T interval, and the T wave inversion. (Compare with Fig. 18-4.)

brings about a more rapid and more forceful myocardial contraction—positive inotropic action. Thus the degree of inhibition of membrane-bound Na^+-K^+-ATPase enzyme by digitalis, which promotes an increase in intracellular Na^+ and Ca^{++}, determines the magnitude of the inotropic effect. (See Fig. 18-1, *E, 1* and *2*.)

Negative chronotropic and negative dromotropic actions. Digitalis has negative chronotropic (decreased heart rate) and negative dromotropic (slowed conduction velocity) effects because it is capable of altering three *electrophysiologic properties* of cardiac tissues:

1. *Automaticity* is a property of cardiac tissue that has the inherent ability to initiate and propagate an impulse. This property affects the rate and rhythm of the heart. Low to moderate doses of digitalis slow the heart rate because the SA node depolarizes less frequently. On the other hand, toxic concentrations of digitalis can directly increase automaticity in all cardiac tissues capable of self-excitation. The result is an increased rate of both action potentials and spontaneous depolarization. This is one of the mechanisms responsible for digitalis-induced ectopic pacemakers. Toxic doses of digitalis

may significantly increase impulse formation in latent or potential pacemaker tissue.

2. *Conduction velocity* is decreased with all concentrations of digitalis. The AV conduction system is particularly affected. This slowing of conduction is partly caused by the direct action of digitalis and also by an increase in vagal action. This is shown on the ECG by a prolonged P-R interval, and in toxic doses it can lead to an increased degree of heart block. (See Fig. 18-5.)

3. *The refractory period* effects of digitalis vary in different parts of the heart. Reduction of the refractory period in the ventricles requires nearly toxic amounts of digitalis. A prolonged refractory period occurs in the AV conduction system, which is very sensitive to digitalis action. This action is partly direct and partly caused by increased vagal tone. Toxic doses of digitalis may prolong the refractory period and depress conduction in the AV conduction system to the point where a complete block occurs. (See section on dysrhythmia for detailed explanation of electrophysiologic properties.)

Pharmacokinetics. The metabolic handling, excretion, and duration of action of the digitalis drugs depend on the glycoside administered. Digoxin, which is becoming most widely used, has a plasma half-life of 36 hours and is excreted mainly by the kidneys; the body loses 37% of its digoxin store every day. On the other hand, digitoxin has a plasma half-life of 5 to 7 days and is metabolized mainly in the liver; the body loses 10% of its store in a day. Clearly then, digitoxin is a very long-acting drug, whereas digoxin remains in the body for a much shorter time. If the daily dose of these drugs exceeds the amount lost, cumulation and digitalis toxicity will result.

Glycoside serum levels are of limited value in establishing therapeutic serum levels but are valuable as an indicator of toxicity:

Drug serum levels	Therapeutic	Toxic
Digoxin	0.8-1.6 ng/ml	>2.4 ng/ml
Digitoxin	14-26 ng/ml	>34 ng/ml

Uses. As stated previously, the primary therapeutic use of digitalis is to treat congestive heart failure. However, digitalis is also a valuable drug in the treatment of atrial fibrillation and in the management of atrial flutter and paroxysmal tachycardia.

Congestive heart failure. Congestive heart failure is also referred to as cardiac insufficiency, heart or pump failure, and cardiac decompensation. Heart failure most often occurs as a late event of various congenital or acquired disorders of the heart or blood vessels, which place the heart under constant stress. A heart in failure is no longer capable of supplying body tissue with adequate oxygen and nutrients or of removing metabolic waste products. When pump failure occurs, there is usually failure of both sides of the heart, although failure of one side may have preceded and precipitated failure of the other side. Most of the signs and symptoms are caused by pulmonary and systemic congestion, the result of inadequate systolic outflow, and delayed venous return. The mortality for congestive heart failure is high.

The positive inotropic effect of digitalis that results in increased myocardial contractility has many important benefits for the patient with a failing heart. The increased force of systolic contraction causes the ventricles to empty more completely. This permits a slower heart rate and more complete filling, which result in the following:

1 Venous pressure falls, and the pulmonary and systemic congestion and their accompanying signs and symptoms are either diminished or completely abolished.
2 Coronary circulation is enhanced, myocardial oxygen demand is reduced, and the supply of oxygen and nutrients to the myocardium is improved.
3 Heart size is often decreased toward normal.

It has been demonstrated that some of the cardiac glycosides have a true but mild diuretic effect. However, marked diuresis in the edematous patient is primarily the result of improved heart action, improved circulation to all body tissue, and improved tissue and organ function including renal function. When digitalis is effective, the patient is noticeably improved and has an increased sense of well-being.

Atrial fibrillation. During atrial fibrillation several hundred impulses originate from the atria, but only a fraction of them are transmitted through the AV node. (See Fig. 18-6 for electrocardiographic pattern of atrial fibrillation.) Digitalis is ideal for slowing the ventricular rate because it increases the refractory period of the AV node and also slows conduction at this site. It is important to know that the purpose of using digitalis in atrial fibrillation is to slow the ventricular rate, which may prevent or eliminate cardiac failure. Digitalis does not convert the fibrillating atria into normally contracting ones.

Protective and prophylactic use. There is no general agreement concerning the value of prophylactic digitalization in the absence of congestive heart failure. Some authorities believe the cardiac glycosides may exert a protective effect on myocardial function in the absence of cardiac failure when (1) an unusual work load is to be placed on the heart or (2) when a patient is to be subjected to the risk of having myocardial function depressed. Patients who may be digitalized in the absence of cardiac failure by the proponents of prophylaxis include prepartum cardiac patients and elderly or cardiac patients who are to undergo the acute stress of anesthesia and major surgery. More extensive studies are needed before the therapeutic effectiveness

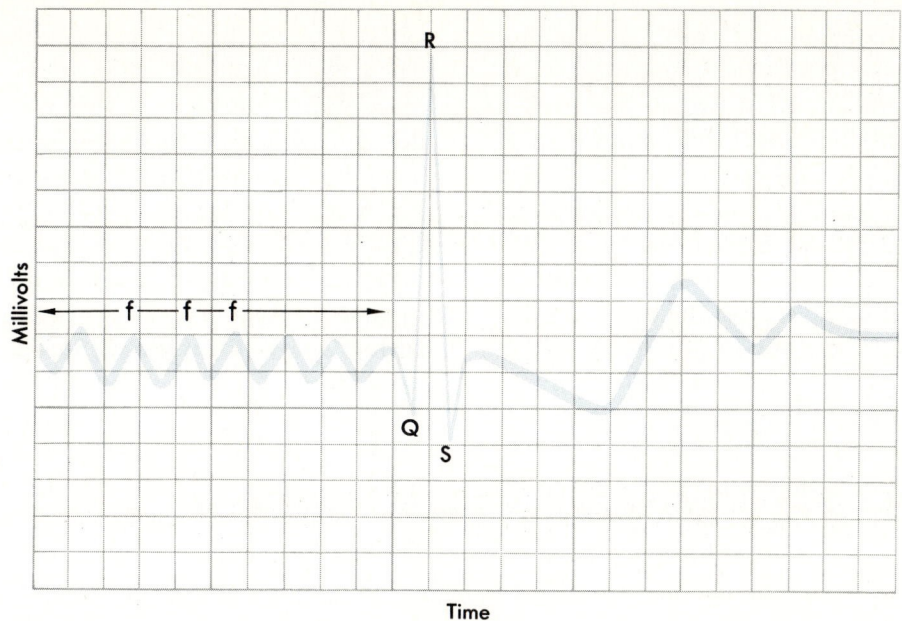

FIG. 18-6. Graphic representation of atrial fibrillation as seen on the electrocardiographic monitor or tracing paper. No true P waves are noted; but f (fibrillation) waves consisting of rapid, small, and irregular waves are noted. The QRS complex is normal in configuration and duration but occurs irregularly.

of prophylactic digitalization can be established.

Preparation, dosage, and administration

Administration. The preferred route of administration of digitalis and the cardiac glycosides for congestive heart failure is oral. Because of variation in rapidity of onset of action, duration of action, and individual response, the oral route is safest to use. It is also least expensive. Local gastric mucosal irritation is decreased by giving the drug with or just after meals.

It is not recommended that digitalis preparations be given subcutaneously because of the local irritating effect of the drugs (producing pain and abscess formation) and uncertain absorption, especially in the presence of congestive heart failure. The intravenous route is usually reserved for cases of emergency (such as patients with pulmonary edema or acute ventricular failure) or when the patient has a condition preventing the use of oral medications (such as vomiting). Rectal administration has been used for patients who have difficulty tolerating the drug orally. However, this is an uncommon route of administration.

Standardization of digitalis preparations.

Preparations of digitalis are assayed biologically. The U.S. Digitalis Reference Standard contains 1 unit of activity in 0.1 g. This is equal to the International Digitalis Standard. While many digitalis preparations must be assayed by the official method in pigeons, the pure glycosides such as digitoxin, digoxin, or deslanoside are assayed colorimetrically.

Digitalization and choice of preparations. In the treatment of heart failure, the aim is to give digitalis until optimal cardiac effects are achieved and most of the signs and symptoms of heart failure have disappeared. When the patient has reached that state in which he has profited all that he can from the drug, he is said to be digitalized. The amount of drug required for digitalization may vary with each patient.

Usually digitalization is accomplished by giving the patient, over a period of hours or days, a total amount necessary to produce the desired cardiac effect—the digitalizing dose—and then keeping him on a smaller daily dose—the maintenance dose—designed to replace the daily loss of the drug from his body by destruction or excretion to maintain the desired effect. For example, a common schedule for an average adult, using whole-leaf digitalis, would include a digitalizing dose of 1 to 1.5 g, given in divided doses over 1 to 2 days, followed by a maintenance dose of 0.1 g daily. Naturally, both the digitalizing and the maintenance doses must be adjusted to the particular patient in terms of toxic reactions and clinical signs of adequate digitalization. If digitoxin were administered orally, 1 to 1.5 mg would constitute an average digitalizing dose of the drug and 0.1 to 0.2 mg the maintenance dose. The rate of drug destruction following adequate digitalization is about one tenth the digitalizing dose per 24 hours. This is the rationale usually used for determining the maintenance dose. Many patients who receive digitalis must continue to take the drug the rest of their lives. In children the dose of digitalis and the rapidity of administration depend on weight and age, body surface, severity of cardiac impairment, and response of the patient.

Differences among the preparations available occur chiefly in absorption from the gastrointestinal tract, local emetic action, and speed of excretion. The glycosides of digitalis are poorly absorbed when the whole drug is administered, which accounts for the fact that only one fifth as much of the intravenous preparation is required as the oral preparation. The digitalis glycosides are irritating to mucous membranes and subcutaneous tissues. Large oral doses of whole drug may produce nausea and vomiting shortly after administration. Smaller doses are less likely to produce emesis from local irritation. The nausea and vomiting occasioned by small doses result from a central effect on the vomiting center. All preparations capable of exerting cardiac effects are capable of emetic action, and this untoward effect cannot be avoided by changing to other members of the digitalis group or by changing the method of administration. All preparations of digitalis or digitalis-like drugs have a cumulative action, although some are more cumulative than others. Digitoxin and digitalis leaf have an especially pronounced cumulative action.

In spite of differences of opinion, the use of the whole drug in the form of digitalis tincture or powdered digitalis has to a certain extent been replaced by the use of refined prepara-

tions or by the use of the crystalline glycosides. These are frequently preferred because they are more stable and can be injected and because dosage can be determined more accurately. They are absorbed much more readily when given orally and cause less gastrointestinal irritation. Several glycosides are available in a high degree of purity, such as digitoxin, digoxin, and lanatoside C. These make rapid digitalization by oral administration possible with a minimum of local irritant action caused by nonabsorbable glycosides.

It should be emphasized that some of the purified digitalis glycosides are extremely potent compounds, and if looked on as poisons they are among the most powerful poisons known. Some of the glycosides have a lethal human dose of about 0.1 mg/kg body weight. The nurse should therefore handle these compounds with great care and respect.

PURPLE FOXGLOVE

Powdered digitalis, prepared digitalis. Powdered digitalis is available in tablets and capsules. Range of maintenance dosage is 50 to 200 mg daily. Onset of action occurs in 2 to 6 hours; maximal effect occurs in 12 to 24 hours. Trade names include Digifortis, Digiglusin, and Digitora.

Digitalis tincture. Digitalis tincture is the only acceptable form of liquid preparation for oral use; 1 ml is equal to 1 digitalis unit. Calibrated medicine droppers or medicine glasses should be used to ensure accuracy.

Gitalin (amorphous). Gitalin is a mixture of glycosides obtained from *Digitalis purpurea.* Its action and uses are the same as those of digitalis, and the same precautions should be taken with its administration. The rate of elimination or destruction is slower than that of digoxin but faster than that of digitoxin. Gitalin is administered orally or intravenously. It is marketed in 0.5-mg tablets. Average maintenance dosage is 0.5 mg daily; range of dose is 0.25 to 1.5 mg daily.

Digitoxin. Digitoxin is the chief active glycoside of *Digitalis purpurea.* It is available in crystalline form and is readily absorbed from the intestinal tract. One milligram of digitoxin has the same effect as 1 g of digitalis when given orally. It is available in tablet form as well as in ampules for intravenous therapy. It is extremely poisonous. Digitoxin is sold under a number of trade names: Crystodigin, Purodigin, and Digitaline Nativelle. *Digitoxin tablets* are available in amounts of 0.1 and 0.2 mg.

Its chief disadvantage is its slow onset of action and prolonged half-life when compared to digoxin. From 2 to 3 weeks may elapse before digitoxin is eliminated from the body. Range of maintenance dosage is 0.1 to 0.2 mg daily. With oral administration onset of action occurs in 2 to 4 hours; maximal effect occurs within 12 to 24 hours. After intravenous injection, onset of action occurs in ½ to 2 hours; maximal effect occurs in 8 to 9 hours. Digitoxin should be avoided in patients with severe liver disease.

WHITE FOXGLOVE

Digilanid. Digilanid is a mixture of the crystallized cardioactive glycosides, lanatoside A, lanatoside B, and lanatoside C, obtained from the leaves of white foxglove, *Digitalis lanata.* The three components are present in this preparation in the same proportion as found in the crude drug. When these glycosides are hydrolyzed, they yield, respectively, digitoxin, gitoxin, and digoxin. The actions and uses of digilanid are similar to those of digitalis. It can be administered orally, intramuscularly, intravenously, and rectally. Dosage is 0.67 to 1.33 mg (two to four tablets). It is usually given daily in tablet form until desired effects are obtained and then one to two tablets are given daily as maintenance dosage. Precautions to be observed are the same as those for any digitalis preparation. It is marketed in solution for injection (0.4 mg/2 ml) and in tablets (0.33 mg).

Acetyldigitoxin (Acylanid). Acetyldigitoxin is a cardiac glycoside derived from lanatoside A. It resembles digitoxin in many ways but has a more rapid onset and a shorter duration of action than digitoxin. It is available in 0.1- and 0.2-mg tablets for oral administration. Onset of action occurs in 1 to 2 hours. Maintenance dose for adults ranges from 0.1 to 0.2 mg daily.

Lanatoside C (Cedilanid). Lanatoside C, a glycoside of *Digitalis lanata,* is thought to be more active, therapeutically, than the other two glycosides of the white foxglove. Lanatoside C is a white powder that is practically insoluble in water. Absorption after oral administration is said to be irregular. It is marketed in tablets for oral administration. Lanatoside C tablets usually contain 0.5 mg of the drug, and 0.5 mg (gr ¹⁄₁₂₀) is the usual dose.

Deslanoside (deacetyllanatoside C, Cedilanid-D). Deslanoside is derived from lanatoside C and has the advantage of being more soluble and more stable than the parent substance. For practical purposes it constitutes the injectable form of lanatoside C. *Deslanoside injection* is marketed in 2- and 4-ml ampules containing 0.4 mg and 0.8 mg of the drug, respectively. Initial loading dose for adults is 0.8 to 1.6 mg. Half the dose may be given immediately with the remainder given in divided doses at 2-hour intervals. Maintenance dosage is 0.25 to 0.5 mg daily until a longer acting preparation can be substituted.

Digoxin (Lanoxin). Digoxin is a hydrolytic product formed from lanatoside C. It has an advantage over digitalis for the patient who must be rapidly digitalized. Some patients seem to tolerate digoxin better than digitalis. The drug may be given intravenously, in which case saturation of the tissues may be accomplished much more rapidly than with digitalis. Digoxin may also be given orally. It should be administered with caution because it is extremely poisonous. After oral administration effects appear in 1 hour, and maximal effect occurs in 6 to 7 hours. After intravenous administration effects occur in 5 to 10 minutes and reach a maximum in 1 to 2 hours. Official preparations of digoxin are available in tablets (0.125, 0.25 and 0.5 mg) and as an injectable solution (0.1 mg in 1 ml and 0.5 mg in 2 ml). Average maintenance dose for adults is 0.25 to 0.75 mg daily. The proprietary name Lanoxin has an advantage in that it helps to differentiate digoxin and digitoxin, which are sometimes mistaken one for the other by the student. Digoxin (Lanoxin) is widely used in pediatrics and is available as an elixir (0.05 mg/ml) for oral administration to children (see Table 18-2).

T A B L E 1 8 - 2   **Dosage of digitalis and cardiac glycosides (adults)**

Preparation (generic name and trade name)	Administration	Usual digitalizing quantity (given in divided doses)	Usual daily maintenance dose
Purple foxglove			
Powdered digitalis (leaf)	Oral	1.5 g (1 to 2 g)	0.1 g (100 to 200 mg)
Digitalis tincture	Oral	10 to 15 ml	1 ml
Cardiac glycosides			
Acetyldigitoxin (Acylanid)	Oral	1.8 mg (0.6 to 2 mg) over 24 hr	0.15 mg (0.1 to 0.2 mg)
Digitoxin (Crystodigin, Digitalline Nativelle, Purodigin)	Oral	1.0 to 1.5 mg over 24 to 48 hr	0.1 to 0.2 mg
	Intravenous	0.5 mg (0.5 to 1.2 mg)	0.1 mg (0.1 to 0.2 mg)
Digoxin (Lanoxin)	Oral	1.5 mg (0.5 to 2 mg)	0.5 mg (0.25 to 0.75 mg)
	Intravenous	1 mg (0.5 to 1.5 mg)	0.5 mg (0.25 to 0.75 mg)
Lanatoside C (Cedilanid)	Oral	8 mg	1.0 mg
Gitalin (Gitaligin)	Oral	6.5 mg (2.5 mg initially and then 0.75 mg every 6 hr)	0.5 mg
	Intravenous	2.5 to 3.0 mg in two injections at 24-hr intervals	2.5 mg two times per week
Ouabain	Intravenous only (slowly)	0.5 mg (0.12 to 0.25 mg)	
Deslanoside (deacetyl-lanatoside C, Cedilanid-D)	Intravenous only (slowly)	1.6 mg (1.2 to 1.6 mg)	0.4 mg (0.2 to 0.6 mg)

Side effects and toxic effects. Not all undesired effects of digitalis are toxic effects. While anorexia, nausea, and vomiting can occur with digitalis toxicity, these symptoms can also be caused by gastric irritation from oral digitalis preparations and stimulation of the vomiting center. These effects are often self-limiting and disappear as the patient adjusts to the drug.

Additional signs and symptoms of digitalis toxicity include diarrhea, headache, visual disturbances, weakness, restlessness, and nervous irritability. These are *extracardiac* manifestations of digitalis excess. These toxic effects, while troublesome to the patient, are rarely serious and are often eliminated by omission of the drug for several days. Once the toxic signs or symptoms are gone, drug therapy can again be reinstituted at a lower dosage.

Almost every type of dysrhythmia can be produced by digitalis toxicity. The type of dysrhythmia produced varies with the age of the patient and other factors. Premature ventricular contractions and bigeminal rhythm (two beats and a pause) are common signs of digitalis toxicity in adults, while children tend to develop ectopic nodal or atrial beats. Digitalis-induced dysrhythmias are caused by depression of the SA and AV nodes. This results in various conduction disturbances (first- or second-degree block or complete heart block). Digitalis may also cause increased myocardial automaticity, producing extra systoles or tachycardias by activating latent pacemakers.

Predisposing factors to digitalis toxicity. Nurses need to be aware of the predisposing factors to digitalis toxicity. The presence of any of these factors in patients indicates the need for close observation of these patients for signs and symptoms of digitalis intoxication.

POTASSIUM LOSS. Hypokalemia is a common cause of digitalis cardiotoxicity. Since potassium inhibits the excitability of the heart, a depletion of body or myocardial potassium increases cardiac excitability. Low extracellular potassium is synergistic with digitalis and enhances ectopic pacemaker activity (dysrhythmias). The following are causes of potassium loss:

1 Hypokalemia occurs if large amounts of body fluids are lost as a result of vomiting, diarrhea, or diuresis from administration of diuretics. The use of various diuretic agents (carbonic-anhydrase inhibitors, ammonium chloride, and thiazide

preparations) induce potassium diuresis along with sodium and water diuresis.
2 Poor dietary intake or severe dietary restrictions decreasing electrolyte intake can cause loss of potassium.
3 Adrenal steroids cause potassium loss and sodium retention.
4 Surgical procedures associated with severe electrolyte disturbances such as abdominoperineal resection, colostomy, ileostomy, colectomy, and ureterosigmoidostomy can cause loss of potassium.
5 Use of potassium-free intravenous fluids can cause hypokalemia.

PATHOLOGIC CONDITIONS. Kidney, liver, and severe heart disease are major factors in digitalis toxicity. From 60% to 80% of the digitalis glycosides are excreted by the kidneys. Therefore renal disease promotes digitalis cumulation and intoxication. Since the liver is the primary organ for inactivating digitalis, any impairment of liver function decreases an individual's tolerance to digitalis. Severe cardiac disease impedes the function of all body organs and increases myocardial sensitivity to digitalis.

ADMINISTRATION OF PURIFIED GLYCOSIDES. Because purified glycosides produce fewer side effects than the whole leaf, there may be continued administration of digitalis without awareness that toxicity is occurring.

SLOWER BODY FUNCTION. Elderly persons have a slowing of body functions and often a decreased tolerance to drug therapy. Older patients often show signs of toxicity with small doses of digitalis.

INTRAVENOUS ADMINISTRATION OF DIGITALIS AND RAPID DIGITALIZATION. The risk of digitalis overdosage is increased by intravenous administration and rapid digitalization.

Treatment of digitalis intoxication. The treatment of digitalis toxicity may consist entirely of omitting administration of digitalis until toxic signs and symptoms have disappeared, or it may include the administration of other drugs such as potassium chloride or rarely disodium ethylenediaminotetraacetic acid (EDTA). Administration of potassium chloride will tend to decrease myocardial excitability and abolish dysrhythmias. EDTA is a calcium chelating

agent. Successful treatment of digitalis toxicity has also been reported with the use of phenytoin and propranolol. There is no specific antidote for digitalis intoxication.

Contraindications and precautions. Digitalis is contraindicated in heart block and usually when ventricular tachycardia is present. Valvular disease, diphtheria, and thyrotoxicosis are not in themselves considered indications for digitalis therapy.

Digitalis must be used with great caution in patients with acute or toxic myocarditis, since the potential for glycoside-induced dysrhythmias is increased in these patients. If congestive heart failure occurs in patients with acute myocarditis, digitalis may be used but in smaller than usual doses and with close observation. Ordinary doses usually do not slow the often associated tachycardia, and high doses produce dysrhythmias. Also, the use of digitalis in the treatment of obesity is unwarranted because of the danger of potentially fatal dysrhythmias.

Ouabain, G-Strophanthin

Ouabain is obtained from *Strophanthus gratus*. For many years it was the standard against which all digitalis preparations were measured. It is not absorbed well from the gastrointestinal tract and hence must be given parenterally (usually intravenously). Its action is relatively rapid. Effects appear within about 30 minutes after intravenous injection, and the peak effect is secured in about 90 minutes. Most of its effects have disappeared within 24 hours. It is one of the preparations of choice for rapid digitalization. It is relatively soluble and not likely to cause venous thrombosis when given intravenously. It is available in 1- and 2-ml ampules containing 0.25 mg/ml solution.

NURSING IMPLICATIONS FOR DIGITALIS PREPARATIONS

Of great importance is the careful observation by the nurse of patients receiving digitalis preparations who have one or more of the predisposing factors to digitalis intoxication. If the patient is being monitored, careful observation should be made of the ECG before and after the institution of or reduction or increase in digitalis dosage. The pulse, preferably apical pulse, should be checked before giving each dose to determine any marked change in rate or rhythm. It is still a safe precaution to report and record a pulse below 60 in the adult or 90 to 110 beats/minute in the child. A decision may be made to withhold the drug.

Understanding on the part of the nurse of the relationship between dosage and potency is fundamental to intelligent cooperation with the physician in the care of the patient who is receiving digitalis or related drugs. When medication is ordered in terms of a small fraction or a decimal fraction, the inference is not only that the drug is potent but also that a mistake in dosage can be especially dangerous even if the amount is small in terms of milligrams. Considerable difference exists among dosages of 1 mg, 0.1 mg, 0.15 mg, and 0.2 mg. Differences of a fraction of a milligram can mean a great deal when administering a potent preparation. The nurse must exert particular care to see that the correct dosage is given.

Antidysrhythmic drugs

Antidysrhythmic drugs are used for the treatment and prevention of disorders of cardiac rhythm. Disturbances in cardiac rhythm result from some aberration in the electrophysiologic properties of the cells of the specialized conduction system or of the cardiac muscle. *Dysrhythmia* may pertain to any disturbance in the regular rhythm, rate, and conduction of the heart. Because the term "dysrhythmia," which means disturbed rhythm, is more accurate than "arrhythmia," which denotes *absence* of rhythm, the former designation will be used here.

A high incidence of dysrhythmia often develops in patients about 4 to 72 hours after the onset of myocardial infarction. In addition, abnormal rhythm may occur as a complication in patients recovering from cardiac surgery or quite frequently in ambulatory patients with coronary heart disease. Also, individuals with extracardiac disorders such as pheochromocytoma, electrolyte imbalance, or thyroid disease generally experience some form of aberration in cardiac rhythm.

CARDIAC DYSRHYTHMIAS

Cardiac dysrhythmia may be defined as any deviation from the normal rhythm of the heartbeat. It originates from some pathologic disorder that modifies the electrophysiologic properties of the cells of the conduction system or cardiac muscle cells.

Disorders in cardiac electrophysiology

Disorders of cardiac rhythm arise as a result of (1) abnormality in spontaneous initiation of an impulse or *automaticity* or (2) abnormality in impulse conduction or *conductivity*. In some conditions, a combination of both processes may occur.

Abnormality in automaticity. A disturbance in automaticity may alter the heart's rate, rhythm, or site of origin of impulse formation. When the rate of pacemaker activity is affected, a decrease in automaticity of the SA node produces sinus bradycardia, whereas an increase in automaticity of the SA node results in sinus tachycardia. On the other hand, *a shift in the site of origin of impulse formation* can generate an abnormal pacemaker or an *ectopic* focus. In an ectopic beat, the impulse originates from an abnormal focus or site, resulting in activation of some part of the heart other than the SA node. This is called an ectopic pacemaker, which may discharge either at a regular or an irregular rhythm. It occurs because the cardiac fibers depolarize more frequently than the SA node. Consequently, abnormal automaticity may develop in cells that ordinarily are incapable of spontaneous initiation of impulses, for example, atrial or muscle cells. Clinical disorders such as hypoxia or ischemia are responsible for activating stimuli that become centers of enhancing automaticity. In addition, ischemic sites are capable of causing impulse disturbances not only in automaticity but also in conductivity, and both manifestations are responsible for ectopic beats. The ectopic beats are classified as escape beats, premature beats or extrasystoles, and ectopic tachydysrhythmia.

Abnormality in conductivity. Altered conduction of the cardiac impulse probably accounts for more dysrhythmia than a change in automaticity. A disturbance in conductivity may be caused by (1) delay or block of impulse conduction or (2) the reentry phenomenon.

Delay or block of impulse conduction. Normally, the SA and AV nodes are poor conductors of impulse transmission. Therefore, under abnormal circumstances, conduction of an atrial impulse to the ventricles may be delayed or blocked in the AV node or structures beyond this region in the conduction pathway. However, impaired impulse transmission generally appears in the AV node or junction and occurs in varying degrees of block. In the first-degree AV block the impulses from the SA node pass through to the ventricles very slowly, and this is noted by a prolonged P-R interval. In the second-degree block some atrial beats fail to pass into the ventricles. Finally, in the third-degree block or complete heart block, no impulses reach the ventricles, in which case the Purkinje fibers initiate their own spontaneous depolarization at a very slow rate. This results in independent ventricular and atrial rhythms referred to as ventricular "escape."

Reentry phenomenon. In addition to a change in automaticity, alteration in conductivity is the second electrophysiologic property causing ectopic beats. The phenomenon of reentry is the mechanism responsible for initiating ectopic beats. *A necessary condition for reentry is unidirectional block.* Normally, when an impulse travels down the Purkinje fiber, it spreads along two branches, and on entry into the connecting branch the impulses are extinguished at the point of collision in the center (Fig. 18-7, *A*). At the same time, other impulses that propagate laterally from the Purkinje fibers produce activation of ventricular muscle tissue. In an abnormal situation the impulse descending from the central Purkinje fiber travels down the left branch normally but in the right branch encounters a block as a result of ischemia or injury (Fig. 18-7, *B*). Therefore a unidirectional block is achieved because the impulse is capable of passing in one direction but not in the other. As a result, in the right branch, where the antegrade impulse is blocked in the forward direction at the site of injury, a retrograde impulse from the ventricular tissue penetrates or *reenters* the depressed region from the other direction, provided that the pathway proximal

to the block is no longer refractory. Subsequently, when the effective refractory period of the blocked area is ended, *reentry* of the impulse from the ventricular muscle into this site affords a potential for the impulse to circulate or recycle repetitively through the loop, resulting in a circus-type movement. Thus a change in conductivity known as *reentry* is capable of sustaining an ectopic tachydysrhythmia. Furthermore, the phenomenon of reentry can occur within any part of the specialized conduction system or the myocardium (Fig. 18-7, *B*).

As shown in Fig. 18-7, *C*, reentry is abolished by certain drug groups such as I-A, IV, and possibly II, which will be explained later in this chapter. *The drugs that decrease or slow conduction velocity possess the ability to convert unidirectional block to a two-way or bidirectional block.* As the impulses traveling in the antegrade or forward direction and those appearing in a retrograde or reverse direction are blocked at the injured site, the reentry pathway is interrupted, thereby abolishing the ectopic beats. In Fig. 18-7, *D*, the conditions required for eradicating reentry by another mechanism are also illustrated. *The Group I-B drugs, which either increase or have no effect on conduction velocity, eliminate reentry by abolishing unidirectional block entirely.* Consequently the normal impulse conduction along the right and left branches of the Purkinje fibers is again restored.

CLASSIFICATION OF ANTIDYSRHYTHMIC DRUGS

In recent years an increasing number of antidysrhythmic drugs have necessitated their classification into more discrete categories with respect to their fundamental mode of action on cardiac muscle. Such a grouping of antidysrhythmic mechanisms should prove of value in predicting its therapeutic efficacy as well as its potential toxic effects in a given clinical cardiac condition. Drugs belonging to a particular class do not necessarily possess actions that are identical in every respect. In some cases a given agent may have subsidiary properties (extracardiac effects) that alter the basic electrophysiologic actions on the cardiac muscle. The currently available antidysrhythmic drugs are classified into four discrete cate-

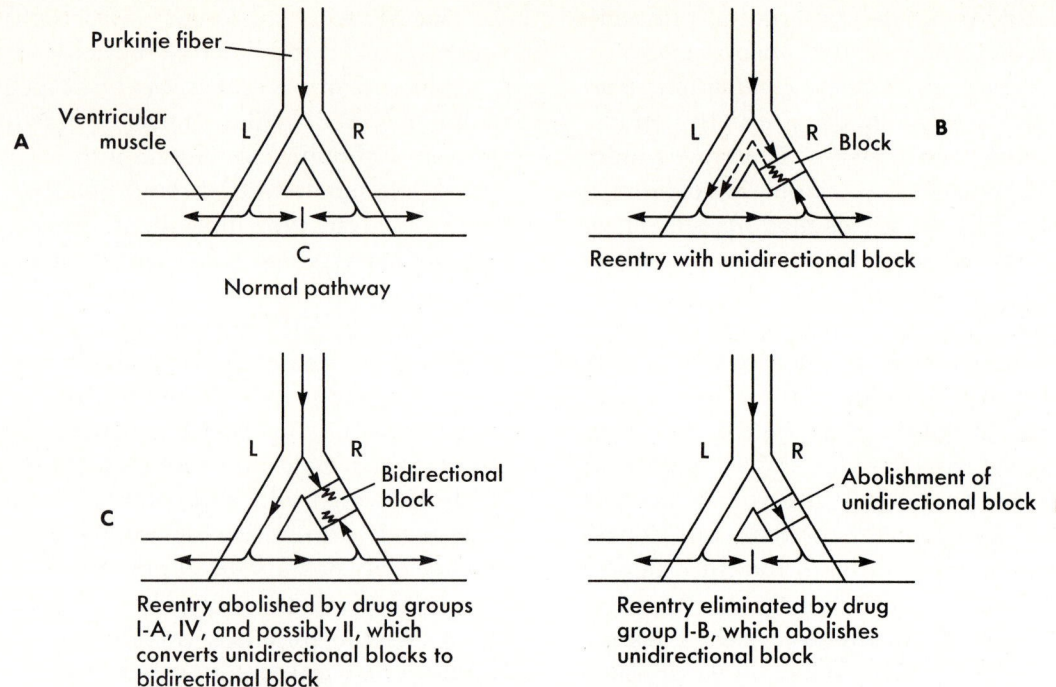

FIG. 18-7. Diagrammatic illustration of unidirectional block in reentry showing a branched Purkinje fiber terminating on the ventricular muscle. **A,** In the normal pathway, the impulse travels down the Purkinje fiber and is conducted along the left *(L)* and right *(R)* branches. In the connecting branch, the impulses are extinguished at the point of collision in the center *(C)*. The propagation of impulses that travel laterally from the Purkinje fiber results in activation of the ventricular muscle. **B,** In the abnormal situation, the impulse in the left branch descends normally from the central Purkinje fiber, but in the right branch the impulse encounters a block caused by ischemia or injury. This is a *unidirectional block* because the impulse is capable of passing in the left branch but not in the right. Therefore, this block creates a condition for *reentry*. As a result, the antegrade impulse is still blocked in the forward direction, but a retrograde impulse from the ventricular tissue penetrates or *reenters* the injured site from the other direction. As long as the pathway proximal to the block is no longer refractory, *reentry* of the impulse can occur and by recycling repetitively through the loop, a circus type of movement is established. In **C,** reentry is abolished by drug groups IA, IV, and possibly II because of a decrease in conduction velocity. Thus these agents convert unidirectional block into bidirectional block by inhibiting the flow of impulses from two directions—the antegrade or forward direction and the retrograde or reverse direction, thereby abolishing the ectopic beats. In **D,** reentry is eliminated by drug group I-B which, by either increasing or not affecting conduction velocity, abolishes the unidirectional block. This process leads to restoration of normal impulse conduction, a condition that enhances the removal of ectopic beats.

gories according to their mechanisms of action (Table 18-3). However, these drugs have one major electrophysiologic property in common: they all have the ability to suppress automaticity. Group I compounds are subdivided into Groups I-A and I-B to reflect the similar electrophysiologic effects of each subgroup. Group I-A drugs include quinidine, procainamide, and disopyramide, all of which decrease conduction velocity, whereas Group I-B drugs such as lidocaine and phenytoin either increase or have no effect on conduction velocity. Propranolol is considered a Group II drug because of its beta adrenergic blocking action. Otherwise its direct membrane effects are similar to that of the Group I drugs. The principal action of bretylium, a Group III compound, involves primarily its antiadrenergic properties. Unlike the other drugs in this category, it has a decidedly positive inotropic action. The last category, which is identified as Group IV agents, is characterized by a selective calcium antagonistic action. For this reason, verapamil is classified independently of other conventional compounds. (See

T A B L E   1 8 - 3   **Classification and comparative mechanisms of action of antidysrhythmic drugs**

Group	I-A Quinidine Procainamide	I-A Disopyramide	I-B Lidocaine Phenytoin	II Propranolol	III Bretylium	IV Verapamil
Electrophysiologic effects						
Automaticity	↓	↓	↓	↓		↓
Conduction velocity	↓	→ or ↓	→ or ↑	↓	→	→ or ↓
Effective refractory period	↑	→ or ↑	↓	↓	↑	→ or ↑
Inotropic effect	↓	↓	→	↓	↑	↓
Autonomic effect	Vagolytic action	Vagolytic action	No vagolytic action	Beta adrenergic blocking action	Adrenergic blocking action	
ECG effects						
P-R interval	→ or ↑	→ or ↑	→ or ↓	→ or ↑	↑	↑
QRS complex	↑	→ or ↑	→	→	→	
Q-T interval	↑	→ or ↑	→ or ↓	↓	↑	
Hemodynamic effects						
Cardiac output	↓	↓	→ or ↓	↓		
Blood pressure	↓	↓	→ or ↓	→ or ↓	↓	

↑, increased; ↓, decreased; →, no change.
P-R interval refers to conduction through the AV node.
QRS complex indicates intraventricular conduction.
Q-T interval refers to repolarization phase of the action potential.

Table 18-3 for comparative mechanisms of action.)

GROUP I-A DRUGS
Quinidine

Like quinine, quinidine is contained in cinchona bark and was used by Peruvian Indians for the treatment of malaria. It was introduced as an antidysrhythmic drug early in the twentieth century following a demonstration by a patient of Wenckebach's that he could control his atrial fibrillation by self-administration of quinine. It was not until 1962 that the electrophysiologic mechanisms of quinidine were identified.

Action and results. The main effect of quinidine is attributed to its direct action on the cardiac cell membrane. This involves alteration of such electrophysiologic properties as automaticity, excitability, conduction velocity, and effective refractory period. The drug stabilizes the cell membrane by preventing ready movement of sodium influx and potassium efflux across this cellular barrier. Thus the inhibition of cation exchange results in a decrease in the rate of diastolic depolarization from resting potential during phase 4 and an increase in the threshold potential (the voltage shifts toward 0)

(Fig. 18-8). By decreasing impulse generation, this effect on automaticity at ectopic sites in the atria, AV junction, and Purkinje fibers is responsible for the ability of quinidine to suppress or abolish dysrhythmias. Fortunately, abnormal or ectopic pacemaker tissue appears to be more sensitive to quinidine than normal pacemaker tissue (SA node). Consequently, this permits the SA node to reestablish control over cardiac impulse formation in the heart. Again, by preventing exchange of ions across the cell membrane, quinidine depresses excitability of both atrial and ventricular myocardium, an important attribute in counteracting dysrhythmia. In addition, the drug slows conduction velocity in all cardiac tissues, namely, atria and ventricles, including the specialized conduction system. Widening of the QRS complex indicates a decrease in intraventricular conduction, and lengthening of the P-R interval represents slower conduction through the AV node, which are changes observed on the ECG. Thus caution must be used when the drug is administered to individuals with intraventricular conduction disorders. Perhaps the most significant action of quinidine is its ability to prolong the effective refractory period of atrial and ventricular fibers. A delay in completion of repolar-

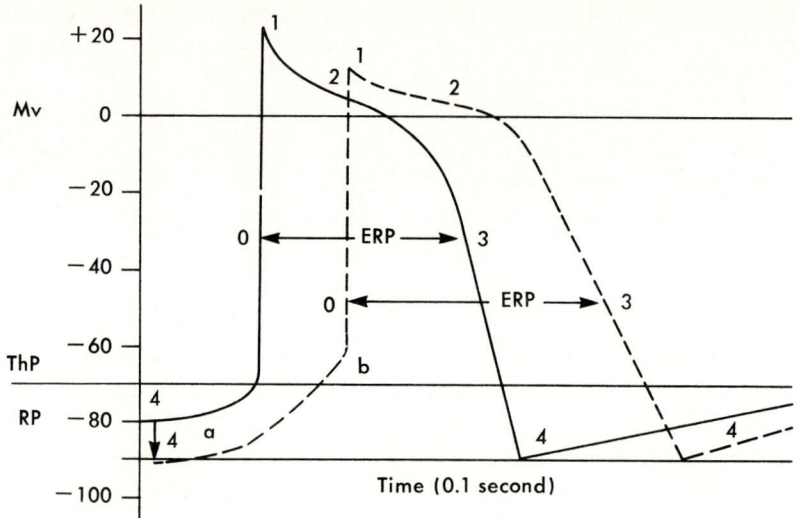

FIG. 18-8. The effect of quinidine on resting membrane potential of a single Purkinje fiber.

The solid line depicts the normal Purkinje fiber during the phases *(0 to 4)* of the action potential; the broken lines show how quinidine alters the action potential of the Purkinje fiber. The use of quinidine suppresses automaticity by effecting a decrease in the rate of depolarization from the resting potential *(RP)* during diastole (phase 4) shown at *a* and an increase in the threshold potential *(ThP)* toward 0 mv indicated at *b*. The effective refractory period *(ERP)* is also prolonged with the use of quinidine. (Modified from Mason, D.T., and others: Clin. Pharmacol. Therap. **11**:460, 1970.)

ization probably exerts an important antifibrillatory action. Since the tissue remains refractory for a period of time after full restoration of the resting membrane potential, this property is believed to influence the conversion of unidirectional block to bidirectional block, thereby abolishing the reentry type of dysrhythmia (Fig. 18-7, *C*).

The indirect anticholinergic effect of quinidine inhibits vagal action on the SA and AV nodes. This exerts an atropine-like effect that permits the sinus node to accelerate and often may provoke a dangerous sinus tachycardia. Moreover, quinidine should be used with caution in atrial flutter because its vagolytic action could facilitate AV conduction and suddenly increase the ventricular rate, particularly in myocardial infarction. Therefore digitalis, which slows conduction at the AV node, usually is administered before quinidine to prevent the adverse effect of ventricular acceleration while attempting to convert atrial fibrillation to normal sinus rhythm. Finally, the chief noncardiac action of quinidine is exerted on the vascular smooth muscle by which its alpha adrenergic blocking effect produces peripheral vasodila-

tion. The combined effect of a decrease in peripheral vascular resistance and a reduced cardiac output caused by depressed myocardial contractility contributes to the development of hypotension, a condition that may reach serious proportions during quinidine therapy.

Pharmacokinetics. After oral administration, quinidine is almost completely absorbed from the intestine, which has an alkaline pH. When an intramuscular injection is given, the deltoid muscle is recommended rather than other regions to promote rapid absorption of the drug. The peak plasma levels are produced within 1 to 2 hours with both oral and intramuscular injection routes. In patients with cardiac failure, absorption may be poor, making it necessary to frequently check serum levels if the dysrhythmia is unresponsive to quinidine. Of the quinidine found in the blood, nearly 80% is bound to plasma albumin. In patients with hepatic disorders this binding is decreased and instead there exists a higher level of free or unbound pharmacologically active drug available for the transport to the myocardium. Consequently, during maintenance therapy with quinidine, dosage may need to be reduced to prevent toxicity in patients with liver disease. Therapeutic plasma concentrations are in the range of 3 to 5 μg/ml. The normal half-life of quinidine is 4 to 8 hours. The major route of elimination is by way of hepatic metabolism. Since almost 20% of the drug is excreted unchanged in the urine, the dose should be decreased in patients with renal failure.

Uses. Quinidine is indicated for treatment of atrial and ventricular dysrhythmia. The major use of the drug, however, is to prevent recurrent atrial fibrillation in patients who have been successfully converted to a normal sinus rhythm by direct current cardioversion or by other drugs. As a preventive agent, quinidine is also given for supraventricular dysrhythmias, which include any abnormal rhythm rising above the ventricles in any portion of the conduction system. These patients are placed on a maintenance regimen of quinidine to prevent the recurrence of tachycardia. Although this drug has been successfully used to correct ventricular premature beats and tachycardia, it is no longer given as the drug of first choice.

Preparation, dosage, and administration. The maximal effect of an oral dose of quinidine occurs within 1 to 3 hours after administration, and the effect persists for 6 to 8 hours. Quinidine sulfate is used for oral administration, and the hydrochloride, lactate, gluconate, or sulfate preparations are used for intramuscular administration. It is recommended that quinidine only be given orally, since there are other drugs available that can be more safely used intravenously. When given intravenously, the drug causes severe hypotension. Quinidine should not be given rectally because it has a severe irritating effect on rectal mucosa.

Quinidine sulfate. Quinidine sulfate is available in 100-, 200-, and 300-mg capsules, and 100-, 130-, 200-, and 325-mg tablets. Quinidine sulfate is given orally in doses of 200 to 300 mg and repeated every 2, 4, or 6 hours. When given every 2 hours, peak blood levels are usually achieved after the fifth dose; when given orally every 4 hours, peak blood levels are achieved within 48 to 72 hours; when given every 6 hours, or four times a day, peak blood levels may not be reached until the fifth day of administration. The oral maintenance dose is usually

from 200 to 600 mg daily. The dosage for children is 6 mg/kg body weight every 4 to 6 hours.

Quinidine gluconate. Quinidine gluconate is sometimes administered intramuscularly. The initial dose is from 300 to 500 mg. The drug begins to act within 15 to 30 minutes; maximum effect is reached within 1 to 3 hours. Quinidine gluconate is also given orally. In acute situations, 200 mg of quinidine gluconate in dilute solution may be given intravenously, very slowly, with continuous monitoring of the ECG and blood pressure.

Side effects and toxic effects. Quinidine is a potentially hazardous drug. A number of sudden deaths have been reported in patients undergoing quinidine therapy.

The toxic effects of quinidine in approximate order of frequency of occurrence include cinchonism (nausea, vomiting, diarrhea, tinnitus, vertigo, and visual disturbances), thrombocytopenic purpura, rashes and urticaria, hypotension, and ventricular fibrillation.

Some of these effects, such as thrombocytopenic purpura, are thought to be a true allergic hypersensitivity to the drug. Therefore some clinicians give a test dose of the drug before instituting intensive therapy.

The most frequent and serious toxic effects of quinidine involve cardiovascular abnormalities such as complete heart block, ventricular disorders, and hypotension.

The first important toxic manifestation of quinidine is associated with the various degrees of AV block. This may occur as a consequence of slowed conduction through the AV node that eventually may lead to cardiac standstill (asystole). Plasma concentration of quinidine above 6 μg/ml indicates overdosage, and this value correlates with ECG changes. The slowing of conduction through the AV junction prolongs the P-R interval, and a decrease in conduction velocity through the ventricles widens the QRS complex. If the duration of the QRS complex is prolonged to 25% of the premedication value, there is cause for concern. A 50% increase should prompt a reduction of dosage or discontinuation of the drug.

The second adverse effect of quinidine is the occurrence of a ventricular disorder known as premature ventricular contraction (PVC) not noted before drug administration. This appears as an ectopic foci that may develop from a reentry phenomenon. If this warning is neglected, PVC may subsequently lead to ventricular tachycardia or fibrillation, which is difficult to treat and can result in cardiac standstill. Bretylium tosylate has been used successfully in some patients with this disorder. Another form of ventricular disorder that has already been mentioned is "quinidine syncope" caused by ventricular tachycardia or fibrillation. The extremely rapid ventricular rate decreases the cardiac output and thereby diminishes blood flow to the brain. This results in a feeling of faintness, eventual loss of consciousness, and ultimately sudden death.

Quinidine overdosage can also weaken the force of myocardial contraction and cause congestive heart failure. The early symptoms of this complication are fatigue, ankle edema, and dyspnea. Patients using oral doses of quinidine at home should report these signs of toxicity to the physician. Finally, the large doses of quinidine depress the circulation by reducing arterial pressure. The combined effects of peripheral vasodilation and depressed myocardial contractility are responsible for the development of hypotension.

Precautions and contraindications. Quinidine should be used with caution in atrial fibrillation or atrial flutter. Because of its vagal blocking effect, the drug may increase the number of atrial beats conducted across the AV junction, resulting in a sudden acceleration in ventricular rate. Prior administration of digitalis to slow AV conduction reduces the hazard of ventricular tachycardia. An additional hazard that exists following conversion of atrial fibrillation to normal sinus rhythm is the formation of embolism. Because the fibrillating atria do not contract, thrombi often develop in the left atrium. After resumption of atrial contraction, the dislodging of the thrombi may often lead to a stroke.

Quinidine is contraindicated in patients with conduction defects. In the presence of any degree of block, the drug may cause complete atrioventricular block. "Quinidine syncope," which is associated with ventricular tachydys-

rhythmias produced by the drug, is a condition that leads to loss of consciousness in patients on maintenance quinidine therapy. When this complication occurs, the drug should be discontinued. Quinidine is contraindicated in patients who are hypersensitive to this agent. Finally, the drug should not be given to patients with myasthenia gravis, a condition in which skeletal muscle weakness occurs because of impaired acetylcholine production. The curarelike action of quinidine blocks acetylcholine needed for impulse transmission, and thus a more serious muscle weakness ensues. When the respiratory muscles are affected, respiratory distress usually develops.

Drug interactions. The following drug interactions may occur:

1 The action of anticoagulants may be enhanced since quinidine prolongs prothrombin time.
2 Quinidine may potentiate the hypotensive effect of antihypertensive drugs and diuretics.
3 Quinidine has a weak curare-like action and therefore it may intensify the action of neuromuscular blocking agents (for example, tubocurarine) and enhance the action of drugs that can depress conduction at the myoneural junction (for example, polymyxin B, neomycin, kanamycin).
4 Quinidine may antagonize the action of neostigmine, physostigmine, and related drugs.
5 The concomitant use of quinidine with reserpine or other Rauwolfia alkaloids may produce dysrhythmias.

Nursing implications. Patients with liver disease, congestive heart failure, or renal insufficiency should be closely observed for toxic reactions, since interference with metabolism of quinidine or its excretion from the body can greatly increase the body's response to any given dose of the drug.

Since the drug can cause thrombocytopenic purpura, patients undergoing quinidine therapy should be closely observed for bleeding tendencies, petechiae, or ecchymotic or purpuric areas. Patients with decreased platelets require protection from injury that could result in hemorrhage.

Early evidence of quinidine toxicity is best detected by having the patient monitored electrocardiographically and observing for changes in the patient's cardiac electric activity pattern. Abnormal prolongation of the QRS complex, evidence of second-degree or complete heart block, or appearance of premature ventricular contractions precludes continued quinidine administration.

It is recommended that the patient's blood pressure be checked before administration of quinidine. If hypotension is noted, the physician should be notified.

Procainamide hydrochloride (Pronestyl)

Procainamide is a synthetic drug that is an effective antidysrhythmic agent with fewer toxic effects than quinidine. Procainamide is the result of investigations to produce a drug similar to the local anesthetic procaine but with fewer central nervous system effects. It had been demonstrated that topical application of procaine to the myocardium reduced the occurrence of premature cardiac contractions during thoracic surgery.

Action and results. Procainamide, an amide derivative of the local anesthetic procaine, has electrophysiologic properties resembling those of quinidine. This drug depresses automaticity by decreasing the rate of diastolic depolarization in the atrial and ventricular fibers. This accounts for its use in treating ectopic dysrhythmias. It also reduces conduction velocity in all cardiac tissues. Its ability to lengthen the effective refractory period exerts a major antifibrillatory action at the atrial and ventricular level that may be important in preventing reentrant types of dysrhythmias. Procainamide is identical to quinidine in lowering excitability in the atria and ventricles. In therapeutic concentrations procainamide depresses myocardial contractility, producing a negative inotropic effect. However, its indirect anticholinergic effect is somewhat weaker than that of quinidine but in high concentrations may be responsible for the development of cardioacceleration.

Pharmacokinetics. An oral dose of procainamide is well absorbed from the small intestine where an alkaline pH exists. The peak plasma level is usually attained within 1 hour after administration. Intramuscular injection produces a peak blood level within 25 minutes, and when given intravenously, its action begins almost immediately. Only about 15% of the drug is bound to plasma albumin, and since 85% of the drug is free, a liver disorder such as cirrhosis has little effect on blood levels. In patients with normal cardiac, renal, or liver function the elimination half-life of the drug averages 3½ hours. This means that about 4 hours after administration only about 45% of the drug remains in the body. Effective therapeutic serum concentration of procainamide is 4 to 8 µg/ml, and at levels above 12µg/ml the drug is potentially toxic.

In the liver approximately 25% to 30% of a dose of procainamide is metabolized by acetylation forming N-acetylprocainamide (NAPA), a major metabolite that exerts the same amount of pharmacologic activity on the heart as the drug itself. As a consequence, measurement of only the procainamide level may provide an erroneous indication of the total concentration of the drug. The half-life of NAPA is 6 hours in patients with normal renal function, and this is prolonged in individuals with renal failure. Therefore dosage should be reduced to avoid high plasma concentration of procainamide and NAPA. Approximately 50% to 60% is eliminated in the urine as unchanged drug, the remainder is excreted as metabolites by the same route.

Uses. Because of its side effects, procainamide is not the drug of first choice for the treatment of atrial or ventricular dysrhythmias. Generally, this agent is indicated as a second-line drug after control by lidocaine has been established. Procainamide is useful in treating ventricular tachycardia and premature ventricular contractions in patients with most types of heart disease. However, as a prophylactic agent its use is contraindicated because of its high incidence of toxic effects. Prevention of premature ventricular contraction and ventricular tachycardia is now being treated by a safer drug, disopyramide.

Preparation, dosage, and administration. Procainamide is available in 250- and 500-mg capsules and in solution for injection (100 mg/ml). It is usually administered orally or intravenously, although it can be administered intramuscularly. A continuous intravenous drip of procainamide in 5% glucose in water may be used to control acute dysrhythmias.

The usual oral dose for adults is 250 to 500 mg four times daily; for children it is 50 mg/kg body weight daily in divided doses.

Procainamide is safer than quinidine for intravenous use.

Side effects and toxic effects. Cardiac electrophysiologic toxicity to procainamide is similar to that of quinidine. To avoid severe hypotension the patient must be supine during intravenous infusion. Blood pressure should be taken frequently, and a fall of more than 15 mm Hg indicates overdosage. The infusion should be stopped if the ECG shows signs of toxicity. This is caused by slowing of ventricular conduction time and is observed as widening of the QRS complex by 25%. As with quinidine, procainamide can exert a vagolytic action so that patients with atrial flutter or fibrillation may suddenly experience an excessive increase in ventricular rate. These patients may also have gastrointestinal and central nervous system disturbances.

Following chronic use of procainamide for more than 6 months, the most common side effect is the development of systemic lupus erythematosus (SLE)-type syndrome. The rate of acetylation or metabolism of procainamide in the liver influences the development of the SLE-like reaction to the drug. Individuals who are genetically slow acetylators of the compound tend to have a higher plasma concentration of procainamide than of NAPA. Thus patients with this metabolic difference tend to develop antinuclear antibodies, which produce the lupuslike reaction. This syndrome is accompanied by fever, arthralgia, pleuritic pain, and insomnia. The condition is reversible after discontinuation of the drug. Meanwhile, measurement of antinuclear antibody (ANA) and LE preparations determine the feasibility of continuing drug therapy. These tests remain positive for some time after symptoms have subsided and the drug has been discontinued. Another problem includes agranulocytosis, a hypersensitive reaction that may occur in the early weeks of therapy. Complaints of sore throat require prompt evaluation to avoid fatal infection. Thus frequent differential blood counts should be performed regularly during the course of procainamide therapy.

Contraindications. Procainamide is usually contraindicated in patients with severe heart damage and shock, since increasing the hypotension may result in fatality. It is also contraindicated in patients with complete heart block and in patients manifesting allergic reactions. Increased widening of the QRS complex caused by procainamide contraindicates further administration of the drug.

Drug interactions. Procainamide may enhance the action of drugs with neuromuscular blocking action (curariform drugs and various antibiotics such as neomycin). This interaction may cause respiratory depression.

Procainamide may also potentiate the hypotensive effect of antihypertensive drugs and thiazide diuretics.

Nursing implications. When the drug is given intravenously, eletrocardiographic and blood pressure monitoring is required. Further administration of the drug should be questioned when hypotension, progressive widening of the QRS complex, or undesirable changes in the ECG pattern occur. Vasopressors, such as norepinephrine, should be readily available if hypotension occurs. Patients should be observed for and told to report symptoms of arthralgia and fever (lupus syndrome).

Disopyramide phosphate (Norpace)

Disopyramide, a synthetic agent discovered in 1962, is chemically unrelated to any of the conventional antidysrhythmic agents presently used.

Action and results. Disopyramide has a pharmacologic profile almost similar to that of quinidine and procainamide. It decreases automaticity of ectopic cardiac pacemaker cells. In addition, it lengthens the effective refractory period of the atrial and ventricular muscle cells. However, unlike quinidine and procainamide, disopyramide does not change the effective refractory period of the AV node. Also, the conduction time of the AV node and the His-Purkinje system is usually unaltered. On the ECG the P-R interval is not changed as much as with quinidine or procainamide, and the QRS rarely increases by more than 20% when therapeutic concentrations of the drug are given. This drug also exerts an anticholinergic or atropine-like effect. It is a myocardial depressant. Because it also blocks postganglionic sympathetic nerve transmission, it produces orthostatic hypotension.

Pharmacokinetics. The oral preparation of disopyramide is absorbed almost completely from the intestinal tract. The usual therapeutic plasma levels are 2 to 4 µg/ml, and the mean plasma half-life is about 6½ hours. Approximately 50% to 60% of a dose is excreted unchanged, mainly in the urine. In patients with impaired renal function a reduction in dosage is adjusted in accordance with the creatinine clearance levels. Also, individuals with hepatic disorders require a lower dosage of the drug.

Uses. The oral form of disopyramide is indicated for suppression and prevention of premature ventricular contractions and ventricular tachycardia. Since its approval by the Food and Drug Administration in 1977, this drug has rapidly established itself as an effective antidysrhythmic agent in the prophylactic treatment of patients with ventricular dysrhythmias.

Preparation, dosage, and administration. Disopyramide phosphate is available as an oral preparation in hard gelatin capsules that contain 100 or 150 mg of the drug. In the United States only the oral preparation of this agent is approved by the FDA. The usual oral dosage ranges 100 to 150 mg every 6 hours, and the maximal daily dose is 800 mg. When rapid control of dysrhythmia is required, an initial loading dose of 300 mg is given before administration of maintenance therapy.

Side effects and toxic effects. The most distressing side effects of the drug are caused by its anticholinergic properties, and these include dryness of the mouth, blurring of vision, and urinary retention. Therefore the drug should be avoided in patients with prostatic hypertrophy or glaucoma.

Precautions and contraindications. Despite the fact that little effect has been shown on the AV nodal conduction time, disopyramide should not be used on patients with greater than first-degree block. If second- or third-degree block occurs during therapy, the drug should be discontinued. Moreover, disopyramide is contraindicated in the presence of cardiogenic shock or known hypersensitivity to the drug.

GROUP I-B DRUGS
Lidocaine (Xylocaine), lignocaine hydrochloride

Lidocaine is better known and extensively used as a local and topical anesthetic agent. However, in recent years it has become one of the most frequently used drugs, and in some institutions it is the drug of choice, in the treatment of ventricular dysrhythmias. It has gained considerable acclaim as an effective antidysrhythmic agent. Lidocaine apparently does not depress conduction in the heart, and it has less negative inotropic action than either quinidine or procainamide.

Action and results. Originally introduced as a synthetic local anesthetic, lidocaine has been found to have pharmacologic actions that make it useful for the treatment of cardiac dysrhythmias. Its electrophysiologic properties are almost similar to that of quinidine and procainamide. Lidocaine exerts its most important cardiac effect by depressing excessive automaticity of ectopic pacemakers in the His-Purkinje fibers. Thus it is useful in suppressing premature ventricular contractions, a dysrhythmia that may be provoked by hypoxic or ischemic cells in myocardial infarction. Ischemia is a condition that favors the development of an ectopic pacemaker, discharging faster than the normal pacemaker in the SA node. In some cardiac disorders, premature ventricular contractions may eventually precipitate ventricular tachycardia or fibrillation. Therefore it is essential to provide effective treatment immediately.

In contrast to the findings with quinidine and procainamide, lidocaine has little, if any, effect on conduction velocity (phase 0) or on the effective refractory period in the AV node and the Purkinje fibers. The absence of these properties possibly prevents reentrant types of dysrhythmia. For this reason the drug may play a part in improving AV conduction in the digitalis-intoxicated heart. Also, the potential for development of heart block, cardiac asystole, or ventricular ectopic rhythm is minimized with the use of lidocaine. On the ECG the

P-R or Q-T intervals may not shorten, and the QRS is not prolonged. Unlike quinidine and procainamide, lidocaine has no vagolytic properties nor does it influence cardiac output and arterial pressure. Also, it does not depress myocardial contractility and thereby provides no potential for the development of congestive heart failure. Since it exerts limited if any effect on the SA node and atrial myocardium, the drug has no use in the treatment of supraventricular tachycardias. Because electric activities are primarily limited to the ventricular cells, the major use of lidocaine is in abolishing ventricular dysrhythmias.

Pharmacokinetics. The oral administration of lidocaine fails to reach therapeutically effective levels in the blood because much of the drug is metabolized in the liver during its first hepatic pass. In addition, this route causes nausea, vomiting, and gastrointestinal discomfort, and therefore lidocaine is only given parenterally. Intramuscular administration of the drug into the deltoid muscle promotes more rapid absorption than injection into the vastus lateralis or gluteus maximus. When given intravenously, lidocaine is quickly distributed by the blood to the myocardium. Onset of action occurs within 10 to 90 seconds, with a duration of action lasting 20 minutes. Since the true half-life of the drug is 2 hours, repeated bolus injections (such as every 20 minutes) eventually result in accumulation of toxic levels in the plasma. The therapeutic plasma concentration of lidocaine is 1.5 to 5 μg/ml. Levels above 5 μg/ml increase the risk of toxicity.

The drug is metabolized primarily in the liver. The presence of liver disease or of reduced hepatic blood flow as in cardiac failure decreases the rate of metabolism and thereby promotes toxic accumulation of lidocaine in the plasma. In patients with either one of these conditions a reduction in dosage is indicated. Moreover, the active metabolite monoethylglycinexylidide (MEGX) formed in the liver may also contribute to toxicity, since this compound is almost as potent as lidocaine itself. Since the liver is the major route of elimination of the drug, dose adjustment must be a constant concern in individuals with impaired liver function.

Uses. The primary use of lidocaine is to treat ventricular tachycardia. It is particularly useful in patients with recent myocardial infarction because it has an advantage over quinidine and procainamide in not causing a drop in blood pressure. Again, unlike quinidine and procainamide, it can also be used to treat digitalis toxicity since it has little or no effect on conduction velocity and is less likely to cause conduction defects. Lidocaine actually suppresses ventricular dysrhythmia of any origin, including that associated with cardiac surgery. However, its effect on atrial dysrhythmia is limited. The efficacy of intramuscular injection of lidocaine to prevent ventricular fibrillation in patients with acute myocardial infarction is still a matter of dispute.

Preparation, dosage, and administration. Lidocaine supplied for the treatment of dysrhythmia contains *no* preservatives. Preparations of lidocaine intended for use as a local anesthetic contain *epinephrine* and should *not* be used for treating dysrhythmias. The route of administration of lidocaine includes intravenous infusion, either by bolus or by continuous method, or intramuscular injections. For bolus injection the preparation may be in the form of prefilled syringes or 5-ml ampules that contain 100 mg of the drug. To prevent the return of the dysrhythmia, the initial bolus injection is usually followed by continuous intravenous drip. Lidocaine is available in a variety of ampule and multiple-dose vial solutions for injection. A 2% solution without epinephrine is available in 5- and 50-ml containers for use in cardiac dysrhythmias. Lidocaine is administered intravenously, 1 mg/kg body weight, and by slow intravenous injection or continuous intravenous drip. The onset of action of lidocaine occurs within 2 minutes. Duration of action of a single dose is 10 to 20 minutes. If an injection of 50 to 100 mg does not produce a desired response, additional injections may be given every 20 minutes until the cumulative maximum of 5 mg/kg body weight is reached. For intravenous infusion, lidocaine is added to 1 liter of 5% dextrose in water and infused at a rate of 15 to 45 μg/kg per minute. Therapeutic blood levels for lidocaine range from 1.5 to 5 μg/ml. Lidocaine may be given intramuscularly into the deltoid muscle. Intramuscular administration is controversial. It may be of value when a patient with acute myocardial infarction and ventricular premature beats is seen at home and is to be transported to the hospital. Otherwise, the routine prophylactic use of lidocaine in impending myocardial infarction is a matter still awaiting more study.

Side effects and toxic effects. Drowsiness is a very common side effect but this is often desirable, particularly in patients with acute myocardial infarction.

Some investigators report central nervous system disturbances (agitation, disorientation, muscle twitching, and convulsions), heart block, and hypotension, particularly with high dosage or rapid rate of administration. Blurred vision, nausea, paresthesias, tinnitus, euphoria, respiratory depression, bradycardia, and respiratory and cardiac arrest may occur. Toxic effects rapidly disappear on discontinuance of drug administration.

Patients undergoing infusion of lidocaine should be carefully monitored for cardiac depressant effects. On the ECG, signs of excessive depression of cardiac conductivity appear as prolongation of P-R interval and QRS complex. Prompt cessation of drug administration is indicated. The blood pressure should be checked for hypotensive effect, and the patient should be carefully observed for other undesirable effects. Lidocaine must be used cautiously in patients with congestive heart failure or severe liver disease since cumulative effects can occur.

Precautions and contraindications. Since the drug is metabolized mainly in the liver, caution must be employed with repeated dose therapy in patients with liver disease or low cardiac output. To prevent the possible toxic accumulation of lidocaine and its metabolites, the dosage is usually reduced in these individuals. The drug is contraindicated in patients with bradycardia and conduction defects.

Phenytoin sodium (Dilantin)

Phenytoin (formerly known in the United States as diphenylhydantoin) was introduced over 30 years ago for control of epilepsy. In 1950 phenytoin was found effective in controlling

dysrhythmias in experiments on dogs. During the 1960's the drug was found useful for treating dysrhythmias in humans.

The structure of phenytoin is related to that of the barbiturates.

Action and results. Phenytoin depresses automaticity at ectopic pacemakers and in the digitalis-intoxicated heart. Depending on the initial condition of cardiac fibers, phenytoin resembles lidocaine by either causing no change or producing an actual increase in the rate of conduction through the atrioventricular tissues and Purkinje fibers. This effect may be observed in the ECG as a shortening of the Q-T interval. Moreover, in contrast with the Group I-A type drugs, the refractory period of the AV node may accelerate AV conduction time, a property that actually improves conduction in patients with digitalis overdosage when the dysrhythmia is caused by partial AV block. It must be noted that digitalis slows conduction through the AV node. Furthermore, since phenytoin depresses ventricular automaticity, it is found to be effective in the treatment of ventricular dysrhythmia occurring in acute myocardial infarction.

Pharmacokinetics. The rate of absorption of phenytoin following oral administration is slow (approximately 6 hours) and variable with individual patients. The drug is widely distributed to all tissues with highest concentrations in the liver and adipose tissue. Phenytoin is highly bound to plasma albumin—70% to 95%. Binding is decreased in patients with cirrhosis, hypoalbuminemia, or uremia. These patients, therefore, are subject to toxicity, since they have a higher concentration of unbound drug in the plasma. In this situation a lower dosage is indicated. The effective serum level of phenytoin for controlling antidysrhythmic activity is 10 to 20 μg/ml. The therapeutic effect corresponds with the unbound phenytoin concentration. This drug has a long elimination half-life of around 18 to 24 hours so that it permits once daily dosing in many patients. Metabolism of phenytoin occurs in the liver, and 75% of inactive metabolites are excreted in the urine. Less than 5% is excreted unchanged by the same route.

Uses. Phenytoin is effective in the treatment

of ventricular dysrhythmias, particularly those produced by overdoses of digitalis. It is also used in patients unable to tolerate quinidine or procainamide. Phenytoin is ineffective in atrial fibrillation, flutter, and atrial and AV junctional premature beats.

Preparation, dosage, and administration. For oral use, phenytoin is available in tablets, chewable tablets, extended release tablets, and oral suspensions. For injection, the drug is available in 100- and 250-mg vials with ampules of special diluents. Phenytoin may be given orally or intravenously. The intramuscular route is seldom used because absorption is too unreliable. Subcutaneous injections are very irritating to the tissue and therefore should be avoided.

In emergency situations intravenous administration of phenytoin can be given slowly as a bolus (at a rate of 50 mg/minute) at a dosage of 100 mg every 5 minutes for a total of 700 to 1000 mg. Since prolonged infusion irritates the vein, the bolus route of administration is preferred. During this time the ECG should be monitored constantly, and the drug should be stopped as soon as a therapeutic effect is noted or signs of toxicity such as hypotension appear. To maintain suppression of dysrhythmia, oral phenytoin may be given on a daily basis at a dosage of 100 to 200 mg every 8 hours per day.

For parenteral use, it is recommended that phenytoin be diluted with the special diluent supplied by the manufacturer. The vehicle has a high alkaline pH of about 11. The drug should not be mixed with dextrose and water or with other acidic solutions because a fine precipitate may result.

Side effects and toxic effects. The drug's ability to depress conduction may result in heart block; its ability to reduce the sinus rate and to cause vasodilation may result in bradycardia and hypotension. Rapid intravenous administration may result in cardiac or respiratory arrest. Phenytoin may cause extracardiac toxic effects including nervousness, confusion, drowsiness, ataxia, tremors, visual disturbances, cutaneous eruptions, and hyperplasia of the gums after prolonged administration.

Heart block or bradycardia caused by phenytoin may be reversed with intravenous administration of atropine.

The common toxic effects occur with blood levels of greater than 20 μg/ml and include nystagmus and ataxia. Toxicity is most likely to occur in the elderly and in hemodynamically unstable patients who should probably receive a much lower dosage. Because the diluent in which it is supplied for parenteral use is highly alkaline, it can produce a precipitous drop in blood pressure. For this reason phenytoin administered intravenously must always be given slowly. Megaloblastic anemia has been observed in some patients. Administration of folic acid and cyanocobalamin (vitamin B_{12}) has resulted in a favorable response.

Precautions and contraindications. This drug may elevate blood glucose levels, particularly when larger doses are used. Patients with diabetes mellitus or renal insufficiency may be more susceptible to hyperglycemia.

Phenytoin is contraindicated in patients with bradycardia or second-degree or complete heart block.

Drug interactions. If phenytoin is given with coumarin or phenylbutazone, the plasma concentration of each of the drugs will rise. If an anticoagulant is indicated, phenindione should be used instead of coumarins because it does not interfere with phenytoin metabolism.

GROUP II DRUG
Propranolol hydrochloride (Inderal)

Action and results. Propranolol, a beta adrenergic blocking agent, is used to control cardiac dysrhythmias caused by excessive sympathetic nerve activity. The stimulation of the sympathetic fibers releases norepinephrine which activates the beta$_1$ receptors on the cells of cardiac tissues. The receptors also respond to circulating norepinephrine and epinephrine. These actions result in rapid heart rate, acceleration of impulse conduction especially through the AV node, and increased force of myocardial contraction.

As an antidysrhythmic agent, propranolol is unique because it controls disturbances in cardiac rhythm by two mechanisms: (1) it blocks beta receptors by competitively inhibiting the access of catecholamines to these sites, and (2) it exerts a direct membrane action by affecting the electrophysiologic properties of the cardiac cell. By the first mechanism, propranolol decreases heart rate and myocardial contraction. Furthermore, it reduces automaticity of pacemakers, which slows the sinus rate and suppresses ectopic beats. In addition, the beta blocking effect decreases conduction velocity and prolongs the effective refractory period of the AV node. The depressed action of the AV node reduces ventricular response to atrial fibrillation. By the second mechanism, the direct membrane action is similar to that of the so-called quinidine-like property that reduces automaticity and conduction velocity. However, unlike its beta adrenergic blocking action, this mechanism shortens the refractory period. The second mechanism of propranolol is considered to be of less importance in exerting antidysrhythmic effects on the heart. Indeed, the principal action of propranolol is associated with its ability to *inhibit adrenergic stimulation* of the heart. Therefore dysrhythmias precipitated by increased sympathetic discharge are effectively blocked by the beta adrenergic action of propranolol.

Pharmacokinetics. The pharmacokinetics of propranolol are complex and varies markedly with the individual. After oral administration, the drug is completely absorbed, provided it is given with no food. The drug is widely distributed in the body tissues and even crosses the blood-brain barrier and placental barrier. After initiating therapy, the plasma half-life is only 3 hours because part of the drug is metabolized or sequestered by the liver during its first pass. Hence, a loading dose of 60 to 80 mg may often be necessary to overcome the hepatic first pass effect of the drug. With continued administration, the half-life appears to increase to a mean of 4 to 6 hours. Effective therapeutic plasma levels of propranolol are shown to be 0.04 to 0.1 μg/ml, but these concentrations may not be as useful a guide to therapy because of individual variability. Moreover, smoking decreases plasma concentration. The drug is metabolized extensively in the liver and is eliminated almost entirely in the urine both as a metabo-

lite and in the free form (about 5%). In patients with liver disease, lower dosage adjustment may be necessary to prevent toxicity.

Uses. The beta adrenergic blocking effect of propranolol makes the drug useful in managing dysrhythmias caused by increased sympathetic activity or excessive catecholamine release such as hyperthyroidism or pheochromocytoma. Propranolol is also used for the control of supraventricular tachycardia. It is effective in this case because the beta blocking action of the drug reduces conduction velocity and prolongs the refractory period, thereby slowing the ventricular response to atrial flutter or fibrillation. The drug may be indicated for treating ventricular tachycardia associated with surgical anesthetic agents, particularly cyclopropane. Otherwise, propranolol is not the drug of first choice in treating ventricular tachycardias because of its myocardial depressant action. Although the drug may produce good results with digitalis-induced ventricular tachycardia, the undesirable side effects such as bradycardia or cardiac arrest limit its use.

Preparation, dosage, and administration. Propranolol is available in tablet form for oral use and 1-ml ampules containing 1 mg of drug for intravenous use. Oral dosage is 10 to 40 mg three to four times a day. Intravenously, 1 to 3 mg may be given at a rate not exceeding 1 mg/minute. A second dose may be given after 2 minutes; additional doses may be given at 4-hour intervals. Patients should be monitored by ECG. Propranolol increases the P-R interval without affecting the duration of the QRS interval. Following oral dosage, blockade occurs within 30 minutes and lasts about 3 to 6 hours. After intravenous administration, onset of action occurs in 2 minutes and peak action in 3 to 5 minutes; duration of action is 2 to 4 hours.

Sudden withdrawal of propranolol in patients with angina pectoris can exacerbate angina, cardiac dysrhythmia, and acute myocardial infarction. Therefore dosage should be gradually reduced, and withdrawal is recommended over a 2-week period.

Side effects and toxic effects. Side effects of propranolol include nausea, vomiting, and diarrhea. In some patients central nervous system effects have been observed, and they include hallucinations, insomnia, dizziness, and depression. Rash, fever, and purpura indicate an allergic response and require discontinuation of the drug.

During therapy, patients should be observed for symptoms of impending cardiac failure, hypotension, bradycardia, and hypoglycemia. The drug may cause an increase in blood urea nitrogen and SGOT levels. Atropine and isoproterenol are antagonists of propranolol. Atropine is given for excessive bradycardia, and isoproterenol improves the circulation if myocardial contractility is severely diminished.

Precautions and contraindications. Propranolol should be used with caution in patients with heart disease because its negative inotropic effect decreases cardiac output, which may result in acute heart failure. In addition, patients with an inadequate cardiac output may develop hypotension and shock. This agent is contraindicated in patients with sinus bradycardia and in those individuals with greater than first-degree block or with right-sided heart failure secondary to pulmonary hypertension. Because of its beta adrenergic blocking effect on smooth muscle, the drug can aggravate bronchial constriction. Therefore propranolol is not administered to patients with bronchial asthma or allergic rhinitis during the pollen season. In patients with thyrotoxicosis propranolol may give a false impression of improvement. In addition, it may mask the clinical signs of developing hyperthyroidism. Abrupt withdrawal of the drug should be avoided because it may exacerbate symptoms of hyperthyroidism including thyroid storm. Labile diabetic patients treated with insulin or oral hypoglycemic agents must be observed carefully, since propranolol masks signs of hypoglycemia such as increased blood pressure and pulse rate. The safe use in women during pregnancy and lactation has not been established.

Drug interactions. The use of adrenergic augmenting psychotropic drugs such as monoamine oxidase inhibitors (which increase the catecholamine level) is counteracted by the beta adrenergic blocking effect of propranolol. Therefore the concomitant use of these two drugs is contraindicated. Patients receiving the catecholamine-depleting drug, namely, reserpine, should be closely observed because excessive reduction in sympathetic tone can occur when reserpine is given with propranolol, which additionally blocks adrenergic action.

GROUP III DRUG
Bretylium tosylate (Bretylol)

Originally, bretylium was introduced for the treatment of hypertension but because of the rapid development of tolerance, the drug was found unsatisfactory for this purpose. In 1965 the antidysrhythmic effects of bretylium were recognized. However, the electrophysiologic properties of this drug differ markedly from the ones previously discussed.

Action and results. Unlike other antidysrhythmic agents, bretylium does not suppress automaticity. In addition, it has no effect on conduction velocity. The only direct electrophysiologic action on the heart appears to be prolongation of the action potential duration and a lengthening of the effective refractory period. It is believed that this mechanism helps to terminate dysrhythmias caused by the reentry phenomenon. As an antidysrhythmic agent, the significant effect of bretylium is related primarily to its *adrenergic blocking action*. The drug is taken up and concentrated in the adrenergic nerve terminals where it *prevents* the release of norepinephrine. This sympatholytic action significantly increases the threshold, producing an antifibrillatory response in the ventricles. The drug exerts no influence on vagal reflexes. Furthermore, in contrast to other agents in this category bretylium produces a positive inotropic effect, increasing myocardial contractility. With long-term treatment, the drug shows increased responsiveness to circulating epinephrine and norepinephrine, which may account for the increased myocardial contractility.

Pharmacokinetics. Because of its erratic absorption from the gastrointestinal tract, oral use of bretylium is still under investigation. After intramuscular administration, peak plasma concentration is attained within an hour, presumably reflecting its adrenergic blocking action. On the other hand, intraveous injection achieves an antifibrillatory effect within minutes. The drug is eliminated almost entirely in an unchanged form by the kidneys without the formation of metabolites. Its half-life varies from 6 to 10 hours. In patients with renal insufficiency the half-life is longer, therefore dosage should be decreased.

Uses. Currently, bretylium tosylate is indicated only for the treatment of life-threatening ventricular dysrhythmias that are unresponsive to lidocaine and procainamide. The drug is also useful in the treatment of ventricular fibrillation that fails to respond to repeated DC countershock. At present, this agent should not be considered a first-line drug because of its serious side effects.

Preparation, dosage, and administration. Only the intravenous and intramuscular uses of bretylium tosylate are approved in the United States. The preparation is available in 10-ml ampules and should be diluted to a volume of 50 ml or more for intravenous use. The dosage of 5 to 10 mg/kg body weight should be infused over a period of 10 to 30 minutes. In an emergency such as cardiac resuscitation a dose of 5 mg/kg of undiluted solution can be given intravenously with repeated doses that should not exceed a total of 30 mg/kg. For intramuscular administration 5 to 10 mg/kg of undiluted bretylium is given every 6 hours. During treatment, the patient is maintained in a supine position and observed for postural hypotension.

Side effects and toxic effects. The most frequently reported adverse effect of bretylium is hypotension. Following its administration, peripheral adrenergic blockade regularly results in postural hypotension despite an increase in myocardial contractility. This causes dizziness, light-headedness, or syncope. In addition, some degree of hypotension occurs in individuals while in the supine position. Patients should be kept in the supine position until tolerance to the hypotensive effect develops. However, if supine systolic pressure falls below 75 mm Hg, an infusion of dopamine may be required. On occasion, initiation of dysrhythmias such as premature ventricular contractions may also occur in some patients. This is caused by the initial

effect of the drug, producing an early release of norepinephrine from adrenergic postganglionic nerve terminals.

With parenteral use of bretylium, some patients may experience transient nausea and occasional vomiting.

Precautions and contraindications. In disorders with a fixed cardiac output such as severe aortic stenosis, bretylium should be used with caution because in this condition cardiac output may not be able to compensate for the increased intravascular volume produced by the drug. Presently, there are no known contraindications for its use in life-threatening ventricular dysrhythmias.

Drug interaction. The unique properties of bretylium prevent its use in combination therapy with digitalis.

GROUP IV DRUG
Verapamil (Isoptin, Calan)

Action and results. Verapamil, a calcium antagonist, is a new antidysrhythmic drug with electrophysiologic actions that are strikingly different from those of the conventional agents. During membrane depolarization, calcium current is selectively inhibited without affecting Na^+ influx in myocardial cells. This action on transmembrane Ca^{++} movement impairs excitation-contraction coupling in myocardial fibers resulting in a negative inotropic action. The inhibition of membrane calcium transport accounts for the antidysrhythmic effect of verapamil. Furthermore, impedance of membrane transport of Ca^{++} in vascular smooth muscle cells of the coronary arteries leads to coronary vasodilation, thereby decreasing myocardial oxygen demands and improving left ventricular performance. Also, the effect of verapamil slowing AV nodal conduction is responsible for reducing the ventricular rate in atrial flutter and fibrillation. However, the preceding properties contraindicate the use of verapamil in patients with AV block and in conditions of reduced myocardial contractility.

In atrial dysrhythmias, the onset of action on the AV node occurs 1 to 5 minutes following rapid intravenous administration. The drug also produces a hypotensive effect during that time and it lasts for 10 to 20 minutes.

Preparation, dosage, and administration. Verapamil is highly effective when given intravenously to treat supraventricular dysrhythmias caused by AV nodal reentry impulses. This is attributed to the fact that slowing of the AV node interrupts the reentrant circuits. This drug also slows the ventricular rate in patients with atrial fibrillation and atrial flutter. The intravenous dosage of verapamil is 10 mg.

Side effects. Side effects include bradycardia and hypotension, particularly in patients with poor myocardial function or sick sinus syndrome.

Antianginal drugs
CORONARY VESSELS

The entire blood supply to the myocardium is provided by the right and left coronary arteries, which arise from the base of the aorta (Fig. 18-9). The right ventricle and atrium are supplied with blood from the right coronary artery. The left coronary artery divides into the anterior descending branch and the circumflex branch and supplies blood to the left ventricle and atrium. These main coronary vessels con-

tinue to divide, forming numerous branches. The result is a profuse network of coronary vessels. The major arterial vessels are located on the external surface of the ventricles. Arterial branches penetrate the myocardium toward the endocardial surface.

Increased oxygen delivery to the myocardium is supported almost exclusively by increased coronary blood flow. When there is increased demand for oxygen and nutrients by body tissues, the heart must increase its output. At the same time, the heart itself must be supplied with enough oxygen and nutrients to replace the energy expended. In other words, a balance must be maintained between energy expenditure and energy restoration.

During systole the myocardial contraction compresses the coronary vascular bed. This restricts coronary inflow but increases coronary outflow. Coronary inflow occurs primarily during diastole when the ventricles have relaxed and the coronary vessels are no longer compressed. Blood is driven through the coronary arteries by aortic pressure, perfusing the myocardium.

A change in heart rate is accomplished by shortening or lengthening diastole. With tachy-

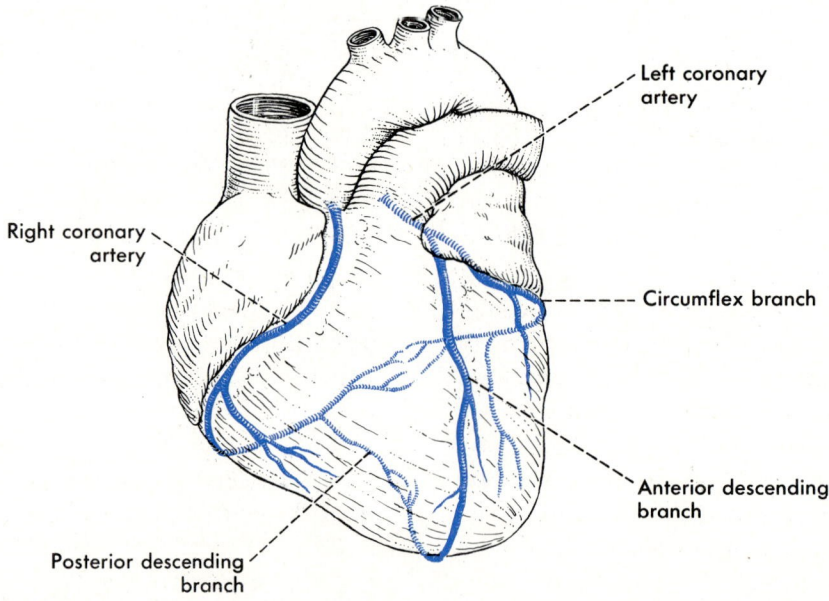

FIG. 18-9. Coronary blood supply to the heart. Dark shaded vessels are those located on the external surface of the ventricles; light shaded vessels show penetration of arterial branches toward the endocardial surface.

cardia the increased amount of time required for the increased number of systolic contractions per minute reduces the time available for diastole and coronary inflow. There is also an increase in the metabolic needs of the rapidly beating heart. Coronary dilation occurs in an attempt to overcome restricted blood inflow. With bradycardia, the decreased number of systolic contractions per minute prolongs the diastolic period. There is a decrease in resistance to coronary flow and a decrease in the metabolic requirements of the myocardium.

Whenever the delivery of oxygen to the myocardium is inadequate to meet the heart's oxygen consumption needs, myocardial ischemia occurs. One of the major causes of ischemia is coronary artery disease.

ANGINA PECTORIS

The term "angina pectoris" refers to intermittent myocardal ischemia (temporary interference with the flow of blood, oxygen, and nutrients to heart muscle). Angina is characterized by substernal pain usually occurring with exercise or stress and relieved by rest. *Angina pectoris occurs when the work load on the heart is too great and oxygen delivery is inadequate.* Since coronary flow is very responsive to oxygen requirements of the heart, inadequate myocardial oxygenation implies inadequate coronary flow in relation to need. Therefore the characteristic syndrome of angina pectoris is usually associated with myocardial ischemia. When coronary blood flow is inadequate, hypoxia causes an accumulation of pain-producing substances such as lactic acid (anaerobic metabolite) and other chemical irritants such as potassium ions, kinins, and prostaglandins. These products then stimulate the cardiac sensory nerve endings, after which the impulses transmitted to the central nervous system produce the typical anginal pain response.

Inadequate oxygenation may be caused by coronary atherosclerosis or even vasomotor spasm of the coronary vessels. Other causes of anginal pain may be associated with pulmonary hypertension and valvular heart disease. Individuals with severe anemia, even with minimal coronary artery disease, may suffer from anginal attacks because of inadequate oxygen supply. The presence of carbon monoxide hemoglobin in smokers who suffer from a reduction in available blood oxygen is another factor in causing angina pectoris. During an attack induced by an exercise test, the severity of the coronary disease appears to be directly proportional to the depth of depression of the S-T segment observed in the ECG; the greater the depth, the greater the severity of the disease.

Drug therapy of angina pectoris is based on the belief that relaxation of coronary smooth muscle will bring about coronary vasodilation, which in turn will improve blood flow to the myocardium. However, coronary arteries narrowed by disorders such as sclerosis and calcification cannot respond to any coronary vasodilator. Actually, when a highly effective vasodilator is used in this type of condition, the blood is diverted from the narrowed vessels to the ones capable of dilating. As a consequence, the occurrence of diminished perfusion to the diseased area produces a further increase in regional myocardial ischemia. This condition, therefore, necessitates the use of nonnitrate vasodilator drugs. There are three therapeutic objectives for the use of antianginal drugs:

1 To decrease the duration and intensity of pain during an attack
2 To prophylactically decrease frequency of attacks and improve work capacity even though angina may occur
3 To prevent or delay the onset of myocardial infarction

While evidence exists that the first objective may be achieved, less evidence exists that the second objective can be attained, and no real proof exists that the third objective is attainable. The ideal antianginal drug would:

1 Establish a balance between coronary blood flow and the metabolic demands of the myocardium
2 Have a local rather than a systemic effect (It would act directly on coronary vessels to promote coronary vasodilation with absence of effects on other organ systems.)
3 Promote myocardial oxygen extraction from arterial flow
4 Have oral effectiveness with sustained action
5 Have absence of tolerance

No drug at the present time meets these criteria. Drugs presently available provide only temporary relief. Evidence is increasing that the nitrites exert their effect not so much by coronary vasodilation but by lowering blood pressure and decreasing venous return and cardiac work.

NITRATE VASODILATOR DRUGS
Nitrites

Certain members of the nitrite group of drugs have been used clinically for more than 100 years. Organic and inorganic nitrites and organic nitrites possess the pharmacologic effect of vasodilation. However, the exact mechanism of action of the organic nitrates remains obscure.

Since the nitrites and organic nitrates exert similar qualitative effects on the blood and circulatory system, the term "nitrite" as used in the following discussion will include both nitrates and nitrites.

Action and uses. The nitrites have a direct cellular action that causes relaxation of most smooth muscles in the body including bronchial, biliary, ureteral, uterine, and gastrointestinal smooth muscle. The most important pharmacologic effects are on vascular smooth muscle. The nitrites dilate all large arteries (temporal, radial, and coronary arteries) as well as arterioles (retinal, skin, meningeal, and splanchnic), capillaries, and venules. For this reason they can be called universal vasodilators. The nitrites are used extensively for patients with angina pectoris.

Because of the vasodilating effect, there is a reduction in vascular resistance and blood pressure, resulting in decreased work load on the heart. In patients with advanced coronary arteriosclerosis there may be an absence of response to the nitrites; no change in coronary resistance is noted, since blood vessel elasticity has been severely diminished.

Uses. The rapid-acting nitrites (nitroglycerin) remain the drugs of choice for treatment of angina pectoris.

Side effects. The side effects of the nitrites result from their vasodilator action. Severe headache, flushing of the skin, nausea and vom-

iting, hypotension, and vertigo may occur. Nitrites should be used with caution in patients with glaucoma, since dilated retinal vessels may increase intraocular pressure.

Tolerance. Tolerance to the nitrites is easily developed and necessitates the employment of the smallest dose of the drug that will give satisfactory results so that dosage may be increased as tolerance develops. Tolerance begins to appear within a few days and is well established within a few weeks. On the other hand, tolerance is rather easily broken by stopping administration, and the patient is again susceptible to the effects of the drug.

Preparation, dosage, and administration. The following are available preparations of nitrates.

Nitroglycerin tablets; glyceryl trinitrate tablets. Nitroglycerine is available in 0.3-, 0.4-, and 0.6-mg tablets for sublingual administration, and in 2.5- and 6.5-mg timed-release capsules for oral administration. The usual sublingual dose is 0.4 mg (gr $\frac{1}{150}$) and may be repeated several times during the day. Oral dosage is 2.5 or 6.5 mg at 8- or 12-hour intervals. Hypodermic tablets of this preparation are used when it is desirable to give the drug subcutaneously.

When taken sublingually, the drug appears in the blood in about 2 minutes; peak blood level is reached in 4 minutes; the effect begins to disappear in 10 minutes and is virtually dissipated within 30 minutes. Fall in blood pressure occurs in 1 to 5 minutes after administration and maximal fall occurs in 5 to 10 minutes. There is a return to initial blood pressure readings within 15 to 40 minutes.

During an acute anginal attack, if pain is not relieved within 5 to 10 minutes, the dose may be repeated. If pain persists after two or more tablets have been taken, the physician should be notified. However, some patients take as many as 30 tablets per day without harm.

For prophylactic use the patient should be instructed to insert a nitroglycerin tablet sublingually prior to undertaking any effort that may cause him to have an anginal attack. ECG patterns are unchanged by nitroglycerin. Oral preparations should be taken on an empty stomach.

TABLE 18-4 Coronary vasodilators

Generic name	Trade name or synonym	Route of adminis- tration	Dose*	Onset of action	Duration
Amyl nitrite	—	Inhalation	0.3 ml	30 to 60 sec	3 min
Nitroglycerin	Glyceryl trinitrate	Sublingual	gr $\frac{1}{150}$; 0.4 mg	2 min	15 to 30 min
		Oral	2.5 to 6.5 mg	30 to 60 min	8 to 12 hr
Pentaerythritol tetranitrate	Peritrate	Sublingual	10 mg	10 min	30 min
	Pentritol	Oral	60 mg	30 min	12 hr
	Pentafin	Oral	10 to 20 mg	30 to 60 min	4 to 5 hr
	Vasitol	Sustained- release	80 mg	30 to 60 min	12 hr
Erythrityl tetranitrate	Cardilate	Sublingual	5 to 30 mg	5 to 10 min	2 to 4 hr
	Tetranitrol	Oral	5 to 30 mg	30 min	4 hr
	Erythrol tetranitrate	Oral	5 to 30 mg	30 min	2 to 4 hr
Isosorbide dinitrate	Isordil	Sublingual, oral	5 to 10 mg	2 min	1½ to 2 hr
			5 to 30 mg	15 to 30 min	4 hr
Trolnitrate phosphate	Metamine	Oral	2 to 10 mg	Slow, 3 days	Up to 1 week
Dipyrimadole	Persantin	Oral	25 to 50 mg	2 to 5 min	20 to 30 min

*Single dose only; dose may be repeated three or four times a day or as necessary.

Nitroglycerin readily deteriorates, for it is inactivated by time, light, heat, air, and moisture. Patients should be instructed as follows:

1 A *fresh* supply of drug should be kept on hand. A fresh supply should be obtained at least every 3 months.
2 The drug should always be kept in a dark, airtight container.
3 All but a few days' supply of drug should be kept refrigerated.
4 The drug should not be kept close to the body to protect it from body heat.
5 Do not leave cotton or a label or package insert in the container; these articles may absorb some of the drug, resulting in less potent tablets.

Ineffectiveness of nitroglycerin may be caused by failure to adhere to these few simple rules.

Nitroglycerin ointment (Nitro-Bid). Nitroglycerin ointment is used for prevention and treatment of anginal attacks, especially at night. It contains 2% nitroglycerin in a lanolin-petrolatum base. A special dose-measuring applicator is provided for measuring the amount of and spreading the ointment on the skin; this prevents absorption through the fingers during application. A thin layer of ointment is applied over the chest, abdomen, or anterior thighs without rubbing it in. Nitroglycerin is continuously absorbed through the skin into the circulation producing prolonged vasodilation. The ointment may be applied every 3 to 4 hours and at bedtime. Dosage is usually 1 to 2 inches of ointment. The ointment is available in 60-g tubes, which should be kept tightly closed and stored in a cool place. Discontinuation of treatment should be gradual over a period of 4 to 6 weeks to prevent sudden withdrawal reactions. If headache and postural hypotension occur, dosage should be reduced.

Mannitol hexanitrate. Mannitol hexanitrate is one of the longer acting nitrites. It is given orally, and the usual dosage range is 16 to 64 mg every 4 to 6 hours. It is available in 32-mg tablets.

Pentaerythritol tetranitrate (Peritrate, Pentritol, Quintrate, Vasitol, Pentafin). Pentaerythritol tetranitrate is available in 10- and 20-mg tablets and in sustained-release preparations of 60 and 80 mg. The usual oral dosage is 10 to 20 mg four times a day, or one sustained-release tablet on arising and another 12 hours later. Onset of action of the tablets occurs within 30 to 60 minutes and disappears in 4 to 5 hours. Sustained-release preparations persist for about 12 hours. Tolerance rapidly develops with continuous administration.

Amyl nitrite. Amyl nitrite is available in glass ampules (pearls) that are fitted into a loosely woven material so that the pearl can be crushed and the drug inhaled. Each pearl contains about 0.3 ml (5 minims). It has a strong unpleasant odor, and the patient should not inhale more than two or three times to prevent overdosage. The drug is effective within 30 to 60 seconds; effects last about 3 minutes. Amyl nitrite is very flammable. It is more likely to cause a throbbing headache, facial flushing, nausea, vomiting, hypotension, and reflex tachycardia than nitroglycerin.

Erythrityl tetranitrate (Cardilate, Erythrol Tetranitrate, Tetranitrol). Erythrityl tetranitrate is available in 5-, 10-, and 15-mg tablets for oral or sublingual use. Initial dosage is usually 5 to 10 mg three times a day. Dosage may be increased to 30 mg three times a day. When taken sublingually, onset of action occurs within 5 to 10 minutes, orally within 30 minutes. Duration of action for either route is 2 to 4 hours. The oral route is less likely to cause headache.

Isosorbide dinitrate (Isordil). Isosorbide is available in 2.5- and 5-mg sublingual tablets and 5- and 10-mg tablets for oral use. Dosage range is 5 to 30 mg four times daily. Onset of action sublingually is 2 minutes; orally it is 15 to 30 minutes and lasts about 4 hours. Sustained-release tablets of 40 mg are also available (Isordil Tembids). These provide onset of action in 30 minutes with the effect lasting for 12 hours.

Trolnitrate phosphate (Metamine, Nitretamin). Trolnitrate is marketed as 2- or 10-mg tablets for oral use only, one to two tablets four times a day. Sublingual administration produces stomatitis. Sustained-release tablets are also available.

NONNITRATE ANTIANGINAL DRUGS
Ethyl alcohol

It has been common practice to permit and even recommend the use of alcoholic drinks for patients with angina. The beneficial action of alcohol probably results from its sedative action; there is no evidence that alcohol dilates the coronary arteries.

Xanthines

The xanthine derivatives (caffeine, theobromine, theophylline, and aminophylline) have been widely used for many years for treatment of angina. However, their use in angina has been steadily decreasing.

Propranolol hydrocholoride (Inderal)

Propranolol, a beta adrenergic blocking drug, has produced beneficial effects in patients with angina pectoris. Because of its serious side effects, it is recommended that the drug be reserved for the patient with disabling pain who does not respond to other treatment. Propranolol decreases sympathetic stimulation of the heart by blocking access to beta adrenergic receptors that release the catecholamines. This causes a decrease in both heart rate and myocardial contraction, reducing oxygen requirements for the ischemic myocardium. By lessening the work of the heart, the beneficial effects reported include decreased frequency of attacks, decreased intensity of pain, and increased tolerance to exercise.

Preparation, dosage, and administration. Propranolol is available in 10-, 40-, and 80-mg tablets. Used as an antianginal agent, dosage range is from 40 to 320 mg in four divided doses.

Side effects. Side effects include nausea, vomiting, light-headedness, diarrhea, constipation, rash, and mental depression. Hypotension and bradycardia may also occur. There is some evidence that propranolol can induce congestive heart failure in patients with low cardiac reserve. It is also not recommended for patients with a history of obstructive lung diseases.

Sudden withdrawal of propranolol in patients with angina pectoris can exacerbate angina. Therefore dosage should be gradually reduced, and withdrawal is recommended over a 2-week period.

Nadolol (Corgard)

Nadolol is a synthetic nonselective beta adrenergic receptor blocking agent that recently has been approved for clinical use in the United States.

Action and results. The drug competes with beta adrenergic receptor agonists for available beta receptor sites by inhibiting both $beta_1$ and $beta_2$ receptor effects. The prevention of catecholamine release reduces heart rate and cardiac output during both rest and on exercise. The resultant decrease in the oxygen requirement of the heart makes this drug useful for long-term management of angina pectoris.

Absorption of oral dosage of nadolol is variable, and the presence of food in the gastrointestinal tract does not affect the extent of absorption. It is excreted unchanged in the urine. The half-life ranges between 20 and 24 hours, permitting once daily dosage. In patients with renal impairment, lower dosage adjustment is essential.

Preparation, dosage, and administration. Nadolol is available for oral administration in 40-, 80-, and 120-mg tablets. For treatment of angina pectoris, the usual daily maintenance dose is 80 to 240 mg.

When discontinuing long-term use of nadolol, particularly in patients with ischemic heart disease, dosage must be gradually reduced over a 1- to 2-week period to avoid exacerbation of angina pectoris and possible occurrence of myocardial infarction.

Side effects and toxic effects. The major adverse reactions of nadolol are similar to that of propranolol. They include bradycardia, AV conduction block in patients with preexisting AV block, and bronchospasm in individuals suffering from chronic obstructive pulmonary disease. Diabetic patients receiving insulin or oral hypoglycemic drugs may experience hypoglycemia. This drug is contraindicated in individuals with AV conduction defects, uncontrolled congestive heart failure (because of its negative inotropic effect), and pulmonary obstructive lung disease.

Antilipemic drugs

From both clinical and experimental studies there is evidence that an important relationship exists between *atherosclerosis* and high levels of circulating blood lipids or fats (triglycerides, phospholipids, and cholesterol). Atherosclerosis is a causative factor in coronary artery disease and myocardial infarction, in cerebral arterial disease that results in senility or cerebrovascular accidents, in peripheral arterial occlusive disease (which may cause gangrene and loss of limb), and in renal arterial insufficiency. It is also a factor in hypertension. There-

fore there is intensive research to develop antilipemic drugs. If serum lipid levels could be controlled within normal limits, the development and progression of atherosclerosis might be inhibited or prevented.

That a positive relationship exists between high serum lipid levels and atherosclerosis is controversial; some individuals with high serum lipid levels have no objective evidence of atherosclerosis, whereas others with marked atherosclerotic signs and symptoms have normal serum lipid levels. However, more persons with high blood lipid levels have atherosclerosis than those with so-called normal blood lipid levels. Consequently, some researchers and clinicians believe that if lipid levels can be controlled, so can the atherosclerotic process. At the present time the available antilipemic drugs are also controversial, and their place in drug therapy requires more long-term critical studies. None of the antilipemic drugs is thought to have any effect on reversing the atherosclerotic process once it has begun. Means of preventing atherosclerosis remain obscure. Multicausative factors are undoubtedly involved and include dietary saturated fats, faulty fat metabolism, genetic influence, and other factors as yet unknown.

Hyperlipemia is a metabolic condition that is characterized by increased concentrations of cholesterol and triglycerides. The major serum lipids in the body include the triglycerides, cholesterol, and phospholipids. These compounds do not circulate freely in the plasma, but rather are transported in combination with proteins called lipoproteins. Hyperlipoproteinemia is always associated with an increased concentration of one or more lipoproteins. The major families of lipoproteins are classified into five types and are listed according to their lipid composition and drug therapy (Table 18-5).

The total cholesterol in the body reflects the amount of cholesterol that is contained in the lipoproteins. Low-density lipoproteins (LDL) contain the major portion of cholesterol in blood and are the most harmful. On the other hand, high-density lipoproteins (HDL) contain about 20% cholesterol and 5% triglycerides and appear to be beneficial. The higher the HDL

T A B L E   1 8 - 5   Classes of lipoprotein and drug therapy

Type	Lipid components		Other features	Drug therapy
	Cholesterol (%)	Triglycerides (%)		
I Chylomicrons	5	90	Originates in intestine from dietary fat	None; controlled by limiting dietary intake of triglycerides
IIa Low-density lipoproteins (LDL)	50	10	Elevated levels correlated with incidence of coronary heart disease (derived from breakdown of VLDL in circulation)	Cholestyramine, dextrothyroxine, probucol, nicotinic acid
IIb LDL and very low–density lipoproteins (VLDL)			Combination of LDL and VLDL	Same as type IIa plus clofibrate
III Intermediate-density lipoproteins (IDL)	30	40	Excess concentrations associated with high incidence of coronary disease	Clofibrate, nicotinic acid
IV VLDL	12	60	Primarily triglycerides associated with high carbohydrate diet	Chlofibrate, nicotinic acid
V VLDL and chylomicrons			Combination of type I and IV; uncommon	Nicotinic acid, clofibrate

concentration, the lower is the risk of cardiovascular disease. By contrast the very low–density (VLDL) and the intermediate-density lipoproteins (IDL) tend to be atherogenic. HDL is protective because it picks up cholesterol from the body cells and carries it back to the liver from which it is then excreted. This transport mechanism, therefore, prevents the accumulation of lipids in the arterial walls, resulting in protection against the development of coronary artery disease. In addition, it has now been found that exercise increases the HDL level, providing another form of prevention against atherosclerosis.

In addition to dietary modification, drugs are currently available to reduce plasma lipid levels. Diagnosis of the type of lipoprotein present is essential in the selection of the appropriate agent. There are three categories of hypolipemic drugs: (1) those that involve the intravascular metabolism of lipoproteins, for example, clofibrate; (2) those that involve removal of lipoproteins from the blood, for example, cholestyramine; and (3) those that affect the production of lipoproteins, for example, nicotinic acid.

Clofibrate (Atromid)

Clofibrate is a preparation of p-chlorophenoxyisobutyric acid. It is particularly effective in lowering serum triglycerides, serum cholesterol, and phospholipids. The exact mode of action of clofibrate is unknown, but the drug appears to block the synthesis of cholesterol and increases catabolism of LDL. It is administered orally in doses of 500 mg two to four times daily. Several weeks or even 2 or more months of therapy are required before the serum lipid level is reduced to the desirable level. Clofibrate has also been shown to enhance the action of anticoagulants. Side effects reported include nausea, abdominal discomfort, urticaria, abnormal liver function tests, and alopecia. Further clinical trials are necessary before the role of clofibrate in the control of atherosclerosis can be determined. It is used in the treatment of types III and IV hyperlipoproteinemia.

Cholestyramine resin (Cuemid, Questran)

Cholestyramine is a chloride salt of a quaternary ammonium anion exchange resin. In the intestinal lumen it exchanges chloride ions for bile acids. Since the resin and the bile acids bound to the resin are nonabsorbable, there is increased fecal excretion of bile acids. To compensate for this loss of bile acids, the body increases the rate of oxidation of cholesterol to convert the sterol to bile acids. This in turn lowers serum cholesterol levels.

Cholestyramine was originally introduced for the treatment of pruritus associated with biliary stasis. It is now used clinically in the treatment of type II hyperlipidemia.

Preparation, dosage, and administration. Cholestyramine is available as a powder for oral administration. The powder should be mixed with fruit juice, soup, milk, water, or pureed fruit before administration and given with the patient's meal. Adult dosage is 4 g (one packet) given three or four times daily. It should not be given simultaneously with other drugs, particularly acid drugs such as aspirin, because of its ability to bind acids. A period of 1 to 4 hours should intervene between the administration of cholestyramine and other oral medications.

Side effects. Side effects from cholestyramine include nausea, vomiting, constipation, diarrhea, and skin reactions. Bleeding tendencies have been noted during prolonged treatment with cholestyramine. This effect is thought to be caused by hypoprothrombinemia associated with vitamin K deficiency. It is recommended that fat-soluble vitamins be given intramuscularly to patients receiving cholestyramine.

Niacin; nicotinic acid

Nicotinic acid decreases serum lipids. Its exact mode of action is unknown. Niacin is the generic name now used for nicotinic acid. It reduces the level of triglycerides and cholesterol in types II, III, IV, and V hyperlipoproteinemia.

Reductions in serum lipids have been sustained for 2 to 5 years with nicotinic acid therapy. However, with discontinuance of therapy, serum lipid levels return to pretreatment levels within 2 to 6 weeks. Resistance to nicotinic acid therapy occurs in about 25% of patients.

Preparation, dosage, and administration. Nicotinic acid is available in tablets of varying strengths for oral administration. The usual adult dosage is 1 to 2 g daily with or after meals.

Side effects. Numerous and often disagreeable side effects may occur from nicotinic acid. Common side effects include severe gastrointestinal upset, flushing, pruritus, nervousness, and urticaria. The drug should be used cautiously in patients with allergies and peptic ulcers, since nicotinic acid causes a release of histamine and stimulates hydrochloric acid secretion. Giving the drug with meals or with antacids may reduce the incidence and severity of side effects. Prolonged treatment with niacin has resulted in hepatic disease.

Dextrothyroxine sodium (Choloxin, D-thyroxine)

It has long been known that a definite relationship exists between thyroid function and serum cholesterol levels. Hypothyroidism is associated with high serum cholesterol levels, and administration of thyroid hormones lowers serum cholesterol. Dextrothyroxine apparently increases the rate of oxidation of cholesterol, increases biliary excretion of cholesterol, and promotes intestinal excretion of cholesterol and other lipids.

However, its numerous side effects and the suspicion that it may have caused mortalities when used in a coronary research project has made it an unpopular drug.

Dextrothyroxine also tends to elevate blood sugar levels in diabetic persons, which necessitates increased dosage of insulin or hypoglycemic agents.

Because dextrothyroxine increases the metabolic rate, it must be used cautiously in patients with angina pectoris; the drug may precipitate attacks. An increase in incidence or severity of anginal attacks indicates the need to discontinue the use of dextrothyroxine.

This drug is contraindicated for patients with advanced liver or kidney disease, hypertension, or organic heart disease and in pregnant women and nursing mothers.

Probucol (Lorelco)

Probucol is a new agent that has recently been introduced in the United States. It is most effective in reducing cholesterol levels in patients with elevated concentration of low-density lipoproteins. It is believed to act by enhancing removal of lipoproteins from the circulation. The drug is employed in the treatment of type II hyperlipoproteinemia along with dietary control measures.

The recommended dosage is 500 mg twice daily with morning and evening meals. Side effects include diarrhea, flatulence, abdominal pain, nausea, and vomiting. If these symptoms persist, the physician should be notified before the patient discontinues the drug.

Summary of nursing considerations

The cardiovascular system is comprised of the heart and blood vessels. Because it functions as a unit, this system provides uninterrupted circulation of blood flow, which is continuously regulated according to varying tissue demands. To balance blood flow through the body's billions of capillaries requires an efficient cardiac pump, effective vascular resistance, and an adequate circulating blood volume.

The rhythmic contractions of the heart provide the energy necessary to drive the blood through the peripheral vascular system. In various types of cardiac disorders drugs are used to modify the action of three major tissues of the heart. Cardiac glycosides improve cardiac output by acting on the myocardium to increase the force of contraction; the antidysrhythmic drugs affect the specialized conduction system by abolishing the abnormal rate and rhythm of the heart; the antianginal drugs produce coronary vasodilation or lessen work of the heart to enhance a more adequate supply of nutrients required for myocardial function.

The pumping action of the heart depends on the contractile properties of the cardiac muscle or myocardium. Anatomically, the myocardium forms the walls of the two atria and the two ventricles. Furthermore, it is composed of interconnecting branching fibers (cells) of which the ultimate contractile unit is the sarcomere. The sarcomeres themselves are composed of two primary contractile proteins: myosin, the thick

filament, and actin, the thin filament. Between these two strands of actin and myosin, the biochemical and biophysical interactions ultimately generate force and shortening of muscle fiber.

The autonomic nervous system has an important role in the regulation of the rate, rhythm, and force of myocardial contraction of the heart. Acetylcholine, the neurotransmitter secreted by the parasympathetic system, acts on muscarinic receptors to decrease heart rate and possibly ventricular contraction. By contrast, stimulation of the sympathetic fiber is mediated by the release of norepinephrine, which acts on the beta$_1$ receptors in the cardiac tissue. Circulating epinephrine released from the adrenal medulla also acts on the beta$_1$ receptors. These neurohormones, norepinephrine and epinephrine, increase both the heart rate and the force of myocardial contraction.

Cardiac glycosides (digitalis and digitalis-like drugs) are among the oldest, most effective therapeutic agents available for treatment of congestive heart failure (cardiac insufficiency and cardiac decompensation). They are also useful in the treatment of atrial fibrillation and management of atrial flutter and paroxysmal tachycardia. All cardiac glycosides are composed of a sugar, a steroid, and a lactone; however, they differ in absorption and rate of elimination, time of onset of action, and duration of action.

Digitalis is the dried leaves of purple foxglove and affects cardiac function through two important mechanisms. First, the positive inotropic action increases the strength of myocardial contraction. Associated with this mechanism is the effect of digitalis on both the cell membrane (sarcolemma) and the chemical composition within the myocardial cell. On depolarization, sodium enters and potassium leaves the cell. The binding of digitalis to the sarcolemma inhibits the activity of the Na$^+$-K$^+$ ATPase pump, causing intracellular sodium to accumulate. This ionic action then effects an exchange of intracellular sodium for calcium. Because digitalis increases the influx of calcium to the contractile proteins, the fibers shorten faster with a more forceful contraction. Thus the increase in cardiac output improves the myocardial efficiency of the failing heart. Other therapeutic benefits include a reduction in venous pressure, decreased heart size, and relief of edema. Second, by altering the electrophysiologic properties of the heart, digitalis causes a negative dromotropic action (slowed conduction velocity) and a lengthened effective refractory period through the AV node. The prolonged P-R interval indicates an increasing degree of heart block. This action can also slow ventricular response in atrial fibrillation and atrial flutter. In addition, digitalis produces a negative chronotropic action (decreased heart rate) as a result of both vagal stimulation and direct membrane effect.

Oral administration of digitalis and the cardiac glycosides is safest and least expensive. Subcutaneous injection is not recommended because of local irritating effect; intravenous injection is usually reserved for emergencies and for those patients whose conditions prevent oral administration.

Digitalis is contraindicated in heart block and usually in ventricular tachycardia. It must be used with great care in patients with acute or toxic myocarditis.

Although anorexia, nausea, and vomiting can occur with digitalis toxicity, these symptoms may be caused by gastric irritation from oral digitalis preparations and often disappear as the patient adjusts to the drug. Other extracardiac manifestations of digitalis toxicity include diarrhea, headache, visual disturbances, weakness, restlessness, and nervous irritability. Digitalis toxicity can produce almost every kind of dysrhythmia, depending on the age of the patient and other factors.

Nurses need to be aware of the predisposing factors to digitalis toxicity, including (1) hypokalemia; (2) kidney, liver, and severe heart disease; (3) administration of purified glycosides; (4) slower body functions, and (5) intravenous administration of digitalis and rapid digitalization. Careful evaluation of the electrocardiogram should be made before and after any change in dosage. Pulse, preferably apical, should be checked prior to giving each dose.

Antidysrhythmic agents are used to prevent and treat disorders of cardiac rhythm. Most are cardiac depressants that can produce dangerous effects. The specialized conduction system normally generates and conducts impulses in the heart. Its electrophysiology centers around the action potential that is associated with automaticity, velocity of conduction, and refractory periods.

The antidysrhythmic drugs are classified into four discrete categories: Group I drugs are subdivided into Group I-A and Group I-B compounds. Group I-A drugs include quinidine, procainamide, and disopyramide, all of which decrease conduction velocity. Lidocaine and phenytoin are Group I-B drugs, and these along with other antidysrhythmic effects either increase or have no effect on conduction velocity. Propranolol is a Group II drug because of its beta adrenergic blocking action. Bretylium is a Group III drug that is characterized by its antiadrenergic properties. Finally, the Group IV drug, verapamil, exerts a selective calcium antagonistic action in restoring the heart to normal rate and rhythm. All these agents with the exception of bretylium have one major electrophysiologic property in common: they all are capable of suppressing automaticity.

Changes in the heart's electric activity can be readily determined by electrocardiographic monitoring. A knowledgeable, observant nurse can use ECG tracings to assess the effectiveness of drug therapy in cardiovascular disease.

Antianginal agents are used to produce coronary vasodilation to increase the supply of oxygen and nutrients to the myocardium and other tissues of the heart or they can lessen the workload of the heart. The most commonly used coronary vasodilators are the nitrites administered for angina pectoris (intermittent myocardial ischemia). Their exact mechanism of action is obscure; however, they do decrease the duration and intensity of pain during an attack by dilating all large arteries as well as arterioles, capillaries, and venules. Nitrites may produce severe headache, flushing of the skin, nausea and vomiting, hypotension, and vertigo. They should be used cautiously in patients with glaucoma. Instruction of the patient concerning care and storage of the drug is critically important, since nitroglycerin is inactivated by time, light, heat, air, and moisture.

Propranolol, a beta adrenergic blocking agent, has also produced beneficial effects in patients with angina pectoris. In addition, alcoholic drinks have occasionally been recommended for patients with angina.

Antilipemic agents are designed to reduce the levels of circulating blood cholesterol and triglycerides. The total cholesterol in the body reflects the amount of cholesterol that is contained in the lipoproteins. Low-density lipoproteins contain the major portion of cholesterol in the blood and are the most harmful; high-density lipoproteins contain much less (about 20%) cholesterol and appear to be beneficial.

In addition to dietary modification, drugs are currently available to reduce plasma lipid levels. The antilipemic drugs include clofibrate, cholestyramine, and nicotinic acid.

QUESTIONS

FOR STUDY AND REVIEW

1 Explain the meaning of the following terms:
 a inotropic
 b chronotropic
 c dromotropic
2 How does digitalis exert its inotropic action?
3 Explain the various methods for digitalizing a patient.
4 Why is digoxin more popular than other digitalis preparations?
5 What symptoms should alert the nurse to the possibility that a patient may be experiencing digitalis toxicity?
6 How does potassium loss from the body enhance ectopic pacemaker activity?
7 Explain the effects of digitalis on the ECG tracing or monitor.
8 Which digitalis preparations may be given intravenously?
9 Prepare a lesson plan for teaching a patient about digitalis therapy.
10 How does digitalis restore atrial dysrhythmia to normal sinus rhythm?
11 What properties of quinidine account for its antidysrhythmic effects?
12 What ECG findings would indicate quinidine toxicity?
13 Explain how quinidine can cause cardiac arrest. Give the reason why digitalis and quinidine may be used together.
14 Explain the reentry phenomenon. What drugs are used to abolish unidirectional block? How is unidirectional block converted to bidirectional block by Groups I-A and IV drugs?
15 Following chronic use of procainamide, what common side effect may result?
16 What is the clinical use of disopyramide? What caution must be observed during its administration?
17 Explain the mechanism of action of propranolol. What effect does sudden withdrawal have on the patient? For what types of clinical disorders is propranolol contraindicated?
18 How does bretylium differ from the other types of antidysrhythmic agents?
19 Why is nitroglycerin the drug of choice for most patients with angina pectoris?
20 What instructions would you provide a patient on nitrate therapy?
21 What is the rationale for the use of antilipemic agents? What precautions must be taken when antilipemic agents are used?

BIBLIOGRAPHY

GENERAL

A.M.A. drug evaluation, ed. 3, Acton, Mass., 1977, Publishing Sciences Group, Inc.

Andreoli, K., and others: Comprehensive cardiac care, ed. 4, St. Louis, 1979, The C.V. Mosby Co.

Avery, G.S., editor: Drug treatment, ed. 2, Acton, Mass., 1980, Publishing Sciences Group, Inc.

Berne, R., and Levy, M.: Cardiovascular physiology, ed. 4, St. Louis, 1981, The C.V. Mosby Co.

Bowman, W., and Rand, M.: Textbook of pharmacology, ed. 2, London, 1980, Blackwell Scientific Publications.

Deberry, P., and others: Teaching cardiac patients to manage medications, Am. J. Nurs. **75:**2191, 1975.

DiPalma, J.R.: Basic pharmacology in medicine, New York, 1976, McGraw-Hill Book Co.

Goldberger, E.: Treatment of cardiac emergencies, ed. 3, St. Louis, 1982, The C.V. Mosby Co.

Goodman, L.S., and Gilman, A., editors: The pharmacological basis of therapeutics, ed. 6, New York, 1980, Macmillan, Inc.

Goth, A.: Medical pharmacology: principles and concepts, ed. 10, St. Louis, 1981, The C.V. Mosby Co.

Gringauz, A.: Drugs: how they act and why, St. Louis, 1978, The C.V. Mosby Co.

Hurst, W., and others: The heart, ed. 3, New York, 1974, McGraw-Hill Book Co.

Meyers, F.H., Jawetz, E., and Goldfien, A.: Review of medical pharmacology, ed. 5, Los Altos, Calif., 1980, Lange Medical Publications, Inc.

Modell, W., editor: Drugs of choice 1980-1981, St. Louis, 1980, The C.V. Mosby Co.

Mountcastle, V., editor, Medical physiology, ed. 14, St. Louis, 1980, The C.V. Mosby Co.

Prasod, K., and Callaghan, J.C.: Electrophysiologic basis of use of a polarizing solution in the treatment of myocardial infarction, Clin. Pharmacol. Ther. **12:**666, 1971.

Shinn, A.F.: Drug interactions of common CCU medications, Am. J. Nurs. **75:**1470, 1975.

Sodeman, W., and Sodeman, T.: Pathologic physiology: mechanisms of disease, ed. 6, Philadelphia, 1979, W.B. Saunders Co.

Turner, P., and Richens, A.: Clinical pharmacology, Edinburgh, 1973, Churchill Livingstone.

CARDIAC GLYCOSIDES

Arbeit, S., and others: Recognizing digitalis toxicity, Am. J. Nurs. **77:**1935, 1977.

Chidsey, C.: Calcium metabolism in the normal and failing heart, Hosp. Pract. **7:**65, Aug. 1972.

Cutler, P., Talby, R., and Zinn, M.: Digitalis: avoiding the problems of therapy, Curr. Prescribing **4:**78, July 1978.

Doherty, J.E.: Digitalis glycosides: pharmacokinetics and their clinical implications, Ann. Intern. Med. **79:**229, 1973.

Doherty, J.E.: Which patients are prone to digitalis intoxication? Mod. Med. **47:**137, Jan. 30-Feb. 15, 1979.

Doherty, J.E., and Kane, J.J.: Clinical pharmacology and therapeutic use of digitalis glycosides, Drugs **6:**182, 1973.

Ferlinz, J., and Aronow W.: Assessing antiarrhythmic actions. IV. Digitalis, Drug. Therapy **7:**26, Mar. 1977.

Gullner, H.G., and others: Correlation of serum concentrations with heart concentrations of digoxin in human subjects, Circulation **50:**653, 1974.

Jeliffe, R.W.: An improved method of digoxin therapy, Ann. Intern. Med. **77:**891, 1972.

Jeliffe, R.W., and Brooker, G.: A nomogram for digoxin therapy, Am. J. Med. **57:**63, 1974.

Katz, A.: Contractile proteins in normal and failing myocardium, Hosp. Pract. **7:**570, 1972.

Katz, A.: Congestive heart failure: role of altered myocardial cellular control, N. Engl. J. Med. **293:**1184, 1975.

Kumpuris, A., Raizner, A., and Luchi, R.: The role of serum digitalis levels in clinical practice, Heart Lung **8:**711, 1979.

Luchi, R., and others: Use of cardioactive drugs in acute myocardial infarction, Heart Lung **5:**44, 1976.

Mason, D.T.: Digitalis pharmacology and therapeutics: recent advances. Ann. Intern. Med. **80:**520, 1974.

Ogilvie, R.I., and Ruedy, J.: An educational program in digitalis therapy. J.A.M.A. **222:**50, 1971.

Quest, J.A., and Gillis, R.A.: Effect of digitalis on carotid sinus baroreceptor activity, Circ. Res. **35:**247, 1974.

Sanchez, N., and others: Pharmacokinetics of digoxin: interpreting bioavailability, Br. Med. J. **4:**132, 1973.

Smith, T.W., and Haber, E.: Digitalis, Parts I to IV, N. Engl. J. Med. **289:**945; **289:**1010; **289:**1063; **289:**1125, 1973.

Solomon, H.M., and Abrams, W.B.: Interactions between digitoxin and other drugs in man, Am. Heart J. **83:**277, 1972.

Sonnenblick, E.: Myocardial ultrastructure in the normal and failing heart, Hosp. Pract. **5:**35, 1970.

Wagner, J.G.: Appraisal of digoxin availability and pharmacokinetics in relation to cardiac therapy, Am. Heart J. **88:**133, 1974.

Weintraub, M., and others: Compliance as a determinant of serum digoxin concentration, J.A.M.A. **224:**481, 1973.

Wormser, H., and Abramson, H.: A review of digitalis therapy, U.S. Pharmacist, p. 50, Feb. 1977.

ANTIDYSRHYTHMIC DRUGS

Arnsdorf, M.: Electrophysiologic properties of antidysrhythmic drugs as a rational basis for therapy, Med. Clin. North Am. **60:**213, 1976.

Befeler, B., Lazzara, R.: Clinical pharmacology of the antiarrhythmic agent disopyramide phosphate (Norpace), Heart Lung **9:**475, 1980.

Bigger, J.T.: Antiarrhythmic drugs in ischemic heart disease, Hosp. Pract. **7:**69, Nov. 1972.

Bloomfield, S.S., and others: Quinidine for prophylaxis of arrhythmias in acute myocardial infarction, N. Engl. J. Med. **285:**979, 1971.

Collinsworth, K.A., and others: The clinical pharmacology of lidocaine as an antiarrhythmic drug, Circulation **50:**1217, 1974.

Danahy, D., and Aronow, W.: Assessing antiarrhythmic actions. III. Propranolol, Drug Therapy **7:**127, 1977.

Dominic, J., and others: Verapamil plasma levels and ventricular rate response in patients with atrial fibrillation and flutter, Clin. Pharmacol. Ther. **26:**710, 1979.

Ellrodt, G., and Singh, B.: Adverse effects of disopyramide (Norpace): toxic interactions with other antiarrhythmic agents, Heart Lung **9:**469, 1980.

Fors, W.J., Vanderark, C.R., and Raynolds, E.W.: Evaluation of propranolol and quinidine in the treatment of quinidine-resistant arrhythmias, Am. J. Cardiol. **27:**190, 1971.

Gettes, L.S.: The electrophysiologic effects of antiarrhythmic drugs. Am. J. Cardiol. **28:**526, 1971.

Gettes, L.S.: Beta blockers and arrhythmia: how and why they work, Med. Opinion **5:**19, 1976.

Gettes, L.S.: On the classification of antiarrhythmic drugs, Mod. Concepts Cardiovasc. Dis. **48:**13, 1979.

Gorfinkel, H.: Bretylium tosylate: a new antiarrhythmic agent, Drug Therapy **7:**138, Jan. 1977.

Green, K.G., and others: Improvement in prognosis of myocardial infarction by long-term beta-adrenoreceptor blockade using practolol, Br. Med. J. **3:**735, 1975.

Harrison, D.C.: Practical guidelines for the use of lidocaine, J.A.M.A. **233:**1202, 1975.

Heger, J., Prystowsky, E., and Zipes, D.: New drugs for treatment of ventricular arrhythmias, Heart Lung **10:**475, 1981.

Heng, M., Effects of intravenous verapamil on cardiac arrhythmias and on the electrocardiogram, Am. Heart J. **90:**487, 1975.

Hoffman, B., Rosen, M., and Wit, A.: Electrophysiology and pharmacology of cardiac arrhythmias. III. The causes and treatment of cardiac arrhythmias, Part A. Am. Heart, J. **89:**116, 1975.

Hoffman, B., Rosen, M., and Wit, A.: Electrophysiology and pharmacology of cardiac arrhythmias. III. The causes and treatment of cardiac arrhythmias, Part B, Am. Heart J. **89:**253, 1975.

Jung, D., and others: Effect of dose on phenytoin absorption, Clin. Pharmacol. Ther. **28:**479, 1980.

Kessler, K.M.: Individualization of dosage of antiarrhythmic drugs, Med. Clin. North Am. **58:**1019, 1974.

Koch-Weser, J.: Drug therapy: bretylium, N. Engl. J. Med. **300:**473, 1979.

Lemberg, L., and others: The treatment of arrhythmias following acute myocardial infarction, Med. Clin. North Am, **55:**273, 1971.

Levy, R.H., et al.: Dosage regimens of antiarrhythmics. I, Pharmacokinetic properties, Am. J. Hosp. Pharm. **30:**398, 1973.

Mason, D.T., and others: The clinical pharmacology and therapeutic applications of the antiarrhythmic drugs, Clin. Pharmacol. Therap. **11:**460, 1970.

Mason, D.T., and others: Antiarrhythmic agents. I, Mechanisms of action and clinical pharmacology, Drugs **5**:261, 1973.

Mason, D.T., and others: Antiarrhythmic agents. II. Therapeutic considerations, Drugs **5**:292, 1973.

Michaelson, S.: Clinical pharmacology of antiarrhythmic drugs, Today's Clinician, p. 40, Sept. 1978.

Nies, A.S., and Shand, D.G.: Clinical pharmacology of propranolol, Circulation **52**:6, 1975.

Rosowskz, B.D., and others: Long-term use of procainamide following acute myocardial infarction, Circulation **47**:1204, 1973.

Sasyniuk, B.I., and Ogilvie, R.I.: Antiarrhythmic drugs: electrophysiological and pharmacokinetic considerations, Annu. Rev. Pharmacol. **15**:131, 1975.

Shand, D.: Propranolol: resolving problems in usage, Drug Therapy **8**:53, 1978.

Singh, B.: Rational basis of antiarrhythmic therapy: clinical pharmacology of commonly used antiarrhythmic drugs, Angiology, **29**:206, 1978.

Stratford, J., Feiner, J., and Arensberg, D.: Antiarrhythmic drug therapy, Am. J. Nurs. **80**:1288, 1980.

Thompson, P.E., and others: Lidocaine pharmacokinetics in advanced heart failure, liver disease, and renal failure in humans, Ann. Intern. Med. **78**:499, 1973.

Valentine, P.A., and others: Lidocaine in the pre-hospital phase of acute infarction: a double blind study, N. Engl. J. Med. **291**:1327, 1974.

Wasserman, A.J., and Proctor, J.D.: Pharmacology of antiarrhythmias: quinidine, beta blockers, diphenylhydantoin, bretylium, Med. Coll. Va. Q. **9**:53, 1973.

Wilhelmsson, C., and others: Reduction of sudden deaths after myocardial infarction by treatment with alprenolol, Lancet **2**:1157, 1974.

Winkle, R., and Harrison, D.: Beta blockers in the treatment of acute arrhythmias, Heart and Lung **6**:62, 1977.

Winkle, R.A., and others: Pharmacologic therapy of ventricular arrhythmias, Am. J. Cardiol. **36**:629, 1975.

Wit, A., Rosen, M., and Hoffman, B.: Electrophysiology and pharmacology of cardiac arrhythmias. II Relationship of normal and abnormal electrical activity of cardiac fibers to the genesis of arrhythmias, Am. Heart J. **88**:515, 1974.

Zakauddin, V., and others: The role of bretylium in refractory ventricular arrhythmias, Drug Therapy **10**:48, Sept. 1980.

ANTIANGINAL DRUGS

Aronow, W.S.: Clinical use of nitrates. Nitrates as antianginal drugs, Mod. Concepts Cardiovasc. Dis. **48**:31, 1971.

Aronow, W.S.: Drug therapy: management of stable angina, N. Engl. J. Med. **289**:516, 1973.

Cohen, L.: Beta blockers: an alternative to nitrates in treating chest pain, Med. Opin. **5**:32, Sept. 1976.

Franciosa, J.: Nitroglycerin and nitrates in congestive heart failure, Heart Lung **9**:873, 1980.

Fuller, E.: The effect of antianginal drugs on myocardial oxygen consumption, Am. J. Nurs. **80**:250, Feb. 1980.

Goldstein, R.E., and others: Medical management of patients with angina pectoris, Prog. Cardiovasc. Dis. **14**:360, 1972.

Goldstein, R.E., and others: Nitrates in the prophylactic treatment of angina pectoris, Circulation **48**:917, 1973.

Gorlin, R.: Pathophysiology of cardiac pain, Circulation **32**:138, 1965.

Klaus, A.P., and others: Comparative evaluation of sublingual long-acting nitrates, Circulation **48**:519, 1973.

Koch-Weser, J.: Vasodilator therapy of cardiac falure, N. Engl. J. Med. **297**:254, 1977.

Miller, R.R., and others: Propranolol—withdrawal rebound phenomenon: exacerbation of coronary events after abrupt cessation of antianginal therapy, N. Engl. J. Med. **293**:416, 1975.

Needleman, P.: Organic nitrate metabolism, Annu. Rev. Pharmacol. Toxicol. **16**:81, 1976.

Parker, J.O., and others: Effect of nitroglycerin ointment on clinical and hemodynamic response to exercise, Am. J. Cardiol. **38**:162, 1976.

Reichek, N., and others: Sustained effects of nitroglycerine ointment in patients with angina pectoris, Circulation **50**:348, 1974.

Reynolds, J.L.: A practical approach to the management of angina, Drugs **8**:208, 1974.

Symposium: angina pectoris, Circulation **46**:6, 1972.

Thadani, U., and others: Comparison of adrenergic beta-receptor antagonists in angina pectoris, Br. Med. J. **1**:138, 1973.

Thompson, E.J., and others: Angiologic assessment of the hemodynamic effects of sustained release nitroglycerin in patients with angina pectoris, Angiology **24**:508, 1973.

Walton, C., and Hammond, B.: Angina: teaching your patient to prevent recurring attacks, Nursing '78 **8**(2):32, 1978.

Weinblatt, A.B., and others: Prognosis of women with newly diagnosed coronary heart disease—a comparison with course of disease among men, Am. J. Public Health **63**:577, 1973.

ANTILIPEMIC DRUGS

Alfin-Slater, R., and others: Hyperlipidemia: what to do about the lipids to-do, Patient Care **14**:14, Oct. 14, 1980.

Azarnoff, D.L.: Individualization of treatment of hyperlipoproteinemic disorders, Med. Clin. North Am. **58**:1129, 1974.

Castelli, W., and Levitas, I.: New look at lipids—why they're not all bad, Curr. Prescribing **3**:39, June 1977.

Corday, E., and Corday, S.: Prevention of heart disease by control of risk factors, Am. J. Cardiol. **35**:330, 1975.

Coronary Drug Project Research Group: Clofibrate and niacin in coronary heart disease. J.A.M.A. **231**:360, 1975.

Krasno, L.R., and Kidera, G.J.: Clofibrate in coronary heart disease: effect on morbidity and mortality, J.A.M.A. **219**:845, 1972.

Kwiterovich, P.: The cardiovascular implications of hyperlipidemia. Pract. Card. **2**:18, Mar. 1976.

Levy, R.I.: Hyperlipidemia from trial and error toward scientific precision, Consultant **18**:32, Oct. 1978.

Levy, R.I.: Dietary and drug treatment of primary hyperlipidemia, Ann. Intern. Med. **77**:267, 1972.

Levy, R.I., and Rifkind, B.M.: Lipid lowering drugs and hyperlipidaemia, Drugs **6**:12, 1973.

Scott, P.: Lipid lowering drugs and coronary heart disease, Drugs **10**:218, 1975.

Peripheral vascular drugs

Blood pressure

The purpose of arterial pressure is to transmit, under regulated conditions, the output of blood from the heart to the various body tissues wherever and whenever needed. Mean arterial pressure or blood pressure is fundamentally dependent on cardiac output and peripheral resistance; the basic equation for blood pressure (BP) is expressed as the product of cardiac output (CO) and peripheral resistance (PR): BP = CO × PR. However, neither of these factors acts as a primary control mechanism in maintaining normal blood pressure. Instead, each factor, that is, cardiac output or peripheral resistance, is regulated by a multiplicity of mechanisms; when one of these regulatory mechanisms malfunctions, the remaining ones tend to compensate for any deviation from normal pressure. There are two primary mechanisms that control normal blood pressure: (1) a rapidly acting system that involves the baroreceptor reflex and (2) a long-term control system associated with the renin-angiotensin-aldosterone mechanism.

BARORECEPTOR REFLEX

The baroreceptors or pressoreceptors are spray-type nerve endings located in the walls of the internal carotid arteries and the aortic arch. The sensory receptors respond rapidly to changes in blood pressure when they occur in these vessels. Thus any elevation in pressure stretches the receptors from which an impulse is then transmitted along the afferent neuron (vagus nerve) to the vasomotor center in the medulla of the brain. As a result, an inhibition of the center produces two important alterations: (1) a decrease in heart rate and force of myocardial contraction, thereby lowering cardiac output, and (2) a vasodilation of peripheral vessels, producing a decrease in peripheral resistance. The subsequent reduction in blood pressure is attributed to the reflex activity of the baroreceptor mechanism (see Fig. 19-1).

605

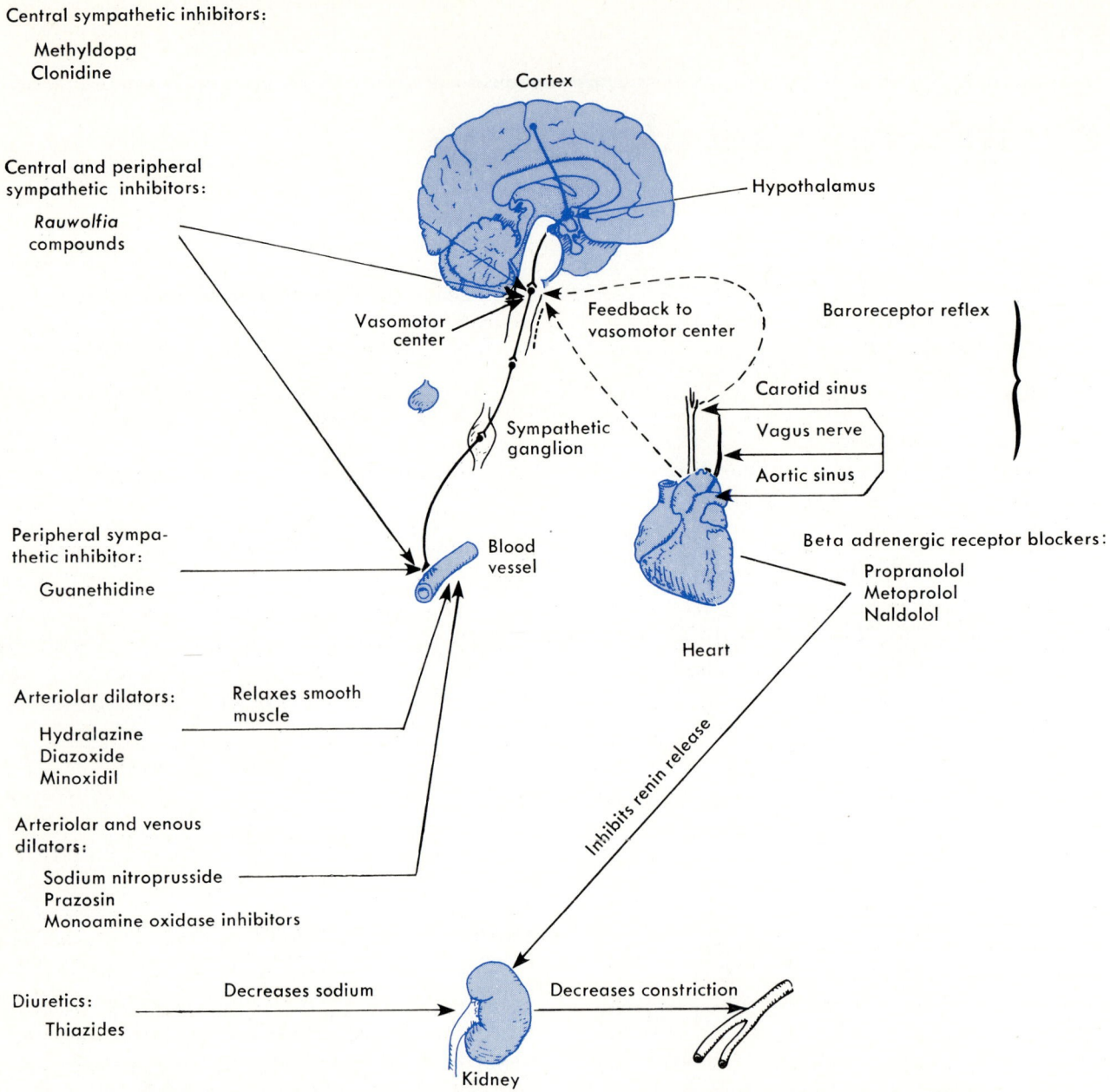

Central sympathetic inhibitors:

Methyldopa
Clonidine

Central and peripheral
sympathetic inhibitors:

Rauwolfia
compounds

Cortex

Hypothalamus

Vasomotor
center

Feedback to
vasomotor center

Baroreceptor reflex

Carotid sinus

Vagus nerve

Aortic sinus

Sympathetic
ganglion

Peripheral sympa-
thetic inhibitor:

Guanethidine

Blood
vessel

Beta adrenergic receptor blockers:

Propranolol
Metoprolol
Naldolol

Heart

Arteriolar dilators:

Hydralazine
Diazoxide
Minoxidil

Relaxes smooth
muscle

Arteriolar and venous
dilators:

Sodium nitroprusside
Prazosin
Monoamine oxidase inhibitors

Inhibits renin release

Diuretics:

Thiazides

Decreases sodium

Decreases constriction

Kidney

FIG. 19-1. Site and method of action of various antihypertensive drugs based on reported clinical and experimental evidence.

This reflex functions as a rapidly acting system with short-term control of blood pressure. It has been demonstrated that over a prolonged period of time the rate of firing of the baroreceptors diminishes even if the blood pressure remains elevated. Therefore in hypertension it has been speculated that these receptors are "reset" to maintain a higher level of blood pressure.

Norepinephrine-epinephrine. The sympathetic nervous system is mediated by two hormones: norepinephrine and epinephrine. Stimulation of the postganglionic adrenergic nerve terminals causes the release of norepinephrine, whereas activation of the adrenal medulla results in secretion of mostly epinephrine and only a small amount of norepinephrine. After leaving the circulation, both of these adrenal hormones influence the activity of the heart and blood vessels. Moreover, norepinephrine

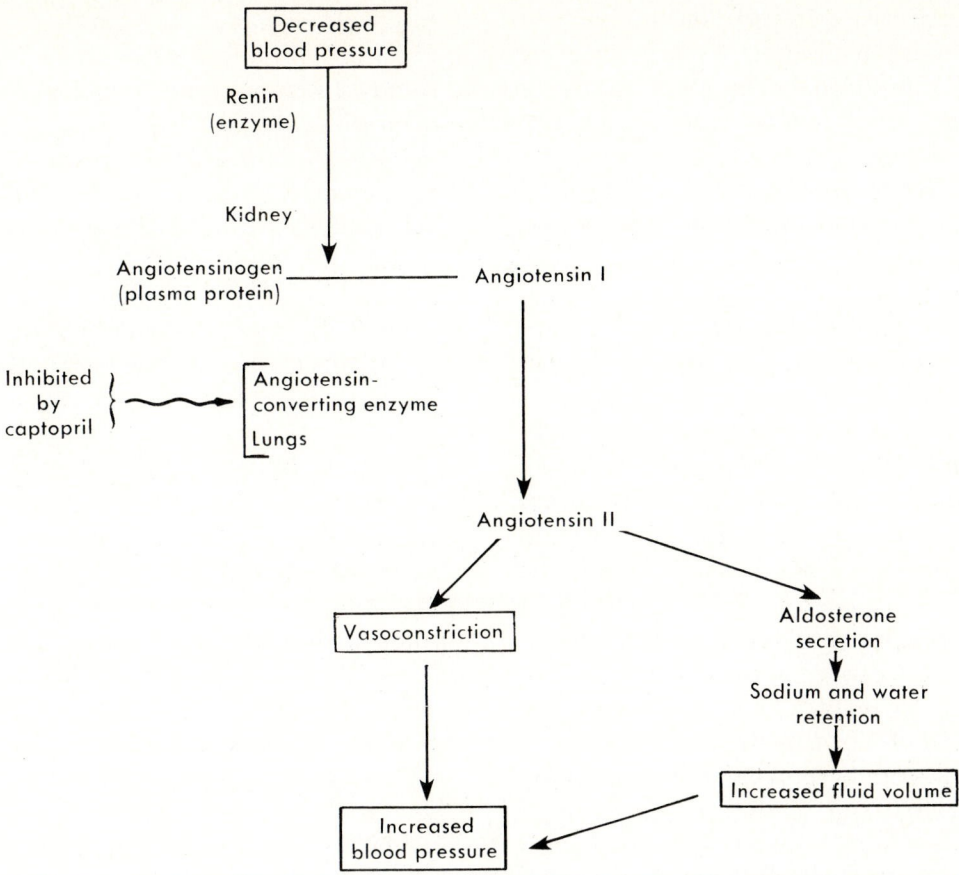

FIG. 19-2. The renin-angiotensin-aldosterone system and its effects on normal blood pressure homeostasis. Note the site of action of captopril, an angiotensin II inhibitor that suppresses the action of the angiotensin-converting enzyme, thereby reducing angiotensin II production and causing a decrease in blood pressure.

acts mainly on alpha adrenergic receptors, and epinephrine acts on both alpha and beta adrenergic receptors. The alpha adrenergic receptors are located in most of the arterioles, and the affinity of norepinephrine for these receptors produces vasoconstriction with a resultant increase in blood pressure. The beta₁ adrenergic receptors prevalent in the heart are also activated by norepinephrine. This response increases both the heart rate and force of myocardial contraction, thereby indirectly causing an elevation in blood pressure. On the other hand, because epinephrine produces dilation of blood vessels, this hormone does not cause any increase in peripheral resistance. However, epinephrine does produce a considerable increase in heart rate and force of myocardial contraction so that the elevation in cardiac output indirectly raises the blood pressure.

RENIN-ANGIOTENSIN-ALDOSTERONE SYSTEM

The renin-angiotensin-aldosterone system regulates blood pressure by increasing or decreasing the blood volume via function of the kidneys. The initiating factor is renin, a proteolytic enzyme secreted by the juxtaglomerular cells located in the afferent arteriolar walls of the nephron. When blood flow through the kidneys is reduced, this decreases renal arterial pressure, which acts as a stimulus for release of renin into the circulation. Here, this enzyme catalyzes the cleavage of a plasma protein to form angiotensin I. Subsequently, angiotensin I is converted to angiotensin II in the small vessels of the lungs. Angiotensin II is one of the most potent *vasoconstrictors* known. It is particularly effective in constricting arterioles, thereby increasing peripheral resistance and raising blood pressure. In addition, angiotensin II acts on the adrenal cortex to stimulate the secretion of aldosterone, a hormone that promotes *reabsorption of sodium by the kidney*. The increased sodium then elevates the osmotic pressure in the plasma, causing a release of antidiuretic hormone from the hypothalamus. Its action on the kidney tubules promotes *reabsorption of water*. By contrast, the excessive fluid retention is controlled by the negative feedback mechanism operating within this system so that fluid balance is again restored to a normal level. Because the renin-angiotensin-aldosterone system involves slow adjustments to changes in fluid volume, the kidneys by far are the most important organs in the body for long-term regulation of blood pressure. When the operation of this system fails, an increase in peripheral resistance and retention of fluid volume produces a combination of hypertensive effects, which is capable of sustaining a continuous elevation of blood pressure (Fig.19-2).

In patients with high plasma renin activity, the retention of fluid volume is perpetuated until the cycle is interrupted by diuretic drugs. The plasma renin levels in individuals vary, and this is classified as low, normal, or high renin activity. In addition, it is now apparent that the cells in the juxtaglomerular apparatus are richly supplied by sympathetic nerves. Thus the stimulation by beta$_2$ adrenergic agonists produces the release of renin. By contrast, the use of a beta$_2$ blocking agent such as propranolol effectively inhibits the secretion of renin, but specifically only in individuals with high plasma renin activity.

Antihypertensive drugs

Hypertension is a circulatory disease that is characterized by a sustained elevation of the systemic arterial pressure. Patients with elevations of blood pressure are frequently asymptomatic, and because there is a steady progression of secondary organ damage that may become fatal, untreated hypertension is known as the "silent killer."

Arterial hypertension is characterized by increased peripheral vascular resistance resulting in a consistent elevation above the accepted range of normal of the systolic pressure (above 150 mm Hg) and diastolic pressure (above 90 mm Hg) with pathologic changes in the retinal arterioles. Hypertension is associated with a variety of cardiac, cerebrovascular, and renal complications and decreased life expectancy. When there is no known cause for the elevated blood pressure (such as no preexisting kidney disease or atherosclerosis), the condition is termed *essential or primary hypertension*. Usually, for this form of hypertension, the only possible means for adequate control is drug therapy.

Evidence is available that a relationship exists between excess salt ingestion and human essential hypertension; susceptibility is undoubtedly on a genetic basis. It is claimed that high blood pressure is more prevalent in cultures with a high salt intake, and it has been demonstrated that children fed large amounts of salt developed hypertension. It is well known that drastic salt restriction or the use of a salt-depleting diuretic like chlorothiazide reduces the blood pressure of some hypertensive individuals. A high salt intake, or retention of sodium and fluids, may cause ionic disturbances in peripheral arterioles, which may in turn increase vascular tone and vascular reactivity (particularly to adrenergic agents).

A drop in blood pressure results in release of renin and the eventual formation of angiotensin II. Its ability to elevate blood pressure is the result of (1) its arteriolar vasoconstricting effect and (2) its ability to stimulate aldosterone release, which causes renal tubular absorption of sodium and an increase in body sodium and water, with a resultant rise in blood volume.

The use of sedatives, diets low in sodium chloride, and weight reduction continue to be advocated for hypertensive patients, although these measures alone are insufficient for many patients. Some patients, such as those with severe renal insufficiency or severe psychiatric disturbance, do not respond well to treatment of hypertension with drugs. On the other hand, many patients benefit from therapy and are spared damage to the heart, kidneys, and brain. The severity of hypertensive disease is sometimes estimated in terms of the level of the diastolic blood pressure and the degree of change in the retinal vessels of the eye.

The judicious use of antihypertensive drugs can effectively control the blood pressure in a majority of hypertensive individuals with less risk of serious complications and intolerable side reactions than was true for older methods of treatment (especially sympathectomy). However, antihypertensive drug therapy remains empirical, since essential hypertension is a disease of unknown origin and the mechanism of action of many antihypertensive drugs also remains unknown.

Most antihypertensive drugs exert their effects by either decreasing sympathetic activi-

TABLE 19-1 Classification of antihypertensive drugs based on their primary site or mechanism of action

Sympatholytic drugs
  Central sympathetic inhibitor drugs
    Methyldopa
    Clonidine
  Central and peripheral sympathetic inhibitor
    drugs
    Rauwolfia derivatives
  Peripheral sympathetic inhibitor drug
    Guanethidine
  Beta adrenergic receptor blocking drugs
    Propranolol (beta$_1$ and beta$_2$ blocker)
    Metoprolol (beta$_1$ blocker)
    Nadolol (beta$_1$ and beta$_2$ blocker)
  Tyrosine hydroxylase inhibitor drug
    Metyrosine (Demser)
Vasodilator drugs
  Arteriolar dilator drugs
    Hydralazine
    Diazoxide
    Minoxidil
  Arteriolar and venous dilator drugs
    Sodium nitroprusside
    Prazosin (alpha adrenergic blocker)
  Monamine oxidase inhibitor
    Pargyline hydrochloride
  Ganglionic blocking drugs
  Mecamylamine hydrochloride
  Trimethapham camsylate
  Hexamethonium chloride
Baroreceptor stimulants
  Veratrum alkaloids
Diuretic drugs
  Thiazides
Renin-angiotensin system antagonists
  Angiotensen II inhibitors
    Captopril
    Saralasin

ty or by promoting the excretion of salt. Decreased sympathetic activity is achieved by many different mechanisms, involving ultimately the decrease of norepinephrine levels. During therapy, most agents produce some degree of postural (orthostatic) hypotension, which means that a precipitous drop of blood pressure occurs when a person suddenly assumes an erect position after reclining or sitting. This usually indicates a need for drug dosage adjustment.

Fig. 19-1 shows the action sites of various antihypertensive drugs.

The ideal antihypertensive drug would:

1 Maintain blood pressure within normal limits for various body positions
2 Maintain or improve blood flow, not compromise tissue perfusion or blood flow to the brain
3 Reduce the work load on the heart
4 Have no undesirable side effects
5 Permit long-term administration without development of tolerance

The currently accepted theory of treatment of hypertension includes the use of drug groups such as sympatholytic, vasodilator, and diuretic agents. Table 19-1 shows the classification of drug groups commonly used to treat hypertension.

Sympatholytic drugs

Drugs that most effectively reduce blood pressure are those inhibiting sympathetic nervous system function. The distinction between depressants of sympathetic function and ganglionic blocking agents is that the former agents do not interfere with parasympathetic innervation. This characteristic explains why clinicians prefer depressants of sympathetic functions to ganglionic blockers for lowering blood pressure.

CENTRAL SYMPATHETIC INHIBITOR DRUGS
Methyldopa (Aldomet)

Action and result. The current theory for the hypotensive effect of methyldopa is associated with a central mechanism that reduces sympathetic outflow from the brain. The central neurogenic mechanism involves the stimulation of alpha receptors in the nucleus tractus solitarius, which control the vasomotor center in the medulla. Moreover, it has been demonstrated that in the central adrenergic neurons, methyldopa is enzymatically converted to a metabolite, alpha-methylnorepinephrine. This compound then acts as a "false" neurotransmitter because it displaces norepinephrine from storage sites. When released, alpha-methylnorepinephrine potently stimulates alpha-adrenergic receptors in the medulla. However, because of its weak neurotransmitter properties, the metabolite lacks the capacity to produce a sympathetic outflow from the brain. Consequently, this reduces peripheral resistance, thereby causing a fall in blood pressure. It is also possible that this "false" transmitter depresses sympathetic transmission peripherally.

Since methyldopa reduces renal vascular resistance, it is often used in patients with renal hypertension and in hypertensive patients with impaired renal function. The drug has little or no effect on cardiac output. Lowered blood pressure occurs in both the lying and standing positions. Although the standing response is greater, the difference between the standing and lying blood pressure is not as great as that obtained with guanethidine or ganglionic blocking agents.

Sedation does occur with methyldopa, since it readily penetrates brain tissue and lowers norepinephrine levels. Methyldopa is absorbed from the gastrointestinal tract and excreted by the kidney.

Uses. Methyldopa may be used for the management of mild or moderate hypertension. It is usually administered in combination with a diuretic because methyldopa does produce sodium and water retention. The combined therapy also prevents the development of tolerance when methyldopa is used as the sole agent. The drug is particularly useful for the treatment of hypertension in patients with impaired renal function. Methyldopa is usually used as a second step in treatment when the effect of a thiazide is inadequate.

Preparation, dosage, and administration. Methyldopa is available in 250-mg tablets for oral use. The usual starting dose is 500 mg daily with increments of 250 mg weekly or biweekly until an optimal blood pressure response is obtained. Daily dosage may range from 500 to 3000 mg (0.5 to 3.0 g). Effect occurs within 4 to 6 hours; duration of action is 8 to 12 hours. On discontinuation of the drug, pretreatment blood pressure levels return within 24 to 48 hours.

Methyldopa is also available in 5-ml ampules containing 50 mg/ml for intravenous use in hypertensive crises. From 250 to 500 mg of the drug is given at 6-hour intervals. Blood pressure begins to fall about 2 hours after injection. The drug may also be given by intravenous infusion in 100 to 200 ml of 5% dextrose in water over a period of 30 to 60 minutes. Frequent blood pressure monitoring is highly recommended. In addition to a diuretic, hydralazine may be added as a third agent to achieve the desired antihypertensive effect.

Side effects. Side effects from the use of methyldopa are sedation, depression, dry mouth, nasal congestion, fever, altered liver function tests (although no liver toxicity has been reported), and decreased white and platelet cell counts. Sodium and water retention occur if a diuretic is not given along with methyldopa. Liver function tests and Coombs' test should be done at regular intervals. Hemolytic anemia occurs in some patients with a positive direct Coombs' test. Discontinuation of the drug may sometimes be indicated. Liver damage may occur within the first 2 or 3 months of therapy as a rare hypersensitivity reaction. Recovery is prompt following withdrawal of the drug. In addition, sudden discontinuation of methyldopa therapy should be avoided to prevent the occurrence of rebound hypertension.

Precautions and contraindications. Methyldopa is contraindicated in patients with liver disease, eclampsia, or a history of mental depression. Cautious use of the drug is indicated in patients with preexisting hepatic impairment. This drug is not to be used in the treatment of pheochromocytoma.

Clonidine hydrochloride (Catapres)

Action and results. Clonidine reduces blood pressure by suppressing the sympathetic outflow from the medulla of the brain. Like methyldopa, this drug stimulates the central alpha adrenergic receptors in the nucleus tractus solitarius, a site that controls the vasomotor center in the medulla. The integrated cardiovascular response that ensues is produced by two actions: (1) vagal stimulation of the cardioaccelerator center decreases cardiac output and heart rate and (2) sympathetic inhibition of the vasoconstrictor center reduces total peripheral vascular resistance.

Clonidine is effective in reducing blood pressure in both the supine and the erect positions and causes only mild postural hypotension. Moreover, by decreasing renal vascular resistance, renal blood flow is preserved and hence renin activity is suppressed. The decreased cardiac output, however, causes sodium retention and edema does occur. This, unfortunately, reduces the antihypertensive effect of clonidine, and therefore a diuretic is needed to correct the extracellular fluid volume retention.

Following oral administration of clonidine, blood pressure is reduced within 1 to 4 hours, and duration of action extends from 6 to 10 hours.

Uses. Clonidine is useful for the control of mild and moderate hypertension. Significant antihypertensive activity could be achieved by a combination of clonidine and a diuretic known as chlorthalidone.

Preparation, dosage, and administration. Clonidine is available as an oral preparation in the form of a scored tablet. Therapy is initiated with a low dose of 0.1 to 0.2 mg daily and is gradually increased to a maintenance dosage of 0.2 to 0.8 mg daily in divided doses. In view of its sodium-retaining property, a diuretic is indicated in the treatment regimen.

Side effects. The most common problems associated with clonidine therapy are similar to those of methyldopa. These central neurogenic effects include sedation and dry mouth. Clonidine-induced sedation, however, is thought to be more common and perhaps more severe than that produced by methyldopa. Both dry mouth and drowsiness are symptoms that gradually diminish with continued use of the drug. Also decreased gastrointestinal secretions and motility can result in constipation. Occasionally, impotence does occur.

Only mild and infrequent postural hypertension is caused by clonidine. However, the reduction of cardiac output and sodium retention makes its use undesirable in patients with congestive heart failure.

Some patients who become depressed as a result of using this drug may voluntarily discontinue therapy. As a consequence, withdrawal reactions could develop within 12 to 48 hours, and the syndrome includes restlessness, insomnia, tremors, tachycardia, headache, salivation, and *rebound hypertension*, which means a *rapid rise in blood pressure*. This phenomenon is due to increased circulating levels of catecholamines following the inhibitory action of clonidine on the medullary centers. The patient, therefore, should be warned that abrupt withdrawal of the drug can set off a fatal potential crisis. It is essential that the patient understand the importance of not missing a dose and having an adequate supply of drug while away from home during vacation. Clonidine is not recommended for use by individuals who are known to be undependable. If the drug is to be discontinued, the dosage should be reduced gradually over a period of 2 to 3 days.

Precautions and contraindications. Clonidine should be used with caution in patients with coronary insufficiency, recent myocardial infarction, cerebrovascular disease, or chronic renal failure. Clonidine is not recommended for use during pregnancy, since animal tests have shown toxicity of the embryo. Also periodic eye examinations should be performed for long-term therapy, since retinal degeneration has been noted in animal studies.

CENTRAL AND PERIPHERAL SYMPATHETIC INHIBITOR DRUG
RAUWOLFIA DERIVATIVES

Rauwolfia serpentina is a large climbing or twining shrub that grows in India and various tropical regions of the world. The botanical name given to a whole group of these plants was *Rauwolfia*, after an early German physician and botanist, Leonard Rauwolf. The root of the shrub from which the drug is obtained resembles a snake, hence *serpentina*. Extracts of the root of the plant have been used for a long time (in countries where the plant is indigenous) for a variety of ills, including snake bites, hypertension, and emotional disturbances. A report of its effectiveness in treating hypertension and mental disorders first appeared in an Indian medical journal in 1931. In 1952 the alkaloid reserpine was isolated. In 1953 western investigators began using the drug and publishing their findings on the sedative and antihypertensive effects of the drug. The *Rauwolfia* compounds are still widely used, particularly for their antihypertensive effect. Their use as sedatives for emotional disorders has declined as other more effective psychotropic drugs have become available.

Individual *Rauwolfia* alkaloids differ in chemical structure and pharmacologic action but in general have similar actions, uses, and cautions. These agents have a cumulative action; maximum response takes several days to 2 weeks after treatment is initiated. On discontinuation of drug administration effects from the drug may last 4 weeks. No tolerance or dependence has been reported.

These drugs are not recommended for patients with peptic ulcer, colitis, or mental depression. Parkinsonian rigidity may occur when large doses are administered. This symptom disappears when administration of the drug is discontinued.

Reserpine (Serpasil, Sandril, Reserpoid, Rau-Sed)

Reserpine is an ester-containing alkaloid obtained from the root of a certain species of *Rauwolfia*. It is a complex heterocyclic compound that was first synthesized in 1956, although the principal source continues to be the plant. It is a whitish crystalline powder, slightly soluble in water and alcohol but very soluble in organic acids such as acetic acid. It is considered the most potent of the alkaloids of *Rauwolfia*.

Action and results. Reserpine lowers blood pressure by depleting storage sites of catecholamine in the brain, heart, and peripheral postganglionic neurons. Norepinephrine is stored in vesicles within sympathetic nerves and in some areas of the central nervous system, particularly the hypothalamus. It is also present in the medulla. The action of reserpine involves a slow release of norepinephrine from the storage vesicles with a resultant depletion. Released

norepinephrine within the nerve is then inactivated intraneuronally by monoamine oxidase. Studies indicate that reserpine alters the ability of storage granules in nerve cells to take up and bind norepinephrine. (See Fig. 13-5 for norepinephrine storage.) Without adequate norepinephrine available for release, discharges of impulses from the sympathetic nervous system produce little or no effect on the effector organ (blood vessels). Since stimulation of vascular smooth muscle is inhibited, vasomotor tone is lowered, vascular relaxation occurs, and blood pressure is decreased. Reserpine is used in the treatment of moderate forms of hypertension.

Reserpine also depletes norepinephrine from various organs. Depletion of brain norepinephrine and serotonin may account for the sedative action of reserpine and also for some of its antihypertensive effects. It does not alter the brain waves (EEG); it produces calm and quietude without undue drowsiness and without mental confusion or difficulty in movement. When given reserpine, hostile and vicious animals become gentle, calm, and manageable, without loss of alertness and muscle coordination. The animal may go to sleep if undisturbed, but it is easily aroused. The drug seems to reduce attention and responsiveness to outside stimuli. It potentiates the central nervous system depressant actions of drugs such as barbiturates and alcohol. Depletion of cardiac norepinephrine results in bradycardia. In addition, there are constriction of the pupils and increased secretion and motility of the gastrointestinal organs. These effects are believed to be the result of suppression of sympathetic centers that allow the activity of the parasympathetic centers to be more prominent and noticeable. Reserpine is not an analgesic, and it does not potentiate the effects of analgesics.

Preparation, dosage, and administration. Reserpine is available in tablets, in sustained-release spansules, as an elixir, and in liquid forms for oral use. It is available in solutions for injection and in preparations containing a thiazide diuretic, potassium chloride, and other antihypertensive agents.

Reserpine is administered orally or by intramuscular or intravenous injection. The usual dosage for adults for mild hypertension is 0.1 to

0.5 mg daily, in two or three divided doses. It is the preparation of choice for most hypertensive emergencies, in which case dosage of 2.5 to 5 mg may be given parenterally every 6 to 12 hours. Blood pressure should be determined before each injection of reserpine to avoid marked hypotension.

Side effects. Reserpine is considered to have a low level of toxicity, but undesirable effects may occur as dosage levels rise. Nasal stuffiness, gain in weight, and diarrhea are common side effects. A parkinsonism state may occur. The drug should not be administered to patients with a history of mental depression. Psychic depression may be severe enough to end in suicide. Other effects include dryness of the mouth, nosebleeds, insomnia, itching, and skin eruptions. The drug sometimes causes gastric irritation, and occasionally it brings about reactivation of old gastric ulcers or causes a new one to form. Also, it remains uncertain whether long-term administration of reserpine is associated with an increased incidence of carcinoma of the breast in women. Postural hypotension may occur after parenteral administration.

Rauwolfia serpentina (Raudixin, Rautina, Rauwoldin)

Rauwolfia serpentina is the powdered whole root of *Rauwolfia serpentina*. It is administered orally. The daily oral dose for adults is 50 to 300 mg. It is usually divided into two doses. If larger doses are required, a more potent antihypertensive drug is indicated. It is available in 50- and 100-mg tablets. It is also available in preparations containing a thiazide diuretic and potassium chloride.

Alseroxylon (Rauwiloid, Rautensin)

Alseroxylon is the fat-soluble alkaloidal fraction extracted from the root of *Rauwolfia serpentina*. It is administered orally. The average adult dose is 2 to 4 mg daily. It is available in 2-mg tablets.

Syrosingopine (Singoserp)

Syrosingopine is a derivative of reserpine. It is the least potent of the *Rauwolfia* derivatives and has minimal central action. It is available in 1-mg tablets. Maintenance dose is 0.5 to 3 mg daily.

Deserpidine (Harmonyl)

Deserpidine's pharmacologic action is like that of reserpine. It is administered orally and is available in 0.1- and 0.25-mg tablets and in combination with a thiazide diuretic. Average daily dose is 0.25 to 1.0 mg.

Rescinnamine (Moderil)

The pharmacologic actions of rescinnamine are indistinguishable from those of reserpine, with the exception that sedation and bradycardia are less common. It is available for oral administration in 0.25- and 0.5-mg tablets. Average initial adult dosage is 0.5 mg once or twice daily for 2 weeks. Maintenance dose is usually 0.25 to 2 mg daily.

PERIPHERAL SYMPATHETIC INHIBITOR DRUG
Guanethidine sulfate (Ismelin)

Action and results. Guanethidine depletes norepinephrine from the heart and other peripheral organs. It causes a release and subsequent depletion of norepinephrine in the postganglionic terminals of adrenergic nerves, thereby inhibiting transmission of nerve impulses at the sympathetic neuroeffector junctions. Unlike the *Rauwolfia* compounds it does not have additional central action since it probably does not penetrate the central nervous system, and unlike the ganglionic blocking agents it does not inhibit the parasympathetic system. Therefore it does not produce a definite sedative effect or the serious side effects of parasympathetic blockade (urinary retention, paralytic ileus).

Guanethidine's blocking actions are very selective. It is a potent antihypertensive agent with fewer side effects than the older ganglionic blocking agents (pentolinium tartrate and hexamethonium chloride). Its prolonged therapeutic effect and the need for only one dose daily make it a clinically advantageous drug in the treatment of severe and malignant hypertension. The drug is only partially absorbed from the gastrointestinal tract and is primarily excreted by the kidney.

Venodilation occurs in addition to arteriolar dilation, which causes blood to pool in the splanchnic and peripheral areas. This results in some reduction in cardiac, renal, cerebral, and coronary flow. It must be kept in mind that these effects are increased in the standing position, and the drug may cause serious side effects in patients with cerebrovascular, coronary, or renal disease.

Uses. Guanethidine is used in the management of severe hypertension. It is usually given with a diuretic, such as a thiazide, to permit a lower dosage of the drug.

Preparation, dosage, and administration. Guanethidine is available in 10- and 25-mg tablets for oral administration. Initial dose is often 10 to 25 mg daily, which is increased by 10 mg weekly until a desirable antihypertensive response is attained. No increased dosage should be given until the patient's blood pressure has been taken in the supine and standing positions and after mild exercise. Average daily dose may range from 10 to 75 mg. Maintenance dose must always be individualized.

The onset of action of guanethidine is slow, and the antihypertensive effect may not be noted for 48 to 72 hours after treatment has been started. The action of the drug is prolonged and the hypotensive effect may persist for 7 to 10 days after drug discontinuation.

A thiazide diuretic is usually given with guanethidine to enhance the antihypertensive effect and to prevent sodium and water retention.

Side effects. The most frequently noted side effects from guanethidine are light-headedness and weakness, especially when the patient first gets out of bed in the morning. This is caused by postural hypotension, the arteriolar and venodilation permitting pooling of the blood in the lower extremities with a reduction in cerebral flow. These symptoms will disappear as the day progresses. (See section on nursing care measures and instructions for patients with postural hypotension.) Some patients receiving guanethidine show marked variation in blood pressure during the day, going from postural hypotension in the morning to severe hypertension by late afternoon or evening. This effect may be alleviated by rest periods during the afternoon or early evening. The postural hypotension actually reflects the therapeutic potency of the drug and is not a true side reaction. This effect may be lessened or eliminated by reduced drug dosage.

Other common side effects are diarrhea occurring after meals and at night and ejaculation failure. Impotence has been reported in a few cases. It appears that ejaculation is a sympathetic function while erection is a parasympathetic function.

Bradycardia occurs with guanethidine, since the drug blocks the sympathetically innervated cardioaccelerator nerves and leaves the vagal influence unopposed. Other side effects include abdominal distress, fatigue, nausea, nasal stuffiness, and weight gain. These symptoms may be relieved by reducing drug dosage. Sodium and water retention occur if a diuretic is not also given.

Precautions. Guanethidine should be used cautiously in patients with coronary insufficiency, recent myocardial infarction, cerebrovascular disease, renal disease with nitrogen retention, or history of peptic ulcer. The increased parasympathetic tone resulting from guanethidine therapy may aggravate these conditions.

In addition, guanethidine should not be used in conjunction with monoamine oxidase inhibitors since these compounds could cause a sharp rise in blood pressure.

BETA ADRENERGIC RECEPTOR BLOCKING DRUGS
Propranolol hydrochloride (Inderal)

Action and results. Propranolol is a nonselective beta adrenergic blocking agent that diminishes sympathetic activity. It exerts its inhibitory effect on both beta$_1$ and beta$_2$ receptors. The exact mechanism of antihypertensive action of propranolol is uncertain. By blocking beta$_1$ receptors in the heart, propranolol inhibits sympathetic stimulation, producing a decrease in myocardial contraction and a reduction in cardiac output. In addition, this agent inhibits the release of renin from the juxtaglomerular cells in the kidney by blocking their beta$_2$ receptor sites. Thus it is possible that the reduction in blood pressure may be related in some way to the combination of these two properties. Since the drug passes the blood-brain barrier, the effects of the central nervous system may also contribute to its antihypertensive action.

Uses. Propranolol is used in the management of mild, moderate, and severe hypertension. However, it generally is used in combination with a thiazide diuretic and hydralazine, a vasodilator, thereby producing a low incidence of side effects.

Preparation, dosage, and administration. Therapy must be individualized. The starting dose should be low—40 mg twice daily with or without another drug. Dosage is increased gradually until adequate blood pressure reduction is reached. The amount given may increase from 160 to 480 mg/day. (See precautions, side effects, and other details of propranolol in Chapter 18.)

Metoprolol tartrate (Lopressor)

Action and results. Metoprolol is a beta adrenergic receptor blocking agent that acts preferentially on the beta$_1$ receptors, particularly in cardiac muscle. This drug provides an advantage over propranolol, which blocks both beta$_1$ and beta$_2$ receptors, in patients with obstructive pulmonary disease for whom bronchodilation is essential. However, the drug is not absolutely beta$_1$ in action because with a relatively large dose beta$_2$ blockade may occur producing bronchoconstriction. Therefore metoprolol should be administered in small doses. Its mechanism of antihypertensive action appears to be similar to that of propranolol. It decreases cardiac output and suppresses renin activity.

Uses. Metoprolol is used to treat hypertension alone or in combination with other agents, especially thiazide-type diuretics or a vasodilating drug such as hydralazine or prazosin.

Preparation, dosage, and administration. The initial dosage is small, and usually 50 mg is administered daily with gradual increases until the desired reduction in blood pressure is obtained. The maintenance dosage is 100 mg twice daily. Abrupt discontinuation of therapy is unwise, since it may produce rapid increase in blood pressure. This is brought about by sudden release of catecholamines that previously had been inhibited by the drug.

Side effects and contraindications. Metoprolol does not produce postural hypotension, and it is effective in controlling hypertension in both supine and standing positions. It is contraindicated in patients with marked bradycardia, congestive heart failure, or chronic obstructive pulmonary disease, particularly if high doses are indicated. Side effects include dizziness, headache, and insomnia.

Nadolol (Corgard)

Nadolol is a nonselective beta adrenergic blocking agent that has received recent approval for clinical use in the United States. This drug is nearly as potent as propranolol. The compound is not metabolized and it is primarily excreted unchanged in the urine. Its relatively long plasma half-life (20 to 24 hours) allows for a once-daily dosage for effective control of hypertension.

For the treatment of hypertension, the initial oral dose is 40 mg/day, and the daily maintenance dosage ranges between 80 to 320 mg. The side effects of this drug appear to be the same as those described for propranolol. (See Chapter 18 for other details.)

TYROSINE HYDROXYLASE INHIBITOR DRUG
Metyrosine (Demser)

Metyrosine blocks the synthesis of norepinephrine and epinephrine by inhibiting the action of tyrosine hydroxylase. This enzyme catalyzes the conversion of tyrosine to dopa, which is the first biosynthetic step in the formation of the catecholamines. (See Chapter 13 for formula on biosynthesis of norepinephrine and epinephrine.) As a result, the synthesis of endogenous levels of catecholamines is reduced, thereby lowering blood pressure. The successful inhibition of tyrosine hydroxylase by the drug usually is measured as a decrease in urinary excretion of catecholamines and their metabolites.

Metyrosine is well absorbed from the gastrointestinal tract, and following oral maintenance dosages of 600 to 4000 mg/24 hours about

53% to 88% is recovered in the urine as unchanged drug.

Uses. Metyrosine is employed for the treatment of patients with pheochromocytoma to reduce blood pressure. In this condition, there is an excessive amount of circulating catecholamines resulting from hypersecretion of tumors, usually located in the medulla of one or both adrenal glands or even outside the glands. If possible, the treatment of choice is surgical removal of these tumors. Metyrosine, therefore, is used for preoperative preparation of patients for this type of surgery. It also is given for the management of patients when surgery is contraindicated or for chronic treatment of individuals with malignant pheochromocytoma. On the other hand, this drug is not recommended for the control of essential hypertension.

Preparation, dosage, and administration. The recommended initial dosage for adults and children over 12 years of age is 250 mg four times daily. This may be increased by 250 to 500 mg every day to a maximum of 4 g/day, which is administered in divided doses. When metyrosine is used for preoperative preparation, the drug should be given at least 5 to 7 days in an optimally effective dosage. This usually ranges between 2 to 3 g/day. By monitoring the clinical symptoms and catecholamine excretion, the desired dosage is established. The addition of an alpha adrenergic blocking agent such as phenoxybenzamine may be required if the patient is not adequately controlled by the use of metyrosine. Patients who respond to this tyrosine hydroxylase inhibitor experience a progressive decrease in blood pressure during the first 2 days of therapy. However, after withdrawal of the drug, blood pressure gradually increases to pretreatment values within 2 to 3 days.

Side effects. The side effects produced by metyrosine may include headache, nausea, sweating, and tachycardia. The most common adverse reaction observed is the presence of moderate to severe sedation. Sedative effects are maximal after 2 to 3 days, and then the condition tends to wane with continued administration. Some patients suffer from drooling, speech difficulty, and tremor. This occasionally has been accompanied by frank parkinsonism.

Additional adverse reactions include depression and hallucinations. These disturbing signs usually can be corrected by a reduction in dosage. Also, diarrhea in some patients may be severe, and if the drug must be continued, antidiarrheal agents may be required. Finally, in a few patients, crystalluria, transient dysuria, and hematuria have been observed. An increase in daily fluid intake is required to prevent crystalluria. When taking doses greater than 2g/day, water intake should be increased to achieve a daily urine volume of 2000 ml or more to minimize the risk of developing crystalluria. Because metyrosine will crystallize as rods, routine examination of the urine should be performed.

Precautions. Caution must be observed when administering metyrosine to patients receiving phenothiazine or haloperidol because the extrapyramidal effects can be potentiated by the inhibition of catecholamine synthesis. The drug is contraindicated if known hypersensitivity to it exists. Presently, there are no well-known studies in pregnant women; if possible, metyrosine use should be avoided, in pregnant women. If the patient suffers from stiffness of the jaw, drooling or speech difficulty, tremors, disorientation, diarrhea, or painful urination, the physician should be notified.

Vasodilator drugs

The vasodilator drugs reduce blood pressure by acting directly on vascular smooth muscle and thereby decreasing peripheral resistance. As a consequence, the sympathetic nervous system via the baroreceptor reflex is activated, producing an increase in heart rate, cardiac output, and force of myocardial contraction. This reflex increase in cardiac action generally causes annoying side effects and may precipitate angina, myocardial infarction, or congestive heart failure. Therefore combined therapy is recommended. To inhibit the sympathetic reflex response, the use of a beta adrenergic blocker such as propranolol has been advocated along with a diuretic to alleviate sodium and water retention that occurs during vasodilator therapy.

There are two types of vasodilators: (1) arteriolar dilators, which exert a selective effect on arterioles (these drugs include hydralazine, diazoxide, and minoxidil), and (2) arteriolar and venous dilators, which lower blood pressure by acting on both arteriolar resistance vessels and venous capacitance vessels (these drugs include sodium nitroprusside and prazosin).

ARTERIOLAR DILATOR DRUGS
Hydralazine hydrochloride (Apresoline)

Hydralazine hydrochloride is an effective antihypertensive agent, particularly when used in combination with other drugs for treating the patient with moderately severe hypertension. Hydralazine is thought to produce its effects by direct action on blood vessels. These actions reduce vascular resistance by producing arteriolar vasodilation and increasing renal blood flow. In combination with propranolol or a thiazide, hydralazine lowers blood pressure by alleviating the increase in heart rate, cardiac output, and fluid retention. Toxic effects from hydralazine are decreased because of smaller dosage.

Preparation, dosage, and administration. Hydralazine hydrochloride is usually administered orally, although it may be given intravenously or intramuscularly when the patient is unable to take the drug orally. It is available in 10-, 25-, 50-, and 100-mg tablets and as a sterile solution for injection of 20 mg/ml. As with other antihypertensive drugs, medication is started with small doses, and the dosage is increased gradually until the desired effects are obtained or symptoms of toxicity appear. The initial oral dosage for patients with moderate to severe hypertension is 10 mg given after meals and at bedtime. Patients may receive larger doses, depending on the severity of the hypertension and their response to the drug. Maximal daily dose is 400 mg, which is usually given in four divided doses. Repeated blood pressure readings must be taken not only to determine the effect of the drug but also to avoid serious side effects.

Side effects and toxic effects. Side effects associated with hydralazine hydrochloride vary from merely unpleasant effects to those that are serious and require cessation of administration. Headache, heart palpitations, anxi-

ety, mild depression, dry mouth, unpleasant taste in the mouth, and nausea and vomiting are symptoms that are unpleasant but may not necessitate discontinuance of administration. More serious symptoms include symptoms of coronary insufficiency, edema, chills, fever, and severe depression. Toxic symptoms that may result from prolonged administration of hydralazine hydrochloride in large doses resemble those of early rheumatoid arthritis or acute systemic lupus erythematosus. The drug should be discontinued if toxic symptoms appear.

Antihistaminic drugs, salicylates, or barbiturates are useful in controlling headache, palpitations, anxiety, and nausea and vomiting. The more severe symptoms require cessation of therapy with this drug. Fortunately, most symptoms subside when the drug is withdrawn. However, the lupoid state may persist for an indefinite period.

Diazoxide (Hyperstat IV)

Diazoxide is a chlorothiazide derivative but it has no diuretic activity. It does have marked antihypertensive action as a result of a direct vasodilator action on peripheral arterioles. Its basic mechanism of action remains uncertain. Diazoxide has been used to effectively treat patients with severe or malignant hypertension refractory to other antihypertensive agents. Some clinicians consider it the drug of choice *for treatment of hypertensive crisis.* Advantages of diazoxide include: (1) it has rapid onset of action, with maximal blood pressure fall usually occurring within 5 minutes after intravenous injection, (2) it does not require continuous infusion, (3) it does not cause extreme hypotension, (4) it does not cause sedation, and (5) drug resistance apparently does not occur.

Preparation, dosage, and administration. Diazoxide is available in solution for intravenous injection containing 15 mg/ml in 20-ml containers. The usual adult dose is 300 mg (20 ml of injectable solution) given intravenously within 30 seconds or less to the recumbent patient. Rapid injection ensures maximal response. Blood pressure should be monitored at 1-minute intervals for the first 5 minutes, then at 5-minute intervals until blood pressure is stabilized, then at hourly intervals. In ambulatory patients blood pressure should be measured with the patient standing before monitoring is completed. The injection may be repeated every 30 minutes for a period of 24 hours if necessary. Oral hypotensive therapy should be started as soon as the blood pressure is stabilized. Dosage for children or adults is 5 mg/kg body weight.

Side effects. Numerous side effects can occur with diazoxide, the more common ones being nausea, vomiting, abdominal discomfort, tachycardia, and a sensation of warmth or burning along the injected vein. Phlebitis and cellulitis may result from extravasation.

Other adverse effects include sodium and water retention and hyperglycemia. Use of a diuretic will help prevent fluid overload and decrease the risk of precipitating congestive heart failure. The hyperglycemic effect is usually mild and subsides without treatment, but oral hypoglycemic agents or insulin may be indicated. Orthostatic hypotension may occur, especially if diuretics are given; it is recommended that these patients remain recumbent for 8 to 10 hours.

Precautions. Blood glucose levels should be monitored in patients with diabetes or a family history of diabetes and in patients requiring multiple injections of the drug. Diazoxide should be used with caution in patients with cerebrovascular or coronary artery disease and those with impaired cardiac reserve. Safe use in pregnancy has not been established; adverse effects on the fetus have been reported. Mothers receiving the drug should not breast feed their infants.

Drug interactions. Diazoxide may increase the action of other hypotensive agents. It displaces warfarin from its protein binding sites, and its use in patients receiving coumarin anticoagulants may potentiate hypoprothrombinemia, necessitating reduction in anticoagulant dosage.

Minoxidil (Loniten)

Minoxidil is a potent and orally effective direct-acting peripheral vasodilator. It reduces elevated systolic and diastolic blood pressure by decreasing peripheral vascular resistance in the arteriolar vessels. The vasodilator effect of minoxidil is considerably greater than that of hydralazine. Like other vasodilators, minoxidil causes an increase in cardiac output, induces sodium retention, promotes development of edema, and increases plasma renin activity. This drug is useful in the treatment of severe hypertension that is refractory to the conventional antihypertensive agents. It also has been effective in the treatment of hypertensive patients who suffer from advanced renal failure. Concomitant administration of a beta adrenergic blocking agent such as propranolol is necessary to prevent the severe reflex tachycardia and postural hypotension. Also, a diuretic agent is essential to counteract sodium retention. Since the drug has only been marketed recently in the United States, treatment of milder degrees of hypertension is not recommended until more information is obtained through wider use.

The initial daily oral dose is 5 mg and this is increased, if necessary, to 40 mg/day. The maximum daily dose may be increased to 100 mg when propranolol and a diuretic are concomitantly used. An important side effect is generalized hypertrichosis, which occurs even with relatively small doses. The excessive hair growth appears over the temples, the malar area, the shoulders, the back, and the forearms. On discontinuation of the drug, hair growth stops. No endocrine abnormalities have been found to account for this distressing effect.

ARTERIOLAR AND VENOUS DILATOR DRUGS
Sodium nitroprusside (Nipride)

Sodium nitroprusside is a potent direct-acting vasodilator used for treatment of hypertensive crisis when immediate reduction in blood pressure is required. This drug relaxes both arteriolar and venous smooth muscle. Because of the latter effect, more venous pooling of blood occurs when the patient is upright, thereby increasing heart rate. Nitroprusside also increases the secretion of renin. It acts rapidly, within 2 minutes, but continuous infusion is necessary to maintain the hypotensive effect. Other antihypertensives should be started as soon as the blood pressure is under control. Solutions are reddish brown in color; deterioration by light is evidenced by a change in color to blue. Solutions that change color should be discarded.

Sodium nitroprusside must be prepared by the hospital pharmacy using 50 mg of drug/500 to 1000 ml of 5% dextrose in water. A fresh solution must be prepared every 4 hours; the solution should be protected from light by covering the bottle with aluminum foil or opaque material. The solution is administered intravenously at a rate of 10 to 30 drops/minute with the aid of an infusion pump. The patient, his blood pressure, and the flow rate must be monitored continuously.

Prazosin (Minipress)

Prazosin reduces blood pressure by decreasing peripheral vascular resistance. Although several mechanisms of action have been proposed, some aspects of how this drug produces a hypotensive effect are still not completely understood. According to the current hypothesis, prazosin is an alpha adrenergic blocking agent. By selectively blocking the postsynaptic alpha receptors on the vascular smooth muscle of both the arterioles and veins, it inhibits the action of norepinephrine when the sympathetic nerves are stimulated. This blocking action thereby causes a decrease in peripheral vascular resistance, lowering blood pressure in both the supine and standing positions. The drug produces no reflex tachycardia nor does it increase renin release as occurs with hydralazine or diazoxide. However, it does produce fluid retention. Prazosin is effective in the treatment of mild to moderate hypertension. When used in combination with a thiazide diuretic and/or a beta blocking agent, it is more effective than when used alone. The initial oral dosage of 1 mg two or three times daily may be slowly increased to a maintenance daily total of 20 mg, which is administered in divided doses. The therapeutic dosages have ranged from 6 to 15 mg daily given in divided doses.

Prazosin is a relatively new antipressor agent that has the ability to lower blood pressure without causing any significant side effects, which include headache, palpitations, drowsiness, and dizziness. Sexual dysfunction occasionally does occur.

It must be noted that in some patients, excessive postural hypotension may occur, causing a sudden loss of consciousness, particularly early in treatment. Syncopal episodes may be avoided by starting the patient on low doses of prazosin and gradually increasing the amount. During intitiation of treatment the patient should be advised to sit or lie down if light-headedness or dizziness occurs. As with all antihypertensive patients, these individuals should be encouraged to be drug compliant, although the full effect of prazosin may not be evident for 4 to 6 weeks.

Monoamine oxidase inhibitor drug

The monoamine oxidase (MAO) inhibitors have the ability to lower blood pressure by blocking the release of norepinephrine at the sympathetic neuroeffector junctions. MAO is an enzyme active in the metabolic breakdown of catecholamines within the adrenergic nerve terminals (see Fig. 13-5). By blocking the enzyme action, MAO inhibitors actually increase the amount of norepinephrine in the adrenergic nerve endings. However, because these drugs interfere with the transmission of the sympathetic nerve impulse, they produce a reduction in peripheral resistance and a decrease in blood pressure.

Since safer and more effective drugs are now available for the treatment of hypertension, there is no reason to use MAO inhibitors for this purpose. Nevertheless, this group of drugs does have a place in the management of mental depression.

Pargyline hydrochloride (Eutonyl)

Pargyline is used for severe hypertension. It is a potent amine oxidase inhibitor that, like guanethidine and ganglionic blocking agents, exerts a predominant postural antihypertensive effect. Onset of action is slow, about 3 to 4 days. It takes 7 days for the cumulative effect to be sufficient to bring about a decrease in blood pressure. Maximum response to the drug may take as long as 3 weeks.

On discontinuation of the drug, blood pressure returns to pretreatment levels in 10 to 14 days.

Preparation, dosage, and administration. Pargyline is available in 10-, 25-, and 50-mg tablets. The usual initial dose is 10 to 25 mg daily. Because of the cumulative effect, drug dosage should be increased slowly by increments of 10 mg at weekly or biweekly intervals until the desired blood pressure response is obtained. The usual maintenance dose is 25 to 75 mg/day. Pargyline is not recommended for children under 12 years of age.

Pargyline is usually used along with an oral diuretic, since this reduces the amount of pargyline required, reduces side effects, and promotes more effective lowering of blood pressure in the supine position.

Side effects. The most common side effects are dry mouth, insomnia, daytime drowsiness, nervousness, weight gain, and impotence or inability to ejaculate. Reducing drug dosage may eliminate these side effects. For some patients a different antihypertensive drug may be needed. Nightmares and psychotic reactions may occur.

Pargyline has been known to exert a euphoric action in some patients; this is particularly helpful for the depressed hypertensive patient.

Precautions. Since pargyline is an amine oxidase inhibitor, the patient must be cautioned against ingesting foods or liquids that contain large amounts of tyramine. The combined effect of the drug and the tyramine-containing foods may precipitate a hypertensive crisis. Since monoamine oxidase inhibitors increase the concentration of norepinephrine and the additional tyramine produces more norepinephrine, a "flooding" of the body with norepinephrine may result. Severe vasoconstriction can occur with marked blood pressure elevation. Several deaths reported in the literature have been attributed to this effect. Foods known to contain high tyramine content are cheese products, particularly cheddar cheese; excluded are cream and cottage cheese. The

more aged and the less acid the cheese, the greater its tyramine content. Some alcoholic beverages, beer and wine (especially chianti), and some meats, fruits, and vegetables have sufficient concentrations of tyramine and tyrosine to cause the patient on MAO inhibitors to have extreme headaches, serious blood pressure elevation, and tachycardia. Since these reactions can occur with the use of pargyline and amphetamines, amphetamines and antidepressants should not be taken concomitantly. Fortunately, these reactions disappear in 1 to 2 hours in most cases, but they may be serious and caution must be exercised.

Since pargyline may potentiate action of drugs affecting the central nervous system, it should not be given with imipramine, amitriptyline, ganglionic blocking agents, or sympathomimetic amines. If barbiturates are used, they must be given in reduced dosage.

Ganglionic blocking drugs

Ganglionic blocking drugs block transmission of both sympathetic and parasympathetic nerve impulses at the ganglia. The parent compound of this group of drugs is a quaternary ammonium compound, tetraethylammonium chloride. It is not well suited for the treatment of hypertension because of its short duration of action, its ineffectiveness when given orally, and its distressing side effects.

In 1950 the methonium derivatives were introduced, and hexamethonium chloride became the drug of choice in managing severe and malignant hypertension. Despite the difficulties in managing patients receiving hexamethonium because of its erratic absorption and action and severe side effects, its use demonstrated that severe hypertension could be controlled with an improvement in mordibity and mortality. Since 1961, however, the ganglionic blocking agents have been seldom used. Newer antihypertensive drugs that have more selective action and less severe side effects are preferred.

Ganglionic blocking agents block the action of acetylcholine on the ganglion cells by competing with acetylcholine at the synapse of autonomic ganglia. This results in reduced transmission of impulses from preganglionic to postganglionic fibers in both sympathetic and parasympathetic nerves. Blocking transmission of impulses through the sympathetic ganglia abolishes vasoconstrictor tone; the blood vessels dilate and arterial pressure falls. This is the desired clinical effect. The greatest antihypertensive effect occurs when the patient stands, since compensatory vasoconstrictor reflexes regulating blood pressure with position change are suppressed. The result is that blood pools in the leg veins, venous return to the heart is decreased, and cardiac output falls. If blood supply to the brain is inefficient, fainting occurs. These are of course undesired effects but a natural result of the drugs' pharmacologic action. Sympathetic block also causes loss of body heat and lowered body temperature as a result of vasodilation in the skin. Sweating is also inhibited.

Major disadvantages in the use of ganglionic blockers result from parasympathetic blockade. This causes dry mouth, reduced gastric secretion, paralytic ileus, constipation, urinary retention, blurred vision, and loss of visual accommodation.

Impotence may also occur, owing to the combined sympathetic and parasympathetic block. Erection is prevented by the latter, while the former prevents ejaculation.

These drugs do not cross the blood-brain barrier and therefore do not exert central nervous system actions.

Mecamylamine hydrochloride (Inversine)

Mecamylamine is marketed in 2.5- and 10-mg tablets for oral administration. The dosage recommended is that which will reduce the blood pressure and maintain it without the appearance of severe side effects. Treatment is usually started with a dosage of 2.5 mg twice daily and is gradually increased. The average total daily maintenance dose is about 25 mg (divided into three portions). Dosage must be determined in relation to blood pressure readings.

Mecamylamine is well absorbed from the intestinal tract. It lowers the blood pressure of both normal persons and hypertensive patients. Its duration of action is 6 to 12 hours. Mecamylamine is absorbed by the central nervous system; confusion, tremors, and psychologic difficulties have been observed in some patients being treated with the drug.

Trimethaphan camsylate (Arfonad)

Trimethaphan is a rapid-acting ganglionic blocking agent that lowers blood pressure in both normotensive and hypertensive persons. The duration of its action is brief. It is used in hypertensive crisis and for initial control of blood pressure in patients with dissecting aortic aneurysm.

This drug is used for the production of controlled hypotension during certain types of surgical procedures in which the production of some degree of hemostasis in capillary beds, arterioles, and venules helps to prevent excessive bleeding and increases visualization and exposure of the surgical field. It is used especially in neurosurgery and cardiovascular surgery.

Preparation, dosage, and administration. Trimethaphan camsylate is administered by continuous intravenous infusion as a 0.1% solution in 5% dextrose in water or in isotonic salt solution. It is available in 10-ml ampules containing 500 mg. Blood pressure returns to normal levels about 5 minutes after administration is stopped.

The use of this drug is recommended for administration only by experienced individuals. Respiratory depression is a complication, particularly when a muscle relaxant has been used. Tachycardia also is a potential complication.

Hexamethonium chloride; hexamethonium tartrate

Hexamethonium is rarely used today except in emergencies. Many of its previous dosage forms are no longer available. It is not given orally since it is poorly and irregularly absorbed from the gastrointestinal tract. When it is given parenterally, its effects are achieved rather promptly and last 4 to 6 hours.

Baroreceptor stimulants

VERATRUM ALKALOIDS

Veratrum viride and *Veratrum album* (green and white hellebore) are two species of plants that contain alkaloids with the capacity to slow the heart and lower blood pressure.

The hypotensive effect of veratrum alkaloids results from their rather unique ability to reflexly depress the vasomotor center and sympathetic activity by stimulating receptors in the carotid sinus and aortic arch. The veratrum compounds also stimulate the vagus, which slows the heart and dilates peripheral blood vessels with a fall in blood pressure.

The veratrum alkaloids all have a central emetic effect and the resulting nausea and vomiting is a serious disadvantage. In addition, the range between toxic and therapeutic dose is narrow. These disadvantages have limited their usefulness.

Veratrum preparations such as alkavervir (Veriloid) or cryptenamine (Unitensin) have been used effectively for hypertensive emergencies. They reduce blood pressure almost immediately on intravenous use. Constant expert supervision and blood pressure monitoring are required to regulate the dose according to blood pressure response and to avoid serious side effects such as respiratory depression and collapse.

Side effects. Side effects of the veratrum preparations include epigastric distress, increased flow of saliva, nausea, vomiting, hiccuping, and slow pulse. These effects may be stopped with atropine. Overdosage causes bradycardia, hypotension, respiratory depression, and collapse. Ephedrine is useful in overcoming the hypotension.

Contraindications. Veratrum products are contraindicated in patients with high intracranial pressure (which is not secondary to hypertension), digitalis intoxication, uremia, or cerebrovascular disease.

Diuretic drugs

The use of diuretics in the treatment of hypertension results in a loss of excess salt and water from the body by their renal excretion. Diuretics exert no antihypertensive effects.

However, they do decrease plasma and extracellular fluid volume, which subsequently depresses vascular reactivity to sympathetic stimulation. This response, therefore, produces an initial decline of cardiac output followed by a decrease in peripheral resistance and a lowering of blood pressure.

THIAZIDE DIURETICS
Chlorothiazide (Diuril); hydrochlorothiazide (HydroDiuril, Esidrix, Oretic)

The effectiveness of chlorothiazide and certain related compounds, when given alone or in conjunction with other antihypertensive agents in the treatment of hypertension, has now been established.

Action. Although introduced and primarily useful as a diuretic agent, chlorothiazide has been found to have significant blood pressure lowering action in hypertensive individuals, perhaps because of its effect in reducing the amount of water, sodium, and chloride in the body and possibly because of certain inherent properties of the drug. It also augments the effects of other drugs used in treatment of hypertension.

Uses. Chlorothiazide is used either alone, in cases of mild hypertension, or in combination with other antihypertensive drugs. This permits lower drug dosage, reduction of unpleasant side effects, and enhanced hypotensive effects.

Preparation, dosage, and administration. Chlorothiazide is available in tablets of 250 and 500 mg for oral administration. When given alone, doses of 500 mg may be prescribed to be given from one to three times daily. When combined with other antihypertensive drugs, the dosage is lower, usually 250 mg twice daily.

Hydrochlorothiazide is available in tablets of 25 and 50 mg for oral administration. There are also tablets containing hydrochlorothiazide and potassium. Some pharmaceutical companies market a combination of this drug and another antihypertensive in the same tablet. The usual antihypertensive dosage is 25 to 50 mg one or two times a day, but doses as high as 200 mg/day may be used.

Side effects. Patients occasionally experience weakness, fatigue, nausea, abdominal pain, distention, and diarrhea. A fairly high percentage of patients has been known to show some disturbance of blood electrolytes. The blood urea nitrogen level may be elevated and the level of serum potassium lowered. Also, hyperglycemia may occur. Chlorothiazide is administered cautiously to patients with renal insufficiency. Some physicians recommend that the patient on prolonged therapy with this drug be given supplemental amounts of potassium chloride. Skin rash has been observed occasionally. Leukopenia, thrombocytopenia, and agranulocytosis have occurred but are rare.

OTHER DIURETIC COMPOUNDS

A number of preparations chemically related to chlorothiazide have been marketed, such as polythiazide (Renese) and bendroflumethiazide (Naturetin).

A loop diuretic such as furosemide (Lasix) is a powerful drug that causes excessive loss of potassium and water and, therefore, is not appropriate for use as an antihypertensive agent. Spironolactone (Aldactone), a distal tubular diuretic, may cause hyperkalemia and so its use is contraindicated in patients with impaired renal function. (See Chapter 21 for more detailed information on individual agents.)

Renin-angiotensin system antagonists

ANGIOTENSIN II INHIBITORS

The recent introduction of a new class of antihypertensive drugs has given rise to a unique approach to the treatment and control of hypertension. This category of agents is known as angiotensin II antagonists, and it is involved with inhibiting the action of the renin-angiotensin-aldosterone system. The importance of this system in maintaining blood pressure and sodium and fluid balance is now well accepted.

Under normal circumstances, the activation of this mechanism is initiated by a decrease in blood flow or blood pressure in the kidneys, which then causes a release of renin into the circulation. The production of renin occurs in the juxtaglomerular cells located in the walls of the afferent arterioles that are immediately proximal to the glomeruli. Renin itself is an enzyme and it catalyzes the conversion of circulating angiotensinogen (plasma globulin substrate) to angiotensin I. Angiotensin I is then transformed by *angiotensin-converting enzyme* to angiotensin II. This latter conversion occurs almost entirely in the small blood vessels in the lungs. Angiotensin II is an extremely potent vasopressor that produces arteriolar constriction and thereby raises the blood pressure back to normal. In addition, angiotensin II performs another function causing the release of aldosterone from the adrenal cortex. This hormone then acts on the kidneys to enhance the reabsorption of sodium. The resultant increase in plasma osmolarity stimulates antidiuretic hormone secretion from the hypothalamus, which also acts on the kidneys to promote reabsorption of water. Both these effects tend to elevate the extracellular fluid volume and help to restore blood pressure to normal (see Fig. 19-2). In summary, the resultant increases in blood pressure, in extracellular fluid volume, and in angiotensin II itself exert a negative "feedback" response that causes renin release from the kidney, thus providing a system for maintaining normal blood pressure homeostasis.

Indeed, it is now apparent that a disturbance of the basic function involving the renin-angiotensin-aldosterone system results in the pathogenesis of hypertension. Furthermore, a damaged kidney that cannot regulate its renin release through normal feedback mechanisms can easily produce an elevation in blood pressure. Fortunately, this evidence has given rise to a new concept in the pharmacologic treatment of hypertension. More importantly, it has led to the development of a new class of drugs, the angiotensin II inhibitors, which blocks the conversion of angiotensin I to angiotensin II. One such drug is captopril, the only orally active compound presently available in the United States. Another drug, called saralasin, is still under investigation. Its safety is limited because of its partial agonist (angiotensin II-like) action that shows some tendency to increase blood pressure. The clinical utility of saralasin is further limited by the fact that it must be administered intravenously.

Captopril (Capoten)

Captopril reduces blood pressure primarily through suppression of the renin-angiotensin-aldosterone system. By inhibiting the action of the *angiotensin-converting enzyme*, it prevents the conversion of angiotensin I to angiotensin II (Fig. 19-2). The interruption of this reaction results in a decrease in the plasma angiotensin II level, producing a reduction in vascular tone and a direct lowering of blood pressure. The blockade of angiotensin II formation also prevents aldosterone release, which in turn reduces sodium retention and indirectly decreases water reabsorption by inhibiting antidiuretic hormone production. The resultant sodium and water excretion is thought to contribute only secondarily to the reduction in blood pressure. Interestingly, in clinical trials, it has been demonstrated that the blood pressure is lowered in hypertensive patients irrespective of whether plasma renin activity is high or low. Although captopril is known as an orally active angiotensin-coverting enzyme inhibitor, the mechanism of its action is still controversial. Further study of the drug is required to clarify the role of the kallikrein-kinin-prostaglandin system, for experimental evidence shows that this system is an integral part of the mechanism mediating the captopril hypotensive effect.

After oral administration, captopril is adsorbed rapidly into the bloodstream, reaching a peak concentration in about 1 hour. It is recommended that the drug be given about 1 hour before meals; the presence of food reduces absorption by 30% to 40%. In a 24-hour period, about 75% of the ingested drug is eliminated in the urine and about 15% in the feces of patients with normal renal function. In normal persons given radiolabeled drug, the apparent elimination half-life for total radioactivity in blood is probably less than 3 hours. In patients with renal impairment, retention of captopril occurs; therefore, adjustment of dosage and dosage intervals is necessary.

Uses. Captopril is an orally effective angiotensin-converting enzyme inhibitor that is used to lower blood pressure in patients with either renovascular or essential hypertension. Al-though this is still controversial, it appears that the response to captopril is likely to be greater in patients with high pretreatment plasma renin activity. On the other hand, it also is capable of lowering blood pressure in many patients with normal or low plasma renin activity. Because of its potential for serious side effects, the drug should be reserved for the treatment of hypertension in patients who have failed to respond satisfactorily to multidrug antihypertensive regimens. The combination of drugs in the multidrug regimens usually include a diuretic, a sympathominetic agent such as a beta blocker, and a vasodilator. While captopril is effective alone, in the population described a marked reduction in blood pressure occurs when it is used in combination with a thiazide diuretic in resistant hypertension.

Administration of captopril is also effective in controlling blood pressure in a small number of patients with hypertension associated with chronic renal failure and scleroderma crisis. Presently, an additional area of interest now involves its use for patients in severe treatment-resistant heart failure. In this type of congestive heart failure, there is often an increase in plasma renin and aldosterone concentration. The hemodynamic changes produced by captopril have resulted in improved cardiac performance. Although further clinical experience is needed to clearly define the long-term effectiveness of captopril this appears to be a promising area of potential use.

Preparation, dosage, and administration. The oral preparation of captopril appears in 25-, 50-, and 100-mg scored tablets. Therapy is individualized and previous antihypertensive drug regimen should be discontinued for 1 week before administering captopril. The starting dose is 25 mg three times a day. If blood pressure reduction is unsatisfactory after 1 or 2 weeks, the dose may be increased to 50 mg three times a day. To enhance absorption, the drug should be given 1 hour before meals without food. The addition of a thiazide diuretic may be required if blood pressure is not controlled after another 1 or 2 weeks. While continuing the diuretic, the dose of captopril may be increased from 100 to 150 mg three times a day if further blood pressure reduction is required. The maximum daily dose should not exceed 450 mg. Because the excretion of captopril is reduced in impaired renal function, patients so affected may respond to smaller and less frequent doses.

Side effects and toxic effects. In about 1% to 2% of patients, proteinuria has been reported. In addition, the nephrotic syndrome has occurred in some individuals with proteinuria. Therefore, caution is needed if captopril is necessary in individuals with preexisting renal dysfunction or in renal transplant patients. Neutropenia and agranulocytosis have also been observed. Some neutropenic patients develop systemic or oral cavity infections. Most of these patients appear to have complex medical histories such as advanced renal failure, systemic lupus erythematosus, or other autoimmune/collagen disorders. Therefore, a few of these individuals may be receiving multiple concomitant drug therapy, including immunosuppressive therapy.

During the first 4 weeks of therapy, rash with pruritus and sometimes fever and eosinophilia occurs in about 10% of patients. The rash is usually mild and disappears with dosage reduction. Angioedema of the face, mucous membranes of the mouth, or the extremities has also been observed. This condition is reversible on discontinuation of therapy. Reversible loss of taste or taste disturbance such as persistent metallic or salty taste may be an additional potential side effect. Finally, postural hypotension has not generally been a problem during captopril therapy. Nevertheless, difficulty in assuming the erect position may occur in sodium-depleted patients.

Since most cases of proteinuria occur by the eighth month of therapy, urinary protein tests should be done before therapy and at monthly intervals for the first 9 months with periodic follow-up thereafter. Furthermore, to prevent the risk of neutropenia, white blood cell counts should be performed every 2 weeks for the first 3 months of therapy and periodically thereafter. Any signs of infection, such as a sore throat or fever, should be reported immediately. Discontinuation of captopril has usually led to

prompt return of white blood count to normal.

Drug interactions. Because captopril decreases aldosterone production, an increase of serum potassium may occur. If the patient has been receiving a potassium-sparing diuretic such as spironolactone, the serum potassium level must be restored to normal before beginning captopril therapy. Additionally, patients receiving potassium supplements must be closely monitored for possible significant increase in serum potassium with captopril therapy. Finally, it should be noted that captopril may cause a false-positive test for urine acetone.

Nursing implications for antihypertensive therapy
INSTRUCTIONS TO PATIENTS TO AVOID OR DECREASE POSTURAL (ORTHOSTATIC) HYPOTENSION

The nurse should give the patient undergoing antihypertensive therapy the following instructions:

1 The patient should rise slowly from a lying to a sitting position and from a sitting to a standing position. This allows for the delay in sympathetic nerve stimulation of the vascular system to occur during the position change. The vasoconstriction of arterioles of the lower extremities prevents pooling of blood and syncope.
2 The patient should never stand perfectly still in one place for any length of time, especially within 2 hours after taking the drug. Standing still causes relaxation of leg vessels with pooling of blood and may result in syncope or weakness. This is particularly true in the early morning, since this is the time when postural hypotension is often most severe. The patient should avoid standing still in church, waiting in line, standing on buses and subway trains, and in telephone booths. The patient should use caution while shaving or showering.
3 If weakness and dizziness occur they can be relieved by muscular activity or recumbency.
 a If standing or sitting, the patient should flex the calf muscles, wiggle the toes, rise up on the toes, and allow the feet to return to flat position. This results in alternate vasoconstriction and vasodilation and prevents blood from pooling in lower extremities.
 b If possible, the patient should lie flat with the legs slightly higher than the head to promote

cerebral flow and decrease pooling of blood in the legs.

4 The patient should be instructed to be careful within 2 hours after taking drugs. The patient should avoid driving a car if blurred vision or hypotension occurs and should be cautious when working with or around heavy and dangerous machinery.

5 The patient should not take prolonged hot baths or steambaths, since this promotes peripheral vasodilation and may cause a hypotensive reaction.

OTHER INSTRUCTIONS TO PATIENT

1 The patient should take precautions in the heat, when in the sun, or at the beach, since heat increases peripheral blood flow through vascular relaxation from heat dissipation, and since some antihypertensive drugs cause decreased sweating, hypotension, heat stroke, and other serious side effects from vasodilation.

2 If impotency occurs, the patient should consult his doctor. Omission of an occasional dose or a decrease in dosage may overcome this effect.

3 The patient should *not suddenly discontinue drug therapy.* If the drug is suddenly discontinued, blood pressure tends to rise higher because of increased sensitivity to pressor substances. *Gradual withdrawal of the drug is therefore necessary.*

4 The patient should carry an identification card with the name of the drug, dosage, and the times the drug is taken.

5 If chest pain occurs after taking the drug, the patient should discontinue taking the drug and consult the physician. This is especially important in patients with a history of angina pectoris.

6 Alcohol in moderation is acceptable.

7 If headache occurs at night or early in the morning, the patient should sleep with the head elevated or in a sitting position.

8 A patient taking a monoamine oxidase inhibitor should be cautioned to avoid foods or beverages high in tyramine or tyrosine to prevent the occurrence of a hypertensive crisis. No medication should be taken unless prescribed by the physician, since drug incompatibilities may occur.

9 Another important aspect is moderation with salt intake or the ingestion of foods high in sodium content. Such foods include bacon, ham, sausage, tuna, crabmeat, various cheeses, crackers, and licorice.

NURSING CARE OF PATIENTS WITH POSTURAL (ORTHOSTATIC) HYPOTENSION

An Ace bandage or an elastic stocking can be used to overcome vascular relaxation in lower extremities. It should be applied with the legs slightly elevated or horizontal. Bandages or stockings should be snug but not excessively constricting. The bandages need be applied only when the patient is up and about; they should be removed when the patient returns to bed.

The patient's blood pressure should be checked in lying, sitting, and standing positions. The readings should be charted and reported. Dosage is often regulated according to blood pressure obtained in the standing or upright position. With some drugs blood pressure is lowest in the standing position and highest in the lying position. Blood pressure in the sitting position may be lower than that obtained in the lying position but higher than that recorded for the standing position. The patient should be upright for at least 3 minutes before the reading is taken. Patients on bed rest should be in a semireclining position with the head of the bed elevated.

NURSING CARE OF PATIENTS WITH SIDE EFFECTS

Visual disturbances may occur with the use of some drugs such as ganglionic blockers. There may be interference with pupillary response and sensitivity to light because of poor accommodation. The patient may need to wear sunglasses and avoid bright lights.

Constipation is a common effect with some antihypertensive drugs such as ganglionic blockers. Daily elimination is very important when antihypertensive drugs are given orally or if the drug is primarily eliminated via the intestinal tract. Constipation may cause either irregular or constant absorption of the drug, and cumulative effects may occur. Adequate diet, liquids, and exercise are important to avoid this effect. Cathartics or enemas may be necessary during the early stages of treatment. The antihypertensive agent may need to be changed if regular and unassisted elimination cannot be established.

Other side effects include diarrhea, urinary retention, and dry mouth and nasal mucosa. Diarrhea is likely to occur with guanethidine therapy. This may require changing the drug or the use of antidiarrheic agents. Urinary retention is likely to occur in the older male with prostatic hypertrophy. These patients should be placed on recorded intake and output. Dry mouth is likely to occur with any drug that inhibits sympathetic activity, since the salivary glands are innervated by the sympathetic nerves. Dry mouth interferes with carbohydrate digestion. In addition, the patient is more prone to oral infections. Good oral hygiene is essential for these patients.

TEACHING THE PATIENT TO TAKE HIS/HER OWN BLOOD PRESSURE

Some authorities believe that the patient should be taught to take, record, and graph his or her own blood pressure at home. This often lessens nonadherence to the therapeutic program and serious side effects from overdosage.

Antihypotensive drugs

Circulatory shock occurs when blood flow to the tissues is inadequate for normal functioning of the body cells. The basic components that regulate normal circulation include (1) sufficient pumping action of the heart, (2) adequate blood volume, and (3) normal vascular tone. The shock syndrome develops as a consequence of impairment of one or more of these factors. Therefore, in any instance of shock, circulation must be improved before the patient's condition deteriorates to the extent that tissue hypoxia occurs.

The drugs used for the treatment of shock include sympathomimetic agents, both alpha and beta receptor agonists. The details of the individual agents appear in Chapter 13. In addition, when volume replacement is indicated, such as whole blood and its components, the description of these agents may be found in Chapter 20.

The use of vasoconstrictors (such as norepinephrine) is considered by researchers to be *contraindicated* in circulatory shock. These drugs will further reduce capillary blood flow and hasten cell death.

In some cases where significant vasoconstriction is present, vasodilators such as phenoxybenzamine or phentolamine have been used to reduce peripheral resistance to blood flow and to increase capillary perfusion. The use of vasodilators plus volume replacement has resulted in a decrease in mortality from circulatory shock.

Since circulatory shock can be more successfully treated than other forms of shock, its prompt recognition and safe management are of great importance.

Dobutamine hydrochloride (Dobutrex)

Dobutamine is a synthetic catecholamine that acts directly on the heart muscle by producing an increased force of myocardial contraction. This activity is attributed to the direct stimulation of the beta$_1$ adrenergic receptors of the heart. In addition, this agent produces comparatively mild chronotropic, hypertensive, dysrhythmogenic, and vasodilator effects. Dobutamine is an effective positive inotropic drug, and because of its minimal influence on heart rate and blood pressure (both major determinants of myocardial oxygen demand) it is of value in patients with low cardiac output syndrome. Like dopamine it is most effective for improving myocardial function in patients with cardiogenic shock. However, in contrast to dopamine, it does not produce renal vasodilation.

Preparation, dosage, and administration. Dobutamine is administered intravenously in the *short-term* management of patients requiring inotropic support. It is employed for use in individuals with low cardiac output resulting from organic heart disease such as myocardial infarction or from cardiac surgical procedures.

Because of its short half-life in plasma (about 2 minutes), dobutamine is administered by continuous intravenous infusion at a usual dose of 2.5 to 10 µg/kg/minute. During therapy, the electrocardiogram and blood pressure should be continuously monitored. Before instituting treatment with dobutamine, it is necessary to correct hypovolemia with a suitable volume expander, particularly if cardiogenic shock and severe hypotension are present. During this procedure, both the pulmonary wedge pressure and cardiac output must be monitored.

Contraindications. Dobutamine is contraindicated in patients with obstruction to cardiac ejection. Thus, its positive inotropic effect prevents its use in idiopathic hypertrophic subaortic stenosis.

Side effects and toxic effects. Adverse reactions include increased heart rate and blood pressure. Dobutamine may produce serious dysrhythmias; however, the incidence usually is low. Since atrioventricular conduction is enhanced by this drug, its use should be avoided in patients with atrial fibrillation. On occasion if the heart rate increases, this effect can be reversed by reducing the rate of administration of the drug. Other side effects include nausea, headache, dyspnea, palpitations, and anginal pain.

Peripheral vasodilator drugs

The use of vasodilating drugs in chronic occlusive arterial disease or peripheral vascular disease has to date been very discouraging. Adrenergic blocking agents are frequently used to treat peripheral vascular diseases.

However, several drugs that are not adrenergic blocking agents have been used with some success in the treatment of these diseases.

The rating for these drugs is *possibly effective* for treatment of peripheral vascular diseases.

Nicotinyl tartrate (Roniacol)

Nicotinyl tartrate is the tartrate salt of nicotinyl alcohol. By its conversion to nicotinic acid in the body, nicotinyl tartrate produces direct peripheral vasodilation and increases blood flow to the extremities. Since it is oxidized slowly, it has a more prolonged effect than nicotinic acid.

Nicotinyl tartrate is used in the treatment of peripheral vascular diseases. It has been reported to be beneficial in relieving intermittent claudication of peripheral arteriosclerosis and thromboangiitis obliterans.

Side effects include flushing of face and neck, gastrointestinal disturbances, and allergic reactions.

It is available in 50-mg tablets and 150-mg timed released tablets and as an elixir, 50 mg/5 ml. It is given in doses of 50 to 150 mg three times a day after meals. Dose of timed-release tablets is 150 or 300 mg morning and evening.

Cyclandelate (Cyclospasmol)

Cyclandelate has a direct relaxation effect on the smoooth muscles of peripheral arterial walls. It increases peripheral circulation of the extremities and digits and elevates skin temperature of the extremities.

The drug is available in 100-mg tablets and 200-mg capsules for oral use. The usual dosage is 100 mg four times a day given before meals and at bedtime.

Side effects include tingling, flushing, sweating, dizziness, and headache.

Isoxsuprine hydrochloride (Vasodilan)

Isoxsuprine hydrochloride has potent inhibitory effects on vascular and uterine smooth muscle. It is used in the treatment of peripheral vascular spasm, Raynaud's and Buerger's diseases, and arteriosclerotic vascular disease.

Side effects are relatively mild and include light-headedness, dizziness, nausea, and vomiting. These effects usually subside with a reduction in dosage. Transient hypotension and tachycardia have also been reported.

It is available in 10- and 20-mg tablets. Oral dosage is 10 to 20 mg three or four times daily. Action occurs within 1 hour and persists for 3 hours after oral administration. An intramuscular preparation of 5 mg/ml in 2-ml containers is also available for acute and severe symptoms of arterial insufficiency. However, for prolonged use oral therapy is preferred.

Nylidrin hydrochloride (Arlidin)

Nylidrin hydrochloride is a beta adrenergic stimulating agent that causes dilation of the arterioles in skeletal muscles. This action is thought to increase the blood supply to the calf muscles of patients with intermittent claudication caused by arteriosclerosis obliterans or thromboangiitis obliterans. The drug is also used for circulatory disturbances of the inner ear, such as primary cochlear cell ischemia.

Oral dosage is 6 to 24 mg four times daily. Side effects include anxiety, palpitations, tachycardia, and postural hypotension.

Summary of nursing considerations

Hypertension is a condition in which blood pressure in the arterial system is persistently elevated above the normal level. Essential hypertension, which has an unknown cause, is characterized by arteriolar constriction and volume overload. These hemodynamic changes usually are associated with an elevation of plasma renin level. By contrast, the cause of secondary hypertension may be attributed to renal or endocrine dysfunctions for which, fortunately, specific surgical or medical treatment is available.

Although a variety of drugs are effectively used for the control of essential hypertension, they are not curative. The antihypertensive agents currently in use include the following drug groups: (1) sympatholytics, (2) vasodilators, and (3) diuretics.

The sympatholytic drugs exert their influence on various sites of the autonomic nervous system. Methyldopa and clonidine act as central sympathetic inhibitors, reducing blood pressure by decreasing sympathetic outflow from the brain. On the other hand, the action of the reserpine compounds is attributed to both a central and a peripheral inhibitory sympathetic response. These drugs deplete the storage sites of catecholamines in the brain, heart, and peripheral postganglionic neurons. The lowering of blood pressure is caused by a depletion of norepinephrine from the storage vesicles at the nerve terminals. Additionally, in the brain, serotonin levels are reduced. As a consequence, peripheral sympathetic nerve impulse transmission to the blood vessels is inhibited causing vasodilation and a lowering of blood pressure.

Unlike the reserpine compounds, guanethidine limits its action to the sympathetic neuroeffector junctions by inhibiting the release of norepinephrine at this site. Its potency makes it one of the agents of choice in the management of severe hypertension. Its most important complication is postural hypotension. An additional type of sympatholytic agent involves the beta adrenergic blocking agents. Propranolol, a nonselective beta adrenergic blocker, reduces cardiac output by suppressing sympathetic nerve stimulation in the heart and decreases fluid volume by inhibiting renin release from the kidneys. This drug is effective in the treatment of hypertension, particularly when used in combination with a diuretic. Unlike other sympathetic inhibitors, propranolol does not cause postural hypotension. Additional adrenergic blockers include metoprolol and nadolol.

The vasodilator drugs represent a group of antihypertensive agents that act directly on vascular smooth muscle to produce vasodilation. There are two categories: (1) arteriolar dilator drugs and (2) arteriolar and venous dilator drugs. The first category includes hydrolazine, diazoxide, and minoxidil, which reduce blood pressure by dilating the arterioles. Their effect is often accompanied by reflex cardiac stimulation; to decrease this side effect, these drugs are sometimes combined with propranolol.

Diazoxide is sometimes considered the drug of choice for treatment of hypertensive crisis because of its rapid onset of action; it does not require continuous infusion or cause extreme hypotension or sedation. Diazoxide can produce sodium and water retention and hyperglycemia. It should be used with caution in patients with diabetes or cerebrovascular or coronary artery disease. It is not safe for use during pregnancy and lactation. Minoxidil recently has been introduced as a potent arteriolar vasodilator. It has been used with success in the treatment of patients with severe or accelerated hypertension and impaired renal function. It is administered orally along with a beta adrenergic blocking agent and a diuretic to prevent reflex tachycardia and counteract sodium retention.

The arteriolar and venous dilator drugs represent the second subgroup of vasodilators. Sodium nitroprusside is an ideal agent for lowering blood pressure in hypertensive emergencies when other drugs have been ineffective. Its potent vasodilator effect exerts an immediate onset of action by acting on both the arteriolar resistance vessels and on the venous capacitance vessels. This drug requires continuous infusion to maintain its effect and should be replaced by other agents as soon as the blood pressure is under control. Prazosin, an alpha adrenergic blocker, also reduces blood pressure by causing arteriolar and venous dilation.

Pargyline, a monoamine oxidase inhibitor, takes 7 days before the cumulative effect is sufficient to lower blood pressure. Its common side effects include dry mouth, insomnia, nervousness, weight gain, and impotence. The patient is cautioned to avoid foods high in tyramine content because that substance releases norepinephrine, which can cause severe vasoconstriction. Pargyline should not be used concomitantly with amphetamines and antidepressants.

An additional method of antihypertensive therapy is based on the use of diuretic agents that lower blood pressure by promoting salt excretion, thereby reducing extracellular fluid volume. Among the oral diuretic drugs the thiazides are usually the agents of choice and generally are the first to be used for the treatment of hypertension. If other drugs are needed, either sympatholytic or vasodilator agents are added to the regimen. This permits control of blood pressure with smaller doses of the more potent agents. Another advantage of combined therapy with diuretics is that both sympatholytic (with the exception of beta adrenergic blocking agents) and vasodilator agents cause plasma volume expansion. Diuretics tend to prevent this uncomfortable secondary effect.

Patient teaching is a critically important part of nursing care for the patient receiving antihypertensive therapy. The patient should be cautioned to rise slowly from lying and from sitting, to avoid standing still for any length of time, to relieve dizziness by muscular activity or recumbency, and to exercise particular caution for 2 hours after taking drugs. It is also helpful to teach the patient to take his own blood pressure.

In the treatment of circulatory shock the *antihypotensive agents* exert their effects either by acting on the blood vessels or by restoring adequate circulatory volume. Vasoconstrictors are *contraindicated* in shock caused by hemorrhage. The use of vasodilators plus volume replacement has decreased mortality from circulatory shock.

The use of *peripheral vasodilator drugs* in chronic occlusive arterial disease has to date been very discouraging. They include nicotinyl tartrate, cyclandelate, isoxsuprine hydrochloride, and nilidrin hydrochloride. These have been used with some success in the treatment of chronic occlusive arterial disease or peripheral vascular disease.

QUESTIONS

FOR STUDY AND REVIEW

1 What is meant by essential hypertension? secondary hypertension? Explain how each type is treated.
2 What are the major groups of antihypertensive drugs? Explain how each group of antihypertensives lowers blood pressure.
3 What instructions should be given to the patient who experiences orthostatic hypotension from antihypertensive therapy?
4 Why do clonidine and methyldopa cause sedation? What is the nursing measure in preventing this condition?
5 Explain why a diuretic such as a thiazide is used as an initial treatment of hypertension? Why is it sometimes used in combination therapy?
6 What is the action of propranolol? In patients with what type of clinical disorders is the drug contraindicated?
7 Name two agents that are used to treat hypertensive crisis. How does each one lower blood pressure?
8 For what type of hypertension is minoxidil indicated? What distressing side effect does it cause?
9 Investigate the price and effectiveness of commercially available blood pressure equipment for the lay person.
10 Check and record your own blood pressure four times daily (for example, 8, 12, 4, and 8 o'clock) for 1 week. Analyze your findings.
11 Under what circumstances would vasoconstrictors be used to treat hypotension accompanying shock? When would vasodilators be used?

12 Of what value is dobutamine in the treatment of cardiogenic shock?

13 Name some drugs that are used as peripheral vasodilators in the treatment of peripheral vascular disease. How does isoxsuprine relieve Raynaud's disease?

BIBLIOGRAPHY

Avery, G.S., editor: Drug treatment, ed. 2, Acton, Mass., 1980, Publishing Sciences Group, Inc.

Bowman, W., and Rand, M.: Textbook of pharmacology, ed. 2, London, 1980, Blackwell Scientific Publications, Ltd.

Goodman, L.S., and Gilman, A., editors: The pharmacological basis of therapeutics, ed. 6, New York, 1980, Macmillan, Inc.

Meyers, F.H., Jawetz, E., and Goldfien, A.: Review of medical pharmacology, ed. 5, Los Altos, Calif., 1980, Lange Medical Publications, Inc.

Modell, W., editor: Drugs of choice, 1980-1981, St. Louis, 1980, The C.V. Mosby Co.

Mountcastle, V., editor: Medical physiology, ed. 14, St. Louis, 1980, The C.V. Mosby Co.

Sodeman, W., and Sodeman, T.: Pathologic physiology: mechanisms of disease, ed. 6, Philadelphia, 1979, W.B. Saunders Co.

ANTIHYPERTENSIVE DRUGS

Aagaard, G.M.: Treatment of hypertension, Am. J. Nurs. **73:**620, 1973.

A.M.A. Committee on Hypertension: Drug treatment of ambulatory patients with hypertension, J.A.M.A. **225:**1647, 1973.

A.M.A. Committee on Hypertension: The treatment of malignant hypertension and hypertensive emergencies, J.A.M.A. **228:**1673, 1974.

Eaton, M.: Methyldopa: heading off adverse reactions, Curr. Prescribing **8:**58, 1977.

Finnerty, F.A.: Hypertensive crisis, J.A.M.A. **229:**1479, 1974.

Frohlich, E.D.: Beta blockers in hypertension: their value and rationale, Med. Opinion **5:**12, 1976.

Frohlich, E.D., and others: Hypertension therapy—1974: symposium, Postgrad. Med. **56:**19, 1974.

Gifford, R.W., Jr.: Managing hypertension, Postgrad. Med. **61:**153, 1977.

Goldberg, L.I.: Current therapy of hypertension: a pharmacologic approach, Am. J. Med. **58:**489, 1975.

Grim, C., and others: Rapid blood pressure control with minoxidil, Arch. Intern. Med. **139:**529, 1979.

Halberstam, M.: The limits of hypertension: how they affect treatment, Mod. Med. **47:**11, Aug. 15-Sept. 15, 1979.

Holland, O.B., and Kaplan, N.M.: Propranolol in the treatment of hypertension, N. Engl. J. Med. **294:**930, 1976.

Kaplan, N.: Salt, diuretics and hypertension, Urban Health **9:**37, 1980.

Kilcoyne, M.: The developing phase of primary hypertension, Mod. Concepts Cardiovasr. Dis. **49:**19, 1980.

Kincaid-Smith, P.: Treatment of hypertension—the place of vasodilators, Clin. Ther. **1:**285, 1978.

Koch-Weser, J.: Hypertensive emergencies, N. Engl. J. Med. **290:**211, 1974.

Koch-Weser, J.: Individualization of antihypertensive therapy, Med. Clin. North Am. **58:**1027, 1974.

Koch-Weser, J.: Vasodilator drugs in the treatment of hypertension, Arch. Intern. Med. **133:**1017, 1974.

Kosman, M.E.: Evaluation of clonidine hydrochloride (Catapres): a new antihypertensive agent, J.A.M.A. **233:**174, 1975.

Kosman, M.E.: Evaluation of a new antihypertensive agent: prazosin hydrochloride (Minipress), J.A.M.A. **238:**157, 1977.

Long, M.L., and others: Hypertension: what patients need to know, Am. J. Nurs. **76:**765, 1976.

Maloney, R.: Helping your hypertensive patients live longer, Nursing '78, **8:**26, 1978.

Martin, J.D.: The management of hypertensive disease of pregnancy, Drugs **8:**125, 1974.

Materson, B.: Beta-adrenergic blocking agents in hypertension: pro and con, Consultant, **18:**98, Oct. 1978.

McKinstry, D.N., Willard, D.A., and Vukovich, R.A.: Antihypertensive and hormonal effects of the converting-enzyme inhibitor, captopril, alone or combined with hydrochlorothiazide, Clin. Pharmacol. Ther. **25:**237, 1979.

Moser, M., chairman: Report of the Joint National Committee on Detection, Evaluation, and Treatment of High Blood Pressure: a cooperative study, J.A.M.A. **237:**255, 1977.

Nies, A.S.: Adverse reactions and interactions limiting the use of antihypertensive drugs, Am. J. Med. **58:**495, 1975.

Onesti, G., and Brest, A., editors: Hypertension: mechanisms, diagnosis, and treatment, Philadelphia, 1978, F.A. Davis Co.

Owens, C.: Sustained release beta-blockade, Clin. Ther. **1:**319, 1978.

Palmer, R.F., and Lasseter, K.C.: Sodium nitroprusside, N. Engl. J. Med. **292:**294, 1975.

Putnam, P.: Clonidine (Catapres): a new antihypertensive agent, Heart Lung, **5:**457, 1976.

Ram, C.: Newer antihypertensive drugs, Heart Lung, **6:**679, 1977.

Riddlough, M.: Preventing, detecting and managing adverse reactions of antihypertensive agents in the ambulant patient with essential hypertension, Am. J. Hosp. Pharm. **34:**465, 1977.

Rodman, M.: Drug therapy today: how to cope with those new antihypertensive drugs, R.N., **42:**109, 1979.

Rubin, B., and Antonaccio, M.J.: Captopril, In Scriabine, A., editor: Pharmacology of antihypertensive drugs, New York, 1980, Raven Press, pp. 21-42.

Sambhi, M.P., and others: Essential hypertension: new concepts about mechanisms, Ann. Intern. Med. **79:**411, 1973.

Simpson, F.O.: β-Adrenergic receptor blocking drugs in hypertension, Drugs **7:**85, 1974.

Swartz, C., and others: Drug therapy of hypertension: current management and future agents, Medicine/Genesis **1:**12, 1975.

Vidt, D.G.: Management of hypertensive emergencies, Clin. Med. **82**(2):35, 1975.

Vidt, D.: Combination therapy in hypertension: a rational approach, Drug Therapy, p. 78, Aug. 1978.

ANTIHYPOTENSIVE DRUGS

Goldberg, L.I.: Dopamine—clinical uses of an endogenous catecholamine, N. Engl. J. Med. **291:**707, 1974.

Karliner, J.S.: Dopamine for cardiogenic shock, J.A.M.A. **226:**1217, 1973.

Molyneux-Luick, M., and Knecht, J.: The emergency that supercedes all other duties: hypovolemic shock, Nursing '77 **7**(11):32, 1977.

Reid, P.R., and Thompson, W.L.: The clinical use of dopa-mine in the treatment of shock, Johns Hopkins Med. J. **137:**276, 1975.

Wiley, L.: Staying ahead of shock, Nursing '74 **4**(4):19, 1974.

Wiley, L.: Shock. II. Different kinds—different problems, Nursing '74 **4**(5):43, 1974.

CHAPTER 20

Hematologic drugs

The drugs and agents discussed in this chapter include only those used to treat certain anemias, to influence blood clotting, and to replace blood volume.

Blood

The primary function of blood is to circulate through the tissues of the body and act as a transport system. Blood carries oxygen, nutrients, hormones, and other essential materials to the tissues and at the same time serves as a medium for the removal of carbon dioxide and additional waste products to organs of excretion.

Blood is classified as a liquid connective tissue. It consists of plasma, the liquid portion, and cellular elements that include red blood cells, white blood cells, and platelets. The white blood cells (leukocytes) are important for combating the invasion of foreign organisms. The platelets (thrombocytes) and plasma contain all the factors necessary for blood clotting. The red blood cells (erythrocytes) are vital for oxygen transport from the lungs to the tissues and carbon dioxide transport from the tissues to the lungs.

The blood cell concerned with various types of anemia is the erythrocyte. The term "anemia" implies that there is a relative deficiency of red cells or hemoglobin or both. The deficit may be caused by inadequate formation of erythrocytes, blood loss, abnormal destruction of erythrocytes, or a combination of these factors. The building materials necessary for normal red cell maturation include vitamin B_{12}, folic acid, and intrinsic factor from the stomach mucosa. Iron is important for the formation of hemoglobin. The absence of any one of these factors can lead to failure of normal development of the red blood cell and thereby cause some form of anemia.

Production of the normal red blood cell

The red blood cells have a life span of 120 days, after which time they break down and are replaced by new cells. To maintain normal quantities of erythrocytes required for the transport of oxygen to the tissues, the body must continuously generate new mature cells. After birth, the formation of blood cells takes place solely within the red bone marrow.

ERYTHROPOIESIS

The process of red blood cell formation is termed "erythropoiesis." This is associated with the substance called *erythropoietic stimulating factor* or *erythropoietin*, a glycoprotein that is synthesized in the kidney. Because patients with chronic renal failure have a decreased production of this hormone, anemia almost always becomes an accompanying clinical problem.

Erythropoietic action. Erythropoiesis is initiated by tissue hypoxia resulting from either decreased oxygen tension or decreased oxygen content of arterial blood. Hypoxia provides the stimulus to release erythropoietin from the kidneys. The hormone then enters the bone marrow, where it increases the rate of production of red blood cells. Erythropoietin appears to exert its major effect on the stem cells by accelerating their differentiation into erythroblasts. (See Fig. 20-1, *A*, for erythropoietic action.)

Genesis of the red blood cell. The stem cells or hemocytoblasts are the initial cells that later differentiate into proerythroblasts. Both of these cell types contain a round nucleus. As maturation continues, a gradual development of hemoglobin in the cytoplasm of the erythroblast begins. Following this, the nucleus of the cell shrinks and the normoblast is formed. When the nucleus is finally extruded from the cell, it becomes a reticulocyte. The cell contains a dense fibrous network of threads, and during this stage the reticulocyte is released into the circulation. By now a large quantity of iron-containing hemoglobin has been synthesized. Following disappearance of the reticulum, the cell finally becomes a mature erythrocyte. (See Fig. 20-1, *B*, for normal maturation of the red blood cell.)

Materials required. The formation of red cells and hemoglobin is a complex process, and deficiency in any one of a number of constituents may result in failure to produce the needed number of red cells or an adequate amount of hemoglobin.

Some factors that promote formation of red blood cells are:

1 A diet adequate in essentials for production of mature red blood cells; namely, the antianemic factor (vitamin B_{12}), folic acid, and iron
2 Normal gastrointestinal tract activity to ensure adequate digestion and absorption of needed essentials
3 A liver able to store iron as well as vitamin B_{12}. It has been observed that chronic disease of the liver leads to anemia. Much of the iron needed for synthesis of hemoglobin is salvaged from erythrocytes.
4 Normal activity of blood-forming tissues, particularly the red bone marrow of the adult

Vitamin B_{12}. The development of red cells requires vitamin B_{12}, a cobalt-containing molecule essential for maturation of the nucleus of the cell. By promoting the conversion of ribose nucleotide into deoxyribose nucleotide, the vitamin acts as a coenzyme required for deoxyribonucleic acid (DNA) synthesis. The nucleus contains large quantities of DNA, which functions in cell division and thus promotes the formation of greater numbers of red cells. By contrast, a deficiency of vitamin B_{12} results in the cell's inability to divide at a normal rate and to mature in a normal form. Consequently, fewer but larger and less mature cells are formed.

Since vitamin B_{12} is not synthesized in the body, adequate dietary intake is necessary. However, maturation failure of the red cell also may occur because of inability to absorb the vitamin from the gastrointestinal tract. Absorption of vitamin B_{12} requires *intrinsic factor*, a mucoprotein secreted by the parietal cells in the stomach. Intrinsic factor facilitates absorption by binding to the ingested vitamin B_{12} *(extrinsic factor)* in the stomach. The resulting complex travels to the ileum and becomes adsorbed to specific receptor sites on the brush border membranes of the mucosal cells. After

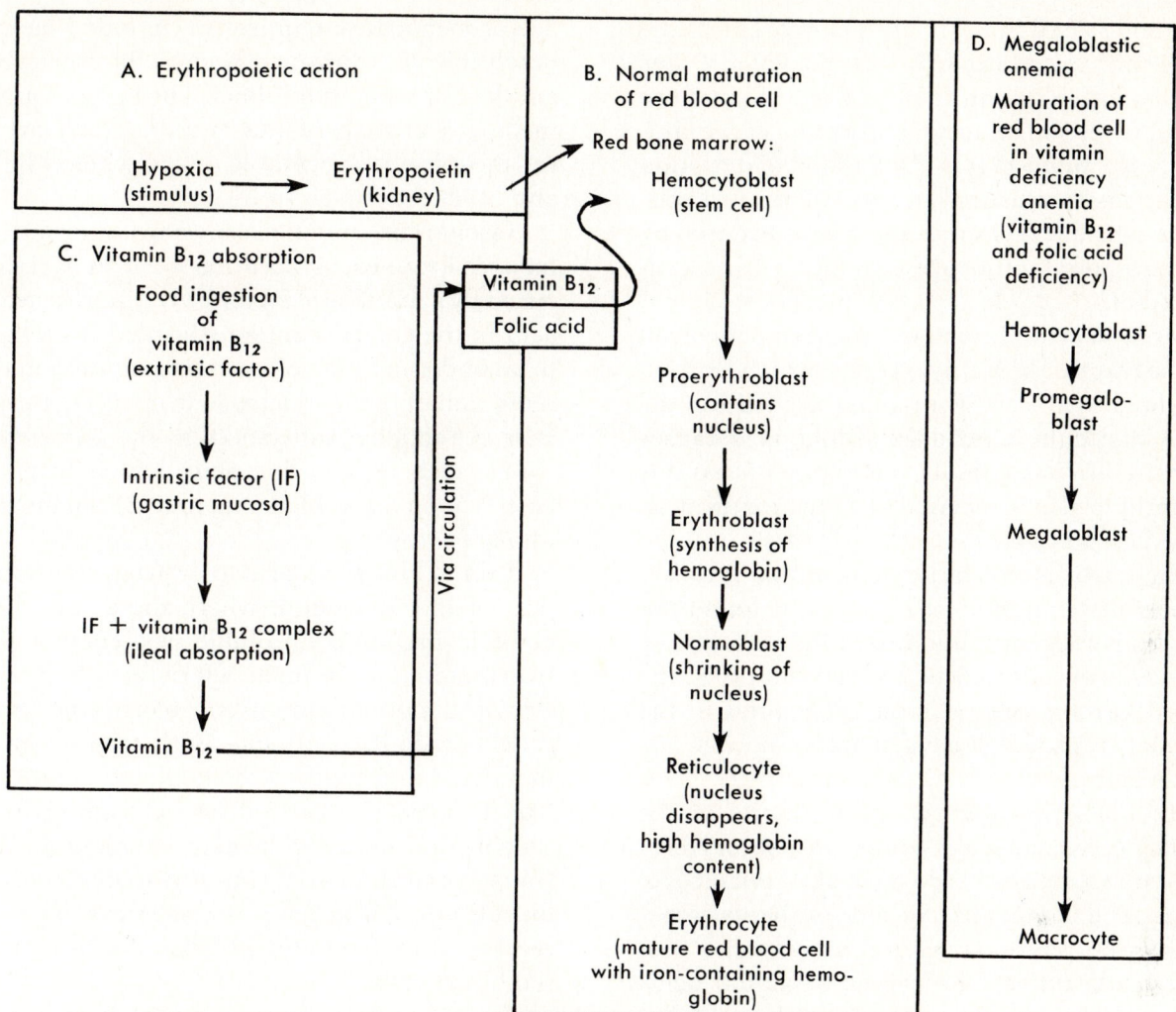

FIG. 20-1. Production of the normal red blood cell.

A. Erythropoietic action: Hypoxia stimulates the release of erythropoietin from the kidney. This hormone activates the red bone marrow to initiate the differentiation of the hemocytoblast, the stem cell. The development of the cell then progresses to the formation of the erythroblast.

B. Normal maturation of red blood cell: The genesis of the red blood cell shows the steps of development from the hemocytoblast to the erythrocyte, the mature red blood cell containing hemoglobin.

C. Vitamin B₁₂ absorption: Dietary vitamin B_{12}, when ingested, combines with the intrinsic factor *(IF)*, a mucoprotein secreted by the parietal cells in the gastric mucosa. This complex is transported to the ileum and becomes adsorbed to the receptor sites on the brush border membranes of the mucosal cells. After transport across the membrane, vitamin B_{12} is released into the circulation and is stored in the liver. It enters the bone marrow as needed for maturation of the red cell. Folic acid is required for DNA synthesis and also is essential for the maturation of the red cell.

D. Megaloblastic anemia: Deficiency of vitamin B_{12} and folic acid results in faulty maturation of the red blood cell. Because DNA replication is impaired, fewer and larger cells are formed. The erythroblastic cells of the bone marrow become larger than normal, developing into megaloblasts. Rather than the mature erythrocyte, the macrocyte is formed.

the complex is transported across the membrane, vitamin B_{12} is released into the circulation and stored in the liver. It slowly enters the bone marrow as needed. (See Fig. 20-1, *C*, for absorption of vitamin B_{12}.) Lack of intrinsic factor results in failure of absorption of the vitamin. Also, much of it is lost because of digestion by the gastrointestinal enzymes. Therefore during a deficiency, vitamin B_{12} is administered by the parenteral route to bypass the gastrointestinal tract.

Folic acid. Folic acid is a coenzyme involved in the transfer of methyl groups, which leads to the final synthesis of thymine needed for the DNA molecule. Since lack of folic acid causes impaired DNA synthesis, it is apparent that this vitamin is also associated with the maturation of red blood cells.

Iron. Iron is a metallic element that is rather widely distributed in the body. It is found not only in hemoglobin but also in the cytochrome pigments of cells and as a reserve supply in the blood-forming organs. Iron is essential to the normal transport of oxygen and to normal tissue respiration.

In the bone marrow the synthesis of the hemoglobin molecule begins in the erythroblasts and continues through the reticulocyte stage. The compound consists of the iron-containing porphyrin structure, *heme*, and a protein made up of four chains of amino acids called *globin*. Each molecule of hemoglobin consists of four molecules of heme. Thus one molecule of hemoglobin contains four atoms of iron, one in each heme group, and is able to unite four molecules of oxygen. Molecular oxygen is bound reversibly by the iron of the hemoglobin for transport throughout the body. On arrival at the tissue, oxidation of the iron causes hemoglobin to give up its oxygen.

IRON REQUIREMENTS IN HUMANS. Since much of the iron salvaged from worn-out red cells is reused in the body, only a small amount (1 to 2 mg) must be absorbed from the diet to maintain a positive iron balance. During periods of rapid growth and development the body's need for iron is correspondingly increased. Pregnancy, early childhood, early adolescence (especially in girls), and menopause constitute periods when the iron content should probably be increased either by increased dietary intake or medicinal iron or both. Women up through the age of menopause require two to four times as much iron as adult men because of pregnancy and loss of menstrual blood. The body requirements are ordinarily met by a diet adequate in red meats, green vegetables, eggs, whole wheat, and other foods rich in iron.

ABSORPTION, METABOLISM, AND EXCRETION OF IRON COMPOUNDS. Absorption of iron is influenced by a number of factors: (1) the presence of acid in the gastric content (the acid is thought to favor dissociation of iron compounds and the reduction of ferric to ferrous iron), (2) the presence of reducing substances in the alimentary canal, such as ascorbic acid, which helps to keep iron in a soluble form, and (3) the dietary intake of iron.

Iron is absorbed primarily from the upper part of the duodenum where the acidity prevents formation of insoluble iron compounds. Iron is stored in the form of ferritin or hemosiderin in bone marrow, liver, spleen, and other reticuloendothelial tissue. Both forms can be mobilized and used for hemoglobin synthesis. Iron transport is carried on by transferrin, a specific iron-binding protein in plasma. The transfer of iron to maturing erythrocytes occurs by release of iron from transferrin to specific receptor sites on the membranes of immature red blood cells.

Most iron used for new erythrocyte formation comes from disintegrated red blood cells, whose life span is about 120 days. Approximately 25 mg of iron daily comes from this source. At best the amount of iron actually absorbed from the gastrointestinal tract is small, about 1 to 2 mg daily. This is usually adequate since the body is extremely protective of its iron supply.

Iron is not readily eliminated from the body; that which is eliminated was probably not absorbed. It is excreted primarily via the intestinal tract. Only minute traces of iron are excreted via the urinary tract.

Deficiency of iron results in interference with the synthesis of a normal amount of hemoglobin. This leads to the development of smaller or microcytic cells. As synthesis of hemoglobin is further restricted, the microcytic cells lack pigment and become hypochromic. For this reason iron-deficiency anemia is sometimes called hypochromic microcytic anemia.

Antianemic drugs

An anemic state is one in which the concentration of hemoglobin in the red blood cell falls below the normal range. One cause of anemia may be a deficiency of factors essential for normal blood formation. As already discussed, these factors include iron, vitamin B_{12}, and folic acid.

Although an adequate diet is the preferable way to acquire the essential constituents for blood formation, various disease conditions require treatment that brings about more rapid results than can be obtained from diet alone.

Antianemic drug therapy is aimed at eliminating the cause of anemia or at symptomatic relief. Vitamin or hormonal deficiency may lead to anemia; specific examples are deficiency of ascorbic acid or of thyroid or adrenocortical hormones. Replacement of any of these missing substances can be considered specific therapy for the corresponding anemia.

The major antianemic drugs discussed here include those used to treat iron-deficiency anemia and vitamin-deficiency or megaloblastic anemia (deficiency of vitamin B_{12} and folic acid). Inadequate absorption of vitamin B_{12} results in pernicious anemia.

IRON-DEFICIENCY ANEMIA

Iron deficiency results in a form of anemia in which the red blood cells are hypochromic and microcytic—the red blood cells contain less hemoglobin (and therefore have a low color index) and are smaller than normal. It occurs following *hemorrhage* or in persons with an *inadequate supply of iron*. The major and only significant way of losing iron from the body to such an extent that anemia develops is by blood loss resulting from a sudden acute large hemorrhage or a slow insidious loss from menorrhagia, hemorrhoids, or a silent ulcer or tumor of the gastrointestinal tract.

Iron is used prophylactically in pregnancy, for premature infants, and for those whose diet contains an inadequate amount of iron, (such as a diet for peptic ulcer) to prevent anemia from occurring.

Iron-deficiency anemia is associated with symptoms of low vitality, pallor of the skin and mucous membrane, fatigue, and poor appetite. It is treated with iron, which results in an increased rate of production of red blood cells. Within about 3 days of treatment, the concentration of hemoglobin and hematocrit, begins to increase.

IRON PREPARATIONS

Action and results. Iron preparations cause various effects after ingestion to treat iron-deficiency anemia. These effects can be grouped as local effects and systemic effects.

Local effects. When inorganic iron compounds are administered orally, iron acts as an irritant and astringent. It reacts with tissue proteins and forms an insoluble iron compound. Irritation and astringent effects along the gastrointestinal tract may cause nausea and vomiting, constipation or diarrhea, and abdominal distress. Solutions of ferric iron are sometimes used for their strong astringent properties. They are applied externally as styptics. Organic forms do not cause the same irritation because they dissociate with difficulty.

Systemic effects. The action for which iron is most often administered is its hematopoietic one. If iron reserves of the body are depleted, they are restored when ample amounts are administered. It is believed that the action of iron in conditions of deficiency is largely to supply that which is needed for the hemoglobin molecule. Iron is of value only in hypochromic anemias or those in which the color index is low. Iron therapy in this condition can be expected to result in increased vigor on the part of the patient, increased resistance to fatigue, improved condition of the skin and nails, improved appetite, and general feeling of well-being. In other words, it brings about a tonic effect. When administered to individuals with normal blood values, it does not bring about an increase in the hemoglobin but only increases the reserve supply of iron in the body.

In the case of hypochromic anemias maximum response may be expected between the second and the fourth week. Favorable response may, however, be inhibited by vitamin deficiency, infection, achlorhydria, hepatic disorder, or disorders of absorption in the intestine. If the iron deficiency is a severe one, other forms of therapy may be needed to supplement the iron therapy. Blood transfusion will restore the blood more rapidly than anything else that can be done. The physician is likely to maintain that the major medical indication, apart from replacing iron, is to find the source of blood loss. Leading hematologists have criticized treating iron-deficiency anemia without investigating the possible cause.

Chlorosis, an iron-deficiency condition in its classic form, has largely disappeared, but a similar although mild grade of anemia in girls of adolescent years (ages 14 to 20) is still a common finding. It responds well to iron therapy.

Preparation, dosage, and administration. It is widely accepted that ferrous salts are better absorbed than ferric salts and that oral administration is preferable to parenteral. Large doses of iron are usually given, since only 15% of an oral dose is absorbed. Oral preparations are best absorbed when taken between meals. However, administration after meals tends to reduce gastrointestinal irritation. The concomitant administration of orange juice or ascorbic acid is sometimes used, since either acts as a reducing agent to aid absorption.

ORAL IRON PREPARATIONS

Ferrous sulfate (Feosol, Mol-Iron). Ferrous sulfate is the most widely used form of iron and is very economical. It is always given orally as a tablet, extended-release capsule, or elixir. The tablets are often enteric coated, since ferrous sulfate rapidly oxidizes in air to form ferric sulfate. The average dose of ferrous sulfate for adults is 300 mg to 1.2 g daily. Dosage range for infants and children is usually 75 to 600 mg daily. Dosage must be individually determined according to the severity of anemia.

Ferrous gluconate (Fergon). Ferrous gluconate is available in tablet, capsule, and liquid forms. Dosage is usually 320 to 640 mg daily; dosage for children is 100 to 300 mg daily. It is said to have less tendency to cause gastric distress and is better tolerated by some patients than is ferrous sulfate.

Ferrous fumarate (Ircon). It is claimed that ferrous fumarate is better tolerated than either the sulfate or gluconate preparations. It is available as tablets, chewable tablets, and sustained-release forms. The usual adult dose is 600 to 800 mg three or four times daily.

Ferrocholinate (Chel-Iron, Ferrolip). Ferrocholinate is a chelated (bound) form of iron that is believed to be less toxic and better tolerated than some of the older preparations such as ferrous sulfate and ferrous gluconate. At the same time it is said to be clinically effective in the treatment of iron-deficiency anemia. It is administered orally and can be given between meals. It is available in tablets, as a syrup, and as a solution. The proposed dose is 330 to 660 mg three times daily for adults.

Side effects and toxic effects. Long-continued administration of iron may cause headache, loss of appetite, gastric pain, nausea, vomiting, and constipation or diarrhea. Patients should be forewarned of the possibility of abdominal cramps and diarrhea when taking certain preparations of iron. If only the latter symptoms develop, the drug can be stopped for a day or two and then resumed. Patients should also be told that oral preparations will usually cause the stool to be dark red or black. If many untoward symptoms develop, it may be necessary to take a longer rest period before resuming administration. Tolerance to iron is apparently not developed.

Serious acute poisoning can result from ingestion of large doses of iron compounds. Most cases of severe poisoning have occurred in young children who have swallowed many tablets of ferrous sulfate. Some deaths have been reported. Preparations of iron should be kept out of the reach of children. The signs and symptoms of poisoning are those of gastrointestinal irritation, destruction of tissue, and shock.

Precautions. To avoid injury or staining of the teeth, solutions should be well diluted with water or fruit juice and taken through a glass tube or straw. Iron stains on linen and clothing may be removed with oxalic acid.

PARENTERAL IRON PREPARATIONS

The preferable route of administration of iron is usually the oral one. However, the following conditions are indications for parenteral administration: (1) for patients with hypochromic anemia who do not tolerate oral iron preparations, (2) for those who do not absorb iron well from the gastrointestinal tract or who have gastrointestinal complications such as ulceration or severe diarrhea, (3) for those who for one reason or another cannot be relied on to take the iron orally, such as certain aged or the mentally disturbed, and (4) for those in whom a maximal rate of hemoglobin regeneration is needed, such as patients with severe iron deficiency (patients before surgery for which there is immediate need or patients in the last trimester of pregnancy).

Iron-dextran injection (Imferon). Iron-dextran injection is a colloidal suspension of ferric hydroxide in complex with partially hydrolyzed low molecular weight dextran. The preparation is stable, has a pH of 6, and contains 50 mg elemental iron/ml. It is available in 2- and 5-ml ampules and in 10-ml vials. It is *effective* for treatment of iron-deficiency anemia. Total dosage is calculated by determining the approximate extent of the hemoglobin deficit and adjusting the daily dose accordingly. The initial dose is usually 50 mg on the first day, and amounts up to 250 mg may be given every day or every other day thereafter until the amount needed has been given. Dosage for children is 25 to 100 mg daily. The intramuscular preparation is given by deep injection into the gluteal muscle. The Z-track technique is recommended to avoid brown staining of tissue. The subcutaneous tissue should be pushed aside before insertion of the needle to prevent leakage along the tract of the needle. Occlusion of the injection site occurs when the tissues return to their natural position. The initial intravenous dose is 15 to 30 mg; this is increased by 10 mg daily until the hemoglobin level returns to normal. The maximum dose is 100 mg. It should be given slowly, 1 ml in 2 minutes, and the patient should rest 15 to 30 minutes after each dose. The total dose may also be infused in 500 to 1000 ml 5% dextrose solution over a 12-hour period.

Iron sorbitex (Jectofer); iron sorbitol. Iron sorbitex is an intramuscular preparation of iron in combination with sorbitol and citric acid. It is available in 2-ml ampules that contain 50 mg

iron/ml. Iron sorbitex is rapidly absorbed (50% to 70% within 3 hours and up to 95% within 24 hours after injection). It is primarily excreted in the urine, and the urine of patients receiving this drug may turn dark. Dosage must be determined individually for each patient.

Side effects. Side effects from parenteral administration of iron include headache, nausea, vomiting, muscle ache, fever, and mild urticaria. Severe anaphylactic reactions can also occur. Parenteral iron should not be administered concomitantly with oral iron preparations.

Pain sometimes occurs at the site of intramuscular injection, and there may be permanent brownish discoloration of the skin at the injection site. Injection of an iron preparation outside a vein may cause a severe local reaction. When iron is administered orally there is a limit to which it will be absorbed, but when it is injected into the bloodstream an overdose may be serious, partly because there is no satisfactory way for the body to excrete the ingested amount that exceeds what the body can use or can store as a normal reserve. It is deposited in organs such as the liver or pancreas and may cause hemochromatosis.

IRON ANTIDOTE

Deferoxamine (Desferrioxamine B, Desferal). Deferoxamine is a polyhydroxamic acid found in combination with iron in certain microorganisms. Deferoxamine is an iron-chelating agent; that is, it has great affinity for iron, removes iron from its tissue storage form (ferritin), binds the iron, and blocks its absorption.

Deferoxamine is used to treat iron overloading that may result from ingestion of large quantities of iron over a long period of time or from a metabolic abnormality that permits absorption of large amounts of iron from the diet, thereby increasing iron storage. This condition is termed hemosiderosis if no tissue damage occurs and hematochromatosis if tissue damage results. Deferoxamine is also used to treat iron poisoning.

Deferoxamine may be given intramuscularly or intravenously and by direct instillation into the stomach via gastric tube. Rapid urinary excretion of iron occurs after parenteral administration.

MEGALOBLASTIC ANEMIAS

In megaloblastic anemia, the deficiency of either vitamin B_{12} or folic acid results in faulty cell division and maturation. The rate of red cell production therefore is decreased because of slower and less frequent mitosis than normal. This deficiency also leads to the formation of larger and less mature cells. Because DNA replication is impaired, the erythroblastic cells of the bone marrow become larger than normal, developing into megaloblasts and in place of the mature erythrocyte, the macrocyte is formed. (See Fig. 20-1, *D*, for the changes in red blood cell formation that occur in megaloblastic anemias.)

VITAMIN PREPARATIONS

Vitamin B_{12} (cyanocobalamin)

One of the major developments in nutrition in the past 50 years began with the recognition by Minot and Murphy in 1926 that a substance in liver could cure the hitherto fatal disease pernicious anemia. Their discovery led to the eventual isolation by other scientists of the pure compound, at first called "antianemic factor" in 1948, and in 1956 the elucidation of the structure of this molecule—vitamin B_{12}. Vitamin B_{12} is an antipernicious anemia vitamin. It is an extremely complex and large organic molecule containing the metal cobalt. It has a structure similar to that of heme, the iron-bearing porphyrin in the hemoglobin molecule.

There is no lack of vitamin B_{12} in a normal diet. Even without a dietary supply, evidence shows that there is sufficient formation of the vitamin by bacteria normally present in the intestine of humans and other mammals. The patient with pernicious anemia therefore, in a sense, starves in the midst of plenty, since there is a lack of intrinsic factor necessary for absorption of vitamin B_{12}. The deficiency of intrinsic factor can occur in gastric malignancy because of atrophy of cells in the gastric mucosa that produce the compound.

For this reason, it is also possible to supply the vitamin indirectly by giving the patient a preparation of dried gastric mucosa containing intrinsic factor and thereby enabling him to absorb his own vitamin B_{12} from the diet. The surest way of remedying a deficiency, however, is to give the vitamin directly by injection, and this is the most common way of treating pernicious anemia.

When the body is deficient of vitamin B_{12} over a period of time, a series of characteristic symptoms and pathologic changes develops. The onset is gradual, and the early symptoms are usually fatigue, sore tongue, and achlorhydria. The patient has a peculiar yellowish pallor and complains of increasing weakness, breathlessness, itching, dyspepsia, and diarrhea. Degenerative changes in the nervous system also occur, giving rise to incoordination of movement, loss of vibratory sense (as a result of changes in the dorsal columns of the spinal cord), peripheral neuritis, optic atrophy, and, sometimes, psychosis. Death may result from the changes associated with pernicious anemia unless the changes are arrested, which is accomplished effectively with the administration of vitamin B_{12}.

Uses. Pernicious anemia is one of the megaloblastic anemias for which the administration of vitamin B_{12} is effective either as the pure vitamin or in a preparation of liver. It constitutes a form of replacement therapy, and administration must be continued indefinitely. It corrects the abnormalities of the red blood cells, relieves the sore mouth and tongue, restores normal function of the peripheral nerves, and arrests the progression of changes in the central nervous system. In some cases the changes in the nervous system are reversed if the irreversible stage of degeneration has not been reached. Vitamin B_{12} is also used in certain nutritional macrocytic anemias and for tropical and nontropical sprue. Beneficial effects have been reported in a number of neurologic disorders and in anemia occurring after gastrectomy because the cells that produce the intrinsic factor have been removed.

Preparation, dosage, and administration. Cyanocobalamin is a red crystalline substance that contains cobalt; it is obtained from cultures of *Streptomyces griseus* as a by-product in the manufacture of antibiotics. Because there is a group of closely related B_{12} factors, the activity of any preparation coming from natural sources may result from several members of this group. Before the availability of pure vitamin B_{12}, liver was administered extensively, since it contains vitamin B_{12}. This is now considered scientifically obsolete, since liver preparations have no advantage over the pure vitamin but have several distinct disadvantages—liver is more expensive, may be painful to receive, and is allergenic in some persons.

Cyanocobalamin is available in a variety of preparations for injection. The parenteral dosage for adults is 100 to 1000 µg daily for 1 week followed by the same dose one to three times weekly until remission occurs. The remission maintenance dose is 100 to 1000 µg every 4 weeks. For patients with neurologic damage, 1000 µg may be given one or more times weekly for several months, then once or twice weekly for a year. If neurologic damage is not reversed by that time, it is probably irreversible. The dosage for children is 1000 to 5000 µg given in doses of 100 µg over a period of 2 or more weeks, then 30 to 50 µg every 4 weeks. Oral doses are inadequate for treating pernicious anemia.

Side effects and toxic effects. No serious side effects or toxic effects have been reported following administration of vitamin B_{12}, even after large parenteral doses. Allergic reactions have occurred rarely and were probably caused by the preservatives or impurities in the preparation.

Hydrochloric acid

Since nearly all patients with pernicious anemia have a lack of hydrochloric acid in the stomach, full doses of the official dilute hydrochloric acid may be prescribed for the patient. This is given with meals not only to aid digestion but also to act as a gastric antiseptic. The usual dose is ½ to 1 fluidram, which is well diluted with water (one-third to one-half glass) and sipped through a tube to avoid damage to the teeth.

Folic acid (Folvite)

The chemical name for folic acid is pteroylglutamic acid. It is a member of the vitamin B complex and can be prepared synthetically. It is found only in small amounts in the free state in a number of foods.

Folic acid is an important maturation factor for a large number of cells. As previously mentioned, it participates in the synthesis of amino acids and DNA during the early phases of maturation of the erythrocyte. DNA deficiency interferes with cell mitosis, and this may result in the development of large cells (megaloblasts) that are characteristic of megaloblastic anemias.

Folic acid has been used as a supplement to therapy in the treatment of pernicious anemia. It produces a response in blood similar to that produced by iron therapy. The hemoglobin and red cell levels increase to normal, and bone marrow returns to its normal state. The appetite improves, and the patient feels better in general. In most patients the blood response is apparently maintained indefinitely with folic acid. It does not, however, prevent the development or the progression of neurologic changes that are often a part of the disease, and it may in fact make them worse. Because of this, it cannot be recognized as adequate therapy for pernicious anemia and cannot replace vitamin B_{12}. It is therefore dangerous when used alone for this condition, and the presence of folic acid in many multivitamin preparations adds to the hazard of this type of irrational therapy when it is used in the treatment of an undiagnosed anemia.

Uses. This drug is used for therapy of megaloblastic anemia caused by deficiency of folic acid. Although folic acid should not be employed in the treatment of pernicious anemia except possibly as a supplement to adequate therapy with vitamin B_{12}, it is used for the treatment of selected cases of megaloblastic anemias and of nutritional and metabolic disorders associated with such anemias. It frequently is useful in the treatment of an anemia of pregnancy. It is sometimes used in the treatment of anemia associated with tropical sprue and celiac disease, although there is some question as to whether it constitutes complete therapy.

Preparation, dosage, and administration. Folic acid is marketed in 0.25- and 1-mg tablets for oral administration, and as a solution for injection, 5 mg/ml. The usual oral and parenteral dose for adults and children is 0.25 to 1 mg daily. Folic acid injection is the same as sodium folate. It is the preparation preferred for parenteral therapy. Folic acid is nontoxic, but allergic reactions may occur.

Agents affecting blood coagulation

Hemostasis

Hemostasis is a process that spontaneously arrests blood loss from damaged blood vessels. Blood is normally fluid while circulating in the vessels, but on injury it rapidly clots when shed. To maintain normal liquid blood flow in the vascular system, a dynamic balance exists between clot dissolution involving anticoagulant factors and clot formation implicating procoagulant factors. Following any injury to the blood vessel, hemostasis is achieved by three sequential steps: (1) blood vessel constriction to retard blood flow from the injured area, (2) platelet plug formation to seal the leaking vessels, and (3) blood coagulation to plug openings within the damaged vessels and wounds to prevent further bleeding.

Blood vessel constriction. Immediately after a blood vessel is injured, vascular constriction occurs as a reflex response. This local myogenic contractile response instantaneously retards the flow of blood from the ruptured vessel.

Platelet plug formation. Platelets (thrombocytes) originate from giant cells called megakaryocytes found in the bone marrow. When giant cells disintegrate into minute colorless oval disks, they are released into the blood as platelets. Following injury to a blood vessel, interruption of the continuity of its endothelial lining exposes the collagen (a fibrous protein) in the underlying connective tissue. Immediately, platelets adhere to the exposed collagen to form a dense aggregate, a process known as *platelet adhesion*. This attachment triggers the release of adenosine diphosphate (ADP), which causes the outer surface of the platelets to become extremely sticky so that other adjacent platelets adhere to one another at the damaged site (platelet aggregation). This process gives rise to the eventual formation of the *platelet plug*. Because this plug is relatively unstable, it can stop bleeding quickly as long as the damage to the vessel is minute. However, for long-term effectiveness, the platelet plug must be reinforced by fibrin. This involves a chemical mechanism called blood coagulation.

Blood coagulation. Blood coagulation represents the final stage of an exceedingly complex succession of events occurring in hemostasis. The process ultimately results in the formation of a stable fibrin clot, which is composed of a meshwork of fibrin threads that entraps platelets, blood cells, and plasma. Thus the physical formation of a *blood clot* or *thrombus* plays a key role in hemostasis by permanently closing the hole in the injured vessel to prevent further bleeding.

The chemical events in the blood coagulation mechanism involve two distinct pathways: the intrinsic pathway and the extrinsic pathway.

Intrinsic pathway. Because all the chemical substances involved in coagulation are normally found within the circulating blood, this pathway is referred to as the intrinsic system of coagulation. In this pathway, activation of specific blood coagulation factors is initiated by injury to the endothelial lining of the blood vessel wall. When blood comes in contact with the exposed underlying collagen, this activates the Hageman factor (factor XII) by enzymatically converting it to the active form (factor XIIa). The simultaneous damage of platelets also causes the release of platelet phospholipid (platelet factor 3), which is required later in the coagulation process. Factor XIIa then activates factor XI to XIa. The reaction of factor XIa with factor IX requires calcium ions to form activated factor IX. In the presence of calcium ions and platelet phospholipid, factor IXa interacts with factor VIII and thrombin to form a complex, and this combination then accelerates the activation of factor X. Factor Xa combines with factor V, Ca^{++}, and platelet phospholipid to form a complex known as the prothrombin activator (factor IIa). Factor IIa initiates the cleavage of prothrombin to form thrombin, which then enzymatically converts fibrinogen into fibrin, forming an unstable clot. The final step involves the action of factor XIII (a fibrin-stabilizing factor), thrombin, and Ca^{++}, which catalyze

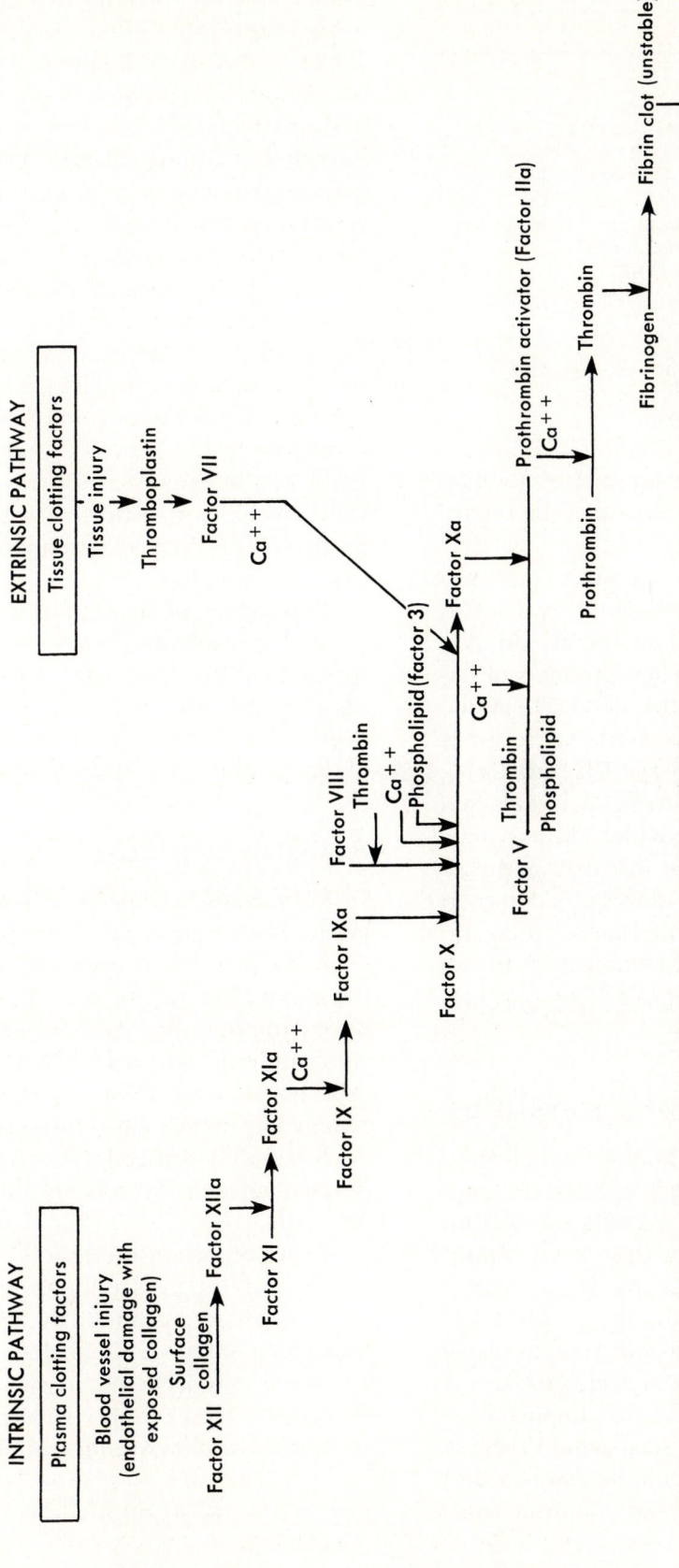

FIG. 20-2. Coagulation mechanism showing the steps in the intrinsic pathway and the extrinsic pathway for initiating blood clotting. The protein factors are present in plasma as inactive precursors. The letter *a* following a Roman numeral indicates an activated factor. See Table 20-1 for synonyms of coagulation factors.

T A B L E 2 0 - 1 Blood coagulation factors and synonyms

Factor	Name or synonym
I	Fibrinogen
II	Prothrombin
III	Tissue thromboplastin
IV	Calcium
V	Proaccelerin (labile factor, accelerator globulin)
VII	Proconvertin (stable factor, serum prothrombin conversion accelerator [SPCA])
VIII	Antihemophilic factor (AHF)
IX	Plasma thromboplastin component, Christmas factor
X	Stuart-Prower factor
XI	Plasma thromboplastin antecedent (PTA)
XII	Hageman factor
XIII	Fibrin stabilizing factor

the formation of a stronger, stabilizing clot. Fig. 20-2 summarizes the main events of the intrinsic pathway.

Extrinsic pathway. The extrinsic pathway begins with trauma to the vascular wall or to the tissues outside the blood vessels. In this pathway, clotting occurs when products of tissue damage gain access to the blood. The tissue factor thromboplastin is released and becomes part of a complex with factor VII and Ca^{++}. This combination of components activates factor X, which is the step at which the extrinsic pathway covergcs with thc intrinsic pathway and coagulation continues through a common route with the resultant formation of a final stable clot. (See Fig. 20-2 for the extrinsic pathway and Table 20-1 for synonyms of blood coagulation factors.)

Blood coagulation abnormalities

Diseases associated with abnormal clotting within vessels take a great toll of lives. It is estimated that over a million persons suffer from thrombosis or embolism in the United States each year. Diseases caused by intravascular clotting include some of the major causes of death from cardiovascular sources—coronary occlusion and cerebrovascular accidents. Drugs that inhibit clotting are therefore important.

Local trauma, vascular stasis, and systemic alterations in coagulability of blood are considered the principal etiologic factors in the initiation of thrombosis.

Basically, the coagulation mechanisms are responsible for forming two kinds of thrombi: arterial thrombi and venous thrombi. Arterial thrombi are most frequently associated with atherosclerotic plaques, high blood pressure, and turbulent blood flow that damages the endothelial lining of the blood vessel and causes platelets to stick and aggregate in the arterial system. Arterial thrombi are platelet or white thrombi and their formation is associated with the intrinsic pathway of the coagulation mechanism.

Venous thrombi occur most often in areas where blood flow is reduced or static. This appears to initiate clotting and produce a red thrombus in the venous system. Its formation involves the extrinsic pathway of the coagulation mechanism. Current anticoagulants are more effective in preventing venous rather than arterial thrombi.

Prevention of arterial thrombi requires a drug that controls platelet aggregation, and, experimentally at least, several drugs can accomplish this. Such drugs include aspirin, dipyridamole (Persantin), and some prostaglandins.

Anticoagulant drugs

Anticoagulant therapy is primarily prophylactic. These agents act (1) by preventing fibrin deposits, (2) by preventing extension of a thrombus, and (3) by preventing thromboembolic complications. Anticoagulation therapy is still empirical and is based largely on clinical experience. Long-term anticoagulant therapy remains controversial. Nevertheless, there is evidence that anticoagulant therapy reduces the incidence of thrombosis and therefore prolongs life.

Anticoagulation therapy is directed toward preventing intravascular thrombosis by decreasing blood coagulability. This therapy has no direct effect on a blood clot that has already formed or on ischemic tissue injured by an inadequate blood supply because of the clot.

Anticoagulants are indicated in:

1 Occlusive vascular disease such as thromboangiitis obliterans

T A B L E   2 0 - 2   Comparison of characteristics of anticoagulant drugs

	Heparin	Coumarin and indandione derivatives
Onset of action	Immediate	Slow (24 to 48 hours)
Route of administration	Parenteral	Oral
Duration of action	Short (less than 4 hours)	Long (approximately 2 to 5 days)
Laboratory test for dosage control	APTT,* clotting time	Prothrombin time
Antidote	Protamine sulfate	Vitamin K, whole blood, or plasma
Cost	Expensive	Inexpensive

*APTT, activated partial thromboplastin time.

2 Sudden arterial occlusion
3 Venous thrombosis
4 Pulmonary embolism
5 Cerebrovascular thrombosis
6 Coronary artery occlusion or myocardial infarction
7 Disseminated intravascular coagulation (DIC)

The last-named is a syndrome marked by both coagulation and hemorrhage occurring concurrently. During an episode, the activation of the blood coagulation mechanism is followed by consumption of clotting factors and fibrinolysis. Since DIC is a secondary disorder, effective treatment is based on an accurate diagnosis of the underlying cause, which may be bacterial or viral infection, obstetric trauma, or certain neoplasms.

Anticoagulants are used prophylactically in:

1 Major surgery when there is previous history of thrombosis or when prolonged immobilization will be necessary
2 Pelvic surgery in the male or female, since pelvic surgery is notorious for its high incidence of postoperative thrombophlebitis
3 Patients who have had bed rest for more than 2 or 3 days, since this predisposes them to vascular stasis
4 Rheumatic heart disease

Anticoagulants are also used to prevent clotting of blood to be used for transfusion, laboratory, or experimental work. Table 20-2 gives a comparison of actions of the anticoagulants, heparin, coumarin, and indandione derivatives. For effective anticoagulant therapy the manner of use of both heparin and coumarin derivatives is important. They can be used to complement each other. In some instances the administration of both heparin and one of the synthetic anticoagulants such as dicumarol is started simultaneously. The heparin is discontinued as soon as the prothrombin activity has been sufficiently reduced and the coumarin compound is producing a full therapeutic effect. Heparin is needed when a rapid anticoagulant effect is required or when adequate facilities for determining the prothrombin time are unavailable (this prevents the use of one of the synthetic anticoagulants).

In certain conditions when a rapid but not immediate anticoagulant effect is desired, dicumarol and ethyl biscoumacetate are given together on the first day of therapy and only the former drug is given on successive days.

PARENTERAL ANTICOAGULANT DRUGS
Heparin sodium

Heparin (derived from the Greek word *hepar* meaning liver) is a mucopolysaccharide that is strongly acidic because of the presence of sulfate groups in the molecule. Heparin, as the name implies, was first found in the liver and subsequently in the lungs and intestinal mucosa. It is formed in especially large amounts in the mast cells of these tissues. It also has been found in the tunica intima of blood vessels. For drug use, heparin is obtained from beef lung and mucosal lining of pig intestine.

Heparin produces its anticoagulant effect by combining with antithrombin III, a naturally occurring anticlotting factor in the plasma. This compound is unrelated to factor III, which is involved in blood coagulation. The normal function of antithrombin III is to maintain intravascular fluidity of the blood. Thromboembolism frequently occurs in individuals with acquired or congenital deficiency of this plasma protein. Therefore, in the absence of antithrombin III, heparin has no effect on clot formation.

The binding of heparin with the plasma cofactor antithrombin III forms a complex that retards thrombin activity and neutralizes factors IXa, Xa, XIa, and XIIa in the coagulation mechanism. Furthermore, by inhibiting the activation of factor XIII, heparin prevents the formation of a stable fibrin clot. However, the most important action of this complex is to inhibit thrombin synthesis, especially by accelerating the neutralization of factor Xa.

Heparin is also known to be antilipemic; that is, it reduces blood lipids or fats.

Pharmacokinetics. Because of its large molecular size and polarity, heparin is not absorbed from the gastrointestinal tract. For this reason, the drug is given only by the parenteral route. In addition, the chemical configuration of the drug hinders its passage across the placental membrane as well as into maternal milk.

Once absorbed, heparin is bound to antithrombin III and to low-density lipoprotein. The serum half-life of the drug is dose dependent; higher doses lead to more prolonged elimination from the plasma. Thus, when 100 units/kg is administered intravenously, the half-life of the drug is 1 hour. When 400 units/kg is given by the same route, the half-life is extended to 2½ hours. Heparin is metabolized in the liver, and the metabolic products are excreted in the urine. In patients with hepatic cirrhosis or renal failure, the drug has a significantly longer anticoagulant activity.

Laboratory control. Variability in plasma clearance of heparin among patients is sufficiently important to make laboratory control of heparin dosage necessary. The *activated partial thromboplastin time* (APTT) is a good test to determine the response to heparin therapy. The normal APTT ranges between 30 to 35 seconds. For patients undergoing heparin therapy it should be about twice the baseline level. If the APTT is too long (over 120 seconds) a dose of the drug may be omitted, or if it is too short, the dose may be increased.

A less specific test for measuring coagulation is the *clotting time*. It takes 3 to 6 minutes for normal blood to clot in a test tube. The clotting time should be prolonged from 2 to 2½ times the normal range in patients undergoing heparin therapy.

Uses. Heparin is employed in the prevention and treatment of all types of thromboses and emboli. It is also administered to patients with disseminated intravascular coagulation. Heparin is used prophylactically to prevent clotting in surgery of the heart or blood vessels. In addition, it is used during blood transfusions and in hemodialysis to prevent blood clotting. The benefits of using heparin in patients with myocardial infarction still have not been established.

Heparin is the drug of choice for sudden arterial occlusion, since its action is immediate and readily reversible if surgery becomes necessary for clot removal. In thrombophlebitis there is evidence that heparin is superior to the coumarin drugs in preventing pulmonary complications. It is also preferred for treating thrombophlebitis occurring during pregnancy, since it does not cross the placental barrier. Heparin is not excreted in the mother's milk. Since coumarin drugs can go through these channels, they can cause fetal complications and hemorrhage in the newborn.

Heparin is usually used *when rapid anticoagulant action is desired. It is used before the use of oral anticoagulants* (coumarin derivatives). Heparin approaches the ideal anticoagulant—it is rapidly absorbed, readily excreted, and almost nontoxic. Its main disadvantages are its short action, high cost, need for parenteral injection, and local reactions at injection sites. (See Table 20-2.)

Preparation, dosage, and administration. Heparin is inactive orally and must be administered parenterally. It is obtained commercially from domestic animals slaughtered for food. It may be given by a single injection or continuous intravenous drip. The response to heparin occurs almost immediately and lasts for a relatively short time (3 to 4 hours) unless the dose is repeated. When administration is discontinued, the clotting time returns to normal rather quickly, and there is danger of massive clot formation should the drug be discontinued too soon. The dosage must be determined for each individual patient and is based on the APTT or the clotting time (see "Laboratory control" for time). The potency of heparin sodium is expressed in units. When it is given intravenously at spaced intervals, 50 mg (5000 units) may be given at a time. For continuous drip, 100 to 200 mg (10,000 to 20,000 units) is added to 1000 ml of 5% sterile glucose solution or to isotonic saline solution and the flow is started at about 20 to 25 drops/minute. When heparin is administered intermittently, a heparin lock is usually secured in the vein.

Subcutaneous injections of 10,000 to 12,000 units every 8 hours or 14,000 to 20,000 units every 12 hours are also acceptable. Different injection sites should be used to avoid producing a massive hematoma. After withdrawal of the needle, light pressure but no massage should be applied to the injection site. The patient should be observed for bleeding.

Intramuscular injection of heparin in a slowly absorbed medium repository form has been used, and this does reduce the frequency of the injections to one every 48 hours. The dosage for the repository form is 20,000 to 40,000 units. There are accompanying disadvantages, however. The injections may be painful and the absorption may not be even, so that sometimes there is inadequate heparinization and at other times an excessive effect may be obtained. Nurses should check the injection site carefully because of the possibility that a local hematoma will develop, which may result in tissue slough. Actually, this route of administration should be avoided, since it also may produce bleeding into the muscle.

Side effects and toxic effects. Bleeding tendencies constitute the most important side effect of heparin. Hematuria, epistaxis, ecchymosis, bleeding gums, and tarry stools may occur. Hypersensitivity to heparin is rare, but allergic reactions have been reported. Alopecia may occur, but it is reversible after withdrawal of the drug. Osteoporosis has been reported in patients taking large doses of heparin for long periods of time (6 months or more). This occurs because the drug potentiates parathyroid hormone activity, producing bone resorption. Other than hemorrhage reactions to heparin are rare.

Precautions and contraindications. Caution must be used in administering heparin to patients with any condition in which there is a possibility of hemorrhage.

Contraindications to the use of anticoagulants include blood dyscrasias, liver disease (with hypoprothrombinemia), kidney disease, peptic ulcer, chronic ulcerative colitis, and active bleeding. Patients undergoing spinal cord or brain surgery should not use anticoagulants, since even minor bleeding may cause serious consequences.

The use of heparin is also contraindicated in patients with continuous drainage of the stomach or small intestine, threatened abortion, subacute endocarditis, severe hypertension, or hypersensitivity to the drug.

Drug interactions. Certain drugs such as salicylates, cincophen, phenylbutazone, and reserpine increase the risk of bleeding and should not be given with anticoagulants. Also, antihistamines, digitalis, and tetracyclines should not be given with heparin because they partially antagonize the anticoagulant effect of heparin.

Protamine sulfate (Heparin antidote)

Protamine sulfate is a protein-like substance derived from the sperm and mature testes of the salmon and other fish. Protamine by itself is a very weak anticoagulant but will cause prolongation of clotting time; it is an antithromboplastin but is not as active as heparin. When protamine is given in the presence of heparin, they form a combination, and each neutralizes the anticoagulant activity of the other. Because protamine is a basic protein (many free amino groups), it is able to combine with the sulfuric acids of heparin and inactivate them.

Uses. Protamine is used as a heparin antagonist to combat the bleeding tendency from an overdosage of heparin.

When given intravenously to treat the bleeding tendency resulting from an overdose of heparin, protamine acts almost instantaneously, and its effects persist for about 2 hours. Its availability is therefore essential for safe management of a patient having anticoagulant therapy with heparin. It has been used experimentally to treat certain bleeding states believed to be characterized by increased amounts of heparin or heparin-like substances in the circulation.

Preparation, dosage, and administration. Protamine sulfate is administered intravenously and, occasionally, intramuscularly. In the treatment of overdosage of heparin, the extent of the overdosage can be determined from the amount of heparin given over the previous 3 or 4 hours; the amount of protamine needed is approximately equal to the amount of heparin overdosage. The commercial preparation of protamine sulfate consists of a solution containing 10 mg/ml.

Sodium citrate

Sodium citrate is used as an anticoagulant in blood that is to be used for a transfusion or that is to be stored for a time. Anticoagulant sodium citrate solution is a sterile solution of approximately 4% sodium citrate in water. It is used as an anticoagulant for blood plasma and for blood for fractionation. Anticoagulant citrate dextrose solution is used as an anticoagulant for storage of whole blood. Sodium citrate acts by binding plasma calcium and preventing the formation of thrombin.

ORAL ANTICOAGULANT DRUGS
COUMARIN DERIVATIVES

When cattle are allowed to eat improperly cured sweet clover, they may develop a hemorrhagic disorder believed to be caused by a deficiency of prothrombin. In 1941 Link and his associates at the University of Wisconsin were able to show that the substance responsible for the prothrombin deficiency was a coumarin derivative. These workers later synthesized dicumarol, and since that time other coumarin derivatives have been synthesized. These compounds differ mainly in their speed and dura-

tion of action. (See Table 20-3 for comparison of various coumarin and indandione derivatives.)

Action and result. Although the coumarin drugs are referred to as anticoagulants, they do not appreciably affect coagulation time or bleeding time when they are administered in therapeutic amounts. Dosage is computed on the basis of the plasma prothrombin time. Decreased prothrombin activity seems to act as a deterrent to intravascular clotting. Adequate and safe therapy therefore depends in part on accurate determinations of the patient's plasma prothrombin time.

Coumarin derivatives are prothrombin depressants, and they depress hepatic synthesis of factors II, VII, IX, and X. These agents probably compete with vitamin K, which functions enzymatically in the clotting process.

Vitamin K and a coumarin compound such as dicumarol show similarity of structure. This has led to the supposition that the coumarin compounds act as competitors to prevent the utilization of vitamin K by the liver. Thus, the antagonist to the anticoagulant effect of coumarin agents is vitamin K.

Laboratory control. Coumarin drugs depress factors other than prothrombin, and this may account for unexplained bleeding at "safe" levels of prothrombin. Since it is impractical to measure each factor separately, and since it is not known which factor when excessively depressed results in bleeding, *Quick's prothrombin test* remains the standard test in most clin-

T A B L E   2 0 - 3   **Comparison of various coumarin and indandione derivatives**

Generic name	Trade name	Peak effect (hours)	Recovery	Average initial dose (mg)	Average maintenance dose (mg)	Route of administration
Acenocoumarin	Sintrom	24 to 48	48 hr.	16 to 28	2 to 10	Oral
Anisindione	Miradon	36 to 72	24 to 72 hr.	300	25 to 250	Oral
Dicumarol	—	24 to 72	7 to 9 days	200 to 300	25 to 150	Oral
Diphenadione	Dipaxin	48	20 days	20 to 30	3 to 5	Oral
Ethyl biscoumacetate	Tromexan	18 to 24	48 hr.	1500 to 1800	600 to 900	Oral
Phenindione	Danilone Hedulin Eridone	18 to 24	24 to 48 hr.	200 to 300	50 to 100	Oral
Phenprocoumon	Liquamar	36 to 48	7 to 14 days	24	0.75 to 6	Oral
Warfarin sodium	Coumadin Sodium Panwarfin	12 to 18	5 to 7 days	20 to 60	2 to 10	Oral Intramuscular Intravenous

ical laboratories. This test measures the time in seconds required for a sample of the patient's plasma to clot when mixed with tissue thromboplastin and calcium. The normal clotting time ranges from 11 to 14 seconds and this time is used as the control. The therapeutic aim for patients undergoing anticoagulant therapy is to produce a prolongation of the prothrombin time within 1½ to 2½ times the control.

Uses. Coumarin derivatives are the drugs of choice for long-term anticoagulant therapy to protect against sudden acute arterial occlusion or thromboembolic phenomena from any predisposing factor that may cause loss of limb or life. They are the drugs of choice for recurrent phlebitis, chronic occlusive arterial disease, and myocardial infarction.

Major advantages of these drugs are the following: (1) they are effective with oral administration, (2) they are inexpensive, and (3) they need be given only once a day when the maintenance dose has been established. (See Table 20-3.)

The use of coumarin derivatives is contraindicated for the same conditions as those of the parenteral anticoagulant heparin. In addition, the precautions to be observed and the side effects of these drugs are similar to those of heparin. However, osteoporosis does not occur with the use of oral anticoagulants. Instead, diarrhea is a common problem, and occasionally leukopenia may develop.

Oral anticoagulant antidote. Hemorrhage may develop as a consequence of oral anticoagulant therapy. Bleeding episodes often occur even when the prothrombin time is within the expected therapeutic range. Treatment consists of immediate withdrawal of the drug and the oral administration of vitamin K_1. If bleeding is excessive, fresh whole blood or plasma may be required. The advantage of infusion of fresh plasma is that it provides the clotting factors that have been suppressed during anticoagulant therapy. Careful assessment of the clinical status of the patient must be made before resuming anticoagulant therapy. (See details of vitamin K in this chapter.)

Drug interactions. Many drugs interact with coumarin derivatives, resulting in an alteration of anticoagulant activity. Drugs that increase coumarin anticoagulant activity may cause a decrease in intestinal absorption of vitamin K and an alteration of the bacterial flora of the intestine that synthesize the vitamin. Another contributing factor may be associated with a change in platelet activity. Drugs that may cause a significant increase in anticoagulant activity include broad-spectrum antibiotics, anabolic steroids, clofibrate, phenylbutazone, and thyroid preparations. By contrast, drugs that may significantly decrease anticoagulant activity include barbiturates, estrogens, and oral contraceptives.

Use of barbiturates and oral anticoagulants is somewhat hazardous; discontinuance of the barbiturate with continued administration of the anticoagulant may result in active bleeding. In the presence of barbiturates, higher doses of the anticoagulants are required for optimum effect. Unless the anticoagulant dosage is reduced when barbiturates are discontinued, excessive loading of the anticoagulant may occur, resulting in toxic or bleeding effects.

Dicumarol (dicoumarin, bishydroxycoumarin)

Official preparations of dicumarol are available in 25-, 50-, and 100-mg tablets and also in capsules. It is administered orally. The usual initial dose is 200 to 300 mg daily. Subsequent dosage for a day or two depends on the prothrombin time of the patient and may vary from 50 to 200 mg. Some authorities attempt to keep prothrombin activity between 10% and 30% of normal and others between 15% and 25% of normal. In most patients, 25 to 150 mg daily is required as maintenance dosage. Dosage is determined not only by the prothrombin time but also by the direction in which it is changing. Dicumarol requires 24 to 72 hours for its action to develop, and its action persists 24 to 72 hours after its administration is discontinued.

Ethyl biscoumacetate (Tromexan)

Ethyl biscoumacetate is a synthetic derivative of dicumarol and produces a similar anticoagulant action. It is available in 150- and 300-mg tablets for oral administration. Its action and uses are similar to those of dicumarol, but it is more rapidly absorbed, acts over a shorter period of time, is detoxified and excreted faster, and has less cumulative effect than dicumarol. The average initial dose for a 24-hour period is 1.5 g given at one time or in divided dosage. Subsequent daily doses of 600 to 900 mg are usual, but maintenance dosage is regulated by determinations of prothrombin activity. This compound is more expensive than dicumarol.

Warfarin sodium (Coumadin Sodium, Panwarfin)

Warfarin sodium is available in 5-, 10-, and 25-mg tablets for oral administration and as a powder from which a solution is made for injection (intravenous and intramuscular). Its action is more rapid and prolonged than that of dicumarol. The initial oral and intravenous dose is 20 to 60 mg, then 2 to 10 mg daily, depending on prothrombin activity.

Acenocoumarin (Sintrom)

Acenocoumarin is a synthetic coumarin type of anticoagulant. Its action is faster than that of dicumarol but less rapid than that of ethyl biscoumacetate. It is available in 4-mg tablets for oral administration. The initial dose is 16 to 28 mg on the first day of therapy followed by 8 to 16 mg on the second day. The average maintenance dose is 2 to 10 mg daily, depending on the response of the patient as measured by frequent determinations of the prothrombin time.

INDANDIONE DERIVATIVES
Phenindione (Danilone, Hedulin)

Phenindione is a synthetic anticoagulant similar in action to dicumarol but unrelated chemically. It acts more promptly than dicumarol and in smaller doses. Therapeutic levels are generally obtained within 18 to 24 hours, and the prothrombin time usually returns to normal 24 to 48 hours after administration of the drug has been discontinued.

This drug may produce an orange or reddish discoloration of the urine that patients may mistake for hematuria. Phenindione is administered orally in initial doses of 200 to 300 mg; half is given in the morning and half at bedtime. Continued dosage is adjusted as determinations of prothrombin activity indicate.

Periodic examinations of the blood, liver, and kidneys have been recommended because this drug has been known to cause agranulocytosis and hepatic and renal damage.

Diphenadione (Dipaxin)

Diphenadione is closely related to phenindione and is one of the most potent and long-acting depressants of prothrombin activity. It is therefore effective in smaller doses than most oral anticoagulants. The initial dose is 20 to 30 mg orally, followed by 10 to 15 mg on the second day. Subsequent dosage is determined in accordance with the prothrombin time. The precautions to be observed for these drugs are much the same as those for the coumarin derivatives.

NURSING IMPLICATIONS FOR ANTICOAGULANT DRUG THERAPY

The following are aspects of care for patients taking anticoagulant drugs.

1 Patients should be observed for bleeding
   a Nosebleeds or bleeding gums
   b Petechiae, purpura, or ecchymotic areas
   c Blood in urine or stools
2 Patients undergoing anticoagulant therapy should be instructed to carry an identification card that lists the patient's and physician's names and phone numbers and the name and dosage of drug.
3 Dietary factors, especially the ingestion of fat, are associated with increased tendency to thrombosis. It may be of benefit to advise the patient to follow a diet with moderate to low fat content.
4 Patients should be advised to protect themselves from injury.
5 When heparin is used, blood should be drawn for APTT or clotting time when heparin activity is least, just before another injection of heparin is to be given.
6 Vitamin K should be readily accessible if bleeding occurs. Outpatients should carry vitamin K with them, and 5 to 20 mg should be taken at once if bleeding occurs. Statistics show that bleeding occurs in approximately 10% of all patients on long-term anticoagulant therapy. However, fatalities are rare.
7 Patients undergoing long-term therapy must be instructed to take their medication as prescribed and to report without fail for their blood tests. Cooperation of the patient is important for safe and effective anticoagulation therapy. Some phy-

sicians do not advocate long-term anticoagulant therapy for unreliable patients—those patients who do not eat properly; go on alcoholic binges, which cause decrease in vitamin K; do not take their medicine as directed; and do not report for the test of their prothrombin activity (prothrombin time) as they have been directed to do.

Antiplatelet drugs

The platelet phase of clotting involves the intrinsic pathway of blood coagulation and is responsible for causing arterial thrombotic disorders. Antiplatelet or antithrombotic drugs interfere with this action by inhibiting the adherence of platelets to exposed collagen at sites of vascular injury. These drugs apparently prevent the release of adenosine diphosphate (ADP) from platelets and thereby hinder platelet aggregation, which leads to the eventual formation of a thrombus. Since most arterial thrombi consist of platelet plugs, it appears that drugs which interrupt this process would be useful. Nevertheless, the efficacy of antiplatelet drugs is still under investigation, and results of some extensive clinical trials require further evaluation. The drugs that inhibit platelet adhesiveness or platelet aggregation include acetylsalicylic acid, dipyridamole, sulfinpyrazone, and dextrans.

Acetylsalicylic acid (aspirin) has been used in a long-term study to prevent cerebral or myocardial infarction. The efficacy of aspirin as an antithrombotic agent has still to be demonstrated. *Dipyridamole (Persantine)* has been used to prevent thrombi in patients with prosthetic heart valves. Individuals with heart valve replacement, particularly those with the ball valve and disk valve type of devices, have an increased risk of thromboembolism. When the clots form at the replaced valve, they either interfere with the valve's function or become dislodged and travel to the brain, heart, kidney, or other organs of the body. Dipyridamole is administered in combination with warfarin to prevent thromboembolic complications. *Sulfinpyrazone (Anturane)* is used to treat gout because of its uricosuric properties. This drug also has been employed in clinical trials as an antiplatelet drug to prevent thromboembolism in patients after an attack of myocardial infarction. However, definitive data are required before sulfinpyrazone can be recommended as an antiplatelet agent. *Dextran 75* and *dextran 70* are glucose polymers that are used as plasma volume expanders. In addition, these agents can coat not only erythrocytes but also platelets and intimal surfaces of blood vessels. Thus platelet adhesiveness and aggregation may be decreased. Dextran is currently being studied for its efficacy in preventing postoperative thromboembolic disease in surgical patients. (Dextran is discussed later in this chapter.)

Thrombolytic (fibrinolytic) drugs

Thrombolytic drugs are used for the treatment of acute thromboembolic disorders. These agents are responsible for dissolving clots via the endogenous fibrinolytic system. This mechanism involves the conversion of a plasma protein, plasminogen, to plasmin (fibrinolysin). The activated plasmin then functions as an enzyme that digests fibrin threads and fibrinogen, thereby resulting in lysis of the blood clot. Moreover, the thrombolytic enzymes act by causing dissolution of thrombi *after* their formation rather than by *preventing their extension* as the anticoagulants do. Furthermore, thrombolytic enzyme therapy alters the hemostatic capability of the patient more profoundly than does anticoagulant therapy. Consequently, when bleeding occurs, it is more severe and very difficult to control.

Streptokinase (Streptase)

Streptokinase is an enzyme of bacterial origin. It acts by increasing the concentration of plasmin within a clot, thereby promoting its dissolution. Streptokinase is used to treat acute pulmonary embolism and deep vein thrombosis. It is administered intravenously at a loading dose of 250,000 international units (IU) over a 30-minute period. This is followed by 100,000 IU/hour for 24 to 72 hours. Therapy is monitored according to the thrombin time, which should be prolonged by two to five times the control value. After completion of treatment with streptokinase, heparin therapy followed by an oral anticoagulant regimen is recommended. Streptokinase is antigenic so that anaphylactoid reactions may occur from the formation of antibodies. Fever is an additional problem resulting from the use of this drug.

Urokinase (Abbokinase)

Urokinase is a proteolytic enzyme derived from human urine. Urokinase directly activates plasminogen, which in turn is converted to plasmin. Indications for use are similar to those for streptokinase. It has been shown to be effective in acute pulmonary embolism and deep vein thrombosis. An initial loading dose of 4400 IU/kg is given intravenously over a period of 10 minutes. This is followed by a continuous infusion of 4400 IU/kg/hour for 12 hours. Urokinase therapy does not require the monitoring of thrombin time during treatment. However, this test should be performed before instituting a heparin regimen. Moreover, the patient should be placed on heparin and then oral anticoagulant therapy following the completion of urokinase administration. The major advantage of this drug is that it is nonantigenic so that serious allergic reactions are rare. Because of the high cost, it is used as an alternative thrombolytic drug for patients who are allergic to streptokinase. Currently, a course of treatment of urokinase costs about $3000, whereas that of streptokinase is $250.

Antifibrinolytic drug
Aminocaproic acid (Amicar)

Aminocaproic acid is a synthetic compound that inhibits fibrinolysis when excessive bleeding is encountered. This drug acts as a competitive antagonist of plasminogen, preventing the generation of plasmin and thereby inhibiting the dissolution of clots. Aminocaproic acid is used as a specific antidote for an overdose of thrombolytic drugs such as streptokinase and urokinase. It is also used in patients with hemophilia when fibrin formation is deficient. The usual dose of 5 g may be administered orally or intravenously, followed by 1.25 g/hour until

bleeding is brought under control. Intravenous administration of the drug should be slow to prevent hypotension and bradycardia during therapy.

Antihemophilic agents

Hemophilia is a hereditary disorder caused by a deficiency of one or more plasma protein clotting factors. This condition usually leads to persistent and uncontrollable hemorrhage after even minor injury. The symptoms include excessive bleeding from wounds and hemorrhage into joints, urinary tract, and on occasion even the central nervous system. There are two types of hemophilia: hemophilia A, the classic type in which factor VIII activity is deficient, and hemophilia B or Christmas disease, in which factor IX complex activity is deficient. In recent years a correct diagnosis of the coagulation disorder has led to specific factor replacement therapy, and this medical advance has resulted in effective management of the patient at home.

Factor VIII (Factorate, Hemofil, Humafac, Koāte, Profilate)

In the intrinsic pathway of the coagulation mechanism, antihemophilic factor (AHF) or factor VIII is required for the transformation of prothrombin to thrombin. In the treatment of hemophilia A, administration of factor VIII is based on replacement of this missing plasma clotting factor. Thus AHF specifically corrects or prevents bleeding episodes in patients with only hemophilia A.

Dosage of factor VIII must be individualized according to the patient's weight, severity of the deficiency, and the amount of hemorrhage. The prophylactic dose is 250 units/day for patients weighing less than 50 kg and 500 units/day for heavier individuals. During hemorrhage, the dosage is adjusted so that a level of at least 40% of normal can produce hemostasis. The drug is administered by the intravenous route only. A plastic syringe is used because with a glass syringe, the solution may bind to the surface of ground glass. Since factor VIII is prepared from human plasma, the risk of transmitting hepatitis exists. Side effects include mild allergic reactions, bronchospasm, urticaria, chills, and nausea. Patients who develop inhibitors to factor VIII may not respond to factor VIII therapy. After careful evaluation of the patient, the administration of anti-inhibitor coagulant complex may be indicated to correct this condition.

Factor IX complex (Konȳne, Proplex)

Factor IX complex is a concentrated preparation that contains factors II, VII, IX, and X. These are known as the vitamin K coagulation factors. This agent is used for therapy in patients with a deficiency of these factors during hemorrhage or before surgery. It is also indicated for hemophilia B in which factor IX is deficient. The dosage is individualized according to the patient's coagulation assay, which is performed before treatment. Indiscriminate use of this agent is not recommended because of the high risk of viral hepatitis.

Hemostatic agents

Hemostatic agents are used to hasten the clotting of blood. In some instances natural clotting factors of blood may be applied topically. In other situations hemostatic drugs act systemically, for example, vitamin K, which is administered by the oral or parenteral routes. The purpose of these agents is to control rapid loss of blood.

SYSTEMIC HEMOSTATIC AGENTS
Vitamin K

Vitamin K was discovered by Dam of Copenhagen in 1935 as a result of a study of newly hatched chicks that had a fatal hemorrhagic disease. This condition, he found, could be prevented and cured by the administration of a substance found in hog liver and in alfalfa. It was later discovered that the delayed clotting time of the blood was caused by deficiency of prothrombin content. Vitamin K occurs naturally in two forms known as K_1 and K_2. Both have a naphthoquinone nucleus and exhibit similar physiologic properties.

In natural vitamin K (K_1 or K_2), R is a long alkyl chain of 20 or 30 carbons. In synthetic vitamin K (Menadione, vitamin K_3), R is only hydrogen. These compounds are called naphthoquinones from the parent nucleus. The synthetic analogs greatly resemble the natural vitamin. Certain of the analogs are water soluble, whereas the natural vitamin is fat soluble. The fat-soluble vitamin requires the presence of bile in the intestine to ensure adequate absorption after oral administration. This is not essential for the water-soluble preparations.

Vitamin K is widely found in foods such as liver, egg yolk, fish, cheese, cabbage, cauliflower, spinach, and tomatoes. The enteric bacteria act on these foods to synthesize vitamin K. Dietary deficiency of vitamin K is rare.

Action and result. Vitamin K is essential to the hepatic synthesis of prothrombin and factors VII, IX, and X. It contributes to the activation of an enzyme necessary to the formation of prothrombin. Deficiency of vitamin K leads to hypoprothrombinemia and hemorrhage.

Prothrombin deficiency may occur because of inadequate absorption of vitamin K from the intestine (usually because of biliary disease in which bile fails to enter the intestine) or because of destruction of intestinal organisms, which may occur with antibiotic therapy. It is also encountered in the newborn, in which case it is probably caused by the fact that the intestinal organisms have not yet become established. It may result from therapy with certain anticoagulants.

Uses. Vitamin K is useful only in conditions in which the prolonged bleeding time is the result of low concentration of prothrombin in the blood, which is not in turn the result of damaged liver cells. Vitamin K is routinely administered to newborns to help prevent hemorrhage. Although prothrombin may be normal at birth, it declines until about the sixth day, when the liver is able to form prothrombin. Vitamin K may be given to the mother before delivery.

Vitamin K is also indicated in the preoperative preparation of patients with deficient prothrombin, particularly those with obstructive jaundice. In addition, it is given as an antidote for overdosage of systemic anticoagulants such as bishydroxycoumarin, as well as for hemorrhagic disorders and hypoprothrombinemia secondary to large doses, or overdosages, of drugs such as salicylates, quinine, sulfonamides, arsenicals, and barbiturates. Hemorrhagic conditions not caused by deficiency of prothrombin are not successfully treated with vitamin K.

The natural concentrates have, to a great extent, been replaced by the synthetic preparations. It is important that the prothrombin activity of the blood be measured frequently when the patient is receiving a preparation of vitamin K. Parenteral preparations should be administered if for some reason the intestinal absorption is impaired.

Preparation, dosage, and administration. The following are the preparations of vitamin K available.

Menadione. Menadione is a synthetic substitute for natural vitamin K. The presence of bile is essential for adequate absorption after oral administration. Menadione tablets and menadione injection are official preparations. The usual dose is 2 to 10 mg daily.

Menadione sodium bisulfite (Hykinone). Menadione sodium bisulfite is similar to menadione, but it is water soluble and oral doses need not be accompanied by bile salts. It is available in solution for subcutaneous, intramuscular, and intravenous injection. Menadione sodium bisulfite injection and menaphthone sodium bisulfite injection are official preparations for injection. The average daily dose is 2.5 to 10 mg. The dosage is determined in relation to the prothrombin level of the blood.

Chlorophyll complex perles. Chlorophyll complex perles is natural chlorophyll extracted from alfalfa and pineapple plants and is a rich source of fat-soluble vitamin K. The dose is 3 to 6 perles/day.

Menadiol sodium diphosphate (Synkayvite). Menadiol sodium diphosphate is a derivative of menadione and has the same action and uses as other analogs of vitamin K. It is water soluble and is adequately absorbed after oral administration without bile salts. It is administered orally, subcutaneously, intramuscularly, and intravenously. The dosage is approximately

three times that of menadione. It is available in 5-mg tablets for oral administration and in solution for injection. The usual dose is 5 to 75 mg.

Phytonadione (vitamin K$_1$, Mephyton, Konakion); phytomenadione. Phytonadione acts more promptly and over a longer period of time than the vitamin K analogs. It is a fat-soluble vitamin, and the presence of bile salts in the intestine is essential to adequate absorption. It will stop bleeding 3 to 6 hours after intravenous administration and produces a normal prothrombin level in 12 to 14 hours. It is useful to reverse the effects of anticoagulant therapy that have produced a serious deficiency of prothrombin in the blood. Phytonadione is available in 5-mg oral tablets and as an emulsion for intravenous injection. The emulsion is diluted with isotonic salt solution or sterile water before it is injected. The dosage varies greatly; 2.5 to 20 mg may be given daily, although much larger doses have been given in emergency situations. However, small doses of vitamin K$_1$ orally administered will effectively correct the reduced prothrombin activity induced by certain anticoagulants (coumarin drugs). The effects are said to be less predictable when severe liver damage is present. The dosage must be determined according to the level of prothrombin activity, the length of time during which the patient has received anticoagulant therapy, and the hazard of restoring the risk of thrombosis. Large doses of vitamin K$_1$ are said to make subsequent regulation of anticoagulant therapy with coumarin drugs more difficult.

Phytonadione solution (AquaMEPHYTON, Konakion). Phytonadione solution is a water-soluble form of vitamin K$_1$ that may be given subcutaneously or intramuscularly.

TOPICAL HEMOSTATIC AGENTS
Absorbable gelatin sponge (Gelfoam)

Absorbable gelatin sponge is a specially prepared form of gelatin having a porous nature. It is used to control capillary bleeding and may be left in place in a surgical wound. It is completely absorbed in 4 to 6 weeks. It should be well moistened with isotonic saline solution or thrombin solution before it is applied to a bleeding surface. Its presence does not induce excessive scar formation.

The hemostatic action is the result of its action as a tampon and liberation of thromboplastin from damaged platelets traumatized by contact with the sponge.

Human fibrin foam

Human fibrin foam is a sterile dry preparation of human fibrin that, when applied to a bleeding surface, acts as a mechanical coagulant. In combination with thrombin it gives a chemical as well as a mechanical matrix for coagulation. It is used in surgery of organs such as the brain, liver, or kidneys when ordinary methods for the control of bleeding are ineffective or inadvisable. It is absorbed within a short period of time and need not be removed after bleeding has stopped.

Oxidized cellulose (Oxycel, Hemo-Pak)

Oxidized cellulose is a specially treated form of surgical gauze or cotton that exerts a hemostatic effect but is absorbable when buried in the tissues. The hemostatic action is caused by the formation of an artificial clot by cellulosic acid. Absorption of oxidized cellulose occurs between the second and the seventh day following implantation, although absorption of large amounts of blood-soaked material may take 6 weeks or longer. Oxidized cellulose is of value in the control of bleeding in surgery of organs such as the liver, pancreas, spleen, kidney, thyroid, and prostate. Its hemostatic action is not increased by the addition of other hemostatic agents. It should not be used as a surface dressing except for the control of bleeding, because cellulosic acid inhibits the growth of epithelial tissue. Since it interferes with bone regeneration, it should not be implanted in fractures.

Thrombin

Thrombin is a preparation isolated from bovine plasma. It catalyzes the conversion of fibrinogen to fibrin. It is intended as a hemostatic agent for *topical application* to control capillary bleeding. It may be applied as a dry powder or dissolved in sterile isotonic saline solution. It is not injected.

Replacement of blood volume and blood components

Physiologic factors such as whole blood or blood components can be replaced in the body by means of nondrug therapy. Transfusions of whole blood are of value not only to replace red cells but also to restore blood volume and blood pressure. The latter value is seen particularly in the treatment of shock.

Blood transfusion plays an important although passive role in the treatment of anemic conditions. Transfusions apparently do not stimulate the bone marrow to greater activity, but in crises they may save the patient's life when the patient cannot wait for iron or liver to become effective.

For blood transfusions to be used satisfactorily, it is important that the blood be readily available and of the suitable type. It is also essential that a careful technique be developed and strictly followed to help prevent reactions. The blood should be administered slowly, particularly if the patient's anemia is severe. Sometimes one transfusion of whole blood will suffice, but under other conditions a series of small transfusions may accomplish better results.

Blood

Whole blood

Whole blood is used primarily to treat acute hemorrhage or trauma when volume and erythrocytes have been lost. In this situation an adequate circulating volume is usually more important than an adequate red cell mass. Administration of 2 units of whole blood will raise the hemoglobin by 2 to 3 g in the average (70-kg) adult.

Whole blood is also used for exchange transfusion in the treatment of erythroblastosis fetalis.

Administration of incompatible blood can cause a rapid destruction of the patient's own red blood cells. The signs and symptoms of this hemolytic reaction include chills, fever, headache, and chest and lower back pain. The nurse should discontinue the transfusion immediately to avoid dangerous adverse effects. Also, the physician should be notified. A urine specimen should be sent to the laboratory for analysis, and a record of the intake and output must be kept. In addition, the remaining blood or container should be returned to the blood bank with a report detailing the patient's reaction.

Human packed red blood cells

The human red blood cell is the only component removed from the plasma. Its use is indicated when red blood cell replacement is necessary but an increase of plasma volume is unnecessary or undesirable. It is used for treating certain types of anemia to improve the oxygen-carrying capacity of the blood. Since patients who are chronically anemic have a normal or increased blood volume, only packed red blood cells are required.

Blood plasma

Blood plasma is the fluid part of the blood that may be procured by separating the blood cells from the whole citrated blood. Plasma may be given irrespective of the donor's group. This is particularly useful when whole blood is unavailable or cannot be properly cross matched. Many authorities believe that blood plasma, since it contains fibrinogen, albumin, gamma globulins, hemagglutinins, prothrombin, sugar, and salts, is an ideal transfusion medium to restore effective blood volume in the treatment of peripheral circulatory failure associated with severe burns, traumatic shock, or hemorrhage. It is also used to maintain colloid osmotic pressure and to supplement blood proteins. Blood plasma can be used as it is for transfusions, or it can be concentrated, dehydrated, and stored for long periods of time without deterioration. The addition of sterile distilled water is all that is needed to make it ready for immediate use. Plasma in the dried form is particularly stable and useful when transportation, storage, and contamination are problems that must be considered.

Normal human plasma. Normal human plasma is obtained by pooling equal parts of citrated whole blood from eight or more adults who qualify as donors by virtue of their having passed physical examinations and various clinical tests. Procedures are carried out under definite aseptic conditions, and the cell-free plasma is obtained by centrifugation or by sedimentation. It is dispensed in liquid, dried, or frozen form. The usual amount given whole or restored is 500 ml. It is administered to combat surgical and traumatic shock, in the treatment of burned persons when much plasma has been lost, and in cases in which whole blood is not immediately available for the treatment of hemorrhage.

A serious problem with the use of pooled human plasma is the transmission of viral hepatitis. Since plasma from one infected donor may appear in many bottles of plasma, the incidence of transmitting viral hepatitis is far greater than when whole blood is used.

Normal human serum albumin. Normal human serum albumin is a brownish, viscous, clear, relatively odorless liquid obtained from the blood of healthy human donors. It is made free of the hazard of the virus of serum hepatitis by heating at 60° C for 10 hours. It is available in a solution (25 g in 100 ml) or as a dried preparation. The normal unit is composed of 25 g of human albumin to which sterile water or physiologic saline solution can be added before use. This is then equivalent to about 500 ml of whole human plasma, in terms of protein osmotic pressure. It is used in the treatment of shock when it is undesirable to expand plasma volume and in situations in which it is important to raise the serum protein of the blood, such as burns, hypoproteinemia, hepatic cirrhosis, and cerebral edema. It is administered intravenously.

PLASMA SUBSTITUTES
Dextran (Expandex, Gentran); dextran 70

Dextran is a glucose polymer made by the action of special bacteria *(Leuconostoc mesenteroides)* on sucrose. The resulting polysaccharide does not easily pass through capillary walls. The molecules are like those of serum albumin and have a molecular weight of about 75,000.

Uses. Dextran is used to expand plasma volume and maintain blood pressure in emergency conditions resulting from shock and hemorrhage. It is not a substitute for whole blood or its derivatives when the latter are needed for the treatment of anemia secondary to hemorrhage or when it is essential to restore blood proteins after traumatic injuries, burns, and so forth. It has no oxygen-carrying property. The effect of an injection of 500 to 1000 ml of dextran (6%) usually persists for a period of 24 hours. From 30% to 50% is excreted in the urine, and the remainder is metabolized in the body.

Preparation, dosage, and administration. Dextran is administered intravenously in isotonic solution of sodium chloride. The usual dose is 500 ml of 6% solution infused at the rate of 20 to 40 ml/minute. Repeated infusions can be given when necessary, if blood or its derivatives are not at hand or if their use is not indicated. Solutions of dextran do not require refrigeration and are easily stored. The 6% solution of dextran is osmotically equivalent to serum albumin.

Although high molecular weight dextran is effective in replacing lost blood volume, it has been shown clinically and experimentally that this form of dextran has an adverse effect on flow in minute vessels and capillaries because it increases blood viscosity. Another disadvantage of this form of dextran is that it interferes with normal clotting by coating platelets.

Side effects and toxic effects. Untoward effects are rare with the exception of an antigen-antibody type of reaction in certain persons. It has been established that bleeding time of recipients may be increased because dextran interferes with platelet function. This seems to be a temporary effect. Patients with cardiovascular disease who receive dextran infusions should be watched for congestive heart failure and pulmonary edema caused by circulatory volume overload. Temporary depression of renal tubule functioning has been reported; the cause is unknown.

Dextran 40 (LMD, Rheomarcrodex)

Low molecular weight dextran with a molecular weight of 40,000 is a less effective expander of plasma volume than high molecular weight dextran. However, it has been used effectively to restore flow in the microcircula-

tion and to improve tissue perfusion by reducing blood viscosity and sludging and preventing intravascular coagulation.

Dextran 40 is also used as a priming agent for pump oxygenators or bypass machines used for open-heart surgery.

Action. Dextran 40 may reduce blood viscosity by drawing fluid from the tissues into the vascular system, and therefore patients should be watched for signs of dehydration (warm dry skin and mouth, thirst, rise in body temperature). Prevention of intravascular clotting is theorized by some researchers to result from the ability of dextran 40 to maintain the electronegativity of red blood cells, which causes the cells to repel one another. In addition, red blood cell rigidity may be decreased, which promotes flow of red cells through the small blood vessels.

Absorption and excretion. Dextran 40 is rather rapidly excreted by the kidneys in patients with normal renal function. The viscosity and specific gravity of the urine may be increased during the administration of dextran 40 and throughout the duration of its effects, particularly in patients with decreased urine flow. A low specific gravity of urine with dextran 40 may indicate inability of the kidneys to remove dextran and is an indication for discontinuance of therapy. This drug should not be used in patients with renal disease. Its use is not contraindicated in patients with reduced urine output caused by shock. However, its use should be discontinued if no improvement in urine flow occurs. Unexcreted dextran is slowly degraded to glucose, which is then metabolized to respiratory carbon dioxide and water.

Preparation, dosage, and administration. Dextran 40 is available for intravenous injection as a 10% solution in 500- and 1000-ml bottles in combination with dextrose 5% or sodium chloride 0.9%. When dextran-40 is used in shock therapy, total dosage in the first 24 hours should not exceed 2 g/kg body weight (10 ml of a 10% solution equals 1 g of dextran). Thereafter, total dosage should not exceed 1 g/kg/24 hours. It is not recommended that therapy be continued for longer than 5 days.

Side effects and toxic effects. Adverse effects to dextran 40 include urticarial reactions, nausea, vomiting, wheezing, a tight feeling in the chest, and hypotension. However, these are not common reactions but are anaphylactoid.

6% Hetastarch (Hespan)

Hespan is a plasma volume expander that was introduced in 1980. It is an artificial colloid that closely resembles human glycogen and is available at about one third of the cost of albumin. A 6% solution of hetastarch has approximately the same osmotic pressure as that of human albumin. Its advantages over dextran are that it does not interfere with blood group determinations and it is reported to be less liable to produce anaphylactoid reactions.

Uses. Hespan is employed as a plasma volume expander in the treatment of shock caused by hemorrhage, surgery, burns, sepsis, and other trauma.

Preparation, dosage and administration. Hespan is available in 500-ml bottles containing 6% hetastarch in a 0.9% sodium chloride solution. This preparation is administered intravenously and the usual adult dose is 0.5 to 1.5 liters.

Side effects and toxic effects. Vomiting, fever, chills, itching, parotid gland enlargement, headache, muscle pain, and peripheral edema may occur. Hetastarch is nonantigenic. However, some mild sensitivity reactions have been reported.

Precautions and contraindications. Caution should be used in administering hespan to patients with pulmonary edema and congestive heart failure because of the possibility of circulatory overload. Patients with impaired renal clearance must be observed carefully, since hetastarch is eliminated by renal excretion. This agent is not to be used in individuals with preexisting severe bleeding disorders, severe congestive heart failure, or renal failure associated with oliguria or anuria.

TREATMENT OF HYPOVOLEMIC SHOCK

Adequate blood volume is absolutely essential to maintain viability of cells, normal tissue function, and life itself. Extensive trauma and hemorrhage that seriously lower blood volume usually require blood replacement. Whenever 30% of the blood volume is lost, prompt treat-

ment is essential. Fresh whole blood replaces not only blood volume but vital clotting factors (platelets) and essential cellular elements (red and white blood cells). Stored blood rapidly loses its platelets and clotting factors. In cases of severe and continued blood loss, it may be necessary to administer blood under pressure and even through more than one infusion route. Need for blood volume replacement may be determined not only by estimating blood loss when hemorrhage is visible and blood loss is measurable, but also by severity of shock, serial measurement of arterial blood pressure and blood volume, central venous pressure, hematocrit, pulse, and hourly urine output. Blood pressure alone, without the use of other physiologic parameters, is a very unreliable criterion for the presence or severity of shock. Prompt control of bleeding as well as blood replacement is essential.

It is important, of course, that blood used for replacement match the patient's specific type of blood. Therefore, before giving a transfusion, routine testing for antigens—ABO and $D(Rh_o)$—should always be performed in donors and recipients. Although blood may not always be the fluid of choice for volume replacement, it is usually the most dependable. If the loss of blood volume is the result of hemorrhage, whole blood replacement is the therapy of choice, along with control of hemorrhage. Whole blood contains all the necessary fluid-holding constituents and does not pass out of the vascular system as rapidly as most parenteral fluids. The use of plasma expanders and noncolloid fluids, such as isotonic saline, offers only temporary support. Blood should not be used for transfusion if more than 21 days have passed since it was obtained from the donor. With massive transfusions, hypocalcemia may occur from the citrate used to prevent the blood from clotting. Citrate binds and inactivates calcium. Calcium gluconate is given to replace the calcium content.

If lost blood volume is replaced promptly with adequate amounts of blood, there is no problem. However, if treatment is delayed, more and more blood is required to maintain blood pressure and other vital signs. Actually more blood will be required than has been lost from hemorrhage. The reason for this is that some of the blood remaining in the circulatory system becomes trapped in the capillaries and small blood vessels, particularly in the liver and splanchnic area. The trapped cells may form microclots or small thrombi. Trapping is probably caused by increased resistance to blood flow from compensatory vasoconstriction. In addition, with decreased velocity of flow, there is increased viscosity. As blood viscosity increases, the plasma cannot keep red cells in suspension, and they settle out of the plasma causing sludging or aggregation of cells in the microcirculation. As blood flow slows and red blood cells bump into one another in the small vessels, a sticky substance forms on the outside of the red blood cell, and this further promotes sludging or red cell aggregation.

The use of high molecular weight dextran (or hetastarch) may further increase viscosity as well as red blood cell aggregation. Clinical studies have shown that low viscosity dextran infusions help to mobilize noncirculating red cells, thus it is used along with whole blood for treatment of shock caused by hemorrhage.

Avoidance of sludging. Following are methods used to avoid aggregation of red blood cells:

1 Adequate mechanical respiratory movements should be maintained by encouraging the patient to breathe deeply and regularly or by using mechanical assistance. These respiratory movements help to bring blood into the thorax and assist blood flow. (From 30% to 50% of the patients who die following shock show signs of pulmonary insufficiency and pulmonary emboli.)
2 Muscle movement is promoted by having the patient contract and relax the muscles in his extremities, shoulders, and buttocks. Circulation can be assisted by massaging and moving the patient's muscles and by position movement of the patient (if this is not contraindicated by his condition).

Summary of nursing considerations

The formation of both red cells and hemoglobin is a complex process, and deficiency in any one of a number of constituents may result in anemia because of failure to produce the needed number of red cells or an adequate amount of hemoglobin. Although an adequate diet is the preferable way to acquire the essential constituents for blood formation, various disease conditions require treatment to bring about more rapid results than can be obtained from diet alone.

Antianemic drugs are used to eliminate the cause of anemia or to provide symptomatic relief. The major antianemic substances used in replacement therapy for the corresponding anemia are iron, vitamin B_{12}, and folic acid.

Anticoagulants inhibit blood clotting and are used to prevent intravascular thrombosis by preventing (1) fibrin deposits, (2) extension of a thrombus, and (3) thromboembolic complications. Long-term anticoagulant therapy remains controversial, and even short-term use of these drugs holds great potential for serious side effects, drug interactions, and toxic complications. Among the anticoagulants currently used are heparin, coumarin derivatives, and indandione derivatives.

Patients receiving anticoagulant therapy should be carefully monitored for bleeding tendencies. Blood should be drawn for clotting time or APTT before heparin is to be injected. Protamine sulfate is used as an antidote to combat bleeding in case of heparin overdose; vitamin K is used as an antidote for overdose of coumarin derivatives. Patients must be instructed concerning diet, medication, follow-up visits, and other critical aspects of self-care.

Hemostatic drugs reduce blood clotting time. Useful preoperatively and postoperatively, these substances include absorbable gelatine sponge, human fibrin foam, oxidized cellulose, thrombin, and natural and synthetic vitamin K.

Whole blood or blood components can be replaced in the body by means of nondrug therapy. Adequate blood volume is essential to maintain viability of cells, normal tissue function, and life itself. When blood is lost through trauma and hemorrhage, it must be replaced promptly to maintain blood pressure and other vital signs. Fresh whole blood that matches the patient's specific type replaces not only blood volume but vital clotting factors (platelets) and essential cellular elements (red and white blood cells). If treatment is delayed, blood flow slows and red cells settle out of plasma, causing sludging or aggregation. Low viscosity dextran, a glucose polymer, is used along with whole blood to help mobilize red cells and avoid sludging.

When whole blood is unavailable for transfusion, blood plasma may be used. Plasma is the fluid part of the blood obtained by separating the cells from the whole citrated blood and can be given to any patient regardless of blood group. Certain proteins in blood plasma can be separated out and effectively used in specific treatment situations. These include albumin, thrombin, fibrinogen, and human antihemophilic human factor.

QUESTIONS

FOR STUDY AND REVIEW

1 Why are different drugs used in the treatment of hypochromic anemia and pernicious anemia?
2 Name two oral preparations of iron that are better tolerated than ferrous sulfate.
3 How should a liquid form of iron be prepared for oral administration? Why?
4 What is the action of heparin? What are the uses of heparin?
5 Why, when, and how is vitamin K used to promote blood coagulation?
6 Compare the use, effects, and administration of heparin with coumarin derivatives.
7 What should a patient who is to undergo long-term anticoagulant therapy with dicumarol have in the way of instruction before treatment is begun?
8 Why are the coumarin or phenindione drugs the drugs of choice for long-term anticoagulant therapy?
9 Discuss the use of blood transfusions in hypovolemic shock.
10 Compare the uses and effects of dextran 70 and dextran 40.

BIBLIOGRAPHY

GENERAL

Avery, G.S., editor: Drug treatment, ed. 2, Acton, Mass., 1980, Publishing Sciences Group, Inc.
Bowman, W.C., and Rand, M.J.: Textbook of pharmacology, ed. 2, London, 1980, Blackwell Scientific Publications.
Goodman, L.S., and Gilman, A., editors: The pharmacological basis of therapeutics, ed. 6, New York, 1980, Macmillan, Inc.

Meyers, F.H., Jawetz, E., and Goldfien, A.: Review of medical pharmacology, ed. 5, Los Altos, Calif., 1980, Lange Medical Publications.
Modell, W., editor: Drugs of choice 1980-1981, St. Louis, 1980, The C.V. Mosby Co.
Mountcastle, V.B., editor: Medical physiology, ed. 14, St. Louis, 1980, The C.V. Mosby Co.
Sodeman, W., and Sodeman, T.: Pathologic physiology: mechanisms of disease, ed. 6, Philadelphia, 1979, W.B. Saunders Co.

ANTIANEMIC DRUGS

Beal, R.W.: Haematinics I: patho-physiological and clinical aspects, Drugs **2**:190, 1971.
Beal, R.W.: Haematinics II: clinical pharmacological and therapeutic aspects, Drugs **2**:207, 1971.
Forget, B.: Hemolytic anemias: congenital and acquired, Hosp. Pract. **15**:67, 1980.
Hoffbraud, A.V., editor: Megaloblastic anemia, Clin. Haematol. **5**:471, 1976.
Nienhuis, A., and Benz, E.: Regulation of hemoglobin synthesis. I, N. Engl. J. Med. **297**:1318, 1977; II, N. Engl. J. Med. **297**:1371, 1977.
O'Malley, K., and Stevenson, I.H.: Iron deficiency anaemia and drug metabolism, J. Pharm. Pharmacol. **25**:339, 1973.
Smith, R., and LoBuglio, A.: An approach to patients with anemia, Med. Opinion **6**:14, 1977.
Wasserman, G.S., Martens, D.O., and Green, V.A.: Early aggressive treatment of iron poisoning, Am. Fam. Physician **15**:125, 1977.

ANTICOAGULANT DRUGS AND OTHER MISCELLANEOUS AGENTS

Adar, R., and Salzman, E.W.: Treatment of thrombosis of veins of the lower extremities, N. Engl. J. Med. **292**:348, 1975.
Anticoagulants in acute myocardial infarction: results of a cooperative clinical trial, J.A.M.A. **225**:724, 1973.
Brogden, R.N., and others: Streptokinase: a review of its clinical pharmacology, mechanisms of action and therapeutic uses, Drugs **5**:357, 1973.
Clagett, G.P., and others: Prevention of venous thromboembolism in surgical patients, N. Engl. J. Med. **290**:93, 1974.
Cooperative Clinical Trial: Anticoagulants in acute myocardial infarction, J.A.M.A. **225**:724, 1973.
Copans, H., and Lakier, J.: Commonly encountered problems in anticoagulant therapy, Prac. Cardiol. **6**:23, 1980.
Douglas, A.S.: Management of thrombotic diseases, Semin. Hematol. **2**:175, 1973.
Drapkin, A., and others: Anticoagulant therapy after acute myocardial infarction: relation of therapeutic benefit to patient's age, sex, and severity of infarction, J.A.M.A. **222**:541, 1972.
Franco, L.: Acute disseminated intravascular coagulation, Cardiovasc. Nurs. **15**:22, 1979.
Gallus, A.S., and others: Small subcutaneous doses of heparin in prevention of venous thrombosis, N. Engl. J. Med. **288**:11, 1973.
Genton, E.: Guidelines for heparin therapy, Ann. Intern. Med. **80**:77, 1974.

Glazier, R.: Small-dose prophylactic heparin: does it prevent venous thrombosis? Mod. Med. **45:**37, Oct. 30, 1977.

Gross, H., and others: Anticoagulant therapy in myocardial infarction, an overview of methodology, Am. J. Med. **52:**421, 1972

Hanson, R.: Heparin-lock or keep-open I.V.? Am. J. Nurs. **76:**1102, 1976.

Hirsh, J., and others: Anticoagulants in pregnancy: a review of indications and complications, Am. Heart J. **83:**301, 1972.

Hirsh, J., and others: Using the antithrombotic agents, Patient Care **14:**62, 1980.

Kakkar, V.V., and others: Prevention of fatal postoperative pulmonary embolism by low doses of heparin: an international multicentre trial, Lancet **2:**45, 1975.

Lewis, J., Spero, J., and Hasiba, U.: Coagulopathies, D.M. **23:**2, 1977.

Martyn, D.T., and others: Continuous intravenous administration of heparin, Mayo Clin. Proc. **46:**347, 1971.

McCullough, J., and Crosby, W.: Hematology, J.A.M.A. **243:**2188, 1980.

Mitchell, A.A.: Smoking and warfarin dosage, N. Engl. J. Med. **287:**1153, 1972.

Moore, K., and Maschak, B.: How patient education can reduce the risks of anticoagulation, Nursing '77 **7**(9):24, 1977.

Nyman, J.E.: Thrombophlebitis in pregnancy, Am. J. Nurs. **80:**90, 1980.

O'Brian, B.S., and Woods, S.: The paradox of DIC, Am. J. Nurs., **78:**1878, 1978.

O'Reilly, R.A.: Vitamin K and oral anticoagulant drugs as competitive antagonists in man, Pharmacology **7:**149, 1972.

Quick, A.J.: Quick on Quick's test, N. Engl. J. Med. **288:**1079, 1973.

Rosenberg, R., and Rosenberg, J.: The anticoagulant function of heparin, Drug Therapy **9:**26, 1979.

Scarlato, M.: Blood transfusions today; what you should know and should do. Nursing '78 **8**(2):68, 1978.

Shapiro, R.: Anticoagulant therapy, Am. J. Nurs. **74:**439, 1974.

Sherry, S.: Streptokinase—use it to lyse clots, Mod. Med. **46:**93, May 30-June 15, 1978.

Stein, R.: Hypercoagulable states, Curr. Prescribing **5:**82, July 1979.

Wessler, S.: Anticoagulant therapy, J.A.M.A. **228:**757, 1974.

Wessler, S., and others: Theory and practice of minidose heparin in surgical patients: a status report, Circulation **47:**4, 1973.

Westphal, R.G.: Rational alternatives to the use of whole blood, Ann. Intern. Med. **76:**987, 1972.

CHAPTER 21

Diuretics

MARY ANNE TOLL and SARA J. WHITE

The kidney

Classification of diuretics

    Proximal tubule diuretics
    Diluting segment diuretics
    Loop diuretics
    Distal tubule diuretics

Miscellaneous diuretics

    Osmotic diuretics
    Water
    Xanthine diuretics
    Acid-forming salts

Summary of nursing considerations

Diuretics are among the most commonly used chemotherapeutic modalities. These drugs represent the mainstay in the treatment of hypertension and are an integral part of drug therapies in edematous conditions such as cirrhosis, nephrotic syndrome, and congestive heart failure. Diuretics are used because of their role in influencing water and electrolyte balance, particularly sodium, in the body. This action is exerted on tubular function of the kidney rather than on glomerular filtration. It generally involves the inhibition of solute reabsorption and consequently water reabsorption, since water passively diffuses across the tubular membrane when sodium transport occurs. This inhibition results in a diuresis, or loss of body water via urination. To better understand the specific action of the diuretic agents, it will be necessary to review some basic kidney physiology.

The kidney

The kidney is composed of millions of individual units called nephrons. Each nephron consists of a glomerulus and a tubular system. The volume and composition of urine as a result of concentration and dilution depend on three major processes in the kidney: glomerular filtration, tubular reabsorption, and tubular secretion.

Glomerular filtration. Glomerular filtration occurs as a result of plasma flowing across a capillary bed called the glomerulus. The heart works to create hydrostatic pressure in the blood vessels, which in turn provides the force necessary to accomplish glomerular filtration. Blood flow to the kidney is 1200 ml/minute, which is 20% to 25% of cardiac output. The hydrostatic pressure within the glomerular capillaries is about 60% of arterial pressure. Systemic blood pressure has to be significantly reduced before glomerular filtration is greatly altered. Usually some degree of filtration will exist if the mean blood pressure remains above 50 mm Hg. Maintenance of the glomerular hydrostatic pressure is aided by the ability of the afferent and efferent arterioles to effectively alter vessel resistance. In the absence of disease the glomerular membrane does not filter plasma proteins greater than 100 A, such as hemoglobin and albumin and the small amount of protein-bound substances. The glomerular filtrate is otherwise almost identical to plasma. The rate of filtration in an average adult is approximately 125 ml/minute; 99% of this tubular filtrate is ultimately reabsorbed throughout the tubule.

Tubular reabsorption. Tubular reabsorption involves both active and passive transport of substances into the tubular epithelial cell and into the extracellular fluid compartment.

One such transport mechanism is the capacitance gradient, which demands that a certain amount of a substance in the glomerular filtrate be absorbed rather than a constant percentage. In the case of glucose, usually all is reabsorbed in the proximal tubule unless an extra load is presented. Once the gradient is satisfied, the remainder is excreted in the urine. Other gradients exist to satisfy electrical, osmotic, and chemical differences between tubular fluid and the interstitium. For example, in the proximal tubule sodium is *actively* transported across the tubular cell membrane from tubule filtrate. Chloride follows passively because of an electromagnetic gradient. Water in turn follows passively in response to an osmotic gradient established by sodium chloride solute. Then passive diffusion of 60% of urea content occurs to maintain a chemical gradient. Depending on the pK_a of a drug and pH of the tubular fluid, weak acids and weak bases may be reabsorbed by nonionic back diffusion.

Tubular secretion. Tubular secretion affects the composition of urine by allowing compounds such as penicillin, probenecid, methotrexate, and thiazides to enter into tubular fluid from peritubular or interstitial capillaries. This is accomplished via specific transport mechanisms for secretion of organic acids, organic basis, and EDTA in the proximal tubule. Other very important examples of tubular secretion include that of the hydrogen ion, ammonia, and potassium.

• • •

Diuretics mainly have their effect on tubular function in the nephron. Understanding of their action requires knowledge of the events that take place along each of the tubular segments. These segments include the proximal tubule, the descending and ascending limbs of the loop of Henle, the distal convoluted tubule, and the collecting duct.

Proximal tubule. Most of the glomerular filtrate is reabsorbed in the proximal tubule and returned to the bloodstream. Approximately 60% to 70% of salt and water is reabsorbed rapidly, maintaining nearly the same osmolality between tubular fluid and interstitial fluid at the end of the proximal tubule. The general mechanism for sodium, chloride, water, and urea reabsorption has previously been described under tubular reabsorption with respect to gradient transport. There is *no* dilutional or concentration changes of these ions in the proximal tubule.

Other substances reabsorbed at this site include glucose, amino acids, phosphate, uric acid, and a major portion of potassium. Nearly 90% of bicarbonate in tubular filtrate is reabsorbed as carbon dioxide if hydrogen ion is secreted in the tubular lumen. Plasma carbon dioxide is hydrolyzed in the tubular cell to form carbonic acid, which dissociates to give bicarbonate and hydrogen ion. This reversible reaction is catalyzed by carbonic anhydrase. The hydrogen ion secreted into the lumen combines with bicarbonate of glomerular filtrate to form carbonic acid in the lumen. This again dissociates to give water and carbon dioxide, which are reabsorbed. This reaction is again catalyzed at both steps by carbonic anhydrase. Proximal tubule reabsorption is usually constant in spite of moderate changes in glomerular filtration rate. There are several factors, however, that decrease reabsorption. Saline infusions increase the concentration of sodium and chloride ions in the lumen, which negates the solute gradient for water reabsorption. This osmotic diuresis decreases reabsorption of calcium ions in a therapeutic manner. Osmotic diuretics such as mannitol and urea decrease proximal tubule reabsorption. Acetazolamide achieves the same effect by inhibiting the enzyme carbonic anhydrase. Conversely, extracellular fluid depletion and sodium restriction are factors that increase reabsorption at the proximal tubule.

Tubular secretion is another important function of the proximal tubule. Common drugs as well as hydrogen ion are secreted and include acetazolamide, hydrochlorothiazide, ethacrynic acid, furosemide, penicillin, aspirin, quinine, and morphine. It becomes very important to consider the effect of competition on secretion with respect to increased serum levels; for example probenecid increases and prolongs penicillin blood levels.

Descending loop of Henle. This portion of the nephron is permeable to water; water is passively taken up to equilibrate medullary interstitial osmolality. This produces a hypertonic filtrate at the tip of the loop of Henle, the papilla. There is very low sodium and urea permeability in this segment.

Ascending loop of Henle. Water permeability is almost nil in the ascending limb of the loop of Henle, whereas sodium and chloride permeability is high. Approximately 20% to 25% of sodium load in glomerular filtrate is reabsorbed in this segment. Chloride is *actively* reabsorbed and sodium *passively* follows. Consequently, two very important situations occur. The concentration of tubular filtrates becomes very dilute, or hypotonic; this is often termed "free water production." Meanwhile, the medullary interstitium becomes hypertonic, which is necessary to the concentration capacity of the countercurrent multiplier. The concentration gradient established across the tubular epithelium becomes multiplied in a longitudinal direction, resulting in a large osmotic gradient between isosmotic renal cortex and hyperosmotic medulla and papilla. The ascending limb of the loop of Henle is not responsive to any hormones as are other segments.

Distal convoluted tubule. Between 5% and 10% of sodium reabsorption *actively* takes place in the distal tubule. This uptake is largely determined by the presence of a hormone called aldosterone. When the extracellular fluid volume is decreased, the renin-angiotensin system is involved, stimulating the release of aldosterone. Increased levels of aldosterone act to increase the active reabsorption of sodium. Although an increase in potassium secretion is seen, a simple Na^+-K^+ exchange pump is no longer recognized. It is in this portion of the nephron that spironolactone, amiloride, and triamterene act to minimize potassium loss.

Collecting duct. The hypotonic fluid entering the collecting duct may be altered in the medullary portion by the presence of antidiuretic hormone (ADH). Fluid is lost because of the osmotic gradient set up by hypertonic medullary interstitium. Thus the collecting duct is responsible for urine concentration.

Classification of diuretics

Therapeutically, drug selection is facilitated if each diuretic is presented according to the

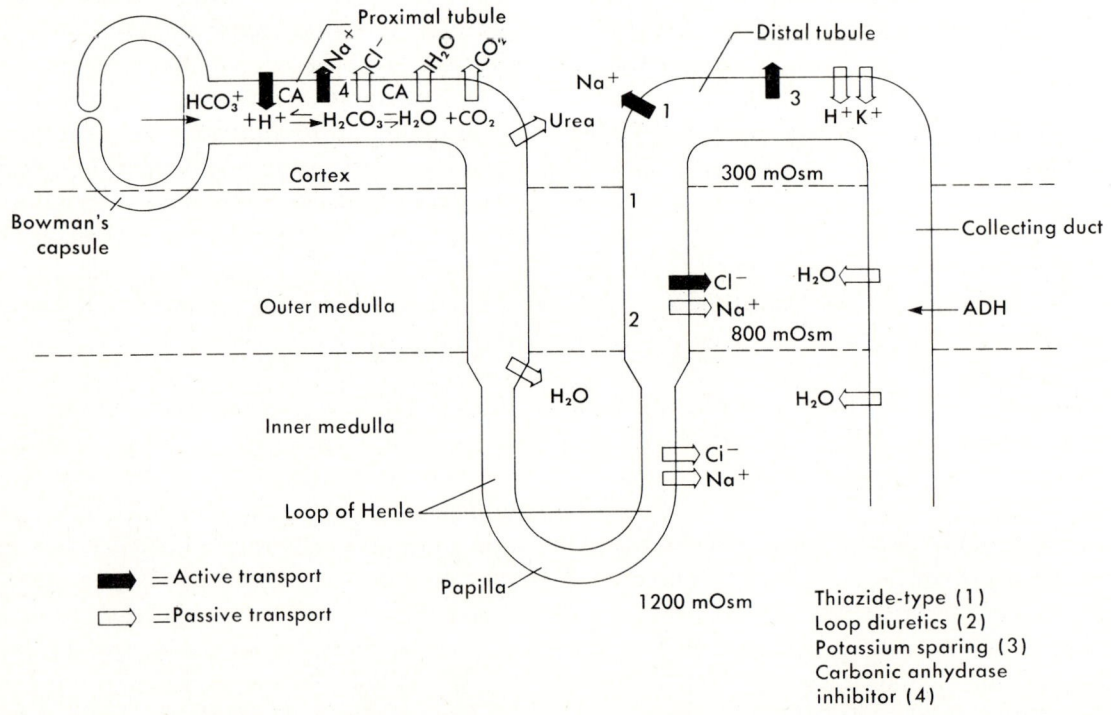

FIG. 21-1. Diuretics. Site of action via water and electrolyte transport.

major site of action. This approach does not preclude drug effect at other sites in the nephron. Fig. 21-1 shows the various sites of action of diuretic groups via water and electrolyte transport system in a kidney nephron.

PROXIMAL TUBULE DIURETICS
Carbonic anhydrase inhibitors

Carbonic anhydrase inhibitors have acetazolamide as their prototype. These agents are not useful therapeutically as diuretics. Their sodium excretion is minimal and temporary because of the metabolic acidosis from continued use. A carbonic anhydrase inhibitor prevents the secretion of hydrogen ion in the proximal tubule and to a lesser extent in the distal tubule. Alkaline urine is produced, which inhibits bicarbonate reabsorption. Urine resulting from the use of carbonic anhydrase inhibitors has sodium, potassium, and bicarbonate but no

TABLE 21-1   Thiazide and thiazide-type diuretics

Generic name (Brand name)	Availability	Usual daily dose (maximum)	Duration of action (hours)
Benzothiadiazines			
Chlorothiazide (Diuril)	250, 500 mg	500-1000 mg (2000 mg) in one or two doses for hypertension 1000-2000 mg as one or two doses in edema	6-12
Hydrochlorothiazide			
(Hydrodiuril)	25, 50, 100 mg	75-100 mg (200 mg) in one or two doses for edema	12
(Esidrex)	25, 50, 100 mg		
(Oretic)	25, 50 mg	50-100 mg in two doses for hypertension	
Bendroflumethiazide (Naturetin)	2.5, 5, 10 mg	2.5-5 mg in single dose	18-24
Methyclothiazide			
(Enduron)	2.5, 5 mg	2.5-10 mg in single dose	24
(Aquatensen)	5 mg	2.5-5 mg (10 mg) in single dose	
Hydroflumethiazide (Saluron)	50 mg	25-200 mg in one or two doses for edema 50-100 mg in one or two doses for hypertension	12
Benzthiazide (Exna)	50 mg	50-200 mg in two doses	12
Polythiazide (Renese)	1, 2, 4 mg	1-4 mg in single dose for edema	
		2-4 mg in single dose for hypertension	18-24
Cyclothiazide (Anhydron)	2 mg	1-2 mg in single dose for edema 2 mg in single dose for hypertension	18-24
Trichlormethiazide			
(Naqua)	2, 4 mg	2-4 mg in single dose for hypertension	18-24
(Metahydrin)	4 mg	1-4 mg in single dose for edema	
Phthalimidines			
Chlorthalidone (Hygroton)	50, 100 mg	50-100 mg in single dose	54
Quinazolines			
Quinethazone (Hydromox)	50 mg	50-100 mg (150 mg) in one or two doses	18-24
Metolazone (Zaroxolyn)	2.5, 5, 10 mg	5-10 mg (20 mg) in single dose for edema	
		2.5-5 mg in single dose for hypertension	12-24

chloride ions because of reabsorption in the ascending limb of the loop of Henle. Acetazolamide is not filtered in the glomerulus, a result of protein binding, but is presented to the proximal tubule by tubular secretion.

DILUTING SEGMENT DIURETICS
Thiazides and thiazide-type drugs

The thiazides, the major diuretics active within the diluting segments of the kidney, are synthetic drugs chemically related to the sulfonamides; chlorothiazide and hydrochlorothiazide are the two most commonly used thiazides. Since quinethazone, metolazone, and chlorthalidone—other common diluting segment diuretics—are pharmacologically and structurally similar to the thiazides, all of the diluting segment diuretics will be described collectively as the thiazide-type diuretics. Important differences will be mentioned later. Table 21-1 presents these diuretics, their availability, dosage, and duration of actions.

Mechanism of action. The thiazide-type diuretics have variable but clinically insignificant diuretic action as inhibitors of carbonic anhydrase. Their primary action and site of action appear to be inhibition of sodium reabsorption at the cortical diluting segment of the nephron, including portions of the thick ascending loop of Henle and the distal convoluted tubule. The exact mechanism of these drugs is unclear. They are less potent than the loop diuretics, since the maximum portion of the sodium load they can affect at the distal tubule is less than 10% of the glomerular filtrate. The thiazide-type diuretics therefore primarily promote the excretion of sodium, chloride, and water. Especially important is their ability to impair free water clearance with no effect on concentration ability. The initial natriuretic effect lasts for about 1 week and then resets at a lower level. This diuretic tolerance occurs because of increased aldosterone levels and a decreased sodium load at the distal tubule.

As an increased sodium load is presented to the distal tubule, a corresponding increase in potassium secretion is recognized. In addition, as the extracellular fluid volume decreases, plasma renin activity and aldosterone levels increase, with resulting potassium loss. Potassium is the most common electrolyte lost; with loss occurring in 30% to 50% of patients. This loss is dose-related, usually intermittent, not harmful, and generally not clinically recognized. Potassium loss may become a severe problem in patients with myocardial disease who are taking digitalis preparations, since it can precipitate serious arrhythmias. Hypokalemia in a cirrhotic patient may predispose to hepatic encephalopathy and coma. The hypokalemia may be reversed with potassium supplementation either by an increase in dietary intake, which is unreliable and may tend to alter other electrolytes, or by oral medication. The oral medication route is met with an outstanding lack of compliance because of the unpleasant taste.

The potassium loss may also be reversed by the addition of potassium-sparing diuretics acting to inhibit potassium loss at the distal tubule. However, potassium replacement is usually not necessary in 80% to 90% of patients taking the thiazide diuretics, particularly in the treatment of nonedematous states. It should be remembered potassium replacement may be dangerous in the elderly, in renal dysfunction, and when used in combination with potassium-sparing diuretics.

The thiazide-type diuretics are noted to increase serum uric acid in 40% of men and less often in women. The 1 to 2 mg/100 ml increase in serum uric acid is persistent and probably results from inhibition of tubular secretion of uric acid. This effect is reversible on discontinuation of the drugs. In the absence of gout or genetic predisposition the hyperuricemia is usually no problem and requires no treatment. However, in a patient with a history of gout the use of allopurinol or probenecid is suggested.

Carbohydrate tolerance may be impaired by these diuretics, but the degree is usually not significant. The thiazide diuretics are not contraindicated in diabetes. Only rarely has severe hyperglycemia been induced, and this may have been associated with potassium depletion.

The thiazide-type diuretics affect the transport of other ions. Transient calcium excretion may be seen initially, but long-term use of these diuretics causes a hypocalciuric response. Hypercalcemia is rare, although serum calcium, both total and ionized, may be increased. This effect on calcium may be a result of increased hemoconcentration, decreased calcium excretion, increased bone resorption, or possibly enhancement of parathyroid or vitamin D action. The excretion of bicarbonate is increased only with very high doses of the thiazide-type diuretics and thus produces no significant change in urine pH. The effectiveness of these diuretics is not affected by changes in acid-base balance. Magnesium, bromide, iodide, and phosphate excretion are enhanced.

Azotemia, seen as an increase in BUN and serum creatinine, may be precipitated with the thiazide diuretics. This may be caused by volume depletion or a direct effect on the renal vasculature. The resultant decrease in glomerular filtration rate makes these diuretics, with the exception of metolazone, ineffective at creatinine clearance of less than 20 ml/minute. The thiazide-type diuretics have been reported to elevate serum lipids, including cholesterol and triglycerides. This effect is persistent and may occur within 7 days of thiazide use.

Pharmacokinetics. The thiazide-type diuretics are absorbed rapidly on oral administration and produce a diuresis within 2 hours. Their peak effect is usually seen at 3 to 6 hours. When these drugs are given in equivalent dosages, they are equally effective under normal kidney function and share the same adverse effects. The thiazides differ in their relative potency and duration of action (see Table 21-1). Drug selection may be influenced by cost and patient compliance with respect to single daily dosing. Dose-versus-response data supply a flat curve, suggesting that when dosage exceeds the maximal range, little increase in effectiveness is seen and side effects are more frequent. The duration of action of the thiazides is influenced by the relative degree of protein binding and corresponding decrease in excretion rate. Chlorthalidone is almost 90% bound to protein or red blood cells and has a duration of approximately 54 hours. The thiazide-type diuretics are primarily excreted unchanged in the urine by glomerular filtration and proximal tubule secretion via organic acid transport. Competition of

the latter with probenecid and some antibiotics may be responsible for certain drug interactions. These drugs rapidly cross the placental barrier to the fetus and are found in breast milk. Diuretic activity of the thiazide-type diuretics is directly related to their solubility ratios in water and lipids. The duration effect is greater with increased lipid solubility because of increased volume of distribution. Lipid solubility may facilitate drug access to the site of action.

Side effects and toxic effects. The major side and toxic effects of the thiazide-type diuretics have been previously described in terms of electrolyte alterations. Other effects reported infrequently are gastrointestinal, including gastric irritation, anorexia, cramping, constipation, jaundice, and rare cases of pancreatitis in which the role of the thiazides is unclear. Central nervous system toxicity may include headache, vertigo, paresthesias, and xanthopsia. Effects on the blood are very infrequent and may present as neutropenia, thrombotic purpura, agranulocytosis, and immune hemolytic anemia. Because these drugs are sulfonamide derivatives, allergic manifestations are possible, especially in those patients known to be sensitive to the sulfas. The allergic response may be recognized as photosensitivity, rash, urticaria, or the rare immune hemolytic anemia.

Indications. The thiazide-type diuretics are indicated in the management of disorders associated with edema by virtue of their ability to excrete sodium and water. They are the diuretic of choice initially in right-sided heart failure, mild to moderate left-sided heart failure, congestive heart failure, and chronic lymphedema. They are helpful in treating edema of pregnancy when renal dysfunction is present, but continued use is not recommended. Preeclampsia may require a more potent diuretic. Edema resulting from renal failure and estrogen or steroid use may be relatively resistant to the thiazides. In combination with spironolactone, they are indicated in the treatment of the nephrotic syndrome, cirrhosis with ascites, and idiopathic water-retention syndrome.

The thiazide-type diuretics are most useful in the initial treatment of all stages of essential hypertension when normal renal function prevails. Malignant hypertension requires a more potent diuretic and additional hypotensive agents. The thiazide-type diuretics can be expected to lower the blood pressure by 10 to 15 mm Hg. Their role in hypertension is ascribed to their ability to produce a direct vasodilator effect on arterioles and enhance other antihypertensives that tend to increase sodium and plasma volume. The onset of the vasodilator effect is seen after 3 to 4 days of therapy and ceases within a week after drug removal. Paradoxically thiazide-type diuretics decrease urine volume in diabetes insipidus by 50% and are especially the drugs of choice in nephrogenic diabetes. These drugs are also indicated in the treatment of idiopathic hypercalciuria, which may lead to renal stone formation. Sodium intake should not be rigidly restricted to induce hyponatremia, but some reduction is important in preventing thiazide tolerance.

Drug interactions

1 Digitalis glycoside toxicity may occur in the presence of hypokalemia induced by the thiazides.
2 Severe hypokalemia may result with concommitant use with other drugs that deplete potassium, such as steroids and amphotericin.
3 Lithium clearance is decreased by thiazides, predisposing to toxicity.
4 The hyperglycemic, hypotensive, and hyperuricemic effects of diazoxide may be potentiated.
5 The hypotensive effects of other hypotensive agents such as alcohol, methyldopa, and guanethidine may be increased.
6 The slight alkalinization of the urine that may occur with the thiazides may decrease the effectiveness of methanamine compounds, which require a pH of 5.5 or less.
7 Thiazides should be administered 1 hour before cholestyramine resins to prevent binding and decreased absorption.
8 Probenecid blocks tubular secretion of thiazides and thiazide-induced uric acid retention.

Exception

Metolazone. Metolazone shares the pharmacologic actions of the thiazide-type diuretics, but it does not significantly decrease glomerular filtration rate or renal plasma flow. Metolazone may produce a diuresis in a patient with a creatinine clearance less than 20 ml/minute.

Metolazone has been shown to be synergistic in combination with furosemide and to produce a diuresis in patients who did not respond to either agent alone. This combination may result in excess loss of extracellular fluid volume and electrolytes. Doses of 5 to 20 mg daily, plus large doses of furosemide, have been shown to reverse edema refractory to furosemide. Metolazone does not show any carbonic anhydrase inhibition. Additional adverse reactions reported with metolazone include abdominal bloating, palpitation, chest pain, and chills.

LOOP DIURETICS

Furosemide and ethacrynic acid are the classic examples of the loop diuretics, so called because they exert their action in the loop of Henle. These drugs for the most part are very similar to the thiazide-type diuretics in pharmacology and in the side effects they produce. Thus, to avoid unnecessary repetition, only the differences are presented. Furosemide and ethacrynic acid exhibit their major effect by inhibiting active *chloride* transport in the thick portion of the ascending limb of the loop of Henle. The resulting passive sodium transport is also inhibited. The maximal effect of the loop diuretics is their indirect influence on urine concentration rather than on urine dilution. Furosemide and ethacrynic acid are more potent diuretics than the thiazides because they have the potential for altering 20% to 25% of the filtered sodium load, which is presented to the ascending limb of the loop of Henle. The loop diuretics do not inhibit carbonic anhydrase, except when furosemide is administered in very high doses. Carbohydrate intolerance may occur but is less frequent. Rather than the hypocalciuric effect of the thiazides, the loop diuretics (particularly furosemide) promote calcium excretion. Furosemide in combination with normal saline infusion is the treatment of choice in hypercalcemia. Ethacrynic acid has little or no direct effect on glomerular filtration rate, whereas furosemide exhibits a renal vasodilator effect, resulting in less vascular resistance and increased renal blood flow. In addition, in severe renal dysfunction furosemide can convert to increase liver metabolism and excretion. Furosemide is therefore useful in renal failure, although it is contraindicated in anuria.

The loop diuretics also differ from the thiazides in that they have an infinite dose-response curve. Increasing the dose continues to produce greater responses; hence they are referred to as "high-ceiling" diuretics. Both furosemide and ethacrynic acid given intravenously exert an effect within 5 minutes, show a peak effect at 15 to 20 minutes, and have a duration of response less than 3 hours. Oral administration shows an onset in 30 minutes, a peak effect at 1 to 2 hours, and a duration of 6 to 8 hours. Indications for use of the loop diuretics are edematous conditions showing resistance to the thiazides, acute and severe left-sided heart failure, and pulmonary edema. In these instances the loop diuretics may be almost too effective in their induction of a rapid and severe volume depletion, particularly in a patient with severe heart failure. The patient should be monitored for decreased blood pressure, tiredness, and lethargy. The loop diuretics are not as effective as the thiazides in treating hypertension. Additional drug interactions for the loop diuretics include the following.

1 Rarely, ototoxicity is produced and is associated with high doses administered very rapidly, usually to a patient with renal dysfunction or a patient on concomitant therapy with an agent known to be ototoxic, such as an aminoglycoside antibiotic.
2 The loop diuretics are highly protein bound, and ethacrynic acid is particularly incriminated in displacing warfarin-like drugs from receptor sites, thus increasing their effect.
3 Furosemide is reported to potentiate the nephrotoxicity of drugs such as cephaloridine.

Furosemide (Lasix)

Furosemide is a sulfonamide derivative and shares the same potential for allergic response, photosensitivity, and marrow depression as do the thiazide diuretics. It is available in 20- and 40-mg tablets and 20- and 100-mg ampules for injection. The usual oral adult dose in the treatment of edema is 20 to 80 mg daily as a single dose. The dose may be titrated upward gradually and has reached 600 mg daily in certain cases of severe edema. As a diuretic, the usual intravenous or intramuscular dose is 20 to 40 mg, administered slowly; 20-mg increments may be added every 2 hours if needed. A 40-mg dose of furosemide is slowly administered and may be repeated once if needed in the treatment of acute pulmonary edema.

Side effects include nausea and vomiting, diarrhea, dermatitis, pruritus, blurring of vision, and postural hypotension, resulting primarily from marked diuresis and electrolyte imbalance. Furosemide is contraindicated in pregnancy and nursing mothers, and like other diuretics, in states of anuria, hepatic coma, and electrolyte depletion.

Ethacrynic acid (Edecrin)

Ethacrynic acid is not a sulfonamide derivative but is more closely related to the mercurial diuretics. It is associated with less photosensitivity. Ethacrynic acid is not used as often as furosemide, probably because of the increased frequency of gastrointestinal toxicity, the need for reconstitution before use, the potential for thrombophlebitis, and marketing prejudice. It is available in 25- and 50-mg tablets and a 50-mg vial for injection. The usual oral adult dose in edema is 50 mg daily for several days with gradual increases as needed thereafter; 50 mg of the sodium salt may be given intravenously with care and may be repeated once if needed.

Bumetanide

Bumetanide is a loop diuretic shown to behave like furosemide with regard to action, effectiveness, and side effects. It is more potent on a milligram basis, with 1 mg of bumetanide equivalent to 40 mg of furosemide. This drug is not available for clinical use in the United States.

Mercurial diuretics

These diuretics have been shown to inhibit tubular reabsorption of sodium at most sites throughout the nephron but primarily in the ascending limb of the loop of Henle. The mercurial diuretics are administered only by the parenteral route, are associated with more severe toxicities, and elicit no better response than the thiazides and loop diuretics. For these reasons, furosemide and ethacrynic acid are not often used today.

DISTAL TUBULE DIURETICS
Spironolactone (Aldactone)

Spironolactone is a synthetic steroidal compound used to antagonize the effect of aldosterone by competitively binding to the protein that permits potassium secretion at the distal tubule. This response is directly related to the amount of circulating aldosterone in the serum. Spironolactone produces a very mild diuresis of sodium and water at the distal tubule via this mechanism. It does not interfere with renal tubule transport of sodium or chloride and does not inhibit carbonic anhydrase. Spironolactone has no effect on uric acid or glucose tolerance. This drug is not effective until metabolized in the liver to its active metabolite, canrenone. Canrenone usually has an elimination half-life of 12 to 24 hours, which is prolonged in congestive heart failure and chronic liver disease. In spite of prolonged excretion, blood levels are not changed and no dose alteration is necessary in liver disease. The mild diuresis produced by spironolactone has a gradual onset, with a peak effect occurring after 3 days.

Preparation, dosage, and administration. Spironolatone is available in 25-mg tablets. Although treatment may range from 50 to 800 mg daily, usually 100 mg daily is employed in edema and 50 to 100 mg daily in hypertension. The daily dose is usually given in two doses. There are important drug interactions with spironolactone and potassium salt substitutes and potassium-rich diets; these should be avoided to prevent hyperkalemia. Six hundred milligrams of aspirin is reported to block the action of spironolactone, but the clinical significance of this is not known. Spironolactone falsely represents a fourfold to ninefold increase in cortisol levels on fluorometric tests.

Side effects and toxic effects. Side effects of spironolactone include minor gastrointestinal distress (anorexia, nausea, vomiting, diarrhea) and occasional headache, drowsiness, ataxia, and mental confusion. In the male, androgen-like effects present as hirsutism, deepening of the voice, impotence, and decreased libido. Gynecomastia (excessive enlargement of male mammary glands) is more commonly seen, occurring in a few weeks or as late as 2 years; it may involve tender lumps in the breast. This side effect is slowly reversible on stopping the drug, sometimes over several months. The gynecomastia is usually seen with moderate to high doses but may occur at doses as low as 50 mg/day. The female may experience breast soreness and menstrual irregularities. The most serious side effect is hyperkalemia, which can be expected when spironolactone is used in renal impairment (the drug is contraindicated if BUN is greater than 40 mg/100 ml) or in combination with potassium supplements.

Since a mild diuresis is produced, spironolactone is usually used in combination with thiazide-type or loop diuretics because of the additive sodium excretion and especially for its effect in preventing potassium loss. In combination with the thiazide-type diuretics, spironolactone is employed in edematous conditions such as congestive heart failure, nephrotic syndrome, cirrhosis with ascites, and idiopathic water retention syndrome, all of which involve elevated aldosterone levels. It is recommended that cirrhotic patients be pretreated for several days with spironolactone alone before starting combination therapy.

Triamterene (Dyrenium)

Triamterene directly depresses the renal tubular transport of sodium in the distal tubule independent of the presence of aldosterone. Excretion of sodium, chloride, bicarbonate, magnesium, and calcium is increased. The increased loss of bicarbonate, which may slightly alkalinize the urine, is not a result of carbonic anhydrase inhibition. The decreased serum bicarbonate levels could possibly produce a metabolic acidosis. More important is the ability of triamterene to decrease the secretion of potassium at the distal tubule. Unlike the thiazide-type diuretics, triamterene does not inhibit uric acid excretion, although elevated serum levels have been reported, particularly in patients with a history of gout. Cardiac output is decreased, as is the glomerular filtration rate, which may result in an increased BUN and a decreased creatinine clearance.

Triamterene is rapidly absorbed and metabolized in the liver and excreted renally via glomerular filtration and tubular secretion. A diuresis ensues within 2 to 4 hours, with a maximal duration of 12 to 16 hours. Although more potent than spironolactone, triamterene as a single agent is a mild diuretic. Therefore, triamterene is usually employed in combination with other diuretics for its additive natriuretic effect and primarily because of the inhibition of potassium loss. It is used in combination therapy for the treatment of edema in congestive heart failure, nephrotic syndrome, and cirrhosis with ascites.

Triamterene is also indicated in idiopathic edema, steroid-induced edema, and edema of secondary aldosteronism. It has little usefulness in the treatment of hypertension.

It is available as 50- and 100-mg capsules. Usual daily doses of 100 to 200 mg are given in two doses.

Triamterene has few toxic effects. Gastrointestinal effects are less frequent than with spironolactone. However, the most serious toxic effect is hyperkalemia, mainly seen in renal impairment and with large, prolonged dosages. The concomitant administration of potassium as a salt substitute or a diet high in potassium is to be avoided. Triamterene should not be used concomitantly with spironolactone. Because of triamterene's structural similarity to folic acid, a causal relationship with megaloblastic anemia has been suggested.

Amiloride

Amiloride is structurally and pharmacologically similar to triamterene. It is used in combination with the thiazide diuretics to promote sodium excretion while sparing the loss of potassium in the urine. This drug is not available for use in the United States.

Miscellaneous diuretics

There are four groups of miscellaneous diuretics discussed here: (1) osmotic diuretics, (2) water, (3) xanthine diuretics, and (4) acid-forming salts.

OSMOTIC DIURETICS

Osmotic diuretics include mannitol and urea. These agents exert diuresis by adding to the solutes already present in the tubular fluid. With higher concentration of solutes present in the tubular fluid, sodium and water are not reabsorbed and are excreted in the urine. Additional water is pulled into the tubular fluid to equalize the higher solute content. These agents are not very efficient and require high doses.

Urea

Urea, although normally present in body fluids, serves as an osmotic diuretic when given in sufficiently large amounts. In a person with normal kidneys it is rapidly eliminated and is not toxic. It should not be administered when there is renal disease characterized by retention of nitrogen. Since a large amount of it is not reabsorbed by the tubular cells, it prevents the reabsorption of a proportional amount of water.

At present urea is not widely used because of the large dosage required, its bitter taste, and its ineffectiveness in terms of net sodium removal.

Sterile preparations are available from which solutions can be prepared for intravenous administration. The dosage is 0.1 to 1 g/kg body weight.

Mannitol (Osmitrol)

Mannitol is a sugar alcohol that occurs naturally in a number of plants and fungi and is also synthesized. Since mannitol is not reabsorbed by the tubules, it is excreted along with the water that is bound to it. It is considered to be the most effective osmotic diuretic. Mannitol is also used to test kidney function.

Mannitol is used for its diuretic action to relieve cerebral edema and to reduce elevated intraocular pressure, to treat oliguria resulting from transfusion reactions and trauma, and to promote excretion of toxic substances resulting from overdosage of sedatives.

Preparation, dosage, and administration. Mannitol is available in 5%, 10%, 15%, and 20% solutions in bottles of 500 and 1000 ml and as a 25% solution in 50 ml for intravenous injection. A preparation of mannitol and sodium chloride is available in various concentrations for injection. The adult dosage is 50 to 200 g infused over 24 hours. The dose for children is 0.75 g/kg body weight. Dosage must be regulated according to the patient's fluid and electrolyte balance, urinary output, and clinical signs.

Side effects. Side effects include headache, nausea, chills, mild chest pain, and low sodium and chloride blood levels. Fatal convulsions and anaphylaxis have also been reported.

Precautions. Mannitol should not be administered to patients with severe congestive heart failure or to patients with chronic edema regardless of cause. Its use in patients with impaired renal function should be preceded by administration of a test dose of 200 mg/kg body weight over 3 to 5 minutes. Mannitol may be given if the patient produces 40 ml or more of urine within 1 hour for 2 to 3 hours. Extravasation should be prevented, since local edema and tissue necrosis may occur. Mannitol crystallizes at a cool room temperature; it should always be administered with a filter. If crystals do form in the bottle, warm water run over the bottle will redissolve them.

WATER

Water is a physiologic diuretic. Fluid intake is frequently forced to increase urine output. The barrier to water reabsorption presented by the tubule cells appears to be related to the concentration of the posterior pituitary secretions in the blood. When fluid intake is increased, posterior pituitary activity is decreased, less water is removed from the urine, and diuresis results. Water is not a diuretic in the sense that it causes the excretion of edema fluid from the tissues. However, it has been shown that 5 to 8 liters of water daily can remove a considerable amount of edema in conjunction with an acid-ash diet. Excessive use of water can cause electrolyte imbalance. It frequently is considered unnecessary to restrict fluids for edematous patients, provided there is a restriction placed on intake of sodium. Therefore, it is important to know the sodium content of the tap water used.

XANTHINE DIURETICS

Xanthine diuretics include caffeine, theobromine, and theophylline, all of which exert similar actions in the body but differ in degree of effect on various tissues and organs. Caffeine exerts a marked action on the central nervous system but is relatively weak in its action on the kidney. Theobromine and theophylline are weak in their action on the nervous system but have a somewhat greater effect on the kidney and cardiovascular system.

Xanthines produce their diuretic effect by (1) improving glomerular function by increasing renal blood flow (especially with caffeine and theobromine); (2) improving renal blood flow as a result of their ability to stimulate heart action and improve cardiac output, which enhances their slight direct action on the kidneys; and (3) inhibiting tubular reabsorption of sodium and chloride (most pronounced with theophylline).

The effects of the xanthine diuretics are inferior to those that can be obtained from other diuretics. The oral forms of the xanthines are seldom used as diuretics, since more effective oral drugs are available. At present, aminophylline is used more commonly in the treatment of asthma than as a diuretic.

Tolerance to these drugs develops with repeated dosages. Xanthines are contraindicated in patients with renal insufficiency.

ACID-FORMING SALTS

Agents that increase renal excretion of sodium include the acid-forming salts and the plasma expanders (discussed in the next section). Diuretics that produce acidosis exert only transient action. The acidifying diuretics are chiefly ammonium chloride, ammonium nitrate, and calcium chloride. Of these, only ammonium chloride continues to be used with any regularity.

Ammonium chloride

Action. After absorption, the ammonium portion of the compound is converted in the liver to urea, with the liberation of hydrogen ions and chloride ions. Neutralization of the hydrogen ions is accomplished by a shift in the buffer system, with a compensatory loss of carbon dioxide via the lungs and a loss of available base to the excess of chloride ions. A state of acidosis results.

The number of chloride ions reaching the renal tubules is greatly increased, causing an increase in the urinary loss of chloride wih an equivalent amount of cation (chiefly sodium) and water. By achieving a net loss of water and electrolytes (sodium chloride), ammonium chloride promotes the movement and excretion of edema fluid.

The action of ammonium chloride would soon deplete the body of sodium if several compensatory mechanisms did not effect a return to a state of equilibrium. The diuretic effect of this compound is therefore greatest during the first or second day of administration. The principal compensatory mechanisms include increased renal excretion of cations (hydrogen and potassium) and the formation of ammonia by the renal cells with the recovery of corresponding amounts of sodium ions.

Preparation, dosage, and administration. Ammonium chloride is available in 500-mg and 1-g enteric-coated tablets or capsules for oral administration. The dose varies, although 4 to 12 g is sometimes given daily in divided doses. It may cause gastric irritation, nausea, and vomiting. It should not be used if renal function is seriously impaired because of the danger of causing uncompensated acidosis. The chief value of ammonium chloride as a diuretic is observed when it is used in combination with the mercurial diuretics.

Summary of nursing considerations

The kidneys are the primary organs that excrete water-soluble substances from the body, including products of metabolism, electrolytes, and foreign substances. They play an important part in maintaining the osmotic pressure of the blood and optimum concentrations of individual constituents of plasma and other body fluids.

The many functional units of the kidney are called nephrons. Within each nephron is a tuft of capillary vessels, the glomerulus, which is attached to a tubule divided into several segments: proximal convoluted tubule, descending and ascending limbs of the loop of Henle; distal convoluted tubule, and collecting duct.

These renal tubules regulate the substances excreted into the urine by glomerular filtration, tubular reabsorption, and tubular secretion. Diuretics increase the flow of urine by modifying one of the first two processes.

Diuretics act in various sites to (1) increase glomerular filtration, (2) inhibit reabsorption of sodium and chloride by direct action on the tubules, and (3) inhibit reabsorption of sodium by an indirect mechanism.

Thiazides are synthetic drugs chemically related to the sulfonamides. They appear to act directly on the distal tubule to decrease reabsorption of sodium, potassium, chloride, bicarbonate, and water; decrease urinary diluting capacity; decrease hypertension; and reduce elimination of bicarbonate. They potentiate antihypertensive drugs but have no serious effects on diseased kidneys.

Thiazides are potent drugs that may produce hypokalemia, precipitating digitalis toxicity, or may aggravate diabetes mellitus. They are useful for relief of practically all kinds of fluid retention in the body. Chlorothiazide is the prototype thiazide. These relatively inexpensive drugs have certain advantages over older diuretics: convenience of oral administration, low toxicity, low incidence of side effects over long periods, and equal or greater effectiveness than organic mercurial diuretics.

Furosemide is a powerful diuretic that finds its greatest application in congestive heart failure, cirrhosis of the liver, and nephrosis. Its potency demands careful monitoring of patients for signs of dehydration and reduction of blood volume that can precipitate vascular collapse, thrombosis, and embolism.

Ethacrynic acid is a powerful diuretic, similar in effect and side effects to furosemide. Patients with congestive heart failure and acute pulmonary edema who are unresponsive to other diuretics may respond to ethacrynic acid. Diuretics with primary action in distal tubules include potassium-excreting diuretics (the thiazides) and potassium-sparing diuretics.

Potassium-sparing diuretics include spironolactone and triamterene. Spironolactone blocks aldosterone competitively, causing the excretion of sodium and chloride and the retention of potassium. It is expensive, poorly absorbed from the gastrointestinal tract, and may produce skin rash, drowsiness, and ataxia. Its action is potentiated by other diuretics, and it may potentiate the action of antihypertensive drugs. Triamterene is used for purposes similar to spironolactone, but it is not as powerful. Diarrhea, nausea and vomiting, weakness, headache, dry mouth, and rash may occur.

Among the remaining diuretics that act on the distal tubule are the osmotic diuretics such as urea and mannitol, the xanthines, and the acid-forming salts. These are rarely used because superior results may be obtained with other agents.

Nursing implications for patients receiving diuretic therapy include recorded intake and output, daily weight record for the first few days of therapy followed by once or twice weekly weight recording, and careful assessment for edema, hypokalemia, and signs and symptoms of drug interactions and electrolyte imbalance.

QUESTIONS

FOR STUDY AND REVIEW

1 Explain the important nursing care aspects for patients receiving diuretic therapy.
2 Explain the mode of action of the thiazide diuretics.
3 Explain how antialdosterone compounds promote diuresis.
4 Explain the need for caution when diuretics are administered to patients receiving digitalis preparations.
5 Explain the most frequent side effects occurring with diuretic therapy.
6 From a survey of patients' charts (hospital, clinic, nursing home), determine which diuretics are most commonly prescribed and for which conditions. What is the range of dosage and the frequency of administration? How do these factors relate to age and sex? Do a comparison of costs of these drugs.

7 Explore a local pharmacy and compile a list of over-the-counter diuretic preparations. From an analysis of (a) major ingredients, (b) recommended dosage, and (c) precautions, is there additional information that should be provided to persons purchasing these products?

BIBLIOGRAPHY

Amery, A. and others: Glucose intolerance during diuretic therapy, Lancet, Apr. 1, 1978, p. 681.

Beyer, K.H., Jr.: The pharmacological basis for modern diuretic therapy, Ration. Drug Ther. **12**(2):1, 1978.

Burg, M.: Mechanisms of action of diuretic drugs. The kidney, Philadelphia, 1976, W.B. Saunders Co.

Carriere, S., and others: Bumetanide, a new loop diuretic, Clin. Pharmacol. Ther. **20**:424, 1976.

Davies, D.L., and Wilson, G.M.: Diuretic: mechanism of action and clinical application, Drugs **9**:178, 1975.

Diuretic, American Society of Hospital Pharmacy Formulary Service, Sec. 40, p. 28, Washington D.C., 1980, American Society of Hospital Pharmacists, Inc.

Epstein, M., and others: Potentiation of furosemide by metolazone in refractory edema, Curr. Ther. Res. **21**(5):656, 1977.

Gifford, R.W., Jr.: A guide to the practical use of diuretics, J.A.M.A. **235**:1890, 1976.

Kassirer, J.P., and Harrington, J.T.: Diuretics and potassium metabolism: a reassessment of the need, effectiveness, and safety of potassium therapy, Kidney Int. **11**:505, 1977.

Kelleher, M.: Diuretic therapy, Apothecary, May/June 1980, p. 21.

Kokko, J.P.: Renal concentrating and diluting mechanisms, Hosp. Prac., February, 1979, p. 110.

Mangini, R.J., and Young, L.Y.: Edema. In Applied therapeutics for clinical pharmacists, San Francisco, 1978, Applied Therapeutics, Inc.

Mead, G.M., and others: Drug associated primary acute pancreatitis, Lancet, Apr. 1, 1978, p. 706.

Morgan, T.O.: Diuretics: basic clinical pharmacology and therapeutic use, Drugs **15**:151, 1978.

Mudge, G.: Drugs affecting renal function and electrolyte metabolism—introduction, and Diuretics and other agents employed in the mobilization of edema fluid. In Goodman, L., and Gilman, A., editors: The pharmacological basis of therapeutics, ed. 6, New York, 1980, Macmillan, Inc.

Fluids, electrolytes, and nutrients

The student who stops to consider the place of certain drugs in the body economy will quickly recognize that in some instances substances given as medications are not foreign to the body but are provided as replacement therapy. They stand in contrast to a large number of drugs, the "foreign" compounds such as the anesthetics, antibiotics, and antihistamines, given to achieve a desirable pharmacologic effect. This "normal" group of drugs are natural constituents of the body or diet that are required in certain quantities to preserve healthy function. When absent, as in nutritional deficiency diseases, they must be replaced if the disease is to be cured. However, they may also be given when a deficiency is not present to obtain physiologic actions available only at high blood levels.

Fluids

Water

In humans water comprises from 45% to 75% of the total body weight, depending on the amount of adipose tissue present. Infants and young children have more water per unit of body weight than adults, and female adults have less water content than male adults. The greatest amount of body water (up to 45% of body weight) is to be found in the *intracellular fluid*, that is, the fluid inside the cells. It is in this fluid that the chemical reactions of all metabolism so essential to life occur. The remainder of body water is located in the *extracellular fluid*, that is, the fluid surrounding the cells (Fig. 22-1). This extracellular fluid consists of plasma, interstitial fluid, and lymph, and extracellular portions of dense connective tissue, cartilage, and bone. The volume of fluid in the two body fluid compartments varies with age and differs in the sexes. It is in this fluid that metabolic exchanges between cells and tissues and the external environment occur.

The importance of body water is highlighted by the facts that (1) it is the medium in which all metabolic reactions occur, and (2) precise regulation of volume and composition of body fluid is essential to health. In the healthy individual body water remains remarkably con-

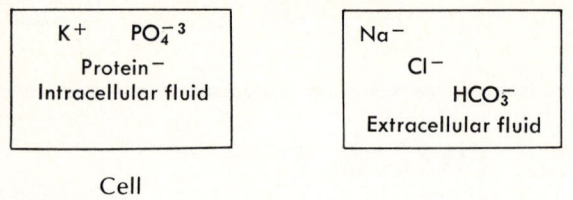

FIG. 22-1. Principal ions in intracellular and extracellular fluid.

stant, maintained by a balance between intake and excretion—the water gained each day is equal to the water lost. If the water gained exceeds the water lost, there will be *water excess*, or *overhydration* and edema. If the water lost exceeds the water gained, there will be a *water deficit*, or *dehydration*. The importance of body water is further emphasized by the fact that if 20% to 25% of body water is lost, death usually occurs.

Water is an excellent solvent that permits many substances to be dispersed through it. It also has a high dielectric constant, which permits ionization of electrolytes. These electrolytes are important in maintaining body fluid volume and distribution. They include the cations sodium (Na^+) for extracellular fluid, and potassium (K^+) and magnesium (Mg^{++}) for intracellular fluid; and the anions chloride (Cl^-) and bicarbonate (HCO_3) for extracellular fluid, and phosphate ($PO_4^=$) and protein for intracellular fluid. Intracellular ions also occur in the extracellular fluid but in smaller amounts.

Water is also an excellent lubricant between membranes, and it functions well as a heat insulator and heat exchanger.

As previously stated, water balance must be maintained between the amount of water taken in and the amount of water excreted. Water intake occurs primarily by (1) drinking fluids, (2) ingesting food containing moisture (most foods contain a high percentage of water), and (3) water formed by the oxidation of hydrogen in the food during metabolic processes. This latter method produces about ½ liter of water per day.

Water is lost from the body in five principal ways: (1) via the kidneys as urine, (2) through the skin as insensible perspiration and sweat, (3) through expired air as water vapor, (4) through feces, and (5) through the excretion of tears and saliva. Urine excretion accounts for 50% to 60% of the total daily water loss. Urine output, of course, varies with the amount of water ingested.

Water loss by the kidney varies with the solute load and the antidiuretic hormone (ADH) level. The kidney excretes sufficient urine to transport the solutes into the bladder if an increase in solute load occurs (for example, in diabetes mellitus or following ingestion of excessive amounts of food). The reabsorption of water in the distal convoluted tubules is controlled by ADH. An increase in ADH levels will lead to an increase in water reabsorption, which produces a more concentrated urine. ADH (vasopressin) is secreted by the posterior pituitary gland. This secretion is regulated by osmoreceptors located in the supraoptic nucleus. ADH has an action on specific vasopressin receptors on the medullary tubular cell to stimulate cyclic AMP (cAMP) production in this cell. The cAMP activates an enzyme that alters protein structure in the cell membrane to increase tubular cell permeability to water. This will increase water resorption and increase urine osmolality.

In humans, some daily intake of water is essential to maintain water balance. During starvation humans can go several weeks without food but can survive only a few days without water. The average volumes of water consumed daily are as follows: 120 to 150 ml/kg body weight in neonates and infants, 120 to 130 ml/kg in children, and 30 ml/kg in adults.

Thirst, the subjective desire to ingest water, helps to maintain water balance. Although thirst is complex and not well understood, it is induced by a decrease in saliva and dryness of the mouth and throat. It may be that dehydration of thirst receptors leads to their stimulation.

Abnormal states of hydration

A dynamic relationship exists in the human body between water and sodium, and abnormal states of hydration can be classified as (1) dehydration (volume depletion), (2) overhydration (hypervolemia or volume excess), (3) loss of water in excess of sodium ("hypernatremia"), and (4) loss of sodium in excess of water ("hyponatremia").

DEHYDRATION

Isotonic dehydration, or volume depletion, is the excessive loss of water and sodium in nearly equivalent proportions. This may result from vomiting, diarrhea, or fistula drainage. An isotonic solution of sodium chloride (0.9%) is often used to correct this condition. Flow rate of intravenous isotonic solutions is usually 125 ml/hour, or about 2 ml/minute. However, the flow rates may vary, depending on the patient's age, body surface area, ability to assimilate fluid, and cardiac and renal function.

Sodium chloride injection

Sodium chloride injection is available as a 0.9% isotonic solution (normal saline) containing 154 mEq sodium and 154 mEq chloride per liter or a "½ normal saline solution," which is 0.45% (hypotonic) with 77 mEq sodium and 77 mEq chloride per liter. It is administered intravenously to replace water and electrolytes that have been depleted in isotonic, or equivalent, proportions. The infusion is continued until signs of dehydration are corrected. It is also given during and after surgery to patients with normal renal function to maintain stable circulation and to reduce the need for blood transfusions by helping to maintain adequate circulating fluid volume. It is not used with patients limited by strict sodium restrictions (for example, in hypertension). It is the fluid of choice in initiating and terminating transfusions of red blood cells (glucose solutions will cause hemolysis and should never be administered with blood transfusions), since it decreases adherence of red blood cells and lessens impedance of infusion flow. It should be used with caution if the patient has congestive heart failure, circulatory insufficiency, hypoproteinemia, or renal dysfunction.

If the patient can take fluids orally, he may be given a solution to drink containing 3 to 4 g sodium chloride and 1.5 to 3 g sodium bicarbonate per liter.

Simple dehydration involving water loss without electrolyte loss, such as that caused by insufficient water intake, can be remedied by giving water orally or by giving a 2.5% to 5% dextrose solution intravenously.

Dextrose 5% in water

Dextrose solution is almost isotonic with blood and provides about 170 calories/liter. It should not be used as a diluent in transfusions of red blood cells because it does not ionize in solution and it causes hemolysis of the red blood cells. In the body the dextrose is oxidized to yield water. If the patient has normal renal function, he may receive from 2 to 3 liters of fluid per day. This will provide a liberal fluid intake. The rate of administration may be 1 liter over a 3½- to 5-hour period. Exceeding 3 liters/day is not recommended and therefore rarely ordered because of the danger of circulatory overload. Caution is observed in diabetic patients when urine testing for dextrose is employed.

Dextrose 5% or sodium chloride 0.11% to 0.45% (½ normal saline) with dextrose 5% in water is the preferred solution when there has been a loss of water in excess of sodium.

Subcutaneous administration of dextrose solutions is not recommended, since they are irritating and may cause fluid and electrolytes to be drawn into interstitial areas causing edema and possibly necrosis.

Balanced electrolyte injection

After dehydration has been corrected and the serum sodium level is normal, the extracellular fluid is further increased by the injection of balanced electrolyte solutions approaching that of normal blood plasma. These solutions contain sodium, potassium, magnesium, chloride, aceate, and gluconate. Once dehydration is corrected, the use of oral fluids will serve to improve hydration status.

OVERHYDRATION

Overhydration results in increased volume of body fluid and decreased concentration, or dilution, of plasma electrolytes and protein. This condition, also known as water intoxication, produces symptoms of headache, nausea, vomiting, muscular pains, abdominal cramps, weakness, stupor, coma, and convulsions.

Water excess may also result from administering excessive amounts of fluids parenterally, impaired renal and cardiac function, or administration or excessive secretion of antidiuretic hormone. It is also seen in complex endocrine disturbances.

The basic treatment is water restriction. However, if there is also a deficit of sodium, saline solutions are usually given to promote movement of intracellular fluid into the extracellular space.

The most common form of water excess occurs after extensive losses of water and electrolytes by sweating, followed by drinking large amounts of plain water. Its prevention and treatment involve normalizing the tonicity of body water by increasing the intake of salt, often in the form of salt tablets, to balance the amount of water ingested.

HYPERNATREMIA

Increased concentration of extracellular sodium may be caused by water loss without equivalent sodium loss (simple dehydration); excessive sodium administration or intake without adequate water intake; or retention of sodium because of heart failure, cirrhosis of the liver, or nephrosis.

Treatment must be based on serum sodium levels. If hypernatremia is the result of water deficit, treatment consists of replenishing body water either orally or by giving dextrose and water intravenously. Administration of drugs containing sodium may also be withheld, and the patient may be placed on a sodium-restricted diet. The natriuretic diuretics may be administered to increase sodium excretion.

HYPONATREMIA

Decreased concentration of sodium may result from loss of sodium, which can occur with vigorous diuretic therapy, prolonged or excessive sweating, renal insufficiency, Addison's disease, and loss of gastrointestinal fluid. This type of hyponatremia may be treated with 0.9% sodium chloride solution or Ringer's solution with or without lactate. If the sodium deficit is severe, a 3% or 5% sodium chloride solution may be administered.

A change in the concentration of sodium normally will stimulate a pituitary response by the antidiuretic hormone (ADH). ADH promotes water reabsorption in the distal tubules and has an effect on the concentration of extracellular sodium. The adrenal gland secretes aldosterone, which is the naturally occurring inhibitor of renal sodium excretion influencing sodium balance.

Sodium chloride in 3% or 5% solution

Solutions of 3% or 5% sodium chloride are recommended for treatment of severe sodium deficits. The 3% solution contains 513 mEq sodium/liter; the 5% solution contains 855 mEq sodium/liter. These solutions must be used with caution because of the danger of increased fluid load, which may lead to pulmonary edema. Extreme caution is required if administered to patients with cardiovascular or renal disease. These solutions should be administered slowly and in small volumes (200 to 400 ml). The patient's central venous pressure should be monitored.

Intravenous fluid therapy

Intravenous solutions are used to supply electrolytes, nutrients, and water. Electrolytes contained in intravenous solutions include sodium, potassium, calcium, ammonium chloride, bicarbonate, and phosphate. These solutions can be grouped into single salt and multiple salt solutions. Intravenous fluid therapy has become routine therapy before, during, and after surgery. Fluid loss during these times is estimated and replaced by the proper solution; the consequences of using the wrong solution can be disastrous.

SINGLE SALT SOLUTIONS

The following single salt solutions are used for replacement therapy. Sodium chloride solution has already been discussed.

Ammonium chloride injection

Ammonium chloride injection is available as a 2.14% solution (0.14 mEq/ml); 100 to 500 ml is infused over a 3-hour period. It must be infused slowly (125 ml/hour of the 2% solution) to allow for metabolism of ammonium ions by the liver and to avoid ammonia toxicity. It is effective for treatment of chloride loss caused by vomiting, fistula drainage, gastric suction, or excessive use of alkalinizing drugs or mercurial diuretics. When used to treat metabolic alkalosis, it should be given with potassium chloride and sodium chloride to prevent potassium and sodium depletion.

Calcium gluconate

Calcium gluconate solution is available for intravenous injection as a 10% solution (1 g contains 90 mg [4.5 mEq] calcium) in 10-ml vials for rapid replacement of calcium ions. It is the drug of choice for severely hypocalemic tetany. It must be administered slowly (0.5 ml over 1 minute), and care should be taken to prevent infiltration into surrounding tissues and tissue necrosis. If diluted to 1000 ml with 0.9% normal saline, it may be administered over a 12- to 24-hour period.

Potassium chloride injection

Potassium chloride is available for intravenous injection in 10 to 40 mEq solutions. It should not be administered as a bolus undiluted but rather at a moderate rate (10 mEq/hour) in solutions containing 40 to 60 mEq liter (not more than 80 mEq/liter). Rapid administration may cause pain or burning at the infusion site or serious cardiac dysrhythmias. Infusions should be regulated by ECG monitoring and repeated serum potassium determinations. It is effective for treatment of potassium deficiency when oral therapy is not feasible. It is dangerous in renal insufficiency or if urine output is less than 500 ml/day since hyperkalemia and cardiac arrest may result.

Sodium bicarbonate injection

Sodium bicarbonate injection is the drug of choice in the treatment of metabolic acidosis. It is available as a 7.5% solution in a 50-ml ampule or additive syringe to be added to 1 liter of solution. The 7.5% solution (hypertonic 3.75 g or 44.6 mEq/50 ml) may be administered at a rate of 1 mEq/kg body weight over 1 to 3 minutes in cardiac arrest. Repeated doses are determined by response, condition, blood pH, Po_2 and Pco_2. The usual rate of administration

in a nonarrest situation should not be in excess of 50 mEq/hour. It is also available as an isotonic solution (1.5%), as a hypertonic solution (2% to 5%), and in a 0.15% to 0.30% solution in combination with sodium chloride (0.3% to 4%). This drug is used to restore the bicarbonate ion and elevate the pH of the blood. Giving excessive amounts of sodium bicarbonate may cause metabolic alkalosis. This drug must be used very cautiously in patients with cardiac or renal disease, since large amounts of sodium can intensify these disorders.

Sodium lactate injection

Sodium lactate injection is available in 50 mEq as a 2.5 mEq/ml solution to be added to 1 liter of solution and premixed as 1 liter of ⅙ molar (167 mEq/liter each sodium and lactate ions) solution, which is to be given at a rate not exceeding 300 ml/hour. It is also available as a 44.8% (4 molar) solution. It is used in the treatment of metabolic acidosis when there is no evidence of an elevated lactic acid level. Since sodium lactate must be metabolized to sodium bicarbonate, the patient with lactic acidosis should be given sodium bicarbonate solution. This conversion of lactate to bicarbonate is impaired in hepatic disease.

MULTIPLE SALT SOLUTIONS

Ringer's lactate solution was the first multiple salt solution introduced for replacement therapy. At the present time there are 12 additional multiple salt solutions on the market. These solutions contain two or more cations. Multiple salt solutions can be classified as high, medium, or low electrolyte content solutions based primarily on their sodium content.

Multiple salt solutions are used to replace lost salt and to help correct electrolyte balance in patients unable to ingest food and water. The composition of electrolytes in various solutions is summarized in Table 22-1.

PARENTERAL NUTRITION

Parenteral nutrition therapy maintains a patient on the calories, amino acids, fats, trace elements, and other essential nutrients needed for growth, weight gain, and wound healing. This form of intravenous feeding should be

TABLE 22-1 Multiple salt solutions for intravenous administration

Generic name	Trade name or common name	Cations mEq/liter					Anions mEq/liter				
		Na$^+$	K$^+$	Ca^{++}	Mg^{++}	NH$_4^-$	Cl$^-$	HCO$_3^-$	PO$_4^-$	Lactate	Acetate
High electrolyte content											
Ringer's solution		147	4	5			156				
Lactated Ringer's solution	Hartmann's solution	130	4	3			109			28	
Sodium lactate	Ionosol D-CM	138	12	5	3		108	50		27	23
	Normosol-R	140	5		3		98	50			
	Plasma-Lyte	140	10	5	3		103	55		8	47
	Polysal	140	10	5	3		103				55
Medium electrolyte content											
Sodium, potassium-	Ionosol B	57	25			5	49		13	25	
ammonium	Normosol-M	40	13		3		40				16
chloride in dextrose	Electrolyte-2	55	23		5		55		12	26	
5%	Polysal-M	40	16	5	3		40			12	12
Low electrolyte content	Ionosol MB	25	20		3		22		3	23	
in dextrose 5%	Electrolyte-48	25	20		3		22		3	23	
	Isolyte P	25	20		3		22		3		23

employed when the patient cannot eat, should not eat, refuses to eat, or is unable to eat enough. The following list provides some of the indications for parenteral nutrition:

Acute and chronic renal failure
Alimentary tract anomalies
Alimentary tract fistula
Burns
Chronic diarrhea
Chronic vomiting
Complicated trauma or surgery
Diverticulitis
Failure to thrive
Gastrointestinal obstruction
Granulomatous enterocolitis
Hypermetabolic states
Indolent wounds and decubitus ulcers
Malabsorption
Malignant disease (adjunct to chemotherapy)
Malnutrition
Nonterminal coma
Pancreatitis
Postoperative gastrointestinal ulcer disease
Protein-losing gastroenteropathy
Reversible liver failure
Severe anorexia nervosa
Short bowel syndrome
Ulcerative colitis

The information in this section on parenteral nutrition is focused on the adult patient's requirements; however, some reference will be made to the pediatric patient.

Parenteral nutrition enables the intestinal tract to rest and provides an opportunity for more rapid healing of gastrointestinal lesions.

Those patients with hepatic function impairments or renal failure are provided support by special formulated solutions. Parenteral feeding provides calories in addition to oral or tube feedings for major burn patients. Applications in pediatric patients may be catastrophic gastrointestinal abnormalities, during the postoperative adjustment periods of surgically staged repair, malabsorption or malnutrition leading to nonspecific intractable diarrhea, and low birth weight infants.

Debilitation from nutritional deprivation may impair wound healing, reduce collagen synthesis, reduce essential protein production (for example, albumin, fibrinogen, and hemoglobin), reduce hormones, and reduce digestible enzymes. Parenteral nutrition solutions are metabolized in all body tissue that requires protein and energy.

During mild to moderate starvation the cellular changes in biochemistry are similar to those of malnutrition. Some of the more prominent cellular changes are as follows: glycogen (a carbohydrate) stores in the liver are diminished in less than 1 day; the protein stores are reduced as a result of gluconeogenesis because amino acids are converted into glucose as an energy source; the intestinal mucous membranes, liver, pancreas, and tubular epithelium of the kidney have proteins with short half-lives and are placed at risk because of dietary deprivation; muscle proteins are used to provide energy as a result of the lowered nutrition; adipose tissues are metabolized to produce free fatty acids for energy substrates; the by-products of oxidation of the fatty acids are ketones that provide energy for the brain after extensive starvation. A high rate of protein catabolism to produce amino acids exists after surgical procedures and trauma. These amino acids are converted to glucose to provide the increased energy requirements to meet these needs.

Parenteral nutrition assists in the rehabilitation of the patient who cannot tolerate or utilize enteral (oral) nutrition. When parenteral nutrition is to be withdrawn, small enteral feedings are begun slowly, and the parenteral nutrition is reduced gradually over a period of several days or longer. The process is slowly achieved. While the patient is on parenteral nutrition, carbon dioxide (from the lungs), water, and urea (from the kidneys) are excreted; however, the stomach and bowel are reduced in size, and the bowel is in a state of rest or reduced state of peristalsis.

Each patient is assessed to determine his nutritional status. The following measurements are necessary in determining the patient's needs: gross assessment, body weight, fat stores, lean body mass, blood proteins, immune function, nitrogen balance, net protein utilization, protein, and caloric requirements.

Some general guidelines for calories for the patient who is a candidate for parenteral nutrition are (1) weight maintenance (not acutely stressed), 30 to 35 kcal/kg/day and amino acid requirements of 0.7 g/kg; (2) weight maintenance (acutely stressed), 55 to 60 kcal/kg/day; (3) weight maintenance (extremely stressed), greater than 55 to 60 kcal/kg/day, as in burn patients, and amino acid requirements in excess of 3.25 g/kg; (4) weight gain, only 55 to 60 kcal/kg/day. Calorie and protein requirements are influenced by factors that affect the metabolism of amino acids. An increase may be caused by injury, sepsis, or stress, and a decrease may result from liver dysfunction or renal failure.

Types of parenteral nutrition

Postoperative protein-sparing therapy. Postoperative protein-sparing therapy provides the patient with substrates of energy or amino acids to reduce the body protein loss. This therapy is used for short periods of up to 5 days in previously adequately nourished patients. For periods in excess of 5 days total parenteral nutrition (TPN) should be employed. An amino acid solution (3% to 3.5%) is used in the peripheral vein with no carbohydrate calories. The patient usually receives 1 to 1.7 g/kg/day of amino acids on this therapy. The 5% to 8.5% may also be used when appropriately diluted with fluids and electrolytes.

Hyperalimentation therapy. Hyperalimentation(HA) therapy is the administration of hypertonic solutions of dextrose, amino acids, vitamins, and electrolytes through a central venous catheter. Before hyperalimentation the conventional intravenous feeding only provided a supplement to enteral (oral) nutrition. These standard intravenous solutions are administered by peripheral vein; the concentration of nutrients cannot be excessive, since sclerosis, thrombosis, and phlebitis will occur in the peripheral vein. The volume of fluid must not exceed the daily requirements or it will cause fluid overload complications.

A central high-flow, large-bore vein (preferably the superior vena cava via the subclavian) is used to administer hyperosmotic solutions because effective and efficient dilution occurs as a result of the large flow and volume of blood in the vena cava. Placement of this catheter is a surgical procedure and carries a risk of incorrect catheter placement; a roentgenogram is essential to ensure proper catheter positioning. Furthermore, the risk of bacterial contamination *(Candida)*, which could produce sepsis, exists in the catheter tract. The potential for essential fatty acid deficiency (EFAD) syndrome and trace element (zinc, chromium, and so forth) deficiencies exists. This is discussed later in the chapter.

Total parenteral nutrition. Total parenteral nutrition (TPN) therapy is described as the central or peripheral venous infusion of amino acids, dextrose, electrolytes, fat, trace elements, and vitamins. This method is indicated when the duration of parenteral nutrition exceeds 7 days. The goal of TPN is to provide the essential nutrients of the normal diet in similar ratios. This can be designed to provide adequate nutritional needs for considerable time periods (for example, over 22 months) with a positive nitrogen balance and oral intake. Total parenteral nutrition by a peripheral vein has advantages over the central venous route. Two of these advantages are the minimization of risks associated with central venous catheterization and the fact that no special or unique catheter insertion techniques are required. Basic nutritional support is provided by using isotonic solutions of amino acids and dextrose plus fat emulsions in the peripheral vein which may provide approximately 1600 kcal.

Parenteral nutrition for septic patients. An interesting application of parenteral nutrition may be seen in the septic patient. The prognosis of septic patients may be improved by treating them with glucose, insulin, and branched chain amino acids via the parenteral nutrition technique.

Sepsis is a catabolic insult culminating in modifications of carbohydrate and fat metabolism, which lead to an increased breakdown of muscle and nitrogen loss. During sepsis insulin resistance may develop in peripheral tissues (mainly muscle) and may decrease glucose utilization, but plasma insulin levels remain elevated and prevent lipolysis, which leads to a further energy deficit. Insulin resistance and inability to use fat lead to increased muscle proteolysis. Muscle proteolysis leads to an increased release of high levels of amino acids (aromatic and sulfur containing) into the blood. The aromatic amino acids are phenylalanine and tyrosine, and the sulfur-containing amino acids are taurine, cystine (cysteine), and methionine. During sepsis there is a limited availability of fuels as muscle proteolysis, gluconeogenesis, and amino acid oxidation are used as energy sources.

Survival of septic patients has been correlated with higher levels of branched chain amino acids and alanine and lower levels of aromatic and sulfur-containing amino acids. It has been demonstrated that infusion of a branched-chain amino acid mixture (leucine, isoleucine, and valine) with low amounts of aromatic amino acids may result in normalizing the deranged amino acid pattern, leading to a better prognosis for those patients having septic metabolic coma.

Parenteral nutrition ingredients

Amino acids. The substrates needed for protein synthesis are provided by amino acids, and individual patient requirements vary with the condition of each patient. The normal adult has a daily average protein requirement of 0.5 to 0.7 g. The protein must be of high biologic value per kilogram of body weight. This requirement is significantly increased (almost six times) in a traumatized patient or a seriously ill patient, since this patient's daily need is approximately 3 g/kg body weight. A nonprotein source of calories must be provided with the amino acids to offset their use as an energy source. The currently recognized infused calories to nitrogen ratio exceeds 150 to 180 calories to 1 g of nitrogen for the patient who has not undergone starvation.

Protein is composed of amino acids identified as essential and nonessential. Eight amino acids are essential in adults. In infants, however, 10 amino acids are termed essential because arginine and histidine are considered essential in infants but not in adults. The term "essential" indicates that it is not capable of being synthesized. The semiessential amino acids (arginine and histidine) are not synthesized in adequate amounts during growth. The nonessential amino acids are synthesizable from a nitrogen source (amino acids, ammonium salts, and urea). All natural amino acids are needed for growth and development and must be present concurrently in the proper amounts for protein synthesis to occur. The adult can endogenously synthesize all but eight of these amino acids; therefore protein synthesis is totally dependent on an exogenous source for the balance and is further limited by the smallest amount of an available essential amino acid. Table 22-2 provides the classification of amino acids.

Carbohydrates. Under most normal circumstances dextrose has become the carbohydrate source of choice. Fructose, a carbohydrate normally found in the blood, does not require insulin for peripheral utilization. However, fructose administration has produced elevated lactic acid levels, and deaths have occurred in patients with hereditary fructose intolerance.

Fructose can intensify existing metabolic

TABLE 22-2   Classification of amino acids

Essential	Nonessential	Semiessential
Isoleucine	Alanine	Arginine
Leucine	Aspartic acid	Histidine
Lysine	Cysteine	
Methionine	Glutamic acid	
Phenylalanine	Glycine	
Threonine	Proline	
Tryptophan	Serine	
Valine	Tyrosine	

acidosis, deplete liver adenine nucleotides, and dehydrate through its osmotic diuretic effect.

Alcohol is another substrate providing 7 kcal/g, and it does not require insulin for peripheral utilization. To provide enough calories would necessitate a quantity of alcohol that would produce intoxication and hepatotoxicity potential. Dextrose is an inexpensive and readily available caloric source that provides 4 kcal/g (1 kcal of heat is necessary to raise the temperature of 1 kg of water 1° C). Because of large amounts of dextrose in the parenteral nutrition solutions, it is necessary to carefully monitor serum and urine glucose and electrolytes. Exogenous insulin may be administered subcutaneously to control this. Generally a 20% to 25% dextrose solution is used. The dextrose used is derived from corn sugar; however, a small portion of the population may be sensitive to corn derivatives, and for these patients invert sugar from cane or beet sugar is the only reasonable alternative.

Fat (Intralipid [10%, 20%] and Liposyn [10%] as fat emulsions). Fat constitutes 40% to 50% of the total calories supplied in the average North American diet. The two functions of intravenous fat emulsion in parenteral nutrition are to supply essential fatty acids and to furnish energy. The clinical usefulness, if given in small amounts, is to have the fat emulsion act as a source of linoleic acid to treat and to prevent essential fatty acid deficiency (EFAD). If the fat emulsion is administered in larger amounts, it will partially replace glucose as the major source of energy in parenteral nutrition. The fat emulsion serving as a source of extra calories supplies 9 kcal/g. The concurrent use of fat and carbohydrates permits the reduction of

dextrose load or reinforcement of the caloric needs. The 10% fat emulsion is isotonic, providing 1.1 kcal/ml, and is less likely to cause vein irritation. Fat emulsions break down when mixed with amino acid and dextrose solutions so they are administered from separate containers and flow into the same vein as the dextrose and amino acid solutions via a Y connector positioned just in front of the infusion site. No filters are used on the fat emulsion line and no additions are made to the fat emulsion. It is important to note that the fat emulsion limb of the Y connector must be higher (6 inches) than the amino acid limb because the fat emulsion has a lower density.

The fat emulsion provides the following fatty acids: linoleic, oleic, palmitic, and linolenic acids. The fat emulsions currently available are either safflower oil (Liposyn) or soybean oil (Intralipid) emulsions. The fat emulsion particles are thought to be metabolized from the bloodstream circulation in a manner similar to that of the chylomicra, which appear in the blood postprandially. No more than 60% of the total daily caloric needs of the patient should be provided by fat emulsions. The fat emulsions may prevent hyperglycemia, hyperinsulinemia, and hyperosmolar syndrome, often occurring in patients given glucose as the only source of parenteral caloric nutrition. Fat emulsions pose some dangers, including their use in patients with severe liver disease, pulmonary disease, anemia, and blood coagulation disorders; the dangers of fat emboli and of accumulation of intravascular fat in lungs of premature, preterm, or low-birth-weight infants (infusion rate not to exceed 1 g/kg in 4 hours) must also be kept in mind. A normal diet should be 40% fat, 40% protein, and 20% carbohydrate.

Trace elements (minerals). The commercial hyperalimentation solutions contain trace elements (zinc, copper, and manganese). Zinc was found to be in the highest concentrations. Patients placed on a long-term regimen should be evaluated for trace element deficiencies. Trace element solutions for addition to total parenteral nutrition are being prefabricated in many hospitals, and commercial solutions are available in the United States (Abbott and Travenol manufacturers). The trace element solutions being prefabricated as separate trace elements or in combination (M.T.E.-4 by Travenol) contain the following cations: zinc, copper, manganese, and chromium. Zinc deficiencies seen during parenteral nutrition are present as diarrhea, apathy, and depression. Perianal and elbow skin lesions are examples of the dermatitis that is followed by alopecia when plasma zinc levels are below 20 μg/100 ml. These are associated with a decrease in zinc intake and an increase in excretion during parenteral nutrition therapy. Trace element deficiencies exist for copper, manganese, and chromium.

Some other essential trace elements are cobalt, fluoride, iodide, molybdenum, nickel, selenium, silicon, tin, and vanadium. Some trace elements have an identified deficiency syndrome, function, and metabolism.

Exact trace element requirements have not yet been determined. Some hospitals use plasma protein fractions or simple plasma infusions as a source of trace elements.

Multiple electrolytes are to be monitored also, including the cations of sodium, potassium, calcium, and magnesium and the anions of phosphate, bicarbonate, chloride, and acetate. Iron is administered intramuscularly by the Z track technique or injection and is added to the patient's regimen accordingly by monitoring individual patient response. The iron is not added to the parenteral nutrition solutions.

Vitamins. Some vitamins may be supplied in the parenteral nutrition solution, whereas others are administered directly. There are commercially available multiple vitamin preparations that provide most fat-soluble (A, D, and E) and water-soluble (B_1, B_2, B_6, C, niacin, pantothenic acid, and biotin) vitamins. Folic acid, vitamin B_{12}, and vitamin K cannot be included in the parenteral nutrition solution, since these are not stable in such an acid solution.

Nursing implications

Paramount nursing responsibilities in a parenteral nutrition regimen are catheter care, solution setup, very close patient observation, and critical monitoring of the patient. Parenteral nutrition rates of flow are described as follows. The nurse must have the patient hydrated

before inserting the central venous catheter, since this increases the ease of catheter placement. The nurse may begin with dextrose 5% in 0.45% saline and run at a rate of 125 to 150 ml/hour before catheter insertion.

The parenteral nutrition solution is initially set to flow at 50 ml/hour; this is increased to 75 to 100 ml/hour in 12 hours and increased again by 25 to 50 ml in another 12 hours. The urine should be tested for glycosuria, and blood glucose is to be checked. Testing of blood glucose is indicated at 6-hour intervals, since this is critical if any signs of diabetes mellitus or the presence of glycosuria is evident. The patient's weight must be taken accurately and recorded. Blood urea nitrogen is tested daily for 3 to 5 days then every other day as needed. An SMA 12/60 should be done weekly with tests for protein, PTT, and CBC, along with strict intake and output monitoring.

The daily recording of the data and the communication of any incongruity in these data to the attending physician are critical. These data include blood glucose in excess of 200 mg/100 ml; weight loss; urine glucose in excess of 1+ (glycosuria); an increase in pulse and blood pressure and sweating; elevated temperature; swelling and edema over the puncture site or on the head, neck, or face; low serum electrolytes; distended veins in the neck, arms, and hands; convulsions; coma; or radical changes in the patient. The nurse is the key to the success or failure of this therapy, which is based on close monitoring and observations. The importance of a nurse-oriented aseptic protocol for changing dressings cannot be stressed enough. The nurse must be aware of potential complications arising from parenteral nutrition that may be caused by subclavian catheterization, infection, and sepsis and its attendant metabolic complications. The accompanying box lists potential complications that will be further discussed under "Nursing Implications for Intravenous Therapy."

Protein hydrolysate injection (Amigen, Travamin); amino acid solution (FreAmine, Travasol, Aminosyn, Veinamine)

Protein hydrolysates may be prepared from pure proteins such as casein or lactalbumin or

Complications of parenteral nutrition

Complications arising from infection and sepsis

Catheter seeding from blood-borne or distant infection

Contamination of catheter entrance site during insertion or long-term catheter placement

Solution contamination

Complications that are metabolic in origin

Azotemia

Dehydration from osmotic diuresis

Electrolyte imbalance

Hyperammonemia

Hyperosmolar, hyperglycemic, nonketotic coma (HHNC)

Hyperphosphatemia and hypophosphatemia

Hypocalcemia

Hypomagnesemia

Rebound hypoglycemia on sudden cessation of parenteral nutrition

Trace element deficiencies

Complications arising from subclavian catheterization

Air embolism

Arteriovenous fistula

Brachial plexus injury

Cardiac perforation, tamponade

Catheter embolism

Catheter misplacement

Central vein thrombophlebitis

Endocarditis

Hemothorax

Hydromediastinum

Hydrothorax

Pneumothorax

Subclavian artery injury

Subclavian hematoma

Subcutaneous emphysema

Tension pneumothorax

Thoracic duct injury

other sources of protein such as blood, liver, or yeast with the aid of acids, alkalis, or enzymes. Determinations are made of the amino acid content, and pure amino acids are added or excesses removed so that only those amino acids considered essential to human nutrition are contained in the solution. These solutions also contain varying amounts of electrolytes. About 60% of the amino acids are free, the rest are peptides that are excreted unchanged.

Amino acid solution contains synthetic amino acids but no peptides. Patients unable to tolerate protein hydrolysate may be able to tolerate amino acid solution.

Dextrose is usually administered with these solutions because of the protein-sparing action of carbohydrates. If the protein is administered without adequate calories in the form of carbohydrate, the protein will be used for the body's caloric need rather than for repair and regeneration of tissue.

Side effects. Protein hydrolysates may cause nausea and vomiting, headache, flushing, hypotension, abdominal pain, convulsions, thrombosis, phlebitis, and edema at the site of injection. Hyperpyrexia (fever) may occur after the solutions have been administered for a few days. These solutions must be used with caution in patients with liver or renal impairment. Solutions that are cloudy or contain a sediment should not be used. If administration of the solution is interrupted, the remaining solution must be discarded.

NURSING IMPLICATIONS FOR INTRAVENOUS THERAPY

Intravenous therapy is such a common, everyday phenomenon in hospitalized patients that nurses are often less attentive to the problems and complications of intravenous therapy than is necessary if the therapy is to be effective and safe. Many of the complications of intravenous therapy can be avoided if the nurse is a keen observer, knowledgeable, and skillful.

The recommended system for surveillance and reporting of problems with large-volume parenteral solutions in hospitals has been delegated to the National Coordinating Committee on Large-Volume Parenterals. The Committee is composed of legally recognized standards-setting bodies, enforcement agencies, and national groups with a major influence over the manufacture and use of large-volume parenterals. Organizations represented on the Committee are the American Hospital Association, American Medical Association, American Nurses' Association, American Society of Hospital Pharmacists, Centers for Disease Control, Food and Drug Administration, Joint Commission of Accreditation of Hospitals, National Association of Boards of Pharmacy, National Association for Practical Nurse Education and Service, Parenteral Drug Association, The United States Pharmacopeial Convention, and major large-volume parenteral manufacturers (Abbott, Cutter, McGraw, and Travenol). The mission of the Committee is to find workable solutions to those large-volume parenteral problems judged to have the greatest clinical significance and potential for finding a solution.

The recommendations have covered the areas of a system for surveillance and reporting of problems with large-volume parenterals in hospitals, methods for compounding intravenous admixtures in hospitals, recommendations to pharmacists for solving problems with large-volume parenterals, labeling of large-volume parenterals, procedures for in-use testing of large-volume parenterals suspected of contamination or of producing a reaction in a patient, and recommendations for filter selection used on large-volume parenterals.

The nurse should be aware of the options available in selecting a filter for the intravenous infusion. There are several different intravenous filter products designed for different filtration needs. The filters are available in a range of sizes and in an add-on or in-line form. The following provides an overview of filter selection:

1 A 5-μm filter removes "particulate" material and is designed to filter gross particulate matter. The smallest particle visible to the unaided eye is approximately 30 μm across.
2 0.5-μm filter is considered a bacteria-retention filter, which is designed to prevent passage of most particulate matter and certain fungi and bacteria (a yeast cell is approximately 3 μm in diameter).
3 The 0.22-μm filter is called a "sterilizing" filter, since it is designed to prevent passage of virtually all particulate matter and most bacteria for at least 24 hours. Bacteria range in size from 0.2 to 2 μm in diameter. Travenol Laboratories and other manufacturers provide these filters to be used with the add-on or in-line systems. The nurse should select a 0.22-μm filter for parenteral nutrition solutions.

Complications. Complications of intravenous therapy include the following.

Infiltration. Infiltration occurs when the needle is dislodged from the vein permitting the solution to enter the surrounding tissues causing pain and edema of the area. Patients or relatives should be informed to notify the nurse if pain or swelling occurs at the infusion site. In addition, nurses should frequently check the infusion site for signs of infiltration. The infusion should be stopped if infiltration occurs. Restarting the intravenous therapy usually requires a new infusion site.

Extravasation. This occurs when fluids in the vein escape through the vascular wall into the tissues surrounding the vein. This may occur because of (1) changes in osomotic pressures, (2) the type of fluid being infused, (3) overdistention of the vein caused by too rapid a flow rate, or (4) stretching of the venipuncture site permitting fluids to escape. In the last case there is no longer a closed system, and microorganisms may invade the venous system. Sterile aseptic technique should be followed and the infusion restarted at a different site.

Thrombosis. An intravascular blood clot occurs when platelets agglutinate and fibrin strands and red and white blood cells adhere to the platelet mass. A thrombus may form any time a blood vessel is injured, including injury by venipuncture. A thrombus may form around the needle or catheter plugging the lumen; if this occurs the infusion stops. The infusion should be restarted at a new site with a new needle or catheter. Attempts to unplug the needle by forcing a bolus of solution through the needle into the vein is not a wise or safe practice. The thrombus may become an embolus and lodge in a vital organ causing more serious complications such as pulmonary embolus.

Thrombophlebitis. Blood clot formation and inflammation of the vein may result from a number of factors; prolonged duration of infusion, use of contaminated equipment or contaminated solutions, irritation from drugs in the infusion, toxicity and pH of the solution, site of administration, and infection. Thrombophlebitis is manifested by pain, heat, swelling, redness, and loss of motion of the affected part. When this occurs, the infusion should be stopped, the needle withdrawn, and the condition reported and recorded immediately. Treatment usually consists of the application of moist heat to the affected area; anticoagulant therapy may also be ordered. Nurses should take the necessary precautions to prevent occurrence of thrombophlebitis by (1) using sterile aseptic technique with proper cleansing of skin before insertion of the needle; (2) being certain equipment is not contaminated; (3) checking solutions for precipitation, debris or sediment, or change in color before and during intravenous therapy; (4) ascertaining that no intravenous bottle is left in place for more than 24 hours, since some organisms proliferate at room temperature in intravenous fluids (for open intravenous therapy, 250-ml bottles should be used); (5) changing the administration set every 24 hours to reduce the possibility of sepsis; and (6) administering irritating drugs slowly.

Pain at administration site. Pain occurs when the needle touches the venous wall, when there is too much tension on the needle or tubing, and when irritating drugs are administered too rapidly. Adjusting the needle, relieving the tension by readjusting the needle support or relaxing the pull on the tubing, and administering irritating drugs at a slow rate may alleviate the pain and discomfort.

Necrosis. Death and sloughing of tissue can occur when irritating drugs or solutions, such as levarterenol, infiltrate into the tissues. The infusion should be stopped *immediately.* If the infiltration contains levarterenol, the antidote phentolamine (Regitine) should be injected subcutaneously in minute amounts at many sites in the edematous area immediately on discovery.

Pulmonary edema. Pulmonary edema occurs when the circulatory system is overloaded with fluids. Central venous pressure monitoring (particularly in cardiac patients) can help to prevent this hazardous complication.

Pyrogenic reactions. Pyrogenic reactions occur when pyrogens are introduced into the circulatory system. Pyrogens are fever-producing substances. Bacterial pyrogens are filtrable thermostable products of bacterial origin and activity that may accumulate and tend to cause a severe rigor when injected into the body. Pyrogenic reactions are characterized by fever and chills, malaise, headache, nausea, and vomiting. The infusion should be stopped *at once.* The intravenous solution may contain the pyrogens. The solution should not be discarded but sent to the pharmacist. The stock number should be noted, since an entire batch of solutions may be contaminated. Pyrogenic reactions must be reported and recorded.

Electrolytes
Potassium

Potassium is the major positively charged ion in the intracellular fluid. The amount of potassium in the intracellular fluid is 150 mEq/liter; the amount in the plasma is 3.5 to 5 mEq. Even though this latter amount appears to be quite low, it is of great importance, since serum potassium must be maintained between 3.5 and 5 mEq/liter for survival. The diet of most individuals contains from 35 to 100 mEq of potassium daily. Normally, any excess potassium is excreted by the kidney in the urine. Potassium plays an important part in (1) muscle contraction, (2) conduction of nerve impulses, (3) enzyme action, and (4) cell membrane function. High and low concentrations of potassium affect these physiologic functions.

HYPOKALEMIA

Potassium deficit, or hypokalemia, can be caused by the following:

1 Reduced dietary intake (rare)
2 Poor absorption because of steatorrhea, regional enteritis, or short bowel syndrome
3 Loss of gastrointestinal secretions (which are rich in this ion) as a result of vomiting, diarrhea, gastrointestinal suction, or fistula drainage
4 Kidney disease
5 Diuretic therapy (potassium depleting)
6 Infusions of solutions containing little or no K^+
7 Extensive burns
8 Excessive amounts of adrenocortical hormone

Unlike sodium, which is reabsorbed when serum sodium level is low, potassium ions continue to be excreted in the urine when the serum potassium level is low. As potassium loss continues, the patient's condition deteriorates until potassium intake is increased and normal levels are reestablished.

With hypokalemia there is impaired muscle function. Impairment of skeletal muscle function may cause profound weakness or paralysis, including paralysis of the respiratory muscles.

Impaired smooth muscle function may result in ileus.

Cardiac effects of hypokalemia include increased sensitivity to digitalis with potential toxicity and ECG changes such as ST segment depression, U waves, and T wave flattening, depression, or inversion. For example, early potassium deficiency may be detected by the use of the electrocardiogram. The T wave tends to flatten when serum potassium levels are below 3.5 mEq/liter. The T wave tends to vertically elongate when the serum potassium level is 5.8 mEq/liter or higher. Atrioventricular block and cardiac arrest may occur.

Hypokalemia also causes movement of Na^+ and H^+ from extracellular fluid and the excretion of H^+. This elevates the plasma pH, which results in *metabolic alkalosis*. Other effects are decreased water reabsorption in the renal tubule, resulting in polyuria, and hypochloremia.

Treatment. Hypokalemia is treated by replacing potassium orally or parenterally. A hazard of parenteral correction of potassium deficit is the production of potassium poisoning, or hyperkalemia. Administration of potassium salts intravenously must be performed cautiously to avoid reaching a concentration that can cause bradycardia, asystole, or cardiac arrest. The patient should be monitored, since the ECG will show changes more rapidly than will serum potassium levels. Urinary output and urinary loss of potassium should also be measured. Potassium should not be given in the immediate postoperative period until urine flow is established.

Potassium salts are contraindicated in severe renal impairment, untreated Addison's disease, acute dehydration, and hyperkalemia from any cause. They must be used with caution in cardiac patients.

Potassium acetate, potassium bicarbonate, potassium chloride, potassium citrate, and potassium gluconate are available alone or in combinations for oral administration. Potassium acetate, potassium chloride, and potassium phosphate are available as parenteral solutions. In addition, potassium chloride is a component in a number of multiple electrolyte intravenous fluids (for example, Ringer's solution).

Liquid preparations are preferred for oral therapy and most contain 10, 20, or 40 mEq K^+/ 15 ml. These preparations must be diluted with fruit juice or water before ingestion and taken after meals with a full glass of water to minimize gastric irritation. Powdered preparations (such as K-lor and Kato) should be dissolved according to the manufacturer's instructions. Ingestion of potassium-rich foods may also be helpful.

Approximately 45 mEq potassium may be added to the diet by consuming 2 medium sized bananas and an 8-ounce glass of orange juice; 40 mEq of potassium may be derived from eating 20 large dried apricots, and a cup of dates will yield 36 mEq of potassium. A salt substitute (KCl) may provide 60 mEq of potassium per level teaspoon.

Uncoated tablets are not recommended by the AMA because they cause gastric irritation; enteric-coated tablets are not recommended because their rate of absorption is undependable and they cause small bowel ulcerations in the duodenum. Small bowel ulcerations and strictures are reported in a sustained-action (matrix formulation) potassium chloride (available in tablets having 6.67, 8, and 10 mEq potassium chloride). There is a very limited application for these tablets including conditions where dietary adjustment is not practical, where the potassium supplements in a liquid form are undesirable, and when the patient is only compliant if a solid dosage form is available. The practitioner must always keep in mind the potential for potassium chloride—induced ulcerations when ingestion is in the solid dosage form. The purpose of this formulation of sustained action—matrix tablets is to slowly release the potassium chloride as it passes through the gastrointestinal tract.

Preparation, dosage, and administration. The dosage of potassium supplements depends on individual requirements. The approximate minimum daily requirement for adults is 40 to 50 mEq; for infants it is about 2 to 3 mEq/kg body weight daily. Oral dosage is usually gradually increased over a 3- to 7-day period to avoid producing hyperkalemia.

Intravenous administration of potassium is based on serial ECG and serum electrolyte determinations; intravenous fluids should not contain more than 80 mEq/liter potassium, and as a guide the maximum rate of administration should be 10 mEq/hour if the serum potassium is greater than 2.5 mEq/liter and 40 mEq/hour if the serum potassium is less than 2.0 mEq/liter. The nurse should know how fast the solution is to run; rapid infusion causes pain or burning at the infusion site and may cause cardiac dysrhythmias.

Potassium chloride injection. Potassium chloride injection is available in sterile solutions containing 10, 20, 30, 40, 60, and 100 mEq K^+ and Cl^- for injection (2 mEq/ml).

Potassium chloride oral solution. Potassium chloride oral solution contains 20 mEq potassium/15 ml.

Potassium acetate. Potassium acetate is available in 30-ml vials, containing 3 and 4 mEq K^+, and as a powder.

Potassium bicarbonate (K-Lyte). Potassium bicarbonate is available as effervescent tablets, which, when dissolved in 3 to 4 ounces of water, produce a liquid containing 25 mEq K^+. It has also been used as a gastric antacid and to alkalinize the urine.

Potassium citrate. Potassium citrate is available in powder and tablet form containing varying amounts of potassium.

Potassium gluconate (Kaon). Potassium gluconate is available as a powder, an elixir containing 6.7 mEq K^+/5 ml, as chewable tablets containing 1.1 mEq K^+, and as tablets containing 2.1 or 5 mEq K^+. This drug may be used for patients who cannot tolerate potassium chloride.

Potassium phosphate, dibasic. Dibasic potassium phosphate is available as a powder and as an injection containing 2 mEq K^+ and 1 mEq HPO_4^-/ml in 30-ml vials.

HYPERKALEMIA

Potassium excess, or hyperkalemia, can be caused by the following:

1 Acute or chronic renal failure; severe oliguria as a result of trauma whereby the kidney fails to excrete K^+
2 Release of large amounts of intracellular K^+ such as occurs in burns, crush injuries, or severe infections
3 Overtreatment with potassium salts
4 Metabolic acidosis, causing a shift of potassium from the cells into the extracellular fluid

Hyperkalemia causes interference with neuromuscular function, which can produce weakness and paralysis. Abdominal distention and diarrhea also occur. Cardiac effects caused by hyperkalemia result from impaired conduction. The ECG shows widening and slurring of the QRS complexes, peaked T waves, depressed ST segments, and possibly disappearance of P waves. Ventricular fibrillation and cardiac arrest may occur.

Treatment. Hyperkalemia is treated by withholding potassium and administering sodium polystyrene sulfonate (Kayexalate), a cation exchange resin. The drug is usually given orally or by stomach tube. It may also be given by high retention enema, although this is not a reliable method of administration.

In the intestines, particularly the colon, the sodium of the resin is in part replaced by potassium, approximately 3.1 mEq potassium per gram of resin. The potassium is eliminated from the body when the resin is eliminated with the feces or enema. Laxatives must be used when the drug is given orally. Since its action is slow, up to 24 hours, other treatment is indicated if ECG changes indicate advanced potassium intoxication. Administration should be discontinued when the serum potassium level falls to 4 or 5 mEq/liter.

Side effects of sodium polystyrene sulfonate treatment include anorexia, nausea, vomiting, hypokalemia, hypocalcemia, constipation, and fecal impaction. The latter can be prevented by the use of laxatives.

Preparation, dosage, and administration. Oral dose for adults is 15 g up to four times daily in 150 to 200 ml of water. Rectal dose for adults is 30 to 80 g suspended in 150 to 200 ml of 1% methylcellulose solution, 10% dextrose solution, or water. This dose may be given one to three times daily. The solution should be retained for 4 to 10 hours if possible, followed by a cleansing enema.

Calcium

Calcium, a positively charged ion (Ca^{++}), is essential for:

1 Growth and ossification of bone
2 Neuromuscular transmission
3 Cell membrane permeability

4 Maintaining excitability of nerve fibers
5 Hormone secretion and action
6 Muscle contraction
7 Maintenance of cardiac and vascular tone
8 Many enzyme activities
9 Normal coagulation of blood

Almost all of the 1000 to 1200 g calcium present in the normal adult is in the skeletal tissue, and only about 1% of the total body calcium is in solution in body fluids. About half of the calcium in plasma is bound to serum proteins; a small portion is bound to complex organic anions (for example, bicarbonate and phosphate). Almost all unbound serum calcium is ionized. Normal serum calcium concentration is 4.5 to 5.5 mEq/liter or 9 to 11 mg/100 ml.

The recommended dietary allowance of calcium for adults is 800 to 1200 mg daily. Pregnant or lactating women need 1.2 g; children age 6 to 18 years need 0.8 to 1.2 g. The intake of calcium in a balanced diet is sufficient for normal body needs. Absorption of calcium depends on how well it is kept in solution in the digestive tract. An acid medium favors calcium solubility; thus calcium is absorbed mainly in the upper intestinal tract. Absorption is decreased by the presence of alkalies and large amounts of fatty acids with which the calcium forms insoluble soaps. Adequate intake of vitamin D appears to promote calcium absorption. Calcium is excreted in the urine and feces; it is also excreted in perspiration.

Maintenance of normal concentration of serum calcium depends on the interactions of three agents: parathyroid hormone, vitamin D, and calcitonin. Parathyroid hormone and vitamin D mobilize the removal of calcium from bone, the principal source of calcium for extracellular fluids. Parathyroid hormone also promotes renal tubular reabsorption of calcium and a slight increase in intestinal absorption of calcium. Calcitonin is synthesized in the thyroid gland; it moderates or decreases the rate of removal of calcium from the bone.

HYPOCALCEMIA

A decrease in serum calcium results from (1) hypoparathyroidism, (2) chronic renal insufficiency, (3) rickets and osteomalacia, (4) malabsorption syndrome, and (5) deficiency of vitamin D. Hypoparathyroidism may follow thyroidectomy, since several of the parathyroid glands are frequently removed by this operation. If the function of the remaining gland(s) is impaired, the result is depressed parathyroid activity.

Patients who are bedridden tend to develop a negative calcium balance because the ion is lost from bones and is excreted. This effect is likely to be serious only when long immobilization of the patient is necessary.

Hypocalcemia causes increased excitability of the nerves and neuromuscular junction, which leads to muscle cramps, muscle twitching, and tetany. Numbness and tingling of the fingers, toes, and lips occur. The hypertonicity of muscle may cause tonic contractions of the hands and feet (carpopedal spasm). The increased neural excitability may cause convulsions, abnormal behavior, and personality changes. In children, prolonged hypocalcemia has resulted in mental retardation. Other effects of hypocalcemia include dyspnea, laryngeal spasm, diplopia, abdominal cramps, and urinary frequency. Diminished cardiac contractility may occur. The ECG shows a prolonged QT interval and an inverted T wave. In prolonged hypocalcemia defects can occur in the nails, skin, and teeth; cataracts may appear, and calcification of the basal ganglia may occur.

Treatment. Regardless of the underlying cause, severe hypocalcemia is treated initially with the intravenous administration of rapidly available calcium ions. For latent tetany, mild symptoms of hypocalcemia, and maintenance therapy, a calcium salt is given orally. Vitamin D may be given. Parathyroid injection is now considered obsolete and is not used for therapy; its biologic activity is uncertain. Overdosage of calcium may cause hypercalcemia, which results in anorexia, nausea, vomiting, weakness, depression, polyuria, and polydipsia. Calcium must be administered cautiously to patients on digitalis therapy, since calcium potentiates the effect of digitalis and may precipitate arrhythmias. ECG monitoring of the patient is recommended.

Preparation, dosage, and administration. Calcium salts are used as a nutritional supplement, particularly during pregnancy and lactation. They are specific in the treatment of hypocalcemic tetany. They have also been used for their antispasmodic effects in cases of abdominal pain, tenesmus, and colic resulting from disease of the gallbladder or painful contractions of the ureters. The basic salts of calcium are used as antacids.

Calcium chloride. Calcium chloride is a salt of calcium irritating to tissues when given parenterally other than by intravenous injection. It is available as a 10% solution. Care must be taken that the needle does not slip out of the vein and cause serious tissue irritation. Calcium chloride may be given orally but tends to cause gastric disturbance. When administered orally, it is best given in capsules. It is an acidifying salt and for that reason promotes the absorption of calcium. It may evoke acidosis. The average adult dose for oral administration is 1 g (gr 15) four times a day.

Calcium gluconate. Calcium gluconate is a white, crystalline or granular powder, which is odorless and tasteless. It has an advantage over calcium chloride, since it is more palatable for oral administration and can be given parenterally. It should not be administered intramuscularly, since there is danger of abscess formation and tissue slough. For severe hypocalcemic tetany, calcium gluconate injection is administered slowly in a 10% solution, intravenously (5 to 30 ml). A 0.3% solution (30 ml of a 10% solution in 1 liter of sodium chloride injection) may be given by slow drip infusion throughout the day. For mild hypocalcemic tetany, calcium gluconate may be given orally, 5 g three times a day 1 to 1½ hours after meals. Dosage for children is 500 mg/kg body weight in divided doses. It is available in tablet form for oral administration.

Calcium lactate. Calcium lactate is given orally. Its physical properties are similar to those of calcium gluconate. The usual adult dose is 5 g, which may be repeated three or four times a day. For children, dosage is 500 mg/kg body weight in divided doses. It is marketed in 300- and 600-mg tablets. Calcium lactate is more soluble in hot water than in cold and should be dissolved in hot water before it is given to the patient. Calcium lactate is not given parenterally. Some hospital pharmacies prepare a solution of calcium lactate for oral administration (1-liter bottles containing 2 g in 40 ml of water).

Calcium gluceptate. Calcium gluceptate is available in a 1.8% solution (18 mg/ml) in 5-ml ampules. It is used in the treatment of severe hypocalcemia. Intravenous dosage for adults and children is 90 to 360 mg. The rate of administration may be 1 ml or less over 1 minute. It may also be given intramuscularly; dosage for adults and children is 36 to 90 mg in the gluteal region or lateral aspect of the thigh; for infants, dose is 36 to 90 mg in the lateral thigh. Mild local irritation may occur.

Calcium phosphate, dibasic; calcium phosphate, tribasic. Dibasic and tribasic calcium phosphate salts are administered orally for treatment of mild and latent hypocalcemic tetany and for maintenance therapy. They are not used if the patient has renal insufficiency accompanied by hyperphosphatemia. These drugs are particularly useful for supplying calcium and phosphorus to pregnant and lactating women and to children. Oral dose is 1 to 2 g three times daily with meals.

Dihydrotachysterol. (Hytakerol). Dihydrotachysterol is an irradiated form of vitamin D used to treat hypocalcemia. When compared to ergocalciferol, dihydrotachysterol produces almost as great phosphate excretion, less absorption of calcium from the intestine, and more rapid rise in serum calcium levels. Dilhydrotachysterol has a shorter duration of action and less potential for accumulation and hypercalcemia than ergocalciferol. It may act more rapidly than vitamin D_2 or D_3. Tolerance or refractoriness does not seem to occur.

Dihydrotachysterol is effective when taken orally. Overdosage produces hypercalcemia, anorexia, nausea, vomiting, headache, renal calculi, and stupor. These symptoms disappear with withdrawal of the drug.

Dosage should be determined by frequent determinations of serum calcium levels. Initially, dosage is 0.75 to 2.5 mg daily; maintenance dose is 0.25 to 1.75 mg once or twice weekly.

HYPERCALCEMIA

Hypercalcemia may be caused by neoplasms with or without bone metastases. Carcinoma of the ovary, kidney, or lung can synthesize and secrete a parathyroid-like hormone causing hypercalcemia. Other common causes are hyperparathyroidism, thiazide or diuretic therapy, multiple myeloma, sarcoidosis, and vitamin D intoxication.

Clinical manifestations. Clinical manifestations of hypercalcemia are highly variable and involve many organ systems. Calcium may be deposited in various body tissues.

Gastrointestinal system. Symptoms are anorexia, nausea and vomiting, constipation, and abdominal pain. Hyperchlorhydria may occur, and 15% to 25% of the patients develop peptic ulcer. Antacids containing calcium should not be used.

Central nervous system. Symptoms include apathy, depression, amnesia, headaches, and drowsiness. In severe cases disorientation, syncope, hallucinations, and coma may occur.

Renal system. Polyuria and polydipsia occur from loss of renal concentrating ability. Kidney stones may be formed. Nephrocalcinosis may occur, seriously impairing renal function. This may lead to edema, uremia, and hypertension, which may be irreversible.

Neuromuscular system. Neural excitability is diminished causing weakness and muscle flaccidity.

Cardiovascular system. Elevated serum calcium causes increased cardiac contractility, ventricular extrasystoles, and heart block. ECG changes include a short QT interval and characteristic signs of heart block. In severe calcium toxicity, cardiac arrest in systole may occur.

Treatment. Treatment is variable and aimed at controlling the underlying disease. If hypercalcemia is caused by thiazide diuretic therapy, the diuretic is discontinued; the serum calcium returns to normal levels in about 1 month.

Renal excretion of calcium can be promoted with a number of drugs. Infusions of sodium chloride may be given to increase sodium excretion, which in turn increases calcium excretion. Natriuretic drugs, such as furosemide (Lasix) or ethacrynic acid (Edecrin), may be used. Chelating, or binding, agents, such as disodium edetate, increase renal excretion of calcium by forming soluble complexes with the calcium that are not reabsorbed by the renal

tubules. Inorganic phosphates may be given orally or intravenously to foster deposition of calcium in bone, thereby decreasing serum levels. An antineoplastic drug, mithramycin, also reduces serum calcium levels.

Preparation, dosage, and administration

Phosphate salts. Monobasic or dibasic sodium or potassium phosphate may be used to treat mild to moderate hypercalcemia when other forms of therapy are ineffective. The mechanism of action of phosphate salts is not known. However, they decrease serum levels of calcium probably by depositing calcium phosphate in the tissues; if there are bone lesions, these show improvement.

Oral administration for adults consists of 24 ml of 1 m dibasic sodium phosphate or a mixed salt solution four times daily to supply 3 g of phosphorus. Oral doses may cause nausea and vomiting.

The intravenous dose is 1 liter of a 0.1 m solution of phosphate salts (0.081 mole of dibasic sodium phosphate and 0.019 mole of monobasic potassium phosphate). This dose is administered over a period of 6 to 12 hours. Intravenous doses may cause hypotension, acute renal failure, and even myocardial infarction. Deaths have been reported. Overdosage will cause tetany.

The use of phosphate is hazardous, and patients should be carefully observed and monitored if possible.

Magnesium

Magnesium (Mg^{++}) is an important activator ion for the function of many enzymes. Normal serum concentration is 1.5 to 2.5 mEq/liter with one third bound to protein and two thirds as free cation. A toxic blood level is greater than 4 mEq/liter. About 50% of the total body magnesium exists in an insoluble state in bone, 45% is intracellular cation, and 5% extracellular cation. The normal dietary intake of magnesium has a range of approximately 8 to 24 mEq/24 hours in the adult (recommended dietary allowance is 300 to 400 mg daily). Magnesium is excreted via the kidney. Magnesium has physiologic effects on the nervous system similar to those of calcium.

HYPOMAGNESEMIA

A deficit of magnesium may be encountered in chronic alcoholism, severe malabsorption, starvation, diarrhea, prolonged gastrointestinal suction, vigorous diuresis, diseases causing hypocalcemia and hypokalemia, acute pancreatitis, and primary aldosteronism.

Hypomagnesemia is characterized by increased irritability of the nervous system, which may lead to disorientation and convulsions. Increased neuromuscular irritability and contractility also occur. There may be coarse tremor, muscle spasm, delirium, athetoid movements, and nystagmus. Tetany may occur. Hypomagnesemia also causes tachycardia, hypertension, and vasomotor changes. The use of intravenous fluids containing from 3 to 5 mEq magnesium/liter may avert magnesium deficiency that arises from prolonged administration of intravenous solutions that do not contain magnesium.

Treatment. Hypomagnesemia is treated with intravenous fluids containing magnesium, 10 to 40 mEq/day for severe deficit followed by 10 mEq/day for maintenance. Table 22-3 presents a list of minerals, mineral deficiencies, and appropriate treatments.

HYPERMAGNESEMIA

Hypermagnesemia occurs primarily in patients with chronic renal insufficiency. An excess of magnesium causes depression of the central nervous system, which leads to sedation and confusion. Blockade of the myoneural junction occurs by inhibiting acetylcholine release and diminishing muscle cell excitability. This causes muscle weakness. Respiratory muscle paralysis may occur causing death. Hypermagnesemia also causes blockade of sympathetic ganglia and has a direct vasodilating effect that results in a decrease in blood pressure.

Excess magnesium has a cardiac inhibitory effect. Conduction time is increased and the ECG will show a lengthened PR interval and a prolonged QRS complex. If the Mg^{++} concentration continues to increase, cardiac arrest in diastole may occur. Third-degree atrioventricular block may also occur.

Treatment. An excess of Mg^{++} may require dialysis. Since calcium acts as an antagonist to Mg^{++}, calcium salts may be given parenterally.

Nutrients
Vitamins

Vitamins have great biochemical importance because they are essential for maintenance of normal metabolic function, growth, and health. The name *vitamin* means "vital for life." Originally the word was spelled with an "e" on the end (vitamine), since it was believed that these substances were amines; the "e" was dropped on recognition that all vitamins were not amines.

Only a few vitamins are synthesized in the body; vitamin K is formed by bacteria in the gut, and vitamin D is produced by exposure of the skin to sunlight. Thus most vitamins must be ingested in food or in their pure form as dietary supplements. Only small amounts of the vitamins are necessary for growth and health, and an adequate and varied diet will provide all the vitamins needed except during pregnancy and infancy. Restricted diets as a result of cultural or idiosyncratic beliefs, alcoholism, poverty, ignorance, or disorders of the gastrointestinal tract that interfere with absorption will lead to vitamin deficiency. In these cases, vitamin preparations are therapeutic. In the United States and Canada, mild forms of avitaminosis are more common than the pronounced deficiency states of beriberi, pellagra, rickets, or scurvy.

Vitamins are classified as being *fat soluble* or *water soluble*. Fat-soluble vitamins are A, D, E, and K. They are stored in the liver and fatty tissue in large amounts, and a deficiency in these vitamins occurs only after long deprivation from an adequate supply or disorders preventing their absorption. Water-soluble vitamins include the B group and C. These vitamins are not stored in the body in large amounts, and short periods of inadequate intake can lead to a deficiency. Vitamins are important components of enzyme systems that catalyze the reactions for protein, fat, and carbohydrate metabolism.

The sale of vitamins in the United States constitutes a multimillion-dollar business. They are widely used, and often unjustifiably, primarily because of successful advertising that vitamins will improve even normal health. The

T A B L E 2 2 - 3 **Minerals, mineral defiencies, and treatment**

Mineral	Source	Daily requirements in adult male	Specific functions	Deficiency clinical state

Sodium	Common salt
	Citrate and tartrate
	  in fruits
		1.3 to 3.3	Control of body water
			Electrophysiology of nerve,
			  muscle, gland cells
			Regulation of pH, isotonicity
				Hyponatremia
				  Lassitude, hypotension,
				    vomiting, cramps,
				    hemoconcentration

Potassium	Present in all plant
	  and animal food
		1.8 to 5.6	Necessary for electrophysi-
			  ology of cell membranes
			Regulation of pH, isotonicity
				Hypokalemia
				  Mental changes,
				    loquacity, hallu-
				    cinations
				  Limp, soft, weak
				    muscles
				  ECG: prolonged
				    QT, depressed ST,
				    inverted T

Calcium	Milk, cheese,
	  sardines,
	  salmon
		800 mg	Calcification of bones and
			  teeth, blood clotting,
			  excitation-coupling
			  mechanisms, cofactor in
			  enzyme reactions
				Hypocalcemia
				Tetany
				Osteomalacia

Magnesium	Fruit, peas, beans,
	  nuts
		350 to 400 mg	Electrophysiology, enzyme
			  reactions
				Neuromuscular disorders

Iron	Meat, liver, kidney,
	  fruits, vegetables,
	  cereals
		10 mg	Hemoglobin	Iron-deficiency anemia

Copper	Liver, oysters, salmon, fruits	2 to 3	Hemoglobin synthesis	Anemia

indiscriminate use of vitamins is not likely to decline in the near future.

The potency of vitamins A and D, when described on a label, must be in USP units, but the vitamin content of ascorbic acid, thiamine, riboflavin, nicotinic acid, nicotinamide, pyridoxine, and menadione and other vitamin K preparations, when expressed, must be in terms of milligrams.

The FDA proposed regulations dividing vitamin-mineral products into three categories:

1 *Supplement*—all ingredients are within established limits
2 *O-T-C/Proprietary*—the vitamin-mineral contents exceed the limits established for supplement use but not excessively
3 *Prescription status*—contents exceed the upper limit for O-T-C/proprietary products

Many multivitamin capsules and tablets vary in their contents. Some contain ingredients such as biotin and pantothenic acid for which evidence as to their essential role in human nutrition is inconclusive. However, the presence of such ingredients in these preparations is not permitted. The amounts of vitamins A and D in oral nonprescription vitamin preparations are limited to not more than 10,000 IU vitamin A and not more than 400 IU vitamin D.

"Optional vitamins" (E, B_6, folic acid, pantothenic acid, and B_{12}) may or may not be included as ingredients in over-the-counter, multivitamin preparations. However, the most popular OTC multivitamin preparations are those that contain all vitamins needed by humans. Most OTC vitamin preparations are designed to fulfill daily body needs completely without regard for the amount of various vitamins contained in the daily diet.

Stability of vitamins is of great importance, since vitamin preparations may be on the pharmacy or grocery shelf for months before being purchased and used. Vitamins may lose as much as one third of their potency in 1 month and 80% of their potency in 6 months. If the

Treatment	Excess clinical state	Treatment
Ringer's solution Sodium chloride 0.9% solution	*Hypernatremia* Edema, hypertonicity	Dextrose and water intravenously
Potassium chloride oral solution or injection	*Hyperkalemia* Central nervous system stimulation and paralysis ECG: peaked T waves, prolonged QRS, PR interval Listlessness, weakness, numbness	Intravenous glucose and insulin Extracorporeal dialysis Calcium gluconate
Intravenous calcium chloride or calcium gluconate Oral calcium lactate or calcium gluconate	Hypercalcemia Renal calculi	Calcitonin EDTA—very cautiously owing to liver damage IV infusion of saline Sulfate and citrate salts Dialysis Corticosteroids Furosemide
Magnesium ion replacement	Diminished excitability of muscle fibers Hypotension Respiratory paralysis	Intravenous injection of calcium salts Artificial respiration
Ferrous sulfate and gluconate	Hemosiderosis	Chelating agent

label is not dated concerning potency expiration, vitamins should preferably be purchased at stores with high sales volume. Patients should be instructed not to purchase a large amount of vitamin preparations at one time and to discard old vitamin preparations.

FAT-SOLUBLE VITAMINS
Vitamin A

Vitamin A, the fat-soluble, growth-promoting vitamin, is essential for growth in the young and for maintenance of health at all ages. The chemistry of this vitamin has been established and is related to the carotenoid pigments of plants, especially carotene. In fact, the term "vitamin A" may be applied to vitamin A, alpha-carotene, beta-carotene, gamma-carotene, and cryptoxanthin. The last four factors are formed in plants and are precursors of vitamin A in the body. Beta-carotene in the body is hydrolyzed to form two molecules of vitamin A.

Chemists have failed to discover vitamin A in any plant foodstuff. The carotene of plants, therefore, seems to supply the provitamin from which the body tissues prepare vitamin A. The amount of chlorophyll in the plant is a rough indication of the amount of carotene present. Animal fats, such as those found in butter, milk, eggs, and fish liver, are sources of the carotenoids; they were originally derived from plants and stored in animal tissue.

Vitamin A is essential in humans to promote normal growth and development of bones and teeth and to maintain the health of epithelial tissues of the body. Its function in relation to normal vision and the prevention of night blindness has been carefully studied. Vitamin A actually makes up a portion of one of the major retinal pigments, rhodopsin, and is thus required for normal "rod vision" in the retina of humans and many of the animals.

Vitamin A is also functional in conversion processes resulting in corticosterone and cholesterol.

Absorption, storage, and excretion. Vitamin A and carotene are readily absorbed from the normal gastrointestinal tract. Efficient absorption depends on fat absorption and, therefore, on the presence of adequate bile salts in the intestine. Certain conditions, such as obstructive jaundice, some infectious diseases, and the presence of mineral oil in the intestine, may result in vitamin A deficiency in spite of the fact that the amount ingested was normal.

Vitamin A is stored in the liver to a greater extent than elsewhere. The liver also functions in changing carotene to vitamin A; this function is inhibited in liver diseases and in diabetes. The amount of vitamin A stored depends on the dietary intake. When intake is high or excessive, the stores formed in the liver may become sufficient to last a long time. Vitamin A is lost chiefly by destruction. Little is lost through the ordinary channels of excretion.

Uses. Vitamin A is used to treat or relieve symptoms associated with a deficiency of vitamin A (avitaminosis), such as night blindness (nyctalopia), hyperkeratosis, retarded growth, xerophthalmia, keratomalacia, weakness, and increased susceptibility of mucous membranes to infection. It is effective in the treatment of vitamin A deficiency.

The diet low in vitamin A should be corrected with foods rather than with drugs. It appears that large doses of vitamin A may be given with no apparent harm to the adult, although excessive doses have been known to produce toxic effects in rats and in young children.

There are times when vitamin A concentrates have a legitimate use as supplements to the diet. Increased need occurs during pregnancy and lactation, in infancy, and in conditions characterized by lack of normal absorption and storage of vitamin A.

Daily requirement. It has been conclusively established that the vitamin A daily requirement is a rather large one, if optimal conditions of nutrition are to be maintained. The minimum daily requirements for vitamin A are 400 to 420 units for infants, 400 to 1000 units for children, and 800 to 1000 units for adults. During pregnancy and lactation, requirements equal 1000 to 1200 units, respectively. Thera-

peutic dosages may be three times these amounts. Although larger doses have been used in experimental studies, there is no evidence that justifies the use of more than 25,000 units/day. It has not been shown that excess dosage over and above the daily requirement is of value in the prevention of colds, influenza, and so on. Large dosages are injurious to infants. Symptoms of hypervitaminosis A include anorexia; altered liver function; brittle nails; cracked and bleeding lips; dry, itchy, and scaly skin; hyperirritability; and neurologic symptoms. Symptoms disappear after cessation of ingestion of the vitamin. Oral contraceptives increase plasma vitamin A levels.

When the vitamin A requirement is met in the form of carotene or the provitamin A, twice as many units of the carotene are required to produce the same effect.

Preparation, dosage, and administration. The following are preparations of vitamin A and combinations of vitamins A and D.

Vitamin A. Vitamin A is either fish liver oil, fish liver oil diluted with vegetable oil, or a solution of vitamin A concentrate in fish liver oil or vegetable oil. Vitamin A capsules are available containing 5000, 10,000, 25,000, or 50,000 USP units. The usual follow-up therapeutic dose is 10,000 to 25,000 units daily for 60 days.

Water miscible vitamin A (Aquasol A). Water miscible vitamin A is available in 25,000- and 50,000-unit capsules and in a parenteral form containing 50,000 units/ml. Absorption is greater for aqueous preparations. Intramuscular injections should be given deep and slow.

Oleovitamin A and D capsules. Oleovitamin A and D capsules contain 5000 units of vitamin A and 100 units of vitamin D.

Vitamin A ester concentrate. Vitamin A ester concentrate contains not less than 485,000 units of vitamin A activity in each gram.

Cod liver oil. Cod liver oil is partially destearinated. The usual dosage is 4 ml orally, which contains 3000 USP units of vitamin A and 300 USP units of vitamin D. This is one of the least expensive sources of vitamin A and D.

Halibut liver oil. Usual daily prophylactic dose for infants and adults is 0.1 ml (1½ minim). Halibut liver oil contains in each gram not less than 30,000 units of vitamin A and between 2500 and 3500 units of vitamin D. In 0.1 ml there are 5000 units of vitamin A.

Halibut-liver oil capsules. Each capsule contains 4500 units of vitamin A activity. The dose is one to three capsules daily.

A and D ointment. A and D ointment is a preparation containing both vitamins in a lanolin-petrolatum base. It is used in treatment of epithelial lesions, such as diaper rash, superficial burns, and excoriations.

Vitamin D

Vitamin D is a term applied to two or more substances that affect the proper utilization of calcium and phosphorus in the body. Two forms of naturally occurring vitamin D have been isolated. One of these forms is obtained as one of the products of irradiated ergosterol and is known as vitamin D_2 or ergocalciferol. Ergosterol has therefore been shown to be a precursor of vitamin D. Further investigation has shown that there are a number of precursors that can be changed by irradiation into compounds that have vitamin D activity. Irradiation of 7-dehydrocholesterol results in the formation of vitamin D_3 (cholecalciferol) which is stored in the body. It is formed also in skin exposed to sunlight. Irradiated ergosterol (calciferol) is the active constituent in various vitamin preparations such as viosterol and irradiated yeast.

Vitamin D_2 and vitamin D_3, as well as other products of irradiated ergosterol, are capable of antirachitic activity. The metabolic activation of vitamin D will be discussed below.

Although vitamin D is an essential vitamin, it is contained in only a few foods (milk, bread, cereals) of the average American diet. Small amounts are present in herring, sardines, salmon, tuna fish, eggs, and butter. Vitamin D is found in high concentrations in a number of fish oils (cod, halibut).

At present, milk is the chief commercial food product enriched by the addition of vitamin D concentrate. By federal regulation, milk products are standardized at 400 International Units per quart, which represents a day's requirement of vitamin D.

Action and result. The exact mechanism by which vitamin D functions in the metabolism of calcium and phosphorus is not known. There is evidence that a complex relationship exists between vitamin D and parathyroid hormone, but this is not yet conclusive. The vitamin seems to be concerned directly with the absorption of calcium and phosphorus from the intestinal tract and their deposition in bone and teeth. In the absence of vitamin D the amount of these substances absorbed from the bowel is diminished to such an extent that even though the calcium and phosphate intake is adequate, rickets results in the child and osteomalacia in the adult.

An enzyme called alkaline phosphatase exists in the body and is closely related to phosphorus metabolism. It is distributed widely in the animal body and is particularly active in ossifying cartilage. When rickets is present, the level of phosphatase in blood serum is high. This is thought to be caused by leakage from the diseased bone. Administration of vitamin D causes the enzyme to return to normal slowly.

It has been shown that vitamin D is converted into hydroxy-vitamin D in the liver, and then to dihydroxy-vitamin D (the active form of vitamin D) by the kidney when blood calcium is low. The dihydroxy compound is more potent than vitamin D and greatly increases the absorption of calcium from the digestive tract. When serum calcium becomes normal, this conversion ceases and calcium absorption declines. A discussion of this 1,25-dihydroxy form and the 25-hydroxy form are found in the "preparation, dosage, and administration" section.

Symptoms of deficiency. The chief indication of vitamin D deficiency is rickets, characterized by irritability, craniotabes, prominent frontal bones, delayed closing of the fontanels, soft bones, pigeon breast, rachitic rosary, flaring ribs, epiphyseal enlargement at wrists and elbows, muscular weakness, protruding abdomen, bowed legs, delayed eruption of teeth, abnormal ratio of calcium and phosphorus in the blood, and tetany.

Daily requirement. It is thought that either the human requirement of vitamin D is relatively low or else it is met by the action of sunlight on the skin. A daily intake of 400 units is considered adequate to meet the ordinary requirements of all age groups.

Older children and adults who live in a climate where they do not have access to abundant sunshine need to supplement their vitamin D intake. The amount supplied probably should be up to the minimum requirements for the infant. To prevent the development of rickets, it is important to start the administration of vitamin D early in the infant's life, and full dosage should be given by the second month.

Uses. The prevention of rickets in young children is one of the most justified uses of vitamin D. The initial dose should be about 200 units daily, with an increase in dosage up to 800 units by the second month. Premature infants or those who seem to be especially susceptible to the development of rickets need a larger intake (800 to 1200 units usually). When children already have rickets, the dosage is also greater. The average daily dose usually is about 1200 to 1500 units, but in some instances it may be increased to as much as 60,000 or more units daily. Vitamin D–resistant rickets is a condition that does not respond to usual doses of vitamin D but requires unusually large doses. If nausea or anorexia appears, the vitamin should be discontinued temporarily. Hypervitaminosis D causes hypercalcemia, which may lead to calcification of soft tissues.

In adults osteomalacia also calls for large doses of vitamin D, improved dietary and living conditions, and more exposure to sunlight.

Patients suffering from bone fractures, especially elderly individuals, may benefit from the administration of vitamin D, thus promoting optimal conditions for bone healing.

Vitamin D may be administered in a number of conditions such as arthritis, psoriasis, diarrhea, and steatorrhea, if there is good evidence that a deficiency of this vitamin exists.

Preparation, dosage, and administration

Ergocalciferol (vitamin D_2, Calciferol, Drisdol), cholecalciferol (vitamin D_3). The preparation of this vitamin is available in capsules, each containing 50,000 USP units (1.25 mg) and in solution, 0.25 mg (10,000 USP units)/g for oral administration. The average therapeutic dose for rickets is 1200 USP units (30 μg). The normal daily intake for adults is 400 USP units (10 μg). This preparation is especially suitable for severe or refractory rickets. Therapeutic dosage varies from 30 μg to 5 mg.

Calcitriol (1,25-dihydroxycholecalciferol, Rocaltrol). Calcitrol is a potent, prompt-acting vitamin-hormone involved in calcium absorption and used in the treatment of hypocalcemia in patients with chronic renal failure for osteodystrophy and hypocalcemia of hypoparathyroidism where failure of 1-hydroxylation has resulted in functional deficiency of vitamin D.

Rocaltrol is available commercially in 0.25-μg and 0.5-μg capsules. The usual maintenance dose is 0.5 to 1 μg daily. It is of paramount importance to initially monitor serum calcium levels because of hypercalcemia, which is a side effect. Antacids of the aluminum carbonate or gel type may be administered to initiate phosphate binding in the lower gastrointestinal tract as a result of hyperphosphatemia, since the rising serum calcium will combine with phosphate and create ectopic calcifications, thus impairing renal function.

Dietary vitamin D in the liver is hydroxylated by microsomes to the active 25-hydroxycholecalciferol (calcifediol, Calderol), and finally the mitochondria of the kidney convert it to the 1,25-hydroxy form. Calcitriol bound to the intestinal mucosa may lead to the formation of calcium-binding protein that affects increased calcium absorption from the low gastrointestinal tract. Apparently, calcitriol along with parathyroid hormone is involved in the transfer of calcium ion to the extracellular fluid, following absorption from bone and glomerular filtrate.

Calcifediol (Calderol; 25-hydroxycholecalciferol; 25-hydroxyvitamin D_3; 25-HCC; 25-OHCC; 25-OHD$_3$). Calcifediol is identical to the natural circulating vitamin D metabolite produced in the liver. The other principal circulating vitamin D metabolite is the kidney product, calcitriol. Calcifediol (the liver product metabolite) has beneficial effects on uremic bone disease; it is effective in the treatment of renal osteodystrophy in patients undergoing long-term hemodialysis, in patients with renal failure undergoing dialysis, and in the management of metabolic bone disease associated with chronic renal failure. Calcifediol improves calcium absorption in the absence of renal tissue, which suggests that the conversion to the calcitriol form may not be essential for the calcifediol effect on the gastrointestinal tract of uremic patients to increase intestinal calcium absorption.

Humans derive natural vitamin D from the ultraviolet rays of the sun by converting 7-hydrocholesterol synthesized in the skin to vitamin D_3 (cholecalciferol). Vitamin D_3 is first converted to calcifediol by an enzyme of the liver (25-OHase) and is the major transport form of vitamin D_3. Calcifediol is then converted to calcitriol by renal mitochondria in the kidney. Calcifediol activity is dual in that it possesses intrinsic activity and is converted to other metabolites. Calcifediol is rapidly absorbed from the intestine after oral administration, and peak serum concentrations occur after 4 hours; it is transported in the blood and bound to a specific plasma protein and has a serum half-life of 16 days (far in excess of calcitriol).

As with calcitriol, aluminum carbonate or hydroxide gels are to be used to control serum phosphorus levels in patients undergoing dialysis. Caution is used in patients receiving digitalis preparations because hypercalcemia may precipitate cardiac dysrhythmias. The patient should be informed about compliance and adherence to dosage, diet, calcium supplementation, phosphate binding (aluminum carbonate/hyroxide gels), and the symptoms of hypercalcemia. The early and late signs and symptoms of vitamin intoxication associated with hypercalcemia are:

1 Early—weakness; headache; somnolence; nausea; vomiting; constipation; dry mouth; muscle pain; bone pain; and metallic taste
2 Late—polyurea; polydipsia; anorexia; irritability; weight loss; nocturia; conjunctivitis; pancreatitis; photophobia; rhinorrhea; pruritus; hyperthermia; decreased libido; elevated BUN, SGOT and SGPT; albuminuria; hypercholesterolemia; ectopic calcification; hypertension; cardiac dysrhythmias; and rarely overt psychosis

The capsules are available in 20-μg and 50-μg strengths. In patients with chronic renal failure undergoing dialysis the initial dose is 300 to 350 μg weekly on a daily or alternate-day schedule and individually titrated to response at 4-week intervals with weekly serum calcium levels to ensure normocalcemia. Most patients respond to 50 to 100 μg daily or 100 to 200 μg on alternate days.

Side effects and toxic effects. Certain pathologic changes have been noted in animals after the administration of excessive doses of vitamin D_1. This vitamin represents the exceptional case of a vitamin in which excessive dosage can cause disease. Symptoms of hypervitaminosis D include anorexia, nausea, vomiting, weakness, weight loss, diarrhea, vague aches, stiffness, and drowsiness. Doses greatly in excess of the usual therapeutic level can so increase the renal excretion of phosphate and calcium that these elements are withdrawn from bone, producing demineralization and calcium deposition in soft tissues. It is curious that both a lack and an excess of vitamin D may produce softening of the bones, although by different mechanisms. Elevation of serum calcium above 12 mg/100 ml is considered a danger signal, and dosage should be reduced or temporarily discontinued.

Vitamin E (tocopherol)

Vitamin E is a fat-soluble vitamin, the richest source of which is wheat germ oil, although it occurs in other vegetable oils such as cottonseed oil and peanut oil. It is also found in green leafy vegetables.

A number of compounds have been found that exhibit vitamin E activity. The most active of these are the tocopherols, of which three are naturally occurring compounds known as alpha-, beta-, and gamma-tocopherol. The most biologically potent of these compounds is alpha-tocopherol.

In laboratory animals a lack of vitamin E manifests itself by infertility or failure of the female to carry a pregnancy to term, muscular dystrophy, paralysis of the hindquarters, and cardiac lesions. In humans a deficiency of vitamin E results in hemolysis of erythrocytes. Vitamin E plays an important role in heme synthesis. The requirement for vitamin E increases with the intake of polyunsaturated fats. Daily requirement for adults is 8 to 10 alpha-tocopherol equivalents.

Vitamin E in human physiology does not appear to be of value in the treatment of sterility or the prevention of abortions.

Preparation, dosage, and administration

Vitamin E (Aquasol E, E-Ferol). Official capsules contain 30 to 1000 IU of vitamin E in the form of alpha-tocopherol. Injectable forms contain 100 or 200 IU/ml. It has been successfully used to treat anemia unresponsive to iron or other drugs.

Vitamin K

Vitamin K is also a fat-soluble vitamin that has been presented in Unit VI.

WATER-SOLUBLE VITAMINS
VITAMIN B COMPLEX

The vitamin B complex refers to a group of vitamins that are often found together in food, although they are chemically dissimilar and have different metabolic functions. Grouping them together is based largely on the historical basis of their having been discovered in a sequential order. They have little in common other than their sources and the fact that they are water soluble. There is a sensible and increasingly popular trend to discard such names as vitamins B_1 and B_2 and to refer to these vitamins as thiamine and riboflavin. Vitamin B complex includes thiamine, riboflavin, nicotinic acid, pyridoxine, pantothenic acid, biotin, choline, inositol, and para-aminobenzoic acid.

Thiamine (vitamin B_1)

Thiamine is also known as the antineuritic or antiberiberi vitamin. It was first synthesized in 1937. It is found abundantly in yeast, in whole grain cereals, and in pork and liver.

Thiamine is believed to play an essential role in the intermediate steps of carbohydrate metabolism. Specifically, thiamine is a major portion of the coenzyme decarboxylase necessary for the normal metabolism of pyruvic acid and other compounds as well. Thus it plays a part in the metabolism of all living cells.

Thiamine deficiency is recognized as being of fundamental importance in beriberi. This disease is still found in Asia but is seldom encountered in the United States and Europe except in persons whose dietary pattern is abnormal. The symptoms of thiamine deficiency are particularly related to changes in the nervous and cardiovascular systems and include muscular weakness, disturbances of sensation, tenderness over nerve trunks, polyneuritis, loss of appetite, dyspnea, epigastric disorders, and irregularities of heart action. Milder symptoms may consist of muscular aches and pains, anorexia, tachycardia, irritability, and mental depression. Deficiency states in the United States are much less common since white flour has been enriched with thiamine.

Daily requirement. It has been estimated that adult females require 1 mg of thiamine chloride daily. The recommended amount for males is from 1.2 to 1.5 mg. For the infant, 0.3 to 0.5 mg is the optimal daily dose, increasing to 1.2 to 1.4 mg between the ages of 10 and 18 years. Requirements are increased during pregnancy and lactation and when the metabolic rate is increased or the body is unable to absorb or utilize the vitamin. Treatment of thiamine deficiency states requires several times the amount ordinarily needed. Thiamine is found to some extent in all body tissues but, like all B vitamins, exists in high concentrations in the liver. It is absorbed from the gastrointestinal tract as well as from parenteral sites of administration.

Uses. The only therapeutic value of thiamine is in the treatment or prevention of thiamine deficiency. Since deficiency in one of the vitamin B factors may be accompanied by deficiency in others, some authorities prefer to give several components of the vitamin B complex. Treatment is best accomplished by an adequate diet or preparations rich in the B factors, such as brewers' yeast. Thiamine is indicated for treatment of beriberi and polyneuritis and for the relief of symptoms that accompany milder forms of thiamine deficiency.

Thiamine replacement is necessary for patients receiving nourishment parenterally and only in the form of dextrose. Carbohydrate metabolism is increased and, therefore, requires additional amounts of thiamine.

Preparation, dosage, and administration

Thiamine hydrochloride. Thiamine hydrochloride is marketed in tablets for oral administration and in solution for injection. When injected, thiamine hydrochloride is usually

T A B L E 2 2 - 4 Vitamins and human nutrition

Vitamin	Source	Daily requirements in adult male	Specific functions	Deficiency	Therapeutic source
A	Dairy products, carrots, green vegetables, liver, kidneys, eggs	1000 IU*	Visual pigments Maintenance of epithelial tissue	Nightblindness Corneal softening Hyperkeratosis	Halibut liver oil Cod liver oil
C	Fruit, fresh green vegetables, corn, tomatoes, rose hips	50 to 60 mg	Oxidation-reduction processes Maintenance of normal connective tissue Adrenocortical function	Scurvy Swelling, redness, and bleeding of gums Petechiae Capillary fragility Anemia	Ascorbic acid tablets and injection Decavitamins
D	Egg yolk, butter, milk, fish liver oils, shrimp, salmon	400 IU	Absorption of calcium from intestine Deposition of mineral in bone	Rickets in children Osteomalacia in adults	Cod liver oil Halibut liver oil Calciferol tablets Sunlight
E	Wheat germ, egg yolk, liver, vegetable oils	8 to 10 IU	Essential for normal hematopoiesis	Hemolytic anemia†	Multivitamins Tocopherol capsules and tablets
B complex Thiamine (B₁)	Cereal grains, yeast, meat, peas, beans	1.2-1.5 mg	Carbohydrate metabolism	Central and autonomic nervous system disturbances Fatigue Neuritis Beriberi	Thiamine hydrochloride tablets or injection Multivitamins
Riboflavin (B₂)	Yeast, meat, liver, green leafy vegetables	1.4 to 1.6 mg	Coenzymes for metabolism of respiratory proteins	Glossitis Dermatitis Stomatitis	Riboflavin tablets and injection Decavitamins
Niacin (nicotinic acid)	Yeast, lean meat, liver	16 to 19 mg		Pellagra	B complex vitamins
Pyridoxine (B₆)	Yeast, cereal grains, egg yolk, liver, nuts, peas, potatoes, meat, fish	1.8 to 2.2 mg	Formation of aminobutyric acid, an inhibitory transmitter substance Metabolism of amino acids, nucleic acids, protein	Convulsions Hyperirritability Neuritis Edema	Pyridoxine tablets Decavitamins
Pantothenic acid	Liver, eggs, wheat germ, cheese	4 to 7 mg	Component of coenzyme A	Neurologic disturbances Irritability Fatigue Muscle cramps Dry, scaly skin Adrenal hypofunction	Decavitamins
Biotin	Egg yolk, liver, nuts, cereals	100 to 200 mg	Coenzyme for carbon dioxide fixation	Anorexia Malaise Dermatitis	Multivitamin preparations

*IU, International Units, which are identical to USP units.
†Not well established.

administered subcutaneously, or it may be added to intravenous fluids. The usual dosage of thiamine hydrochloride is 1 to 50 mg daily. It is marketed under a number of trade names such Betalin S.

Thiamine mononitrate. Thiamine mononitrate is available in 3-, 5-, 10-, and 25-mg tablets.

Dried yeast. Dried yeast must contain in each gram not less than 0.12 mg thiamine hydrochloride, 0.04 mg riboflavin, and 0.30 mg niacin. The usual dose is 10 g four times a day.

Side effects and toxic effects. Large doses of thiamine when given intravenously have been known to cause anaphylactic shock, probably because of allergic responses to the preparation. However, the incidence of toxicity is so low as to be almost nonexistent.

Riboflavin (vitamin B₂)

Crystals of riboflavin are an orange-yellow color and are slightly soluble in water. Thiamine contains sulfur; riboflavin does not. Riboflavin was identified first in milk. Later it was identified in other substances and was called lactoflavin because of its intense yellow color. Its relationship to the vitamin B complex was not appreciated until it was observed that concentrates of vitamin B₂ had a yellow color, the intensity of which was related to the potency of the concentrate. At present, vitamin B₂ is synthesized and all doubt of its identity has been removed. It was named riboflavin because of the presence of ribose in its structure.

Metabolic function. Riboflavin seems to function in cellular respiration and is a constituent of all cells. It is slightly water soluble and heat stable. Many enzymes contain the riboflavin molecule as an essential portion of their molecule. These so-called flavo-enzymes include a number of oxidizing enzymes such as those that oxidize the common amino acids to ketoacids. In addition, flavo-enzymes form part of the chain of "electron transport" by which the energy obtained from oxidizing foodstuff is stored as chemical energy in the form of adenosine triphosphate (ATP). The flavo-enzymes can carry out their function because the riboflavin molecule can be easily oxidized and reduced (loss and gain of electrons) so that it

can act as a link in the bridge by which electrons are removed from organic compounds and transferred to oxygen.

The functions of flavo-enzymes are therefore so extensive and important that it becomes difficult to pinpoint single specific reactions that result from a riboflavin deficiency.

Symptoms of deficiency. Deficiency in human beings is associated with superficial fissures about the angles of the mouth (cheilosis) and nose at the junction between the mucous membrane and the skin, visual disturbances, glossitis, and a peculiar red color of the tongue. Actual tissue changes in the eye may occur. Riboflavin deficiency is likely to occur along with a deficiency of other members of the B complex.

Milk is one of the most important sources of riboflavin. Other sources include yeast, liver, kidney, eggs, lean meat, and leafy vegetables. The addition of riboflavin to white flour has helped to increase the intake of this vitamin for many persons.

Daily requirement. The requirement of riboflavin does not appear to be related to caloric intake or to muscular activity, but there does seem to be a relationship to body weight. The Food and Nutrition Board of the National Research Council in 1980 recommended 1.2 to 1.3 mg for women and 1.4 to 1.7 mg for men as a daily requirement for optimal nutrition. During pregnancy and lactation the recommended allowance should be increased by 0.3 to 0.5 mg/day. For infants the recommended daily allowance is from 0.4 to 0.6 mg and for children ages 1 to 18 the daily recommended allowance is from 0.8 to 1.7 mg.

Uses. Riboflavin is used to prevent and to treat deficiency states and is used along with niacin in the treatment of pellagra.

Preparation, dosage, and administration

Riboflavin (Lactoflavin). Riboflavin is usually administered orally because it is well absorbed from the gastrointestinal tract. Tablets of 5, 10, and 25 mg are available for oral administration. Riboflavin injection, 0.5 to 50 mg/ml, can be given subcutaneously. The usual therapeutic daily dose is 5 mg, although 2 to 20 mg daily may be needed, depending on the degree of deficiency. It is effective for treatment of riboflavin deficiency. Yeast preparations are also given for their riboflavin content.

Side effects and toxic effects. Riboflavin is completely nontoxic and reactions to it do not seem to occur. No side effects have been noted after relatively large doses.

Niacin (nicotinic acid)

Niacin is related chemically to nicotine but possesses none of the latter's pharmacologic properties. Niacin is converted in the body to niacinamide, a dietary essential, the lack of which is responsible for the symptoms of pellagra. Pellagra is characterized by disturbances of the gastrointestinal tract, skin, and nervous system. In a milder degree of deficiency, patients are nervous or irritable and have indigestion, diarrhea or constipation, and abnormal skin pigmentation.

Pellagra occurs among persons of low economic means and has been noted especially among peoples who eat a good deal of corn (maize) but whose total diet is limited in protein. It is also seen as a result of dietary fads and disease of the gastrointestinal tract in which there is poor intestinal absorption.

Lean meats, poultry, and fish have been found to be a better source of niacin than vegetables and fruits. Milk and eggs are good sources of the precursor substance, tryptophan. The enrichment of white flour has made an appreciable contribution to the increase of niacin in the average diet in the United States.

Unlike some of the other water-soluble vitamins, niacin can be synthesized in the body from the essential amino acid, tryptophan. Diets low in both niacin and tryptophan are the most likely to produce clinical deficiency.

Metabolic function. As in the case of riboflavin, a large group of enzymes depends for their function on coenzymes containing niacin. The vital oxidation-reduction coenzymes, diphosphopyridine nucleotide and triphosphopyridine nucleotide, are required for the early reactions of many metabolic pathways.

Both contain the nicotinamide molecule as part of their structure. No biologic role of niacin is known except for its presence in coenzymes, but so many metabolic processes depend on the pyridine nucleotides that this is ample to explain the widespread symptoms caused by niacin lack.

Daily requirement. The National Research Council (USA), in its 1980 revision of Recommended Dietary Allowances, states the daily niacin requirements in terms of niacin equivalents, assuming that 60 mg of tryptophan will supply 1 mg of niacin. Requirements are estimated on the basis of body weight and caloric intake and then increased by 50% to provide for varying physiologic needs and dietary situations. The niacin requirement for women is given as 13 to 14 mg daily and for men it is 16 to 19 mg daily. For pregnancy and lactation an increase of from 2 to 5 mg/day is recommended. For infants the daily recommended intake is 6 to 8 mg. The recommended allowance for children ages 1 to 18 is 9 to 18 mg daily.

Uses. Both nicotinic acid and nicotinamide are used in the treatment and prophylaxis of pellagra, but since pellagra is a disease associated with multiple vitamin deficiencies, riboflavin and thiamine are also indicated. Optimal treatment of the disease must include the administration of all members of the vitamin B complex as well as a diet adequate in animal protein. Results of therapy are frequently dramatic. Some positive results have been noted when niacin has been administered to patients with a variety of diagnoses, ranging from sprue to Meniere's syndrome. It has been used to reverse some characteristics of aging, in lowering cholesterol levels, and in psychiatric contexts to differentiate between psychoses of dietary and nondietary origin.

Preparation, dosage, and administration. The following are available preparations of niacin.

Niacin; nicotinic acid. Nicotinic acid is available as a powder and in tablet form of 25, 50, or 100 mg for oral administration.

Niacin injection. Niacin injection is available in 10-ml ampules containing 100 mg of the drug for parenteral use.

Niacinamide; nicotinamide. Official preparations of niacinamide include tablets of 25, 50, 100, and 500 mg and ampules containing a solution for injection. The concentration of the solution is 50, 100, or 200 mg/ml.

These vitamins are usually given orally but

they may also be given parenterally. The dose for the treatment of pellagra may be as much as 500 mg daily by mouth in divided doses or 100 to 200 mg by injection. The dose must be determined by the degree of deficiency.

Side effects and toxic effects. The administration of large doses of nicotine acid (especially when given intravenously) causes flushing of the face and neck, which may be associated with burning and pruritus. This does not occur after the administration of nicotinamide, which is therefore preferred for parenteral administration. In spite of this transient reaction, niacin is considered a nontoxic substance.

Pyridoxine hydrochloride (vitamin B_6)

Vitamin B_6 occurs as a group of chemically related compounds—pyridoxine, pyridoxal, and pyridoxamine. In the body tissues these compounds can be converted from one form to another. Pyridoxine is changed into pyridoxal, which seems to be especially active. Pyridoxal phosphate functions as a coenzyme and is involved in changing tryptophan to the nicotinamide portion of the pyridine coenzymes. It plays an important role in the metabolism of amino acids and fatty acids and is said to participate in energy transformation in the brain and nerve tissues. In large doses pyridoxine opposes the actions of levodopa by promoting its extracerebral decarboxylation.

Pork and glandular meats are said to be especially rich in the vitamin B_6 group of enzymes, although these substances are found in many different foods.

Although no specific deficiency disease has been recognized in humans, convulsive disorders have been observed in infants who were fed a diet deficient in vitamin B_6, and adults who have received a vitamin B_6 antagonist have developed seborrheic dermatitis, lesions on mucous membranes, and peripheral neuritis. Patients with an unusual type of hypochromic anemia have responded well to the administration of vitamin B_6.

Daily requirement. The daily recommended allowance of vitamin B_6 is from 0.3 to 0.4 mg for infants and from 0.6 to 1.6 mg for children ages 1 through 14. The requirement is 2 mg for adolescents and adults. An increase of 0.5 mg daily

is recommended during pregnancy and lactation.

Uses. Pyridoxine hydrochloride is used as an adjunct in the treatment of nausea and vomiting of pregnancy and irradiation sickness. Research evidence indicates that pyridoxine may block lactation by inhibition of breast milk secretion in nursing mothers. The mechanism for this has been postulated as pyridoxine suppression of the normally elevated prolactin hormone levels that stimulate milk production.

Isoniazid, an antituberculosis drug, acts as an antagonist of vitamin B_6, and when used over a period of time it may produce a vitamin deficiency unless additional amounts of vitamin B_6 are administered. This has also occurred with penicillamine.

Preparation, dosage, and administration. Official preparations are available in 5-, 10-, 25-, and 50-mg tablets for oral administration and in solution (concentrations varying from 50 to 100 mg/milliliter) for intramuscular or intravenous injection. The usual dosage is 5 mg daily, although as much as 25 to 100 mg has been administered. It is effective for treatment of pyridoxine deficiency.

Pantothenic acid

Pantothenic acid is widely distributed in nature. It is believed to be a constituent of coenzyme A, which plays an important role in the release of energy from carbohydratres, and in the release of energy from carbohydrates, and in the synthesis and degradation of fatty acids, sterols, and steroid hormones. Pantothenic acid is believed to be essential for human beings, although what constitutes the daily requirement is uncertain. An average American diet is said to provide 8.7 mg daily. It is known to prevent nutritional dermatosis in chicks and to promote normal growth in rats. Calcium pantothenate is available in 10- and 30-mg tablets. It is included in many multivitamin preparations. The usual dose is 10 mg.

Biotin

Biotin is a substance that plays a role in metabolism as a coenzyme with an important function in carbon dioxide fixation. Deficiency states have been reported in humans only when they are fed a diet containing a large amount of raw egg white. Avidine, a protein found in egg white, binds the biotin and prevents its absorption from the intestine. This results in the development of anorexia, malaise, and dermatitis. Daily administration of 150 to 300 µg will prevent the development of these symptoms in human beings. This amount is found in an average American diet.

Choline; inositol; para-aminobenzoic acid

Choline, inositol, and para-aminobenzoic acid have been included in the vitamin B complex, but their status is uncertain. Choline and inositol have been found to have a lipotropic (exhibiting an affinity for fat) effect. The lipotropic effect of choline was first noted in the liver, and this led to its use for the treatment of fatty infiltration of the liver and other disorders of fat metabolism. However, the evidence to support claims for clinical usefulness is questionable. Choline is a precursor of acetylcholine.

Vitamin B$_{12}$; folic acid

Vitamin B$_{12}$ and folic acid (pteroylglutamic acid) were discussed in Chapter 10.

ASCORBIC ACID (VITAMIN C)

Scurvy was formerly common among sailors deprived of fresh fruits and vegetables during long voyages. The well-known effects of lemon and orange juices in curing this disease led to attempts to concentrate the active principle by chemical means. Crystalline ascorbic acid in large amounts has been prepared from Hungarian red pepper. Biologic tests show that ascorbic acid is pure vitamin C, which is not synthesized on a commercial scale. Ascorbic acid is a powerful reducing agent and is therefore sensitive to oxidation. It is relatively stable in an acid medium but quickly oxidized in an alkaline medium. It is believed to be concerned in the oxidation-reduction reactions of living cells.

However, less is known about its function than is known about many of the other water-soluble vitamins already discussed. Ascorbic acid is concerned with the formation of collagen in all fibrous tissue, including bone, and with the development of teeth, blood vessels, and blood cells. It is also involved in carbohydrate metabolism. It is believed to stimulate the fibroblasts of connective tissue and thus promote tissue repair and the healing of wounds. It is said to help maintain the integrity of the intercellular substance in the walls of blood vessels, and the capillary fragility associated with scurvy is explained on this basis.

A deficiency in the intake of vitamin C results in scurvy, the chief symptoms of which are spongy, bleeding gums; loosened teeth; hemorrhagic tendencies in regions subjected to trauma or mechanical stress; sore, swollen joints; fatigue; pallor; and anemia. Vitamin C deficiency is thought to be a contributory factor in dental caries, pyorrhea, and certain oral infections.

Foods rich in vitamin C include citrus fruits (orange, lemons, limes, and grapefruit) as well as tomato juice, raw cabbage, broccoli, and strawberries.

Daily requirement. Vitamin C is constantly being destroyed in the body, probably through the process of oxidation. If deficiency is to be avoided, daily requirements must be met. The optimal daily intake of ascorbic acid for adults is 50 to 60 mg; for infants, 35 mg; and 45 mg for children. During pregnancy and lactation the requirement is 20 to 40 mg.

Uses. The specific use of vitamin C is in the prevention and treatment of scurvy and for the subclinical manifestations of this disease. An optimal amount of ascorbic acid should be supplied for individuals of all ages to prevent the development of scurvy. In the absence of vitamin C changes occur in the collagen of fibrous tissues, in the matrix of tooth substance (dentin), in bone and cartilage, and in the endothelium of blood vessels. Since vitamin C is not stored to any appreciable extent, deficiency can develop easily. Patients who do not eat well or who do not receive a diet adequate for their needs or those who must be fed intravenously for a long time may develop a deficiency unless they are given ascorbic acid as a dietary supplement. Vitamin C deficiency may result in delay in wound healing, or it may actually cause a breakdown in the healing process. Its prophylactic use to prevent colds is highly controversial.

The administration of vitamin C is not considered specific treatment for pyorrhea, dental caries, and certain gum infections, unless these symptoms are associated with vitamin C deficiency. In fact, bleeding gums are a rather common finding among otherwise healthy individuals. Vitamin C deficiency to the extent necessary to cause capillary bleeding is quite rare. It is therefore most unreasonable to treat bleeding gums with an increased and supernormal intake of ascorbic acid.

Nurses who instruct young parents should stress the importance of not heating orange juice or adding vitamins to formula before it is heated, because heat destroys the vitamin C.

Preparation, dosage, and administration. The following are available preparations.

Ascorbic acid. Ascorbic acid is available in 25-, 50-, 100-, 250-, and 500-mg tablets. A number of multiple-vitamin preparations also contain vitamin C.

Ascorbic acid injection. This is a preparation of ascorbic acid, 50 to 500 mg/ml, suited for parenteral administration.

Ascorbic acid may be given orally because it is well absorbed from the intestinal tract, or the injectable form may be given intramuscularly or added to intravenous fluids. The therapeutic dose for adults is 500 mg daily. High doses may cause diarrhea.

MULTIPLE-VITAMIN PREPARATIONS

The daily intake of principal vitamins recommended by the Food and Nutrition Board of the National Research Council (1980 revision) is as follows for adults who are normally vigorous and living in a temperate climate: vitamin A, 1000 units for men, 800 units for women; vitamin D, 400 units; thiamine (vitamin B_1), 1 to 1.5 mg; riboflavin, 1.2 to 1.7 mg; niacin, 13 to 19 mg; ascorbic acid (vitamin C), 50 to 60 mg.

Many of the multiple-vitamin preparations that have come into extensive use in recent years contain amounts of the aforementioned vitamins that bear no relation to established therapeutic dosage or to normal daily requirements. In addition, many such preparations contain purified vitamins that are not yet known to be represented by any known deficiency diseases.

Certain multiple-vitamin preparations not only have excessive amounts of each vitamin but also contain vitamins whose importance in human nutrition is open to question. The cost of "overstuffed" vitamin preparations is unnecessarily high. Vitamin requirements may be abnormally high, for a time in individuals who are acutely and severely ill, but that is another matter.

Decavitamin capsules, decavitamin tablets

Decavitamin capsules and tablets contain not less than 1.2 mg (4000 USP units) vitamin A, 10 μg (400 USP units) vitamin D, 70 mg ascorbic acid, 10 mg calcium pantothenate, 1 μg cyanocobalamin, 50 μg folic acid, 20 mg niacinamide, 2 mg pyridoxine hydrochloride, 2 mg riboflavin, and 2 mg thiamine hydrochloride. The usual daily dose is one capsule or one tablet. These preparations are the only official multiple-vitamin therapeutic drugs.

Minerals

Oral sources of minerals may be found commercially individually or combined within a multivitamin and mineral combination. The United States Recommended Daily Allowance (US RDA) for labeling purposes for adults of the following minerals is as follows: calcium, 800 to 1200 mg; phosphorus, 800 to 1200 mg; iodine, 150 μg; iron 10 to 18 mg; magnesium 300 to 400 mg; copper, 2 to 3 mg; and zinc, 15 mg. The amounts and the minerals vary with each commercially available product as do individual requirements.

Summary of nursing considerations

Depending on the amount of adipose tissue present, water makes up from 45% to 75% of the total body weight. Water is found in the fluid both inside and surrounding body cells. In this fluid metabolic exchanges between cells and tissues and the external environment occur. Precise regulation of volume and composition of body fluid is essential to health. Death usually occurs if 20% to 25% of body water is lost.

Water is a solvent that permits many substances to be dispersed through it. It has a high dielectric constant that permits ionization of electrolytes, cations, and anions important in maintaining body fluid volume and distribution. Water is also an excellent heat insulator and lubricant between membranes.

Abnormal states of hydration can be classified as (1) dehydration (volume depletion), (2) overhydration (hypervolemia or volume excess), (3) loss of water in excess of sodium (hypernatremia), and (4) loss of sodium in excess of water (hyponatremia). Sodium chloride and dextrose solutions are used as treatment for these conditions.

Intravenous solutions are used routinely before, during, and after surgery to supply electrolytes, nutrients, and water. Single salt solutions include ammonium chloride, calcium gluconate, potassium chloride, sodium bicarbonate, and sodium lactate. Table 22-1 indicates multiple salt solutions for intravenous administration. Parenteral nutrition is the intravenous feeding of protein hydrolysate, vitamins, trace elements, fat emulsion, amino acid solution, or high-calorie solutions to patients unable to eat, digest, or absorb nutrients for prolonged periods of time. Parenteral feeding is also used to provide nutritional support to help sustain life in malnourished and burned patients. Such intravenous feeding may cause adverse effects. The nurse should be alert and watch for the following possible complications of intravenous therapy: infiltration, extravasation, thrombosis, thrombophlebitis, pain at the administration site, necrosis, pulmonary edema, and pyrogenic reactions.

Potassium is the major cation in intracellular fluid. It plays an important part in muscle contraction, conduction of nerve impulses, enzyme action, and cell membrane function. Potassium deficit (hypokalemia) and potassium excess (hyperkalemia) affect these physiologic functions.

The electrolyte calcium is essential in maintaining much of the growth and ossification of bones and the function of cells, nerves, hormones, muscles, enzymes, and the cardiovascular system. A decrease in serum calcium (hypocalcemia) or an excess in serum calcium (hypercalcemia) affects these physiologic functions.

Magnesium is an important activator ion for the function of many enzymes. Magnesium has physiologic effects on the nervous system similar to those of calcium. A deficit in magnesium (hypomagnesemia) and an excess of magnesium (hypermagnesemia) affect these functions.

Vitamins are essential for maintenance of normal metabolic function, growth, and health. Vitamins are classified as being fat soluble or water soluble. Fat-soluble vitamins are A, D, E, and K. They are stored in the liver and fatty tissue in large amounts, and a deficiency in these vitamins occurs only after long deprivation from an adequate supply or from disorders preventing their absorption. Water-soluble vitamins include the B group and vitamin C. These vitamins are not stored in the body in large amounts, and short periods of inadequate intake can lead to a deficiency. Vitamins are important components of enzyme systems that catalyze the reactions for protein, fat, and carbohydrate metabolism.

QUESTIONS

FOR STUDY AND REVIEW

1 Discuss the importance of the following electrolytes:
   a sodium
   b potassium
   c calcium
   d magnesium
2 Select a clinical unit where intravenous solutions are being administered. Determine which solutions are being given, why, and how often. Are your findings congruent with medical literature recommendations? Explain.
3 Explain how the complications of intravenous therapy can be prevented or modified by the nurse.
4 Explain the difference between fat-soluble and water-soluble vitamins.
5 Interview 10 adults to determine whether or not they take vitamins on a daily basis, which vitamin preparations they use and why, and if the vitamins were prescribed. Analyze your findings.
6 Interview the parents of five nonrelated infants to determine if the infants receive vitamin preparations and why, the preparation(s) used and how they are administered, and cost and methods of storage. Compare your findings with those of your classmates. Analyze the overall findings.

7 What are the advantages and disadvantages of one-a-day multiple vitamin preparations?

8 What is parenteral nutrition? Why is a large vein selected for the administration of a hyperosmotic solution?

BIBLIOGRAPHY

GENERAL

AMA drug evaluations, ed. 4, New York, 1980, John Wiley & Sons, Inc.

Gahart, B.L.: Intravenous medications, ed. 3, St. Louis, 1980, The C.V. Mosby Co.

Goodman, L.S., and Gilman, A., editors: The pharmacological basis of therapeutics, ed. 6, New York, 1980, Macmillan, Inc.

Goth, A.: Medical pharmacology: principles and concepts, ed. 10, St. Louis, 1981, The C.V. Mosby Co.

Meyers, F.H., Jawetz, E., and Goldfien, A.: Review of medical pharmacology, ed. 4, Los Altos, Calif., 1974, Lange Medical Publications, Inc.

Modell, W., editor: Drugs of choice 1980-1981, St. Louis, 1980, The C.V. Mosby Co.

Moss, N.H., and Mayer, J., editors: Food and nutrition in health and disease, Ann. N.Y. Acad. Sci. **300:**1, 1977.

Osol, A., and Pratt, R.: The United States Dispensatory, ed. 27, Philadelphia, 1973, J.B. Lippincott Co.

Taylor, W.H.: Fluid therapy and disorders of electrolyte balance, ed. 2, London, 1974, Blackwell Scientific Publications, Ltd.

Turner, P., and Richens, A.: Clinical pharmacology, Edinburgh, 1973, Churchill Livingstone.

FLUIDS AND ELECTROLYTES

Conway, A., and Williams, T.: Parenteral alimentation, Am. J. Nurs. **76:**574, 1976.

Data, J.L., and Nies, A.S.: Dextran 40, Ann. Intern. Med. **81:**500, 1974.

Dudrick, S.J.: Rational intravenous therapy, Am. J. Hosp. Pharm. **28:**82, 1971.

Elbaum, N.: Detecting and correcting magnesium imbalance, Nursing '77 **7**(8):34, 1977.

Geyer, R.P.: Symposium: artificial blood, Fed. Proc. **34:**1429, 1975.

Gruber, U.F., editor: Shock, Triangle **13:**81, 1974.

Hall, R.C.W., and Joffe, J.R.: Hypomagnesemia; physical and psychiatric symptoms, J.A.M.A. **224:**1749, 1973.

Hutchin, P.: Metabolic response to surgery in relation to calorie, fluid and electrolyte intake, Curr. Probl. Surg., April 1971.

Inglott, A.S.: I.V. additive review. Part I. Drug Intell. Clin. Pharmacol. **6:**28, 1972.

Inglott, A.S.: I.V. additive review. Part II. Drug intell. Clin. Pharmacol. **6:**69, 1972.

Johnston, I.D.A., editor: Advances in parenteral nutrition, Lancaster, England, 1978, MTP Press.

Kee, J.L., and Gregory A.P.: The ABC's (and mEq's) of fluid balance in children, Nursing '74, **4:**(6):28, 1974.

Klotz R., and Sherman, J.O.: Preparation of hyperalimentation solutions for the pediatric patient, Am. J. Hosp. Pharm. **28:**102, 1971.

Kramer, W.: Precipitates found in admixtures of potassium chloride and dextrose 5% in water, Am. J. Hosp. Pharm. **27:**518, 1970.

Krumlovsky, F.A.: Hyponatremia, Ration. Drug Ther. **9:**1, 1975.

Kurdi, W.J.: Refining your I.V. therapy techniques, Nursing '75 **5**(11):41, 1975.

Lamb, J.: Intra-arterial monitoring: rescinding the risks, Nursing '77 **7**(11):65, 1977.

Moore, F.D., and Brennan, M.F.: Intravenous feeding, N. Engl. J. Med. **287:**862, 1972.

Moses, A: Diabetes insipidus and ADH regulation, Hosp. Pract., p. 37, July 1977.

Moses, A.M., and Miller. M.: Drug induced dilutional hyponatremia, N. Engl. J. Med. **291:**1234, 1974.

Newmark, S.R., and Forte, L.R.: Hyperkalemia and hypokalemia, J.A.M.A. **231:**631, 1975.

Rocchio, M.A., and others: Role of electrolyte solutions in treatment of hemorrhagic shock, Am. J. Surg. **125:**488, 1973.

Scarlato, M.: Blood transfusions today: what you should know and do, Nursing '78 **8**(2):68, 1978.

Share, L., and others: Regulation of body fluids, Annu. Rev. Physiol. **34:**235, 1972.

Shils, M.E.: Guidelines for total parenteral nutrition, J.A.M.A. **220:**1721, 1972.

Turco, S., and Davis, N.: Clinical significance of particulate matter: a review of the literature, Hosp. Pharmacol. **8:**137, 1970.

Turco, S., and Davis N.: Glass particles in intravenous injections, N. Engl. J. Med. **287:**1204, 1972.

Westphal, R.G.: Rational alternatives to the use of whole blood, Ann. Intern. Med. **76:**987, 1972.

NUTRIENTS

Anderson, T.W., and others: Winter illness and vitamin C: the effect of relatively low doses, Can. Med. Assoc. J. **112:**823, 1975.

Avioli, L.V., and Haddad, J.G.: Vitamin D: current concepts, Metabolism **22:**507, 1973.

Axelrod, A.E.: Immune processes in vitamin deficiency states, Am. J. Clin. Nutr. **24:**265, 1971.

Bollag, W.: Vitamin A and vitamin A acid in the prophylaxis and therapy of epithelial tumours, Int. J. Vitam. Nutr. Res. **40:**299, 1970.

Calcitriol, Med. Lett. Drugs Ther. **21:**50, 1979.

Coulehan, J.L., and others: Vitamin C prophylaxis in a boarding school, N. Engl. J. Med. **290:**6, 1974.

Deluca, H.F., and Suttie, J.W.: The fat-soluble vitamins, Madison, 1970, University of Wisconsin Press.

Dykes, M.H.M., and Meir, P.: Ascorbic acid and the common cold: evaluation of its efficacy and toxicity, J.A.M.A. **231:**1073, 1975.

Frennd, H.R., Ryan, J.A., and Fischer, J.E.: Amino acid derangements in patients with sepsis, Ann. Surg., p. 423, Sept. 1978.

Greentree, L.B.: Dangers of vitamin B_6 in nursing mothers, N. Engl. J. Med. **300:**141, 1979.

Katsikas, J.L., and others: Disorders of potassium metabolism, Med. Clin. North Am. **55:**503, 1971.

Laflamme, G.H., and Jowsey, J.: Bone and soft tissue changes with oral phosphate supplements, J. Clin. Invest. **51:**2834, 1972.

Muenter, M.D., and others: Chronic vitamin A intoxication in adults, Am. J. Med. **50:**129, 1971.

Olson, R.E.: The mode of action of vitamin K, Nutr. Rev. **28:**171, 1970.

Owens, J.A.: Focus on calcitriol, Hosp. Form. **14**(10):882, 1979.

Pace, H.B., and Barnes, B.A.: Vitamins. In Griffenhagen, G.B., and Hawkins, L.L., editors: Handbook of non-prescription drugs, Washington, 1973, American Pharmaceutical Association.

Raisz, L.G.: A confusion of vitamin D's, N. Engl. J. Med. **287**:926, 1972.

Recker, and others: Efficacy of calcifediol in renal osteodystrophy, Arch. Intern. Med. **138**:857, 1978.

Ritchie, J.H., and others: Edema and hemolytic anaemia in premature infants: a vitamin E deficiency syndrome, N. Engl. J. Med. **279**:1185, 1968.

Rivlin, R.S.: Riboflavin metabolism, N. Engl. J. Med. **283**:463, 1970.

Roels, O.A.: Vitamin A physiology, J.A.M.A. **214**:1097, 1970.

Rosenberg, L.E.: Vitamin-dependent genetic disease, Hosp. Pract. **5**:59, 1970.

Rovner, D.R.: Use of pharmacologic agents in the treatment of hypokalemia and hyperkalemia, Ration. Drug Ther. **6**:1, 1972.

Rutherford, W.E., and others: Effect of 25-hydroxycalciferol on calcium absorption in chronic renal disease, Kidney Int. **8**:320, 1975.

Schwartz, P.L.: Ascorbic acid in wound healing—a review, J. Am. Diet. Assoc. **56**:497, 1970.

Wecksler, W.R., Mason, R.S., and Norman, A.W.: Specific cytosol receptors for 1,25-dihydroxy vitamin D_3 in human intestine, J. Clin. Endocrinol. Metab. **48**:715, 1979.

Wilson, C.W.M.: Colds, ascorbic acid metabolism, and vitamin C, J. Clin. Pharmacol. **15**:570, 1975.

Wilson, C.W.M., and Loh, H.S.: Vitamin C metabolism and the common cold, Eur. J. Clin. Pharmacol. **7**:421, 1974.

UNIT SEVEN

DRUGS USED IN INFECTIOUS DISEASES

CHAPTER 23

Antimicrobial agents

KAY SEE-LASLEY

Infectious diseases include a wide spectrum of illnesses caused by pathogenic microorganisms. Some common pathogens and their most likely sites of infection in the body are listed in Table 23-1. A few of the disease states that these pathogens cause are pneumonias, urinary tract infections, upper respiratory infections, venereal disease, vaginitis, tuberculosis, and candidiasis.

Microorganisms are divided into several groups: bacteria, mycoplasmas, spirochetes, fungi, and viruses. Bacteria are classified according to shape and capacity to be stained. Gram's stain is the most well-known staining method. It is a sequential procedure that involves crystal violet and iodine solutions, followed by alcohol.

Antimicrobial therapy

The approach to the treatment of an infectious disease caused by a microorganism depends on the group to which the microorganism belongs; different groups of antimicrobial

TABLE 23-1 Primary organisms causing infectious diseases, and their common sites of infection

Organism	Infection site
Gram-positive cocci	
Staphylococcus aureus	Burns, skin infections, decubitus and surgical wounds, paranasal and middle ear (chronic sinusitis and otitis), lungs, lung abscess, pleura, endocardium, bone (osteomyelitis), and joints
Non-penicillinase-producing	
Penicillinase-producing	
Streptococcus pneumoniae	Paranasal and middle ear, lungs, pleura
Streptococcus pyogenes (group A β-hemolytic)	Burns, skin infections, decubitus and surgical wounds, paranasal and middle ear, throat, bone (osteomyelitis), and joints
Streptococcus, viridans group	Endocardium
Gram-positive bacilli	
Clostridium tetani	Puncture wounds, lacerations, and crush injuries; toxins affect nervous system
Corynebacterium diphtheriae	Throat, upper part of the respiratory tract
Gram-negative cocci	
Neisseria gonorrhoeae	Urethra, prostate, epididymis and testes, joints
Neisseria meningitidis	Meninges
Enteric gram-negative bacilli	
As a group (*Bacteroides, Enterobacter, Escherichia coli, Klebsiella pneumoniae, Proteus mirabilis, other Proteus, Salmonella, Serratia, Shigella*)	Peritoneum, biliary tract, kidney and bladder, prostate, decubitus and surgical wounds, bone
Bacteroides	Brain abscess, lung abscess, throat, peritoneum
Enterobacter	Peritoneum, biliary tract, kidney and bladder, endocardium
Escherichia coli	Peritoneum, biliary tract, kidney and bladder
Klebsiella pneumoniae	Lungs, lung abscess
Other gram-negative bacilli	
Haemophilus influenzae	Meninges, paranasal and middle ear, lungs, pleura
Pseudomonas aeruginosa	Burns, paranasal and middle ear (chronic otitis media), decubitus and surgical wounds, lungs, joints
Acid-fast bacilli	
Mycobacterium tuberculosis	Lungs, pleura, peritoneum, meninges, kidney and bladder, testes, bone, joints
Mycoplasmas	
Mycoplasma pneumoniae	Lungs
Spirochetes	
Treponema pallidum (syphilis)	Any tissue or vascular organ of the body
Fungi	
Aspergillus	Paranasal and middle ear, lungs
Candida species	Skin infections, throat, lungs, endocardium, kidney and bladder, vagina
Viruses	
Herpes virus or varicella-zoster virus	Skin infections (herpes simplex or zoster)
Enterovirus, mumps virus, and others	Meninges, epididymis, and testes
Respiratory viruses (including Epstein-Barr virus)	Throat, lungs

agents are used for treating different groups of microorganisms. Table 23-2 lists a few of the antimicrobial agents of choice in the treatment of diseases caused by various microorganisms.

Antimicrobial agents have made it possible to cure or control most infections caused by microorganisms. But this has not always been true. The first major group of antimicrobial agents were limited to antibiotics. They were substances derived from certain organisms used against infections caused by other organisms. As a result of research, there are now many synthetic and semisynthetic antibiotics, and antimicrobial agents now include not only antibiotics but also the sulfonamides, urinary tract antiseptics, and antimycobacterial, antifungal, and antiviral agents. In this chapter, these drugs' common characteristics and distinct differences will be discussed.

TABLE 23-2 **Antimicrobial drugs of choice**

Organism	Drug
Gram-positive cocci	
Staphylococcus aureus	
Non-penicillinase-producing	Penicillin G or V
Penicillinase-producing	Cloxacillin or dicloxacillin
Resistant infections	Methicillin, nafcillin, or oxacillin
Streptococcus pneumoniae	Penicillin G or V
Streptococcus pyogenes	Penicillin G or V
(group A β-hemolytic)	
Streptococcus viridans group	Penicillin G with or without streptomycin
Gram-positive bacilli	
Clostridium tetani	Penicillin G
Corynebacterium diphtheriae	An erythromycin
Gram-negative cocci	
Neisseria gonorrhoeae	Tetracycline, penicillin G or amoxicillin
Neisseria meningitidis	Penicillin G
Enteric gram-negative bacilli	
Bacteroides	Penicillin G
	Clindamycin
Enterobacter	Gentamicin or tobramycin
Escherichia coli	Gentamicin or tobramycin
Urinary tract infections	Sulfisoxazole, ampicillin, or amoxicillin
Klebsiella pneumoniae	Gentamicin or tobramycin
Proteus mirabilis	Ampicillin
Other *Proteus*	Gentamicin or tobramycin
Other gram-negative bacilli	
Haemophilis influenzae	Chloramphenicol, ampicillin, or amoxicillin
Pseudomonas aeruginosa	
Urinary tract infections	Carbenicillin or ticarcillin
Other infections	Tobramycin or gentamicin with carbenicillin or ticarcillin
Acid-fast bacilli	
Mycobacterium tuberculosis	Isoniazid with ethambutol, with or without rifampin
Mycoplasmas	
Mycoplasma pneumoniae	An erythromycin or a tetracycline
Spirochetes	
Treponema pallidum (syphilis)	Penicillin G
Fungi	
Aspergillus, Candida species	Amphotericin B
Viruses	
Herpes simplex	Vidarabine

Mechanisms of action

The goal of antimicrobial therapy is to destroy or to suppress the growth of infecting microorganisms so that normal host defense mechanisms can gain control of the infection, resulting in its cure. In order to exert their effects, antimicrobial agents must first gain access to target sites. Usually this can be accomplished by absorption of the drug into and distribution via the circulatory system. Sometimes, as in the case of infections of the skin and eyes, local application to the infected area may be necessary. Once the drug has reached its site of action, it can have bacterio-static or bactericidal effects, depending on its mechanism of action (see Table 23-3).

Bacteriostatic agents inhibit bacterial growth, allowing host defense mechanisms additional time to remove the invading microorganisms. *Bactericidal agents*, on the other hand, cause bacterial cell death and lysis, superimposing the killing effect of the drug on the effects of host defenses. Antimicrobial agents may be divided into bacteriostatic and bactericidal categories, with the sulfonamides as an example of the former and the penicillins exemplifying the latter. Such categorization is not always valid or reliable, however, since the

TABLE 23-3   Classification of antimicrobial agents by mechanism of action

Inhibit cell wall synthesis
  Penicillins
  Cephalosporins
  Vancomycin
  Bacitracin
  Cycloserine
  Ristocetin
Alter membrane permeability
  Amphotericin B
  Nystatin
  Polymyxin
  Colistin
Inhibit protein synthesis
  Impede replication of genetic information
    Nalidixic acid
    Griseofulvin
    Novobiocin
    Rifampin
    Pyrimethamine
  Impair translation of genetic information
    Chloramphenicol
    Tetracycline
    Erythromycin
    Aminoglycosides
    Lincomycins
Antimetabolites
  Sulfonamides
  Sulfones
  PAS
  INH
  Ethambutol

Adapted from Kagan, B. M., editor: Antimicrobial therapy, ed. 2, Philadelphia, 1980, W. B. Saunders Co.

TABLE 23-4   Summary of some major allergic and toxic effects of antimicrobial agents

Penicillin	Anaphylaxis
Chloramphenicol (low incidence but high mortality) Sulfonamides (low incidence)	Hematologic effects
Polymyxins Aminoglycosides Sulfonamides (low incidence with newer drugs)	Nephrotoxicity
Polymyxins Aminoglycosides	Potential for neuro-muscular block-ade
Aminoglycosides	Injury to eighth cranial nerve

abolic substrates. Agents causing these effects can be either bacteriostatic or bactericidal.

3 Inhibition of protein synthesis. Antimicrobial agents may induce the formation of defective protein molecules; such agents are bactericidal in their action. Antimicrobial agents that inhibit specific steps in protein synthesis are bacteriostatic.

4 Inhibition of synthesis of essential metabolites. Antimicrobial agents that work in this manner structurally resemble physiologic compounds and act as competitive inhibitors in a metabolic sequence. With the exception of isoniazid, they are bacteriostatic.

General adverse reactions to antimicrobial agents

While the development of antimicrobial agents represents one of the most important advances in drug therapy, these drugs are not free of adverse and toxic effects. The list of side effects and toxic effects of each specific drug group is long and varied. Table 23-4 presents some of the major allergic and toxic effects of a few antimicrobial agents. All antimicrobial agents, however, are capable of producing three general types of adverse reactions of which the nurse must be aware.

1. Allergic or hypersensitivity reactions. Allergic or hypersensitivity reactions occur in response to all presently available antimicrobial agents. Allergic reactions may range from mild responses, such as rash, fever, or urticaria with pruritus, to the extreme of anaphylactic shock, simultaneously or in some sequence.

same antimicrobial agent may have either effect depending on the dose administered and the concentration achieved at its site of action. Tetracycline, for example, is generally bacteriostatic but may be bactericidal in high concentrations.

Antimicrobial agents may exert their bacteriostatic or bactericidal effects in one of four major ways:

1 Inhibition of cell wall synthesis in bacteria. Unlike host cells, bacteria are not isotonic with body fluids. Their contents are under high osmotic pressure and their viability depends on the integrity of the cell walls. Any compound that inhibits any step in the synthesis of this cell wall causes it to be weakened and the cell to lyse. Antimicrobial agents having this mechanism of action are bactericidal.

2 Disruption or alteration of membrane permeability, resulting in leakage of essential bacterial met-

When untoward effects are more severe than a rash, therapy with the drug is usually discontinued. Allergic reactions have become more of a serious problem in antimicrobial therapy because sensitization to antimicrobial agents may occur in a patient without any history of previous administration of the drug in question. Sensitization has been known to occur through exposure to a drug that is not obvious, such as drinking milk from cows treated for mastitis with penicillin.

Treatment of allergic reactions includes the use of antihistamines and epinephrine, which serve to block or to counteract the effects of the vasoactive mediators of allergy, and the use of corticosteroids, which may reduce tissue injury and edema in the inflammatory response.

2. Resistance. Resistance is defined as the ability of a microorganism previously sensitive to an antimicrobial agent to withstand the effects of that drug. Resistance can develop either gradually or suddenly in response to high drug concentrations. Bacterial resistance is suspected when the infectious process becomes less responsive and/or the patient's condition regresses. Bacterial resistance is generally the result of genetic events leading to the development of mutants of the microorganism that are drug resistant and that proliferate in the presence of the drug, becoming the predominant bacterial form. Mutants resist the activity of an antimicrobial agent by (1) elaboration of specific inactivating enzymes, (2) restriction of uptake of the drug, or (3) alteration or elimination of binding of the drug to its target site. As a rule, microorganisms resistant to a certain drug will tend to be resistant to all other chemically related antimicrobial agents, a phenomenon known as *cross-resistance*. For example, bacteria unresponsive to tetracycline will also be resistant to oxytetracycline and chlortetracycline.

3. Superinfection. Superinfection may occur when the normal microbial flora of the body is disturbed, thereby allowing entry to an organism that normally would be unable to penetrate. Superinfection may be defined as the appearance of bacteriologic and clinical evidence of a new infection during the chemotherapy for a primary one. It is relatively common and potentially very dangerous because the microorganisms responsible for the new disease are often *Proteus* strains, drug-resistant staphylococci, *Pseudomonas*, *Candida*, or the true fungi, any of which may be very difficult to eradicate with presently available antimicrobial agents. The proper management of superinfections includes (1) discontinuation of the drug being given, (2) culture of the suspected infected area, and (3) administration of an antimicrobial agent effective against the new offending organism.

General principles

Several important principles guide the judicious and optimal use of the antimicrobial agents. Causes of adverse reactions to antimicrobial agents and of therapeutic failures are often related to lack of adherence to the following principles of antimicrobial therapy.

IDENTIFICATION OF INFECTING ORGANISM

Because most antimicrobial agents have a specific effect on a very limited range of types of microorganisms, the physician must attempt to formulate a specific diagnosis about the organism most likely to be causing a given infectious process. The drug most likely to be specifically toxic against the suspected microorganism can then be selected. This objective is most validly and reliably accomplished by obtaining specimens from the infected area if possible (for example, urine, sputum, wound drainage) or by obtaining venous blood specimens and sending them to the laboratory for culture and identification of the causative organism. The recovery of a specific microorganism from appropriate specimens is always a significant factor in the determination of antimicrobial therapy. When a significant microorganism has been isolated, laboratory tests for antimicrobial susceptibility (sensitivity) to various antimicrobial agents are often also requested.

It is always desirable to receive culture and sensitivity reports before initiating antimicrobial therapy. In some situations, however, it is not practical to await these laboratory results. For example, antimicrobial therapy must be initiated without delay in acute, life-threatening situations such as peritonitis, septicemia, or pneumonia. In such situations, the choice of antimicrobial agent for initial use must be based on tentative identification of the pathogen. It is known, for example, that microorganisms commonly isolated in acute adult infections of the lung include pneumococci, streptococci, and staphylococci. Antimicrobial agents specifically toxic to those organisms may be administered temporarily. The drugs can then be changed, if necessary, after laboratory reports have been received. When even tentative identification is difficult, *broad-spectrum* antibiotics, which are effective against a wide range of microorganisms, can be prescribed or several antimicrobial agents may be prescribed for simultaneous administration.

It must be noted here that some infections are most effectively treated with the use of only one antibiotic. In other situations, such as the one described above, *combined antimicrobial drug therapy* may be indicated. Other indications for the simultaneous use of two or more antimicrobial agents include (1) treatment of mixed infections, in which each drug may act on a separate portion of a complex microbial flora; (2) need to delay the rapid emergence of bacteria resistant to one drug; and (3) need to reduce the incidence or intensity of adverse effects by decreasing the dose of a potentially toxic drug. Indiscriminate use of combined antimicrobial drug therapy should be avoided because of expense, toxicity, and higher incidence of superinfections and resistance.

ASSESSMENT OF HOST DEFENSE MECHANISMS

No antimicrobial agent will effect the cure of an infectious process if host defense mechanisms are inadequate. Such drugs act only on the causative organisms of infectious disease and have no effect on the defense mechanisms of the body, which need to be assessed and supported. Many infections do not require drug therapy and are adequately combatted by individual defense mechanisms such as antibody production, phagocytosis, interferon production, fibrosis, or gastrointestinal rejection (vomiting, diarrhea). However, host defense

mechanisms may be diminished, as, for example, in diabetes mellitus, neoplastic disease, and immunologic suppression. The therapeutic problem may be complicated, requiring therapy for preexisting disease conditions as well as supportive care in adequate oxygenation, fluid and electrolyte balance, and so on, before antimicrobial therapy can be optimally effective. In some situations surgical intervention is also necessary. In general, in the presence of a substantial amount of pus, necrotic tissue, or a foreign body, the most effective treatment is a combination of an antimicrobial agent plus an appropriate surgical procedure.

The status of the host's defense mechanisms will also influence choice of therapy, route of administration, and dosage. If an infection is fulminating, for example, parenteral (preferably intravenous) administration of a bactericidal drug will be selected rather than oral administration of a bacteriostatic drug. Large "loading" doses of antimicrobial agents are often administered at the beginning of treatment of severe infections, to achieve maximum blood concentrations rapidly. However, factors influencing drug dosage are also related to the status of a patient's renal function. Because many antimicrobial agents are metabolized and/or excreted by the kidneys, a major management problem exists in regard to patients with compromised renal function. Drug doses are then generally reduced in parallel with the patient's creatinine clearance levels. Hemodialysis may further alter the therapeutic regimen.

In short, the administration of an antimicrobial agent specifically toxic to the isolated microorganism is not the only important measure in antimicrobial therapy. An additional and very important determinant of the effectiveness of an antimicrobial agent is the functional state of the host's defense mechanisms.

PROPER DOSAGE AND DURATION OF THERAPY

Administering antimicrobial drugs in adequate dosage and for long enough periods of time is an important principle of infectious disease therapy. Failures in antimicrobial therapy are not infrequently the result of drug doses being too small or being given for too short a period of time. Generally, antimicrobial therapy should not be discontinued until the patient has been afebrile and clinically well for 48 to 72 hours. Follow-up cultures should be obtained to assess the effectiveness of therapy. Discontinuing treatment as soon as the patient is asymptomatic usually promotes development of resistance and/or results in a disease process characterized by repeated remissions and exacerbations.

Antimicrobial agents currently being used will be discussed as chemically related groups of drugs, in order to help the nurse or the nursing student think of them in an organized manner. The nurse should be familiar with the general characteristics of each drug group or category and with one or two prototype drugs in each group.

Antibiotics

Antibiotics used primarily against gram-positive bacteria

PENICILLINS

The penicillins are antibiotics derived from a number of strains of *Penicillium notatum* and *P. chrysogenum*, common molds often seen on bread or fruit (see Fig. 23-1). Introduced into clinical practice in 1941, the penicillins constitute a large group of antimicrobial agents that remain the most effective and least toxic of all available antimicrobial drugs. Table 23-5 lists the penicillins used in current therapeutic practice and their routes of administration. Penicillins encompass true antibiotics as well as many newer, semisynthetic compounds that share a common chemical nucleus and a common mechanism of action.

Action and results. The penicillins specifically inhibit synthesis of bacterial cell walls, probably by interfering with the biosynthesis of mucopeptides and preventing linkage of structural components of the cell wall. They are bactericidal for a wide variety of gram-positive and some gram-negative organisms. Bacterial species considered highly susceptible to the penicillins include *Diplococcus pneumoniae*, group A β-hemolytic streptococci, *Neisseria meningitidis*, *N. gonorrhoeae*, non-penicillinase-produc-

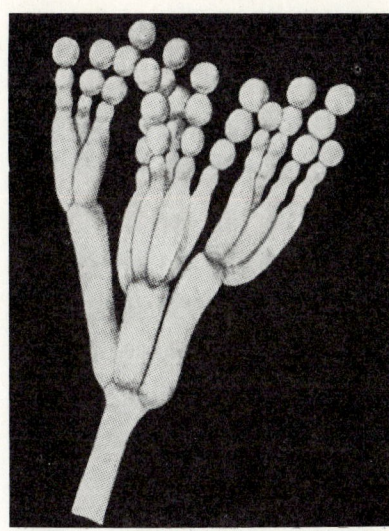

FIG. 23-1. Typical penicillus of *Penicillium notatum;* Fleming's strain. (From Raper, K.B., and Alexander, D.F.: J. Elisha Mitchell Sc. Soc. **61**:74, 1945.)

ing *Staphylococcus aureus, Clostridium tetani, Clostridium perfringens, Corynebacterium diphtheriae, Actinomyces,* and *Treponema pallidum* and other spirochetes. Most penicillins are much more active against gram-positive than gram-negative bacteria. There are exceptions, however. Gram-negative gonococci, for example, are penicillin susceptible.

Pharmacokinetics. Absorption of the penicillins after oral administration is incomplete, being limited by gastric acidity and binding to food. The penicillins are completely and rapidly absorbed after parenteral administration and achieve wide distribution throughout the body. They do not readily enter cerebrospinal fluid when meninges are normal, but do achieve therapeutically effective levels in cerebrospinal fluid when meninges are inflamed. The penicillins cross the placenta. They are excreted primarily by the kidneys, although some excretion occurs into sputum and milk. Their renal excretion is rapid but can be therapeutically delayed by concurrent administration of probenecid (Benemid), which partially blocks tubular transport of penicillin, resulting in higher and more prolonged blood levels.

Uses. The penicillins remain by far the most effective and most widely used antibiotics. Their clinical effectiveness encompasses the

TABLE 23-5   Penicillins

Generic and brand names	Route
Penicillin G and closely related compounds	
Benzathine penicillin G (Bicillin)	Oral, intramuscular
Penicillin G potassium (various)	Oral, intramuscular, intravenous
Penicillin G sodium (various)	Intramuscular, intravenous
Procaine penicillin G (Wycillin, various)	Intramuscular
Penicillin V (V-Cillin)	Oral
Potassium penicillin V (Pen-Vee-K, V-Cillin K, various)	Oral
Semisynthetic penicillins (penicillinase resistant)	
Cloxacillin sodium (Tegopen, Cloxapen)	Oral
Dicloxacillin sodium (Pathocil, Dynapen, various)	Oral
Methicillin sodium (Staphcillin, Celbenin, Azapen)	Intramuscular, intravenous
Nafcillin sodium (Nafcil, Unipen)	Oral, intramuscular, intravenous
Oxacillin sodium (Prostaphlin, Bactocill)	Oral, intramuscular, intravenous
Semisynthetic penicillins (not penicillinase resistant)	
Amoxicillin trihydrate (Amoxil, various)	Oral
Ampicillin anhydrous or trihydrate (Amcill, Omnipen, Polycillin, various)	Oral
Ampicillin sodium (Amcill-S, Omnipen-N, various)	Intramuscular, intravenous
Bacampicillin hydrochloride (Spectrobid)	
Carbenicillin disodium (Geopen, Pyopen)	Intramuscular, intravenous
Carbenicillin indanyl sodium (Geocillin)	Oral
Cyclacillin (Cyclapen)	Oral
Hetacillin (Versapen)	Oral
Hetacillin potassium (Versapen-K)	Oral
Ticarcillin (Ticar)	Intramuscular, intravenous

treatment of pneumococcal pneumonia; streptococcal infections such as pharyngitis, tonsillitis, scarlet fever, otitis media, rheumatic fever, and bacterial endocarditis; meningococcal meningitis, gonorrhea, syphilis, and salmonella infections. The penicillins are not useful in the presence of bacteria producing enzymes capable of destroying penicillins, such as penicillin-ase-producing *S. aureus*, *E. coli*, indole-positive *Proteus*, or *P. aeruginosa*. However, semisynthetic penicillins that are not destroyed by penicillinase have been introduced.

Studies of the prophylactic use of penicillin have shown it to be of value in (1) treatment of persons exposed to group A *Streptococcus pyogenes*, (2) prevention of rheumatic fever recurrences, (3) prevention of gonorrhea and syphilis, and (4) prevention of subacute bacterial endocarditis in patients with valvular heart disease who must undergo surgical or dental procedures.

Side effects and toxic effects. The penicillins are virtually nontoxic for mammalian cells, and their use has been attended only by minor cases of skin rashes, mild gastrointestinal disturbances, and local irritation following parenteral administration. It must be noted, however, that all penicillins have potential central nervous system toxicity and are capable of producing CNS excitation and convulsions when administered in very high doses, especially to patients with preexisting renal disease.

There is some evidence that the semisynthetic penicillins may have inherent toxicity not found in the parent compound, benzylpenicillin.

Despite their unquestioned value, the penicillins have three distinct disadvantages that are not direct toxic effects: (1) they are readily destroyed by gastric acid, rendering their oral absorption unpredictable; (2) they are rendered inactive by penicillinase,* making them useless against microorganisms that elaborate this substance; (3) their use is characterized by a relatively high incidence of allergic reactions; and (4) they have a somewhat "limited" antibacterial spectrum, especially in relation to gram-negative bacteria.

Allergic reactions to penicillin, which are thought to be the most common type of drug allergy, are a significant problem. Acute anaphylactic reactions constitute the most important immediate danger associated with the use

---

*Penicillinase is an enzyme secreted by a number of bacteria; it hydrolyzes a portion of the penicillin molecule and produces a derivative (penicilloic acid) that is inactive against bacteria. Penicillinase is believed to have little or no antigenic or allergenic activity.

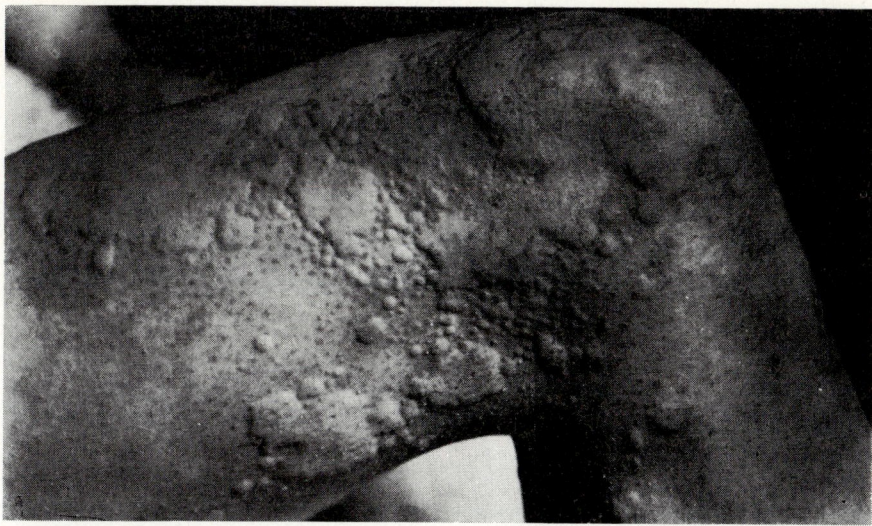

FIG. 23-2. Urticaria such as may be seen in patients who are sensitive to penicillin.

of penicillin. Among all the antimicrobial drugs, the penicillins are most often responsible for anaphylaxis. In more mild allergic reactions to penicillin, skin rashes, contact dermatitis (especially among physicians, nurses, and pharmacists), oral lesions, fever, and eosinophilia have been observed. (See Chapter 15.)

Semisynthetic penicillin derivatives have been produced in an attempt to overcome these serious disadvantages. Consequently, many preparations of natural penicillins and semisynthetic penicillins are available. The various preparations of penicillins are obtained by chemical or biologic modification of the 6-aminopenicillanic acid nucleus. The semisynthetic preparations are characterized by increased stability in gastric acid, increased penicillinase resistance, or extended bacterial spectrum properties. Only the most widely used preparations will be discussed.

PENICILLIN G AND CLOSELY RELATED COMPOUNDS

Penicillin G potassium; benzylpenicillin. This is one of the most potent of all antimicrobial agents on a weight-for-weight basis and is the prototype form of all penicillins. It is unpredictably absorbed from the gastrointestinal tract; therefore, the dose administered must be from three to five times that which would be given parenterally. It is available in tablets and liquid form in doses ranging from 50,000 to 500,000 units and as aqueous penicillin G for parenteral administration by means of subcutaneous, intramuscular, intravenous, or intrathecal injection.

Penicillin G procaine. This form of penicillin G can be given only by the intramuscular route. It has the advantage of slow absorption with prolonged effectiveness; it needs to be administered only every 12 hours. Blood levels of the drug are somewhat lower than those obtained following intramuscular injection of aqueous penicillin. The usual adult dose is 300,000 units every 12 to 24 hours.

Penicillin G benzathine (Bicillin). This is the longest lasting form of penicillin. Oral tablets contain 200,000 units. A single injection of 1.2 million units is absorbed so slowly that it can provide therapeutic effects for as long as 1 month. Disadvantages of this drug form include very low blood levels of the drug, local pain attendant to the injection, and risk of severe and sometimes prolonged allergic reactions.

Penicillin V potassium; phenoxymethylpenicillin. The antibacterial spectrum of this semisynthetic penicillin is identical to that of penicillin G. Its advantage is that it is both insoluble and stable at a low pH, escaping destruction in gastric juice. It is available for oral use in tablet and liquid forms. It is more expensive and less active against some bacteria than penicillin G. The usual adult dose is 250 mg every 6 hours.

SEMISYNTHETIC PENICILLINS

Penicillinase resistant. An increasing number of penicillin cogeners have been developed that resist hydrolysis by penicillinase and, by virtue of their resistance to this enzyme, exert remarkable antistaphylococcal activity.

Methicillin sodium (Staphcillin, Celbenin). Since this drug is inactivated by gastric acid, it must be administered parenterally. It is more expensive than penicillin G but has the advantage of having bactericidal activity against nearly all strains of *S. aureus,* including penicillinase-producing strains. It is not as effective as penicillin G against other gram-positive organisms. It has been recommended that its use be reserved for treatment of patients hospitalized with severe staphylococcal infections. The usual adult dose is 1 g every 4 to 6 hours intramuscularly or 1 g every 6 hours intravenously.

Acid and penicillinase resistant. Acid and penicillinase resistant semisynthetic penicillins possess greater stability in gastric acid as well as resistance to penicillinase.

Oxacillin sodium (Prostaphlin). Oxacillin is stable in acid media as well as resistant to destruction by penicillinase. Its advantages over methicillin include oral administration and greater effectiveness against gram-positive organisms other than staphylococci. The usual adult dose is 500 mg every 6 hours.

Cloxacillin sodium (Tegopen). This analog of oxacillin is identical in its pharmacologic and therapeutic properties to the parent compound. Its advantages over oxacillin are said to be more uniform gastrointestinal absorption, achievement of higher blood levels, and more sustained action. The usual adult dose is 250 to 500 mg every 6 hours.

Dicloxacillin sodium (Dynapen). Dicloxacillin is appreciably more active against penicillinase-producing *S. aureus* than either oxacillin or cloxacillin. Well absorbed from the gastrointestinal tract, dicloxacillin is available for oral use in capsule and suspension form. The usual adult dose is 250 mg every 6 hours.

Nafcillin sodium (Unipen). Nafcillin is highly resistant to penicillinase and is more effective than methicillin against penicillin G–resistant *S. aureus.* It is inactivated to a variable degree in gastric acids, and its absorption after oral administration is somewhat irregular. It is available for oral and parenteral use; the usual adult dose is 250 mg to 1 g every 6 hours.

Non-penicillinase-resistant (broad-spectrum).

Ampicillin (Omnipen, Polycillin). Ampicillin differs from other semisynthetic penicillins because of its broad-spectrum antimicrobial effects. It was the first of the semisynthetic penicillins to provide increased activity against some of the gram-negative bacilli, including *H. influenzae, Salmonella, Shigella, E. coli,* and *P. mirabilis.* Ampicillin is not penicillinase resistant. It is available in both oral and parenteral forms. The average dose for infections caused by gram-negative organisms in adults is 2 to 4 g daily, given in divided doses. Ampicillin has been popular in pediatric practice, especially in the treatment of otitis media and meningitis.

Bacampicillin hydrochloride (Spectrobid). A new oral semisynthetic penicillin, this drug has the same bacterial spectrum and side effects as ampicillin. It is more completely and rapidly absorbed than ampicillin. After absorption it is metabolized into its parent compound, ampicillin, with peak serum levels being three times that of ampicillin alone. Its tissue and body serum levels are also higher. Therefore frequency of administration can be limited to twice a day. The usual dose of bacampicillin is 400 to 800 mg every 12 hours. It is available in 400-mg tablets.

Hetacillin (Versapen). Hetacillin is metabolized in the body into ampicillin and acetone. It has no antibacterial activity itself and, of course, has the same antibacterial spectrum as ampicillin. It has no advantages over ampicillin.

Amoxicillin. Amoxicillin is also a congener of ampicillin. It produces consistently higher blood levels of antibiotic than do comparable doses of ampicillin, probably because of better gastrointestinal absorption. The usual adult dose is 125 to 250 mg every 6 hours.

Cyclacillin (Cyclapen). Cyclacillin has less in vitro activity than the other broad-spectrum penicillins, but studies show that is is effective for the recommended indications for this group. Its use against *E. coli* and *P. mirabilis,* however, is restricted to urinary tract infections (unlike ampicillin, hetacillin, and amoxicillin). It also cannot be used effectively in *N. gonorrhoeae* or *N. meningitidis* infections. Cyclacillin is given orally, usually in doses of 250 to 500 mg four times daily.

Carbenicillin. Carbenicillin has attracted attention because of its bactericidal activity against a number of gram-negative bacteria, especially *P. aeruginosa* and some strains of *Proteus* resistant to ampicillin. It is less active than penicillin G and ampicillin against gram-positive organisms and less active than ampicillin against many of the gram-negative bacilli. Since carbenicillin is not absorbed from the gastrointestinal tract, it must be administered parenterally. Its major use is to treat urinary tract infections. The usual adult dose is 200 mg/kg/day given in divided doses.

Ticarcillin (Ticar). Ticarcillin is closely related to carbenicillin and has a similar antibacterial spectrum except that it is more active in vitro against *E. coli, Klebsiella, Enterobacter, Proteus,* and *P. aeruginosa.* It is also active against *Bacteroides fragilis.* Ticarcillin can be given only parenterally; the usual dose is 200 to 300 mg/kg/day.

CEPHALOSPORINS

The cephalosporin antimicrobial agents, which were introduced in the early 1960s, are a group of semisynthetic derivatives of cephalosporin C, an antibiotic produced by the fungus *Cephalosporium acremonium.* (Table 23-6 lists the cephalosporins currently being used in clinical practice.) This group of antimicrobial drugs is similar in many ways to the penicillins: (1) they have similar, but not identical, chemical structures; (2) they have the same mechanism of action; and (3) they exhibit a similar bacterial spectrum. Their advantage over the penicillins lies in the fact that they are resistant to hydrolysis by the penicillinases. It has also been claimed that the cephalosporins can be

TABLE 23-6 Cephalosporins

Parenteral
 Cefamandole (Mandol): intramuscular, intravenous
 Cefazolin (Ancef, Kefzol): intramuscular, intravenous
 Cefotaxime (Claforan): intramuscular, intravenous
 Cefoxitin (Mefoxin): intramuscular, intravenous
 Cephacetrile (Celospor): intramuscular, intravenous
 Cephaloridine (Loridine): intramuscular, intravenous
 Cephalothin (Keflin): intramuscular, intravenous
 Cephapirin (Cefadyl): intramuscular, intravenous
Oral and parenteral
 Cephradine (Anspor, Velosef): Oral, intramuscular, intravenous
Oral
 Cefadroxil (Duricef)
 Cephalexin (Keflex)
 Cephaloglycin (Kafocin)

administered to persons allergic to penicillin without fear of reaction. At present, however, this claim is controversial, and it is not clear whether the cephalosporins have cross-sensitivity with the penicillins.

There appears to be no universally agreed upon, single, firm indication for the use of cephalosporins. They are effective in numerous situations, but in no case are they the outstanding drug of choice at present. Diseases produced by *S. aureus,* group A *S. pyogenes,* some non–group A streptococci, *Diplococcus pneumoniae,* and *Clostridium welchii* respond very favorably to proper doses of these agents. Infections caused by a number of gram-negative bacilli, such as *E. coli, Klebsiella,* and *Proteus,* also respond to cephalosporins. The new cephalosporins—cefamandole, cephamycin, and cefoxitin—are also active against *Enterobacter* species and indole-positive *Proteus* species.

Side effects and toxic effects. Toxic reactions to the cephalosporins include the development of a positive Coombs test when large doses are administered, reversible renal tubular necrosis, and pain and sterile abscesses at injection sites. Diarrhea and eosinophilia have been observed after the oral administration of cephaloglycin and cephalexin.

PARENTERAL CEPHALOSPORINS

Cephalothin sodium (Keflin). Cephalothin is not absorbed after oral administration and therefore must be given parenterally. It is usually injected intravenously, after being dissolved in 25 to 50 ml of 5% dextrose in water, and administered over a 30-minute period. Usual adult doses range between 4 and 12 g/day. Because of its rapid excretion, necessitating repeated doses at 4- to 6-hour intervals, and the necessity for parenteral administration, cephalothin is used mainly in the treatment of hospitalized patients.

Cephaloridine (Loridine). Cephaloridine, like cephalothin, is not well absorbed from the gastrointestinal tract and must be administered parenterally. It appears to be more soluble and less irritating than cephalothin, rendering it more appropriate for intramuscular injection. It differs from other members of the penicillin-cephalosporin family because of its potential to cause serious nephrotoxicity. The usual adult dose is 0.5 to 1 g three times daily. When larger doses are necessary, cephalothin is preferred in order to avoid nephrotoxicity.

Cephapirin (Cefadyl). Cephapirin's bacterial spectrum is identical to cephalothin's. Cephapirin is equal to cephalothin in effectiveness; when a decision is made about which to use, the cost of the antibiotic determines the choice. Cephapirin's usual dose is 500 mg to 1 g every 4 to 6 hours.

Cephacetrile (Celospor). Like cephapirin, cephacetrile's properties are the same as cephalothin's. Cephacetrile likewise is chosen based on its cost in comparison to cephalothin's. The usual dose of cephacetrile is 500 mg to 1 g every 4 to 6 hours.

Cefazolin (Ancef, Kefzol). Cefazolin is more active against *E. coli* and less active against staphylococci than cephalothin. It is often chosen over cephalothin because of its longer half-life and because it causes less pain during intramuscular injection. Its dosage ranges from 250 to 500 mg every 8 hours (for mild infections) to 6 to 8 g daily (for life-threatening infections).

Cefamandole (Mandol). Cefamandole is effective against a broader spectrum of gram-negative bacilli, such as *Enterobacter* and indole-positive *Proteus* organisms, than cephalothin, but it is less active against staphylococci and streptococci than cephalothin. Cefamandole is also less painful at the injection site when given intramuscularly. Because of its high cost, it is usually reserved for the treatment of cephalothin-resistant gram-negative bacilli. Its usual dose is 500 mg to 1 g every 4 to 8 hours. In life-threatening infections, up to 2 g may be given every 4 hours.

Cefotaxime sodium (Claforan). This new cephalosporin causes greater inhibition of cell wall synthesis of bacteria than does penicillin or other cephalosporins. It is stable in the presence of beta-lactamases, penicillinases, and cephalosporinases of both gram-negative and gram-positive bacteria. Cefotaxime has a broad spectrum of activity; it is effective against most gram-positive and gram-negative bacteria as well as some anaerobes. Its usual dose is 1 g every 6 to 8 hours, given intramuscularly or intravenously. Cefotaxime is available in vials and infusion bottles in strengths of 500 mg, 1 g, and 2 g.

Cefoxitin (Mefoxin). Cefoxitin is a beta-lactam antibiotic that is closely related to cephalosporins; it is classified as a cephamycin. Its bacterial spectrum is similar to that of cefamandole. Cefoxitin too is reserved for the treatment of infections caused by cephalothin-resistant gram-negative bacilli. Its usual dose is 1 g every 6 to 8 hours.

ORAL CEPHALOSPORINS

Cephalexin (Keflex). Cephalexin is well absorbed from the gastrointestinal tract. It appears to be somewhat less active than the parent compound, cephalothin. Cephalexin is useful in the treatment of urinary tract infections that are resistant to other antibiotics. The usual adult dose is 1 to 4 g daily in divided doses.

Cephaloglycin (Kafocin). Cephaloglycin is poorly absorbed orally and cannot be used for systemic infections. Its use is limited. Cephaloglycin has largely been replaced by other oral cephalosporins.

Cefadroxil (Duricef). Cefadroxil is similar to cephalexin in its activity and pharmacologically, except that it has a longer half-life. It is commonly given in doses of 500 mg to 1 g every 12 hours.

Cefaclor (Ceclor). Cefaclor is more active than most cephalosporins against *H. influenzae*, including ampicillin-resistant strains. It has a broader spectrum than the other oral cephalosporins. Cefaclor is well absorbed. The commonly given dose is 250 mg every 8 hours.

ORAL AND PARENTERAL CEPHALOSPORIN

Cephradine (Anspor, Velosef). Cephradine is the only cephalosporin that can be given by the oral route and the parenteral route. It is clinically and pharmacologically equivalent to cephalexin. Parenteral administration consists of 2 to 4 g daily in divided doses, with a maximum of 8 g. The usual oral dose is 250 to 500 mg every 6 hours or 500 mg to 1 g every 12 hours.

NURSING IMPLICATIONS SPECIFIC TO PENICILLINS AND CEPHALOSPORINS

In addition to performing nursing measures common to all types of antimicrobial drug therapy, the nurse must be especially cognizant of several factors when penicillins or cephalosporins are prescribed.

Because allergic reactions are a significant problem in the use of penicillins, the nurse must meticulously assess the patient's previous drug experiences. For infants less than 3 months old, a history of penicillin allergy in the mother should be sought. If at all possible, no penicillin preparation of any kind should be prescribed for or administered to a patient with a history of allergic reaction to the drug. Because of possible cross-sensitization, it also seems wise to avoid the use of cephalosporins in patients with severe or immediate allergic reactions to penicillins.

In administering penicillins, the nurse should remember that oral penicillins are bound to food and that they are poorly absorbed in acid media. Their administration, therefore, should not be preceded or followed by food for at least 1 hour, in order to minimize binding. It is also recommended that penicillins not be taken with acidic fruit juices, because they may facilitate decomposition of penicillins.

In administering penicillins intravenously, the nurse should note that most penicillins in clinical use are sodium or potassium salts. Significant amounts of cation can be administered when these drugs are given intravenously in

T A B L E 2 3 - 7 Macrolide and lincosamide antibiotics

Generic and brand names	Route
Macrolides	
Erythromycin (E-Mycin, Ilotycin, various)	Oral
Erythromycin estolate (Ilosone)	Oral
Erythromycin ethylsuccinate (EES, various)	Oral
Erythromycin glucept ate (Ilotycin Glucept ate)	Intravenous
Erythromycin lactobionate (Erythrocin Lactobionate, IV)	Intravenous
Erythromycin stearate (Erythrocin Stearate)	Oral
Troleandomycin (TAO)	Oral
Lincosamides	
Clindamycin hydrochloride (Cleocin)	Oral
Clindamycin palmitate hydrochloride (Cleocin)	Oral (pediatric)
Clindamycin phosphate (cleosin)	Intramuscular, intravenous
Lincomycin (Lincocin)	Oral, intramuscular, intravenous

massive dosage. For example, 20 million units of potassium penicillin G contains 33 mEq of potassium ion. Fatalities have occurred because of the toxic effect of potassium on the heart following administration of such large doses in the presence of renal insufficiency. Signs and symptoms of hyperkalemia and hypernatremia should be duly noted and reported.

MACROLIDES, LINCOSAMIDES, AND VANCOMYCIN
MACROLIDES

The macrolide antibiotics constitute a large group of substances that were introduced in the early 1950s. They are bacteriostatic, since they inhibit protein synthesis, but in high concentrations they may also be bactericidal. The macrolides are effective against gram-positive cocci, especially pneumococci, streptococci, and staphylococci. *Corynebacteria*, *Neisseria*, *Haemophilus*, and *Mycoplasma* are also susceptible to the macrolides.

Table 23-7 summarizes the drugs in this group and their routes of administration. The most important of the macrolide antimicrobial drugs is erythromycin. One other that is available for clinical use is troleandomycin.

Erythromycin (Ilotycin, Erythrocin); erythromycin estolate (Ilosone); erythromycin stearate (Erythrocin); erythromycin lactobionate

Erythromycin is an antibiotic obtained from *Streptomyces erythreus.*

Pharmacokinetics. Erythromycin is readily absorbed from the gastrointestinal tract. Because it has a bitter taste and is destroyed by gastric acid, it is administered in enteric-coated tablets or in the form of insoluble preparations that are slowly hydrolyzed. Erythromycin diffuses through most of the body but is not found in appreciable amounts in the cerebrospinal fluid. It passes from the maternal blood to the fetus in amounts sufficient to be antibacterial. It is concentrated in the liver and excreted in the bile and urine.

Uses. Erythromycin is probably the drug of choice in some *Corynebacteria* infections, such as erythrasma and diptheria, and in disease caused by *Mycoplasma pneumoniae.* The effectiveness of erythromycin in the treatment of infections caused by group A beta-hemolytic streptococci also has been firmly established. Otherwise, erythromycin is most useful as a penicillin substitute in persons allergic to penicillin. Unfortunately, staphylococci develop resistance to erythromycin rapidly, and penicillin-resistant strains also are often erythromycin resistant.

Side effects and toxic effects. Erythromycin administration is accompanied by relatively few adverse reactions. The most frequently encountered adverse effect is gastrointestinal disturbance with nausea, vomiting, and diarrhea. Allergic reactions may occur. Hepatotoxicity resulting in cholestatic hepatitis has occurred with erythromycin estolate and with troleandomycin.

Preparations. Erythromycin is available for oral, topical, intramuscular, and intravenous use in a wide variety of commercial preparations. The usual adult dose of any of the forms of erythromycin is 250 to 500 mg every 6 hours.

Troleandomycin (TAO). Troleandomycin has been shown to be effective against much the same spectrum of organisms as erythromycin. Troleandomycin is a derivative of oleandomycin; it differs from the parent compound in that it is more active after oral administration because of better absorption from the gastrointestinal tract. Adverse reactions to troleandomycin include hepatic changes. The most common adverse reactions are hypersensitivity and gastrointestinal upset. In clinical practice, troleandomycin has limited usefulness. Indications for its use are essentially the same as for erythromycin, and it seems to offer no special advantages. Usual adult doses range from 250 to 500 mg, given four times daily.

LINCOSAMIDES
Lincomycin hydrochloride (Lincocin); clindamycin hydrochloride (Cleocin)

Lincomycin, an antibiotic produced by *Streptomyces lincolnensis,* was made available in the early 1960s. Primarily bacteriostatic, it exerts its action by inhibiting protein synthesis in sensitive bacteria. Its antibacterial spectrum and pharmacologic properties are similar to those of erythromycin, but its chemical structure is different. The antibacterial spectrum of this drug includes most gram-positive cocci.

Clindamycin, a derivative of lincomycin, offers the advantage of more complete and predictable absorption from the gastrointestinal tract, and it is said to cause diarrhea less frequently.

Lincomycin has been used successfully in the treatment of a variety of ear, nose, throat, respiratory, dental, skin and soft tissue, bone and joint, and septicemic infections caused by streptococci, staphylococci, and pneumococci. It is useful primarily as an alternative antibiotic to the penicillins and cephalosporins.

Lincomycin produces few adverse effects, with diarrhea appearing to be the most frequent after oral administration. Severe hemorrhagic colitis has occurred following the use of clindamycin. Allergy is not common. Superinfections in the intestinal tract may occur. Cardiopulmonary arrest after rapid intravenous injection has been reported.

The recommended adult oral dose of lincomycin is 500 mg every 6 or 8 hours. Lincomycin may also be administered intramuscularly or intravenously. Clindamycin is available for oral administration; recommended dosage is 0.15 to 0.3 g every 6 hours.

• • •

Vancomycin hydrochloride (Vancocin)

Vancomycin, discovered in 1956, is produced by *Streptomyces orientalis*. It is not related to any other antimicrobial agent, and its exact structural formula is not known. Vancomycin is bacteridal for many gram-positive bacteria because it inhibits bacterial cell wall synthesis. It is not absorbed from the gastrointestinal tract; it must be administered intravenously, because intramuscular injection is painful. Vancomycin is widely distributed in the tissues, and it is excreted primarily through the kidneys. If renal function is impaired, vancomycin may accumulate, with increased risk of toxicity.

The drug possesses significant ototoxicity and nephrotoxicity and may also produce allergic reactions. It is highly irritating to tissues and may result in pain and thrombophlebitis after intravenous injection. Because other, less toxic drugs are available, the principal clinical indication for the use of vancomycin is serious gram-positive infection in which other drugs cannot be given. Vancomycin can be very useful in the treatment of serious staphylococcal infection or enterococcal endocarditis not responding to other treatment. For staphylococcal enterocolitis, 3 to 4 g is administered orally daily. For staphylococcal septicemia, 0.5 g is injected intravenously over a period of 20 to 30 minutes every 6 to 8 hours in adults.

Antibiotics used against both gram-positive and gram-negative bacteria

AMINOGLYCOSIDES

The aminoglycosides are a group of drugs sharing chemical, antimicrobial, pharmacologic, and toxic characteristics. The drugs presently included in this category are streptomycin, kanamycin, gentamicin, neomycin, paromomycin, tobramycin, and amikacin. Table 23-8

TABLE 23-8 Aminoglycosides

Generic and brand names	Route
Amikacin sulfate (Amikin)	Intramuscular, intravenous
Gentamicin sulfate (Garamycin)	Intramuscular, intravenous
Kanamycin sulfate (Kantrex)	Oral, intramuscular, intravenous
Neomycin sulfate (Mycifradin Sulfate, Myciguent, Neobiotic)	Topical, oral, intramuscular
Paromomycin sulfate (Humatin)	Oral
Streptomycin sulfate	Intramuscular
Tobramycin sulfate (Nebcin)	Intramuscular, intravenous

shows their normal routes of administration. These drugs are especially alike in mechanism of action, metabolism, and toxicity. They differ in clinical uses.

Action and results. The aminoglycosides act on the bacterial ribosome to induce specific misreading of the genetic code. By virtue of irreversible inhibition of protein synthesis, they are bactericidal against a wide range of gram-positive and gram-negative species and mycobacteria. Their widespread clinical use has resulted in some resistant strains, and these drugs manifest a high degree of cross-resistance.

Pharmacokinetics. The aminoglycosides are generally poorly absorbed after oral administration, but they are well absorbed following intramuscular injection. They are moderately well distributed except for the central nervous system. They do cross the placenta. Excretion is primarily by glomerular filtration. In the presence of renal damage, cumulation of the aminoglycosides to toxic levels can occur.

Side effects and toxic effects. Aminoglycosides can cause varying degrees of ototoxicity and nephrotoxicity. They all damage both the vestibular and the auditory branches of the eighth cranial nerve, resulting in deafness, vertigo, and loss of balance. Vestibular damage may be partially reversed after the drugs are discontinued, but auditory damage is often permanent and may progress even after discontinuation of the drug. Ototoxicity is more frequent in older patients and in patients with renal failure.

The nephrotoxicity of the aminoglycosides varies in degree according to the particular drug used. Neomycin is the most toxic; kanamycin is intermediate; streptomycin and gentamicin are generally mild. Nephrotoxicity is usually manifested by proteinuria and nonprotein nitrogen retention. Because of this nephrotoxic tendency, these drugs are not administered in combination and, if administered to patients with renal insufficiency, only in greatly modified doses.

Neuromuscular blockade leading to respiratory arrest has been observed with use of high doses of aminoglycosides. It is particularly likely to occur in the presence of renal failure; when these drugs are used concurrently with neuromuscular blocking agents or anesthetic agents, such as ether, tubocurarine, succinylcholine, and decamethonium; when the drugs are administered to patients with myasthenia gravis; or when the drugs are rapidly injected intravenously or applied directly to serosal surfaces. The process can be reversed with neostigmine or with calcium gluconate. Peripheral neuritis and allergic reactions are less common but do occur.

Streptomycin sulfate

The isolation of streptomycin from *Streptomyces griseus* was reported in 1944. It was the first agent to be useful against a broad spectrum of gram-negative bacteria and mycobacteria, and it revolutionized the treatment of tuberculosis. Because of the rapid emergence of resistant bacterial strains, the use of streptomycin alone is rarely indicated. The majority of strains of certain gram-negative pathogens, such as *Proteus vulgaris*, *Pseudomonas aeruginosa*, and *Aerobacter aerogenes*, now being isolated in infections are streptomycin resistant. In addition, many organisms, with the exception of the tubercle bacillus, that are sensitive to streptomycin are also sensitive to the tetracyclines. The latter are safer to use, and organisms usually do not acquire resistance to the tetracyclines as rapidly as they do to streptomycin. Therefore, many authorities recommend that streptomycin be limited to the treatment of tuberculosis and to infections in which the

bacteria are resistant to other, safer antibiotics but susceptible to streptomycin.

In the treatment of tuberculosis, streptomycin is used in combination with other tuberculostatic drugs such as para-aminosalicylic acid (PAS), isoniazid (INH), ethambutol, or rifampin. It is believed best not to give streptomycin and isoniazid together except in extreme need, so that resistance to both drugs will not develop at the same time, depriving the patient of the two most powerful antituberculosis drugs. To prevent toxicity during treatment of tuberculosis, the dosage of streptomycin is carefully regulated. The dosage schedule is adjusted according to the severity of the disease and the other drugs given.

One other important use of streptomycin has been as an adjunct to penicillin G in the treatment of subacute bacterial endocarditis caused by *Streptococcus faecalis*. Tularemia and plague are among the few diseases for which the drug may be used alone with a high degree of specificity and effectiveness. Generally, the need for streptomycin in the therapy for other nontuberculous infections has decreased as other, less toxic drugs have emerged, but for systemic infections streptomycin may be given in doses of 0.5 to 1.0 g two to four times daily.

Although streptomycin is usually administered by intermittent, deep intramuscular injection, it can be administered intravenously, and the intrathecal route may be used in patients with meningitis caused by organisms susceptible to streptomycin. Intramuscular administration of streptomycin commonly produces pain at the site of injection and may produce sterile abscesses.

Neomycin sulfate (Myciguent)

Neomycin is obtained from *Streptomyces fradiae*. It is severely toxic and rarely used parenterally. It has been used widely for topical treatment of skin infections, including burns, wounds, ulcers, and infected dermatoses, in the form of 0.5% ointment or solution. Oral administration of neomycin has been used in preoperative preparation of the bowel and in the treatment of hepatic coma—for reducing intestinal flora and subsequently decreasing blood ammonia levels. In the treatment of hepatic coma, 4 to 8 g can be administered daily in divided doses. When used as a bowel preparatory agent, neomycin in doses of 1 g every 4 to 6 hours is combined with a low-residue diet and cleansing enemas for 2 or 3 days preoperatively. Following oral administration, intestinal malabsorption with a sprue-like syndrome may occur. Absorption of neomycin into the bloodstream may be facilitated in the presence of impaired gastrointestinal motility or mucosal ulceration, and prolonged topical application of the drug has also resulted in toxic effects.

Paromomycin sulfate (Humatin)

Paromomycin has been used in place of neomycin to reduce bacterial flora for preoperative preparation of the bowel and in the treatment of hepatic coma to control the nitrogen-fixing bacteria in patients with elevated blood ammonia levels. It has also been effective in the treatment of bacillary dysentery. Paromomycin is available in 250-mg capsules and as a pediatric syrup.

Kanamycin sulfate (Kantrex)

Kanamycin, an antibiotic derived from *Streptomyces kanamyceticus*, was first isolated in 1957. It resembles neomycin and paromomycin but is slightly less toxic than neomycin. It is of greatest usefulness in the treatment of systemic infections caused by gram-negative bacilli, except for *Salmonella typhosa* and *Pseudomonas*. It has been used in "sterilization" of the bowel prior to surgery. Like other aminoglycosides, kanamycin is quite toxic and it should not be used for treatment of infections known to be sensitive to less toxic drugs. Because of its toxicity, it has been largely replaced by gentamicin.

Gentamicin sulfate (Garamycin)

Gentamicin, which is derived from *Micromonospora purpura*, was introduced in the early 1960s. It possesses rapid bactericidal activity for many gram-positive and gram-negative bacteria.

Gentamicin has been very effective in the treatment of bacteremia resulting from species

of *Klebsiella*, *Enterobacter*, *E. coli*, and *Serratia*, and it has been found to be of great clinical usefulness in the treatment of infections caused by *Proteus* species and by *Pseudomonas*. In these severe infections, gentamicin is employed in doses of 2 to 3 mg/kg/day intramuscularly in divided doses for 7 to 10 days. While it is effective against penicillin-resistant staphylococci, the semisynthetic penicillins and the cephalosporins are less toxic and remain the drugs of choice for these organisms. Gentamicin is available for intramuscular injection or as a cream, an ointment, or a solution containing 0.1 to 0.3% gentamicin sulfate for treatment of infected burns, wounds, or skin lesions.

Tobramycin (Nebcin)

Tobramycin is similar to gentamicin in bacterial spectrum and pharmacology but appears to have a more marked activity against *Pseudomonas aeruginosa* and less activity against *Serratia marcescens*. Tobramycin is usually reserved to treat gentamicin-resistant organisms. It may have a use in long-term treatments, since it has less renal toxicity than gentamicin. It is administered in the same doses as gentamicin.

Amikacin (Amikin)

Amikacin is a semisynthetic derivative of kanamycin. Its bacterial spectrum, which is broader than that of kanamycin, includes *P. aeruginosa* and many gentamicin-resistant gram-negative bacilli. Like tobramycin, amikacin is reserved for the treatment of gentamicin-resistant infections. Its usual administration in severe infections consists of 15 mg/kg/day in three divided doses given intramuscularly or intravenously.

NURSING IMPLICATIONS

Because the aminoglycosides characteristically exhibit toxicity, the nurse should make the following assessments of patients receiving these drugs:

1 Observe carefully for beginning signs and symptoms of toxicity to the eighth cranial nerve, such as tinnitus, vertigo, hearing loss, and ataxia.
2 Observe carefully for beginning signs and symptoms of nephrotoxicity. Intake and output should

be monitored, and periodic urinalysis and renal function tests (for example, creatinine clearance) may be necessary in long-term treatment.

3 Be alert to the neuromuscular blocking potential of the aminoglycosides, especially when these drugs are used in any of the following ways:

   a. Administered concurrently with other neuromuscular blocking agents, such as muscle relaxants or sedatives

   b. Administered to patients with myasthenia gravis

   c. Injected rapidly into the venous system

   d. Applied to serosal surfaces

4 The toxic potential of the aminoglycosides is greater in the presence of renal impairment, prematurity, old age, or dehydration, or when they are used simultaneously with potent diuretics. Patients to whom any of these citeria apply should be observed carefully.

TETRACYCLINES

The tetracyclines, introduced in 1948, were the first truly broad-spectrum antibiotics (Fig. 22-3). They include a large group of drugs with a common basic structure and chemical activity. Table 23-9 lists those currently being used in clinical practice.

Action and results. The most important mechanism of action of the tetracyclines is their blocking of the binding of the transfer RNA–amino acid complex to the ribosome. Thus no amino acid is available to the messenger RNA to produce polypeptides; therefore,

TABLE 23-9 **Tetracyclines**

Generic and brand names	Route
Chlortetracycline hydrochloride (Aureomycin)	Oral, intramuscular, intravenous, topical
Demeclocycline hydrochloride (Declomycin)	Oral
Doxycycline hyclate (Vibramycin, Vibramycin IV, various)	Oral, intravenous
Methacycline hydrochloride (Rondomycin)	Oral
Minocycline hydrochloride (Minocin, Minocin IV)	Oral, intravenous
Oxytetracycline (Terramycin, Terramycin IM, Terramycin IV, various)	Oral, intramuscular, intravenous
Tetracycline hydrochloride (Achromycin V, Achromycin IM, Achromycin IV, various)	Oral, intramuscular, intravenous, topical
Tetracycline phosphate complex (Tetrex)	Oral

protein synthesis is prevented. The tetracyclines are bacteriostatic for many gram-negative and gram-positive organisms, including anaerobes, and they strongly inhibit the growth of mycobacteria, rickettsiae, mycoplasmas, agents of the psittacosis–lymphogranuloma venereum–trachoma group, and some protozoa. *Proteus* and *Pseudomonas* are generally resistant. Complete cross-sensitivity and cross-resistance among all tetracyclines is the rule.

Pharmacokinetics. The tetracyclines are readily but incompletely absorbed from the gastrointestinal tract. Their absorption is inhibited by food, milk, and milk products and by concurrent administration of antacids with aluminum, magnesium, or calcium bases. The tetracyclines are well distributed throughout the body with the exception of cerebrospinal fluid. They diffuse into brain, saliva, synovial tissues, placenta, and fetal tissues. They are readily bound to calcium deposited in newly formed bone and to certain malignant tissues. Because of their binding to newly formed bone and teeth in the fetus, these drugs should not be administered during pregnancy. Also, the binding of the drug during calcification of bones and teeth in small children can lead to tooth discoloration, enamel dysplasia, and bone deformity. The drug is excreted in both urine and feces and also appear in the milk of lactating patients. Patients with impaired renal function require dose reduction in order to avoid serious side effects.

Uses. Because of their broad spectrum, tetracyclines are most valuable in the treatment of mixed infections, such as chronic bronchitis and peritonitis. They are drugs of choice, however, for only a few bacterial infections: cholera, granuloma inguinale, chancroid infection, and gastrointestinal infection with *Bacteroides*. Tetracyclines are the best drugs for treatment of rickettsial disease such as Rocky Mountain spotted fever, Q fever, and typhus, and they are also effective in the treatment of psittacosis, lymphogranuloma venereum, trachoma, and inclusion conjunctivitis. Long-term therapy with the tetracyclines have been effective in decreasing the severity and frequency of febrile episodes in chronic bronchitis and bronchiectasis and in the treatment of acne vulgaris. For acne vulgaris, tetracyclines are used in low doses daily for periods of months to years. They act by excretion into the sebum, resulting in the reduction of the number and frequency of skin lesions.

Side effects and toxic effects. The tetracyclines are relatively nontoxic, the most common side effects being gastrointestinal disturbances, which are manifested as epigastric burning, nausea, vomiting, and diarrhea. Allergic reactions may be manifested as rash, urticaria, anaphylaxis, angioneurotic edema, or simulated lupus erythematosus, but they are relatively rare. Phototoxicity may occur with the administration of demeclocycline. Large doses of these drugs (more than 2 g/day parenterally) may produce liver damage. Administration during pregnancy and in children under age 7 may produce discoloration of teeth and depression of bone growth. Superimposed infections, especially caused by *Monilia* and staphylococci, represent a serious hazard to patients receiving long-term therapy. The tetracyclines are also irritative when given intravenously; they can cause thrombophlebitis.

Preparations, dosage, and administration. The tetracycline family is represented by so many dosage forms for each member that a detailed description is not possible here. In general, when a tetracycline is indicated, an oral preparation should be used. Parenteral tetracyclines are available but should be used only for initial treatment of severe infections. Besides these major dosage forms, there are ophthalmic and otic solutions and ointments, powders, tablets, troches, vaginal tablets, and dental paste.

The tetracyclines may vary somewhat in the intensity of their action on different strains of bacteria, as well as in frequency of dose, absorption, and rate of excretion. Aside from these variations, the tetracycline preparations do not differ significantly in clinical effectiveness.

Chlortetracycline and oxytetracycline were the first drugs of this class to be introduced. Newer drugs, such as demeclocycline, doxycycline, and minocycline, produce longer-lasting antimicrobial activity and can be administered in lower and less frequent doses.

Tetracycline hydrochloride (Achromycin, Panmycin, Tetracin). This drug is primarily excreted by the kidneys. The usual adult dose is 250 mg every 6 hours.

Chlortetracycline hydrochloride (Aureomycin). The usual adult dose is 250 mg every 6 hours.

Oxytetracycline hydrochloride (Terramycin). The usual adult dose is 250 mg every 6 hours.

Demeclocycline (Declomycin). The antibacterial potency of this drug is about twice that of the other tetracyclines. It produces blood levels of drug that are higher and more sustained than equal doses of the preceding tetracyclines. The usual adult dose is 100 to 300 mg every 6 to 12 hours. This drug demonstrates a phototoxic effect that is much less common with other tetracyclines.

Doxycycline (Vibramycin). Doxycycline is better absorbed than other tetracyclines when administered orally, and blood levels are sustained longer. This drug is excreted by the kidneys much less than are other tetracyclines; therefore doxycycline should be the drug of choice when it is necessary to administer a tetracycline to a patient with renal insufficiency. The usual adult dose is 50 to 100 mg every 12 to 24 hours.

Minocycline (Minocin). Minocycline, like doxycycline, is a long-lasting tetracycline. This drug is also excreted by the kidneys much less than other tetracyclines. The usual adult dosage is 50 to 100 mg every 12 hours.

Methacycline (Rondomycin). Methacycline is an analog of oxytetracycline. It has a prolonged half-life (15 hours) and is less likely to cause photosensitivity than other tetracyclines. Administration consists of 600 mg daily in two or four divided doses.

NURSING IMPLICATIONS

In addition to nursing measures common to all types of antimicrobial drug therapy, the nurse should observe the following measures when patients are receiving drugs of the tetracycline family:

1 The tetracyclines should not be administered with milk, milk products, antacids, or iron preparations, because they combine with metal ions to form nonabsorbable compounds.

2 Gastrointestinal side effects may be controlled by concurrent administration of food (not milk products).

3 The tetracyclines should not be administered to pregnant women or to children under age 7, because they can delay bone growth and produce discoloration of teeth.

4 Because the potential for superinfections is greater in tetracycline therapy than in therapy with other antimicrobial agents, patients should be observed carefully for signs and symptoms of secondary infections, especially monilial infections. Meticulous oral and perineal hygiene is helpful in preventing monilial superinfections.

5 Tetracyclines decompose with age, exposure to light, and when stored in extreme heat and humidity. Because the resulting products may be toxic, the nurse should store (or instruct the patient to store) these drugs properly. Manufacturers' expiration dates on tetracycline containers should be duly noted and outdated drugs discarded.

6 Patients receiving tetracyclines should be instructed to avoid intense exposure to sunlight or to artificial ultraviolet light.

7 Tetracyclines will delay blood coagulation.

CHLORAMPHENICOL
Chloramphenicol (Chloromycetin)

The antimicrobial agent chloramphenicol was derived from *Streptomyces venezuelae* in 1947. A potent inhibitor of protein synthesis, this drug is bacteriostatic for a wide variety of gram-negative and gram-positive organisms as well as rickettsiae.

Pharmacokinetics. Chloramphenicol is readily absorbed from the gastrointestinal tract. It is widely distributed throughout the body, diffusing into cerebrospinal fluid and passing the placental barrier. It is bound to plasma albumin and rapidly excreted by the liver and kidneys.

Uses. Because of its broad spectrum and apparent lack of toxicity, chloramphenicol was widely used between 1948 and 1951, before its serious toxicity was documented. In spite of its significant therapeutic effectiveness, controversy now exists regarding the use of chloramphenicol, because of its infrequent but severe hematologic side effects. It is now possibly the drug of choice for only a few types of infections: (1) typhoid fever and other salmonelloses, (2) occasional bacteremia caused by gram-negative bacteria expected to be resistant to other drugs, and (3) severe rickettsial infections. The drug should be used primarily for hospitalized patients, and therapy must be stopped at the first sign of adverse reaction.

Side effects and toxic effects. The most important toxic effect of chloramphenicol is the occurrence of blood dyscrasias, most notably bone marrow depression, anemia, and leukopenia. Aplastic anemia that may be irreversible and fatal has been known to occur with the use of this drug. Frequent periodic blood counts must be performed during chloramphenicol therapy, and the drug must be discontinued if agranulocytosis, leukopenia, or thrombocytopenia appear. In newborn infants, chloramphenicol toxicity may be manifest as the "gray baby" syndrome. This often fatal syndrome consists of vasomotor collapse, hypothermia, rapid and irregular respirations, diarrhea, and an ashen gray color. Other toxic effects include gastrointestinal disturbances and optic neuritis.

Preparation and dosage. Chloramphenicol may be administered orally, intramuscularly, intravenously, as an ophthalmic ointment, and as an otic solution. The usual adult dose is 2 to 4 g daily.

POLYMYXINS

The polymyxins, a small group of antimicrobial agents, were discovered in 1947. All but two of the original polymyxins have been discarded from clinical use because of excessive nephrotoxicity. Polymyxin B sulfate and polymyxin E sulfate (colistin) are the agents currently available for clinical use. Table 23-10 lists their salts and routes of administration.

Action and results. Polymyxins act by disrupting the cytoplasmic membrane by means of a detergent-like effect, thereby causing

TABLE 23-10   Polymyxins

Generic and brand names	Route
Colistimethate sodium (Coly-Mycin M)	Intramuscular, intravenous
Colistin sulfate (Coly-Mycin S)	Oral
Polymyxin B sulfate (Aerosporin sulfate)	Intramuscular, intravenous, intrathecal, topical

immediate cell death. They are bactericidal for many gram-negative bacteria including most *Pseudomonas* species and *E. coli*, as well as many *Klebsiella, Enterobacter, Salmonella, Shigella,* and *Haemophilus* species.

Pharmacokinetics. The polymyxins are not absorbed after oral administration. If administered orally, the drugs exert their antibacterial effects in the lumen of the bowel and are then excreted in the feces. Parenterally injected polymyxins do not diffuse into cerebrospinal fluid. The polymyxins are strongly protein-bound and also strongly bound by cell debris, acid phospholipids, and purulent exudates. The drugs are excreted by the kidneys.

Uses. Since other antibiotics have been developed that are either more potent or less toxic than the polymyxins, these drugs are not drugs of choice now for the treatment of any systemic infection. The polymyxins are often used in the treatment of *Pseudomonas* infections that are resistant to other antimicrobial drugs. They have also been effective in the treatment of urinary tract infections caused by *Pseudomonas* or other gram-negative bacilli. Infections of the skin, mucous membranes, eye, and ear due to polymyxin-sensitive organisms have responded well. The drugs have been used to suppress *Shigella* in bacillary dysentery and other gram-negative members of bacterial flora.

Side effects and toxic effects. The most serious toxic effects of the polymyxins include renal damage, peripheral neuropathy, and respiratory arrest. Nephrotoxicity is manifested in proteinuria and hematuria. Neurotoxic effects include paresthesias, vertigo, flushing, and incoordination. All of these signs and symptoms usually disappear when the drugs are discontinued and are excreted. Respiratory arrest has occurred after administration of polymyxins to patients receiving anesthetics or muscle relaxants and to patients with myasthenia gravis. The drugs should be administered parenterally only to hospitalized patients.

Preparation, dosage, and administration
Polymyxin B sulfate (Aerosporin Sulfate). Polymyxin B sulfate is available as a topical powder, an otic solution, as tablets, and in vials for parenteral use. When given intramuscular-

ly, the drug is routinely mixed with procaine hydrochloride to decrease pain accompanying the injection. The total daily intramuscular dosage is 1.5 to 2.5 mg/kg body weight, injected in divided doses.

Colistin sulfate (Coly-Mycin S); colistimethate sodium (Coly-Mycin R). These drugs are marketed for oral and parenteral use. Unlike polymyxin B, colistin cannot be administered intraspinally or intravenously unless special preparations are used. It may be given in doses varying from 2 to 5 mg/kg/day for adults.

Miscellaneous antibiotics

This group of antibiotics consists largely of those used in topical preparations such as bacitracin, the gramicidins, and the tyrocidines (see also Chapter 30). Two other antibiotics, however, are included in this group: spectinomycin and metronidazole hydrochloride.

Spectinomycin (Trobicin)

Spectinomycin is an aminocyclitol elaborated by *Streptomyces spectabilis* and *Streptomyces flavopersicus.* It was marketed in 1971, with the sole therapeutic indication being the treatment of infections caused by *N. gonorrhoeae.* It is largely bacteriostatic and quite effective in the treatment of uncomplicated gonorrhea, acute gonorrheal urethritis, and proctitis. Spectinomycin is given intramuscularly and offers an advantage over most other agents in that it is a single-dose treatment administered at the time of diagnosis. Spectinomycin has been used successfully in patients who are allergic or unresponsive to penicillin. The dose is 2 g for males and 4 g for females.

Metronidazole hydrochloride (Flagyl IV)

This drug has recently been approved for use for serious anaerobic infections, particularly endocarditis and infections of the central nervous system such as meningitis or brain abscesses. It is also being used to treat *Bacteroides fragilis* infections that are resistant to other drugs. The most frequent adverse effects are nausea, dry mouth, and a metallic taste. A loading dose of 15 mg/kg, infused over an hour, followed by 7.5 mg/kg every 6 hours, also infused over an hour, is usually given. When the patient is able to take oral medication 7.5 mg/kg every 6 hours can be given. Metronidazole (intravenous form) is available in 500-mg vials.

Synthetic antibacterial agents

SULFONAMIDES

The sulfonamides were the first effective chemotherapeutic agents to be available in safe therapeutic dosage ranges. More specifically, they are antiinfective agents that were originally used as the mainstay of therapy of bacterial infections in humans before the penicillins were introduced. At present, antimicrobial therapy, which began with the production of penicillin in 1941, has replaced the sulfonamides. Yet sulfonamides are still among the

TABLE 23-11 **Sulfonamides and related compounds**

Generic and brand names	Route
Short acting	
Sulfadiazine	Oral
Sulfadiazine sodium	Intravenous
Sulfamethizole (Thiosulfil)	Oral
Sulfisoxazole (Gantrisin)	Oral, topical
Sulfisoxazole diolamine (Gantrisin)	Intravenous, subcutaneous
Trisulfapyrimidines (Triple Sulfa, various)	Oral
Intermediate and long acting	
Sulfamethoxazole (Gantanol)	Oral
Sulfamethoxydiazine (sulfameter) (Sulla)	Oral
Sulfamethoxypyridazine (Kynex, Midicel)	Oral
Topical sulfonamides	
Mafenide acetate (Sulfamylon)	Topical
Silver sulfadiazine (Silvadene)	Topical
Sulfacetamide sodium (Sulamyd)	Topical
Sulfonamide combinations	
Sulfamethizole, oxytetracycline hydrochloride, and Phenazopyridine (Urobiotic-250)	Oral
Sulfamethoxazole and phenazopyridine (Azo Gantanol)	Oral
Sulfamethoxazole and trimethoprim (Bactrim, Septra)	Oral
Sulfisoxazole and phenazopyridine (Azo Gantrisin)	Oral

most widely used antibacterial agents in the world, chiefly because of their low cost and their effectiveness in treating common bacterial infections. All the sulfonamides used therapeutically are synthetically produced and contain the para-amino-benzene-sulfonamide group, which gives them their common characteristics. Table 23-11 lists the sulfonamides used currently in clinical practice.

Action and results. The sulfonamides are primarily bacteriostatic in concentrations that are normally useful in controlling infections in the human being. They act as antimetabolites of para-aminobenzoic acid (PABA), which is required by susceptible microorganisms in order to form folic acid, an essential vitamin in the production of purines. Sulfonamides can enter into the reaction in place of PABA, compete for the enzyme involved, and form nonfunctional analog of folic acid. Consequently, further growth of the microorganisms is prevented. The presence of pus, necrotic tissue, and serum interferes with the activities of the sulfonamides, since PABA is present in such materials. Among the microorganisms highly susceptible to sulfonamides are group A β-hemolytic streptococci, pneumococci, *Neisseria meningitidis*, *N. gonorrhoeae*, *E. coli*, *Pasteurella pestis*, *Bacillus anthracis*, *Shigella* species, *H. influenzae*, and microorganisms causing granuloma inguinale, lymphogranuloma venereum, psittacosis, and actinomycosis.

Pharmacokinetics. All of the sulfonamides are absorbed from the gastrointestinal tract, although some are more readily absorbed than others. They are distributed widely to tissues and body fluids, including the central nervous system and cerebrospinal fluid, placenta, and fetus.

Acetylation is the major process by which the sulfonamides are metabolically inactivated. This change is probably caused by the action of the liver. Acetylation is important to the physician when choosing a drug: the acetylated forms are believed to be nontherapeutic, and they may produce toxic symptoms.

Excretion of the sulfonamides occurs chiefly by way of the kidney, where both the free and the acetylated forms of the drug are filtered through the glomerulus. Most sulfonamides are reabsorbed to some extent in the kidney. Some of the sulfonamides, and especially their acetyl derivatives, are relatively insoluble in neutral or acid media, and as the kidney concentrates the urine and it becomes acid in reaction, there is some danger that such a sulfonamide will precipitate out of solution, causing crystalluria, hematuria, and even renal shutdown. The forcing of fluids to keep the urine dilute and the administration of an alkaline substance such as sodium bicarbonate help to keep a number of the sulfonamides in solution in the urine. However, sulfonamide precipitation is no longer a great clinical problem. Newer sulfonamides, such as sulfisoxazole and sulfacetamide, are quite soluble even in acid urine. The problem of solubility in the urine can also be dealt with by administration of combinations of small doses of two or three different sulfonamides. In this way the saturation point of each is not reached and each drug remains in solution. The "insoluble" sulfonamides are poorly absorbed from the gastrointestinal tract and are excreted largely in the feces. Their action is mainly on intestinal floral; they are used to inhibit bacterial growth in the colon.

Uses. The therapeutic importance of the sulfonamides has been continually modified with the introduction of new antimicrobial agents. Many infections that were formerly treated with sulfonamides are now being treated with other agents that offer special advantages. Some infectious processes, however, are more susceptible to sulfonamides, or sulfonamides plus an antibiotic, than to antibiotics alone. Among these are acute urinary tract infections caused by *E. coli*, *Proteus*, or *Klebsiella*; chancroid; nocardiosis; toxoplasmosis; falciparum malaria; trachoma; inclusion conjunctivitis; lymphogranuloma venereum; ulcerative colitis; and dermatitis herpetiformis. The sulfonamides are also therapeutically effective in rheumatic fever prophylaxis, preoperative intestinal "antisepsis," prevention and treatment of *Pseudomonas* infections of burns, and (in topical form) treatment of ophthalmic and vaginal infections. In general, the application of sulfonamides to the skin, in wounds, or on mucous membranes is undesirable because of these drugs' low activity and the high risk of allergic

sensitization. An exception to this rule may be the use of sulfonamides in the treatment of burns or conjunctival infections.

Side effects and toxic effects. The sulfonamides can produce a wide variety of side effects, the most common being gastrointestinal and urinary tract disturbances. Anorexia, nausea, and vomiting are the most common manifestations of gastrointestinal disturbances. Urinary tract disturbances, such as crystalluria, hematuria, and obstruction, may be due to the insolubility of many sulfonamides in acid urine. Other toxic effects include hematologic effects (anemia, granulocytopenia, thrombocytopenia), dermatologic effects (such as rashes, photosensitivity, contact dermatitis, Stevens-Johnson syndrome, erythema multiforme), and hypersensitivity effects. Long-term treatment with "insoluble" sulfonamides can greatly reduce the bacterial population of the bowel and may lead to vitamin K deficiency. This possibility should be considered in patients who exhibit any bleeding tendency while taking these drugs.

SHORT-ACTING SULFONAMIDES

Short-acting sulfonamides are rapidly absorbed after oral administration, and therapeutic blood levels are maintained by administering these drugs every 4 to 8 hours. Short-acting sulfonamides are the preparations of choice for treatment of systemic and urinary tract infections. Several commonly used preparations are described. In the *British Pharmacopoea* the sulfa prefix is "sulpha."

Sulfisoxazole (Gantrisin). Sulfisoxazole is the most popular agent for the treatment of urinary tract infections. Compared to other sulfonamides it is relatively more soluble in urine and only infrequently produces crystalluria or hematuria. It is available for oral, topical, and parenteral use. The usual adult dose (oral) is 1 to 2 g every 4 to 6 hours.

Sulfisoxazole with phenazopyridine hydrochloride (Azo Gantrisin). This drug combines the bacteriostatic properties of the sulfonamide with the mucosal analgesic properties of phenazopyridine. It is specifically used for urinary tract infections accompanied by urgency, frequency, and dysuria. It gives the urine an orange-red color that should not be mistaken for blood.

Sulfadiazine. Sulfadiazine is rapidly absorbed from the gastrointestinal tract and is preferred for general use in systemic infections. Because therapeutic levels are attained in the cerebrospinal fluid within 4 hours, it is particularly recommended for treatment of meningitis caused by susceptible organisms. It is available for oral and parenteral administration. Dosage depends on the severity of the infectious process.

Sulfamethizole (Thiosulfil). This highly soluble, rapidly excreted sulfonamide is similar to sulfisoxazole and sulfadiazine in its properties. It is one of the preferred sulfonamides for the treatment of urinary tract infections. It is commonly given in the combination drug Urobiotic-250.

Trisulfapyrimidines. These sulfonamide mixtures are designed to minimize or prevent renal damage from the systemic use of this class of drugs. The combinations take advantage of the fact that each drug behaves as though it were alone in solution as far as solubility is concerned. Antibacterial effects of the three drugs contained in the mixtures (sulfadiazine, sulfamerazine, and sulfamethazine) are additive. These mixtures may also be made up of sulfadiazine in combination with any other short-acting sulfonamide. They are available for oral administration only.

INTERMEDIATE-ACTING SULFONAMIDES

Intermediate-acting sulfonamides are excreted more slowly than the short-acting drugs, and it may be necessary to administer them only twice daily. They are particularly useful when prolonged therapy is necessary, as in chronic urinary tract infections.

Sulfamethoxazole (Gantanol). This drug is a close congener of sulfisoxazole, but it is absorbed and excreted more slowly. It is employed for both systemic and urinary tract infections. Precautions must be observed because it has a greater tendency to cause crystalluria.

Trimethoprim-sulfamethoxazole (Bactrim, Septra). This synthetic antibacterial agent is a combined drug that produces its effects by

blocking two consecutive steps of protein synthesis in susceptible bacteria. One step is blocked by sulfamethoxazole and the other by trimethoprim. Thus this agent exerts synergistic bacteriostatic effects. Since it is rapidly absorbed but slowly excreted, it is administered only twice daily. This agent is used in the treatment of urinary tract infections, otitis media, and *Pneumocystis carinii* pneumonitis. Its administration to pregnant women, nursing mothers, and neonates is not advised.

LONG-ACTING SULFONAMIDES

Long-acting sulfonamides are absorbed relatively rapidly, but their excretion is so slow that therapeutic blood levels may be maintained for several days.

Sulfamethoxypyridazine (Kynex, Midicel). This very toxic drug should not be employed without special indication. Its greatest value is in prophylactic therapy or in long-term suppressive therapy, as in chronic urinary tract infections. Great care must be taken not to exceed the safe dosage range, and the patient must be closely observed for toxic reactions. Most reactions are not serious, and they subside with discontinuation of the drug. However, severe episodes of Stevens-Johnson syndrome have resulted from its use, and deaths have resulted from severe allergic responses.

Sulfamethoxydiazine (Sulfameter, Sulla). This drug is used in treatment of urinary tract infections, but has been largely replaced by the short-acting sulfonamides. It should not be used to treat acute infections.

TOPICAL SULFONAMIDES

Topical sulfonamides are used in the treatment of burns and ophthalmic infections. The following are suitable for topical application.

Mafenide acetate (Sulfamylon). This drug is one sulfonamide that presently can be recommended for application to the skin and that is effective in the presence of pus and necrotic tissue. It is an agent of choice in the treatment of burns for prevention and eradication of *Pseudomonas* infections. The hydrochloride was initially used and sometimes resulted in hyperchloremic alkalosis because of some systemic absorption. The current preparation is the acetate, which seems to be more effective and less toxic. A major disadvantage of mafenide is the severe pain that may follow topical application. It is available as 8.5% cream, to be applied to the skin twice daily, 1 mm thick.

Silver sulfadiazine (Silvadene). This silver salt of sulfadiazine appears to be comparable to mafenide in the treatment of burns. It does not cause pain on application, and it is less toxic than mafenide.

Sulfacetamide sodium (Sulamyd). This drug is used primarily in the treatment of ophthalmic infections. It is also marketed as a lotion, in combination with hydrocortisone and sulfur, for the treatment of acne.

NURSING IMPLICATIONS

In addition to instituting the nursing measures common to all types of antimicrobial therapy, the nurse should observe these precautions for patients receiving sulfonamides:

1 Because renal toxicity may still present a potentially serious problem, the nurse should monitor the hospitalized patient's urinary output and assure that it amounts to at least 1200 ml in 24 hours. Maintenance of urinary output at this level decreases the tendency for crystals to form. Patients who are not hospitalized should be instructed to drink large amounts of liquids. The urine should be visually examined for the presence of crystals, and in long-term sulfonamide therapy periodic urinalysis should be done to determine if crystal accumulation and renal irritation are present.
2 The patient should be carefully observed for toxic effects, such as rash, sore throat, or purpura. Non-hospitalized patients should be instructed to report these symptoms to their physicians and to discontinue taking the drug. In prolonged sulfonamide therapy, periodic blood counts should be performed to assess the occurrence of hematologic side effects.

T A B L E   2 3 - 1 2   Urinary tract antiseptics

Generic and brand names	Route
Cinoxacin (Cinobac)	Oral
Nitrofurantoin (Cyantin, Furadantin, Macrodantin)	Oral, intravenous
Nalidixic acid (NegGram)	Oral
Methenamine mandelate (Mandelamine)	Oral
Phenazopyridine hydrochloride (Pyridium)	Oral

3 Administration of sulfonamides is contraindicated during the last trimester of pregnancy, in nursing mothers, and in infants.
4 Although cross-sensitization is not as severe as among penicillins, it is safer to avoid all sulfonamides in patients who develop hypersensitivity to any one agent.
5 Sulfonamides should not be administered with antacids because the latter inhibit their action by decreasing absorption. Sulfasuxidine and sulfathalidine should not be administered with mineral oil because the oil prevents drug absorption.

URINARY TRACT ANTISEPTICS

Urinary tract antiseptics are drugs that exert antibacterial activity in the urine but have little or no systemic antibacterial effects. Their usefulness is limited to the treatment of urinary tract infections. Table 23-12 lists the urinary tract antiseptics that are currently used in medical practice.

Nitrofurantoin (Furadantin, Macrodantin)

Nitrofurantoin, a synthetic nitrofuran, is bacteriostatic and bactericidal against a wide variety of gram-positive and gram-negative organisms, protozoa, and fungi. Nitrofurantoin is rapidly and completely absorbed from the intestine. Resulting blood concentrations are low, but sufficient bactericidal concentrations are attained in the urine. Most organisms are sensitive to levels attained in the urine, with the exception of *Pseudomonas*. Nitrofurantoin is therapeutically used in pyelonephritis, pyelitis, and cystitis. While it is not the drug of first choice in the treatment of urinary tract infections, it is often valuable if other agents fail.

Hypersensitivity and gastrointestinal disturbances occur in a number of patients receiving nitrofurantoin. This drug will produce yellow-brown discoloration of the urine because of the formation of inactive metabolites. It is available for oral and intravenous administration. The usual adult dose is 100 to 150 mg four times daily.

Cinoxacin (Cinobac)

Cinoxacin, a new oral synthetic antibacterial agent, has a broad spectrum of antibacteral activity against gram-negative bacteria that commonly cause urinary tract infections, including most strains of *E. coli*, *Klebsiella*, *Enterobacter*, *Proteus mirabilis*, and *P. vulgaris*. Its early clinical trials have shown a low incidence of side effects—the most common being nausea and hypersensitivity reactions, either or both of which occur in less than 3% of patients. The usual adult dose is 1 g/day, which can be administered in two or four divided doses, for 7 to 14 days. Cinoxacin is available in 250 and 500-mg capsules.

Nalidixic acid (NegGram)

Nalidixic acid is a urinary antiseptic chemically unrelated to other antimicrobial agents. It is a naphthyridine derivative that is active primarily against gram-negative organisms, except for *Pseudomonas*. Unlike many other drugs, it is active against infections caused by *Proteus* species. It is useful in treating acute and chronic urinary tract infections caused by sensitive bacteria. However, resistance develops frequently and rapidly. The incidence of toxicity is low, with nausea, vomiting, rashes, and urticaria most frequently reported. Occasional central nervous system disturbances have been reported, including headache, drowsiness, vertigo, visual disturbances, and convulsions in patients with preexisting convulsive disorders. Nalidixic acid is available in 250- and 500-mg tablets. The recommended dosage is 4 g daily in divided doses for 10 to 14 days. Nalidixic acid potentiates the anticoagulant effect of coumarin drugs, leading to an increase in prothrombin time.

Methenamine mandelate (Mandelamine)

Methenamine mandelate combines the action of methenamine and mandelic acid; it is used for treatment of urinary tract infections. Its effectiveness depends on the release of formaldehyde, which requires an acid medium. Thus it is ineffective if the urine is alkaline. Because of its fairly wide bacterial spectrum, its low toxicity, and a low incidence of resistance, methenamine mandelate is often the drug of choice in long-term suppression of infections. It is available for oral administration; the drug is given four times daily in the

average dose of 1 g. It should not be used with sulfonamides, since an insoluble precipitate forms in the urine.

Phenazopyridine hydrochloride (Pyridium)

This drug is a synthetic azo dye that was once used as a urinary antiseptic, but is now used more frequently as a urinary tract analgesic. It is used in the treatment of cystitis accompanied by burning, urgency, and frequency. It is also useful in producing surface analgesia in urologic surgical procedures and after diagnostic tests necessitating instrumentation. It causes the urine to be orange or red in color, and patients should be informed of this so they do not become alarmed. It is available in 100-mg tablets; 600 mg is administered daily in divided doses.

Antimycobacterial agents (antituberculous agents)

The chemotherapy for tuberculosis requires a long course of treatment (12 to 36 months). This prolonged treatment presents several problems: (1) Drugs that are effective against the tubercle bacillus may produce serious toxic effects after prolonged administration. (2) The chance of the emergence of drug-resistant organisms increases with the length of treatment. (3) Tubercle bacilli multiply in poorly vascularized caseous lesions, which do not always receive high levels of the drugs. As a consequence, drug therapy may be complex. Drugs are often given initially in the highest tolerated dosages and in combination with other drugs in efforts to delay the emergence of resistance and to increase tuberculostatic effects. Dosage and time intervals between doses must be carefully regulated. Table 23-13 lists the antimycobacterial agents currently used in the treatment of tuberculosis.

Streptomycin was the first antimicrobial drug to exhibit striking action against tubercle bacilli. It remains an important agent in the management of severe tuberculosis. Other important antituberculosis drugs include para-aminosalicylic acid, isoniazid, ethambutol, and rifampin. In some instances, the use of a single drug is sufficient therapy; the drug then employed is usually isoniazid. Combination therapy is significantly more effective than the use of any single drug. For example, concurrent use of streptomycin, isoniazid, and ethambutol is more tuberculostatic than the use of any of these agents alone and also decreases the chance of the emergence of resistance.

If these drugs do not produce an effective therapeutic response, less common and generally more toxic drugs must be employed. These include such drugs as ethionamide, pyrazinamide, cycloserine, kanamycin, and viomycin.

Appropriate chemotherapy is the most important aspect of treatment for tuberculosis, but surgery and adjunctive measures may be necessary. Progress is evaluated by means of periodic examinations, x-rays, and sputum cultures.

Some patients require antituberculosis drug therapy despite the absence of clinical symptoms or positive sputum cultures. Patients who have a positive tuberculin test or have recently converted to PPD-positive and who are under 20 years of age, in contact with patients with active tuberculosis, or have diseases such as leukemia, silicosis, measles, or diabetes mellitus should receive prophylactic treatment. The drug most commonly used in chemoprophylaxis of tuberculosis is isoniazid.

PRIMARY DRUGS
Isoniazid (INH, isonicotinic acid hydrazide)

Isoniazid, introduced in 1952, is the most potent tuberculostatic drug available presently, being superior to streptomycin. The mechanism of action of INH is not known. Isoniazid is readily absorbed after either oral or parenteral administration. It penetrates freely into cerebrospinal fluid and into caseous tissue. Metabolism of the drug varies, and two groups of people ("metabolizers") have been identified—the "slow" and the "rapid" inactivators of the drug. Isoniazid is excreted chiefly by the kidneys.

The most common and important toxic effects of isoniazid are manifested as disturbances of the peripheral and central nervous

TABLE 23-13 Antimycobacterial agents

Generic and brand names	Route
Primary drugs	
Aminosalicylic acid (para-aminosalicylic acid or PAS)	Oral
Ethambutol (Myambutol)	Oral
Isoniazid (INH) (Nydrazid)	Intramuscular, Oral
Rifampin (Rifadin, Rimactane)	Oral
Streptomycin	Intramuscular
Secondary drugs	
Cycloserine (Seromycin)	Oral
Ethionamide (Trecator SC)	Oral
Kanamycin (Kantrex)	Oral, intramuscular, intravenous
Pyrazinamide (PZA)	Oral
Viomycin (Viocin)	IM

systems. Peripheral neuritis is probably a result of pyridoxine deficiency, since it can be controlled by daily administration of the vitamin. "Slow" metabolizers tend to develop polyneuritis more often than "rapid" metabolizers. Headache and vertigo have been reported, and large doses of isoniazid have been known to provoke convulsions in patients with preexisting seizure disorders. Other side effects include gastrointestinal dysfunction, allergic reactions, and hepatic dysfunction.

The present trend in the treatment of tuberculosis is toward the simultaneous use of INH with PAS, ethambutol, or streptomycin.

Isoniazid is available for oral and parenteral administration. Usually 2 to 8 mg/kg body weight is administered twice daily, but higher doses are necessary for the treatment of miliary tuberculosis and tuberculous meningitis. The dose should be adjusted according to 6-hour serum drug levels. Pyridoxine in doses of 50 to 100 mg also may be administered daily to prevent peripheral neuritis.

Ethambutol (Myambutol)

Ethambutol, a tuberculostatic drug introduced in the early 1960s, has been used with considerable success in the management of treatment failures. It has been so successful that it is now also being used for primary treatment.

Ethambutol is well absorbed from the gastrointestinal tract. It is well tolerated and causes little toxicity. When given in conjunction with other tuberculostatic agents, it acts to delay the emergence of resistance. Since mycobacterial resistance to ethambutol emerges fairly rapidly when the drug is used alone, it is best administered in combination with other drugs, most commonly INH. The chief toxic effect of ethambutol is retrobulbar neuritis with loss of visual acuity and disturbances in color discrimination. A decrease in the ability to perceive red and green is an early sign of toxicity. Discontinuation of the drug usually results in complete recovery. Ethambutol is available in 100- and 400-mg tablets. The usual adult dose is 15 to 25 mg/kg body weight, administered once a day.

Rifampin

Rifampin is a semisynthetic derivative of rifomycin, an antibiotic produced by *Streptomyces mediterranei*. It is the most important of the rifomycins and has been available in the United States since 1971. Rifampin is active against many gram-negative and gram-positive bacteria, as well as *Mycobacterium tuberculosis* and other mycobacteria. It acts by inhibiting RNA synthesis in bacteria and chlamydiae. Rifampin has been used mainly in the treatment of tuberculosis. It is administered in conjunction with other tuberculostatic drugs and has given results comparable to those obtained with INH and streptomycin. A number of patients in whom other therapy has failed have been treated successfully with rifampin and ethambutol.

Rifampin is well absorbed from the gastrointestinal tract, although the presence of food in the stomach appears to delay its absorption. The drug is well distributed throughout the body. It has been found in cerebrospinal fluid and diffuses into milk and saliva. It is eliminated primarily in the bile. Toxic effects of rifampin are unusual. Some gastrointestinal disturbances have been reported, as well as liver dysfunction, blood abnormalities, and a "flulike" syndrome that occurs when administration of the drug is stopped and then resumed. Rifampin may produce a harmless reddish color of the urine, sputum, and lacrimal fluid. Administration during pregnancy and in infancy is not recommended.

Rifampin must be used in combination with other tuberculostatic drugs. It is administered orally in a single daily dose of 8 to 12 mg/kg body weight.

Aminosalicylic acid (para-aminosalicylic acid, PAS)

Para-aminosalicylic acid has some bacteriostatic activity against the tubercle bacillus, but this drug is less potent than either streptomycin or isoniazid. The chief value of PAS lies in the fact that it apparently competes with isoniazid for acetylation in the liver, thereby establishing higher blood levels of isoniazid. It also acts to delay the emergence of bacterial resistance to both streptomycin and isoniazid, making it an important ancillary agent in the treatment of tuberculosis.

PAS is well absorbed from the gastrointestinal tract and diffuses rapidly into pleural fluids and into various tissues. It is excreted chiefly by way of the kidneys; however, it is not effective in the treatment of tuberculosis of the urinary tract, since it is subject to change in the liver and the resulting metabolic products are therapeutically inactive.

Gastrointestinal intolerance to PAS, manifested as nausea, vomiting, anorexia, gaseous distention, and diarrhea, occurs frequently and constitutes the principal toxic effect. It may be diminished by administering the drug with meals or antacids or by reducing the dose. Allergic reactions often occur during PAS therapy, necessitating discontinuation of the drug either temporarily or permanently. Allergic reactions appear to be most common between the second and seventh weeks of treatment. Hematologic disturbances include leukopenia, agranulocytosis, eosinophilia, lymphocytosis, and thrombocytopenia.

PAS is available in 0.5-g capsules, tablets, and enteric-coated pills, as a syrup, and as a powder from which solutions can be made for use in cavities and sinuses. The drug should be used only when freshly prepared, and discolored preparations should be discarded. Solutions are stable for only 24 hours and only if stored in a dark place or in light-resistant containers and refrigerated. The usual adult dosage is 8 to 12 g daily in divided doses.

SECONDARY DRUGS
Ethionamide (Trecator SC)

Ethionamide has about one-tenth the potency of isoniazid. It is well absorbed into the body, especially into the central nervous system. Its use is limited because of its severe side effects; patients are seldom able to tolerate therapeutic doses. Gastrointestinal disturbances such as nausea, vomiting, and anorexia are frequent. They are thought to be caused by the drug's central nervous system toxicity rather than by its effects on the gastrointestinal tract. Ganglionic blockage and hepatotoxicity may also be seen. The usual dose is 10 to 12 mg/kg/day, with a maximum of 3 g/day.

Pyrazinamide (PZA)

Pyrazinamide is a synthetic drug made from nicotinamide. It is less effective than streptomycin and isoniazid but more effective than cycloserine and viomycin. Pyrazinamide is considered an effective drug, especially when given with isoniazid for short-term therapy, such as that which precedes surgery in patients in whom the causative organism is resistant to other drugs. Tubercle bacilli develop resistance to the drug relatively quickly. It is available in 500-mg tablets for oral administration. A dose of 1.5 to 2 g daily (after meals) in two or three equally divided portions is recommended.

Hepatic toxicity is the most common untoward effect. All patients being treated with pyrazinamide should have hepatic function studies performed prior to and periodically during treatment. If hepatic dysfunction becomes apparent, the drug must be discontinued.

Cycloserine (Oxamycin, Seromycin)

Cycloserine, an antibiotic produced from *Streptomyces orchidaceus*, was isolated in 1955. It has been employed in the treatment of tuberculosis in conjunction with other tuberculostatic agents, but it is not as effective as INH or streptomycin. Cycloserine is slowly but completely absorbed from the gastrointestinal tract and widely distributed throughout the body. It penetrates well into cerebrospinal fluid, passes through the placenta, and is secreted in the milk of lactating women. It is excreted in the urine. It is more toxic than other drugs used in the treatment of tuberculosis and may produce serious central nervous system toxicity, manifested as somnolence, headache, tremor, vertigo, acute psychosis, and convulsions. Seizure precautions are advisable. Resistance to the drug develops rapidly. The usual adult dose is 10 mg/kg body weight, given in two or three divided doses orally. Cycloserine is supplied in 250-mg capsules.

Viomycin sulfate (Viocin)

Viomycin was isolated from *Streptomyces puniceus* in 1951. It inhibits the growth of a number of bacteria, but its use is confined to the treatment of tuberculosis when streptomycin and isoniazid resistance has occurred. Because absorption of viomycin from the gastrointestinal tract is limited, the drug is administered intramuscularly. Distribution to cerebrospinal fluid is poor. Viomycin toxicity is greater than that of streptomycin, manifesting itself in renal damage, electrolyte disturbances, and impaired vestibular function.

NURSING IMPLICATIONS

1 The nurse should attempt to administer these drugs with consideration for the patient's comfort. For example, gastrointestinal disturbances following administration of PAS can be reduced by concurrent administration of food or antacids.
2 It is imperative that patient take prescribed medications regularly and without interruption. If a patient is responsible for self-medication, he should be instructed about the necessity to take these drugs according to the prescribed regimen and not to discontinue them when he feels better.
3 Patients responsible for self-medication also should be instructed about the necessity for periodic medical evaluations.
4 Because of the long-term nature of drug therapy in tuberculosis, patients may need support in maintaining the therapeutic regimen and in tolerating side effects of the tuberculosis drugs.

Antifungal agents

Antifungal chemotherapy has not developed to the same degree that antibacterial chemotherapy has developed. Most fungi are completely resistant to the action of chemicals at concentrations that can be tolerated by the

TABLE 23-14 **Antifungal agents**

Generic and trade names	Route
Systemic infections	
Amphotericin B (Fungizone)	Intravenous, intrathecal
Flucytosine (5-fluorocytosine, Ancobon)	Oral
Candidal infections	
Amphotericin B (Fungizone)	Oral, topical, intravaginal
Candicidin (Candeptin, Vanobid)	Intravaginal
Clotrimazole (Gyne-Lotrimin, Mycelex-G)	Intravaginal
Miconazole (Monistat 7)	Intravaginal
Nystatin (Candex, Mycostatin, Nilstat, various)	Oral, intra-vaginal, topical
Dermatophytic infections	
Clotrimazole (Lotrimin, Mycelex)	Topical
Griseofulvin (Fulvicin, Grifulvin V, Grisactin, various)	Oral
Haloprogin (Halotex)	Topical
Iodochlorhydroxyquin (Vioform)	Topical
Miconazole (Micatin)	Topical
Selenium sulfide (Exsel, Selsun)	Topical
Tolnaftate (Tinactin, Aftate)	Topical
Triacetin (Enzactin)	Topical
Undecylenic acid (Desenex, Cal-desene)	Topical

host, and only a few antifungal compounds are currently available for use internally. As a result, most antifungal drugs are used topically. Table 23-14 lists the antifungal agents most commonly used in clinical medicine. All topical preparations will be discussed in Chapter 30. The following discussions will include only those agents that are taken by oral or parenteral routes.

Amphotericin B (Fungizone)

The antibiotic agent amphotericin B was derived from *Streptomyces nodosus* in 1956. It is used in the treatment of disseminated mycotic infections, including coccidioidomycosis, cryptococcosis, disseminated moniliasis, histoplasmosis, and North American blastomycosis. The antibiotic is both fungistatic and fungicidal and has no effect on bacteria or viruses. It is the only effective drug for the treatment of deep fungal disease.

Very little amphotericin B is absorbed following oral, subcutaneous, or intramuscular administration. An oral tablet containing 250 mg amphotericin B is designed for treatment of candidal enteritis and as concurrent therapy in the local treatment of vaginal candidiasis. The drug is usually administered by the intravenous route; the dose is increased in small increments until a total daily dose of 1 mg/kg body weight is attained. Intravenous injection usually produces chills, fever, vomiting, and headache. These side effects may be minimized by reducing the dosage temporarily, administering corticosteroids, or discontinuing the drug for several days.

Therapeutic doses of amphotericin B also produce hepatic and renal dysfunction and may result in anemia. Shock-like hypotension, electrolyte disturbances, and a variety of neurologic symptoms may also occur.

All patients receiving amphotericin B must be hospitalized, and renal and hepatic function tests must be performed frequently during therapy with the drug.

Nursing applications. Amphotericin B should not be used if there is any evidence of precipitate or foreign matter in the vial. It should not be mixed with any other drug unless absolutely necessary. Administration of the drug on alternate days may reduce the incidence of some side effects. Frequent renal function tests, blood counts, and electrolyte level determinations are necessary during therapy.

Flucytosine (5-fluorocytosine, Ancobon)

Flucytosine is an antifungal substance that is effective against a number of yeasts and yeast-like organisms, especially *Cryptococcus neoformans* and *Candida albicans*. It is fungistatic and slowly fungicidal. It has been used in the treatment of meningitis caused by *Cryptococcus* and of systemic infections caused by *Candida*. Its one disadvantage is that resistance to the drug develops rapidly during therapy of these infections.

Flucytosine is well absorbed from the gastrointestinal tract and diffuses into cerebrospinal fluid. It is generally well tolerated, although abdominal bloating and diarrhea have been noted. It is less toxic than amphotericin B, even though nausea, vomiting, rash, vertigo, hallucinations, reversible blood dyscrasias, and hepatotoxicity have been observed with its use. The recommended daily adult dose is 150 mg/kg body weight in four equally divided doses.

Nystatin (Mycostatin)

Nystatin, an antibiotic obtained from *Streptomyces noursei,* is primarily useful in the treatment of infections caused by the monilial organism *Candida albicans.* It is administered topically in creams, powders, and ointments that contain 100,000 units of nystatin per gram; it is also available in suppository form. Nystatin may be administered orally for the suppression of *Candida* of the bowel, especially during tetracycline administration. Untoward effects of nystatin are not common. Mild gastrointestinal discomfort may occur after oral administration.

Nursing applications. Unused portions of nystatin should be preserved in light-resistant containers.

Griseofulvin (Fulvicin, Grifulvin)

Griseofulvin, a fungistatic agent obtained from *Penicillium griseofulvum,* inhibits the growth of dermatophytes, including *Epidermophyton, Microsporum,* and *Trichophyton.* It is used in the treatment of mycotic disease of the skin, hair, and nails.

After absorption following oral administration, griseofulvin is bound to keratin and deposited in diseased epidermis, hair, and nails. The infected fungus is not killed, but its growth into new cells is prevented. As the keratinized structures are shed, they tend to be replaced by normal, uninfected ones. The drug is absorbed when taken with a high-fat meal and when taken in the ultrafine particle form. It is poorly distributed to other tissues, and the bulk of orally ingested griseofulvin is eliminated unchanged in the feces. The drug is more effective for chronic fungal infections than for acute ones. It is not recommended for deep or systemic fungal infections.

The incidence of toxic effects associated with the administration of griseofulvin is relatively low. Hepatotoxicity, photosensitivity, and mental and neurologic difficulties have been reported. Headache may be severe at the beginning of therapy but usually abates. Leukopenia may occur but reverses itself as therapy is continued.

Griseofulvin is administered in dosages of 1 to 2 g/day for the regular preparation or 0.75 g/day for the micronized preparation. The absorption of griseofulvin is enhanced by concurrent administration of milk and other fatty foods. The duration of treatment is determined by the rate of complete turnover of the cells in the infected area.

Concurrent administration of phenobarbital reduces the effectiveness of griseofulvin. Griseofulvin interferes with the effectiveness of coumarin anticoagulant therapy and may precipitate acute porphyria.

Nursing applications. Because treatment with griseofulvin may last several months, and because symptoms may abate soon, the patient needs to be taught the importance of adhering to the prescribed dosage schedule. Frequent shampoos and clipping of the hair and nails will support the therapeutic effect of the drug. Frequent blood counts during therapy may be necessary to monitor leukopenia, and periodic renal and hepatic function tests also may be ordered.

Antiviral agents

Chemotherapy for viral diseases has been more limited than chemotherapy for bacterial diseases, because development and clinical application of antiviral drugs are difficult. In many viral infections, the replication of the virus in the body reaches its peak before any clinical symptoms appear. By the time signs and symptoms of illness appear, the multiplication of the virus is ending and the subsequent course of the illness has been determined already. In order to be clinically effective, therefore, antiviral drugs would have to be administered in a chemoprophylactic manner—that is, prior to the appearance of disease. A second factor limiting the development of antiviral drugs is that viruses are true parasites; they replicate within the mammalian cell and utilize the host cell's enzyme systems. Thus drugs that would inhibit virus replication would also disturb the host cells and, therefore, would be too toxic for use.

Table 23-15 lists the common antiviral agents available.

Amantadine hydrochloride (Symmetrel)

Amantadine, a synthetic agent introduced in the middle 1960s, exerts a prophylactic action on certain myxoviruses (influenza A, rubella, and some tumor viruses) by inhibiting their penetration into susceptible host cells. The drug is well absorbed from the gastrointestinal tract and is excreted in the urine. The only antiviral use of amantadine is for the prevention of A2 influenza. Its use is recommended in the presence of a documented influenza A2 epidemic, especially for high-risk patients.

The most marked untoward side effects are central nervous system disturbances, including hyperexcitability, insomnia, slurred speech, vertigo, and ataxia. Doses higher than those recommended may produce convulsions. The drug should be administered cautiously to patients with any disease affecting the central nervous system and should not be administered to pregnant women. The recommended daily dosage for adults is 200 mg in divided doses.

Idoxuridine (Dendrid, Herplex, Stoxil)

Idoxuridine inhibits the replication of certain viruses, probably by inhibiting synthesis of DNA. It has been used primarily in the treatment of herpes simplex keratitis. The drug is available as a 0.1% solution or ointment. One drop should be instilled into the conjunctival sac every hour during the day and every 2 hours during the night, until definite improvement is noted, after which the dose can be decreased. The drug should then be applied every 4 hours during the day. (See Chapter 17.)

Vidarabine (Vira-A)

Vidarabine, a purine nucleoside, is thought to work by the inhibition of DNA polymerase. Its antiviral spectrum includes the herpesviruses, some poxviruses, and the Rous sarcoma leukovirus. It is used topically to treat ocular herpes simplex and skin and mucous membrane herpetic infections. The drug is given parenterally to treat herpes simplex encephali-

T A B L E 2 3 - 1 5   Antiviral agents

Generic and brand names	Route
Amantadine hydrochloride (Symmetrel)	Oral
Idoxuridine (Dendrid, Herplex, Stoxil)	Topical
Vidarabine (Vira-A)	Intravenous, topical

tis. Because of poor solubility and absorption, the drug cannot be given by the intramuscular or oral routes, but only intravenously. Parenteral administration consists of slow, continuous infusion of 15 mg/kg body weight daily for 10 days. Topical ocular application consists of ½ inch of ointment placed into the lower conjunctival sac five times daily at 3-hour intervals. After reepithelialization, 7 days of twice-daily treatments is recommended.

Summary of nursing considerations

Antimicrobial agents destroy or inhibit the growth of microorganisms. Some of these agents are derived from living organisms; others are synthetic and semisynthetic chemical compounds. The goal of chemotherapy for infectious diseases is to destroy or suppress the growth of infecting microorganisms so that normal host defense mechanisms can gain control in their efforts to eliminate the infecting organisms. Among the microorganisms that can be controlled by these drugs today are most bacteria, many fungi, and a few viruses.

In order to exert their effects, antimicrobial agents must first gain access to target sites, usually by absorption of the drug into and distribution through the circulatory system. Then they have bacteriostatic or bactericidal effects, depending on the mechanism of action. Bacteriostatic agents such as sulfonamides inhibit bacterial growth, allowing host defense mechanisms additional time to remove the invading microorganisms. Bactericidal agents, such as the penicillins, cause bacterial cell death and lysis, superimposing the killing effect of the drug on the effects of host defenses. Antimicrobial agents may exert their bacteriostatic or bactericidal effects by inhibition of cell wall synthesis in bacteria, disruption or alteration of membrane permeability, inhibition of protein synthesis, or inhibition of synthesis of essential metabolites.

The nurse must be aware of three general types of adverse reactions from antimicrobial agents: allergic or hypersensitivity reactions, resistance, or superinfection. Several important principles guide the judicious and optimal use of the antimicrobial agents: (1) determination of the infecting organism, (2) assessment of host defense mechanisms, and (3) proper dosage and duration of therapy.

Hundreds of antimicrobial agents are marketed currently, and it is impossible for the nurse to be infinitely knowledgeable about each drug. However, in spite of the numerous and varied drugs available, there are still only a few drug categories to remember. Knowledge of general characteristics of each drug category and of general principles of antimicrobial drug therapy should enable the nurse to function effectively.

In addition to the antibiotics, which include penicillins, cephalosporins, macrolides, lincosamides, vancomycin, aminoglycosides, tetracyclines, chloramphenicol, and polymyxins, major groups of antiinfective drugs include sulfonamides, urinary tract antiseptics, and antimycobacterial, antifungal, and antiviral agents. Table 23-3 gives a brief summary of some major allergic and toxic effects of antimicrobial agents.

Nursing interventions in antimicrobial drug therapy generally relate to (1) assisting in the identification of the infecting organism, (2) actual administration of the drug, (3) assessment of the patient's response to the drug, (4) patient teaching, and (5) prevention and treatment of adverse responses, including pharmacologic and chemical drug-drug interactions.

Assisting in identification of infecting organism. Obtaining cultures of the infected areas is frequently the nurse's responsibility; it should be performed early so that antimicrobial therapy can be instituted without delay. It is very rare that a nurse cannot take a few minutes necessary to obtain cultures. In the event that orders for an antimicrobial agent have been given, the nurse should obtain cul-

tures before administering the first dose of the drug ordered. Specimens obtained for culture should be taken directly to the laboratory and not allowed to stand. Delay may cause the death of fastidious organisms and allow contaminating organisms to overgrow the pathogen.

Administration of antimicrobial drugs. Since the consistent administration of an antimicrobial drug at prescribed dosage intervals is necessary to prevent the emergence of resistance, the nurse should administer such a drug according to prescribed times as accurately as possible. This may mean awakening sleeping patients and ensuring that patient tests or therapies do not interrupt this schedule.

When antimicrobial agents are administered intravenously, the nurse must observe additional precautions: (1) the drugs should be administered in neutral solutions (pH 7.0 to 7.2) of isotonic sodium chloride (0.9%) or 5% dextrose in water; (2) the drugs should be administered without the admixture of any other drug, in order to avoid chemical or physical incompatibilities; (3) the drugs should be administered by intermittent addition to intravenous infusions, to avoid inactivation (for example, by temperature) and prolonged vein irritation from high drug concentration; and (4) the infusion site must be changed every 48 hours to reduce the chances of superinfection.

Assessment of patient's response to drug. Assessment of the patient for therapeutic responses to antimicrobial agents is also the nurse's responsibility. The nurse should observe the patient for signs and symptoms such as decreased fever, decreased purulence of drainage (if appropriate), decreased white blood cell count, and a subjective feeling of increased well-being.

Patient teaching. Patients should be taught principles of antimicrobial therapy clearly enough to understand that these drugs should never be taken without medical supervision and should be taken in strict accordance with physicians' prescriptions. This is especially important because many patients receiving antimicrobial drugs are not hospitalized and are responsible for self-medication. Patients should be taught, for example, not to take "left-

TABLE 23-16 Some antimicrobial pharmacologic drug-drug interactions

Antibiotic	Interfering agent	Effect
Polymyxins	Aminoglycosides	Potentiate the competitive neuromuscular blockade
	Muscle relaxants	
Tetracyclines	Antacids	Form complex with the antibiotic and prevent absorption
	Divalent cations	May potentiate anticoagulant by depressing gastrointestinal flora
	Coumarins	and decreasing vitamin K synthesis
Sulfonamides	Sulfonylureas	Enhance action of the interfering agent by displacement from plasma proteins
	Coumarins	
	Phenylbutazone	Decreased absorption at alkaline pH
	Antacids	May cause crystallization of sulfas in the urine
	Acidifiers	
Aminoglycosides	Polymyxins	Potentiate the competitive neuromuscular blockade
	Muscle relaxants	Enhance antibacterial activity
	Alkalinizing agents	
Nitrofurantoin	Antacids	Decreased absorption at alkaline pH
Furazolidone	MAO inhibitors	Antibiotic potentiates all of these agents
	Catecholamines	
	Phenothiazines	
Griseofulvin	Coumarins	Enzyme induction to cause more rapid metabolism of anticoagulant

From Rosenfeld, M.G., editor: Manual of medical therapeutics, ed. 20, Boston, 1971, Little, Brown & Co.

over" antimicrobial drugs for new illnesses, even if symptoms appear similar; not to stop taking these drugs as soon as symptoms abate; and not to share these drugs with family and friends. Patients who are allergic to an antimicrobial agent should be taught clearly how to protect themselves from future treatment from the drug in question.

PREVENTION AND TREATMENT OF ADVERSE RESPONSES

Allergic responses. Assessment of a patient's previous reactions to drugs and to antimicrobial agents in particular is especially important in avoiding allergic reactions to drugs. Careful questioning of the patient regarding drugs previously taken and his responses to them is an important part of the patient's history. Once drug allergy is known, warnings should be prominently displayed in the patient's record or hospital chart. As additional precautions, the nurse should (1) tell the patient what drug he is receiving; (2) observe the patient for at least ½ hour after administration of the drug (penicillin in particular), especially if it is administered parenterally and the patient has never taken the drug previously; and (3) know what drugs are used for the treatment of allergic responses and where they are kept.

Resistance. The emergence of resistance may be suspected if the infectious process becomes less responsive to drug therapy and/or the patient's condition regresses. The nurse should be vigilant for signs and symptoms indicative of lack of progress or regression.

Superinfection. The emergence of superinfection may be suspected in the presence of new fevers or other new problems, such as vaginal discharge in females or diarrhea. Children, elderly patients, and other patients whose normal host defense mechanisms may be weakened should be especially observed for signs of superinfection. In the course of prolonged antimicrobial drug therapy, periodic cultures of the upper respiratory tract and of feces may be indicated to determine changes in bacterial flora that subsequently may be responsible for secondary infection. The nurse should be careful not to introduce new microorganisms and should emphasize asepsis in contacts with patients receiving antimicrobial therapy.

Stop and renewal orders. The establishment of automatic stop and renewal orders in many hospitals is another precaution against adverse reactions. Such orders restrict the administration of a prescribed antimicrobial agent to a definite time period (for example, 7 days); its continued use past that time requires a new prescription from the physician.

Drug interactions. Because the administration of more than one drug to a patient is the rule rather than the exception in current hospi-

TABLE 23-17 **Some antimicrobial chemical drug-drug interactions**

Antimicrobial drug	Other agent	Results
Amphotericin B	Benzylpenicillin, tetracyclines, aminoglycosides	Precipitate
Cephalosporins	Calcium gluconate or calcium chloride, polymyxin B, erythromycin, tetracyclines	Precipitate
Chloramphenicol	Polymyxin B, tetracyclines, vancomycin hydrocortisone, B complex vitamins	Precipitate
Gentamicin	Carbenicillin	Inactivation
Methicillin	Any acidic solution, tetracyclines	Inactivation in 6 hours
Nafcillin	Any acidic solution, B complex vitamins	Inactivation in 12 hours
Novobiocin	Aminoglycosides, erythromycins	Insoluble precipitate
Oxacillin	Any acidic solution, B complex vitamins	Inactivation in 12 hours
Penicillin G	Any acidic solution, B complex vitamins, amphotericin B, chloramphenicol, tetracyclines, vancomycin, metaraminol, phenylephrine, carbohydrate at pH > 8.0	Inactivation in 12 hours, precipitate
Polymyxin B	Cephalothin	Precipitate
Tetracyclines	Calcium-containing solutions, amphotericin B, cephalosporins, heparin, hydrocortisone, polymyxin B, chloramphenicol, any divalent cations, iron	Chelation, inactivation, precipitate
Vancomycin	Heparin, penicillins, hydrocortisone, chloramphenicol	Precipitate

From Meyers, F.H., Jawetz, E., and Goldfien, A.: Review of medical pharmacology, ed. 4, Los Altos, Calif., 1972, Lange Medical Publications.

tal practice, the possibility of drug interactions must be taken into account if antimicrobial therapy is to be optimally effective. Table 23-16 lists some common drugs that interact biologically with antimicrobial agents. These interactions are often referred to as "pharmacologic drug-drug interactions." Table 23-17 notes chemical incompatibilities between antimicrobial drugs and other agents when they are mixed for intravenous administration. These interactions are commonly referred to as "chemical drug-drug interactions."

QUESTIONS

FOR STUDY AND REVIEW

1 Identify the goal of chemotherapy for infectious diseases.
2 Differentiate between "antibiotic" and "antimicrobial" agents.
3 Differentiate between "bacteriostatic" and "bactericidal" drug effects.
4 Describe the four major ways in which antimicrobial drugs act.
5 Identify and describe the three major adverse effects common to all types of antimicrobial drug therapy.
6 Identify the three major principles of antimicrobial therapy.
7 Explain the pros and cons of obtaining specimens for culture and sensitivity testing before the patient receives his first dose of an antimicrobial drug.

8 Describe several nursing measures that may be taken to prevent allergic reactions to antimicrobial drugs.
9 Identify the six major categories of antibacterial drugs discussed in this chapter.
10 What is the antibacterial spectrum of the penicillins?
11 What is the role of probenecid (Benemid) in drug therapy with the penicillins?
12 Identify the major clinical uses of the penicillins.
13 Identify the three major disadvantages of the penicillins that are not direct toxic effects of the drugs.
14 What are the advantages of semisynthetic penicillins?
15 What is the major clinical use of methicillin?
16 What are the advantages and disadvantages of penicillin G benzathine (Bicillin)?
17 What advantage do the cephalosporins offer over the penicillins?
18 Name the cephalosporins currently in use.
19 Why should a nurse administer oral penicillins at a time when they are not preceded or followed by food for at least one hour?
20 How do the sulfonamides differ from the penicillins in origin and in antibacterial effects?
21 Describe the mechanism of action of the sulfonamides.
22 What are the major clinical uses of the sulfonamides?
23 What are the major adverse effects and toxic effects of the sulfonamides?
24 Why are patients who are going to have intestinal surgery sometimes treated with sulfonamides preoperatively and postoperatively? Why might

vitamin K be administered together with these drugs?

25 What is the advantage of the trisulfapyrimidines?

26 What precautions should the nurse take in regard to the potential renal toxicity of the sulfonamides?

27 Name a specific sulfa preparation used for each of the following conditions:
a. urinary tract infection
b. meningitis
c. bacillary dysentery

28 Define the term "urinary antiseptic" and name several drugs belonging to this category.

29 What is the antibacterial spectrum of the tetracyclines?

30 For what clinical conditions are the tetracyclines currently drugs of choice?

31 Why is the administration of tetracyclines contraindicated during pregnancy and for children under the age of 7?

32 What are the major adverse effects and toxic effects of the tetracyclines?

33 Why should the nurse remember not to administer the tetracyclines together with milk or antacids?

34 Identify the seven drugs included in the aminoglycoside antimicrobial drug category.

35 What are the three major toxic effects of the aminoglycosides?

36 Identify the major clinical uses of the aminoglycosides.

37 What is the major clinical use of spectinomycin?

38 Describe the three major problems attendant to chemotherapy for tuberculosis.

39 Name several nonaminoglycoside drugs used in the therapy for tuberculosis.

40 What is the major function of PAS in the chemotherapy for tuberculosis?

41 What is the major function of INH in the chemotherapy for tuberculosis?

42 What are the most common toxic effects of INH and how are they treated?

43 Why is the chemotherapy for tuberculosis characterized by the concurrent use of several drugs?

44 What is the major function of ethambutol in the chemotherapy for tuberculosis?

45 What is the chief toxic effect of ethambutol?

46 In what kinds of situations should a nurse be especially alert for the neuromuscular blockade potential of the aminoglycosides?

47 Identify the major clinical indications for the use of the macrolide antimicrobial drugs.

48 Identify the two drugs of the polymyxin category that are currently in clinical use.

49 What are the principal toxic effects of the polymyxins?

50 What are the current clinical uses of the polymyxins?

51 Why is chloramphenicol no longer a widely used antibiotic?

52 For what clinical conditions does chloramphenicol remain a drug of choice?

53 Describe the major factors that have limited the development of antiviral chemotherapy.

54 Identify the two antiviral drugs currently available, and name their therapeutic uses.

55 What are the clinical uses of amphotericin B?

56 What are the primary clinical uses of griseofulvin?

57 What is the primary clinical indication for the use of nystatin?

BIBLIOGRAPHY

GENERAL

Barker, B.M., and Prescott, F.: Antimicrobial agents in medicine, Oxford, 1973, Blackwell Scientific Publications.

Bennett, D.R., and others: AMA Drug evaluations, ed. 4, New York, 1980, John Wiley & Sons, Inc.

Boston Collaborative Drug Surveillance Program: Drug-induced deafness, J.A.M.A. **224:**515, 1973.

Caldwell, J.R., and Cluff, L.E.: The real and present danger of antibiotics, Ration. Drug Ther. **7:**1, 1973.

Cohen, S.N., and others: Drug induced nephropathy, J.A.M.A. **227:**325, 1974.

Freitag, J.J., and Miller, L.W. editors: Manual of medical therapeutics, ed. 23, Boston, 1980, Little, Brown & Co.

Glassock, R.J.: Complications of antibiotic therapy. Renal complications, Calif. Med. **117:**31, 1972.

Goodman, L.S., and Gilman, A., editors: The pharmacologic basis of therapeutics, ed. 6, New York, 1980, Macmillan Inc.

Kagan, B.M., editor: Antimicrobial therapy, ed. 2, Philadelphia, 1980, W.B. Saunders Co.

Katstrup, E.K., and Boyd, J.R., editors: Facts and comparisons, St. Louis, 1980, Facts and Comparisons, Inc.

Kucers and Bennett, editors: The use of antibiotics, ed. 3, Philadelphia, 1980, J.B. Lippincott Co.

MacFarlane, M.D., and others: Anaphylactic shock and anaphylactoid reaction: analysis of 62 cases, Drug Intell. Clin. Pharmacol. **7:**394, 1973.

McCracken, G.H.: Pharmacological basis for antimicrobial therapy in newborn infants, Am. J. Dis. Child. **128:**407, 1974.

Pittinger, C.B., and Adamson, R.: Antibiotic blockade of neuromuscular function, Annu. Rev. Pharmacol. **12:**169, 1972.

Schapiro, R.L., and others: Acute enterocolitis: a complication of antibiotic therapy, Radiology **108:**263, 1973.

Tobey, L., and Covington, T.: Antimicrobial drug interactions, Am. J. Nurs. **75:**1470, 1975.

VanOmmen, R.A.: Untoward effects of antimicrobial agents on major organ systems, Med. Clin. North Am. **58:**465, 1974.

Ziment, I., and others: Complications of antibiotic therapy, Calif. Med. **117:**24, 1972.

PENICILLINS AND CEPHALOSPORINS

Boston Collaborative Drug Surveillance Program: Ampicillin rashes, Arch. Dermatol. **107**:74, 1973.

Garrod, L.P.: Choice among penicillins and cephalosporins, Br. Med. J. **3**:96, 1974.

Hansten, P.D.: Cephalothin, gentamicin, colistin hazards, J.A.M.A. **223**:1158, 1973.

Kleinknecht, D., and others: Nephrotoxicity of cephaloridine, Ann. Intern. Med. **80**:421, 1974.

Levine, B.B.: Antigenicity and cross-reactivity of penicillins and cephalosporins, J. Infect. Dis. **128** (Suppl.):364, 1973.

Mandell, G.L.: Cephaloridine, Ann. Intern. Med. **79**:561, 1973.

Neu, H.C.: New broad-spectrum penicillins, Drugs **9**:81, 1975.

Parry, M.F., and others: Nafcillin nephritis, J.A.M.A. **225**:178, 1973.

Ries, K., and others: Clinical and in vitro evaluation of cephazolin, a new cephalosporin antibiotic, Antimicrob. Agents Chemother. **3**:168, 1973.

Stewart, G.T.: Allergy to penicillin and related antibiotics: antigenic and immunochemical mechanism, Annu. Rev. Pharmacol. **13**:309, 1973.

Thrupp, L.D.: Newer cephalosporins and "expanded-spectrum" penicillins, Annu. Rev. Pharmacol. **14**:435, 1974.

Vann, R.L., and others: Twice-a-day penicillin therapy for streptococcal upper respiratory infections, South. Med. J. **65**:203, 1972.

Wise, R.: New penicillins—present and future, J.A.M.A. **232**:493, 1975.

SULFONAMIDES; URINARY TRACT ANTISEPTICS

Brumfitt, W., Hamilton-Miller, J.M., and Kosmidis, J.: Trimethoprimsulfamethoxazole: the present position, J. Infect Dis. **128**(Suppl.):778, 1973.

Craig, W.A., and others: Trimethoprim-sulfamethoxazole: pharmacodynamic effects of urinary pH and renal failure, Ann. Intern. Med. **78**:491, 1973.

Kunin, C.M.: Detection, prevention and management of urinary tract infections, Philadelphia, 1972, Lea & Febiger.

Schiffman, D.O.: Evaluation of an anti-infective combination: trimethoprim-sulfamethoxazole, J.A.M.A. **231**:635, 1975.

ANTIMYCOBACTERIAL AGENTS

Aquinas, M.: Drug treatment of pulmonary tuberculosis, Drugs **9**:5, 1975.

Citron, K.: The chemotherapy of pulmonary tuberculosis, Br. J. Hosp. Med. **12**:731, 1974.

Doster, B., and others: Ethambutol in the initial treatment of pulmonary TB, Am. Rev. Respir. Dis. **107**:177, 1973.

Ellard, G.A., and others: Pharmacology of some slow release preparations of isoniazid, Lancet **1**:340, 1972.

Jenne, J.W., and others: Pharmacokinetics of INH, ethambutol, and rifampin, Am. Rev. Respir. Dis. **107**:1013, 1973.

Johnston, R.F., and others: "State of the art" review. The impact of chemotherapy on the care of patients with tuberculosis, Am. Rev. Respir. Dis. **109**:636, 1974.

Moulding, T.: Chemoprophylaxis of tuberculosis: when is the benefit worth the risk and cost? Ann. Intern. Med. **74**:761, 1971.

Moulding, T., and Davidson, P.T.: Tuberculosis. I. Drug therapy, Drug Ther. **4**:79, 1974.

Rossouw, J.E., and Saunders, S.J.: Hepatic complications of antituberculous therapy, Q. J. Med. **44**:1, 1975.

Schever, P.J., and others: Rifampicin hepatitis, Lancet **1**:421, 1974.

Slagel, W.A.: INH chemoprophylaxis, N. Engl. J. Med. **286**:159, 1972.

ANTIVIRAL AGENTS

Juel-Jensen, B.E.: Virus diseases, Practitioner **213**:508, 1974.

Tilles, J.G.: Antiviral agents, Annu. Rev. Pharmacol. **14**:469, 1974.

Weinstein, L., and Chang, T.W.: The chemotherapy of viral infections, N. Engl. J. Med. **289**:725, 1973.

OTHERS

Barrett-Connor, E.: The epidemiology and control of gonorrhea and syphilis: a reappraisal, Prev. Med. **3**:102, 1974.

Bennett, J.E.: The treatment of systemic mycoses, Ration. Drug Ther. **7**:1, 1973.

Clark, D.O.: Gonorrhea: changing concepts in diagnosis and management, Clin. Obstet. Gynecol. **16**:3, 1973.

Dykers, J.R.: Single-dose metronidazole for trichomonal vaginitis, N. Engl. J. Med. **293**:23, 1974.

Finger, A.H.: Spectinomycin in the treatment of gonorrhea in females and males, Br. J. Vener. Dis. **51**:38, 1975.

Henderson, R.H.: Gonorrhea: recommended treatment schedules, J. Pediatr. **86**:794, 1975.

Kaye, D.: Changes in the spectrum, diagnosis and management of bacterial and fungal endocarditis, Med. Clin. North Am. **57**:941, 1973.

Kim, R.: Tetracycline therapy for atypical mycobacterial granuloma, Arch. Dermatol. **110**:299, 1974.

Klastersky, J., and others: Comparative study of tobramycin and gentamicin with special reference to anti-pseudomonas activity, Clin. Pharmacol. Ther. **14**:104, 1973.

LeFrock, J.L., and others: The spectrum of colitis associated with lincomycin and clindamycin therapy, J. Infect. Dis. **131**(Suppl.):108, 1975.

Phillipson, A., and others: Transplacental passage of erythromycin and clindamycin, N. Engl. J. Med. **288**:1219, 1973.

Stickler, G.B.: How many more treatment trials in otitis media? Am. J. Dis. Child. **125**:403, 1973.

Storey, E.: Tetracyclines and children's teeth, Drugs **6**:321, 1973.

Vandevelde, J., and others: 5-Fluorocytosine in the treatment of mycotic infections, Ann. Intern. Med. **77**:43, 1972.

Wallin, J., and Fosgren, A.: I. Tinidazole—a new preparation for T. vaginalis infections. II. Clinical evaluation of treatment with a single oral dose, Br. J. Vener. Dis. **50**:148, 1974.

CHAPTER 24

Antiseptics and disinfectants

Infections and infectious diseases

Infections and infectious diseases, though differing in type and character, occur in people in all settings—hospitals, institutions, the community at large, and the home.

Nosocomial infections are those that are acquired in a hospital. They have been typified as one of the most significant current ecologic problems in the United States. They are occasionally caused by virulent microorganisms resistant to antibiotics. *Community- or home-acquired infections* are usually fairly benign and relatively responsive to treatment; these include appendicitis, animal bites, lacerations, foreign bodies, and the like.

The emergence of antibiotic-resistant bacteria has become an increasingly important problem, especially in hospitals. Relative virulence of strains of these bacteria tends to change over

time. Burn infections typify this variation. Before 1940, prior to the introduction of antibiotics, group A streptococci represented the major microbial problem. By the mid-1950s, when antibiotics were beginning to proliferate, coagulase-positive *Staphylococcus aureus* predominated. Subsequently, the problem became more complex, with the frequent appearance of aerobic gram-negative bacilli (such as *Pseudomonas*), fungi or yeast such as *Candida albicans*, and herpesvirus hominis. *Serratia marcescens* has also rather quickly become a challenge. Anaerobic organisms such as *Clostridia*, *Bacteroides*, and *Peptostreptococcus* are increasingly common, but the organisms now most frequently responsible for hospital-acquired infections include *Staphylococcus aureus*, *Escherichia coli*, *Klebsiella*, *Enterobacter*, *Pseudomonas*, *Proteus*, *Serratia*, *Providencia*, *Herellea*, and species of *Flavobacterium*. All are common, can survive at room temperature or under refrigeration, and have potential to develop resistance to antibiotics. (See Chapter 23.)

Surgical and medical asepsis

In hospital environments surgical and medical asepsis is employed; these consist of methods to reduce the number and spread of organisms in order to prevent infection or communicable disease. This approach assumes the presence of pathogens or potential pathogens in the immediate environment and seeks to limit their transmission from one location to another. (Pathogens are those organisms capable of inducing disease or infection in human beings.) The major differences are that the methods in surgical asepsis destroy *all* microorganisms; in medical asepsis, only *pathogens* are destroyed or inhibited. The focus in surgical asepsis is to keep *all* organisms out of a designated area (a fresh wound, for example), but in medical asepsis it is to remove or destroy the pathogens in the area and to contain the remaining nonpathogens there by conscious efforts. The former employs practices embodied in "sterile technique" (use of sterile equipment, sterile fields, etc.) and the latter uses "clean technique" (hygienic measures, cleaning agents, antiseptics, disinfectants, barrier fields, etc.). Which is applied in any given situation depends largely on the susceptibility of the host, the organism's virulence, and other factors in the infectious cycle.

STERILIZATION

An object is "sterile" if it is free of *all* forms and types of life. *Sterilization* is any process that destroys all forms of life on an instrument or utensil, in a liquid, or within a substance. It is important to note that living tissue (of patients, nurses, or surgeons) cannot be sterilized by any known means without damage to that living tissue; therefore the process known as sterilization is only applied to objects. It is also important to grasp the concept as put forth by the Council on Pharmacy and Chemistry that use of the terms "sterile," "sterilizer," and "sterilization" can only be used in the absolute sense; there is no acceptable concept of *relative* steril-

ity. However, just because a piece of equipment is labeled "sterilizer" does not mean that is effective for that purpose. Nor does the term "sterilized" testify to an item's current condition of purity.

Three acceptable sterilization methods now exist. Steam under pressure (autoclaving) is preferred as most effective. Ethylene oxide is a gas sterilant used for heat-labile materials, for sharp-edged instruments that could be dulled by steam, for electrical and anesthesia equipment, and for bedding. Hot air ovens are used to sterilize glassware.

Antiseptics and disinfectants

Disinfectants and antiseptics are means, usually chemical, to kill many pathogenic microorganisms within a given population, with the general exceptions of bacterial and fungal spores, many viruses, and some very resistant bacterial strains. As a group, the effects of disinfectants and antiseptics differ from sterilization largely in degree and type of organisms destroyed. Disinfectants and antiseptics kill only pathogens while sterilizing kills all kinds of organisms.

Though some of the literature uses the terms "disinfectant" and "antiseptic" interchangeably, this is erroneous and confusing. Taken separately, disinfectants differ from antiseptics in the matter on which they are used and their degree of ability to destroy organisms. Disinfectants are used only on nonliving objects, while antiseptics are chemicals typically only applied to living tissue. Skin and mucous membranes and wounds cannot tolerate potent disinfectants, which are toxic to living tissue. Antiseptics must be less potent or made more dilute to prevent cell damage. Such lessening of potency, though crucial to viable tissue, does decrease effectiveness accordingly. Some definitions of antiseptics emphasize their inhibiting rather than destructive effects. Antiseptics can markedly differ from disinfectants in chemical composition or may simply be a dilute version of a disinfectant (for example, alcohol) for use on living tissue. Thus some chemical substances may be used both as an antiseptic and as a disinfectant depending on concentration gradient.

Antiseptics and disinfectants are further categorized as *bacteriostatic* or *bactericidal* in character. Antiseptics are most often bacteriostatic. That is, they act to prevent only the growth and replication of bacteria but do not necessarily kill off the entire bacterial population. Disinfectants, on the other hand, as bactericides, actually kill off bacteria, perhaps not all types (depending on the disinfectant, its specificity, and so on), and certainly not fungi, viruses, and spores. Other disinfectants known as *fungicides*, *virucides*, and *sporicides* are targeted specifically at these organisms. *Germicides* is an all-encompassing term for all "germs"—bacteria, fungi, viruses, and spores.

In the box below the organisms are listed according to their sensitivity to disinfectants and antiseptics in general. Factors such as the dormant and impervious spore forms of some bacteria; the waxy envelopes of the tubercle bacilli; and certain properties of some gram-positive bacteria (staphylococci and enterococci), some gram-negative ones (*Salmonella* and *Pseudomonas* species), and hepatitus viruses can make them highly refractory to any form of disinfectant or antiseptic.

Organism sensitivity to disinfectants and antiseptics

Least resistant	Bacteria
	Gram-positive and gram-negative
	Vegetative forms
	Fungi
	Viruses, lipophilic
	Influenza
	Herpes
	Vaccinia
	Rubella
	Mumps
	Varicella
	Tubercle bacilli
	Viruses, hydrophilic
	Enteroviruses
	Rhinoviruses
	Hepatitis viruses, A and B
Most resistant	Bacterial and fungal spores

Ideal antiseptic/disinfectant. The ideal all-around antiseptic/disinfectant does not yet exist. Such an ideal agent would have to:

1 Be destructive to all forms of microorganisms without being toxic to human cells
2 Have a low incidence of hypersensitivity
3 Be active in the presence of organic matter
4 Be stable, noncorrosive, and inexpensive

An *effective* disinfectant kills in 10 minutes all vegetative bacteria (not spores) and fungi, tubercle bacilli, animal parasites, and viruses (but not hepatitis viruses).

To place the concepts of sterilization, disinfection, and antisepsis in perspective, it should be clear that these processes differ in the degree to which they destroy organisms. Thus anything that is sterile can also be considered both disinfected and antiseptic. All of these processes correctly begin with handwashing, even when gloves are worn. It has been repeatedly demonstrated that clean, washed hands are a crucial factor to deter microorganism growth, reproduction, and transmission in any environment.

Mechanisms of action. Antiseptics and disinfectants may act in three ways.

1 They may bring about a change in the structure of the protein of the microbial cell (denaturation), which often proceeds to coagulation of protein with increased concentration of the chemical agent.
2 They may lower the surface tension of the aqueous medium of the parasitic cell. This increases the permeability of the plasma membrane, and the cellular constituents are destroyed by lysis. The cell is unable to maintain its equilibrium in its environment. (The surface-active agents are thought to act this way.)
3 They may interfere with some metabolic processes of the microbial cells in such ways as to interfere with the cell's ability to survive and multiply.

• • •

The following section groups the antiseptics and disinfectant into related chemical groups such as phenol and related compounds, dyes, heavy metals, halogenated compounds, oxidizing agents, surface-active agents, and a miscellaneous group. Each will include individual antiseptics or disinfectants most commonly used in medical asepsis and how they are most commonly employed in nursing practice and health care.

Phenol and related compounds
Phenol (carbolic acid, Lysol, VesPhene, Staphene)

Phenol is believed to exert its germicidal action by altering the structure of the protein in the parasitic cells (denaturation). In high concentrations it precipitates cellular protein. It is not affected much by the presence of organic matter or by high concentrations of bacteria. The use of phenol has declined because better disinfectants have been found that are less irritating, less toxic to human tissues, and more efficient in killing microorganisms.

Solutions of phenol are antiseptic, germicidal, or escharotic (scarring to tissue), depending on the concentration used. Antiseptic solutions are irritating or toxic to tissues, and concentrated solutions may produce death when taken internally or when applied topically to abraded surfaces of the skin. When applied locally, phenol penetrates the skin and exerts a local anesthetic effect on sensory nerve endings. This explains its presence in certain lotions or ointments used to relieve itching (antipruritics).

In aqueous solutions of from 0.1% to 3%, phenol kills bacteria, fungi, and lipophilic viruses, is inconsistently effective against tubercle bacilli, and is ineffective against hydrophilic viruses and spores. Phenol is rapid acting against bacteria but corrosive to equipment and irritating to tissues. It may also be toxic. The 1% and 2% solutions kill all but the hepatitis virus, bacteria, and fungal spores within 20 minutes. However, even the spores are destroyed on smooth, hard surfaces, tubing and catheters, hinged instruments, floors, furniture, and walls for 12 hours after contact with phenol products.

Cresol

Cresol is available as a mixture of the orthometa-, and para-methyl phenols and is derived from coal tar. Cresols are phenols in which one of the hydrogen atoms in the benzene ring has been replaced by a methyl group (CH_3).

Cresol is a thick, heavy, straw-colored liquid with a phenol-like odor. It is two to five times as active as phenol but no more toxic. It is only slightly soluble in water but is soluble in liquid soap. Preparations of cresol are used for disinfecting excreta, sinks, bedpans, toilets, and the like. All are poisonous and should be used for external purposes only or as mentioned. If cresol is accidentally spilled on the skin, a burning sensation will be noted. The area should be washed with copious amounts of water to prevent a painful burn.

Saponated cresol solution. This is a 50% solution of cresol in vegetable oil (saponified). This solution is also known as Lysol.

Lysol forms a milky emulsion in water, but it is more soluble than pure cresol. Its action is not hampered by the presence of organic material. It is used in 2% to 5% strength to disinfect excreta, sinks, toilets, bedpans, and similar utensils. Like the other cresols and phenol, it is poisonous.

Hexachlorophene (hexachlorophane)

Hexachlorophene is a chlorinated diphenol. It is a white to light tan powder and is relatively insoluble in water but soluble in alcohol, fats, and soaps. It is incorporated into detergent creams, oils, soaps, lotions, ointments, shampoos, and other media for topical application to reduce numbers of pathogenic bacteria on the skin and to reduce the incidence of pyogenic skin infections. It is much more effective against gram-positive than against gram-negative bacteria. Optimal effects are secured only when regular and repeated applications are made. If other cleansing agents are substituted, a rapid increase of organisms normally found on the skin may be observed.

Regularly repeated scrubs leave a residual film on the skin that causes a steady decrease in bacterial flora. This antiseptic property permits a 2-minute preoperative scrub.

Antibacterial detergents have been used to prevent and control staphylococcal infections spread by hospital personnel. To control hospital nursery infections a 1% to 3% hexachlorophene preparation can be used for short-term, once daily bathing followed by rinsing.

Hexachlorophene should not be regarded as a substitute for mechanical cleansing of the skin, although products containing this substance are used for preoperative preparation of the skin. It is also used by food handlers and dentists. Its activity is reduced by the presence of organic material and blood serum. Alcohol and other organic solvents should be avoided when hexachlorophene is used.

Precautions. According to the AMA, hexachlorophene should not be used routinely to bathe infants, particularly premature infants, since it can be absorbed and cause neurotoxic effects. In animals it has caused degeneration of the brain. Its use on the skin of any age group should be followed by thorough rinsing.

Cardiovascular disturbances, convulsions, and respiratory arrest have been reported following accidental ingestion or applications of high concentrations (6%) to children.

Preparation

Hexachlorophene liquid soap (pHisoHex liquid soap). pHisoHex is a sudsing skin cleanser that combines several compounds in addition to hexachlorophene. It is bacteriostatic against staphylococci and other gram-positive bacteria. Repeated use leaves an accumulated antibacterial residue that is resistant to solvents, soaps, and detergents for several days. Its action is inhibited in the presence of organic matter or alcohols. The soap contains between 225 and 260 mg hexachlorophene in each 100 ml of 10% to 13% potassium soap base.

USES. pHisoHex is used for routine personnel handwashing, occasionally for patient bathing before surgery, and as a surgical scrub for personnel.

For surgical scrub *without a brush*, a preliminary wash is done for 20 to 30 seconds, adding only a small amount of water; a sudsy 2- to 4-minute scrub is then performed, followed by thorough rinsing. For surgical scrub *with a brush*, the first scrub (as above) is followed by a scrub of varying length using a hand brush (see manufacturer's instructions) depending on the frequency with which pHisoHex has been routinely used by that individual.

PRECAUTIONS. One must rinse off promptly and thoroughly after washing with pHisoHex.

Contact with eyes should be avoided. If any signs of central nervous system irritation occur, use should be discontinued. pHisoHex should not be swallowed or ingested.

CONTRAINDICATIONS. pHisoHex should not be used on mucous membranes or burned or denuded skin. To avoid absorption of this product, it must not be left in contact with skin for any length of time without rinsing (that is, avoid in occlusive dressings, wet packs, lotions, or vaginal packs). It should not be used frequently for bathing, especially of newborns or infants, since it can be absorbed and cause neurotoxicity. Hypersensitivity to any components in this product or halogenated phenol derivatives is a certain contraindication.

SIDE EFFECTS AND TOXIC EFFECTS. Dermatitis, photosensitivity, redness, and drying of skin have been seen. Ingestion may result in anorexia, nausea, vomiting, cramps, diarrhea, dehydration, hypotension, convulsions, shock, or death.

• • •

Hexachlorophene is also found in several other compounds such as Burdeo, a nongreasy gel, and pHisoDerm, pHisoAc, and pHisoDan (the last three are over-the-counter products).

Resorcinol

Resorcinol resembles phenol in effectiveness, but it is less toxic, irritating, and caustic. It is used chiefly as an antiseptic and keratolytic (softening or dissolving the keratin-containing epidermis) in the treatment of acne and various diseases of the skin. It is used in strengths that vary from 2% to 20%. It acts by precipitating cell proteins.

This compound occurs as colorless needle-shaped crystals with a faint odor. It is applied topically as an ointment, lotion, or paste.

Compound resorcinol ointment contains 6% resorcinol in a number of media to make a suitable ointment.

Hexylresorcinol

Hexylresorcinol was first introduced as a urinary antiseptic. Much of its efficiency is the result of its low surface tension. This accounts for the name "ST 37" that is used for a 1:1000 solution of hexylresorcinol in glycerin and water.

Hexylresorcinol is stainless and odorless, but it may be irritating to tissues. Persons who become hypersensitive to it may exhibit allergic reactions. It is used as a topical antiseptic for use on cuts, abrasions, burns, scalds, and sunburns and for mouth care. It also has a mild anesthetic, soothing effect on pain.

Thymol

Thymol is a colorless crystalline solid with an aromatic odor and taste. Chemically, it is related to one of the cresols and is more effective than phenol. It possesses fungicidal properties, and it is an effective anthelmintic for hookworm. Because of its pleasant odor and taste it is an ingredient of many gargles and mouthwashes.

Dyes

Certain dyes are used as antiseptics and antiprotozoal agents as well as to promote the healing of wounds. Because they are rapidly adsorbed on proteins, they exhibit limited ability to penetrate tissues, and their germicidal action tends to be slow.

Triphenylmethane dyes (rosaniline dyes)

Triphenylmethane dyes are a group of basic dyes that include crystal violet, gentian violet, methyl violet, brilliant green, and fuchsin. Solutions of these dyes are used in the form of antiseptic dressings on wounds, serous surfaces, and mucous membranes, or they are applied topically for the treatment of superficial fungous or gram-positive infections of the skin and mucous membranes. Gentian violet is also used in the treatment of certain types of worm infestation. Concentrations of 1:1000 to 1:5000 are used for direct application to tissues. For instillation into body cavities the concentration is decreased to 1:10,000.

Gentian violet; crystal violet. Gentian violet is available in bulk powder and in tablet form containing 10, 15, and 30 mg.

Gentian violet solution. The solution consists mainly of gentian violet with some admixture of the other two violet compounds. It is a 1% solution of the dyes in 10% alcohol.

Carbol-fuchsin solution (Castellani's paint). This Carbolfuchsin solution contains fuchsin, phenol, resorcinol, and boric acid in an acetone-alcohol-water solution. It is used in the treatment of fungous infections. Fuchsin is para-rosaniline chloride and is a red dye.

Heavy metals
MERCURY COMPOUNDS
INORGANIC COMPOUNDS

Inorganic compounds of mercury were among the earliest antiseptics to be used, and they long were regarded as potent germicides. Investigation has shown that their action, in many instances, is bacteriostatic rather than bactericidal, since their effects can be reversed under some conditions and microorganisms have been revived that were previously considered dead. Although the mercuric ion brings about the precipitation of cellular proteins, its bacteriostatic action is said to be the result of inhibition of specific enzymes of bacterial cells. Mercurial antiseptics may also exert toxic effects on the tissue cells of the host when taken internally. The mercurials fall far short of being ideal antiseptics or germicides. The inorganic compounds are irritating to tissues, penetrate poorly, are toxic systemically, are adversely affected by the presence of organic materials, have little or no action on spores, and are corrosive to metals. However, they are effective bacteriostatic agents for certain uses. Some of the organic compounds are more potent than the inorganic ones, especially if they are in alcoholic solution. Some authorities believe that certain organic mercurials are useful antiseptics if used appropriately in proper concentration.

MERCURIAL OINTMENTS

A number of compounds of mercury and metallic mercury are incorporated into ointments for use as antiseptics. The drug slowly dissolves in the tissues to release a low concentration of mercuric ions and thus exerts a prolonged effect.

Ammoniated mercury ointment (White Precipitate Ointment)

The American preparation contains 5% ammoniated mercury and has a base of white ointment and liquid petrolatum. The British preparation contains 2.5% ammoniated mercury and is made with simple ointment. Ammoniated mercury is also used in ointments of 2% to 10% concentrations as antiseptics and local stimulants in cases of suppurating dermatitis, eczematous and parasitic skin diseases, and particularly impetigo.

Ammoniated mercury ophthalmic ointment

Ammoniated mercury ophthalmic ointment contains 3% ammoniated mercury and is applied as an antiseptic to the eyelids.

ORGANIC MERCURIAL PREPARATIONS

Organic mercurial compounds are less toxic and less irritating than the inorganic mercurial antiseptics.

Merbromin (Mercurochrome)

The 2% aqueous solution of merbromin acts as a mild topical bacteriostatic for minor cuts, scratches, burns, and abrasions. Mercurochrome has very low toxicity even if swallowed, but it leaves a bright red stain. It is less effective as an antiseptic than other, newer products.

Thimerosal (Merthiolate)

Thimerosal is a light cream-colored, crystalline powder. It contains about 50% mercury. It is colored red by a coal-tar color so it leaves a red stain after application. It is used as a topical organomercurial bacteriostatic and fungistatic for abrasions or skin and mucous membranes, for wounds, or for surgical preparation of skin. It is also used as a preservative in biologic preparations such as vaccines and tissue grafts. It is available in many pharmaceutical forms including aqueous solutions, tinctures, and ointment. It is contraindicated in patients with hypersensitivity to it or to mercury radicals. Thimerosal is incompatible with acids, heavy metal salts, iodine, and whole blood but is not inactivated by plasma or serum, soaps, cotton materials, organic lipids, or proteins. It may be toxic if swallowed.

Nitromersol (Metaphen); nitromersol tincture

A 0.5% solution of nitromersol in acetone, alcohol, and water is used chiefly as a skin disinfectant. Nitromersol solution is an aqueous solution sometimes used to disinfect instruments in concentrations of 1:1000 to 1:5000; to disinfect the skin it is used in a concentration of 1:1000 to 1:5000; and for irrigation of mucous membranes (eye and urethra) it is used in a concentration of 1:5000 to 1:10,000.

PHENYLMERCURIC COMPOUNDS

Phenylmercuric compounds are active against a variety of pathogenic bacteria and exhibit a low level of toxicity in human tissue. Like other mercurial antiseptics, they cannot be depended on to kill spores. These compounds occasionally cause irritation and poisoning in persons of undue sensitivity. Buffered solutions are odorless, colorless, and stainless and do not react with body proteins. They are noncorrosive to metals with the exception of aluminum, and they do not destroy rubber.

Phenylmercuric nitrate (Merphenyl Nitrate Basic)

This drug is applied topically in 1:1500 solutions for prophylactic disinfection of intact skin and minor injuries and in 1:1500 to 1:24,000 solutions for mucous membranes and wet dressings.

SILVER COMPOUNDS
INORGANIC SALTS

Silver compounds are used in medicine for their antiseptic, caustic, and astringent effects, which are caused by the release of free silver ions. The soluble salts of silver ionize readily in solution, whereas the colloidal silver compounds dissociate only slightly. Silver ions will precipitate cellular protein; inorganic salts of silver are germicidal in solution but colloidal preparations are bacteriostatic. It is thought that silver, like mercury, is capable of interfering with important metabolic activities of microbial cells. Stains on objects such as shoes may be removed with household chlorine bleach.

Silver nitrate

Silver nitrate occurs as flat, transparent crystals that become grayish black on exposure to light and in the presence of organic material. It is odorless and has a bitter, strongly metallic taste. It is freely soluble in water, ionizes readily, and is germicidal. Silver nitrate reacts with soluble chloride, iodides, and bromides to form insoluble salts; therefore, the action of silver salts can be stopped by contact with a solution of sodium chloride. This chemical property also explains why solutions of silver salts penetrate tissues slowly as a result of the precipitation of silver ions in the tissues by chlorides or phosphates. A 1:1000 solution is antiseptic. Weak solutions are astringent on mucous membranes, and strong solutions are caustic when applied to mucous membranes or the skin. Silver salts stain tissues black because of the deposit of silver. This discoloration slowly disappears.

Silver nitrate is used on inflamed mucous membranes and ulcerated surfaces. For diseases of the conjunctiva, solutions varying in strength from 0.2% to 2% may be used. To prevent the development of gonorrheal conjunctivitis in the newborn infant, a drop or two of 1% solution is instilled into each eye as soon as possible after delivery. A stronger solution has been used, but it is dangerous, because strong solutions will kill tissue in a short time and may permit the gonococci to enter and spread into deeper tissues. Blindness has been caused in this way. To stop the action if too much has been used, the eye should be washed with physiologic saline solution. Even a 1% silver nitrate solution produces a chemical conjunctivitis in a rather large number of cases. For this reason, some physicians have advocated the use of penicillin ointment. Silver nitrate is also used as a wet dressing for treatment of burns in a 0.5% solution. Solutions of silver nitrate that vary in concentration from 1:1000 to 1:10,000 are used for irrigation of the bladder and urethra. A 1:1000 solution is germicidal but irritating. Long-continued use of any silver preparation may produce permanent discoloration of the skin and mucous membranes, a condition known as argyria.

Toughened silver nitrate (Lunar Caustic)

Toughened silver nitrate is a white solid generally used in the form of pencils or cones. It is applied as a mild caustic to wounds, ulcers, warts, and granulation tissue. It should be moistened before use and, to avoid blackening the fingers, should be held with forceps. It may be fused on a probe for application to parts with difficult access. The mucous membranes to which solutions of silver nitrate are applied should receive a preliminary cleansing to remove mucus, pus, and food that would interfere with drug action.

Silver sulfadiazine (Silvadene Cream)

Silver sulfadiazine is often used to replace silver nitrate in the topical treatment of extensive burns. Each gram of Silvadene Cream contains 10 mg silver sulfadiazine for the prevention and treatment of infection in second- and third-degree burn wounds. It is bactericidal (to both gram-negative and gram-positive bacteria) and is destructive to yeasts. It may also be bacteriostatic to some organisms resistant to other agents. Other proteolytic enzyme products used along with Silvadene Cream may be inactivated. Burn wounds should be cleansed and debrided before the cream is applied. It should be thinly applied once or twice a day to a depth of approximately $\frac{1}{16}$ inch. Covering dressings are not required. Treatment should be continued until any possibility of infection is past. Contraindications include hypersensitivity to silver or a glucose-6-phosphate dehydrogenase deficiency.

COLLOIDAL SILVER PREPARATIONS

Colloidal preparations do not ionize readily and do not act as corrosives, irritants, or astringents. They penetrate tissue more readily than do the solutions of simple salts of silver. They exert a bacteriostatic effect because of the concentration of silver ions that is gradually produced.

The colloidal preparations of silver are used as antiseptics, particularly on mucous membranes of the nose and throat, the urinary bladder, the urethra, and the conjunctiva. Gonococci are particularly susceptible to the action of silver compounds.

The terms "strong" and "mild" refer to the relative antiseptic values and not to the amount of silver they contain, for the strong preparation contains about 8% silver and the weak contains about 20%. The antiseptic value depends on the extent of ionization in any given liquid. Mild silver protein preparations should be freshly made and dispensed in amber-colored bottles.

Strong silver protein (Protargol)

Strong silver compound contains not less than 7.5% and not more than 8.5% of silver.

Mild silver protein (Argyrol, Silvol)

The mild form contains from 19% to 23% silver. It is entirely nonirritating but it also has less antiseptic action than the strong silver protein. It is usually employed in concentrations of 5% to 25%. A concentration of 5% is commonly used for bladder irrigation, 10% to 15% in the nose, and 20% to 25% in the eye.

Halogens
CHLORINE

Chlorine is a nonmetallic element that occurs in the form of a greenish yellow gas. It has an intensely disagreeable odor. One part of chlorine in 10,000 parts of air causes irritation of the respiratory tract, and exposure to a 1:1000 concentration is fatal after 5 minutes. It causes spasm and pain of the muscles of the larynx and bronchial tubes, coughing, a burning sensation, fainting, unconsciousness, and death. Its extensive use for the purification of water, however, makes it one of the most widely used disinfectants. One part of chlorine in 1 million parts of water will destroy most bacteria in a few minutes. Acid-fast organisms such as *Mycobacterium tuberculosis* are unusually resistant to it. Chlorine is effective against amebas, viruses, organisms of the colon-typhoid group, and many of the spore-forming pathogens. The antibacterial action of chlorine is said to be caused by the formation of hypochlorous acid, which results when chlorine reacts with water. Hypochlorous acid is a rapidly acting bactericidal agent. Its effect is partly the result of its oxidizing action and partly of its effect on

microbial enzymes that are concerned with the metabolism of glucose.

The activity of chlorine and chlorine-releasing compounds is influenced by a number of factors, such as the presence of organic material, the pH of the solution, and the temperature. Chlorine is more effective when there is a minimum of organic matter, when the medium is acid in reaction, and when the temperature is elevated. Chlorine is an efficient deodorant and a strong bleaching agent, and it corrodes many metals.

Gaseous chlorine has limited usefulness because it is difficult to handle. There are a number of compounds that yield hypochlorous acid and that are useful for certain kinds of disinfection.

Sodium hypochlorite solution

This is a 5% solution of sodium hypochlorite. This concentration is too great to be used on living tissues. It is used to disinfect utensils and swimming pools.

Diluted sodium hypochlorite solution, modified
Dakin's solution

This preparation is a 0.5% aqueous solution of sodium hypochlorite. It was once used extensively in the treatment of suppurating wounds. Although it is useful in cleansing wounds, it also interferes with the formation of thrombin, delays clotting of blood, and is irritating to the skin. Dilute solutions have been used to prevent the development of athlete's foot (epidermophytosis). A 0.5% solution of sodium hypochlorite is also used to disinfect walls, furniture, and especially floors. Preparations of sodium hypochlorite are unstable and need to be freshly prepared.

CHLORAMINES

Several compounds are available in which chlorine is linked with nitrogen. The chloramines exert their effects by the release of chlorine to form hypochlorous acid and also by direct action of the parent compound. The chloramines are more stable, less irritating, and slower acting than the hypochlorites. Their action is more prolonged and they are less readily affected by the presence of organic material.

Chloramine-T, chloramine

Chloramine-T is used in 0.1% to 2% aqueous solutions for irrigations of wounds or for dressings.

Halazone

Halazone is available in 4-mg tablets and is employed for the sterilization of drinking water. All pathogens usually found in water will be killed in 30 to 60 minutes by the addition of one or two tablets (4 to 8 mg) per liter of water.

IODINE

Iodine is a heavy, bluish black, crystalline solid that has a metallic luster and a characteristic odor. It is slightly soluble in water but is soluble in alcohol and in aqueous solutions of sodium and potassium iodide. Iodine is volatile, and its solutions should not be exposed to air except during use. The mechanism of disinfectant action is not entirely known. The concentration at which iodine acts as a disinfectant is similar for all bacteria. Iodine is thought to be one of the more efficient chemical disinfectants in present-day usage. Its activity does not vary greatly for vegetative pathogens; it is effective over a wide range of pH, and it is effective against spores, viruses, and fungi. It is not affected by the presence of organic material found in body fluids and exudates. In combination with alcohol, iodine in 0.5% to 1% solution will kill tubercle bacilli. However, iodine does not kill spores readily, and it has the disadvantage of staining skin and clothing. In rare instances, individuals exhibit hypersensitivity reactions to iodine when it is applied to the skin. Iodine is used chiefly for disinfection of small wounds and abraded surfaces in the preoperative preparations of skin surfaces. A fact often overlooked is that aqueous solutions as well as alcoholic solutions of iodine are germicidal. Aqueous solutions are less irritating and are best used on abraded areas of the skin. Iodine penetrates the skin and slight amounts are absorbed.

Another use that may be made of iodine tinc-

ture is the emergency disinfection of water that is suspected of harboring pathogenic amebas. Three drops of iodine tincture to a quart of water will kill amebas and bacteria in 15 minutes without making the water unpalatable.

Iodine stains the skin and linens a brown color. These stains can be removed from the skin with alcohol or ammonia and from fabrics with boiling water.

Iodine tincture

Iodine tincture contains 2% iodine and 2.4% sodium iodide in 46% ethyl alcohol. It has to a great extent replaced the strong iodine tincture. Weak iodine solution contains approximately the same amount of iodine along with potassium iodide and 90% ethyl alcohol.

Strong iodine tincture

This form is an alcoholic solution containing 7% iodine and 5% potassium iodide in 83% ethyl alcohol.

Strong iodine solution (Lugol's Solution)

Strong iodine solution is similar in preparation to strong iodine tincture. The aqueous solution contains 5% iodine and 10% potassium iodide. It is given orally for the treatment of goiter rather than for its antiseptic effect.

Iodine solution

This aqueous solution contains 2% iodine and 2.4% sodium iodide.

IODOPHORS

Iodophors are complex combinations of iodine and a carrier or agent that increases the water solubility of iodine. The word literally means "iodine carrier." The combination contains and slowly releases iodine as it is needed but does not stain as aqueous solutions of iodine do. As used today, it frequently means a combination of iodine and a detergent. *Wescodyne* is one that is said to kill tubercle bacilli as well as other organisms sensitive to iodine. Undecoylium chloride-iodine (Virac) is a combination of iodine and a cationic detergent that is said to make a useful surface-acting agent.

Povidone-iodine solution (Betadine, PVP, Isodine)

Povidone-iodine is an organic iodine and polyvinylpyrrolidone complex. It is water soluble, and when the solution is used as an antiseptic, the complex breaks down on contact with the skin or mucous membranes and free iodine is slowly released. This preparation has the advantage of combining the desirable properties of iodine as a potent germicide with a highly antibacterial, surface-acting agent. It is thought to be superior to soap, hexachlorophene scrubs, and cationic agents as a skin disinfectant but may be somewhat less effective than aqueous or alcoholic solutions of iodine. It is relatively nonirritating, nontoxic, and nonsensitizing to the skin except in those persons sensitive to iodine.

Povidone-iodine is used as an antiseptic on the skin, mucous membranes, and scalp and for surgical preparation of the skin. Available solutions contain 0.75%, 1%, or 1.5% of available iodine.

Oxidizing agents

Certain oxidizing agents are destructive to pathogenic organisms but mild enough to be used on living tissues. Their activity is caused by the oxygen that they liberate. Oxygen combines readily with organic matter and, once combined, it is inert. Oxygen is especially harmful to anaerobic organisms. On the whole, microorganisms vary considerably in their sensitivity to oxygen.

Hydrogen peroxide solution

Hydrogen peroxide solution is a 3% to 6% solution of hydrogen peroxide in water. It is a colorless, odorless liquid that deteriorates on standing. It should be kept in a cool, dark place and should be well stoppered. Hydrogen peroxide decomposes to water and oxygen. This reaction occurs rapidly when the solution is in contact with organic matter. It is an active germicide only while it is actively releasing oxygen. Solutions have a high surface tension and do not penetrate readily. The effervescence (caused by rapid formation of oxygen bubbles) that accompanies decomposition helps to clean suppurating wounds, but it should not be injected into closed body cavities or into abscesses from which the newly formed gas cannot easily escape. The official solution is usually diluted with 1 to 4 parts of water before it is used. It is used for the cleansing of wounds, for repair of cleft lip, and for the treatment of Vincent's infection (trench mouth). In the latter case it is employed full strength for a limited period of time. Nurses use it frequently to remove collections of mucus from the inner cannula of a tracheostomy tube.

Medicinal zinc peroxide

Medicinal zinc peroxide consists of zinc peroxide, zinc carbonate, and zinc hydroxide. On hydrolysis it yields hydrogen peroxide. It has some value in the disinfection and deodorization of wounds, especially those infected with anaerobic organisms. It leaves a residue of zinc oxide that is slightly astringent in effect.

Potassium permanganate

Potassium permanganate occurs as dark purple crystals that are soluble in water (1:15). It decomposes on contact with organic matter and liberates oxygen, which combines with bacteria and inhibits their growth or destroys them. The bactericidal efficiency of solutions of potassium permanganate vary with the type of organism and the amount of organic material present. Solutions stronger than 1:5000 may be irritating to tissues. It is used in vaginal douches in concentrations of 1:1000 to 1:5000 and is applied topically in concentrations of 1:500 to 1:10,000. After potassium permanganate solutions have lost oxygen they appear brown and are inert. Stains may be removed with dilute acids (lemon juice, oxalic acid, or dilute hydrochloric acid).

Potassium permanganate solutions produce irritant, astringent, deodorant, and germicidal effects. It is used much less now than formerly.

Sodium perborate. This is a white powder soluble in water. In solution it forms hydrogen peroxide. It is used as a dusting powder or in 2% solution as an oral antiseptic. Its chief use is in the treatment of Vincent's infection.

Antiseptics and disinfectants   **761**

Chlorhexidine

Chlorhexidine gluconate (Hibiclens, Hibitane Tincture)

Chlorhexidine is a biguanide with potent antiseptic activity. It is effective against both gram-positive and gram-negative bacteria. Its mechanism of action is by disrupting the plasma membrane of the bacterial cell.

Hibiclens is a bactericidal skin cleanser containing chlorhexidine gluconate. It is useful as a surgical scrub, a handwash for personnel, and a skin wound cleanser. As a preoperative skin preparation for patients, Hibiclens is available in tinted or nontinted tinctures combined with isopropyl alcohol. Hibitane Tincture should be applied liberally to the surgical site, swabbed for 2 minutes or more, then the area dried. This routine should be repeated once more and the area allowed to air dry. The tinted tincture will visibly mark the prepared area. Both tinctures have a persistent bactericidal effect against many gram-positive and gram-negative bacteria (such as *Pseudomonas aeruginosa*) and are not affected by the presence of exudate or blood.

For surgical scrub, hands and forearms are scrubbed with approximately 5 ml Hibiclens for 3 minutes without water while using a brush or sponge. After rinsing, the wash is repeated for 3 minutes.

As a handwash, it is used for about 15 seconds. Skin wounds should be washed gently with Hibiclens and rinsed. Hibiclens should be kept out of eyes and ears. (There have been reports of deafness when these products came in contact with the middle ear through a perforated eardrum.) Rare secondary effects include dermatitis, photosensitivity, and irritation of mucosal tissue. These products should be stored below 104° F.

Surface-active agents

Surface-active agents are also known as wetting agents, emulsifiers, and detergents. In some respects, certain of these agents are considered superior to ordinary soap because they can be used in hard water, are stable in both acid and alkaline solutions, decrease surface tension more effectively, and are less irritating to the skin than ordinary soaps. They all lower surface tensions and aid in the mechanical removal of bacteria and soil. Many also exert a bactericidal action. Many are believed to depress metabolic activities of bacteria, but how they do it is not fully known. They have a weak action against fungi, acid-fast organisms, spores, and viruses. Their activity is reduced greatly by the presence of organic matter. If the active portion of the surface-active agent (surfactant) carries a negative electric charge, it is known as an anionic compound; if the active portion carries a positive charge, it is known as a cationic surfactant or surface-active agent.

CATIONIC AGENTS

The most effective cationic agents have been the quaternary ammonium compounds (sometimes referred to as "quats"). These compounds combine detergent and antiseptic action. In general, they are more effective antiseptics than the anionic group of compounds. They inhibit both gram-positive and gram-negative organisms. Soap inactivates cationic detergents and therefore it must be removed before the detergent is used. Hard water also inactivates these agents and causes precipitation. Although they are recomended in the final rinse of laundry materials, they are often ineffective because traces of soap or hard water remain. Cationic detergents cannot be relied on to sterilize instruments and articles that cannot be subjected to heat, but they are sometimes used to preserve sterility of stored materials. They have also been used in aerosols to increase the penetrating power of antibiotics.

Benzalkonium chloride (Zephiran Chloride)

When employed in proper concentration, benzalkonium chloride is a somewhat effective, relatively noninjurious surface disinfectant. It is germicidal for a number of pathogenic nonsporeforming pathogens, including fungi after several minutes of exposure. However, it has no effect on tubercle bacilli. Its viricidal activity is said to be limited. Benzalkonium chloride solutions have a low surface tension and possess keratolytic, detergent, and emulsifying properties. Solutions of soap reduce its germicidal activity unless well rinsed from the area to be disinfected. Seventy percent alcohol serves to diminish the reaction of both the soap and the disinfectant. Alcohol can be used *after* the skin has been prepared with soap and water and *before* the disinfectant is applied.

Solutions of benzalkonium chloride have a relatively low level of toxicity when used as recommended.

It is suitable for prophylactic disinfection of the intact skin and in the treatment of superficial injuries when used in 1:1000 concentration (tincture).

Solutions of 1:1000 are used for preservation of metallic instruments and rubber articles. For disinfection of operating room equipment, solutions of 1:5000 may be used. Although it is noncorrosive, odorless, and stable, its limited effectiveness and documented ability to support growth of contaminants has caused the Centers for Disease Control to recommend other agents (such as alcohols or alcohol-iodine combinations).

Benzethonium chloride (Phemerol Chloride)

Benzethonium chloride is a detergent that exerts an inhibitory effect on the growth activities of commonly occurring bacteria and fungi. Tincture of phemerol chloride 1:500 and benzethonium chloride solution 1:1000 are used full strength as general germicides and antiseptics except for use in the nose and eye. For the latter, the aqueous solution is used and diluted with 4 parts of water.

Cetylpyridinium chloride (Ceepryn Chloride)

Cetylpyridinium chloride is used for preoperative disinfection of intact skin, in the treatment of minor wounds, and for the therapeutic disinfection of mucous membranes. Its effectiveness is reduced by detergents, ordinary soap, and serums and tissue fluids, and it is ineffective against clostridial spores. Strengths used vary from 1:100 for skin preparations, to 1:1000 for minor abrasions, to 1:5000 and 1:10,000 for mucous membranes.

Methylbenzethonium chloride (Diaparene Chloride)

-Methylbenzethonium chloride produces bacteriostasis of urea-splitting organisms. It is used for disinfecting babies' diapers and linen and clothing of incontinent adults; the articles should be free of soap, however, before being rinsed in this disinfectant. It is available in 0.09-g tablets, and the solution is made by dissolving 1 tablet in 2000 ml warm water. This amount is sufficient for rinsing six diapers. They should remain immersed in disinfectant for 3 minutes.

ANIONIC SURFACE AGENTS

Anionic surface agents are the neutral or faintly alkaline salts of acids of high molecular weights. Common soaps and a number of other compounds belong to this group. They are incompatible with cationic compounds. They act best in an acid medium and are most effective against gram-positive organisms.

Tincture of green soap

Tincture of green soap is an alcoholic solution containing about 65% soft soap perfumed with oil of lavender. It is called green because it was first made from oils that contain chlorophyl-like coloring matter. Modern "green soap" may be colorless.

Green soap; soft soap

Green soap is a potassium soap made by the saponification of vegetable oils without the removal of glycerin. Soft soap has little antiseptic value but is used as a cleansing agent.

Hexachlorophene liquid soap

This is a potassium soap to which hexachlorophene has been added.

Sodium tetradecyl sulfate (Sodium Sotradecol)

Sodium tetradecyl sulfate is an anionic surface-acting agent that lowers surface tension of certain antiseptic solutions to which it may be added. It is also used as a sclerosing agent in the treatment of varicose veins and internal hemorrhoids.

• • •

Other anionic surface agents include pHisoDerm, which is a synthetic compound sometimes used as a substitute for soap. It is available as a cream or creamy emulsion. It is sometimes used for certain dermatologic conditions when soap is contraindicated. pHisoHex is pHisoDerm to which 3% hexachlorophene has been added. It exerts a prolonged antiseptic as well as emollient effect when used routinely. pHisoHex is used frequently for preoperative preparation of patients' skin.

Alcohols/aldehydes/acids

ALCOHOLS

Alcohols are organic solvent solutions that are effective in the destruction of gram-positive and gram-negative bacteria, fungi, lipophilic viruses, and tubercle bacilli. They are ineffective against hydrophilic viruses (hepatitis) and spores. Alcohols may be inactivated in the presence of organic matter. They are inexpensive, leave no residue on evaporation, and are noncorrosive to equipment, but they are volatile and drying to the skin.

Preparations include commercially packaged skin preparations, in combination with iodine (for thermometers) or formaldehyde, both effective combinations. Alcohols are also used for disinfection of heat-labile instruments, polyethylene tubing, catheters, implants, prostheses, smooth hard-surfaced objects, hinged instruments, inhalation and anesthesia equipment, and the like. Ethanol may be slightly more effective than the other alcohols against tubercle bacilli, enteroviruses, hepatitis viruses, and spores.

Alcohol, ethanol, ethyl alcohol

Alcohol is one of the oldest and most widely used of the skin disinfectants. Both ethyl alcohol and isopropyl alcohol are used as disinfectants, and their germicidal power is said to be underrated. They are used extensively to prepare the skin prior to venipuncture, subcutaneous and intramuscular injection, and ear or finger pricks for samples of blood. Ethyl alcohol is reported to be most effective in concentrations of 50% to 70%. The growth of some organisms is said to be inhibited by a 1% solution, although the bactericidal action is unreliable when the concentration falls below 20% or is above 95%.

Isopropyl alcohol

Isopropyl alcohol is slightly more antiseptic than ethyl alcohol. It is employed full strength (99%) or as *isopropyl rubbing alcohol,* which is a 70% aqueous solution. It is also used extensively as a 75% aqueous solution for the disinfection and storage of oral thermometers. It can be combined with other disinfectants, such as formaldehyde solution, to make a more effective germicide.

ALDEHYDES
Formaldehyde solution

Formaldehyde in a gaseous form is a powerful parasiticide because of its penetrating power, but it is active only in the presence of abundant moisture. It was used formerly for the fumigation of rooms.

Formaldehyde solution is a 37% solution of formaldehyde (by weight) known as formalin. It is a clear, colorless liquid that, on exposure to air, liberates a pungent, irritating gas. In proper concentration formaldehyde solution is germicidal against all forms of microorganisms. A 0.5% solution will kill all organisms, including spores, in 6 to 12 hours. Higher concentrations are effective in less time. It is not affected by organic matter, and it is effective against viruses. It acts as a precipitant of protein.

Formaldehyde solution hardens tissues, and for this reason it is used as a preservative for specimens and as an astringent. When it is combined with isopropyl alcohol or hexachlorophene, it is probably the most powerful germicidal solution available at the present time. Various modifications of the Bard-Parker germicidal solution are made with formaldehyde solution, isopropyl alcohol, and antirust agents for the disinfection of instruments and articles that cannot be subjected to heat. These solutions are sometimes called "cold sterilization solutions."

The chief disadvantage encountered in using solutions of formaldehyde is that they are irritating to tissues and mucous membranes and have an unpleasant odor.

Glutaraldehyde (Cidex)

The 2% solution of glutaraldehyde with a pH of 7.4 to 8.9 has been found to disinfect against bacteria (works rapidly against both gram-negative and gram-positive bacteria) and their spores (in 3 hours), fungi, and lipophilic viruses. It is not inactivated by organic material. It should be used undiluted as a disinfectant and is especially recommended for use on hinged or lensed instruments, inhalation or anesthesia equipment, tubing and catheters (soak 10 to 20 minutes for chemical disinfection, 10 hours for chemical sterilization), and smooth, hard-surfaced objects. Glutaraldehyde can be corrosive to equipment, however. Disadvantages in its use are that it is explosive, unstable, toxic, and irritating to tissues; has a strong odor; and requires heat and a long exposure to work effectively. Liquid agents such as glutaraldehyde should be used only if neither an autoclave nor ethylene oxide is available or feasible.

ACIDS
Boric acid

Boric acid is a mild antiseptic and astringent. Dilute solutions of boric acid are nonirritating and therefore suitable for use on delicate structures such as the eye. Boric acid is an ingredient of many antiseptic solutions used as washes and gargles. It is still widely used for conditions of the skin in the form of wet dressings, dusting powders, and ointments.

Although boric acid is not customarily considered a toxic substance since it is used externally, serious poisoning and deaths have resulted from its ingestion. Solutions of boric acid should be colored to help prevent accidents. Toxic reactions have occurred from topical application to large denuded areas because of the absorption that took place.

Boric acid solution is a 5% aqueous solution of boric acid.

Miscellaneous agents
Ethylene oxide

Ethylene oxide has come to be used for gaseous sterilization of materials that cannot be subjected to heat or pressure, such as certain plastic parts of machines and optical instruments. It use is more complex and less reliable than steam.

Ethylene oxide is a colorless gas at ordinary temperatures. Its toxicity when inhaled is said to compare with ammonia gas. Temporary exposure to ethylene oxide may irritate skin and mucous membranes and cause upper respiratory problems. As a result of studies correlating ethylene oxide exposure over a long period with the appearance of chromosomal defects and low sperm counts, the Occupational Safety and Health Administration may issue new guidelines that lower the permissible ethylene oxide exposure to 10 parts per million time-weighted average. Proper venting of the exhausted gas away from general ventilation systems is essential.

Ethylene oxide is flammable and when confined is capable of explosive violence. A preparation of 10% ethylene oxide and 90% carbon dioxide is on the market under the name Carboxide. The addition of the carbon dioxide is to reduce the potential for flammability.

Ethylene oxide is apparently effective against all types of microorganisms, including viruses and tubercle bacilli. It is also rapidly effective against spores. Its action is bactericidal rather than bacteriostatic. It is a more expensive form of sterilization than that achieved with heat or other chemical agents, but it has good penetrating power and can be used for many things that would be injured by heat (such as, endoscopes, thermometers, and heart-lung oxygenator parts).

• • •

Beta-propiolactone gas (BPL) is even more rapidly sporicidal but has too many disadvantages to be used as a hospital disinfectant or sterilizer. Several studies have demonstrated its carcinogenic properties as well.

Nursing implications

Assessment of all patients and ongoing monitoring for infection are traditionally and appropriately a role of nurses, who are the only continuous patient observers in all settings. Data collecting should be aimed at assessing susceptibility to, imminence of, or presence of an infection or infectious disease in a patient.

Susceptibility to infection has been proved to be heightened in patients who are either very young (due to underdeveloped and inexperienced immune systems) or elderly (because of limited adaptive defense systems). A patient who has let immunizations lapse, has never been immunized for common illnesses, or has never contracted such an illness is at special risk for contracting it, especially if he or she has small children who are exposed to such illnesses at school. On the other hand, when nutritional status reflects habits of well-selected meals and there is no debilitating disease present, the patient has strengthened protection from infection.

Therapies such as medication by cortisone derivatives, radiation, and chemotherapy for cancer greatly increase potential for infection. A break in the skin, that ultimate barrier to microorganisms, facilitates entry and establishment of infection, so any invasive procedure from intravenous needle insertion to a full surgical procedure naturally exposes the patient to potential infection, though not to the same degree. Attachment or insertion of certain therapeutic appliances or equipment such as indwelling urinary catheters, IPPB tubing, and certain surgical prostheses have been associated with a moderately high rate of infection unless thorough aseptic techniques are used. Complete assessment of all such data culminates in a nursing problem or nursing diagnosis clearly presenting the patient's obvious potential for infection.

Nursing activity related to the actual presence of an already established infectious process is likewise the result of patient data. Systemic infectious processes are typically represented by a temperature over 101° F (38.3° C), aches, pains, headache, and malaise along with symptoms characteristic of the specific illness (such as cough, diarrhea, or sore throat). Local infections are typified by breaks in the skin, especially traumatic wounds and also surgical wounds incurred during prolonged surgery or those that were accidentally contaminated. Manifestations of local infection present at the site of the wound include heat, excessive redness, swelling, tenderness or pain, and/or purulent exudate. Small amounts of clear, straw-colored or pinkish fluid or slight oozing of dark venous blood all fall within the realm of expected wound drainage early in the wound-healing process. Characteristics that differ warrant fur-

ther attention as evidence of a possible infected wound site. A specimen of the exudate should be collected under sterile conditions to be sent for culture and sensitivity to isolate the infecting organism and define treatment. If culture results do not corroborate observations, wound signs may be the more reliable data.

With either a suspected or an established infection a decision to emphasize medical or surgical asepsis needs to be made. An infection control nurse or epidemiologist should be the first individual contacted if an infection is suspected in a hospitalized patient, and plans should be worked out together to detect and contain it by applying infection control measures. Depending on the organism and its characteristics, disinfectants might be used for dishes, thermometers, toilet articles, equipment used in patient care, and linens or for cleaning the floors, walls, and furniture. Antiseptics are applied to a tissue site prior to intravenous needle insertion, total parenteral nutrition dressings, for indwelling urinary catheter insertion, or as a handwash before and after patient care. Antiseptic body scrubs or baths are often prescribed by physicians for patients who are to undergo surgery.

Decisions about the selection of disinfectants for general cleaning and for instruments have usually been made in the institutional setting by other than staff nurses. The Infection Control Committee in concert with a nurse epidemiologist may be the most appropriate body to decide that. However, continued appraisal of disinfectants and antiseptics, their effectiveness, and the factors in the environment that influence effectiveness continues to be a function inherent to nurses who are on the scene.

Several factors weigh in the selection of disinfectants. The type of organism and its relative vulnerability or resistance to the antimicrobial agent are the primary issues. The larger the number of microorganisms and the more heavily contaminated the area (even if the organisms are susceptible to the chosen antimicrobial), the longer the chemical agent will take to work effectively. This phenomenon also illustrates an often-neglected microbiologic principle: once an area or object is exposed, it is indeed considered contaminated, but still needs protection from *further* contamination of all sorts.

Visible dirt and soil, especially of an organic nature, must be removed from the area or object before disinfecting or applying an antiseptic. Adherent soil may physically block access to the area to be cleansed. Organic matter clinging to or surrounding the area acts to absorb and inactivate the agent, leaving very little free chemical.

The effectiveness of the different antiseptic/disinfectant agents varies widely and must be taken into account in each situation. Generally, the stronger the concentration of chemical, the less time it will take to be effective. Of course, the upper limit of concentration is reached earlier when the chemical compounds are used on living tissue than on inanimate objects. The rate of disinfection is often increased when there is an increase in the object's surface temperature or in the temperature of the immediate environment.

Proper application of the germicide in question should closely follow its individual requirements. Some of these chemicals have a fairly narrow range of functioning, and they should not be considered to be interchangeable as random substitutes for one another.

Results of research in testing antiseptic and disinfectant efficacy cannot necessarily be accepted at face value. Laboratory tests merely denote the minimal standards acceptable as criteria for effectiveness. In-use testing to select the best agent for a specific application is more to the point, especially when deciding between antiseptics. Though some such reliable tests exist for floors and anesthetic equipment, many more reliable and less tedious tests need to be developed.

The crucial evaluation, however, is whether or not the patient's potential infection or illness develops or if it worsens—and that depends on a conscientious nursing process with evaluations that are based on patient care outcome criteria or goals.

Summary of nursing considerations

Infections and infectious diseases, though differing in type, occur in patients in all set-tings—hospitals, institutions, community, and the home. Nosocomial infections are hospital acquired and usually are caused by virulent microorganisms. With the emergence of antibiotic-resistant bacteria, it has become an increasingly difficult problem to treat the virulent strains that frequently develop within a relatively short period of time. By contrast, community or home-acquired infections generally are benign and usually are responsive to treatment.

In hospital environments, surgical and medical asepsis is used to reduce the number of organisms in order to prevent the spread of infection or communicable disease. In surgical asepsis, *all* microorganisms are destroyed; in medical asepsis, only *pathogens* are destroyed or their growth is inhibited. Pathogens are organisms capable of inducing disease or infection.

Sterilization is any process that destroys *all* forms of living organisms on surgical equipment that comes in contact with the patient during a surgical procedure. However, other means of destroying pathogenic organisms may be applied when sterilization is not feasible. Chemical agents such as disinfectants and antiseptics are employed beneficially for this purpose. Disinfectants are used on nonliving objects while antiseptics usually are applied to living tissues. Antiseptics are most often bacteriostatic because they inhibit the growth of microorganisms rather than destroy them. They may be used on living tissues such as skin and mucous membranes. On the other hand, disinfectants are bactericidal for they destroy most microorganisms such as bacteria but not fungi, virus, and spores.

There is no ideal chemical agent suitable for all purposes for which antiinfective agents are needed. The ideal disinfectant should not only kill all harmful organisms and have a low incidence of hypersensitivity but should also act in the presence of organic material and be stable, noncorrosive, and inexpensive. Both physical and chemical agents are used in disinfection, but this chapter concentrates on chemical agents. For example, heat, particularly moist heat under pressure (autoclaving), is the method of choice for killing all forms of living organisms. But since not all things that require disinfection can be autoclaved, a need continues for satisfactory chemical disinfectants.

The major groups of chemicals used as disinfectants and antiseptics are phenol and related compounds, dyes, heavy metals, halogens, oxidizing agents, surface-active agents, and miscellaneous agents. Other agents in the highly toxic phenol group include cresol, hexachlorophene, pHisoHex, resorcinol, hexylresorcinol, and thymol. Triphenylmethane, azo, and acridine are dyes used as antiseptics and antiprotozoal agents to promote the healing of wounds. Organic and inorganic compounds of mercury and silver are far from ideal antiseptics. However, silver nitrate has been used successfully to prevent gonorrheal conjunctivitis in newborns and to inhibit infections in treatment of burns. Chlorine and iodine are the halogenous antiseptics. Hydrogen peroxide, medicinal zinc peroxide, chlorhexidine gluconate, and potassium permanganate are oxidizing agents that are destructive to pathogenic organisms but mild enough to be used on living tissues. Benzalkonium chloride and green soap are examples of surface-active agents also known as wetting agents, emulsifiers, and detergents. Alcohol, ethanol, and ethyl alcohol are chemical agents widely used as antiinfectives.

QUESTIONS

FOR STUDY AND REVIEW

1 Explain how antiseptics and disinfectants exert their bacteriostatic or bactericidal action.

2 Make a list of the preparations used as antiseptics or disinfectants in the hospital in which you are obtaining your clinical experience. For what particular purposes are these substances used?
3 Why is silver nitrate solution instilled in the eyes of the newborn? What other uses does silver nitrate have?
4 Which disinfectants and antiseptics would you recommend for home use?
5 Through library research determine the advantages and disadvantages of heat and chemical sterilization.

BIBLIOGRAPHY

Altemeier, W.A., and others, editors: Manual on control of infection in surgical patients, Committee on Control of Surgical Infections of the Committee on Pre- and Postoperative Care, Philadelphia, 1976, J.B. Lippincott Co.

A.M.A. drug evaluations, ed. 3, Littleton, Mass., 1980, PSG Publishing Co., Inc.

Barrett-Connor, E., and others, editors: Epidemiology for the infection control nurse, St. Louis, 1978, The C.V. Mosby Co.

Dineen, P.: Local antiseptics. In Modell, W., editor: Drugs of choice 1980-1981, St. Louis, 1980, The C.V. Mosby Co.

Goodman, L.S., and Gilman, A., editors: The pharmacologic basis of therapeutics, ed. 6, New York, 1980, Macmillan, Inc.

Kimbrough, R.D.: Review of evidence of toxic effects of hexachlorophene, Pediatrics **51**:391, 1973.

Malizia, W.F., and others: Benzalkonium chloride as a source of infection, N. Engl. J. Med. **263**:800, 1960.

Perkins, J.: Principles and methods of sterilization in the hospital, ed. 2, Springfield, Ill., 1969, Charles C Thomas, Publisher.

Reddish, G.F., editor: Antiseptics, disinfectants, fungicides, and chemical and physical sterilization, Philadelphia, 1975, Lea & Febiger.

Spaulding, E.H.: Role of chemical disinfection in the prevention of nosocomial infections, Proceedings of the International Conference of Nosocomial Infections, Atlanta, Georgia, 1970, Centers for Disease Control.

Serums and vaccines

Immunity

In this chapter the control of infectious disease will be discussed from another perspective. Instead of the application of antimicrobial agents (like antibiotics) to attack offending organisms, an artificial means (serum or vaccine) is initiated to augment human resistance to the infectious organisms.

The body itself has an inherited and innate resistance to disease. Over a lifetime it also acquires further immunity by both natural and artificial means (Fig. 25-1). The immunity acquired is of two kinds, active and passive, whether the source is natural or artificial.

When natural resistance is not effective and organisms attack the tissues and live and grow at their expense, the body protects itself by preparing substances destructive to the particular organism making the attack. These substances are called antibodies. They are present in the blood and other body fluids and are carried to the point of infection by the blood and lymph. The antibodies gradually disappear from the blood, but the body has acquired the ability to continue to resist the same organisms. Immunity resulting from these antibodies and the special ability to produce them is known as naturally *acquired immunity*. Since the individual developed the antibodies, the immunity is known as *active immunity*. It is usually present after an attack of an infectious disease such as

smallpox or typhoid fever and may be induced artificially by the injection of substances known as antigens. The antigen may be a suspension of living microorganisms, such as the vaccinia virus, or a suspension of dead microorganisms, such as typhoid vaccine. It may be an extract of the bodies of bacteria, as tuberculosis vaccine, or a soluble toxin produced by bacteria, like diphtheria toxin. This is called artificially acquired active immunity.

Passive acquired immunity against certain diseases is secured by transferring to a person the blood serum of an animal that has been actively immunized by injections with the specific organisms or toxins of those diseases; it may also be secured by injection of the blood serum from an immune person or transferred antibodies from the mother through the placenta to the baby in her womb. Immunity acquired in this way is called *passive immunity* because the recipient's body plays no part in the preparation of the antibodies. The first two examples are passive immunity by artificial means, whereas the last is passive immunity by natural means. The body cells are not prepared to resist infection as they are in active immunity, and as the blood is renewed the antibodies are lost.

The artificially acquired active immunity is of longer duration and results in fewer side effects from the agents used than the artificially acquired passive immunity.

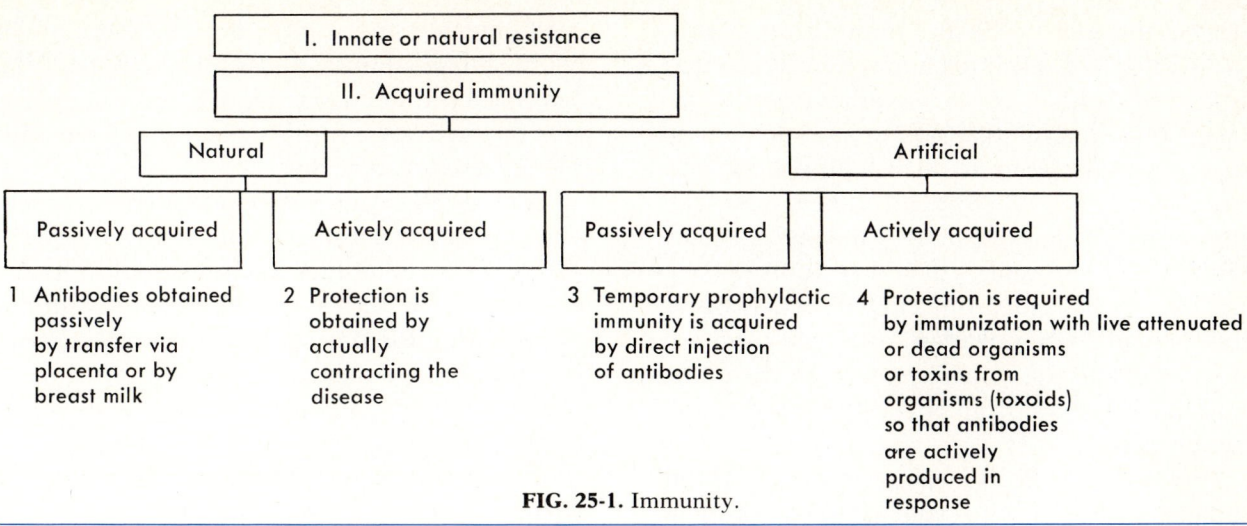

FIG. 25-1. Immunity.

TABLE 25-1 Comparison of active and passive immunity

	Active immunity	Passive immunity
Source	Self	Another human or animal
Effectiveness	High	Moderate to low
Method	Contracting disease itself (clinical or subclinical case)	Method of administration of antibody itself:
	Immunization	Maternal transplacental transfer
	Vaccines (killed or attenuated)	Injection
	Toxoids	
Time taken to develop	5-14 days	Immediate effect
Duration	Relatively long (up to years)	Relatively short (few days or weeks)
Ease of reactivation	Easy, by booster dose	May be dangerous; possible anaphylaxis, especially if animal antiserum used
Purpose	Prophylaxis	Prophylactic and therapeutic

A number of these products used in passive immunity may cause untoward reactions when they are administered as therapeutic or prophylactic agents. Individual sensitivities to animal products, especially horse serum and egg, are primarily responsible for adverse symptoms, and idiosyncrasies toward the products of bacterial metabolism are responsible for the others.

Table 25-1 gives an overview of active and passive immunity that can be acquired by the body over a period of time.

Immunization
THE PRESENT

The critical age period for immunization is 2 months of age through grade school entry and during the school years (several states now require maintenance of immunizations as a criterion for retention in the school system). Several groups are found to be at high risk: adolescents, new parents (unimmunized or with waning immunity, exposed to childhood illness or their vaccinees), and health care providers. Other groups such as migrant workers and recent immigrants to the United States, are predictably at high risk for infectious diseases. International political upheavals in Nicaragua, the Afghanistan invasion, and the Indochinese and Cuban refugee influx to the United States all have pointed up the major problems of these people: diphtheria, measles deaths, hepatitis B, and malaria carrier status. Screening has proved to be the easier problem, preventing outbreaks during the refugee relocation holding period the more difficult. Immunization programs that are taken for granted in the United States and other countries are virtually unheard of in many other countries. Adolescents as a group also seem to be at high risk for preventable infections. Typically, they may lack immunization because of their life-style or their emphasis on present rather than future goals. Of these, certain subgroups may be particularly in need of immunization, such as athletes, heavy drug users, runaways, foreign travelers, and those isolated from or rejecting traditional health care.

Several million children are not immunized against measles, polio, rubella (German measles), mumps, diphtheria, pertussis (whooping cough), and tetanus. These diseases can cause crippling and death, and most are very contagious. Schedules for immunizations of these diseases have been developed as guidelines for the practitioner and for parents to ensure adequate protection for their children (Tables 25-2 and 25-3).

A valid history of clinical disease usually obviates the need for a specific immunization in most cases; however, a proven exposure to the disease does not guarantee immunity. Timely immunization is even more important if the potential for development of the disease is imminent or increased, as it is for persons traveling to foreign countries where diseases unfamiliar to them are endemic. Required and recommended immunizations/prophylaxis for foreign travel are constantly changing and are thus best obtained at the time from the local department of health.

Special assessments must be made when there has been exposure, for example, to measles or tetanus. Measles can be prevented if exposure to the disease is followed within 72 hours by administration of the live measles vaccine. However, people who were vaccinated with the *killed*-virus measles vaccine between 1963 and 1967 and who have never had the disease have now been found to be at considerable risk. They are not protected from measles, and they are at serious risk of developing an atypical type of measles with fever spiking to 104° F (40° C), cough with abnormal infiltrates as seen on roentgenograms, a rash progressing paradoxically from the periphery, and occasionally

cardiomegaly and a mild drop in the platelet count. Nurses should advise all who are over 12 years of age and have not had live measles vaccine or the disease itself to get immunized with the *live* measles vaccine.

Any time a traumatic wound is encountered, especially a puncture wound, the individual's status vis-à-vis tetanus immunization must be assessed. If the person has not been fully immunized within the past 10 years, or if the wound is contaminated and an immunization is more than 5 years old, a booster dose of tetanus toxoid may be in order (Tables 25-3 and 25-4).

In the future it is predicted that vaccines will be available for most of the common bacterial and viral infectious diseases and that measles will be eradicated in the United States (a goal of the Centers for Disease Control). Renewing and reinforcing the public's trust in immunotherapy will be a neccessary corollary to this goal. Most new parents today are too young to know the fear engendered by the very mention of the childhood illnesses a few decades ago. If parents are not convinced, outbreaks of poliomyelitis, for example, may make the argument for us.

Complacency about childhood illnesses and their current and potential threats must be shaken. The initial effects of childhood illnesses can be very serious, and more potential future hazards are currently being discovered, for example, the possible association of mumps with eventual diabetes and chickenpox with "shingles."

During the National League for Nursing–supported Department of Health, Education and Welfare immunization campaign at the end of the 1970s, it was reported that: "Immunization is one of the easiest health services to deliver and to measure. Yet in 1977 nearly 40% of the 52 million children under 15 were not protected against one or more of the vaccine-preventable diseases. This now represents a major national problem."* The campaign focused on vigorous enforcement of state school entry laws and a one-time assessment of all children at *all* grade levels. It sought to allay school officials' fear of a reaction to tougher enforcement with a concerted show of commu-

*From National League for Nursing News **26**:(6), July-Aug. 1978.

TABLE 25-2 Recommended schedule for active immunization of normal infants and children

2 mo	DTP[1]	TOPV[2a]
4 mo	DTP	TOPV[2b]
6 mo	DTP	
1 yr		Tuberculin test[3]
15 mo	Measles,[4] rubella[4]	Mumps[4]
1½ yr	DTP	TOPV
4-6 yr	DTP	TOPV
14-16 yr	Td[5]—repeat every 10 years	

From Report of the Committee on Infectious Diseases, American Academy of Pediatrics, ed. 18, 1977. Reprinted with permission.
[1]DTP—diphtheria and tetanus toxoids combined with pertussis vaccine.
[2a]TOPV—trivalent oral poliovirus vaccine. This recommendation is suitable for breast-fed as well as bottle-fed infants.
[2b]A third dose of TOPV is optional but may be given in areas of high endemicity of poliomyelitis.
[3]Frequency of repeated tuberculin tests depends on risk of exposure of the child and on the prevalence of tuberculosis in the population group. For the pediatrician's office or outpatient clinic, an annual or biennial tuberculin test, unless local circumstances clearly indicate otherwise, is appropriate. The initial test should be done at the time of, or preceding, the measles immunization.
[4]May be given at 15 months as measles-rubella or measles-mumps-rubella combined vaccines.
[5]Td—combined tetanus and diphtheria toxoids (adult type) for those more than 6 years of age, in contrast to diphtheria and tetanus (DT) toxoids which contain a larger amount of diphtheria antigen. *Tetanus toxoid at time of injury:* For clean, minor wounds, no booster dose is needed by a fully immunized child unless more than 10 years have elapsed since the last dose. For contaminated wounds, a booster dose should be given if more than 5 years have elapsed since the last dose.

TABLE 25-3 Primary immunization for children not immunized in early infancy*

Under 6 years of age
First visit	DTP, TOPV, tuberculin test
Interval after first visit	
1 mo	Measles, mumps, rubella
2 mo	DTP, TOPV
4 mo	DTP, TOPV†
10 to 18 mo or preschool	DTP, TOPV
Age 14-16 yr	Td—repeat every 10 yr

6 years of age and over
First visit	Td, TOPV, tuberculin test
Interval after first visit	
1 mo	Measles, mumps, rubella
2 mo	Td, TOPV
8 to 14 mo	Td, TOPV
Age 14-16 yr	Td—repeat every 10 years

From Report of the Committee on Infectious Diseases, American Academy of Pediatrics, ed. 18, 1977. Reprinted with permission.
*Practitioners may choose to alter the sequence of these schedules if specific infections are prevalent at the time. For example, measles vaccine might be given on the first visit if an epidemic is underway in the community.
Measles vaccine is not routinely given before 15 months of age.
†Optional.

TABLE 25-4 Recommended use of tetanus toxoid and tetanus immune globulin (human)—TIG—in wound management*

Type of wound	Immunization status
Unimmunized, uncertain, or incomplete (one or two doses of toxoid)	
Low-risk wound	One dose of Td† or DT‡ followed by completion of immunization; booster every 10 years thereafter
Tetanus-prone wounds and wounds neglected for > 24 hr	One dose of Td† or DT‡ plus 250-500 U TIG followed by completion of immunization. Note: Use separate syringe and sites for TIG and toxoid
Full primary immunization with booster dose within 10 years of wound	
Low-risk wounds	No toxoid necessary
Tetanus-prone wounds	If more than 5 years since last dose, one dose of Td†; if less than 5 years, no toxoid necessary
Wound neglected > 24 hr	One dose of Td plus 250-500 U TIG
Full primary immunization with no booster doses or last booster dose > 10 years	
Low-risk wounds	One dose of Td
Tetanus-prone wounds	One dose of Td
Wounds neglected > 24 hr	One dose of Td plus 250-500 U TIG

From Report of the Committee on Infectious Diseases, American Academy of Pediatrics, ed. 18, 1977. Reprinted with permission.
*Wound definition—It is impossible to categorize all clinical situations by any terminology. In this scheme "tetanus-prone" refers to wounds which yield anaerobic conditions or were incurred in circumstances yielding the probability of exposure to tetanus spores. Examples include severe necrotizing machinery injuries, puncture wounds, wounds heavily contaminated with animal excreta, and so forth. All others are to be considered low-risk from the standpoint of tetanus. Neglected wounds are at greater risk. Wound irrigation, debridement, antibiotics, and other measures should be included in treatment of such wounds as necessary.
†Td—(adult) should be used in individuals more than 6 years old.
‡DT—(pediatric) should be used in individuals less than 8 years old.

nity support. One of the tactics was and is a showing of the film produced by the American Academy of Pediatrics, "A Gift, An Obligation", which is highly acclaimed as a teaching aid.* The Centers for Disease Control (CDC), U.S.

*Available from West Glen Films, 565 Fifth Avenue, New York, N.Y. 10017. Other teaching materials are available from Merck Sharp & Dohme, West Point, Pa. 19486.

Public Health Service, is an excellent source of information for nurses directing or implementing vaccination programs. Free publications are available to health care professionals.*

Requests for exemption from required immunizations for school entry or continued attendance on medical grounds can be obtained from the child's physician. A model form for exemption on religious grounds can be obtained from the Christian Science Committee on Publications. However, it is *theoretically* possible that the right to exempt certain children could interfere with "herd immunity" by sustaining a continued pool of susceptibles, thereby maintaining a hazard that would be unacceptable to other parents who might apply legal and other pressures.

Community health nurses, school nurse-teachers, local public health departments, the Department of Health and Human Services, and the World Health Organization need to work together to share expertise in educating the public, in case finding and reporting, in screening, and in mass immunization programs.

CURRENT AND FUTURE DEVELOPMENTS

The overall picture of immunization shows that currently there is renewed evaluation of the effects and effectiveness of the "vaccine era" during which morbidity and mortality rates of infectious diseases (especially childhood illness, with the exception of pertussis) were significantly reduced by artificially acquired means. Refinements and developments in clinical immunology are advancing while still more dilemmas arise.

1. Live vaccine–related diseases have surfaced as problems. In about 1 case in 11 million live poliovirus vaccinations, the vaccinee suffers the disease itself; about 1 in 4 million of the vaccinees' contacts is found to develop polio of the vaccine type (versus the wild poliovirus type). This is thought to be an outstandingly safe record by comparison with some (the Sovi-

et Union, for example) and a deplorable state by comparison with others. Studies indicate the possibility that mutant strains of neurovirulent polioviruses (especially Type 3 virus) may be excreted in vaccinees' feces. There is now some serious consideration of the renewed use of inactivated poliovirus vaccine (IPV) of the 1950s to avoid this eventuality. This approach must be weighed as to feasibility and risk versus benefits: the probability of a family returning for the necessary booster doses of IPV must be balanced against the probability of their contracting poliovirus as a result of vaccination with TOPV. One recommendation is that intensive campaigns to immunize everyone at one time and then limit vaccine to infants and small children thereafter would cut down on the number of susceptible individuals and diminish potency of mutagenic strains, if any.

The whole question of vaccine safety seems to loom large in the decision-making process of the public. When questioned, only about half the parents interviewed at the close of the 1970s thought vaccines were *very* safe, and only one third thought they were moderately safe. This may partly account for the statistics that, at the same time, only about 68% of 10- to 14-year olds were found to be adequately protected against the common infectious diseases. The other part may be that childhood diseases are just not seen as significant anymore.

2. Pertussis vaccine has been dropped as a required immunization for those under 6 years of age because its value is questionable and the side effects can be serious. This is also true of the killed measles vaccine given from 1963 to 1967; its intended effects are limited and apparently leave the vaccinee more vulnerable to an atypical measles virus with severe side effects. More and more the college-age person or parent is the subject of a relatively virulent form of some childhood disease for which he or she was much earlier immunized or whose antibody titers are waning.

3. Other secondary effects are surfacing: some booster injections seem to increase sensitivity to the antigen, resulting in severe reactions (for example, tetanus). Following the swine flu vaccination program, there were significant reports of apparently vaccine-related

*Public Inquiries, Centers for Disease Control, Atlanta, Ga. 30333; this address may also be used to request *Morbidity & Mortality Weekly Report* (MMWR), containing up-to-date statistics, findings, and instructions about infectious diseases and immunizations worldwide.

cases of Guillain-Barré syndrome. Increasing numbers of liability claims against vaccine producers can be anticipated in our ever more astute population. Children's health care practitioners can increasingly anticipate being objects of a lawsuit or being called as expert witnesses.

Poultry allergy is less of a potential threat than originally supposed, since only minute quantities of potential allergens are found in the vaccines and then only in those grown in egg embryo culture. Reactions to antibiotics and thimerosal allergy must still be dealt with, however.

4. Evidence is building that desired antibody formation from vaccines is subject to interference from concurrent passive transfer via immune serum or antitoxin or maternal transplacental or breast milk transfer of maternal antibodies or interference when one single-virus vaccine is injected simultaneously with another virus vaccine. Such coincidences must be avoided vis-à-vis immunization schedules.

Envisioned for the near future, besides perfection of current vaccines and serums (especially pertussis, cholera, varicella zoster immune globulin [VZIG], rabies, typhoid, and pneumococcal) and standardization of allergen extracts, are the following areas of research:

Bacterial enterotoxoids
Cholera toxoids
Cytomegalovirus vaccine, live
Dental caries vaccine
Gonococcal and syphilis vaccines
Haemophilus influenzae vaccine
Hepatitis virus vaccine, A, B, and C
Herpes simplex virus subunit vaccine
Inactivated and live influenza vaccines
Meningococcal A and B vaccine
Parainfluenza virus vaccines 1 to 3
Production of interferon
Pseudomonas vaccine
Respiratory virus vaccine
Ribosomal vaccines (against tuberculosis, *Salmonella*, pneumococcus)
Rotavirus vaccines
Trachoma vaccine
Tropical diseases and parasite vaccines

The aim of the new World Health Organization campaign is to see that every child is vaccinated against the childhood diseases by 1990 (at a cost of only $3.00 per child).

Genetic engineering using recombinant DNA techniques provides new opportunities for producing large amounts of pure viral components and for creative redesign of viruses for use in live vaccines. Current work is being done on the diarrheal diseases and influenza and hepatitis viruses.

ADMINISTRATION

Before an immunization is given, an interview with the patient and/or family should take place. The individual's age, current physical condition and general resistance to disease, history of exposure to infectious diseases (both past and potential), and previous immunizations should be assessed. A list of the general contraindications to immunizations follows:

1 Current acute or febrile illness
2 Immunosuppressive therapy in progress or immunodeficient state
3 Recent immune serum globulin (ISG), plasma, or blood transfusions
4 Pregnancy—"live" vaccines especially may prove to be teratogenic or cause infection in the conceptus and therefore need to be avoided or given with caution
5 Certain malignancies that leave the individual infection-susceptible (for example, leukemias, lymphomas)
6 Simultaneous administration of another *single* live virus, unless proved safe
7 Prior unusual or allergic reaction to the same or similar vaccine
8 Allergy to antibiotics in vaccine, thimerosal as a preservative, or other constituents

Minor afebrile infections such as the common cold are not usually contraindications to immunization.

Perceptions and misconceptions must be clarified. The relative safety and merits of immunization versus the risks of the disease process itself (both short- and long-range) should be discussed, using statistics where appropriate. Discussion may also include information that a repeat immunization, where memory or records are unclear, is usually not contraindicated; the risk is usually minimal, and future protection is ensured. Unimmunized parents should be identified and probably immunized before their children, especially when TOPV is administered.

Noncompletion of an immunization series

may occasionally be prevented if vaccinees or their parents know that interruption of the series or a prolonged period between phases of immunization makes no difference to eventual antibody levels. A copy of the immunization schedule given to the patient or family also enhances compliance with the immunization series.

Complete written accurate documentation of immunizations with dates is rare even in office records. Nonetheless, it is important to have access to these data; therefore, it is crucial to teach parents or vaccinees that they should also keep careful written records for each vaccination, especially in view of the high mobility of our population. Simple blank forms are available for this purpose and should be given to parents or the vaccinee with an explanation and advice to keep them filled out and in a safe place (for example, with health record files at home or in the family Bible) and to bring them to each appointment.

Almost all immunotherapy is parenteral and must be given by the specified route and with the specified diluent to avoid either local reactions (especially seen when the intracutaneous route is used) or possible anaphylaxis (especially when the intravenous route is used). All needles should be changed after withdrawing the vaccine from the vial, if possible, and 0.2 to 0.3 ml of air should "tail-end" the injection to prevent tracking of irritating substances through local tissues. Aspiration after insertion is, of course, also necessary to prevent the danger of depositing the dose into the bloodstream.

SIDE EFFECTS AND TOXIC EFFECTS

As important as protection from debilitating infectious disease is, even immunization is not without some risk. Side effects, if any, are usually mild and transient: slight fever, sore injection site, or minor rash, but occasionally there are reports of more serious effects such as encephalitis and convulsions. Although serious, the incidence of these effects, when weighed against effects of diseases preventable through immunization, tips the balance in favor of immunization, particularly for these at high risk.

Joint pains and malaise may also be seen, especially after certain live and inactivated vaccines. Rarely, allergy to the egg protein that provided the culture medium for the organism involved, antiserums or antitoxins, the mercury preservative, or contained antibiotics may cause a reaction that is usually controllable by antihistamines. When any unusual or severe reaction occurs, the nurse should contact the practitioner and an informational form should be sent to the Centers for Disease Control. Vaccinees should be given a contact's name in case they get sick and visit a physician, hospital, or clinic within the 4 weeks after immunization. Adverse reaction monitoring is part of a surveillance system to detect uncommon, severe, previously unrecognized, and rare reactions to vaccination. Past examples are the Guillain-Barré syndrome accompanying a small percentage of influenza vaccinations, encephalitis following measles vaccine, and peripheral neuropathy after rubella vaccinations; these are all *very* rare occurrences. Even the report of a large number of benign, expected reactions could indicate a "hot" lot of vaccine, an uncommon event. Data are collected by the Centers for Disease Control for comparison with national data, and they are published in a *Quarterly Adverse Reaction Report*.

Minor expected reactions can be treated with aspirin and rest. Severe fevers (more than 103° F) can be treated with aspirin and sponge baths to reduce the temperature; occasionally a convulsion may accompany a high temperature, and parents need to be so advised. Serum sickness sometimes occurs after repeated serum injections and consists of rash, urticaria, arthritis, adenopathy, and fever starting hours or even days after the injection. Treatment consists of aspirin, antihistamines, ephedrine, or corticosteroids. Rare but serious anaphylactic reactions can cause urticaria, dyspnea, cyanosis, shock, or unconsciousness that occurs within minutes of injection. This is not normal; it is an emergency situation. Therefore any recipient of immunotherapy should be observed by the nurse or someone responsible for up to half an hour after therapy. Treatment for anaphylaxis may involve epinephrine 1:1000 (0.01 ml/kg) in a 1:10 dilution subcutaneously or intramuscularly immediately, administered slowly in a physiologic saline solution. This may possibly be repeated and followed by intravenous administration of epinephrine. Vasopressors and intermittent positive pressure breathing (IPPB) oxygen, antihistamines, and corticosteroids may help. Immunization therapy may cautiously be resumed after all signs of anaphylaxis are gone.

Nurses often find themselves in charge of vaccination programs and clinics. It is important that they keep current on the changes in immunization, since nurses are often the first to be consulted by patients.

NURSING IMPLICATIONS

The role of nurses in implementing immunotherapy begins with knowing when to give immunizations (when "shots are due" as per recommended schedule), when to withhold them, and the discussion of the decision and its rationale with other practitioners and the patient and family. Recording immunizations and any side effects that have already been noted is crucial to continuity of care. Most products must be stored (except for TOPV, which must be frozen) at 2° to 8° C (35.6° to 46.4° F) or potency may be lost. The common practice of storing these compounds on the refrigerator door is negligent, since this has been shown to be the cause of several cases of measles after vaccination in one physician's office.

A crying and wriggling baby or child presents a challenging moving target and must be temporarily restrained. This can often be accomplished just as effectively in the warmth and security of another's arms (possibly the mother's, if feasible) rather than on some hard surface. The needle and syringe and the accompanying short, honest explanation that "this may hurt for just a minute" should be brought out *just* before the actual injection so that less fear builds to potentiate any pain.

Sources of information on immunization include primarily the Public Health Service Advisory Committee on Immunization Practices (ACIP), which advises the public health agencies, and the Committee on Control of Infectious Diseases (the Red Book Committee),

which is drawn from the members of the American Academy of Pediatrics and advises the private health sector. The former can be contacted via the Centers for Disease Control in Atlanta, Georgia. Since the two groups maintain a slightly different perspective, minor inconsequential variations in recommendations may occasionally be noted. Other sources include local public health departments and printed package inserts included with the vaccine or serum. Biologic preparations and accompanying inserts are regulated by the Bureau of Biologics of the FDA. The only constant in immunization practices is change; to read is to keep pace.

Biologic products

In this section the individual serums, vaccines, and toxoids will be presented. An immune serum is the serum of a human being or an animal that has antibodies in the bloodstream.

Serum treatment consists of the transfer of the immune serum into the circulation of the patient. This immune serum contains specific antibodies that act on disease organisms. Tables 25-5 and 25-6 list biologic agents for active and passive immunization.

Summary of nursing considerations

Individuals have natural immunity if microbes causing a disease will not grow in their tissues or the toxins of those microbes are harmless to them. When natural immunity is not effective and organisms attack the tissues, the body protects itself by preparing antibodies. The antibodies empower the body cells with "acquired immunity." Since individuals developed the antibodies themselves, this is considered an "active immunity." It is usually present after an attack of an infectious disease such as smallpox or typhoid fever and may be induced artificially by the injection of substances known as antigens. "Passive acquired immunity" is secured by transferring to a person the blood serum of an animal or a person who has been actively immunized by injections

Text continued on p. 785.

TABLE 25-5 Biologic agents for active immunization

Biologic product	Purpose, preparation, and storage	Alerts
Viral vaccines		
Measles virus (rubeola), live attenuated (Attenuvax) vaccine	Lyophilized preparation of a more attenuated line from Enders' Edmonston strain; produces a modified rubeola infection; given at or after 15 mo of age; no booster needed; offers some protection if given within 72 hr postexposure; CDC predicts eradication of native measles in United States by 1982; store at 10° C (50° F) or less before reconstitution; at 2°-8° C (35.6°-46.4° F) afterward; use within 8 hr; avoid light at all times; inject 0.5 ml reconstituted vaccine subcutaneously	Contraindications: neomycin or chicken product hypersensitivity (however, considered only a *relative* contraindication by DHEW memo of 3/3/78, since there have been no reports of immediate or anaphylactic reactions in 14 yr); active febrile infection; active untreated TB; immunosuppression or immunodeficiency; bone marrow or lymphatic deficiencies; pregnancy (should also be avoided for 3 mo postvaccination) Precautions: give no sooner than 3 mo after transfusion of blood/plasma/human ISG of more than 0.02 ml/lb body weight; give with or after TB skin test; have epinephrine on hand for anaphylaxis; do not give within 1 mo of immunization by other live virus vaccines except one of the M-M-R type or combination Side effects: moderate fever to 102.9° F, rash (in 5-12 days); rare—fever more than 103° F with convulsions; 1 per million occurrences—encephalitis or subacute sclerosing panencephalitis; previous recipients of *killed* virus vaccine—local swelling, redness, vesiculation
Mumps virus vaccine, live (Mumpsvax)	Lyophilized preparation of Jeryl Lynn B level strain of mumps vaccine for 12 mo or older; no need for booster; storage criteria, dosage, and route same as for Attenuvax; no proved association between mumps vaccination and pancreatic damage or subsequent development of diabetes mellitus	Contraindications and precautions same as for Attenuvax with following exceptions in side effects Side effects: mild fever (uncommonly more than 103° F); low incidence of parotitis, orchitis, purpura, allergic reactions (urticaria); very rare—encephalitis and other nervous system reactions
Rubella (German measles) virus vaccine, live, attenuated, (Meruvax II)	Lyophilized preparation of Wistar Institute strain (Wistar RA 27/3 strain) prepared in human diploid cells for immunization from 12 mo of age to puberty; not designed to prevent disease in the recipient, but to protect the unborn from teratogenic effects (blindness/deafness); recommended for children of susceptible pregnant women, for susceptible women in postpartum period, nonpregnant and susceptible postpubertal females, and adolescent or adult males if necessary to control/prevent rubella outbreaks; no booster needed; history of illness usually not reliable enough to preclude immunization; store as for Attenuvax; inject 0.5 ml subcutaneously	Contraindications and precautions as for Attenuvax with the following exceptions: Contraindications: postpubertal females with rubella titers of more than 1:8; pregnancy (also to be avoided for 3 mo postvaccine) Precautions: theoretical possibility of live virus transmission from nose/throat of vacinees Side effects: occasionally mild symptoms of naturally acquired rubella: lymphadenopathy, urticaria, rash, malaise, sore throat, fever, headache, polyneuritis, arthralgias, local pain, swelling, redness; fever rarely more than 103° F; very rarely—encephalitis

TABLE 25-5 Biologic agents for active immunization—cont'd

Biologic product	Purpose, preparation, and storage	Alerts
Measles and rubella virus vaccine, live (M-R-Vax II)	Mixed lyophilized preparation of Attenuvax and Meruvax II for protection against measles and rubella in 15-month-old children (earlier vaccination may result in failed response and may require revaccination at or after 15 mo of age, depending on individual evaluation); storage is as per Attenuvax; inject 0.5 ml subcutaneously	As per individual measles and rubella live vaccines
Rubella (German measles) and mumps virus, live vaccine (Biavax II)	Mixed lyophilized preparation of Wistar strain rubella virus (Meruvax) and Jeryl Lynn B level Mumpsvax; for simultaneous immunization against rubella and mumps virus from 12 mo to puberty; revaccination not necessary unless initial vaccination done *before* 12 mo, on an individual basis; storage as per Attenuvax; inject 0.5 ml subcutaneously	As per individual rubella and mumps virus live vaccines
Measles, mumps, and rubella vaccines, live (M-M-R II)	Mixed lyophilized preparation of Attenuvax, Mumpsvax, and Meruvax; for simultaneous immunization against measles, mumps, and rubella from 15 mo to puberty. No revaccination necessary unless primary immunization done less than 12 mo of age, and then done on individual basis; storage as per Attenuvax; inject 0.5 ml subcutaneously	As per individual measles, mumps, and rubella virus live vaccines
Poliovirus vaccine, live, oral, trivalent (Orimune), TOPV	Mixture of three types of live attenuated polioviruses (Sabin) for routine immunization of those from 6 wk to 18 yr old; evaluated in 1977 by National Academy of Science as preferred for primary vaccination of children and for epidemic control in the United States because it establishes intestinal immunity, is simple to administer, is well accepted by patients, does not require booster doses, and has virtually eliminated disease of wild polioviruses in America; can be given in addition to inactivated polio vaccine (IPV) and simultaneous with M-M-R vaccine; adults usually given IPV if previously unimmunized; store frozen, thaw before use, and agitate before giving 2 drops orally, in chlorine-free water, simple syrup, or milk, or on bread, cake, or cube sugar (using dropper supplied) (see package insert for specific storage advice); given in three spaced doses and one booster at time of school entry; total of three doses in primary series for children and adolescents beyond that age	Contraindications: never administered parenterally nor in acute illness; advanced, debilitated condition; persistent vomiting or diarrhea; immunodeficient or immunosuppressed states Precautions: will not modify/prevent existing or incubating disease Side effects: rarely, paralytic disease after vaccination or after contact with vaccinee; advise unimmunized close contacts of vaccinee to seek immunization as needed

Continued.

T A B L E 2 5 - 5   Biologic agents for active immunization—cont'd

Biologic product	Purpose, preparation, and storage	Alerts
Viral vaccines—cont'd		
Influenza virus vaccine, trivalent types A and B (Fluzone)	Current vaccine is a mixed solution of inactivated influenza viruses (Brazil, Texas, and Hong Kong), which protects only against these three strains. (There is often enough variation within the same subtype of virus over time that vaccination for one strain one year may not be effective protection against the next year. Thus the antigenic composition of the prevalent strains is the criterion for selection of the virus strains to be included in the vaccine.); Public Health Service recommends annual vaccination for adults and children of all ages who have chronic health problems (heart, lung, renal, or diabetic) and for those over 65 yr; shake vigorously before withdrawing the single dose of 0.5 ml for ages 27 and over, and the two doses of 0.5 ml for 13-26 yr, and the two doses of 0.5 ml (split virus only) for 3-12 yr, and the two doses of 0.25 ml (split virus) for 6-35 mo old; inject intramuscularly into deltoid or lateral mid thigh; store at 2°-8° C (frozen vaccine has lost potency, do not use)	Contraindications: hypersensitivity to egg products; individuals who are immunosuppressed; acute febrile illness; do not inject intravenously Precautions: pregnancy; epinephrine on hand; not effective against all possible strains of influenza virus; resterilize jet injection apparatus if contaminated with blood; complete immunizations by November Side effects: local tenderness, redness, induration; fever, malaise, myalgia; rare—allergic skin and respiratory reactions, Guillain-Barré syndrome rare; very rare—encephalopathy
Smallpox vaccine (Dryvax)	Lyophilized vaccine for immunization against smallpox; limited to travelers to countries requiring vaccination as condition for entry (ever fewer in number [a waiver may be obtained]; discontinued as required by United States since 1971) and those few laboratory workers who have contact with the variola virus; last natural smallpox occurrence known developed in 1977; vaccination has high risk of serious complications; injection is by needle punctures through a drop of vaccine on the skin; site should be inspected for presence of desired vesicle after 6-8 days; store dry at 2°-8° C; reconstituted at 0° C	Contraindications: not to be used for treatment of warts or recurrent herpes simplex infections; infants with "failure to thrive" syndrome; anyone with disturbed skin integrity; immunosuppression or immunodeficiency; pregnancy Precautions: blot off excess vaccine; vaccination equipment should be burned, boiled, or autoclaved before disposal Side effects: severe neurologic disorders; generalized rashes; local pyogenic infections (see package insert for details)
Yellow fever vaccine	A live, attenuated virus preparation made from the 17D strain (licensed in the United States) for immunization against jungle yellow fever; recipients as of July 1978 were limited to persons 6 mo of age or older traveling/living in certain parts of Africa and South America and laboratory personnel who might be exposed to virulent yellow fever virus; vaccine is given at an approved Yellow Fever Vaccination Center (see local health department) and an international Certificate of Vaccination is issued; a waiver of vaccination may be sought	Contraindications: pregnancy; altered immune states; hypersensitivity to eggs and certain contained antibiotics Precautions: administer at least 1 month apart from other live virus vaccines Side effects: mild—headache, myalgia, fever; very, very rare—encephalitis

TABLE 25-5 Biologic agents for active immunization—cont'd

Biologic product	Purpose, preparation, and storage	Alerts
Bacterial vaccines		
Bacillus Calmette-Guérin (BCG vaccine)	Attenuated and freeze-dried strain of *Mycobacterium bovis* given as vaccine to protect especially those uninfected persons with repeated exposure to infective cases who cannot or will not obtain or accept treatment; for those who are skin-test negative to 5 US units (5 TU) of tuberculin PPD; may be repeated in 2-3 mo; reconstitute, protect from light, and use within 8 hr; halve dose on label for those under 28 days old and revaccinate with full dose after 1 yr old; intracutaneous route or follow label; strains and efficacy vary among different preparations	Contraindications: altered immune states Precautions: pregnancy; postvaccination sensitivity may mimic positive reaction to tuberculin following a skin test for TB; full, lasting protection from TB cannot be assured postvaccination by BCG (great variance in efficacy among BCG products) Side effects (can occur up to 1 yr later): severe local ulceration, lymphadenitis; very rare—osteomyelitis, lupoid reactions, disseminated BCG infection, death
Pneumococcal vaccine, polyvalent (Pneumovax)	Derived from capsules of 14 mixed types of cultured pneumococci; indicated for immunization against lobar pneumonia and bacteremia caused by included antigens for all who are 2 yr or older and who are at high risk if they develop pneumococcal pneumonia (chronic heart, pulmonary, or renal disease, diabetes, weakened convalescents, and those 50 yr and older); dosage is a single, 0.5 ml subcutaneous or intramuscular injection (preferably in the deltoid or lateral mid-thigh; store at 2°-8° C	Contraindications: hypersensitivity; revaccination more frequently than every 3 years; pregnancy; intradermal administration; intravenous administration; will not protect against antigens not included Precautions: active infection; less than 2 yr old; immunosuppression; severely compromised cardiac and/or pulmonary function; history of pneumococcal infection in the preceding 3 yr; keep epinephrine on hand Side effects: local redness and soreness, induration, fever < 100.9° F; occasionally rare—anaphylactoid reactions
Meningococcal polysaccharide vaccines Group A, Group C, or Groups A and C, bivalent (Menomune)	Monovalent and bivalent polysaccharide vaccines against diseases caused by *Neisseria meningitidis* serogroups A and C (Group B, the commonest strain, is sulfa-sensitive); not for routine vaccinations, but for outbreaks and some travelers (2 yr and older); as adjunct to antibiotics; given in single parenteral dose; see package insert	Contraindications: see package insert for details Precautions: pregnancy Side effects: mild, local erythema
Plague vaccine	Prepared from inactivated *Yersinia pestis* organisms to immunize high-risk persons; personnel working with the organism who are antibiotic-resistant; those engaged in aerosol experiments; those in unpreventable contact (disaster areas), and possibly for laboratory personnel working with the organism or plague-infected rodents; workers living in plague-epidemic rural areas; and anyone who works with wild rodents or rabbits in plague-ridden areas. Primary immunization series: those over 10 yr old, two doses subcutaneously of 0.5 ml each 4 or more wk apart then a third dose of 0.2 ml 4-12 wk after the second injection (in emergencies: three injections of 0.5 ml 1 week apart are acceptable); under 10 yr, see insert; booster may be needed for continued exposure	Side effects: local pain, redness, induration; with repeated doses—fever, headache, malaise; occasionally—sterile abscesses

Continued.

TABLE 25-5   **Biologic agents for active immunization—cont'd**

Biologic product	Purpose, preparation, and storage	Alerts
Bacterial vaccines—cont'd		
Typhoid vaccine	Saline solution of killed *Salmonella typhosa* organisms for active immunization against typhoid fever after intimate exposure to a known carrier or for foreign travel; primary immunization: for those over 10 yr of age, two doses 0.5 ml subcutaneously each at interval of 4 or more wk; under 10 yr old, two doses 0.25 ml subcutaneously each at 4 wk or more interval; in emergencies, three doses may be given at weekly intervals; boosters: over 10 yr old, 0.5 ml subcutaneously, or 0.1 ml intracutaneously; 6 mo to 10 yr, 0.25 ml subcutaneously or 0.1 ml intracutaneously (boosters needed with repeated exposures at least every 3 yr); shake vial well before use	Contraindications: acute infection; allergic reaction to previous dose Precautions: get history of possible hypersensitivity; epinephrine 1:1000 on hand; keep current as to recent literature Side effects: local redness, induration, tenderness; malaise, headache, myalgia, elevated temperature
Cholera vaccine	Suspension of Ogawa and Inaba serotypes of killed *Vibrio cholerae (V. comma)* for active immunization against cholera for those traveling to or residing in countries where cholera is endemic or epidemic; refer to package insert for details	Contraindications: acute illness; severe reaction or allergic response to previous dose; pregnancy evaluated individually Precautions: epinephrine 1:1000; review of hypersensitivity history; knowledge of current related findings in the literature Side effects: redness, induration, pain at site; occasionally malaise, headache, mild to moderate temperature elevations
Diphtheria and tetanus toxoids, and pertussis (whooping cough) vaccine, adsorbed (DTP)	Mixed adsorbed toxoids and a vaccine to immunize against diphtheria, tetanus, and pertussis, given in four doses from 2 mo to 7 yr according to recommended schedules; three primary injections and one booster of 0.5 ml each intramuscularly into deltoid or thigh varying site each time; if immunizations incomplete by 6 yr old along with exposure to any of the antigens, 0.5 ml DTP *or* single antigen dose is advised, (See single antigen vaccine, tetanus toxoid, Td, or TIG for recommended protocol in event of injury for which tetanus prophylaxis is indicated.) *plus* passive immunization, *plus* appropriate antibiotic; store at 2°-8° C (35.6°-46.4° F); see package insert for details	Contraindications: acute infection; previous reactions to an initial dose (all three antigens or only pertussis may be omitted then) such as fever > 103° F (39° C), convulsion, altered consciousness, focal neurologic signs, "screaming fits," shock/collapse, purpura; preexisting neurologic disorder; immunosuppression; over 6 yr old (give Td instead) Precautions: reactions to DTP call for reevaluation and possibly administration of Td only Side effects: usual—local redness, induration, and possible tenderness; possible abscess; mild to moderate fever

TABLE 25-5 **Biologic agents for active immunization—cont'd**

Biologic product	Purpose, preparation, and storage	Alerts
Tetanus and diphtheria toxoids, adsorbed (Td)	Mixed adsorbed toxoids to immunize those over 6yr of age; three basic doses of 0.5 ml intramuscularly (deltoid is preferred site, but sites should be varied each time) with routine boosters no closer than every 10 yr recommended. (See single antigen vaccine, tetanus toxoid, Td, or TIG for recommended protocol in event of injury for which tetanus prophylaxis is indicated); storage 2°-8° C; see package insert for details	Contraindications: administration to those under 6 yr old; acute infection; immunosuppression; hypersensitivity to the product Precautions: epinephrine 1:1000 on hand for allergic reaction Side effects: Occasionally Arthus-type response to high levels of tetanus antibody (antitoxin) in those receiving regular or frequent tetanus toxoid boosters (thus the recommended 10-yr interval between TD booster); response may include significant local symptoms of redness, edema resembling a giant "hive," axillary lymphadenopathy; systemic symptoms can include low fever, malaise, aches and pains, general urticaria, tachycardia, and hypotension; prolonged intervals between primary immunizing doses has no effect on eventual immunity status
Tetanus toxoid, adsorbed (preferred) or fluid	For routine active immunization (although DTP combination is more common) in partially immunized children and adults, especially in case of injury with a wound possibly contaminated by *Clostridium tetani* (TIG may also occasionally be given—see chart "Guide to Tetanus Immune Globulin [Human]); for wounds, recommendations are 0.5 ml tetanus toxoid for the questionably immunized plus 250 units of tetanus immune globulin if wound is neither clean nor minor; for immunization, three doses of 0.5 ml plus booster doses every 10 yr; shake well and give deep intramuscularly, avoiding blood vessels; store at 2°-8° C, do not freeze	Contraindications: not for *treatment* of an actual tetanus infection; any acute infection; immunosuppression Precautions: hypersensitivity; epinephrine on hand; history of cerebral damage, neurologic disorders, or febrile convulsions should be evaluated individually Side effects: as per Td vaccine
Rickettsial vaccine		
Typhus vaccine	Killed vaccine prepared from killed *Rickettsia prowazekii* organisms for protection against louse-borne only (epidemic) typhus, which poses no threat to United States citizens in or out of the United States except in travel to remote highlands of Africa, South America, or mountains of Asia, or in laboratory personnel who work with organism; two subcutaneous injections 4 or more wk apart plus boosters at 6-12 mo intervals as long as exposure exists; see package insert for details	Contraindications: hypersensitivity to eggs Side effects: pain, induration, redness locally; occasionally transient fever, malaise

T A B L E   2 5 - 6   **Biologic agents for passive immunization**

Biologic product	Purpose, preparation, and storage	Alerts
Immune serums		
Tetanus immune globulin, human; TIG (Homo-Tet)	A solution of the gamma globulin fraction of the plasma of persons who have been hyperimmunized with tetanus toxoid; used in the immediate treatment of injuries needing tetanus antitoxin if the injured person has had only one or two tetanus immunizations by vaccination (DTP or Td) and the wound is tetanus prone or neglected or patient is immunosuppressed or immunodeficient; given along with Td immunization at this time (see Table 24-3); give 250 units TIG intramuscularly at a site different from Td site for adults; for children, 2 units/lb body weight or more may be necessary; TIG has also been used in the treatment of clinical tetanus, but results are equivocal; store between 2°-8° C	Contraindications: do not give IV; avoid blood vessels Precautions: keep epinephrine on hand Side effects: occasionally local tenderness, stiffness, allergic or anaphylactic systemic reactions
Immune serum globulin, human; ISG (Gamastan)	Solution of primarily immunoglobin G (IgG) for passive immunization to modify hepatitis A, prevent or modify rubeola, or provide replacement therapy for hypo- or agammaglobulinemia; should be used for prophylaxis of viral hepatitis type B (HBV) *only* when hepatitis B immune globulin not available; ISG may benefit after exposure to rubella in early pregnancy and for passive immunization against varicella if VZIG not available and for travel where hepatitis A is common; usual dose, 0.02 ml/kg intramuscularly (gluteal preferred site) in several muscle sites as needed; store at 2°-8° C; do not freeze; use before expiration date	Contraindications: do not give IV; IgA deficiency (may develop possible anaphylactic reactions to blood products); coagulation disorder; allergy to thimerosal; do not give Gamastan to those with clinical signs of hepatitis A or if exposure within past 2 weeks; vaccination for measles, mumps, polio, or rubella within 3 mo after ISG Precautions: epinephrine should be on hand; avoid blood vessels Side effects: local pain, urticaria, angioedema; rare—anaphylaxis
Zoster immune globulin (ZIG) and varicella-zoster immune globulin (VZIG) for varicella (chickenpox) virus	Investigational substances for passive immunization against the chickenpox virus for those who meet the criteria for age, immunodeficiency and who request it within 72 hr of exposure; available free; contact CDC for information; live vaccine now also available under similar conditions	Contact CDC for information

CHAPTER 26

Chemotherapy of parasitic diseases

KAY SEE-LASLEY

Protozoan infections

Protozoan infections are the most common infections found in the world today. They are especially prevalent in crowded developing countries that have poor sanitation, such as those in Africa, Asia, and South America. These diseases have become more prevalent in the United States since global travel has become commonplace. Thus it is not unusual for the health professional to encounter these diseases and to be faced with their treatment and care. There are four classes of protozoa that have pathogenic organisms:

1 Sarcodina (amebic diseases)
2 Mastigophora (trichomoniasis, giardiasis, leishmaniasis, and trypanosomiasis)
3 Ciliophora (single ciliated organism: *Balantidium coli*)
4 Sporozoa (malaria, toxoplasmosis, pneumocystosis, and isosporiasis)

The antiprotozoan agents used in the treatment of these diseases are grouped and discussed as antimalarial drugs, amebicides, and other antiprotozoan agents in the following paragraphs. Table 26-1 summarizes the agents used in the treatment of protozoan diseases. Only the most commonly used antiprotozoan agents will be discussed in depth in this chapter.

Malaria

Malaria is one of the most prevalent of all diseases in spite of efforts to control the causative parasite and the insect vector. Human malaria can be caused by four species of protozoan parasites: *Plasmodium vivax, P. malariae, P. ovale,* and *P. falciparum.* The first three parasites cause what is termed "relapsing" malarias, because they have a secondary, or persisting, stage of their life cycle. This secondary stage of development provides a reservoir of parasites for the reinfection of erythrocytes that can cause symptoms months or years after clinical cure has been obtained. Treatment for the relapsing malarias must be continued for several weeks after an individual's last exposure to

787

T A B L E   2 6 - 1 **Drugs and drug combinations used in the treatment of protozoan diseases**

Disease	Drug
Malaria	
All plasmodia except chloroquine-resistant *Plasmodium falciparum*	Chloroquine hydrochloride
	Hydroxychloroquine
	Chloroquine phosphate
	Amodiaquine dihydrochloride
	Quinine dihydrochloride
P. vivax and *P. ovale* only	Primaquine phosphate
P. falciparum (chloroquine resistant)	Pyrimethamine + sulfadoxine
	Quinine sulfate + pyrimethamine + sulfadiazine
	Quinine sulfate and tetracycline
	Quinine dihydrochloride
Amebiasis	
Entamoeba histolytica	Diiodohydroxyquin
	Diloxanide-furoate (Furamide)*
	Metronidazole
	Paromomycin
	Dehydroemetine + diiodohydroxyquin
	Metronidazole + diiodohydroxyquin
	Emetine and diiodohydroxyquin
	Dehydroemetine *followed by* chloroquine phosphate and diiodohydroxyquin
	Emetine *followed by* chloroquine phosphate and diiodohydroxyquin
Amebic meningoencephalitis, primary	
Naegleria spp.; *Acanthamoeba* spp.; *Hartmannella* spp.	Amphotericin B
Balantidiasis	
Balantidium coli	Tetracycline (investigational)
	Diiodohydroxyquin (investigational)
Giardiasis	
Giardia lamblia	Quinacrine hydrochloride
	Metronidazole (investigational)
	Furazolidone
Leishmaniasis	
Leishmania braziliensis (American mucocutaneous leishmaniasis)	Stibogluconate sodium*
	Amphotericin B
L. mexicana (American cutaneous leishmaniasis)	Cycloquanil pamoate in oil
L. donovani (kala-azar, visceral leishmaniasis)	Stibogluconate sodium*
	Pentamidine
Pneumocystosis	
Pneumocystis carinii	Trimethoprim-sulfamethoxazole
	Pentamidine
Toxoplasmosis	
Toxoplasma gondii	Pyrimethamine and trisulfapyrimidine
	Spiramycin*
Trichomoniasis	
Trichomonas vaginalis	Metronidazole
	Ornidazol†
	Tinidazole†
Trypanosomiasis	
Trypanosoma cruzi (South American trypanosomiasis, Chagas' disease)	Nifurtimox*
T. brucei gambiense	Suramin sodium*
T. b. rhodesiense (African trypanosomiasis, sleeping sickness	Pentamidine*
	Melarsoprol*
	Tryparsamide† + suramin*

*Drug is available for use only from the Parasitic Disease Drug Service, Centers for Disease Control, Atlanta, GA 30333.
†Not available in the United States.

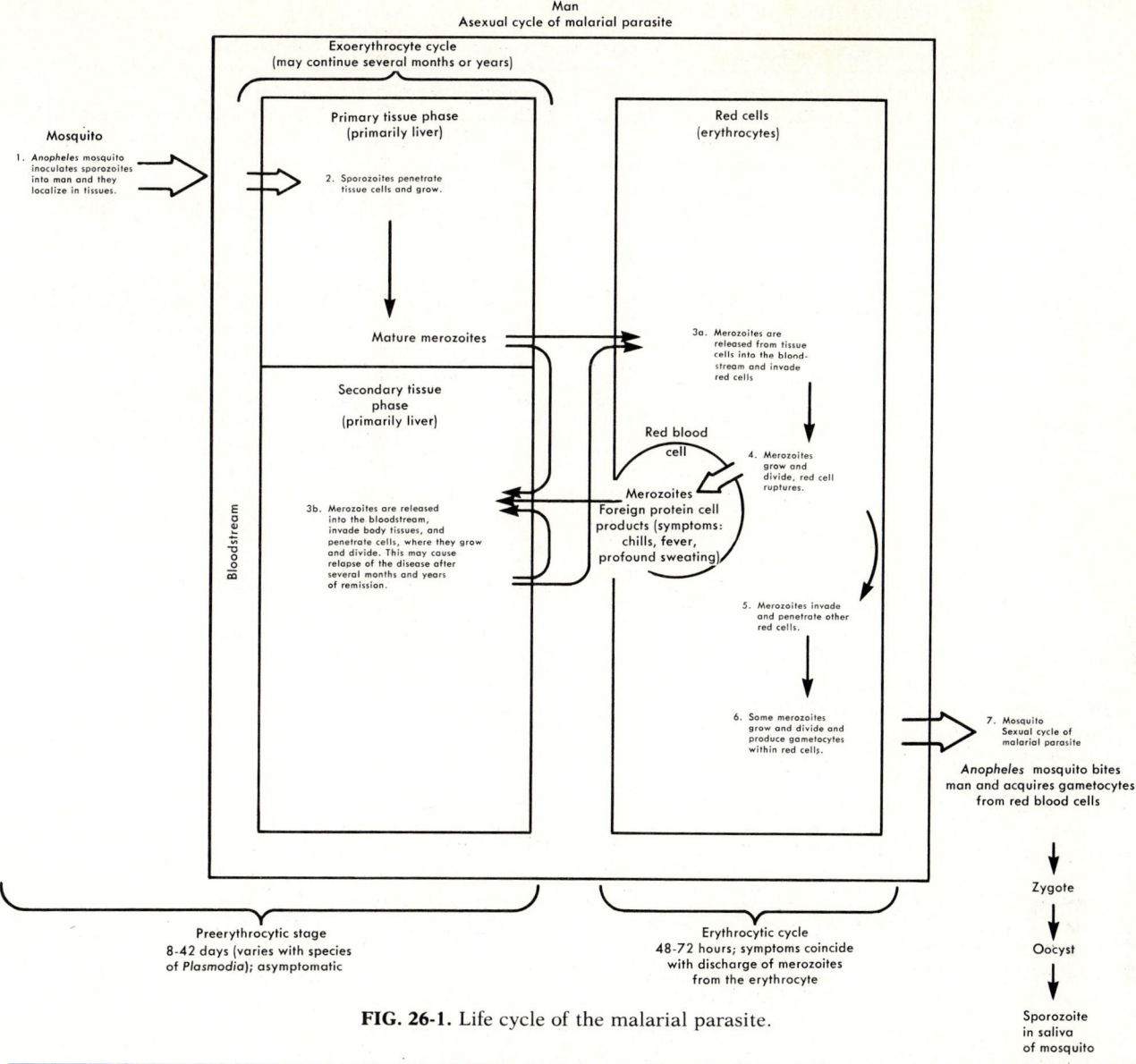

FIG. 26-1. Life cycle of the malarial parasite.

infection. *P. falciparum* is the most lethal form of malaria and has no secondary stages. If the strain is not resistant, it responds readily to treatment, and cure can be achieved.

It is essential to review the life cycle of a malarial parasite to understand the treatment of malaria. Fig. 26-1 presents this cycle in seven basic steps.

The malarial parasite undergoes two phases of development: the sexual cycle, which takes place in the mosquito, and the asexual cycle, which occurs in the human body. The sexual cycle is noted in step 7, Fig. 26-1. The mosquito bites an infected human being and ingests the sexual forms of the parasite, known as gameto-

cytes. In the mosquito the female gametocytes are fertilized by the male gametocyte, forming zygotes, which result in the asexual form, the sporozoites. These are introduced into the blood of human beings by the bite of the *Anopheles* mosquito (step 1, Fig. 26-1). Shortly after the introduction of the sporozoites into the blood, they disappear and enter fixed tissue cells (reticuloendothelial cells of liver) and possibly certain other organs, where development and multiplication take place (step 2). For a period of time (8 to 42 days), which varies with the different plasmodia, the patient exhibits no symptoms, no parasites are found in erythrocytes, and the blood is noninfective. This phase

T A B L E 2 6 - 2 **General treatment of malaria**

Disease state	Drug of choice	Dose	Route	Side effects
Suppression or prophylaxis in endemic areas (except chloroquine-resistant *P. falciparum*)	Chloroquine (Aralen, Resochin) phosphate Hydroxychloroquine sulfate is also effective if chloroquine is not available (400 mg-500 mg chloroquine phosphate)	500 mg (300-mg base) once weekly, continued for 6 weeks after last exposure	Oral	*Occasional:* pruritus, vomiting, headache, confusion, skin eruptions, depigmentation of hair, retinal damage, weight loss, partial alopecia *Rare:* blood dyscrasias, photophobia, deafness, discoloration of nails and mucous membranes of mouth
Prophylaxis after departure of endemic areas and prevention of relapses (*P. vivax* and *P. ovale* only)	Primaquine phosphate	26.3 mg (15-mg base)/ day for 14 days	Oral	*Frequent:* hemolytic anemia in G-6-PD–deficient persons (blacks and Mediterranean peoples) *Occasional:* neutropenia; gastrointestinal disturbances; methemoglobinemia in G-6-PD–deficient persons *Rare:* Central nervous system symptoms, hypertension, dysrhythmias
Acute attack (except chloroquine-resistant *P. falciparum*)	Chloroquine phosphate	1 g (600-mg base); then 500 mg in 6 hours; then 500 mg/day for 2 days	Oral	As above
Severe illness	Chloroquine hydrochoride	250 mg (200-mg base) every 6 hours	Intramuscular	As above

is known as the preerythrocytic stage. The parasites are called primary tissue schizonts, or preerythrocytic forms. After the preerythrocytic stage, the parasites burst from the tissue cells as merozoites, enter the bloodstream, penetrate erythrocytes, and begin the *erythrocytic* cycle of their existence (step 3a). In the case of *P. vivax* (but not *P. falciparum*) some of the merozoites invade other tissue cells to form secondary exoerythrocytic forms (step 3b). The relapses in vivax malaria are believed to be caused by the successive formations of merozoites produced by various secondary exoerythrocytic forms of the parasite. Drugs affecting malarial parasites in the bloodstream do not always destroy those in the exoerythrocytic, or tissue, stage.

After the merozoites bore into the cell, they undergo development and multiplication, and finally cause rupture of the red cell (step 4) to set free many more merozoites. Some of the merozoites may be destroyed in the plasma of

the blood by leukocytes and other agents, but others enter other erythrocytes to repeat the cycle (step 5). The recurring chills, fever, and prostration that are prominent clinical symptoms of malaria occur when the red cells rupture and release the young parasites with foreign protein and cell products. The erythrocytic cycle lasts 48 to 72 hours, depending on the plasmodia involved. After a few cycles, some of the asexual forms of the malarial parasites develop into sexual forms called gametocytes (step 6). When the mosquito bites a person infected with malarial parasites and ingests the sexual forms, the cycle begins again.

Persons who harbor the sexual forms of plasmodia are called carriers, since it is from carriers that mosquitoes receive the forms of the parasite that perpetuate the disease. The asexual forms cause the clinical symptoms of malaria. Carriers should avoid giving blood to blood banks, since it is possible that the recipient of this blood will contract malaria or become a carrier himself.

ANTIMALARIAL DRUGS

Different antimalarial drugs exert their effects at different stages of the parasite's life cycle. They are classified as follows:

1 Primary tissue schizonticides—drugs that destroy preerythrocytic tissue schizonts in the liver soon after infection (for example, primaquine, chloroguanide [Paludrine], and pyrimethamine [Daraprim]). These drugs are usually so toxic that their use as prophylaxis to malaria is avoided. They are termed *causal prophylactic agents.*
2 Blood schizonticides—drugs that suppress symptoms by destroying the asexual forms of the parasite within the blood but permit the continued existence of the exoerythrocytic forms (for example, chloroquine [Aralen], amodiaquine [Camoquin], hydroxychloroquine [Plaquenil sulfate], pyrimethamine [Daraprim], quinine, tetracycline, and combinations of a long-acting sulfonamide with a folic acid antagonist such as pyrimethamine). These drugs are used for prophylaxis of malaria and clinical cures. They are termed *suppressive drugs* or *clinical prophylactic agents.*
3 Secondary tissue schizonticides—drugs used to cure the chronic relapsing fevers resulting from infection by *P. vivax, P. malariae,* and *P. ovale* by destroying the secondary tissue schizonts developing in the liver (for example, primaquine). They are used in *radical cures,* that is, the complete elimination of infection so that relapses cannot occur after treatment has been terminated. They are termed *tissue schizonticides.*

The most effective basic approach to the treatment of malaria is summarized in Table 26-2. Antimalarial drugs such as quinacrine (Atabrine), chloroguanide (Paludrine), cycloguanil pamoate (Camolar), and dapsone either have become obsolete because of new and better agents or are not used extensively because of their toxicity. Quinine, one of the oldest agents, is no longer used extensively because chloroquine and other, newer agents have replaced it in the treatment of malaria. Its primary importance now is in the treatment of chloroquine-resistant falciparum malaria and severe disease states.

A new drug, mefloquine, has been successfully used in the treatment of infections caused by chloroquine-resistant and chloroquine-sensitive falciparum and vivax malaria. It is

expected to be released sometime in the future. It appears that it can also be used effectively in prophylaxis of malaria, since it is a long-acting suppressive agent.

Chloroquine phosphate (Aralen Phosphate); chloroquine hydrochloride (Aralen hydrochloride)

Chloroquine is the drug of choice in the treatment of acute malarial attacks and severe disease and in the prevention or suppression of malaria in persons who are in endemic areas. Table 26-2 summarizes the dosages given in each situation and chloroquine's side effects. Chloroquine is usually given orally except when there is severe nausea and vomiting. Then the hydrochloride salt, the parenteral form, is given. The intramuscular route is preferred.

Chloroquine phosphate is available in 250-mg (150-mg base) and 500-mg (300-mg base) tablets. Chloroquine hydrochloride is available in 5-ml ampuls with a concentration of 50 mg/ml (40 mg/ml base).

The adverse effects of chloroquine are dose related. Most are mild because when the drug is used prophylactically, the doses are low, and when the drug is used in the treatment of an acute attack, the high doses are given over a short period of time. The gastrointestinal disturbances of chloroquine can be minimized by taking the medication with food.

Hydroxychloroquine sulfate (Plaquenil)

Hydroxychloroquine sulfate is an antimalarial drug that is interchangeable with chloroquine in the clinical cure of malarial attacks and prophylaxis of the disease. It has no advantage over chloroquine, and its side effects are the same (Table 26-2).

Hydroxychloroquine is available in 200-mg (155-mg base) tablets. A dosage of 400 mg (310-mg base) hydroxychloroquine is equivalent to 500 mg (300-mg base) chloroquine.

Amodiaquine hydrochloride (Camoquin)

Amodiaquine is a synthetic antimalarial drug that greatly resembles chloroquine both in its effectiveness for treatment of malaria and in its level of toxicity. It is considered the second drug of choice after chloroquine. Like chloroquine, it is effective only in the erythrocytic stages of malaria. It is capable of producing a radical cure only when the infection is caused by *P. falciparum*. It does not effect a similar cure for other forms of malaria, but it is effective in the treatment of an acute attack, it relieves symptoms, and it delays relapse. It is therefore an effective suppressive agent in areas of the world where malaria is endemic.

Amodiaquine hydrochloride is available in 200-mg base tablets for oral administration. the usual single dose for adults during an acute attack of the disease (in terms of base) is 600 mg the first day, and then 400 mg/day for 2 days. For prophylaxis of malaria the usual dose is 400 mg once weekly, continued for 6 weeks after the last exposure in the endemic area.

Side effects include vomiting, diarrhea, and vertigo. When the drug is given for prolonged periods (5 weeks to 6 years), reversible pigmentation of the palate, nail beds, and skin may occur. Rarely agranulocytosis, corneal deposits, retinopathy, polyneuropathy, and liver damage may occur.

Primaquine phosphate

Primaquine phosphate is the drug of choice for the prevention of relapses of malaria caused by *P. vivax* and *P. ovale* and to provide radical cures of these two organisms. Its dosage and side effects are presented in Table 26-2.

Large doses result in hemolytic effects, particularly in persons belonging to the deeply pigmented races, and the drug should be stopped immediately when there is any sign of darkening of the urine or a sudden drop in hemoglobin concentration or leukocyte count. Its main disadvantages are its narrow margin of safety between therapeutic and toxic doses and its ineffectiveness against asexual forms of *P. falciparum*.

Primaquine phosphate is available in tablets containing 26.3 mg of the drug for oral administration. For the treatment of relapsing vivax malaria, one tablet each day for 14 days, given concurrently or consecutively with chloroquine, hydroxychloroquine, or amodiaquine, is considered adequate to produce a radical cure.

Pyrimethamine (Daraprim)

Pyrimethamine is a potent antimalarial agent that is especially valuable as a suppressive agent. It prevents the clinical attacks of all forms of malaria. Unfortunately, when it is used on a large scale, resistance develops quickly. When used in combination with sulfadoxine, it is the drug of choice for the prophylaxis of malaria caused by chloroquine-resistant *P. falciparum*. It is given in doses of 50 mg once every 2 weeks with 1000 mg sulfadoxine. It is also used in the combination of choice for the treatment of acute malarial attacks of chloroquine-resistant *P. falciparum*. This combination consists of quinine sulfate, 650 mg three times a day for 10 to 14 days; pyrimethamine, 25 mg twice a day for 3 days; and sulfadiazine, 500 mg four times a day for 5 days.

Pyrimethamine is available in 25-mg tablets for oral administration. It has a wide margin of safety, and toxic effects are seldom encountered with suppressive antimalarial doses. High doses or prolonged daily doses may produce toxicity, but the development of anemia, thrombocytopenia, and leukopenia can be reversed with concurrent administration of leucovorin calcium, 3 to 9 mg, while still preserving the antimalarial effects of pyrimethamine. Other toxic effects that may appear are folic acid deficiency and, rarely, rash, vomiting, convulsions, and shock.

Quinine sulfate; quinine dihydrochloride

Quinine is available in the oral form quinine sulfate (120-, 200-, 300-, and 325-mg capsules or 300-mg tablets) or the intravenous form quinine dihydrochloride (500-mg vial). The dihydrochloride salt has become the drug of choice in treating severe attacks of chloroquine-resistant *P. falciparum* when absorption of quinine sulfate cannot be assured.

It can be obtained in the United States only from the Parasitic Disease Drug Service of the U.S. Centers for Disease Control in Atlanta. Because of its toxicity, the patient should be changed to the oral form of quinine as soon as possible. Quinine sulfate has become useful in the treatment of acute attacks of chloroquine-resistant *P. falciparum*. When given alone, it is effective in the treatment of the disease, but the patient frequently suffers relapses. When it is combined with pyrimethamine and sulfadiazine or tetracycline, fewer relapses occur. Therefore administrations of these combinations has been established as the optimal therapy for this condition.

Quinine sulfate for the treatment of acute attacks is given in a dose of 650 mg three times a day for 10 to 14 days. In the treatment of severe attacks of malaria caused by chloroquine-resistant *P. falciparum*, the dihydrochloride salt is given intravenously in a dose of 600 mg in 300 ml normal saline solution over a period of at least 1 hour and repeated in 6 to 8 hours (maximum dose, 1800 mg/day).

At the above therapeutic doses quinine frequently causes mild to moderate cinchonism. "Cinchonism" is a collective term that includes the symptoms of tinnitus, headache, altered auditory acuity, blurred vision, nausea, and diarrhea. These symptoms seldom become so severe that therapy has to be discontinued.

Occasionally acute hemolysis, hypoprothrombinemia, thrombocytopenic purpura, agranulocytosis, dysrhythmias, urticaria, or pruritus, with or without a rash, may develop.

Severe side effects rarely develop with quinine, but when they do, plasma levels usually exceed 10 mg/100 ml.

When quinine is given intravenously, hypotension and acute circulatory failure may occur. It should be given slowly. Because its administration can be hazardous to the patient, there should be a constant monitoring of the pulse and blood pressure to detect dysrhythmias or hypotension.

Amebiasis

Amebiasis, or amebic dysentery, is a disease caused by *Entamoeba histolytica*. It may be manifest as (1) an asymptomatic intestinal infection, (2) a mild symptomatic intestinal infection, (3) a severe intestinal infection, or (4) a liver abscess or other extraintestinal infection. The disease is worldwide and is not limited to tropical regions. The parasite occurs in two forms: the active motile form, known as a trophozoite, and the cystic form, which is inactive, resistant to drugs, and present in the intestinal excretions. It replicates in three major locations: (1) the lumen of the bowel, (2) the intestinal mucosa, and (3) extraintestinal sites. When the parasite remains in the lumen of the bowel, the person remains asymptomatic but becomes a carrier of the disease by passing mature cysts of the parasite in formed stools. The infection is then transmitted to others by flies or by contaminated food or water. This state of the disease is called asymptomatic amebiasis.

The trophozoites in the lumen of the bowel, however, may penetrate the mucosa of the walls of the intestine, resulting in diarrhea and abdominal pain. The increased loss of fluid may cause prostration. Also, ulcerative colitis may result. This state of the disease is called intestinal amebiasis and is usually diagnosed as mild to moderate or severe according to the severity of the symptoms and the extent of the disease.

The term "extraintestinal amebiasis" means that the parasites have migrated to other parts of the body, such as the liver or rarely the spleen or lungs. When the parasites are in the liver, "necrotic foci" develop because of the parasites' destructive effect on tissues. When there is liver involvement, the terms "liver abscess" and "hepatic amebiasis" are usually used.

AMEBICIDES

Drugs available for the treatment of amebiasis can be classified according to the site of the previously described amebic action. *Luminal amebicides* act primarily in the bowel lumen, and most are ineffective against parasites in the bowel wall or tissues. *Tissue amebicides* are drugs that act primarily in the bowel wall, liver, and other extraintestinal tissues. The drugs found in each group classification are listed on p. 794.

Luminal amebicides are divided into two groups: (1) the direct amebicidal action drugs and (2) the indirect amebicidal action drugs. The direct amebicidal action drugs are those that kill the trophozoites on contact. Both

---

Classification of amebicides and drugs

Luminal amebicides
   Direct amebicidal action
      Diloxanide-furoate (Furamide)*
      Diiodohydroxyquin (Yodoxin)
      Metronidazole (Flagyl)
      Paromomycin
      Erythromycin
   Indirect amebicidal action
      Tetracycline
      Oxytetracycline (Terramycin)
Tissue amebicides
   Metronidazole (Flagyl)
   Tinidazole†
   Emetine
   Dehydroemetine
   Chloroquine (Aralen)

---

*Drug is available for use only from the Parasitic Disease Drug Service, U.S. Centers for Disease Control, Atlanta, GA 30333.
†Not available for use in the United States.

diloxanide and diiodohydroxyquin are considered the drugs of choice. Metronidazole's main action is as a tissue amebicide, but since a small portion of it is not absorbed by the small intestine, it has some direct amebicidal action. However, it does not have enough effect to be used alone as a luminal amebicide. The antibiotics paromomycin and erythromycin both have amebicidal action, but it is less than that of diloxanide or diiodohydroxyquin. The former are usually used in combination with other drugs. Paromomycin, however, does have sufficient activity to be given alone in some circumstances.

The indirect amebicidal action drugs consist of tetracycline and oxytetracycline. They act in the bowel lumen and wall to alter the flora of the gut and thus deprive the amebae of the environment that is necessary for their survival.

The luminal amebicides are used primarily in the treatment of asymptomatic amebiasis. They are now also being used as adjunctive therapy with the tissue amebicides in the treatment of intestinal and extraintestinal amebiasis to eradicate the intraluminal encysted parasites so that recurrence of the disease is less likely.

The primary tissue amebicide is metronidazole. It has effective action on all tissue sites.

Because of its low toxicity and high degree of effectiveness, it has become the drug of choice in the treatment of both intestinal and hepatic amebiasis.

A new drug similar in structure to metronidazole, tinidazole, appears to be an agent that might soon replace metronidazole. Comparative studies have revealed that is achieves a better response and control of tissue amebiasis and is better tolerated by patients.

Other tissue amebicides are more specific in action (for example, chloroquine is specific for the liver), are less active, are more toxic, or have the disadvantage of having to be given parenterally rather than orally. These amebicides include the parenteral drugs emetine and dehydroemetine and the oral drug chloroquine. They will not be discussed in this chapter.

The general approach to the treatment of amebiasis is summarized in Table 26-3. It is difficult to obtain a complete cure for amebiasis. There are still many unresolved diagnostic and therapeutic questions surrounding this disease.

Diiodohydroxyquin (iodoquinol; Yodoxin)

Diiodohydroxyquin's use, dosage, side effects, and classification are summarized above, left, and in Table 26-3. This drug is an oxyquinoline derivative that contains about 64% iodine. It interferes with thyroid function tests and is contraindicated in patients with liver disease or who are hypersensitive to iodine. It is available in 210- and 650-mg tablets and 25 g powder. It is administered orally as an amebicide and by insufflation for vaginitis.

Diloxanide furoate (Furamide)

Diloxanide is a relatively safe amebicide, and many choose it over diiodohydroxyquin to initiate therapy for asymptomatic or mildly symptomatic amebiasis. Its mechanism is unknown. Discontinuation of diloxanide because of adverse reactions is rarely necessary. Its one disadvantage is that it is available in the United States only from the U.S. Centers for Disease Control. Its use, dose, possible side effects, and classification are summarized above, left, and in Table 26-3.

TABLE 26-3 **General treatment of amebiasis**

Disease state	Drug	Dose	Side effects
Asymptomatic (intra-luminal infection, cysts in bowels, carrier state)	Diiodohydroxyquin (Yodoxin)	650 mg 3 times a day for 20 days	*Occasional:* nausea, diarrhea, cramps, rash, acne, slight enlargement of the thyroid gland *Rare:* optic atrophy and loss of vision in children at high doses for prolonged periods
	or		
	Diloxanide fu-roate* (Furamide)	500 mg 3 times a day for 10 days	*Frequent:* flatulence *Occasional:* nausea, vomiting, diarrhea, urticaria, pruritus
Intestinal disease (intestinal submucosa infection, symptomatic with diarrhea, bloody exudates, etc.)—Mild to moderate and severe disease	Metronidazole (Flagyl) *plus* Diiodohydroxyquin (Yodoxin)	750 mg 3 times a day for 5 to 10 days 650 mg 3 times a day for 20 days	*Frequent:* nausea, headache, metallic taste *Occasional:* vomiting, diarrhea, insomnia, weakness, stomatitis, vertigo, paresthesia, rash, dark urine, dry mouth *Rare:* ataxia, depression, irritability, confusion, mild Antabuse-like reaction with alcohol
Extraintestinal disease (hepatic abscess, other sites)	Treated the same way as intestinal disease		As above

*Drug is available for use only from the Parasitic Disease Drug Service, U.S. Centers for Disease Control, Atlanta, GA 30333.

Metronidazole (Flagyl)

Metronidazole is a nitromidazole found to be effective in the treatment of both intestinal and extraintestinal amebiasis. It is available in a 250-mg tablet. Metronidazole has been found to be carcinogenic in mice and rats, but its carcinogenesis has not been demonstrated in humans. The life-threatening nature of amebiasis, the greater toxicity of other drug combinations, and metronidazole's minimal side effects justify its use in the treatment of this disease. The introductory discussion of amebicides, the box on p. 794, and Table 26-3 summarize its use, dose, side effects, and classification in relation to other amebicides.

Other protozoan diseases

Other common protozoan diseases that may be frequently encountered in medical practice in the United States or that are widespread in other parts of the world are trichomoniasis, toxoplasmosis, pneumocystosis, and trypanosomiasis. The general approach to their treatment is found in Table 26-4, which lists the drugs of choice and their dosages and side effects. In this section, each disease and the pri-

mary antiprotozoan agent used in its treatment will be described.

TRICHOMONIASIS

Trichomoniasis is a disease of the vagina caused by *Trichomonas vaginalis*. Its characteristic presentation consists of a wet, inflamed vagina, a "strawberry" cervix, and a thin, yellow, frothy malodorous discharge. Usually both male and female are infected by this organism which can be identified microscopically from semen, prostatic fluid, or exudate from the vagina. Infections often recur, which indicates that the protozoans persist in extravaginal foci, the male urethra, or the periurethral glands and ducts of both sexes. Metronidazole is the drug of choice, and treatment must be given simultaneously to both sexual partners involved for cure. Two other agents—tinidazole and nimorazole—are being used successfully in its treatment in other countries.

Locally active antiinfective preparations such as povidone-iodine (Betadine) have been used in treatment of trichomoniasis. These locally applied agents, however, do not reach the extravaginal or male sources, and reinfection is likely to occur.

T A B L E 2 6 - 4   General treatment of other protozoan diseases

Disease	Drug	Dose	Side effects
Trichomoniasis	Metronidazole (Flagyl)	1 to 2 g for 1 dose for both male and female, or 250 mg 3 times a day for 7 days	*Frequent:* nausea, headache, metallic taste *Occasional:* vomiting, diarrhea, insomnia, weakness, stomatitis, vertigo, paresthesia, rash, dark urine, dry mouth *Rare:* ataxia, depression, irritability, confusion, mild Antabuse-like reaction with alcohol
Toxoplasmosis	Pyrimethamine *plus*	25 mg/day for 3 to 4 weeks	*Occasional:* blood dyscrasias, folic acid deficiency *Rare:* rash, vomiting, convulsions, shock
	Sulfadiazine	4 g/day for 3 to 4 weeks	*Occasional:* rash, nausea *Rare:* Stevens-Johnson syndrome or Lyell's disease
Pneumocystosis	Trimethoprim-Sulfamethoxazole (Bactrim; Septra)	Trimethoprim, 20 mg/kg/day, with sulfamethoxazole, 100 mg/kg/day, divided in 4 doses for 14 days	*Occasional:* rash, nausea *Occasional:* rash, nausea *Rare:* Stevens-Johnson syndrome or Lyell's disease
Trypanosomiasis *Trypanosoma cruzi* (South American trypanosomiasis, Chagas' disease)	Nifurtimox* (Bayer 2502; Lampit)	5 mg/kg/day orally in 4 divided doses, increasing by 2 mg/kg/day every 2 weeks until dose reaches 15 to 17 mg/kg/day	*Frequent:* anorexia, vomiting, weight loss, loss of memory, sleep disorders, tremor, paresthesias, weakness, polyneuritis *Rare:* convulsions
T. gambiense, T. rhodesiense (African trypanosomiasis, sleeping sickness) Hemolytic stage	Suramin sodium* (Germanin)	100 to 200 mg (test dose), intravenously, then 1 g intravenously on days 1, 3, 7, 14, and 21	*Frequent:* vomiting, pruritus, urticaria, paresthesias, hyperesthesia of hands and feet, photophobia, peripheral neuropathy *Occasional:* kidney damage, blood dyscrasias, shock
Late disease with central nervous system involvement	Melarsoprol* (Mel B; Arsobal)	2 to 3.6 mg/kg/day intravenously for 3 doses; after 1 week 3.6 mg/kg/day intravenously for 3 doses; repeat again after 10 to 21 days	*Frequent:* myocardial damage, albuminuria, hypertension, colic, Herxheimer-type reaction, encephalopathy, vomiting, peripheral neuropathy *Rare:* shock

*Drug is available for use only from the Parasitic Disease Drug Service, U.S. Centers for Disease Control, Atlanta, GA 30333.

TOXOPLASMOSIS

Toxoplasmosis is caused by an intracellular parasite, *Toxoplasma gondii*. This parasite is found worldwide and infects a wide variety of animals including humans. It is often harbored in the host with no evidence of the disease. Toxoplasmosis is contracted by ingesting cysts found in inadequately cooked or raw meat or by accidentally ingesting cysts from cat feces.

The most common form of the disease in the United States is usually subclinical. Symptomatically the patient may experience lymphadenopathy, fever, and occasionally a rash on the palms and soles. The most serious complication of toxoplasmosis is meningoencephalitis. Toxoplasmosis is treated with a combination of sulfadiazine and pyrimethamine, both of which alter the folic acid cycle of the *Toxoplasma* organism, resulting in its death.

PNEUMOCYSTOSIS

Pneumocystosis is a disease found commonly in patients who have impaired immune systems caused by malignancies, collagen vascular diseases, or immunosuppressive therapy. It is caused by the parasite *Pneumocystis carinii.* Characteristically the disease's symptoms initially are vague and generalized and include a dry cough, dyspnea or tachypnea or both, chest discomfort, and marked pallor. Cyanosis is the most common and consistent finding. If untreated, the disease progresses into interstitial plasma cell pneumonia, where its infiltration into the lungs and lung tissue causes a honeycombed appearance. There is a fatality of 50% or more of patients who do not receive treatment at this advanced stage of the disease. Children are more susceptible to pneumocystosis than are adults.

The therapy of choice in treating patients with *Pneumocystis carinii* infection is a combination of sulfamethoxazole and trimethoprim (Bactrim; Septra). In the past, pentamidine, a diamidine drug, was the drug of choice, but because of its toxicities and inconvenience in retrieval from the U.S. Centers for Disease Control, its use has become secondary. Pneumocystosis is more effectively treated in the early stages of the disease process than after it has progressed to the interstitial plasma cell pneumonia stage.

TRYPANOSOMIASIS

Trypanosomiasis is not commonly found in the United States but is found extensively in other parts of the world. There are two types of trypanosomiasis, the African variety and the South American variety.

African trypanosomiasis (sleeping sickness) is caused by *Trypanosoma gambiense* or *T. rhodesiense.* These protozoans are transmitted from host to host by the bite of the tsetse fly. The organism then invades the lymphatic system and causes intermittent attacks of fever, lymphadenopathy, hepatosplenomegaly, dyspnea, and tachycardia. This is called the hemolytic stage of the disease and is treated with suramin sodium, the drug of choice.

As the disease progresses into the central nervous system, the victim experiences head-aches, disturbances in coordination, mental dullness, apathy, and eventually constant sleep, resulting in emaciation and death. This latter stage, with involvement of the central nervous system, has been treated effectively with melarsoprol.

The South American variety of trypanosomiasis is often referred to as Chagas' disease. It is caused by the protozoan *T. cruzi* and is transmitted by the bite of reduviid bugs infected with these parasites. The disease may be either asymptomatic or symptomatic, varying from region to region. Early symptoms may be local swelling (chagoma) at the site of the insect bite, rash, fever, and edema of eyelids and face. The chronic form of the disease may result in visceromegaly, cardiopathy, or meningoencephalitis resulting in death, or the patient may remain asymptomatic. The *T. cruzi* seems to have an affinity for cardiac parenchymal cells and nerve cells in the mesenteric plexus.

Chagas' disease is resistant to most forms of therapy. Recently a new drug, nifurtimox, has shown activity against both extracellular and intracellular parasites that no other drug has demonstrated.

All the agents now used in treating both African and South American trypanosomiasis have severe toxicity. As a result, their usefulness in treating these diseases has been limited. All three agents used in treating trypanosomiasis are available from the U.S. Centers for Disease Control.

Helminthiasis

Anthelmintics are drugs used to rid the body of worms (helminths). The use of anthelmintics (*anti*, against; Gr. *helmins*, worm) is among the most primitive types of chemotherapy. It has been estimated that one third of the world's population is infested with these parasites.

Helminths may be present in the gastrointestinal tract, but several types also penetrate the tissues, and some undergo developmental changes, during which they wander extensively in the host. Because most anthelmintics used today are highly effective against specific parasites, the organism must be accurately identified before treatment is started, usually by finding the parasite ova or larvae in the feces, urine, blood, sputum, or tissues of the host.

Undesirable effects that may result from helminthiasis. Parasitic infestations do not necessarily cause clinical manifestations, although they may be injurious for a number of reasons:

1 Worms may cause mechanical injury to the tissues and organs. Roundworms in large numbers may cause obstruction in the intestine; filariae may block lymphatic channels and cause massive edema; and hookworms often cause extensive damage to the wall of the intestine and considerable loss of blood.
2 Toxic substances made by the parasite may be absorbed by the host.
3 The tissues of the host may be traumatized by the presence of the parasite and made more susceptible to bacterial infections.
4 Heavy infestation with worms will rob the host of food. This is particularly significant in children.

Classification of helminths. Worms that are parasitic to humans may be classified as nematodes, trematodes, and cestodes.

The nematodes are round, unsegmented worms that vary in length from a fraction of an inch to a foot or more. They include *Ascaris lumbricoides* (roundworm), *Necator americanus* and *Ancylostoma duodenale* (two species of hookworm), *Trichuris trichiura* (whipworm), *Trichinella spiralis* (which produces trichinosis), *Enterobius vermicularis* (pinworm), and *Wuchereria bancrofti* (causing filariasis).

The trematodes are flukes, among which are several blood flukes—*Schistosoma mansoni, S. japonicum,* and *S. haematobium*. There are other flukes parasitic to humans, such as the liver and lung flukes. Schistosomiasis is a disease caused by blood flukes. They penetrate the skin of persons who bathe in contaminated water or in some other way come in contact with the infected water in which snails serve as the intermediate host. The adult blood flukes live in the veins of the mesentery and pelvis of humans and accumulate in the portal vein. The liver and spleen are the organs mainly involved.

The *cestodes* are the tapeworms, of which there are four varieties: (1) *Taenia saginata* (beef tapeworm), (2) *T. solium* (pork tapeworm), (3) *Diphyllobothrium latum* (fish tapeworm),

and (4) *Hymenolepis nana* (dwarf tapeworm). As indicated by the name of the worm, the parasite enters the intestine by way of improperly cooked beef, pork, or fish or from contaminated food, as in the case of the dwarf tapeworm.

The cestodes are segmented flatworms with a head and a number of segments, or proglottids, which in some cases may extend for 20 to 30 feet in the bowel. The tapeworms, with the exception of the dwarf tapeworm, spend part of their life cycle in a host other than humans—pigs, fish, or cattle. The dwarf tapeworm does not require an intermediate host.

Anthelmintics

Table 26-5 summarizes the drugs used in the treatment of helminthiasis. Only the drugs of choice for each helminth infection will be discussed further.

DRUGS USED FOR NEMATODE INFECTIONS (ROUNDWORMS)
Pyrantel pamoate (Antiminth)

Pyrantel pamoate is the drug of choice in the treatment of *Ascaris lumbricoides* (roundworm), *Enterobius vermicularis* (pinworms), and *Ancylostoma duodenale* and *Necator americanus* (hookworms). The cure rate for roundworms is approximately 100%, for pinworms 90% to 100%, and for hookworms 92% to 93%. Pyrantel is usually given as one single dose of 11 mg/kg body weight (maximum dose, 1 g). However, many have believed that it is more effective when given in three consecutive daily doses. The dose may be repeated in 1 month if needed.

Pyrantel acts by paralyzing the worms, which are eventually evacuated from the body in the feces. It is poorly absorbed in the gastrointestinal tract, with 50% of the oral dose excreted in the feces.

Pyrantel pamoate is available as an oral suspension of 250 mg/5 ml. Occasionally, it may cause gastrointestinal disturbances, headache, dizziness, rash, or fever.

Thiabendazole (Mintezol)

Thiabendazole is the drug of choice for cutaneous larva migrans (creeping eruption), *Tri-*

TABLE 26-5 Drugs used in treatment of helminthiasis

Class, genus, and species	Drug
Nematoda (roundworm)	
Ancylostoma duodenale (hookworm),	Pyrantel pamoate
	Mebendazole
Ascaris lumbricoides (roundworm)	Pyrantel pamoate
	Mebendazole
	Piperazine citrate
Nematode larvae causing cutaneous	Thiabendazole
larva migrans (creeping eruption)	Ethyl chloride spray
Dracunculus medinensis (guinea worm)	Niridazole*
	Metronidazole
Enterobius vermicularis (pinworm)	Pyrantel pamoate
	Mebendazole
	Piperazine citrate
	Pyrvinium pamoate
Filarial nematodes	
Loa loa	Diethylcarbamazine
Wuchereria bancrofti	
W. (Brugia) malayi	
Acanthocheilonema perstans	
Filariae causing tropical eosinophilia	
Onchocerca volvulus	
Necator americanus (hookworm)	Pyrantel pamoate
	Mebendazole
	Thiabendazole†
Trichinella spiralis (pork roundworm)	Thiabendazole†
Trematoda (flukes)	
Schistosoma japonicum	Niridazole*
	Antimony sodium (antimony dimercaptosuccinate)*
Schistosoma mansoni	Niridazole*
	Oxamniquine
	Antimony sodium (antimony dimercaptosuccinate)*
Cestoda (tapeworms)	
Diphyllobothrim latum (fish tapeworm)	Niclosamide*
Hymenolepis nana (dwarf tapeworm)	Niclosamide*
Taenia saginata (beef tapeworm)	Niclosamide*
	Paromomycin
Taenia solium (pork tapeworm)	Niclosamide*

*Drug is available for use only from the Parasitic Disease Drug Service, U.S. Centers for Disease Control, Atlanta, GA 30333.
†Not available in the United States.

chinella spiralis (pork roundworm), and visceral larva migrans. In the case of cutaneous larva migrans, the drug may be given orally or topically. Orally, it is given in a dose of 25 mg/kg body weight, twice a day for 2 days. For *T. spiralis* and visceral larva migrans, it is given in a dose of 25 mg/kg twice a day for 5 days. Concomitant administration of corticosteroids may be required in these treatments to minimize the severe inflammation caused by the dying larvae.

Thiabendazole is available as an oral suspension, 500 mg/5 ml, and a chewable tablet of 500 mg. Its most frequent side effects are nausea, vomiting, and vertigo. Occasionally leukopenia, crystalluria, rash, hallucinations, and olfactory disturbances may occur. Rarely does one see shock, tinnitus, or Stevens-Johnson syndrome with its administration.

Mebendazole (Vermox)

Mebendazole is the drug of choice in the treatment of *Trichuris trichiura* (whipworm) and has become the alternative drug of choice in the treatment of *Ascaris lumbricoides* (roundworm), *Ancylostoma duodenale* and *Necator americanus* (hookworms), *Enterobius vermicularis* (pinworm), and *Dracunculus medinensis* (guinea worm). It has the broadest spectrum of any anthelmintic drug. In the treatment of infections with whipworm, roundworm, and hookworm, mebendazole is given in a dose of

100 mg twice a day for 3 days. Pinworm infections require only a single dose of 100 mg, which may be repeated after 2 weeks. The guinea worm requires a dose of 250 mg three times a day for 10 days.

Mebendazole is available in 100-mg chewable tablets. It occasionally causes diarrhea and abdominal pain and is considered a relatively safe, nontoxic drug.

Diethylcarbamazine citrate (Hetrazan)

Diethylcarbamazine is a piperazine derivative that has been used for a number of years in the treatment of filariasis. It is the drug of choice for infections with the following parasites: *Wuchereria bancrofti, W. (Brugia) malayi, Loa loa, Acanthocheilonema perstans,* filariae causing tropical eosinophilia, and *Onchocerca volvulus.* In the treatment of *W. bancrofti, W.(B.) malayi, A. perstans,* and *L. loa,* a 21-day schedule is used and consists of 50 mg diethylcarbamazine on day 1; 50 mg three times a day on day 2; 100 mg three times a day on day 3; and 2 mg/kg body weight three times a day on days 4 to 21. In the treatment of tropical eosinophilia the dosage is 2 mg/kg three times a day for 7 to 10 days. Therapy for *Onchocerca volvulus* is initiated with 25 mg/day for 3 days, then 50 mg/day for 5 days, then 100 mg/day for 3 days, and finally 150 mg/day for 12 days.

Diethylcarbamazine citrate is available in 50-mg tablets. Its adverse effects may manifest themselves as headache, lassitude, malaise, anorexia, and nausea and vomiting. Mild to severe allergic reactions are frequent as a result of the release of foreign protein from dying microfilariae or adult worms. If allergic reactions become severe, drug dosage should be reduced or treatment interrupted. Rarely encephalopathy may occur.

DRUGS USED FOR TREMATODE INFECTIONS (FLUKES)
Niridazole (Ambilhar)

Niridazole is considered the drug of choice in the treatment of schistosomiases caused by *Schistosoma japonicum* and *S. mansoni* and is the alternate drug of choice in the treatment of infection with *S. haematobium.* It has also been found to be the agent of choice in the nematode infection *Dracunculus medinensis* (guinea worm). In the treatment of infection with *S. mansoni* or *S. haematobium,* it is given in a dose of 25 mg/kg/day orally for 5 to 7 days, with a maximum dose of 1.5 g to be given during a day. For the treatment of infection with *S. japonicum,* 25 mg/kg/day orally is given for 10 days (maximum dose, 1.5 g). Infection with *D. medinensis* (guinea worm) is treated with 25 mg/kg/day for 15 days (maximum dose, 1.5 g).

Niridazole comes in 500 mg tablets. It produces frequent vomiting, cramps, dizziness, headaches, and immunosuppression. Occasionally diarrhea, slight electrocardiographic changes, rash, insomnia, and paresthesias may be seen. Rarely psychosis, hemolytic anemia in glucose-6-phosphate dehydrogenase–deficient persons, and convulsions will occur. This drug is absolutely contraindicated in patients with hepatocellular disease, portal hypertension, or a history of mental disorders or seizures.

Niridazole is an anthelmintic that is available only through the Parasitic Disease Drug Service of the U.S. Centers for Disease Control.

Metrifonate (Bilarcil)

Metrifonate is an organophosphorus cholinesterase inhibitor that has become the drug of choice in the treatment of *Schistosoma haematobium* infections. It has a cure rate of 90% to 95%. Metrifonate is given in dosages of 10 mg/kg body weight every other week for three treatments. At therapeutic doses it occasionally causes nausea, vomiting, bronchospasms, weakness, diarrhea, and abdominal pain. Metrifonate can be obtained only through the Parasitic Disease Drug Service of the U.S. Centers for Disease Control.

Bithionol (Bitin)

Bithionol has become the drug of choice in the treatment of the liver and lung flukes *Fasciola hepatica* and *Paragonimus westermani.* It is given in dosages of 30 to 50 mg/kg body weight on alternate days for 10 to 15 doses. Bithionol frequently causes photosensitivity skin reactions, vomiting, diarrhea, abdominal pain, and urticaria. It can be obtained only through the Parasitic Disease Drug Service of the U.S. Centers for Disease Control.

DRUGS USED FOR CESTODE INFECTIONS (TAPEWORMS)
Niclosamide (Yomesan)

Niclosamide is the drug of choice in treating tapeworms—*Diphyllobothrim latum* (fish tapeworm), *Hymenolepis nana* (dwarf tapeworm), *Taenia saginata* (beef tapeworm), and *T. solium* (pork tapeworm). It does not require intubation or hospitalization, as previous therapy has done. When it fails, the alternate drug that is used is the antibiotic paromomycin. For the treatment of infections with fish, beef, and pork tapeworms, a single dose of four tablets (2 g) of niclosamide, to be chewed thoroughly, is given.

The dwarf tapeworm requires a single daily dose of four tablets (2 g), to be chewed thoroughly, for 5 days. Niclosamide achieves 86% to 97% cure rates in infections of these tapeworms.

Niclosamide is available in 500-mg chewable tablets from the Parasitic Disease Drug Service of the U.S. Centers for Disease Control. Occasionally a patient may experience nausea and abdominal pain, but in general the drug is considered to be a safe and effective agent.

OTHER ANTHELMINTICS

Numerous other anthelmintics, used as secondary and tertiary treatments, are being developed or used in other parts of the world but are excluded for use in the United States. There are three such agents that should be discussed before concluding the discussion of anthelmintics: oxamniquine, chloroquine phosphate, and a new drug, oxantel-pyrantel.

Oxamniquine (Mansil) is an anthelmintic used in other parts of the world as the drug of choice in the treatment for *Schistosoma mansoni* (blood fluke). Its advantage over other agents is that it can be given both orally and by the intramuscular route, in addition to having a shorter course of therapy. It is considered to have greater activity than niridazole (used in the United States) and has fewer side effects.

Chloroquine phosphate, an antimalarial agent, has also found usefulness as alternative therapy in the treatment for lung and liver flukes. Many believe that it is the drug of choice in the treatment for *Chlonorchis sinensis* (liver fluke) when given in a dose of 250 mg (150-mg base) three times a day for 6 weeks. Even though it does not produce cures, it temporarily suppresses the ova. Other parts of this chapter discuss this drug further.

A new drug, oxantel-pyrantel, is being studied in the treatment of nematode infections. It has been found effective against roundworms, hookworms, and whipworms and is reported more acceptable to patients than mebendazole. Only mild side effects or none at all have been reported for this agent.

Ectoparasitic diseases

Ectoparasiticides are those drugs used against animal parasites. For human use these drugs are more frequently referred to as pediculicides and scabicides (miticides), reflecting the parasite treated with each group.

Pediculosis is a parasite infestation of lice on the skin of a human. Lice infestations have been increasing in North America and western Europe. It was once thought that pediculosis could be attributed to crowded dwellings and poor hygiene, but recently this assumption has proved not to be true. The lice are transmitted from one person to the next by close contact with infested persons, clothing, combs, and towels. There are three different varieties of the infestation: (1) pediculosis pubis, caused by *Phthirus pubis* (pubic louse, or "crabs"), (2) pediculosis corporis, caused by *Pediculus humanus var. corporis* (body louse), and (3) pediculosis capitis, caused by *P. humanus var. capitis* (head louse).

Common findings in a person who is infested include pruritus, nits (eggs of louse) on hair shafts, lice on skin or clothes, and, when there are pubic lice, occasionally sky-blue macules on the inner thighs or lower abdomen. The drug of choice is the pediculicide lindane (Gamma-benzene hexachloride).

A characteristic finding of pediculosis corporis, except in heavily infested individuals, is that the parasite is absent from the body but inhabits seams of clothing that come in contact with the axillae or that are in the beltline or collar.

Scabies is a parasitic infestation caused by

the itch mite, *Sarcoptes scabiei*. It is transmitted from one person to the next by close contact, such as sleeping with an infested individual. It bores into the horny layer of the skin in cracks and folds, causing irritation and pruritus. Itching occurs almost exclusively at night. The infestation is usually generalized over the body except the head and neck regions. The drug of choice is the scabicide, crotamiton.

ECTOPARASITICIDES

The first approach to the treatment of both pediculosis and scabies is identification of the source of infestation. Next, decontamination of clothing and personal articles used by the infested person is necessary. This can be done by washing clothing and bedding with hot, soapy water or by having items dry-cleaned that cannot be washed. Usually all persons involved, such as the whole family, are treated to prevent reinfestation. Table 26-6 summarizes the various topical pediculicides and scabicides used in the treatment of these parasitic infestations.

Lindane (gamma-benzene hexachloride; Kwell)

Lindane is considered both a scabicide and a pediculicide because it is effective in the treatment of both lice and mite infestations. It is available in a 1% cream, lotion, and shampoo. For the treatment of pediculosis pubis and infestations of *Pediculus humanus var. capitis*, the cream or lotion is applied in a sufficient quantity to cover the skin and hair of the infected and surrounding areas. It is left on for 12 hours and then thoroughly washed. It seldom needs to be applied more than once. The shampoo is worked into the hair and left on for 4 minutes. Then the hair is rinsed and dried, and nits (eggs) are combed from the hair shafts. Retreatment is usually not necessary.

For the treatment of scabies, only the cream or lotion is used. If crusted lesions are present, a warm bath preceding the application of lindane is recommended. Lindane is applied over the entire body from the neck down. Again, it is left on for 8 to 12 hours and then washed off. Usually one application is sufficient. It is common to have pruritus after application, but this does

TABLE 26-6 Drugs used in the treatment of ectoparasitic diseases

Disease	Drug
Pediculosis (lice infestation)	
Pediculus humanus var. capitis (head louse)	Lindane (gamma-benzene hexachloride)
Pediculus humanus var. corporis (body louse)	Pyrethrins with piperonylbutoxide
Phthirus pubis (pubic louse)	Copper oleate, 0.03%
Scabies (mite infestation)	
Sarcoptes scabiei	Crotamiton
	Lindane (gamma-benzene hexachloride)
	Benzyl benzoate, 12%-25%
	Sulfur in petrolatum

not indicate a reapplication unless living mites can be demonstrated.

Lindane occasionally will cause an eczematous skin rash. It penetrates human skin and has a potential for central nervous system toxicity, especially in children. Rarely do convulsions or aplastic anemia occur with use of this drug.

Crotamiton (Eurax Cream)

Crotamiton has scabicidal and antipruritic actions. It is massaged into the skin from the chin down, particularly in the folds and creases of the body. It is reapplied in 24 hours, and 48 hours after the second application it is washed from the body surface.

Two applications of crotamiton usually eradicates most mite infestations. In resistant cases it may be applied again 1 week later.

Crotamiton is available as a 10% cream or lotion. Occasionally a skin rash may occur with its application. Rarely allergic or irritant contact dermatitis occur.

Summary of nursing considerations

Protozoan infections are the most common infections found in the world today. They are especially prevalent in crowded developing countries that have poor sanitation, such as countries of Africa, Asia, and South America. These diseases have become more prevalent in the United States since global travel has become commonplace.

Antimalarial drugs are classified into three major groups: (1) primary tissue schizonticides, (2) blood schizonticides, and (3) secondary tissue schizonticides, all corresponding to a stage of the life cycle of the malarial parasite. Most antimalarial agents used are the blood schizonticides such as chloroquine, amodiaquine, hydroxychloroquin, pyrimethamine, and quinine in the treatment and prophylaxis of malaria. Table 26-2 summarizes the general approach to the treatment of malaria.

Primaquine phosphate, a secondary tissue schizonticide, has been found useful in the prophylaxis and treatment of relapsing malarias caused by *Plasmodium vivax* and *P. ovale.*

Amebiasis is a disease caused by *Entamoeba histolytica*. This disease can have three states: (1) asymptomatic, (2) intestinal infection, and (3) an extraintestinal infection, usually referred to as hepatic amebiasis. The amebicides are divided into two groups of agents—the luminal amebicides, which kill the parasite on contact, and the tissue amebicides, which kill the parasites that have penetrated into intestinal and extra-intestinal tissues. Diiodohydroxyquin and diloxanide furoate (Furamide) have become the luminal amebicides of choice, and metronidazole has become the tissue amebicide of choice for intestinal and extra-intestinal amebiasis.

Other common protozoan infections are trichomoniasis, toxoplasmosis, pneumocystosis, and trypanosomiasis (sleeping sickness, or Chagas' disease). Their treatments are summarized in Table 26-4.

Anthelmintics are drugs used to rid the body of worms. Different anthelmintics are used against each of the three different classifications of worms that are parasitic in humans: nematodes, trematodes, and cestodes. Common anthelmintics used in their treatment are pyrantel pamoate (Antiminth), thiabendazole (Mintezol), mebendazole (Vermox), diethylcarbamazine citrate (Hetrazan), niridazole (Ambilhar), metrifonate (Bilarcil), bithinol (Bitin), and niclosamide (Yomesan). Several of these agents can be obtained only through the Parasitic Disease Drug Service of the U.S. Centers for Disease Control.

Ectoparasiticides are those drugs used against animal parasites. For human use these drugs are referred to as pediculicides (drugs used to treat lice infestations) and scabicides or miticides (drugs used to treat mite infestations). Two topical preparations have been found effective in treating scabies: crotamiton and lindane (Kwell).

Pediculosis is effectively treated with lindane in usually a one-time treatment.

QUESTIONS

FOR STUDY AND REVIEW

1 What causes the characteristic recurring chills, fever, and prostration of malaria?
2 Most antimalarial drugs act on what stage of the parasitic cycle? How are they used in the treatment of malaria? Name three drugs used in this manner.
3 Give the general approach to the treatment of malaria, giving drugs, dosages, schedules, and side effects to be aware of in their administration.
4 How is pyrimethamine used in the treatment of malaria?
5 Describe the symptoms of cinchonism that may occur with the use of quinine sulfate.
6 Compare diloxanide and diiodohydroxyquin as the drug of choice in the treatment of asymptomatic amebiasis.
7 Describe the mechanism of action of the indirect amebicidal action drugs.
8 What is the general approach to the treatment of intestinal and hepatic amebiasis? Discuss drugs, dosages, and side effects.
9 What is the anthelmintic of choice in the treatment of hookworms, pinworms, and roundworms? Give dosages.
10 Schistosomiasis is most effectively treated with what agents?
11 The drug of choice in treating tapeworms is what anthelmintic?
12 What is pediculosis and how is it treated?

BIBLIOGRAPHY

GENERAL

A.M.A. drug evaluation, ed. 3, Littleton, Mass., 1980, PSG Publishing Co., Inc.
Goodman, L.S., and Gilman, A., editors: The pharmacological basis of therapeutics, ed. 6, New York, 1980, Macmillan, Inc.
Goth, A.: Medical pharmacology: principles and concepts, ed. 10, St. Louis, 1981, The C.V. Mosby Co.

Kagan, B.M.: Antimicrobial therapy, ed. 3, Philadelphia, Pa., 1980, W.B. Saunders Co.

The Medical Letter on Drugs and Therapeutics: Drugs for parasitic infections, vol. 21, Report No. 26, New Rochelle, N.Y., 1979, The Medical Letter, Inc., pp. 105-112.

Modell, W., editor: Drugs of choice 1980-1981, St. Louis, 1980, The C.V. Mosby Co.

ANTIPROTOZOAN DRUGS

Hall, A.P.: The treatment of malaria, Br. Med. J. **1:**323, 1976.

Hendrickse, R.G.: Dysentery including amoebiasis, Br. Med. J. **1:**669, 1972.

Is Flagyl dangerous? Med. Lett. Drugs Ther. **17:**53, June 20, 1975.

Misra, N.P.: A comparative study of tinidazole and metronidazole as a single daily dose for three days in symptomatic intestial amoebiasis, Drugs **15**(Suppl. 1):19, 1978.

Pittman, F.E., and Pittman, J.C.: Amebic liver abscess following metronidazole therapy for amebic colitis, Am. J. Trop. Med. Hyg. **23:**146, 1974.

Powell, R.D.: Development of new antimalarial drugs, Am. J. Trop. Med. Hyg. **21:**744, 1972.

Powell, S.J.: Therapy of amebiasis, Bull. N.Y. Acad. Sci. **47:**469, 1972.

Report to WHO Scientific Group: Chemotherapy of malaria and resistance to antimalarials, WHO Tech. Rep. Ser., No. 529, 1973.

Rozman, R.S.: Chemotherapy of malaria, Annu. Rev. Pharmacol. **13:**127, 1973.

Rubidge, C.J., and others: Treatment of children with acute amoebic dysentery, Arch. Dis. Child. **45:**196, 1970.

Scott, F., and Miller, M.J.: Trials with metronidazole in amebic dysentery, J.A.M.A. **211:**118, 1970.

Tigertt, W.D., and Clyde, D.F.: Drug resistance in the human malarias, Antibiot. Chemother. **20:**246, 1975.

Weber, D.M.: Amebic abscess of liver following metronidazole therapy, J.A.M.A. **216:**1339, 1971.

Wolfe, M.S.: Non-dysenteric intestinal amebiasis: treatment with diloxanide furoate, J.A.M.A. **18:**1601, 1973.

ANTHELMINTICS

Desowitz, R.S.: Antiparasite chemotherapy, Annu. Rev. Pharmacol. **11:**351, 1971.

Katz, M.: Parasitic infections, J. Pediatr. **87:**165, 1975.

Lee, S.H., and Lim, J.K.: A comparative study of the effect of oxantel-pyrantel suspension and mebendazole in mixed infections with *Ascaris* and *Trichuris*, Drugs **15:**94, 1978.

Miller, M.J., and others: Mebendazole: an effective anthelmintic for trichuriasis and enterobiasis, J.A.M.A. **230:**1412, 1974.

Pena Chavarria, A., and others: Mebendazole: an effective broad-spectrum anthelmintic, Am. J. Trop. Med. Hyg. **22:**592, 1973.

Wolfe, M.S., and Wershing, J.M.: Mebendazole: treatment of trichuriasis and ascariasis in Bahamian children, J.A.M.A. **230:**1408, 1974.

UNIT EIGHT

DRUGS USED IN NEOPLASTIC DISEASES

CHAPTER 27

Cancer chemotherapy (antineoplastic agents)

KAY SEE-LASLEY

Human cancer encompasses a group of over 100 related diseases that constitute the second greatest cause of death in the United States and in western Europe. Although surgery and x-ray therapy are still the most effective treatments of cancer in the early stages of the disease process, great advances have been achieved in antineoplastic drug therapy in the advanced disease process since the 1940s. A variety of drugs can now be used, either alone or in conjunction with surgery and x-ray therapy, to produce palliation of symptoms, regression of the neoplastic process, and prolongation of life. The neoplastic diseases in which a "cure" (or long-term remission) can be achieved include gestational choriocarcinoma, Hodgkin's disease, acute lymphocytic leukemia, Burkitt's lymphoma, embryonal carcinoma of the testes, Wilms' tumor, Ewing's sarcoma, rhabdomyosarcoma, retinoblastoma, osteogenic sarcoma, and histiocytic lymphoma.

Antineoplastic agents, even though they cause damage to both normal and neoplastic cells, have a greater selective toxicity for neo-plastic cells. The reason is that malignant cells are more likely to be in the dividing cycle, consisting of phases G_1, S, G_2, and M (Fig. 27-1). The antineoplastic agents' primary mode of action involves interfering with the supply and utilization of building blocks of nucleic acids, such as enzymes for purines and pyrimidines, as well as interfering with the intact molecules of deoxyribonucleic acid (DNA) and ribonucleic acid (RNA), which are needed for replication and growth. Both normal and malignant cells go through four similar stages of life. The first stage is the dividing cell, which is highly sensitive to antineoplastic agents (Fig. 27-1). The second stage is the temporarily nondividing cell (G_0), which is less sensitive to anticancer drugs. The third stage is the mature cell, which is permanently nondividing; it is highly insensitive to anticancer drugs. The last stage is cell death. Most cells in the body are in the permanently nondividing cell stage, whereas most cells of neoplastic diseases are in the dividing cell stage. The body does, however, have three areas in which the dividing cell stage is ac-

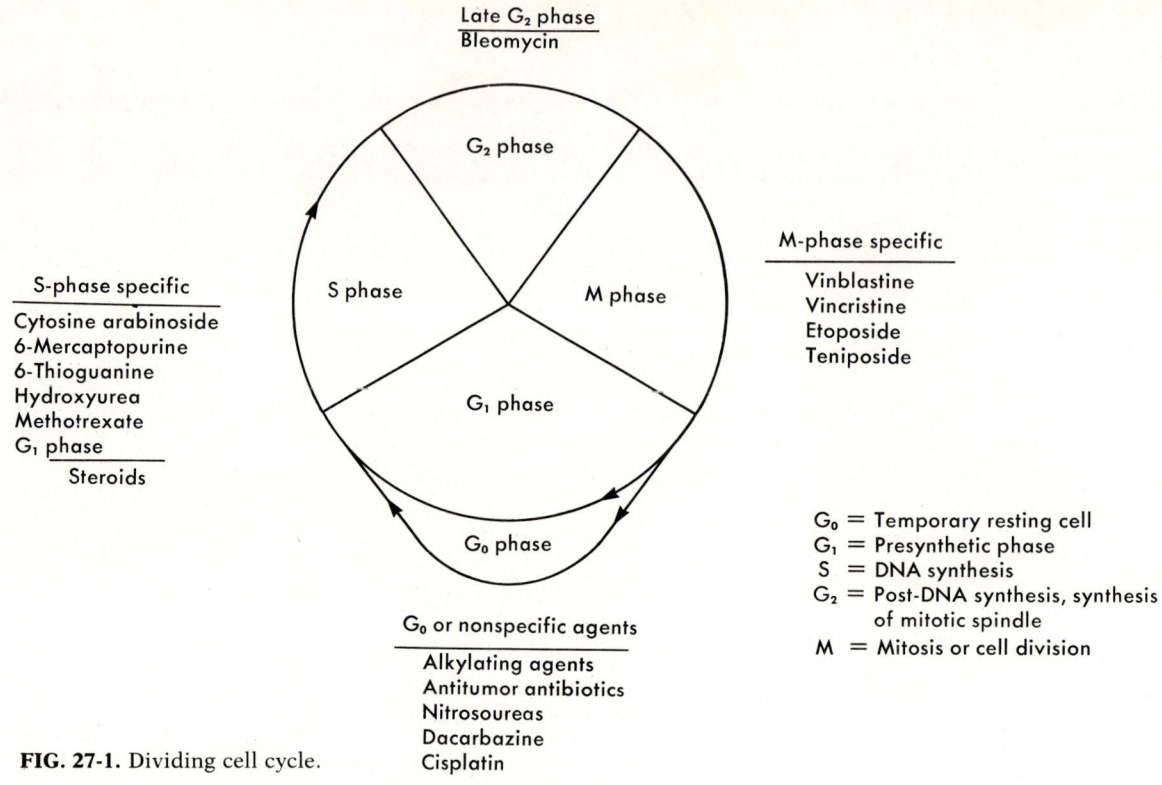

Late G₂ phase
Bleomycin

G₂ phase

S phase

M phase

S-phase specific

Cytosine arabinoside
6-Mercaptopurine
6-Thioguanine
Hydroxyurea
Methotrexate
G₁ phase

Steroids

M-phase specific

Vinblastine
Vincristine
Etoposide
Teniposide

G₁ phase

G₀ phase

G₀ or nonspecific agents

Alkylating agents
Antitumor antibiotics
Nitrosoureas
Dacarbazine
Cisplatin

G₀ = Temporary resting cell
G₁ = Presynthetic phase
S = DNA synthesis
G₂ = Post-DNA synthesis, synthesis
       of mitotic spindle
M = Mitosis or cell division

FIG. 27-1. Dividing cell cycle.

tive: (1) the bone marrow, (2) the hair follicles, and (3) the gastrointestinal tract. These three areas are most affected by the toxicity of anti-cancer drugs. The toxic effects are manifested as bone marrow depression, which predisposes patients to infections and anemias; alopecia; and ulcerations of oral and intestinal mucosa. Most of these conditions are reversible.

Anticancer drugs have different sites of action on the dividing cell cycle. Those agents which are more active on one specific phase are called cell cycle–specific agents. For example, since methotrexate is more active on the S phase of the cell cycle, it would be considered an S-phase cell cycle–specific agent (Fig. 27-1). Agents that are active on both proliferating and resting cells are called cell cycle–nonspecific agents. Examples of this group of agents would be the alkylating agents. Knowledge of sites of action of antineoplastic agents is important to investigators who are selecting agents for combination chemotherapy to maximize therapeutic effects of the drug regimen.

Classification of antineoplastic agents

The antineoplastic drugs can be divided into several classes on the basis of their probable mechanisms of action. These classes and the antineoplastic agents found in each are listed above.

Alkylating agents. The alkylating agents act in a number of ways, but their primary mechanism of action is the alkylation of the nucleic acids, resulting in inactivation of DNA. These agents are also referred to as radiomimetic drugs, since they affect cells in much the same way as does irradiation. Since the initial use of the parent compound of this group, nitrogen mustard, other alkylating agents have been developed in the search for more effective and less toxic drugs. Many of the alkylating agents are interchangeable except for dose, route of administration, and the rapidity and duration of the effect desired. They are primarily used in the treatment of malignancies of the hemato-poietic tissues, neuroblastoma, and dissemi-

Classification of antineoplastic agents

Alkylating agents
Busulfan
Chlorambucil
Cyclophosphamide
Ifosfamide
Mechlorethamine
Melphalan

Antibiotics
Bleomycin
Dactinomycin
Daunorubicin
Doxorubicin
Mithramycin
Mitomycin C
Rubidazone

Antimetabolites
5-Azacitidine
Azathioprine
Baker's antifol
Cytosine arabinoside
 (cytarabine)
Floxuridine
Fluorouracil
Mercaptopurine
Methotrexate
Tegafur
Thioguanine

Hormones
Adrenocorticosteroids
 Dexamethasone
 Hydrocortisone
 Methylprednisolone
 Prednisone
 Antiadrenal agents
  Aminoglutethimide
  Mitotane
   (o, p'-DDD)
Androgens
 Fluoxymesterone
 Methyltestosterone
 Nandrolin
 Propionate
 Testosterone
Antiestrogens
 Nafoxidine
  hydrochloride
 Tamoxifen citrate
Estrogens
 Diethylstilbestrol
 Ethinyl estradiol
Progestins
 Hydroxyproges-
  terone
 Medroxyproges-
  terone

Immune agents
Bacillus Calmette-
 Guerin vaccine (BCG)
Corynebacterium parvum
Levamisole
Methanol extracted
 residue (MER) of BCG

Plant alkaloids
Etoposide (VP 16-213)
Maytansine
Teniposide (VM-26)
Vinblastine
Vincristine

Radioisotopes
Cobalt 60
Gold (^{198}Au)
Iodine (^{131}I)
Phosphorus (^{32}P)

Miscellaneous agents
Alkylator-like agents
 Cisplatin
 Dacarbazine
 Galactitol
 Hexamethylmelamine
Nitrosoureas
 Carmustine (BCNU)
 Lomustine (CCNU)
 Semustine (MeCCNU)
 Streptozocin
Other
 L-Asparaginase
 Hydroxyurea
 Procarbazine
 Razoxane (ICRF-159)

---

nated carcinomas of the lungs, ovaries, testes, and breasts.

Antimetabolites. Antimetabolites are compounds whose chemical structures resemble chemical structures of substances normally used by cells for growth and metabolism. They interfere with the synthesis of nucleic acids, thereby interfering with DNA synthesis and cell growth. They are considered S-phase cell cycle–specific agents. The antimetabolites appear to be most effective in treatment of malignancies that are metabolically very active.

Antibiotics. The antibiotics are antiinfective products found to be too cytotoxic for use in the treatment of infections. They exert their cytotoxic effects by blocking the transcription of new DNA or RNA.

Like the alkylating agents, they are primarily used to treat malignancies of the hematopoietic tissues, neuroblastoma, Ewing's and os-

teogenic sarcomas, and disseminated carcinomas of the lungs, breasts, ovaries, and testes.

Plant alkaloids. This group of drugs derived from various plants has demonstrated an ability to block cell division in metaphase. They have been found useful in the treatment of leukemias; lymphomas; carcinomas of the breasts, lungs, testes, and unknown primary sites; and certain brain tumors.

Immune agents. The agents found in this group are called nonspecific immunoadjuvants. Like bacterial vaccinations, they provoke the stimulation of the immune system to provide minimal protection of the host from the neoplastic disease. The appropriate use of these agents is still under investigation, but they are being employed under the presumption that the immune system, once stimulated, would eradicate any residual neoplastic cells remaining after other modes of therapy.

Hormones. Hormones are used in the treatment of neoplasms that are sensitive to hormonal growth controls in the body. Their exact mechanism against neoplasms is unknown, but it appears that they interfere with growth-stimulating receptor proteins at the cellular membrane. A few drugs, such as aminoglutethimide, block critical biochemical steps in certain tissues (for example, adrenal gland) and interrupt hormone synthesis. Hormones are more specific in their use than other antineoplastic agents. For example, the estrogens are used in androgen-sensitive prostatic carcinomas or in postmenopausal women with breast cancer, and progestins are used in endometrial tumors and renal carcinomas. Androgens are used in the treatment of menopausal women with breast cancer and in prostatic cancer, and antiestrogens are used in breast cancer and endometrial cancer. The antiadrenal agents are applied to adrenal tumors as well as to breast cancer for their palliation.

Because of the ability of the adrenocorticosteroids to retard lymphocytic proliferation, their greatest value lies in the treatment of lymphocytic leukemias and lymphomas. They are also used in conjunction with x-ray therapy to decrease the occurrence of radiation edema in such critical areas as the superior mediastinum, brain, and spinal cord.

Individual drugs belonging to this category are discussed in Chapters 28 and 29.

Radioisotopes. Radioisotopes are used in the treatment of cancer because they liberate highly penetrating beta and gamma rays that destroy cells. Tissues vary in sensitivity to ionizing radiation; cells with a short life and high rate of reproduction are especially vulnerable. Examples are germinal cells of the ovaries and testes, bone marrow, lymphocytes, and the epithelial cells of the gastrointestinal tract. The radioactive isotopes are therefore most useful in hematologic malignancies, in Hodgkin's disease, and for control of localized tumor masses.

Miscellaneous agents. The miscellaneous agents are those agents that cannot be classified by their mechanism of action into any of the other groups previously mentioned. The nitrosoureas and the alkylator-like agents are

often grouped, like the antibiotics, under alkylating agents because of their similar mechanisms of action. The nitrosoureas are unique in their biologic qualities. They are lipid soluble, which permits them to reach neoplasms of the brain and central nervous system. The mechanisms of action of other agents in this group are varied and will not be discussed.

• • •

In the remainder of this chapter the individual agents that are commonly used in cancer chemotherapy will be discussed under each of the classes mentioned above. Additional discussion will consider combination chemotherapy and nursing implications in antineoplastic chemotherapy.

Alkylating agents
Mechlorethamine hydrochloride (nitrogen mustard, Mustargen)

Mechlorethamine hydrochloride is primarily used in combination with other antineoplastic agents in the MOPP regimen (Table 27-1) for the treatment of Hodgkin's disease and non-Hodgkin's lymphomas. It has also been administered intracavitarily to control pleural and other malignant effusions. Mechlorethamine is given by means of IV push in doses of 6 to 8 mg/m² body surface area. Its toxicity is characterized by a rapid onset of severe nausea and vomiting lasting 6 to 12 hours and seldom continuing longer than 24 hours. This side effect is usually minimized, but seldom prevented, by premedication with 10 mg prochlorperazine an hour before administration. Leukopenia and thrombocytopenia also occur, with an onset in 7 to 14 days and complete recovery in 3 to 4 weeks. Amenorrhea and alopecia may also occur, and the patient should be prepared for these toxic effects. Mechlorethamine should be given with caution because it is a vesicant (blistering) chemotherapeutic agent.

Cyclophosphamide (Cytoxan)

Cyclophosphamide has a wide spectrum of clinical uses. It is used extensively in combination chemotherapy and as a single agent in the treatment of acute lymphocytic leukemia, chronic lymphocytic leukemia, breast cancer, Burkitt's lymphoma, Ewing's sarcoma, Hodgkin's disease, lung cancer, multiple myeloma, neuroblastoma, and ovarian carcinoma. Dosage schedule is variable, and the drug may be given as a single agent or in combination with other agents. The daily dose of 2 to 4 mg/kg may be given orally or intravenously. A single intravenous dose of 500 to 1500 mg/m^2 has been effective in patients with lymphomas. Length of therapy is guided by keeping the leukocyte count between 3000 and 4000 mm^3. Hemorrhagic cystitis resulting from interaction of the active metabolites of cyclophosphamide with the bladder wall tissues can be prevented by encouraging patients to drink 1 to 2 liters of fluid on the day of therapy so that there will be frequent urination and flushing of the bladder. Nausea and vomiting are more frequent with the intravenous route than with the oral. The onset is usually within 4 to 6 hours, and the duration is seldom longer than 48 hours. Premedication with 10 mg prochlorperazine usually can prevent such vomiting. Leukopenia, sometimes accompanied by thrombocytopenia, is prevalent, with onset of 10 to 14 days and recovery in 3 to 4 weeks. Alopecia, amenorrhea, azoospermia, and teratogenesis are common, and the patient should be counseled concerning these toxic effects if they occur.

Antimetabolites

Antimetabolites include the folic acid analogs, purine analogs, and pyrimidine analogs.

FOLIC ACID ANALOGS
Methotrexate (Amethopterin)

Methotrexate is the most widely used of the folic acid analogs. It inhibits folic acid reductase, thereby interfering with the synthesis of a coenzyme necessary for DNA synthesis. Methotrexate has a broad spectrum of activity. Its usage has been established as a single agent or in combination with other antineoplastic drugs in the treatment of acute leukemias, trophoblastic tumors, Burkitt's lymphoma, lymphosarcoma, and mycosis fungoides. In high-dose schedules (greater than 100 mg/m^2 body surface area), it is effective in the treatment of osteo-

genic sarcoma; epidermoid carcinoma of the head and neck; lung, breast, and ovarian cancers; and multiple myeloma. The dosage schedules of methotrexate are numerous. The usual starting schedules range from 2.5 mg daily to 50 mg weekly. The intramuscular route is used. High-dose schedules of methotrexate range from 100 mg/m^2 to 10 g/m^2 every 1 to 3 weeks. With high-dose administration, the patient should be well hydrated and serum methotrexate levels taken 24, 48, and 72 hours after administration to anticipate and prevent severe bone marrow aplasia. This condition could result in the death of the patient 5 to 10 days after drug administration. Concurrent leucovorin rescue minimizes the toxicity of methotrexate, resulting in greater selectivity of the methotrexate for neoplastic cells.

The toxicity of methotrexate is naturally greater at higher doses than at lower ones. At normal dosage ranges 2.5 to 50 mg methotrexate has little toxicity. There is some leukopenia and thrombocytopenia. Stomatitis may appear within 4 to 7 days after drug administration, and treatment may or may not be interrupted with its appearance. Hepatotoxicity may also occur after long periods of therapy. At higher doses, bone marrow depression becomes greater, and nausea and vomiting appear with the stomatitis and hepatotoxicity. Alopecia may also occur. When methotrexate is given intrathecally, 10 to 12 mg/m^2, headache, blurred vision, and meningism are commonly seen in 2 to 4 hours and are reversed in about 5 days.

PURINE ANALOGS
Mercaptopurine (6-mercaptopurine; Purinethol)

Mercaptopurine has been found effective in the treatment of acute leukemias and pediatric non-Hodgkin's lymphomas, especially in the maintenance of remissions. It is thought to exert its effects by inhibiting DNA synthesis either by preventing incorporation of the purine into DNA or by utilizing mercaptopurine to form unnatural DNA. Mercaptopurine can be given orally in daily doses of 80 to 100 mg/m^2 body surface area or 2.5 mg/kg body weight (calculated to the nearest 25 mg) for maintenance therapies or intravenously in doses of 500 to 700 mg/m²/day for 5 days for induction therapies in the treatment of leukemias. When given concurrently with allopurinol, which blocks its metabolism, mercaptopurine doses should be reduced to one third or one fourth of the dose that would ordinarily be given. The common toxic effect of mercaptopurine at maintenance doses is leukopenia and is therefore dose limiting. With long-term or sometimes short-term administration, hepatotoxicity may appear. When mercaptopurine is given intravenously at high doses, nausea and vomiting, with anorexia, may appear.

Thioguanine

Thioguanine is similar in its cytotoxic action and dosage requirements to mercaptopurine. It has been used in the treatment of acute leukemia and as an immunosuppressive agent. Its activity is not influenced by allopurinol. Thioguanine is available in 40-mg tablets for oral administration. The average daily dose is 2 mg/kg body weight.

PYRIMIDINE ANALOGS
Fluorouracil

Fluorouracil is used for the palliative treatment of breast, colon, and rectal cancer. Other tumors responsive to this drug include gastrointestinal malignancies and ovarian, bladder, prostatic, and pancreatic carcinomas.

This drug is believed to affect specific steps in pyrimidine metabolism in such a way as to interfere with the synthesis of thymine, an essential part of DNA. It also inhibits the synthesis of RNA and is incorporated into the latter to form a fraudulent molecule of RNA. As a result, synthesis of proteins and proliferation of cancer cells are inhibited. Fluorouracil is available in 10-ml ampules containing 500 mg of the drug for intravenous administration. The recommended dose for an average patient is 12 to 15 mg/kg/day for 4 days, then weekly doses of 15 mg/kg body weight as long as there is evidence of clinical improvement.

It is not uncommon for cancer patients to receive maintenance doses of fluorouracil for months or years and to experience no other side effects to the drug except bone marrow depression. Others may experience, especially at high

doses, stomatitis, diarrhea, anorexia, and nausea and vomiting, all of which can be dose limiting. Alopecia may or may not occur.

Cytarabine (Cytosar-U; Ara-C)

Cytarabine is an antimetabolite that profoundly inhibits biosynthesis of DNA. It is primarily indicated for the induction of remissions in acute granulocytic leukemia. The recommended dosage is 2 mg/kg body weight by rapid injection daily for 10 days or 0.5 to 1 mg/kg by infusion over several hours daily for 10 days.

The primary toxic effect of this drug is manifested by leukopenia and thrombocytopenia. Other toxic manifestations include gastrointestinal disturbances, stomatitis, hepatic dysfunction, and thrombophlebitis at injection sites.

Antibiotics
Dactinomycin (actinomycin D; Cosmegen)

Dactinomycin is an actinomycin antibiotic isolated from a *Streptomyces* culture that has been found to inhibit synthesis of RNA. It appears to be the most effective drug in the treatment in Wilms' tumor. It is also useful in the treatment of soft tissue sarcomas, Ewing's sarcoma, and testicular tumors. The usual dose for children is 15 µg/kg/day intravenously for 5 days. The dose for adults is 0.01 mg/kg body weight for 5 days. Courses of therapy are repeated at 6-week to 3-month intervals. Because it is a vesicant agent, dactinomycin should be given by injection into the tubing of a rapidly flowing intravenous infusion, and great care should be taken to avoid extravasation. Its primary toxic effect is bone marrow depression. Nausea and vomiting, dermal reactions, and follicular acne are common. Alopecia and proctitis may occur.

ANTHRACYCLINES
Daunorubicin (daunomycin); doxorubicin hydrochloride (Adriamycin)

Daunorubicin is an antibiotic very similar in structure and toxicity to doxorubicin and has demonstrated significant activity in the treatment of acute myelocytic leukemia. It is also active in acute lymphocytic leukemia, especially when used together with vincristine and prednisone. It is given intravenously in doses of 30 to 60 mg/m² body surface area weekly.

Doxorubicin, better known as Adriamycin, has a broad spectrum of activity. It has been used in the treatment of many solid tumors, cancers of the lung and bladder, lymphomas, many sarcomas, and metastatic tumors. Doxorubicin is given intravenously in doses of 60 to 75 mg/m² every 3 weeks or 30 mg/m²/day for 3 days every 4 weeks.

Both drugs cause significant bone marrow depression, a high incidence of total hair loss, nausea and vomiting, stomatitis, and possible cardiotoxicity at total cumulative doses greater than 550 mg/m² in adults and 450 mg/m² in children. In the majority of cases the cardiotoxicity is exhibited by dysrhythmias and electrocardiographic changes, but it can progress into congestive heart failure and death. Both drugs are vesicant agents and should be administered with caution to avoid extravasation. The urine is red after these drugs are used, and patients should not be alarmed, since this is the color of the drugs. Doxorubicin commonly causes erythema and hyperpigmentation in previously irradiated areas of the skin.

Bleomycin (Blenoxane)

Bleomycin inhibits cell mitosis and DNA synthesis. It is extremely active in squamous cell skin cancer, testicular tumors, and most lymphomas. The usual dose of bleomycin as a single agent is 10 to 20 units/m² body surface area, once or twice a week, to a total dose of 300 to 400 units. Bleomycin doses are sometimes expressed in milligrams. In such cases 1 unit equals 1 mg. Its toxicity is usually mild but can be severe. A patient may experience nausea and vomiting, fever and chills, alopecia, hypertension, anorexia, hyperpigmentation, leukemia, or hyperbilirubinemia. If doses are greater than 200 mg/m² for a patient who has previously undergone irradiation or has had pulmonary disease, or if the patient is over 60 years of age, there is an 80% probability that pneumonitis will develop within 6 to 8 months after administration of bleomycin. A test dose of 1 or 2 units is usually given to lymphoma patients 24 hours before the main dose, since anaphylaxis and death have been reported a few times.

Mithramycin (Mithracin)

Mithramycin is an antibiotic that also inhibits RNA synthesis and is employed in the treatment of embryonal cell carcinoma of the testes. Its major clinical use, however, is in the treatment of hypercalcemia of malignancies unresponsive to other methods of treatment. Mithramycin is usually given intravenously in doses of 0.025 to 0.050 mg/kg body weight every 2 days for up to eight doses. Common side effects are nausea and vomiting, thrombocytopenia, hypocalcemia, hypokalemia, hepatotoxicity, fever, irritability, headache, lethargy, and some renal toxicity. An important toxic effect is hemorrhagic diathesis, which is life threatening. Mithramycin should be discontinued at the first sign that this condition is present, since it is irreversible.

Mitomycin C (Mutamycin)

Mitomycin is a cytotoxic antibiotic with activity similar to that of the alkylating agents. It is used primarily in the treatment of colorectal, gastric, and pancreatic adenocarcinomas in conjunction with 5-fluorouracil and doxorubicin. Mitomycin C is given intravenously in a dose of 0.05 mg/kg body weight on days 1 to 5 and 8 to 12, inclusively, and is repeated in 2 or 3 weeks if there is no bone marrow toxicity. Its side effects consist of bone marrow depression, nausea and vomiting, and possibly some diarrhea and stomatitis.

Plant alkaloids

Vinblastine and vincristine are two alkaloids derived from the periwinkel plant *Vinca rosea*. The mechanisms of action of these drugs are not well understood currently, but they appear to relate to metaphase arrest.

Vinblastine sulfate (Velban)

The principal use of vinblastine is in the treatment of Hodgkin's disease, in which it produces results that are equal or superior to those of the alkylating agents. Vinblastine also may be effective in the treatment of lymphomas, choriocarcinoma, and embryonal carcinoma of the testis.

Toxic effects occur primarily in the bone marrow, but other toxic manifestations include gastrointestinal disturbances, neurologic disturbances, and alopecia. Recommended dosage is 0.1 to 0.2 mg/kg body weight intravenously, given weekly.

Vincristine sulfate (Oncovin)

Vincristine, in contrast with vinblastine, is very effective in inducing remissions in acute leukemias in children. It is also less toxic to the bone marrow, but it is highly neurotoxic. The neurotoxicity consists of manifestations such as paresthesias, muscle weakness, loss of deep tendon reflexes, headache, vocal cord paralysis, ptosis, diplopia, and paralytic ileus. The neurotoxicity is usually reversed when the drug is withdrawn. Gastrointestinal disturbances and alopecia may also occur.

Commonly employed doses are 1.5 to 2 mg/m² body surface area for children and adults, given weekly.

Miscellaneous antineoplastic agents

NITROSOUREAS
Carmustine (BCNU)
Lomustine (CCNU)
Semustine (MeCCNU)

Carmustine (BCNU) is the most active of the three nitrosoureas and has been found useful in the treatment of brain tumors, colorectal and gastric adenocarcinomas, hepatomas, Hodgkin's disease, malignant melanoma, multiple myeloma, and non-Hodgkin's lymphomas. Both lomustine and semustine have shown activity in the treatment of brain tumors, colorectal adenocarcinoma, and Hodgkin's disease. Lomustine has a unique activity of its own in the treatment of bronchogenic carcinoma. Semustine overlays carmustine's activity in gastric adenocarcinomas and malignant melanoma. Carmustine's usual dose is 100 mg/m² body surface area, given intravenously on days 1 and 2, inclusively, every 6 weeks. Lomustine is given orally, 130 mg/m² as a single dose every 6

weeks. Carmustine has the disadvantage that it can be given only intravenously but must be given slowly to prevent phlebitis and localized pain. All three nitrosoureas have the same side effects: delayed bone marrow depression, nausea and vomiting, and possible hepatotoxicity. Since the myelosuppression of these agents is cumulative, patients should be watched carefully. Deaths caused by bone marrow aplasia have been reported.

ALKYLATOR-LIKE AGENTS
Cisplatin (cis-diamminedichloroplatinum [II]; Platinol)

Cisplatin is a cis-isomer of a platinum molecule. Its cytotoxic action appears to be the inhibition of DNA precursors and to a lesser extent the inhibition of protein and RNA synthesis. Its greatest activity has been shown in the treatment of germinal cell neoplasias of the testis. It has also shown activity in lymphomas, ovarian carcinomas, and squamous cell carcinoma of the head and neck. Cisplatin is usually given in combination with bleomycin and vinblastine in doses of 10 to 20 mg/m²/day for 5 days every 3 to 4 weeks. The maximum recommended single dose, however, is up to 100 mg/m² body surface area once every 3 to 4 weeks. Because this antineoplastic agent is a heavy metal, the patient is usually given a mannitol flush before and after, or concurrently with, its administration to prevent acute tubular necrosis of the kidneys. Nausea and vomiting can be mild to severe. Cisplatin causes a mild and transient bone marrow depression. Some patients have experienced high-frequency hearing loss, which is irreversible after the administration of this drug.

Dacarbazine (DTIC)

Dacarbazine's mechanism of action is not known but is thought to inhibit both RNA and DNA synthesis. The drug's greatest activity and use are in the treatment of malignant melanoma. It is also used in the treatment of Hodgkin's disease, neuroblastoma, and sarcomas. It is commonly given in doses of 250 mg/m²/day for 5 days every 3 to 4 weeks. Dacarbazine causes bone marrow depression and severe nausea and vomiting that may be dose limiting. The patient receiving this drug may also experience a flu-like syndrome of malaise, myalgia, and fever.

OTHER AGENTS
Hydroxyurea (Hydrea)

The primary role of this drug seems to be in the treatment of chronic granulocytic leukemia, but other therapeutic uses are being explored. It is available in 500-mg capsules. Hematopoietic depression is its major toxic effect. Dosage for continuous therapy is 20 to 30 mg/kg/day. When the drug is used in the acute phase of chronic granulocytic leukemia, called "blast crisis" (white count > 100,000/mm^3), a dose of 80 mg/kg body weight is given orally in divided doses every 6 hours for 2 days, until the leukocyte count is lowered so that other drugs or continuous therapy can be given. Nausea and vomiting may or may not occur. Stomatitis is common when high doses are given.

Procarbazine hydrochloride (Matulane)

The greatest effectiveness of procarbazine is in the treatment of Hodgkin's disease, non-Hodgkin's lymphomas, and brain tumors. It seems to lack cross-resistance with other antineoplastic agents. It is supplied in 50-mg capsules and administered in a dosage range of 100 to 300 mg/day. Its principal toxic effects are nausea and vomiting, leukopenia, and thrombocytopenia. Procarbazine is thought to inhibit monoamine oxidase (MAO) and to have an Antabuse-like activity; thus the patient should avoid concurrent use of alcohol, sympathomimetics, antidepressants, tyramine-rich foods, and CNS depressants. These drug-food and drug-drug interactions are rare and have not been reported extensively.

L-Asparaginase (ELSPAR)

L-Asparaginase is an enzyme that inhibits asparagine in tumor cells, which results in the death of the cells. It is used extensively in the treatment of acute lymphocytic leukemia and is usually given in combination with other agents in a dosage of 1000 IU/kg/day for 10 days. Toxic effects include nausea and vomiting, fever, allergy, confusion, hepatic dysfunction, blood dyscrasias, and bone marrow depression. Ana-phylaxis is not uncommon in patients when the drug is given intravenously or after five doses or more. Hyperglycemia and hypocholesterolemia are common. Pancreatitis may occur and is reversible.

Combination chemotherapy

Most neoplastic diseases are treated with a combination of drugs called drug regimens rather than by single agents. Table 27-1 gives a few of the more common regimens found in cancer chemotherapy practice. The rationale for combination chemotherapy is based on two principles: (1) The disease process is more likely to become resistant to a single agent than to a combination of drugs, and (2) combining various agents responsive in the same disease process permits action against the neoplasm at different sites. In addition, drug toxicity may be minimized by varying the toxic effects of the agents, thus enhancing their overall therapeutic effectiveness.

Drug selectivity for these regimens depends on numerous factors, such as the drug's site of action, pharmacokinetics, bioavailability, toxicity, and a dosage schedule that is maximally effective.

Even after a therapeutically effective regimen has been determined by numerous investigational studies, the regimen's effectiveness in the treatment of a patient depends on numerous variables, such as (1) the stage of the patient's disease, (2) the site of the neoplasm, (3) the neoplasm's sensitivity to chemotherapy, (4) prior therapy received by the patient, (5) the patient's performance status, and (6) concurrent organ system dysfunctions. Combination chemotherapy is a complex art of medicine. Even though much is still unknown, investigators have been successful in obtaining "cures" of numerous neoplastic diseases, as mentioned previously in this chapter.

Nursing implications in antineoplastic chemotherapy

Nursing functions related to drug therapy with antineoplastic agents are complex and inseparable from nursing care of the total pa-

T A B L E 2 7 - 1 **Common drug regimens**

Regimen	Disease
VP	Acute lymphocytic leukemia
Vincristine, 2.0 mg/m² body surface area every wk intravenously for 4 to 6 weeks	
Prednisone, 60 mg/m²/day orally for 4 weeks; then taper in week 5-7	
Ara-C + 6-TG	Acute myelogenous leukemia
Cytosine arabinoside, 100 mg/m² every 12 hours intravenously for 10 days	
Thioguanine, 100 mg/m² every 12 hours orally for 10 days	
MOPP	Hodgkin's disease
Mechlorethamine, 6 mg/m²/day intravenously on days 1 and 8	
Vincristine (Oncovin), 2 mg/m²/day intravenously on days 1 and 8	
Procarbazine, 100 mg/m²/day orally on days 1 to 14	
Prednisone, 40 mg/m²/day orally on days 1 to 14; repeat every 28 days for 6 cycles	
CVP	Non-Hodgkin's lymphoma—favorable histology
Cyclophosphamide, 400 mg/m²/day orally on days 2 to 6	
Vincristine, 1.4 mg/m²/intravenously on day 1	
Prednisone, 100 mg/m²/day orally on days 2 to 6; repeat every 21 days for 6 cycles	
CHOP	Non-Hodgkin's lymphoma—unfavorable histology
Cyclophosphamide, 750 mg/m²/day intravenously on day 1	
Doxorubicin (hydroxyldaunorubicin), 50 mg/m²/day intravenously on day 1	
Vincristine (Oncovin), 1.4 mg/m²/day intravenously on day 1	
Prednisone, 100 mg/day orally on days 1 to 5; repeat every 21 to 28 days for 6 cycles	
CMF	Breast cancer
Cyclophosphamide, 100 mg/m²/day orally on days 1 to 14	
Methotrexate, 40 to 60 mg/m²/day intravenously on days 1 and 8	
5-Fluorouracil, 600 mg/m²/day intravenously on days 1 and 8; repeat every 28 days	

tient and the family. The patient may be at any stage of the disease process and may be facing the possibility of impending death. Such a patient will inevitably be under stress. The nurse must recognize this and adapt an approach to the patient that is sensitive and appropriate.

In caring for patients receiving cancer chemotherapy, nurses have several responsibilities in regard to patient assessment. They should assess each patient's degree of acceptance of chemotherapy. They may need to assist the patient to deal with ambivalent feelings. The patient's and family's knowledge of chemotherapy and their expectations should also be assessed. Teaching the patient about drug administration and drug effects may help to ameliorate anxieties. An assessment may reveal that expectations are unrealistic, and the patient and the family may need assistance in accepting a more realistic view of the results of chemotherapy. Expectations of total cure are usually unrealistic in most neoplasms and should not be reinforced, whereas expectations of remissions are usually more acceptable.

In the management of patients receiving antineoplastic agents, the nurse has many responsibilities in dealing with the inevitable side effects of these drugs. Bone marrow depression, for example, greatly increases the patient's vulnerability to infection. The nurse should use strict aseptic technique when in contact with the patient and should protect the patient from individuals harboring harmful microorganisms. Frequent blood counts are necessary, and it is often the nurse's responsibility to ensure that they are taken. Special prophylactic care should be given to patients with thrombocytopenia, including the administration of stool softeners, use of soft toothbrushes, and use of side rails on beds. Intramuscular injections and any soft tissue injury should be avoided. Venipunctures should be done by experienced personnel utilizing strict sterile technique. Platelet transfusions may be necessary in thrombocytopenic patients. Patients with granulocytopenia should also receive stool softeners prophylactically, maintain scrupulous oral hygiene, and receive topical antibiotics for abrasions or scratches.

Alopecia is a side effect extremely distressing to women, even when they have been prepared for it and have cosmetic aids available and even though it is reversible. These patients will need assistance in coping with body image problems. In addition, the vesicant properties of some antineoplastic agents require careful handling of these drugs by both nurse and patient. Common vesicant agents are:

Dactinomycin Mithramycin
Carmustine (BiCNU) Mitomycin C
Daunorubicin Vinblastine
Doxorubicin Vincristine
Mechlorethamine

Other side effects will also require the nurse's interventions. Nausea and vomiting attendant to the use of these drugs can be ameliorated by prior administration of phenothiazines. Stomatitis resulting from these drugs can be very uncomfortable and can interfere with the patient's nutrition. An anesthetic mouth rinse and bland, nonirritating foods may enable the patient to eat in greater comfort. Treatment with hormones may necessitate support for the patient in the event of such side effects as masculinization in female patients and feminization in male patients.

Undoubtedly one of the most important nursing interventions is that of providing emotional support to the patient with a destructive disease who is receiving therapy that is both physically and psychologically distressing. The long periods of therapy, with frequent interruptions and sometimes progress, may compound the patient's anxieties.

Evaluation of drug effects is another integral aspect of nursing function in antineoplastic chemotherapy. The nurse should watch for and report both therapeutic and toxic effects of the antineoplastic agents. This is especially important because there is often no predetermined dosage schedule for antineoplastic agents that is universally therapeutic. Dosage will change according to the patient's response and the toxic effects of the drug. The nurse's evaluation and communication of both drug toxicity and patient response are essential. In evaluating toxic effects, the nurse should be vigilant for very early signs, since progression of toxic effects may have severe and irreversible consequences. Early signs of irritation of the oral mucous membranes, for example, can be noted by frequent examination of the patient's mouth, during which time the nurse observes for erythema, white patchy membranes, and ulceration. Early signs of bone marrow depression may be determined from frequent blood counts, which the nurse should monitor carefully.

Chemotherapy drug administration: double-syringe technique

1. Select site for administration according to following order of preference: forearm, dorsum of hand, wrist, or antecubital fossa.
2. Use a 20- or 21-gauge "butterfly" needle for drug administration. Administer 5 ml normal saline solution and withdraw small amount of blood into tubing to test vein patency. If there is poor blood return, select site other than distal location.
3. Administer vesicant agent over at least 3 minutes, drawing blood back into tubing after every 2 to 3 ml solution.
4. Flush with 3 to 5 ml saline solution after administration.
5. If patient experiences pain at site of injection or an unusual sensation during drug administration, extravasation may have occurred, and a new site for drug injection should be selected.

Summary of nursing considerations

Many drugs can now be used, either alone or in conjunction with surgery and x-ray therapy, to produce palliation of symptoms, regression of the neoplastic process, and prolongation of life. Antineoplastic agents are divided into classes on the basis of their probable mechanisms of action: alkylating agents, antimetabolites, antibiotics, plant alkaloids, immune agents, hormones, radioisotopes, and miscellaneous agents (p. 809). Each agent has its own site of action on the dividing cell cycle. All antineoplastic agents have severe toxic effects that must be monitored closely by health professionals caring for the cancer patient, so that maximal therapeutic results can be achieved. It has been found that combination chemotherapy is more effective in the treatment of neoplasms that are single agents, and its use is extensive today (Table 27-1).

Nursing functions related to drug therapy with antineoplastic agents are complex and inseparable from the nursing care of the total patient and the family. In caring for patients receiving cancer chemotherapy, nurses play a crucial role in helping the patient cope with the physical as well as the emotional side effects.

QUESTIONS

FOR STUDY AND REVIEW

1 Identify the types of malignancies that have been cured with antineoplastic agents.
2 What are the goals of cancer chemotherapy when cure cannot be accomplished?
3 Identify the eight major classes of antineoplastic agents, naming one drug for each class.
4 Describe the major toxic effect that occurs with almost all antineoplastic agents.
5 Name six vesicant agents that require special care in their administration to patients.
6 Give the five steps of the double-syringe technique.
7 How can the severe nausea and vomiting accompanying the use of these drugs be ameliorated?
8 What is the rationale for the use of hormones in the treatment of malignancies?
9 State the rationale for combination chemotherapy.
10 Give the names of three common drug regimens, together with the drugs used and their dosages and schedules.

BIBLIOGRAPHY

Bagley, C.M., and others: Advanced lymphosarcoma: intensive cyclical combination chemotherapy with cyclophosphamide, vincristine, and prednisone, Ann. of Intern. Med. **76:**227, 1972.

Blum, R.H., and others: A clinical review of bleomycin—a new antineoplastic agent, Cancer **31:**903, 1973.

Blum, R.H., and others: Adriamycin: a new anticancer drug with significant clinical acticity, Ann. of Inter. Med. **80:**249, 1974.

Canellos, G.P., and others: Combination chemotherapy for metastatic breast carcinoma: prospective comparison of multiple drug therapy with L-phenylalanine mustard, Cancer **38:**1882, 1976.

Carter, S.K., and others: Chemotherapy of cancer, New York, 1977, John Wiley & Sons, Inc.

DeVita, V.T.: Cell kinetics and chemotherapy of cancer, Cancer Chemotherapy Reports, part 3, vol. 2, Report No. 1, Oct. 1971.

DeVita, V.T., and others: Combination chemotherapy in the treatment of advanced Hodgkin's disease, Ann. of Intern. Med. **73:**881, 1970.

Ellison, R.R., and others: Management of acute leukemia in adults, Med. Pediatr. Oncol. **1:**149, 1975.

Gershwin, M.E., and others: Cyclophosphamide: use in practice, Ann. of Intern. Med. **80:**531, 1974.

Goldin, A.: Rationale of combination chemotherapy based on preclinical experiments, Cancer Chemotherapy Reports, part 3, vol. 4, Report No. 2, March 1973.

Goodman, L.S., and Gilman, A., editors: The pharmacological basis of therapeutics, ed. 6, New York, 1980, Macmillan, Inc.

Goth, A.: Medical pharmacology: principals and concepts, ed. 10, St. Louis, 1981, The C.V. Mosby Co.

Kremer, W.B.: Drugs five years later: cytarabine, Ann. Intern. Med. **82:**684, 1975.

McKelvey, E.M., and others: Hydroxyldaunomycin (Adriamycin) combination chemotherapy in malignant lymphoma, Cancer **38:**1484, 1976.

Mauer, A.M., and others: The current status of the treatment of childhood acute lymphoblastic leukemia, Cancer Treat. Rev. **3:**17, 1976.

See-Lasley, L.K., and Ignoff, R.: Manual of oncology therapeutics, St. Louis, 1981, The C.V. Mosby Co.

Spivack, S.D.: Procarbazine, Ann. Intern. Med. **81:**795, 1974.

Tan, C., and others: Daunomycin, and antitumor antibiotic, in the treatment of neoplastic disease, Cancer **20:**333, 1967.

Wasserman, T.H., and others: Clinical comparison of the nitrosoureas, Cancer **36:**1258, 1975.

UNIT NINE

DRUGS AFFECTING METABOLIC AND ENDOCRINE SYSTEMS

CHAPTER 28

Endocrine hormones

Hormones

The hormones are natural chemical substances that act after being secreted into the bloodstream from the ductless, or endocrine, glands. The word "hormone" is derived from the Greek word *hormaein*, which means "to excite." The word "endocrine" is from the Greek word *endon*, meaning "within."

Hormones have physiologic interrelationships. Hormones from various endocrine glands work in concert to obtain physiologic control of vital processes. Their relationship may be synergistic or antagonistic; this allows for flexibility and control. There are six major areas in which hormones play a crucial regulatory role.

1 Control and coordination of the secretory and motor activities of the digestive tract
2 Control of energy production
3 Control of composition and volume of extracellular fluid
4 Adaptation, such as acclimatization and immunity
5 Growth and development
6 Reproduction and lactation

To maintain the internal environment there must also be control of hormone secretion. This is achieved by a self-regulating series of events known as "negative feedback"; that is, a hormone produces a physiologic effect that, on attaining sufficient magnitude, inhibits further secretion of that hormone, thereby inhibiting the physiologic effect. Increased hormonal secretions may be evoked in response to stimuli from the external environment; cessation of external stimuli terminates the internal secretion response.

Hormones are not "used up" in exerting their physiologic effects but must be inactivated or excreted if the internal environment is to be in dynamic equilibrium. Inactivation occurs enzymatically in the blood or intercellular spaces, in the liver or kidney, or in the target tissues. Excretion of hormones is primarily via the urine and to a lesser extent the bile.

Most hormones are rapidly destroyed, having a half-life in blood of 10 to 30 minutes. However, some, like the catecholamines, have a half-life of seconds, while thyroid hormones

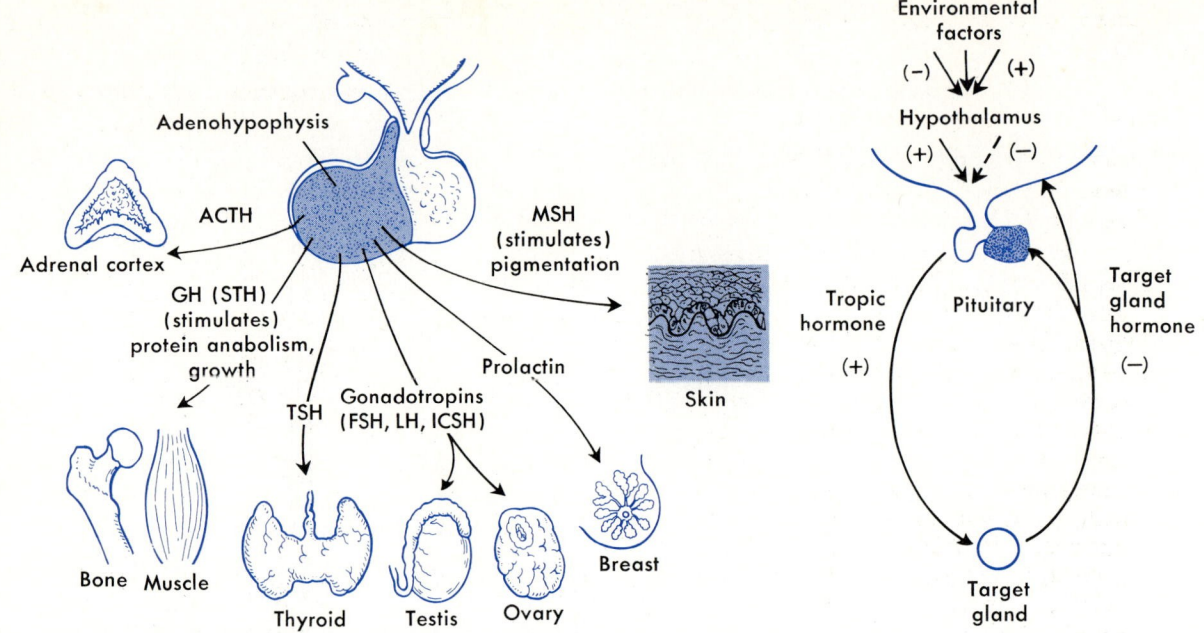

FIG. 28-1. Various internal and external environmental factors may inhibit or stimulate the hypothalamus to secrete inhibitory (−) or releasing (+) factors to control output of hormones from the anterior pituitary and ultimate hormone release from target glands. Hormone secretion from target glands (adrenal cortex, thyroid, etc.), on reaching a critical level, have an inhibitory effect on the secretion of tropic hormones by the anterior pituitary and releasing factors (RF) by the hypothalamus. *ACTH*, Adrenocorticotropic hormone; *GH*, growth hormone; *STH*, somatotropin hormone; *TSH*, thyroid-stimulating hormone; *FSH*, follicle-stimulating hormone; *LH*, luteinizing hormone; *ICSH*, interstitial cell-stimulating hormone; *MSH*, melanocyte-stimulating hormone.

have a half-life measured in days. Some hormones exert their physiologic effects almost instantaneously while others require minutes or hours before their effects occur. In addition, some physiologic effects disappear immediately on the hormone's disappearance from the circulation, while other physiologic responses may persist for hours after hormone concentrations have returned to basal levels. This wide range of onset and duration of hormonal activity contributes to the flexibility of the endocrine system.

Hormones may exert their effects by:

1 Controlling the formation or destruction of some intracellular regulator, such as cyclic AMP
2 Controlling protein synthesis
3 Controlling membrane permeability and the movement of ions and other substances

One of the major developments of this century in the fields of biology and medicine has been the recognition and then the isolation, purification, and chemical understanding of most of the hormones we now know. In addi-

tion, once their chemical structure is known, it becomes hypothetically possible to duplicate them by chemical synthesis. This has been accomplished for some hormones, although not for all.

Exactly what should be called a hormone and what should not is not well defined. A broad definition could be any chemical substance released by one tissue, circulated by the blood, and having characteristic effects on other tissues. This would include many substances not ordinarily classed as hormones, such as carbon dioxide. In common usage, hormones are confined to those well-recognized and chemically specific products of the various endocrine glands that are released in small amounts and that have specific well-defined physiologic effects on metabolism. The list of major hormones includes the products of the secretions of the anterior and posterior pituitary, the thyroid hormone, insulin and glucagon from the pancreas, epinephrine and norepinephrine from the adrenal medulla, several potent steroids from the adrenal cortex, and the gonadal hormones of both sexes.

In medicine these substances are generally used in two ways: (1) for replacement when a patient lacks sufficient endogenous hormone, exemplified by the use of insulin in diabetes or the use of adrenal steroids in Addison's disease, and (2) for pharmacologic effects beyond those of replacement, exemplified by the use of large doses of the adrenal steroids for their antiinflammatory effects.

Pituitary gland

Because the hormones of the pituitary gland exert an important effect in regulating the secretion of other hormones, it is fitting that they be considered first.

The pituitary body is about the size of a pea and occupies a niche in the sella turcica of the sphenoid bone. It consists of an anterior lobe, a posterior lobe, and a smaller pars intermedia composed of secreting cells. The anterior part is particularly important in sustaining life. The function of the pars intermedia is not well known. Oral administration of any part of the whole gland has no visible effect because it is destroyed by proteolytic enzymes as the pituitary hormones are protein or peptide in nature.

Regulation of anterior pituitary function. The pituitary and target glands have a negative feedback relationship. A tropic hormone from the pituitary stimulates the target gland to secrete a hormone that inhibits further secretion of the tropic hormone by the pituitary. When the serum concentration of the target gland hormone falls below a certain level, the pituitary again secretes the tropic hormone until the target gland produces enough hormone to inhibit the pituitary secretion. However, the negative feedback concept alone is not enough to account for changes in serum levels of target gland hormones, especially those caused by changes in the external environment—thus it is theorized that the central nervous system plays a decisive role in regulating pituitary function to meet environmental demands.

Of great research interest is the discovery of various hypothalamic releasing factors (also called hypophysiotropic hormones), which cause the release or inhibition of the various hormones from the anterior pituitary. Among these releasing factors the thyroid-releasing hormone (TRH) is of great interest. Also, somatostatin, a release-inhibiting factor, is receiving clinical trials.

ANTERIOR PITUITARY HORMONES

Present evidence indicates that a number of factors are concerned in the action of extracts of the anterior lobe of the pituitary gland. How many hormones are secreted by the gland is unknown, but at least seven extracts have been prepared in a relatively pure state, and they have definite specific action.

1 A growth factor influences the development of the body. It promotes skeletal, visceral, and general growth of the body. Acromegaly, gigantism, and dwarfism are connected with pathologic conditions of the anterior lobe of the pituitary gland.

Growth hormone or somatotropin somatropin, Assellacrin has been obtained as a small crystalline protein, but thus far the growth hormone has found no established place in medicine except in documented clinical and laboratory evidence of growth hormone deficiency, and its use in various clinical conditions is largely experimental. It tends to increase the blood sugar and antagonize insulin, an it may be the "diabetogenic" hormone postulated some years ago.

2 Follicle-stimulating hormone (FSH) stimulates the growth and maturation of the ovarian follicle, which in turn brings on the characteristic changes of estrus (menstruation in women). This hormone also stimulates spermatogenesis in the male. FSH appears to be a protein or is associated with a protein, but it has not yet been obtained in a highly purified form.

3 Luteinizing hormone (LH), also known as the interstitial cell–stimulating hormone (ICSH), together with FSH (Pergonal) causes maturation of the graafian follicles, ovulation, and the secretion of estrogen in the female. It causes spermatogenesis, androgen formation, and growth of interstitial tissue in the male. Luteinizing hormone also promotes the formation of the corpora lutea in the female.

4 Thyrotropic hormone (TSH) is necessary for normal development and function of the thyroid gland and, if present in excess, is known to produce hyperthyroidism and an increased size of the gland in laboratory animals.

5 A lactogenic factor (prolactin or mammotropin) plays a part in proliferation and secretion of the mammary glands of mammals. This may be identical with the hormone responsible for the devel-

opment of the corpus luteum. In its absence the corpus luteum fails to produce progesterone.

6 Adrenocorticotropic hormone (corticotropin or ACTH) stimulates the cortex of the adrenal gland.

7 Melanocyte-stimulating hormone (intermedin) is probably produced in the intermediate lobe. Its physiologic role is unknown but when injected in humans it will darken the skin.

Although the hormones produced by the anterior lobe of the pituitary gland are important physiologically, a number of reasons explain their limited usefulness. Only in relatively recent times have purified preparations been available, at least for clinical study, and such preparations are both expensive and limited in supply. Increased application of their effects may be expected in the future, however, as chemically defined preparations become available.

Corticotropin

Adrenocorticotropic hormone (corticotropin or ACTH) exerts its action primarily on the cells of the adrenal cortex and causes it to secrete its entire spectrum of hormones. The ultimate effects in the body, therefore, are the effects of the various adrenocortical steroids and, in general, these effects are similar to those of cortisone. Corticotropin is effective only if a functioning adrenal gland is present. The present source of corticotropin is from the pituitary glands of domesticated mammals such as hogs and cattle. The labor involved in the removal of the glands makes this source is an expensive one.

During conditions of stress and strain the activity of the adrenal cortex is increased. This is thought to be the result of an increased secretion of corticotropin. One explanation of the regulation of corticotropic activity is that during stress the tissues of the body utilize more of the adrenal hormones than usual, which results in a decreased concentration of the adrenocortical hormones in the blood. This in turn brings about stimulation of cells in the anterior pituitary gland and the production of more corticotropin. On the other hand, when stress has subsided, the tissues use less of the adrenocortical hormones, their concentration in the blood increases, and this causes activity of the pituitary gland as well as the adrenal cortex to be decreased.

Absorption. Corticotropin is destroyed by enzymes in the gastrointestinal tract and therefore cannot be given orally. It is absorbed readily from sites of injection when given intramuscularly or intravenously. It is said to disappear from the blood rapidly after intravenous injection. Its effects rarely last longer than 6 hours. This necessitates frequent intramuscular injections, administration by slow intravenous drip, or the use of a preparation that is absorbed slowly. Its effectiveness depends on the presence of normal adrenal glands capable of responding to the stimulant made by the pituitary gland.

Uses. Corticotropin is used for many of the same conditions for which cortisone and hydrocortisone are used, such as rheumatic diseases, skin diseases, ocular diseases, and allergic manifestations. But since the corticosteroids are much more convenient, corticotropin is now seldom used, except in diagnostic testing as adrenal function.

Preparation, dosage, and administration. The following are preparations of corticotropin.

Corticotropin injection (Acthar). Corticotropin injection is used for definitive diagnosis of adrenal insufficiency and to establish if the disease is primary or secondary (for example, caused by pituitary disease). Corticotropin is administered intravenously for 2 or 3 consecutive days (over an 8-hour period; 8 AM to 4 PM) and 24-hour urine collections are made to determine the amount of 17-hydroxycorticoids secreted. Patients with normal adrenal function will show a threefold increase in baseline values: patients with primary adrenol cortical deficiency will show a very small increase on the first day with no further increase on remaining days; and patients with secondary insufficiency will show a stepwise increase over the 3-day period.

Corticotropin is also used to manage severe myasthenia gravis. The hormone is given in doses of 100 IU daily until a total of 1000 to 2000 units has been given (1 mg of the International Unit is equal to the activity contained in 1 USP unit). Marked deterioration of muscle strength occurs 2 to 3 days after initiation of therapy; equipment for assisting respiration should be available. Two days to 1 week after completion of treatment muscle strength improves and lasts for an average of 3 months. A second course of treatment may then be given, or a weekly dose of the drug may be given.

When corticotropin is given to diabetic persons, insulin requirements might be increased.

Corticotropin injection is marketed as a powder in 25 or 40 USP units. The average dose of corticotropin for adults is 20 USP units four times daily when given intramuscularly or subcutaneously. When the drug is administered intravenously, 10 to 25 USP units are dissolved in 500 ml to 5% glucose solution, and the solution is administered slowly over an 8-hour period (once daily).

Repository corticotropin injection (Corticotropin Gel, ACTH Gel); corticotrophin gelatin injection. This is corticotropin dissolved in a gelatin solution, which results in slow absorption and more satisfactory clinical effect per unit of activity. Repository corticotropin is administered intramuscularly. Maximum effect occurs in 15 to 18 hours; duration of effect may be as long as 72 hours. A daily injection exerts a prolonged and continuous effect. The usual intramuscular dose is 40 USP units. The maintenance dose is 20 USP units two or three times a week.

Sterile corticotropin–zinc hydroxide suspension; corticotrophin zinc injection. This is purified corticotropin adsorbed on zinc hydroxide. Absorption after parenteral administration is delayed, and thus its action is prolonged. Action of one dose may persist for 3 days. It is administered intramuscularly (deep in gluteal muscle) and is available as a suspension containing 100 to 200 USP units in 5 ml. The usual initial dose is 40 USP units; the maintenance dose is 20 USP units two or three times a week.

Side effects and toxic effects. Effects are much the same as those noted after administration of cortisone or hydrocortisone. Acneiform eruptions have been reported.

Cosyntropin (Cortrosyn)

Cosyntropin is a synthetic peptide subunit of natural corticotropin. A dose of 0.25 mg cosyntropin has the biologic activity of 25 units of natural corticotropin. Cosyntropin is not used as a therapeutic substitute for corticotropin but as a diagnostic agent for adrenocortral insufficiency. After its administration, if the adrenal cortex is able to function, there is an increase in plasma cortisol levels; if no increase occurs 1 hour after 0.25 mg is given intramuscularly, adrenal insufficiency is present. If the latter occurs, 0.25 mg cosyntropin is diluted in saline and injected intravenously over 4 to 8 hours on 2 to 3 consecutive days. If no increase in plasma cortisol level occurs the patient has primary adrenal insufficiency. If pituitary disease is suspected, pituitary functioning can be tested. Urinary excretion of steroids may be used to determine response in place of plasma cortisol levels.

Thyrotropin (Thytropar)

Thyrotropin is an extract of the thyroid-stimulating hormone obtained from bovine anterior pituitary glands. It is not used as a therapeutic agent but to evaluate thyroid function. It is effective for determining low thyroid reserve, for differentiating primary and secondary hypothyroidism, and for evaluating the need for thyroid medication in patients receiving thyroid therapy. Ten units of thyrotropin are injected intramuscularly followed by a tracer dose of radioiodine 18 to 24 hours later. After 24 hours the uptake of iodine by the thyroid increases in a patient with hypopituitarism but does not increase in a patient with primary hypothyroidism.

PITUITARY GONADOTROPIC HORMONES

The pituitary gonadotropic hormones are discussed in Chapter 29.

POSTERIOR PITUITARY HORMONES

When solutions of extracts of the posterior lobes of the pituitary glands of animals (domestic) are administered parenterally, a number of effects have been observed: (1) stimulation of the uterine muscle (oxytocic effect), (2) promotion of the absorption of water in the renal tubules (antidiuretic effect), and (3) stimulation of the muscle of the superficial blood vessels (pressor effect) and of the intestine.

A great advance in the pharmacology of the posterior lobe has been the identification and chemical analysis of two major hormones obtained from the gland in pure form. These compounds, oxytocin and vasopressin (antidiuretic hormone, ADH), are both peptides, each containing eight amino acids. After their isolation and determination it proved possible to synthesize them chemically. Availability of the oxytocic and vasopressor pituitary hormones in pure form has clarified a number of uncertainties about their action and has also encouraged their better-controlled therapeutic use. It is known, for example, that there is a certain overlap of pharmacologic action even in the pure preparation; pure oxytocin has some vasopressor activity, and vice versa. Vasopressin is also the antidiuretic hormone (ADH), its antidiuretic potency being much more marked than its pressor potency. Although the cruder preparations of oxytocic and vasopressor activity are still used, it may be expected that eventually the pure compounds will replace the older extracts.

Oxytocin

Oxytocin is discussed in Chapter 29.

Vasopressin

Vasopressin functions as an antidiuretic hormone (ADH) by enhancing water permeability of the tubular epithelial membranes of the distal convolution and collecting ducts so that water can be absorbed by osmotic flow. Secretion of ADH is influenced by body hydration; if the body is hydrated no ADH can be detected in the urine or plasma, but if the body is dehydrated it is present in both fluids.

The vasopressor effect is a contraction of the smooth muscles in the vascular bed. The vasoconstriction is seen in the portal and splanchnic vessels and to a lesser degree in the peripheral, coronary, cerebral, pulmonary, and intrahepatic vessels. Vasopressin also enhances the motility and tone of the gastrointestinal tract.

Vasopressin is used as an antidiuretic for the symptomatic treatment of polyuria accompanying diabetes insipidus (a condition in which the patient excretes a large amount of urine due to lack of ADH) and is in treatment of esophageal varices.

Vasopressin can be used for rapid testing of renal function. From 5 to 10 units is given intramuscularly, and the specific gravity of urine is determined 1 and 2 hours later. In normal renal function the specific gravity rises to 1.018 or more. No special preparation is required for this test. Vasopressin is not used for its oxytocic or pressor action because of the danger of myocardial depression and ischemia and because better drugs are available for these actions.

Vasopressin is ineffective if given by the oral route. It may be applied topically or given by subcutaneous or intramuscular injection.

Vasopressin injection causes oliguria in 1 to 2 hours, which reaches a peak in 3 hours; duration of action may be as long as 10 hours.

Preparation, dosage, and administration. The following are available preparations of vasopressin.

Vasopressin injection (Pitressin). Vasopressin injection is a purified prepation of antidiuretic and pressor hormone separated from the oxytocic hormone. The usual dose is 0.25 to 0.5 ml (5 to 10 USP units) three or four times daily; for children, dose is 2.5 to 10 units three or four times daily. It is given subcutaneously, intramuscularly, or intravenously.

Vasopressin tannate (Pitressin). Vasopressin tannate is marketed in suspension only for intramuscular injection 0.5 to 1 ml (2.5 to 5 units). It is injected at intervals of 36 to 48 hours. For children the dose is 1.25 to 2.5 units. Its effect is more prolonged than that of vasopressin. It cannot be given intravenously. Prolonged rotation and shaking of the ampule is necessary in order that all of the particles be included in the suspension. Failure to shake the ampule thoroughly can result in inaccurate dosage and inadequate therapeutic response. Vasopressin tannate is effective for the control or prevention of symptoms and complications of diabetes insipidus due to deficiency of the endogenous posterior pituitary antidiuretic hormone.

Lypressin (Diapid). Lypressin is a synthetic polypeptide structurally identical to the antidiuretic hormone found in humans. It is applied as a nasal spray; it is rapidly absorbed from the nasal mucosa. It is effective therapy in controlling the polyuria of diabetes insipidus in mild or moderate cases. Lypressin can be used as adjunctive therapy between injections in more severe cases. It is less likely to cause rhinopharyngitis than posterior pituitary powder. No significant systemic or local allergic reactions have been reported.

One or more sprays are applied to one or both nostrils, one or more times daily. Each spray contains about 2 USP posterior pituitary pressor units. Four sprays in each nostril is the maximal amount that can be absorbed at one time. Lypressin is available in 5-ml containers, which contain 50 pressor units per milliliter.

Posterior pituitary powder. This powder is dried pituitary gland, which can be snuffed into the nose. Absorption from the nasal mucous membrane makes it possible to use it for the relief of symptoms of diabetes insipidus. It is less expensive than the injectable forms. It must be applied several times daily. Irritation of the nasal mucosa limits its use. It may cause sneezing, wheezing, dyspnea, asthmatic attacks, and other hypersensitivity reactions.

Side effects and toxic effects. Vasopressin can cause spasm of coronary arteries, therefore caution is recommended when it is administered to patients with inadequate coronary circulation. Water retention and occasionally water intoxication have been known to occur. The patient with diabetes insipidus will probably have to take the drug the remainder of his life. Large doses may cause intestinal and uterine cramps.

Desmopressin acetate (DDAVP)

Desmopressin acetate is a synthetic analog of the natural hormone arginine vasopressin. Used as a nasal solution, it provides a prompt onset of antidiuretic action with a duration of action from 8 to 20 hours and no vasopressor or oxytocic activity at therapeutic dosages.

The indications are antidiuretic replacement therapy in the management of central (neurogenic) diabetes insipidus and for temporary polyuria and polydipsia associated with trauma to, or surgery in, the pituitary region. It is ineffective for the treatment of nephrogenic diabetes insipidus (renal unresponsiveness to vasopressin).

Preparation, dosage, and administration. Administration of this nasal solution is achieved by blowing the solution in through a calibrated, soft, flexible nasal tube. Dosage is determined for each individual patient and adjusted according to the diurnal pattern of response. Response is estimated by two parameters: (1) adequate duration of sleep and (2) adequate water turnover. Approximately one fourth to one third of the patients may be controlled with a single daily dose. The adult dose range is 0.1 to 0.4 ml daily to one, two, or three doses. Most adults require 0.2 ml daily in two divided doses. The morning and evening doses are adjusted separately for an adequate diurnal rhythm of water turnover. In children the range is 0.05 to 0.3 ml daily in one or two divided doses. The solution is available in vials containing 2.5 ml with applicator tubes. Although it is usually stored at about 4° C, it may be kept at room temperature for 14 days without loss of potency.

Side effects and toxic effects. Adverse reactions include transient headache and nausea; both occur infrequently at higher dosages. Also reported are nasal congestion, rhinitis, flushing, mild abdominal cramps, and vulval pain. If considerable fluid retention occurs a saluretic (such as furosemide) may induce diuresis.

Precautions are used in patients with coronary artery insufficiency and/or hypertensive cardiovascular disease because the higher dosages may slightly elevate the blood pressure. In very young and elderly persons, fluid intake is adjusted to prevent water intoxication and hyponatremia. No studies have been reported in pregnant women.

Potentiation of the antidiuretic effects of desmopressin may be caused by concomitant use with chlorpropamide, clofibrate, and carbamazepine.

Posterior pituitary injection (Pituitrin [obstetric use], Pituitrin-S [surgical use])

Posterior pituitary injection possesses oxytocic, vasopressor, and ADH activity and is used to control postoperative ileus, to promote gas expulsion before pyelography, in surgery to aid in achieving hemostasis in esophageal varices, and to treat diabetes insipidus. For obstetrical use it may be the primary stimulus (rapid and transitory) to uterine contractions after complete placental expulsion and may be used near term with ergot alkaloids to provide prolonged stimulation of uterine tonus.

Parathyroid glands

Lying just above the thyroid, or, in some animals, embodied in it, are a variable number of bean-shaped glands (two pairs in humans) known as the parathyroids. The primary function of the parathyroids is the maintenance of adequate levels of calcium in the extracellular fluid. The most significant function of parathyroid hormone is mobilization of calcium from bone. It also reduces phosphate concentration, permitting more calcium to be mobilized. Hypoparathyroidism leads to manifestations of hypocalcemia and tetany, the symptoms of which include muscle spasms, convulsions, gradual paralysis with dyspnea, and death from exhaustion. Before death gastrointestinal hemorrhages and hematemesis frequently occur. At death the intestinal mucosa is congested and the calcium content of the heart, kidney, and other tissues is increased.

The symptoms of tetany are relieved by administration of calcium salts. It is usually necessary to administer calcium salts intravenously for rapid relief. Large doses of vitamin D are also useful to relieve tetany and to restore the normal level of calcium in the blood. The patient is hospitalized because a frequent check on the blood calcium and phosphate levels is essential. Although parathyroid injection was formerly used to treat tetany, its use is now considered to be obsolete.

Dihydrotachysterol (Hytakerol)

Dihydrotachysterol is effective in raising serum calcium by stimulation of intestinal calcium absorption and bone calcium mobilization in the absence of parathyroid hormone and functioning renal tissue.

The indications are hypocalcemia associated with hypoparathyroidism, both postoperative and idiopathic, and pseudohypoparathyroidism. The major goal of therapy is maintenance of normal serum calcium levels.

Preparation, dosage, and administration. The dosage forms are 0.125-, 0.2-, and 0.4-mg oral tablets and capsules; a solution of 0.25 mg/ml is also available. The initial dose in 0.8 to 2.4 mg daily for several days with a maintenance dose of 0.2 to 1 mg daily as required for normal (9 to 10 mg/100 ml) serum calcium levels. The average dose is 0.6 mg/day, which may be supplemented with oral calcium lactate, using caution in patients with renal stones because of the effect on serum calcium. In patients with renal osteodystrophy (generalized bone changes similar to osteomalacia and rickets or osteitis fibrosa occurring in children or adults with chronic renal failure) accompanied by hyperphosphatemia, dietary phosphate restriction and the administration of aluminum antacid gels (which aid in phosphate binding) will maintain normal serum phosphorus levels and aid in preventing metastatic calcification.

Side effects and toxic effects. Thiazide diuretics administered to hypoparathyroid patients can lead to hypercalcemia, which may cause anorexia, nausea, vomiting, weakness, constipation, lethargy, depression, amnesia, disorientation, hallucinations, syncope, diarrhea, vertigo, headache, polyuria, thirst, and ataxia. The nurse should have the patient report any of these effects to the physician.

The symptoms of overdosage can persist for a month after cessation of therapy, since the toxicity is similar to that caused by large doses of vitamin D and overdosage is manifested by the symptoms of hypercalcemia. Impaired renal function results in polyuria, polydipsia, and proteinuria. Calcification of soft tissue (of heart, blood vessels, kidneys, lungs) is widespread; additionally, death may result from cardiovascular or renal failure.

Calcitonin-salmon (Calcimar)

Calcitonin-salmon is a polypeptide hormone secreted by the parafollicular cells of the thyroid gland in mammals and by the ultimobranchial gland of birds and fish. It acts primarily on bone; however, direct renal effects and gastrointestinal tract effects are also seen. The salmon calcitonin has similar actions to mammalian calcitonins but the milligram potency is greater and it has a longer duration of action.

Use. Single injections of calcitonin-salmon cause a marked transient inhibition of bone resorptive process, but with prolonged use the rate of bone resorption decreases. Possibly by an initial blocking effect on bone resorption, calcitonin-salmon causes a decreased rate of bone turnover.

When given to patients with Paget's disease calcitonin-salmon causes a fall in the serum alkaline phosphatase and urinary hydroxyproline excretion in about 66% of the patients treated. Some patients with Paget's disease having good response initially may later relapse despite continued therapy. Circulating antibodies to calcitonin-salmon are seen in about 50% of the patients with Paget's disease. Calcitonin-salmon may lower elevated serum calcium in patients with carcinoma (with or without metastases), multiple myeloma, or primary hyperparathyroidism (a lesser response). Calcitonin-salmon increases the excretion of filtered phosphate, calcium, and sodium by decreasing their tubular reabsorption. Short-term use decreases the volume and acidity of gastric juice and lowers the volume of trypsin and amylase content in pancreatic juice.

It is suggested that calcitonin-salmon is metabolized rapidly by conversion to smaller inactive fragments in the kidneys, blood, and peripheral tissues and is excreted in the urine.

Preparation, dosage, and administration. Calcitonin-salmon is available as an injection of 200 MRC units*/ml solution in 2-ml vials. The starting dose in Paget's disease is 100 MRC units (0.5 ml)/day subcutaneously or intramuscularly. For hypercalcemia the starting dose is 4 MRC units/kg/12 hours subcutaneously or intramuscularly. The nurse should use multiple sites by the intramuscular route if the volume exceeds 2 ml.

Side effects and toxic effects. Because calcitonin is a protein, a systemic allergic reaction is

*Medical Research Council units, based on assay in comparison from the National Institute for Biological Standard and Control in London, England.

possible, so skin testing with dilute solutions containing about 1 MRC unit may be performed on the inner aspect of the forearm in those with suspected sensitivity. Because of the potential for hypocalcemia tetany, parenteral calcium should be available during administration of the first several doses.

Nausea with or without vomiting is seen in 10% of patients initially and decreases with subsequent doses. Local inflammatory reactions at injection site occur in about 10% of the patients, and facial and hand flushing occurs in about 2% to 5% of the patients.

Etidronate disodium diphosphonate (EHDP, Didronel)

EHDP slows the rate of bone turnover (bone resorption and new bone accretion) in pagetic bone lesions and in the normal remodeling process. The second use for this drug is in heterotopic ossification due to spinal cord injury. EHDP is adsorbed to calcium hydroxyapatite crystals, blocking further crystal growth and mineralization. This is thought to be the mechanism of action that prevents or retards heterotopic bone formation during the active stage.

The absorption is dose dependent. Etidronate is not metabolized, since most of the absorbed drug is cleared from the blood by the kidneys within 6 hours. Within 24 hours about 50% of the absorbed dose is excreted in the urine. The remainder is chemically adsorbed on the bone and eliminated slowly with the unabsorbed portion excreted in the feces.

The first evidence of therapeutic response to therapy is a reduction of urinary hydroxyproline excretion after 1 to 3 months of therapy. The 200-mg tablets of EHDP should be taken with only fruit juice or water on an empty stomach (two hours before meals) because food may interfere with absorption. The patient should be instructed by the nurse to maintain an adequate nutritional status, particularly an adequate intake of calcium and vitamin D, because this drug affects calcium homeostasis.

Preparation, dosage, and administration. Initial treatment for Paget's disease is 5 mg/kg/day for up to 6 months. Doses over 20 mg/kg/day are not recommended. The recommended dose in heterotopic ossification due to spinal cord injury is 20 mg/kg/day for 2 weeks, then 10 mg/kg/day for 10 weeks for a total treatment period of 12 weeks, started immediately following injury, preferably before radiographic evidence of heterotopic ossification is seen.

Precautions. Urinary hydroxyproline excretion and/or serum alkaline phosphatase levels should be monitored periodically during therapy. A 3-month drug-free period must elapse before retreatment for Paget's disease is begun. Signs of biochemical improvement of drug therapy persist for 3 months to 1 year after the drug is discontinued. Increased or recurrent bone pain at existing pagetic sites and/or pain at previously asymptomatic sites has been reported during drug-free periods.

Side effects and toxic effects. Caution is advised in patients with renal impairment. Diarrhea and frequent bowel movements with dosages of 20 mg/kg/day prohibit the use in patients with enterocolitis. It is not known if the drug is excreted in human milk. With doses over 5 mg/kg/day gastrointestinal complaints increase in frequency.

Thyroid gland

The thyroid gland secretes thyroxin and other closely related hormones that are essential for proper regulation of metabolism. The thyroid gland is one of the most richly vascularized tissues in the body; only the lungs and carotid body have a greater blood supply. Blood flow to the thyroid is normally about 5 ml/minute/g, while that for the kidney is about 3 ml/minute/g. Blood flow may increase to as much as 1 liter/minute with extreme stimulation. Blood is supplied to the thyroid via the superior and inferior thyroid arteries, which arise from the external carotids and subclavian arteries. Venous drainage is via superior and middle thyroid veins into the internal jugular veins and via the inferior thyroid vein into the innominate veins. The thyroid also has a rich lymphatic system, which may also serve to distribute hormone to the general circulation. Both sympathetic and parasympathetic fibers from the cervical sympathetic ganglia and the vagus nerve innervate the thyroid gland.

Three hormones are known to be produced by the thyroid gland: thyroxine, triiodothyronine, and calcitonin. Calcitonin helps to regulate calcium metabolism. Thyroxine (tetraiodothyronine, L-thyroxine, levothyroxine) and liothyronine (triiodothyronine) contain four and three atoms of iodine, respectively, and because of this are abbreviated as T_4 and T_3. Thyroxine was isolated by Kendall on Christmas day in 1914. He erroneously thought the hormone was an iodinated oxyindole and proposed the name "thyroxin" for "thyroid oxyindole." The correct structure was identified by Harrington and Barger in 1929, which then permitted them to synthesize thyroxine. Although the name thyroxine is incorrect for identifying the structural formula, it has been retained. Kendall later won the Nobel Prize for his work on adrenal hormones. The large amount of iodine in thyroid hormones and the availability of radioactive iodine has led to fairly detailed knowledge about thyroid physiology and its role in metabolism.

THYROID HORMONES

Iodine is essential for thyroid hormone synthesis. About 1 mg iodine per week is required, most of which is ingested in food, water, and iodized table salt. About two thirds of the iodine ingested is excreted into the urine, with the remaining third being taken up by the thyroid gland for hormone synthesis. This process is aided by the "iodide pump," which takes up the iodide from the extracellular fluid, traps it, and concentrates it to many times that found in plasma. The ratio of iodide in the thyroid gland to that in the serum is expressed as the T/S ratio; normally this ratio is 20:1. In hypoactivity the ratio may be 10:1; in hyperactivity it may be as great as 250:1.

Thyroglobulin is synthesized first. It contains thyrosine, an amino acid that reacts with iodine to form thyroid hormones. The thyroglobulin–thyroid hormone complex is stored in the follicles of the thyroid gland and is termed "colloid"; about 30% of the thyroid mass is stored thyroglobulin, which contains enough thyroid hormone to meet normal requirements for 2 to 3 months without any further synthesis.

Normally, thyroglobulin is not released into

the circulation but undergoes proteolytic digestion, which releases the thyroid hormones T_3 and T_4. Hormone synthesis—iodine trapping, iodination and proteolysis of thyroglobulin, and hormone release—is controlled by the thyroid-stimulating hormone (TSH) from the anterior pituitary. Thyroid secretion is maintained by this TSH secretion. A decreased serum level of T_4 and T_3 stimulate the thyrotropin-releasing hormone (TRH) from the hypothalamus to stimulate the pituitary gland to secrete TSH. TSH secretion is negatively regulated by T_4 and T_3, which directly inhibit the putuitary gland's thyrotropic cells. An increase in free unbound thyroid hormone causes a decrease in TSH secretion and inhibits TRH production, and a decrease in the free unbound hormone causes an increase in TSH secretion and stimulates TRH production—a negative feedback mechanism.

The principal effect of thyroid hormone is an increase in metabolic rate of body tissues, which develops within 48 hours and reaches a maximum in 8 to 10 days, with evidence of full effects in several weeks. Second, thyroid hormones are concerned with growth and tissue differentiation. In the young patient with a deficiency state there is growth retardation and a maturation failure in skeletal and other body systems (especially in failure of ossification in the epiphyses and in the brain's growth and development). Administration of thyroid increases the basal metabolic rate and protein bound iodine in the blood but lowers blood cholesterol levels. A euthyroid patient may tolerate large doses of thyroid without a metabolic increase. Thyroid hormone production is regulated at both thyroidal and peripheral levels.

T_4 is totally a product of the thyroid gland, but T_3 is a product of both the thyroid gland (20%) and the extrathyroidal peripheral enzymatic deiodination accounting for 80% of T_4 to T_3 conversion, which occurs in many tissues (example: liver and kidney). Therefore in the periphery some thyroxine (T_4) is converted to liothyronine (T_3) and a substantial portion of liothyronine originates from thyroxine. Thyroxine has an elimination half-life of 6 to 7 days but liothyronine has an elimination half-life of 12 hours. Liothyronine activity accounts for the primary effect of the thyroid hormone.

The throxine (levothyroxine, T_4) is considered the drug of choice by many clinicians for hypothyroidism because of its purity and the long duration of action (half-life is 6 to 7 days), which compensates for the slow onset and cumulative (3 to 4 weeks) effects. If the hypothyroid patient requires a rapid correction of this state the liothyronine (T_3) is used due to its fast onset and short action (half-life is 12 hours). The long elimination half-life of thyroxine is reflected by the slow onset and slowly disappearing metabolic effects.

About 95% of the hormone in plasma is thyroxine; the remainder is liothyronine. In the plasma, about 99% of the hormones are bound to proteins (thyroxine-binding globulin, TBG) and may be expressed as iodide; thus the term "protein-bound iodine (PBI)." Normal PBI is 4 to 8 μg/100 ml plasma. T_4 is bound more firmly than T_3; this permits a more rapid entry of T_3 into the cells.

Thyroid hormones are primarily metabolized in the liver, excreted into the bile and then into the intestine. The hormone can be reabsorbed from the intestine; that which is not is excreted in the feces. Metabolism of thyroid hormone can also occur in the kidneys and to a small extent in other tissues.

Drugs such as propylthiouracil (PTU), beta blockers (propranolol, nadolol, metoprolol), glucocorticoids, and iodinated contrast media lower the peripheral or extrathyroidal T_4 to T_3 conversion.

Physiologic effects of thyroid hormones

The precise physiologic role of the thyroid hormones is not yet known, although a number of hormonal actions have been identified and studied. Three generalizations can be made about thyroid hormones:

1 They have a diffuse effect and do not seem to have any discrete target organ effect; no special cells or tissues appear to be particularly affected by the thyroid hormones.
2 Their long delay in onset of action and their prolonged action rule them out as minute-to-minute regulators of physiologic function. Instead, their role is more likely to be that of establishing and maintaining long-term functions such as growth, maturation, and adaptation.

3 They are not necessary for survival, although quality of life is affected.

Thyroxine and triiodothyronine appear to have the same physiologic actions, although T_3 is far more potent than T_4. Their primary action is to increase the metabolic rate.

Thyroid hormones have the following physiologic effects:

1 *Growth and maturation.* A normal, functioning thyroid is essential for normal growth. Thyroid hormones stimulate production of messenger RNA molecules, which are involved in the synthesis of various proteins, thus facilitating growth and development. The hormones must be present in the right amounts for growth to occur at the normal rate. In children who are hypothyroid, rate of growth is retarded, which may lead to shortness of stature. Conversely, children who are hyperthyroid may have excessive skeletal growth and become taller than they otherwise would. However, if there is premature closing of the epiphyses because of accelerated bone maturation, stunting of growth results. In the adult, excess thyroid hormone causes increased demineralization of bone and increased loss of calcium and phosphate.

2 *Central nervous system function.* At time of birth through the first year of life thyroid hormone must be present for normal development of the cerebrum; if the hormone is not present, irreversible mental retardation occurs. In the adult, hypothyroidism causes listlessness, a general dulling of mental capacity, decreased sensory capacity, slow speech, impaired memory, and somnolence. Hyperthyroidism in the adult results in hyperexcitability, irritability, restlessness, exaggerated responses to environmental stimuli, and emotional instability. Psychosis can occur in either hypo- or hyperthyroidism.

3 *Basal metabolic rate.* Thyroid hormones increase oxygen consumption in most cells of the body with the exception of the lungs, spleen, gastric smooth muscle, the gonads, and accessory sex organs. In hypothyroidism the basal metabolic rate is subnormal; in hyperthyroidism it may be 40% to 60% above normal.

4 *Carbohydrate and lipid metabolism.* Thyroid hormones accelerate glucose catabolism, increase cholesterol synthesis, and enhance the liver's ability to excrete cholesterol in the bile. Since the effect on cholesterol excretion is greater than that on cholesterol synthesis, the result is a net decrease in plasma cholesterol level. The hormones also stimulate the mobilization of fatty acids from adipose tissue. The hypothyroid individual will have an elevated serum cholesterol level and increased blood levels of phospholipids and triglycerides.

5 *Protein metabolism.* Thyroid hormones are essential for the development of protein mass. In hypothyroidism both the synthesis and the breakdown of protein are diminished, but the effect on protein synthesis is more profound. In addition, there is deposition of mucoproteins in subcutaneous spaces, which osmotically attracts water causing "puffiness." In hyperthyroidism there is increased catabolism of protein, or breakdown of muscle mass, and increased nitrogen excretion.

6 *Gastrointestinal function.* Thyroid hormones increase gastrointestinal motility, absorption of food, and secretion of digestive juices. Hypothyroidism decreases both intestinal absorption and secretion of pancreatic enzymes. Constipation may also occur.

7 *Water and electrolyte balance.* In thyroid hormone deficiency, water and electrolytes accumulate in subcutaneous spaces; administering a thyroid hormone results in diuresis and a loss of fluid and electrolytes from the subcutaneous spaces.

8 *Cardiovascular function.* Since the thyroid hormones increase metabolism, there is increased need in the tissues for oxygen and nutrients and this in turn necessitates increased blood flow. In hyperthyroidism these effects bring about increased cardiac output, increased pulse pressure, and tachycardia. If these effects are prolonged, cardiac hypertrophy and even high-output myocardial failure may occur. Opposite effects occur in hypothyroidism.

9 *Muscle function.* Moderate increases in thyroid hormone makes muscle react with vigor; large increases result in muscle weakness because of excess protein catabolism. A characteristic sign of hyperthyroidism is a fine muscle tremor. Hypothyroidism causes the muscles to be sluggish.

10 *Temperature regulation.* Thyroid hormones must be present for an increase in heat production or a decrease in heat loss to occur. Although the hormones do not initiate the physiologic response to cold, they appear to magnify the body's response to catecholamine effects, which innervate the sympathetic system during cold exposure. In hypothyroidism there is decreased tolerance to cold.

11 *Lactation.* Thyroid hormone is necessary for normal milk production; without it, fat content of milk and total milk production are greatly reduced.

12 *Reproduction.* Thyroid hormone is required for normal rhythmicity in the reproductive cycle.

Regulation of thyroid hormone secretion

A hypothalamic hormone known as "thyroid-releasing hormone" (TRH) was isolated and synthesized. It is believed that TRH has an effect on the pituitary gland and, when released, stimulates the pituitary to release the thyroid-stimulating hormone (TSH), which in turn stimulates the thyroid to release its hormones T_3 and T_4.

THYROID GLAND DISORDERS
Goiter

The synthesis of the thyroid hormones and their maintenance in the blood in adequate amounts depend in large part on an adequate intake of iodine. Iodine ingested by way of food or water is changed into iodide and is stored in the thyroid gland before reaching the circulation. Prolonged iodine deficiency in the diet results in an enlargement of the thyroid gland, known as a simple goiter. When thyroid hormones fail to be synthesized because of a lack of iodine, the anterior lobe of the pituitary is stimulated to increase the secretion of thyrotropic hormone, which in turn causes hypertrophy and hyperplasia of the gland. The enlarged thyroid then mobilizes to remove residual traces of iodine from the blood. This type of goiter (simple or nontoxic) can be prevented by providing an adequate supply of iodine for the young. Iodine is not abundant in most dietary items except fish and seafoods, and iodized salt is frequently the primary resource for iodine in areas where seafood is expensive or not readily available.

Hypothyroidism

Cretinism. Hypothyroidism in the young child is known as cretinism and is characterized by cessation of physical and mental development, which leads to dwarfism and idiocy. Patients with cretinism usually have thick, coarse skin, a thick tongue, gaping mouth, protruding abdomen, thick, short legs, poorly developed hands and feet, and weak musculature. This condition may result from faulty development or atrophy of the thyroid gland during fetal life. Failure of development of the gland may be caused by lack of iodine in the mother.

Myxedema. Severe hypothyroidism in the adult is called myxedema. When it is the last stage of a long-standing inadequately treated or untreated hypothyroidism, a coma appears. Its development is usually insidious and causes a gradual retardation of physical and mental

functions. There is a gradual infiltration of the skin and loss of facial lines and facial expression (a puffy expressionless face). The formation of a subcutaneous connective tissue causes the hands and face to appear puffy and swollen. The basal metabolic rate becomes subnormal, the hair becomes scanty and coarse, movements become sluggish, and the patient becomes hypersensitive to cold.

Hyperthyroidism (thyrotoxicosis)

Excessive formation of the thyroid hormones and their escape into the circulation result in a state of toxicity called thyrotoxicosis. This occurs in the condition known as diffuse toxic goiter or exophthalmic goiter (Graves' disease) or in some forms of adenomatous goiters.

Hyperthyroidism leads to symptoms quite different from those seen in myxedema. The metabolic rate is increased, sometimes as much as a +60 or more. The body temperature frequently is above normal, the pulse rate is fast, and the patient complains of feeling too warm. Other symptoms include restlessness, anxiety, emotional instability, muscle tremor and weakness, sweating, and exophthalmos.

Before the advent of antithyroid drugs treatment was more or less limited to a subtotal resection of the hyperactive gland. Antithyroid drugs provide less rapid control of hyperthyroidism than do surgical measures. Radioactive iodine is one of the more effective antithyroid drugs.

THYROID PREPARATIONS

There is agreement that hypothyroid patients need thyroid replacement therapy. However, considerable controversy has developed over which preparation is the best for substitution therapy. For many years desiccated thyroid served admirably for replacement therapy, and it is still considered to be satisfactory for many patients. A major problem with desiccated thyroid is variation in potency resulting from differences in glands from which it is obtained, variability of preparation, and variability in the rate at which it loses its potency. There is no requirement for metabolic potency, and preparations may not contain enough metabolically active substance to produce desired

TABLE 28-1 Dose equivalents of some thyroid products

Thyroid	65 mg
Liotrix (T_4 and T_3)	T_4—50 µg
	T_3—12.5 µg
Liothyronine (T_3)	25 µg
Sodium levothyroxine (T_4, L-thyroxine)	100 µg (0.1 mg)
Thyroglobulin	65 mg

therapeutic effects even though the drug meets USP requirements. This has led to the present lack of popularity for desiccated thyroid.

Another factor contributing to the thyroid replacement controversy is the availability of synthetic thyroid preparations, such as levothyroxine (Synthroid, Levothroid), liothyronine (Cytomel), and combinations of these two drugs (Liotrix [Euthroid, Thyrolar]). These are chemically pure preparations. The question as to which preparation is superior has not yet been fully answered, but the synthetic preparations have a higher standardization in potency.

Treatment of patients with hypothyroidism or myxedema is aimed at eliminating their symptoms and restoring them to a normal emotional physical state. Clinical response is more important than blood hormone level. However, laboratory assessments of T_3, T_4, and serum cholesterol and TSH levels are used as criteria for adequacy of therapy.

The TSH test, the most sensitive index of hypothyroidism, is elevated in primary hypothyroidism and depressed in secondary hypothyroidism. The free thyroxine index (FTI = $TT_4 \times RT_3U$) is depressed in both primary and secondary hypothyroid patients but elevated in hyperthyroid patients. The T_3 resin uptake (RT_3U) is depressed in pregnancy and in primary and secondary hypothyroid patients but elevated in hyperthyroid patients. The serum T_3 is depressed in both secondary and primary hypothyroidism but elevated in patients with hyperthyroid states and T_3 thyrotoxicosis. The total T_4 (TT_4 Murphy-Pattee) is elevated in pregnancy and hyperthyroidism but depressed in both primary and secondary hypothyroidism. The free T_4 (unbound) is depressed in both primary and secondary hypothyroid states but is elevated in hyperthyroid states.

In children, normal skeletal growth is used as evidence of adequate therapy; an increase in serum alkaline phosphatase indicates that growth will occur. In cretinism, thyroid hormone levels equal to or above those required for the adult must be quickly established (right after birth) to prevent permanent mental and physical retardation. Treatment of the older cretin will not reverse the mental retardation that has already occurred.

Hypothyroid patients need to be informed of their life-long need for replacement therapy. Since hypothyroid individuals respond rapidly to replacement doses, therapy begins with a small dose, which is gradually increased over a period of several weeks until optimal clinical response is obtained. The dose required to maintain this response (maintenance dose) is then taken or given daily, preferably before breakfast.

Other uses. Thyroid hormone is also used to treat nontoxic or nodular goiter. Therapy is aimed at decreasing the goiter or nodules by giving sufficient thyroid hormone to prevent pituitary TSH secretion. In chronic lymphocytic thyroiditis, thyroid hormones are used as replacement therapy and to suppress TSH secretion.

Thyroid may be used to lower serum cholesterol levels in euthyroid (normal thyroid) persons. However, the increased metabolic activity may cause attacks of angina pectoris or congestive heart failure in patients with cardiac disease or hypertension.

Thyroid preparations have been used extensively in the treatment of obesity. This is not an approved use, since (1) most obesity is not caused by hypothyroidism but by overeating, and (2) a state of hyperthyroidism must be induced to achieve weight loss. Thyroid hormone should be regarded as potent drug and should never be used indiscriminately.

Sterility and habitual abortion resulting from hypothyroidism are sometimes successfully treated with thyroid hormone. However, there is no evidence that thyroid hormone is effective in treating most abnormalities of reproductive function.

Side effects and toxic effects. The symptoms of overdosage are, in general, those of hyperthyroidism: cardiac arrhythmias, angina pectoris, dyspnea, nervousness, insomnia, tremor, hyperglycemia, sweating, loss of weight, and the like. It should be remembered that symptoms come on slowly and may last a long time. It is best, therefore, that a small dose be used at first and the patient be watched closely. One of the first symptoms of overdosage that the nurse may have occasion to note is an increase in the sleeping pulse rate and basal metabolism. The pulse should always be counted before the next dose of the drug is given. In some hospitals it is the rule to withhold the drug if the pulse rate has reached 100 beats per minute. For younger children the pulse rate may be higher, yet within the range of safety. The rate will vary with the age of the child. In mild cases withdrawal of the drug will result in return to the normal metabolic level. In severe cases it is important to allow the patient to rest in a comfortable position. A sedative also may be indicated.

Drug interactions. Nurses should be aware of the drug interactions that can occur when thyroid products are administered. Thyroid products prolong the prothrombin time if the patient is stabilized on an oral anticoagulant. This prolonged prothrombin time necessitates a one-third reduction in the anticoagulant dosage at onset of thyroid therapy. The patient taking thyroid and tricyclic antidepressants at the same time incurs the risk of toxicity because of increased plasma levels of the tricyclic antidepressants; patients may exhibit nervousness and tachycardia with related cardiac rhythm disturbances. The diabetic patient controlled with insulin or oral sulfonylureas experiences decreased antidiabetic effects (necessitating an increased dosage of the antidiabetic agent), and by decreasing the thyroid dosage, hypoglycemia may occur if no antidiabetic drug dosage accompanies the change in dosing of thyroid. Both of the antihyperlipidemic agents that are bile acid sequestraints (cholestyramine resin and colestipol) reduce the effect of thyroid products, so the nurse should administer thyroid products not less than 1 hour before or 4 to 6 hours after the dose of these products. If the patient has coronary artery disease and is maintained on a thyroid product, an injection of a catecholamine (such as epinephrine) may create an episode of increased coronary insufficiency. The patient should be cautioned to avoid over-the-counter drug preparations that have sympathomimetic drug ingredients (found in appetite suppressants, and cough, cold, and allergy products). The use of intravenous phenytoin may produce a transient increase of free thyroxine with patients using thyroid compounds.

Thyroid

Thyroid is a yellowish powder obtained from the thyroid glands of domesticated animals used for food by humans. Thyroid is available in tablets containing 16, 32, 65, 98, 130, 150, 195, 260, or 325 mg each for oral administration. After administration there is a lag of 24 to 36 hours before effects are manifested. The usual maintenance oral dose is 60 to 180 mg daily, although the dose must be determined by the response desired and the needs of the patient. Range of dosage for 1 day may be 15 to 180 mg or more. Initial dose for children is 30 mg or less daily, which is increased by 15 to 30 mg at 2-week intervals to a total of 60 mg daily. Dose may then be increased by 30 to 60 mg at 2-week intervals until the desired clinical response is maintained. This is the least expensive preparation of thyroid.

Levothyroxine sodium (Synthroid, Levothroid); thyroxine sodium (T_4), L-thyroxine

Levothyroxine is the sodium salt of the levo isomer of thyroxine. It is given orally (not with food). Usual doses range from 100 to 400 μg daily. Dose for children is quite variable, but it may be 6 μg/kg body weight daily. This may be increased gradually to 100 μg daily. Increase in dosage is made on the basis of patient's response. Tablets are available containing 25, 50, 100, 150, 175, 200, 300, or 400 μg. The parenteral form has 100 μg/ml and is used in myxedema coma or stupor.

It is used cautiously in patients with heart diseae, especially coronary insufficiency.

It enhances the effect of oral anticoagulants.

Liothyronine sodium (Cytomel, T_3)

Liothyronine sodium is the active isomer of triiodothyronine. It exhibits a rapid onset of action, but after administration is stopped the duration of effect is correspondingly brief.

From 5 to 100 μg is given daily for adults being treated for hypothyroid states. Some patients will require higher dosage levels. Initial dose for children is 5 μg daily, which is increased by 5 μg at weekly intervals to a total daily dose of 25 μg; further increase depends on the patient's response. It is available in 5-, 25-, and 50-μg tablets for oral administration. It is also used to differentiate suspected hyperthyroidism from euthyroidism (T_3 suppression test).

Liothyronine (T_3) is more potent than desiccated thyroid and has a more rapid onset of action than T_4 but a higher incidence of cardiac side effects than T_4. It is about four times more costly than thyroid. It is used intravenously to treat myxedema coma because of its rapid onset and short duration of action. Powder for injection can be obtained from the manufacturer upon request. It is effective for treating conditions resulting from inadequate thyroid hormone production.

Thyroglobulin (Proloid)

Thyroglobulin is obtained from a purified extract of hog thyroid. It contains levothyroxine (T_4) and liothyronine (T_3). Its potency is equal to that of thyroid. T_4 and T_3 ratio is 2.5:1. Dosage should be started in small amounts and increased gradually with intervals of 1 to 2 weeks. Oral maintenance dose is 32 to 200 mg daily. It is available in oral tablets containing 16, 32, 65, 100, 130, 200, or 325 mg. It is effective for treatment of inadequate thyroid hormone production.

Liotrix (Euthroid, Thyrolar)

Liotrix is a synthetic mixture of levothyroxine (T_4) and liothyronine (T_3) in a ratio of 4:1, respectively. This combination is preferred by some endocrinologists because of the standardized content of the two hormones, which produces more consistent laboratory test results that are more in agreement with the patient's clinical response.

Liotrix is given orally, usually as a single daily dose before breakfast. The two commercially available liotrix preparations contain different amounts of each ingredient, and patients on one brand should not be changed to the other brand before considering the differences in potency. (Euthroid has 60 μg T_4 and 15 μg T_3, while Thyrolar has 50 μg T_4 and 12.5 μg T_3.) Dosage range is 60 to 180 μg levothyroxine and 15 to 45 μg liothyronine.

IODINE COMPOUNDS

An antithyroid drug is regarded as a chemical agent that lowers the basal metabolic rate by interfering with the formation, release, or action of the hormones made by the thyroid gland. Those that interfere with the synthesis of the thyroid hormones are known as goitrogens. A wide variety of compounds might be included in this category of antithyroid drugs, but only iodine (iodide ion), radioactive iodine, and certain derivatives of thiouracil will be included.

Iodine; iodide

Iodine that has pharmacologic or biochemical significance is either inorganic iodine (iodine ion) or iodine that is bound in an organic compound such as thyroxine. There is thought to be little in common between the physiologic effects of elemental iodine (the iodide ion) and organic compounds that contain iodine in their structure. Confusion seems to have arisen from the incorrect or loose usage of the word *iodine.*

When elemental iodine is administered locally, a certain proportion of it is converted to iodide and is absorbed. This brings about general systemic effects of iodide. Lugol's Solution contains elemental iodine, but it is changed into iodide before absorption. As a result, significant amounts of iodide reach the bloodstream and are effective in the treatment of toxic goiter.

Action and result. Iodide is the oldest of the antithyroid drugs. The response of the thyrotoxic patient frequently is remarkable. The metabolic rate falls at about the same rate as after surgical removal of the gland and many of the symptoms of hyperthyroidism are relieved. Maximum effects usually are attained after 10 to 15 days of continuous administration of iodide. The size of the gland and hyperplasia are reduced, and the gland rapidly stores colloid, which contains highly potent thyroid hormone. During the time when the metabolic rate is somewhere near the normal range, the surgeon may be able to operate on a patient who is nearly normal instead of on a very sick individual.

The mechanism by which iodide accomplishes its beneficial effect is not fully understood. It probably inhibits the organic binding of iodine and the degradation of thyroglobulin. Unfortunately, the beneficial effects from iodine therapy are not prolonged indefinitely. In a few weeks the symptoms are likely to reappear and may be intensified. The thyroid gland has been filled with active hormone that, when released, may plunge the patient into a critical state. Thus patients cannot be maintained on iodine solution therapy.

Uses. The chief use of iodide in the treatment of thyrotoxicosis is in preparation of the patient for thyroidectomy. Patients with severe hyperthyroidism are frequently prepared first with propylthiouracil or a related compound, and during the last part of the treatment, iodide is given to prevent the development of a friable, highly vascular gland, which would increase the hazards of surgery. A certain number of patients, however, may be controlled and prepared for surgery with iodide alone. It is also used to treat "thyroid crisis."

Preparation, dosage, and administration. Convenient preparations are Lugol's Solution and saturated solutions of sodium or potassium iodide; 0.3 ml (0.1 to 1 ml) of these preparations can be given orally three times a day after meals for 2 or 3 weeks before surgery. They should be well diluted in one-third to one-half glass of fruit juice, carbonated beverage, or another vehicle that may be preferred by the patient to improve taste.

Strong iodine solution (Compound Iodine Solution, Lugol's Solution); aqueous iodine solution. This preparation contains iodine (5%) and potassium iodide (10%) (8 mg iodide/drop). Usual dose is 0.3 ml three times daily.

Sodium iodide. Sodium iodide 20%/10 ml and 10%/10 ml may be given for severe thyroid crisis; the intravenous route is usually used, and the range of dose is 1 to 3 g daily. This drug may be given as an expectorant. Dosage ranges from 300 mg to 2 g daily.

Potassium iodide solution: potassium iodide (Saturated Potassium Iodide Solution). Nurses may see this expectorant in a preparation ordered as SSKI, which means "Saturated Solution of Potassium Iodide" (1 g/ml). It is available in 300-mg enteric coated tablets; as a liquid, 500 mg/15 ml; and in unit-dose patient cups of 15 ml. Daily adult dosage is usually 300 mg every 4 to 6 hours (50 mg iodide/drop). The liquid in a dose of 0.3 to 0.6 ml is usually administered four to twelve times, diluted with fruit juice, water, or milk. Since the medication evaporates rapidly, it should not stand open to air for long periods before administration.

Potassium iodide and niacinamide (Iodo-Niacin) may be used for the prophylaxis of goiter, in the management of certain phases of hyperthyroidism, and also as an expectorant. The adult dose is two tables three times daily with water, after meals.

Disadvantages of iodine therapy. The main disadvantage is that other treatments—antithyroid drugs, ^{131}I, and surgery—are much more effective. It has been recommended that iodine solution be used only after very careful consideration because of the following disadvantages:

1 A patient who has received iodine solution cannot be treated immediately with radioactive iodine, since the gland is saturated with iodide and, therefore, will have no affinity for radioactive iodine.
2 Stopping the iodine solution and giving radioactive iodine later may induce an exacerbation of hyperthyroidism. Since iodide causes the gland to store its hormone, destroying the gland by radiation releases the hormone into the circulation, and this may produce severe thyrotoxicosis.
3 Giving iodine solution first and propylthiouracil or another antithyroid drug later may also result in an exacerbation of hyperthyroidism.

Iodine products are contraindicated in patients with demonstrated sensitivity to them. The nurse should remind the patient to discontinue use and notify the physician if any of the following occur: fever, skin rash, metallic brassy taste, swelling of the neck and throat, burning soreness of gums and teeth, head cold symptoms, or severe gastrointestinal distress. These symptoms are characteristic of chronic iodide poisoning (iodism). Iodine products are contraindicated in hyperkalemic states and in patients receiving lithium therapy, since lithium has synergistic hypothyroid activity, resulting in hypothyroidism. Pulmonary tuberculosis is a contraindication to the use of iodines. Abnormal thyroid function or goiter in a newborn has been associated with iodine use by the pregnant mother. The intravenous use of sodium iodide may result in acute iodism, colloidoclastic shock, and pulmonary edema.

ANTITHYROID DRUGS
Radioactive iodine

Sodium Iodide[131] I (Iodotope) is a radioactive isotope of iodine. It is the most commonly used drug for treating hyperthyroidism. It has a half-life of 8.06 days, which means that at the end of about 8 days 50% of its atoms have undergone disintegration and in another 8 days 50% of the remaining amount has disappeared, and so on until an inappreciable amount remains. The radioactivity of this material is therefore dissipated in a relatively short time. The energy liberated during the period of radioactivity is in the form of beta particles (90%) and gamma rays (10%). This radiation brings about the same tissue changes as are secured from radium emanations or from roentgen rays.

Radioiodine is absorbed rapidly from the stomach, and most of the dose is in the blood within the first hour. The cells of the thyroid gland have an unusual affinity for iodine and will concentrate the element to a marked degree. Radioiodine is useful because it may be located even when present in extraordinarily small amounts. Radioiodine behaves exactly as does ordinary nonradioactive iodine; hence, an infinitesimal quantity of it can be used to trace or follow the behavior of any amount of ordinary iodine with which it is mixed. Such tiny doses, appropriately called "tracers," when given to a patient are used to tag all of the ordinary iodine in the patient's body and to permit observers to trace the behavior of the radioiodine. It has become a useful tool with which to study problems of physiology and disease of the thyroid gland. It is also of value in diagnosing functional states of the thyroid gland and in treating selected cases of cancer of the thyroid gland. Some physicians believe that radioiodine is most effective as a therapeutic agent when used in treatment of patients more than

50 years of age, those who have severe complicating disease, those who have recurrent hyperthyroidism after previous resection of the thyroid, and those who have extremely small glands.

After the oral ingestion of a tracer dose of iodine 131, the following determinations are made: (1) the rate and amount of urinary excretion, (2) the rate and amount of uptake of the radioiodine by the gland, and (3) the rate and degree of incorporation of the radioiodine into the hormonal iodine of the blood. These determinations can be of value because they can be used to help differentiate the patient with a normally functioning thyroid gland from the one with hyperthyroidism or hypothyroidism.

Because radioiodine can be taken by mouth and is collected and concentrated by the thyroid tissue, a much greater degree of irradiation can be secured than is possible with radium or roentgen rays. With the latter there is danger of damaging normal tissue, particularly the skin, when large doses are used. The theoretical danger of radiation injury has limited treatment with radioiodine largely to patients over 30 years of age, beyond the child-bearing period, and to those who are considered poor surgical risks. For the latter type of patient this treatment is thought to be superior to the use of other antithyroid drugs. The chief disadvantage of use of radioiodine is that it may promote the formation of depressed hematopoietic system, anemia, or acute leukemia when given in large doses.

When cancer is present in the thyroid gland, the tissue exhibits a variable degree of capacity to collect iodine, depending on the degree of function of the tissue in the tumor. Therefore, the possibility of treating cancer of the thyroid gland with radioiodine appears to be somewhat limited. Metastasis from a malignant tumor of the thyroid gland sometimes can be traced with the use of the Geiger-Müller counter and definite locations of metastatic lesions found. Prolonged treatment with radioiodine may arrest metastatic spread.

Radioactive iodine is effective for treatment of hyperthyroidism and thyroid carcinoma and for diagnosis of thyroid function.

Preparation, dosage, and administration. The following are available radioiodine preparations.

Sodium iodide I^{131} solution. This is a solution containing 7.05 mCi iodine 131 suitable for oral administration. Tracer doses range from 1 to 106 mCi; therapeutic doses range from 1 to 200 mCi. When diagnostic tracer tests are done for evaluation of thyroid function, 1 to 100 mCi iodine 131 is given along with 100 mg nonradioactive sodium iodide as a recommended dosage. This may be given in the morning before breakfast. The test will be invalidated, however, if the patient has been receiving thiouracil or iodine in any form during the preceding week or potassium thiocyanate during the preceding month. Therapeutic dosage is determined by the size of the gland, the severity of the condition being treated, and the results of the preliminary study of the excretion of tracer amounts or the percentage of the tracer dose observed in the thyroid gland.

Sodium iodide I^{131} capsules. These are gelatin capsules that contain a radioactive isotope of iodine (1 to 50 mCi per capsule).

Precautions. Although administration of this substance is in one sense very simple, since it can be added to water and given to the patient to swallow like water (for it has no color or taste), the radiation from this substance is dangerous in the same way and to the same extent as are the effects from radium and roentgen rays. It follows that exposure to radioiodine, like exposure to radium or roentgen rays, should be avoided or minimized as much as possible. Special precautions must be observed, because the drug is frequently in a form that can be spilled on persons or property. The contamination that results from spilling a dose of radioiodine or the urine or other excreta from patients who have received the radioactive substance means that surroundings must be checked and measured with special monitoring instruments, usually by small portable Geiger counters. Nurses and technicians should wear rubber gloves when giving radioiodine to patients and when disposing of their excreta.

Side effects and toxic effects. Radioactive iodine can induce several temporary but potentially serious reactions during the first few days or weeks after therapy. Radioactive thyroiditis may occur causing soreness over the thyroid area. Although incidence of recurrence of hyperthyroidism is low after treatment with radioactive iodine, it may occur and be particularly hazardous in the patient with severe thyrotoxic heart disease. Occasionally, an acute swelling of the thyroid gland can occur; in patients with huge goiters asphyxiation is a possibility.

Follow-up studies on patients who received radioactive iodine reveal that many of them developed hypothyroidism requiring replacement therapy from the first year of treatment to as long as 10 years later (the duration of the study). Thus long-term follow-up is needed to avoid the injurious effects of unrecognized and untreated hypothyroidism.

Radioactive iodine should not be given to pregnant women or nursing mothers.

THIOAMIDES
Propylthiouracil

Propylthiouracil (PTU) interferes with the synthesis of the hormone produced by the thyroid gland and blocks the peripheral conversion of T$_4$ to T$_3$. As a result the gland is depleted of hormone, less hormone reaches the tissues of the body, and the rate of metabolism is lowered. Because of the creation of a thyroid hormone deficiency, the thyrotropic hormone made by the anterior lobe of the pituitary gland is increased, and hyperplasia of the thyroid gland occurs. The inhibition of hormone synthesis is sufficiently effective to make these compounds useful in bringing about relief of symptoms of hyperthyroidism. These drugs inhibit thyroid peroxidase, which is necessary for the iodination of tyrosine. However, after administration of these compounds is stopped, the thyroid gland rapidly regains its ability to synthesize the hormone as well as to store colloid, which contains thyroxin.

Propylthiouracil is used chiefly to control the signs and symptoms of hyperthyroidism in Graves' disease and in toxic nodular goiter and to prepare the patient who must undergo surgery of the thyroid gland. It is true that the gland is made more friable and vascular with their use, but this is overcome with the simultaneous administration of iodide 10 to 15 days prior to the operation.

Propylthiouracil does not interfere with the action of thyroid hormone previously formed and stored in the gland. Because its effects do not appear until this supply of hormone has been used up, it may take several days or weeks before signs of decreased thyroid activity are noted. Patients with severe hyperthyroidism dissipate their stored hormone more rapidly than those with mild hyperthyroidism and thus may respond to therapy more quickly. Duration of treatment necessary to obtain a prolonged remission varies from 6 months to 3 years, with 1 year being the average. It has been reported that prolonged remission occurs in about 50% of patients on long-term antithyroid therapy. If gland enlargement does not stabilize or decrease during therapy, the possibility for prolonged remission is considered to be poor.

Propylthiouracil does not have a permanent effect on the thyroid gland, but it is hoped that long-term antithyroid therapy will foster a spontaneous remission of the disease. It is effective for treatment of hyperthyroidism and for preparation of patients undergoing subtotal thyroidectomy or radioactive iodine therapy.

Preparation, dosage, and administration. Propylthiouracil is readily absorbed from the gastrointestinal tract and is administered by mouth only. To ensure adequate and effective therapy this drug should be administered at evenly spaced intervals during the day. Maintenance doses are determined in accordance with the metabolic rate.

Propylthiouracil is marketed in 50-mg tablets. The initial dose is 300 mg daily. The usual daily dose is 150 mg every 8 hours. In severe hyperthyroidism, initial doses of 400 mg every 8 hours may be required. In some instances much larger doses (600 to 900 mg) are given. Range of dose is 50 to 450 mg. Dose for children 10 years of age and older is 150 to 300 mg daily in divided doses every 8 hours; maintenance dose is usually 100 mg daily divided into two doses every 12 hours. For children ages 6 to 10 the dose initially is 50 to 150 mg daily in divided doses every 8 hours.

Methimazole (Tapazole). Methimazole is one of the most active of the thyroid-inhibiting drugs and its antithyroid activity is 10 times stronger than that of propylthiouracil. It is marketed in 5- and 10-mg tablets. Initial daily dose is 15 mg for mild hyperthyroidism, 30 to 40 mg for moderately severe hyperthyroidism, and 60 mg or more for severe cases. These amounts are given in divided doses every 8 hours. Maintenance dose is 5 to 15 mg daily. For children the dose initially is 0.4 mg/kg body weight divided into three doses; maintenance dose is half the initial dose.

It is effective for treatment of hyperthyroidism in preparation for subtotal thyroidectomy or radioactive iodine therapy.

Side effects and toxic effects. Propylthiouracil and methimazole vary in their capacity to cause toxic reactions. Incidence of adverse effects is dose related; the higher the dose, the greater the incidence of side effects and toxic effects. Thiouracil is most likely to cause toxic effects and has been discarded in favor of propylthiouracil and other less toxic substitutes. However, they are all capable of causing serious untoward effects, which may include leukopenia, skin rash, drug fever, enlargement of the salivary glands and lymph nodes in the neck, hepatitis, loss of the sense of taste, and edema of the lower extremities. The most serious complication is agranulocytosis. Many of the aforementioned reactions necessitate discontinuing administration of the drug and giving appropriate supportive treatment. Patients should be instructed that if they develop sore throat, a head cold, fever, or malaise they should report the symptoms immediately to their physician, for these symptoms signal the onset of agranulocytosis. The nurse should be alert to note warning symptoms as well. The incidence of untoward reactions is said to be between 3% and 5%. The incidence of agranulocytosis is said to approach 0.5%. The need for close medical supervision of patients receiving these drugs is obvious.

Precautions. When given to pregnant women, the smallest effective dose should be used (less than 300 mg daily). Since propylthiouracil crosses the placental barrier, large doses can lead to goiter in the newborn.

Because the drug is excreted in breast milk, mothers who are taking the drug should not nurse their babies.

Drug interactions. Propylthiouracil can cause bleeding and prothrombin deficiency (hypoprothrombinemia), thus increasing the effects of anticoagulants such as coumadin and warfarin. Dosage of anticoagulants should be reduced when the patient is also receiving propylthiouracil. Vitamin K can be administered to prevent bleeding.

Adrenal glands

The adrenal glands are located just above the kidneys and consist of two parts, the inner medulla and the outer cortex.

The adrenal cortex synthesizes three important classes of hormones, which are the glucocorticoids (cortisol), mineralocorticoids (primarily aldosterone), and androgens (primarily dehydroepiandrosterone). The glucocorticoids are primarily synthesized in the zona fasciculata and are under the control of ACTH from the pituitary gland. Although the basal production rate averages 30 mg/24 hours, under conditions of stress (trauma, major surgery, and infection) there is a reserve capacity production of up to 300 mg daily. Increases in glucocorticoid production may be related to proportional increases in release of ACTH by the pituitary.

The mineralocorticoids are synthesized specifically in the zona glomerulosa, with production primarily under the control of both the renin-angiotensin axis system (discussed later) and the blood potassium level. The production of aldosterone is stimulated by salt depletion and causes sodium retention at the kidney distal convoluted tubule in order to preserve the extracellular fluid volume.

The androgens are synthesized in the zona fasciculata and the zona reticularis and essentially control growth of the hair follicles in the skin.

Normally a reaction to serious stress causes a prompt and noticeable increase in cortisol and aldosterone production; these hormones operate together to maintain the cardiovascular tone essential for survival. A patient under stress who has impaired ability to produce these hormones incurs the risk of developing acute adrenal crisis. The production of cortisol is under the control of a continuous feedback mechanism involving the pituitary and ACTH production, which is in turn inhibited by the circulating cortisol levels. Stress acts as a stimulus to override this inhibition and initiates secretion of corticotropin-releasing factor, which culminates in ACTH release and activation of the adrenal cortex leading to an increased production of cortisol.

Adrenocortical steroids

All of the adrenocortical hormones are commercially available as are synthetic analogs of even higher potency. The generic name for these hormones and analogs is *corticosteroids*.

During experimental and clinical investigation it was found that some corticosteroids, such as cortisol, had a profound effect on carbohydrate metabolism, while aldosterone primarily affected mineral (or electrolyte) and water metabolism. Consequently, the corticosteroids were divided into two classes, *glucocorticoids* and *mineralocoticoids* (halogenated glucocorticoids).

Biosynthesis of corticosteroids. Cholesterol, which is used for the biosynthesis of corticosteroids, is synthesized and stored in the adrenal cortex. The adrenal cortex also obtains cholesterol from the blood. This cholesterol may be from dietary sources or synthesized by the liver.

Synthesis of corticosteroids depends on the adrenocorticotropic hormone (ACTH) secreted by the pituitary. The predominent action of ACTH on the adrenal cortex is synthesis of corticosteroids and secretion of glucocorticoids. The exact mechanism for these events is not known.

The release of ACTH by the pituitary is believed to be stimulated by the corticotropin-releasing hormone (CRH) from the hypothalamus, although CRH has not yet been chemically identified. There is some evidence that the corticosteroids can inhibit the adrenal glucocorticoid system by inhibiting the release of

CRH from the hypothalamus and by inhibiting the release of ACTH from the pituitary.

Drug interactions. The interaction of adrenal corticosteroids with other drugs may be achieved by several mechanisms, among which are (1) enzymatic induction, (2) pharmacologic additive effects (potentiation), and (3) pharmacologic opposing activity (antagonism).

1 Patients taking antidiabetic drugs (oral sulfonylureas and insulin) will have increased antidiabetic drug requirements because the glucocortical activity promotes glycogenolysis and gluconeogenesis. This is an example of opposing or antagonistic pharmacologic activity that necessitates additional diabetic monitoring.
2 Patients taking oral anticoagulants should be cautioned about the possibility of decreased prothrombin time response. This would call for frequent checking of prothrombin time (conflicting reports as to potentiation exist).
3 Hypertensive patients receiving potassium-depleting diuretics and corticosteroids will experience increased potassium loss and should be cautioned to look for signs of hypokalemia; this is an example of an additive effect.
4 Patients maintained on digitalis glycoside therapy may experience digitalis toxicity from potassium deficiency (desoxycorticosterone or the glucocorticoids that have high mineralocorticoid properties).
5 The corticosteroids are metabolized by enzyme degradation, and drugs like phenytoin, phenobarbital, ephedrine, and rifampin induce the enzymes that degrade the corticosteroids, resulting in decreased corticosteroid blood levels, lowered therapeutic activity, and a need for increased dosages for steroid maintenance.
6 Aspirin is used with great caution with corticosteroids, since there is an increase in ulcerogenic effect and a decrease in the salicylate effect. Further hypoprothrombinemia may thus develop.
7 If the patient is receiving amphotericin B intravenous therapy, the adrenal corticosteroids (hydrocortisone used to reduce chills and fever) increase the potassium depletion (lower serum potassium levels).
8 Since immunosuppression is seen with vaccines (smallpox and others), high doses of corticosteroids have the potential to cause neurologic complications and an impaired antibody response. This does not apply to those patients receiving corticosteroids as replacement therapy, as in Addison's disease.

GLUCOCORTICOIDS

Glucocorticoid rhythms. Two rhythms appear to influence glucocorticoid function—*circadian* (daily) rhythm and *ultradian* rhythm. Circadian rhythm appears to be entrained by the dark/light and sleep/wakefulness cycles. It has been found that normal persons sleeping in the dark at night will begin to have an increase in their plasma cortisol levels in the early morning hours and reach a peak after they are awake. These levels then slowly fall to very low levels in the evening and during the early phase of sleep. The importance of this rhythm is emphasized by the finding that corticosteroid therapy is more potent when given at midnight than when given at noon.

Ultradian rhythms are periodic or intermittent functions with frequencies higher than once every 24 hours. In humans, from four to eight adrenal glucocorticoid bursts occur in each 24-hour period, which may follow bursts in CRH and ACTH releases. These bursts are clustered closer together and are more pronounced during the circadian rise in plasma glucocorticoid levels in the early hours of the morning than at other times when they may be so widely spaced that adrenal secretion is 0. Consequently, the adrenal cortex secretes glucocorticoids only about 25% of the time in unstressed individuals.

Cortisone; hydrocortisone (cortisol)

Cortisone was isolated from the adrenal gland in 1935 and for a time was known simply as Compound E. Hydrocortisone has been known also as Compound F. The activity of these two adrenal steroids is similar, although hydrocortisone is more potent in its physiologic and antirheumatic effects and is less irritating to synovial membranes when injected into joint cavities. However, it is less soluble in body fluids than cortisone; hence, it is less suited to intramuscular injection.

Sources. Cortisone and hydrocortisone are white, crystalline, odorless powders that are produced synthetically. Cortisone is used in medicine in the form of the acetate ester; the ester enhances stability and may prolong pharmacologic activity. Hydrocortisone differs from cortisone by having the ketone group at carbon 11 reduced to an alcohol group, thereby adding two atoms of hydrogen, hence the name hydrocortisone. Cortisol, however, is a more logical name for hydrocortisone.

Action and result. Cortisone and hydrocortisone affect carbohydrate, protein, and fat metabolism. Large doses over a period of time produce an increased excretion of potassium and retention of sodium. The patient, therefore, must be watched closely to prevent imbalance of electrolytes. Therapeutic doses of cortisone and hydrocortisone depress the function of cells in the adrenal cortex as well as cells of the anterior lobe of the pituitary gland, which produce corticotropin. If administration is prolonged and large amounts of these hormones are given, atrophy of the adrenal cortex will develop. The gland usually recovers, but it must be kept in mind that permanent damage is always a possibility.

Administration of the hormones should be withdrawn gradually rather than abruptly, for while termination of their use does not necessarily bring about symptoms of acute adrenal insufficiency, patients are known to experience muscular weakness, lethargy, and exhaustion after administration has been discontinued. Such symptoms are interpreted to mean that there is depression of cortical function.

Most patients respond to these medications with an elevated mood, which is a result of remission of symptoms or a direct result of central nervous system effects. However, neurosis and psychosis have been noted in patients with Cushing's syndrome.

Both cortisone and hydrocortisone are potent substances that exert widespread physiologic as well as pharmacologic effects in the human body. There is evidence that some of the effects are therapeutically beneficial, others are of no apparent therapeutic significance, and still others are likely to be hazardous to the patient. In most instances, the corticosteroids are used because of their antiinflammatory effect.

Cortisone and the closely related hydrocortisone permit the patient to have certain diseases without having the characteristic symptoms. In spite of the fact that they do not cure the disease, glucocorticoids bring about relief of symptoms in many patients, and in addition they have provided a remarkable research tool for medical science.

Specifically, the glucocorticoids have the following actions:

1 *Antiinflammatory action.* Glucocorticoids can stabilize lysosomal membranes and thus inhibit release of proteolytic enzymes during inflammation. They can also potentiate vasoconstrictor effects.
2 *Maintenance of normal blood pressure.* Glucocorticoids potentiate the vasoconstrictor action of norepinephrine. When glucocorticoids are absent, the vasoconstricting action of the catecholamines is diminished, and blood pressure falls.
3 *Carbohydrate and protein metabolism.* Glucocorticoids help to maintain blood sugar and liver and muscle glycogen content. They facilitate breakdown of protein in muscle and extrahepatic tissues, which leads to increased plasma amino acid levels. Glucocorticoids increase the trapping of amino acids by the liver and stimulate the deamination of amino acids. In addition, they increase the activity of enzymes important to gluconeogenesis and inhibit glycolytic enzymes. This can produce hyperglycemia and glycosuria. These effects can aggravate diabetes, bring on latent diabetes, and cause insulin resistance. Inhibition of protein synthesis can delay wound healing, cause muscle wasting and osteoporosis, and in the young can inhibit growth.
4 *Fat metabolism.* Glucocorticoids promote mobilization of fatty acids from adipose tissue. This increases the concentration of fatty acids in the plasma and their utilization for energy. In spite of this effect, patients taking glucocorticoids may accumulate fat stores (rounded face, buffalo hump). The effect of glucocorticoids on fat metabolism is complex and little known.
5 *Thymolytic, lympholytic, and eosinopenic actions.* Glucocorticoids can cause atrophy of the thymus and decrease the number of lymphocytes, plasma cells, and eosinophils in blood. In addition, they decrease the rate of conversion of lymphocytes into antibodies. These effects can ultimately interfere with the immune and allergic responses. This in turn, along with their antiinflammatory action, makes them useful *immunosuppressants* for delaying rejection in patients with organ or tissue transplants and useful *antiallergenics* for the treatment of acute allergic reactions such as urticaria, bronchial asthma, and anaphylactic shock. However, steroids can be a source of danger in infections by limiting useful protective inflammation. These hormones also inhibit activity of the lymphatic system, causing lymphopenia and reduction in size of enlarged lymph nodes.
6 *Stress effects.* During stress situations (fight or flight phenomena) an acute release of corticosteroids occurs, which is believed to be a protective mechanism. The corticosteroids support blood

pressure and increase blood sugar to provide energy for emergency physiologic actions (for example, running). Patients with decreased adrenal function require increased amounts of steroids during stress periods such as surgery; without steroid administration, hypotension and shock tend to occur.

During stress, epinephrine and norepinephrine are also released from the adrenal medulla, and these catecholamines have a synergistic action with the corticosteroids. However, controversy exists about the physiologic usefulness of the steroids during stress.

Uses. Cortisone and hydrocortisone are used primarily for their antiinflammatory effects. They are also indicated for replacement therapy in conditions of adrenal insufficiency, such as may be found after adrenalectomy, in Addisons's disease, and with hypopituitarism. For these conditions these hormones are lifesaving.

These hormones and their synthetic derivatives may also be used therapeutically for a variety of nonendocrine conditions. It is believed that, by virtue of their antipyretic, antiinflammatory, and mood-elevating properties, they can do more good than harm.

In acute rheumatoid arthritis or arthritic conditions unresponsive to other therapeutic measures, many experts advise glucocorticoid therapy. Intraarticular injection of cortisone has been practiced but with inconclusive results.

In patients with rheumatoid arthritis, there is rapid and marked reduction in the symptoms and signs of the disease. Muscle and joint stiffness, muscle tenderness and weakness, and joint swelling and soreness are diminished. The patient getting the drug for the first time usually notices distinct improvement within a few days. Appetite and weight increase; fever, if present, disappears; and the patient feels more energetic. Sedimentation rates are reduced or become normal and remain so as long as adequate doses of the hormone are given. Anemic patients usually have a rise in hemoglobin and in the number of red blood cells.

However, anatomic changes that have taken place before the administration of the hormones are unaffected, and joint deformities that have resulted from damage to bone and cartilage do not improve. After the withdrawal

of the hormones symptoms generally reappear within a varying period of time, frequently within a short time.

Nephrotic syndrome has been effectively treated with glucocorticoids, as have cerebral edema and chronic ulcerative colitis. Glucocorticoids are also among the most useful therapeutic agents in the treatment of leukemias.

These hormones are used to relieve allergic manifestations such as may be seen in patients with serum sickness, severe hay fever, status asthmaticus, and exfoliative dermatitis. The tissue response to the allergic reaction is somehow modified by the hormones, but the precise mode of action is not understood.

Inflammatory conditions of the eye, such as uveitis, iritis, acute choroiditis, purulent conjunctivitis, allergic blepharitis, and keratitis, are also controlled. Prednisone or prednisolone is considered the steroid of choice in treatment of severe ocular inflammation requiring therapy.

Cortisone and hydrocortisone have been used extensively for the so-called collagen or mesenchymal diseases, such as lupus erythematosus, dermatomyositis, and periarteritis nodosa. In these diseases, particularly lupus erythematosus, a sensitivity seems to have been developed after some acute infection, and the brunt of the sensitivity is borne by the connective tissues of the body. Apparently, the response of connective tissues to mechanical or chemical injury as well as to states of hypersensitivity such as may be produced by disease or by drugs is somehow altered. The reactivity of the connective tissue is suppressed regardless of the cause. This effect of cortisone or hydrocortisone seems to explain their capacity to relieve symptoms in a variety of conditions.

In acute rheumatic fever the muscle tissue of the heart and the connective tissue of the heart valves respond a good deal like other muscle and connective tissues of the body of the patient with rheumatoid arthritis. These hormones suppress the signs and symptoms of the disease, but they neither shorten the natural duration of the disease process nor cure the disease. They do nothing to modify preexisting valvular damage or hypertrophy of the heart. When given especially for antirheumatic effects, the daily dose of the glucocorticoids should be given in approximately equal amounts throughout the 24-hour period. When a dose is due, it should be given promptly so intervals between doses are neither too long nor too short.

Glucocorticoids are also presently being used in shock, specifically shock with gram-negative bacteremia, but also shock from other causes. It has been postulated that the cortisones sometimes lead to "hemodynamic restoration" in circulatory shock when other measures have been futile, although the exact mechanism of action is not clear.

It must be remembered that in all of these conditions the administration of corticosteroids is primarily symptomatic, not curative, therapy.

All of the adrenal steroids used clinically have distinctive and individual qualities. Cortisone is still useful and in some cases is thought to be preferable to other steroids. It is the least costly to synthesize. Hydrocortisone is superior to cortisone, especially for local injection into joints. For prolonged systemic administration, when it is important to avoid disturbances produced by loss of potassium or retention of sodium and to minimize the amount of steroid used, some authorities consider prednisone or prednisolone the steroid of choice.

The production of synthetic compounds has demonstrated that the steroid molecule can be altered to produce compounds with more selective effects and has paved the way for the synthesis of compounds with even greater selectivity of effects.

The degree of adrenal suppression is one of the best indicators of determining relative potency of glucocorticoids. Corticosterone levels reflect steroid-induced adrenal suppression. Other factors to consider are degree of hyperglycemia, growth hormone response, timing of measurements, and disappearance rate from plasma.

Absorption. Cortisone acetate is absorbed effectively after both oral and intramuscular administration. Cortisone and hydrocortisone are metabolized in the liver to inactive products. After degradation 75% of the hormones are excreted in the urine, the remainder being excreted in the feces. The response after oral administration is often more rapid than after intramuscular injection, but the effect is less sustained. Since a constant level of the hormone in the tissues is highly desirable, several doses of intramuscular cortisone may be given during the first days of therapy, after which the size of the maintenance dose is determined. After oral administration the absorption of hydrocortisone is much like that of cortisone. Absorption of hydrocortisone from an intramuscular site of injection, however, takes place much more slowly.

Side effects and toxic effects. Toxic effects resulting from the therapeutic use of corticosteroids fall into two categories: those resulting from withdrawal and those resulting from prolonged administration in large doses (over 20 mg or cortisol equivalent). Side effects do not often constitute a problem when cortisone or hydrocortisone is given for conditions that are benefitted after a short period of administration. This is also true of corticotropin. When large doses or prolonged therapy is necessary, the altered reactions of tissue cells to infections, toxins, and mechanical or chemical injury may bring about serious untoward effects. Healing of wounds may be delayed because of interference with the formation of fibroblasts and their activity in forming ground substance and granulation tissue. Growth of blood vessels into new tissue is also impaired.

Since gastrointestinal ulceration and perforation are effects of short-term (low-dose) use of corticosteroids, they should be administered with caution.

Corticosteroids may suppress the regenerative capacity of stomach mucosa and create a potential increase in injury due to stomach acid. In patients who already have peptic ulcer and have been receiving cortisone, neither fever nor abdominal rigidity occurs when perforation of the ulcer and peritonitis develop. Perforation of the bowel has been reported in patients with chronic ulcerative colitis during treatment with cortisone or corticotropin. Because of the lack of symptoms the diagnosis may be missed, and healing may be impaired seriously because of the effect on new scar-forming tissue. This failure of tissue response also explains a breakdown and active manifestation of tuberculosis in persons in whom the infection has been quiescent.

Other side effects that have been noted include amenorrhea, which presumably is caused by inhibition of the anterior lobe of the pituitary gland; disorders of calcium metabolism, seen particularly after menopause in women who have developed osteoporosis and spontaneous fractures; and increased incidence of thrombosis and embolic formations. Still other symptoms include those associated with Cushing's syndrome—a rounded contour of the face, hirsutism, purplish or reddish striae of the skin, acne, transient retention of salt and water, cervicothoracic hump (buffalo hump), and the appearance of edema. Psychic phenomena have also been observed in the form of restlessness, insomnia, euphoria, and even manic states. The psychic status of a patient is, therefore, considered before these hormones are administered.

Administration of the glucocorticoids may reduce the resistance of the patient to certain infectious processes and to some viral diseases. It is thought, therefore, that acute or subacute infections should be brought under control before starting the administration of these drugs if at all feasible. On the other hand, should an infection occur during the course of treatment with these hormones, it may be necessary to increase the dosage to help cope with the added stress occasioned by the infection.

It is important to remember that any patient who has received a significant amount of cortisone or related glucocorticoids is likely to have a certain amount of atrophy of the adrenal cortex. The amount of hormone that will produce atrophy is not known, nor is it known how long the atrophy will persist, but acute adrenal insufficiency may result from too rapid withdrawal of therapy. Withdrawal syndrome symptoms include weakness, lethargy, restlessness, anorexia, and nausea. Muscle tenderness is common. Withdrawal should be carried out slowly and under close supervision.

The usual rate of withdrawal of systemic corticosteroids is the steroid equivalent of 2.5 mg prednisone every 4 days when the patient is under close and continuous medical supervision. When this is not possible, withdrawal of systemic corticosteroids is slower, approxi-

mately 2.5 mg prednisone (or equivalent corticosteroid dosage) every 10 days. When withdrawal symptoms appear, the previous dose may be resumed for 7 days before continuing a further decrease.

A patient who must undergo surgery and who has received treatment with cortisone should be prepared preoperatively with the administration of cortisone. Its administration should be continued postoperatively in decreasing doses for several days. The nurse should be alert to obtain this type of information. It should be noted whether or not a patient has received treatment with cortisone, and if so, such information should be reported to the physician. It is just possible that it might be overlooked. If patients go to surgery with atrophy of the adrenal gland, it is altogether possible that they will be unable to cope with the stress of such procedure and death may result.

Some physicians recommend that patients who receive cortisone, related adrenocortical steroids, or corticotropin be given cards similar to those carried by diabetic patients, so that in the event of an accident the physician giving emergency treatment may be aware of this fact.

Contraindications. Glucocorticoids are contraindicated for patients with psychoses, peptic ulcer, acute glomerulonephritis, vaccina or varicella, herpes simplex of the eye, and infections uncontrolled by antibiotics. Myasthenic crisis may be induced if these drugs are administered to patients with myasthenia gravis. Pregnancy is an indication for cautious use, if at all, since adrenal insufficiency in both mother and child is a possibility at the time of delivery. Moreover, abnormalities in the fetus are possible. Cautious use is recommended in the presence of hypertension, congestive heart failure, diabetes mellitus, thrombophlebitis, convulsive disorders, renal insufficiency, osteoporosis, and diverticulitis.

Preparation, dosage, and administration. The following are preparations available of cortisone and hydrocortisone.

Hydrocortisone sodium succinate (Solu-Cortef, A-hydroCort). This is a highly soluble salt of hydrocortisone, which lends itself to parenteral therapy in smaller volumes of diluent. It is recommended for short-term emergency therapy. Dosage is 100 to 250 mg intravenously or intramuscularly. It is available in vials containing 100, 250, and 500 mg and 1 g of the powder for injection.

Cortisone acetate (Cortone Acetate). Cortisone is effective for a wide variety of disorders. Official preparations are available in 5-, 10-, and 25-mg tablets for oral administration and as a suspension for intramuscular injection, 25 or 50 mg/ml. There are also available an ophthalmic suspension (0.5% and 2.5%) and an ophthalmic ointment (1.5%). Cortisone acetate is administered parenterally, orally, or topically. Dosage varies greatly with the nature and severity of the disease being treated and with the responsiveness of the patient. In severe disorders as much as 300 mg may be ordered the first day, 200 mg the second day, and 100 mg daily thereafter, reducing the dosage gradually to the minimum amount that will bring about the desired effects. Its use in the treatment of acute self-limiting conditions is usually discontinued as soon as feasible. To avoid undesirable side effects, dosage must be carefully regulated when used for chronic conditions. For rheumatoid arthritis, tolerable doses are frequently less than was considered satisfactory at one time. The patient's age and sex greatly affect the dose. Women, and particularly postmenopausal women, are especially sensitive to adrenocortical steroids. The average maximal daily dose for long-term therapy is 25 to 30 mg for women and 40 to 45 mg for men. The initial dose varies from 25 to 300 mg orally daily or 20 to 300 mg intramuscularly daily. For children, the oral dose is 0.7 mg/kg body weight divided into three doses; intramuscular dose is one third to one half of the oral dose. Once daily or a dose equal to the oral dose every third day.

Hydrocortisone (Cortisol, Cortef, Hydrocortone). Hydrocortisone is available in 5-, 10-, and 20-mg tablets, as a suspension (2 mg/ml) for oral administration, as a 1% lotion for topical application, and as an injection (25 and 50 mg/ml). Additional preparations include a cream (0.5%, 1%, and 2.5%) and an ointment (1% and 2.5%) for topical application. Hydrocortisone is administered orally, intramuscularly, intravenously, and topically. The usual oral dose is 10 to 20 mg three or four times daily; range of dose is usually 10 to 300 mg daily. The usual parenteral dose is one third to one half of the oral dose every 12 hours. The dosage of hydrocortisone is said to be about two thirds to four fifths that of cortisone. Adjustments in dosage are made to meet changes in the needs of the patient. Withdrawal of therapy is sometimes necessary but is avoided when the patient is subjected to additional stress and strain. Hydrocortisone is effective for a wide variety of disorders.

Hydrocortisone acetate (Cortef Acetate, Cortril Acetate, Hydrocortone Acetate). Hydrocortisone acetate is available as a suspension for injection (25 to 50 mg/ml); as an ophthalmic suspension (0.2% to 2.5%); as an ointment (0.5%, 1.5%, and 2.5%); and as an ointment for topical application. The dose for intraarticular injection varies greatly with the degree of inflammation, size of the joint, and response of the patient. Doses vary from 5 to 50 mg. Ophthalmic applications also vary but may be used freely since there is no systemic reaction.

Synthetic antiinflammatory glucocorticoids. Hydrocortisone is considered to be the main steroid with corticoid activity found in the bloodstream. In recent years chemical modifications of the basic steroid structure of the corticoids have been made, with the aim of producing more potent and more selectively acting compounds. If an additional double bond is inserted on ring A of cortisone or hydrocortisone, the compounds called prednisone or prednisolone result.

Prednisone and prednisolone are considerably more active in their antiinflammatory effect but have less salt-retaining action as compared to the parent compounds on a weight basis. Hence, there is less risk of undesirable side actions related to the retention of salt, hypertension, and formation of edema when the newer compounds are used for their antirheumatic activity. The addition of a methyl group in the 6 position of ring B of prednisolone produces an even greater effect. Prednisone is inactive and must be metabolized to prednisolone, and this conversion is impaired in those with liver disease.

Prednisone (Meticorten, Deltasone). Prednisone is available in 1-, 2.5-, 5-, 10-, 20-, and 50-mg tablets for oral administration. Dosage varies with the severity of the disease and patient response. There is wide variation in the dosage for children. A dose of 30 to 50 mg may be required to suppress severe symptoms, although some physicians prefer to start therapy with a relatively small dose. After 2 to 7 days, dosage is gradually reduced and a maintenance dose established. A dose of 5 to 10 mg (or less) daily may suffice for milder conditions. The range of dose is 5 to 60 mg daily. The daily allotment should be divided into installment doses and should be given on a regular 6- or 8-hour schedule. Not only the total daily dose but frequently individual doses in the course of the day must be adjusted to meet the needs of the patient. Patients vary in their need and tolerance to all antirheumatic steroids. The nurse should exert great care that the correct dose is given at the right time. When administration of the drug is to be discontinued, it is usually withdrawn gradually, and in the event of a medical or surgical emergency or period of unusual stress the drug is given again to prevent the possibility of acute adrenal insufficiency. This applies to all cortical steroids given for systemic effects.

Prednisolone (Delta-Cortef). Prednisolone is available in 1-, 2.5-, and 5-mg tablets for oral administration; in addition, many dosage forms are available. It has about the same potency as prednisone. The dosage is approximately the same as prednisone and one fifth that of cortisone.

Prednisolone acetate. This is marketed as an aqueous repository suspension for intramuscular injection. Dosage is 4 to 60 mg daily. Prednisolone acetate is available in 5-mg tablets.

Prednisolone tebutate (Hydeltra-T.B.A.). This compound is marketed as a suspension, 20 mg/ml, for injection into joints, bursae, ganglia, or synovial sheaths. Dosage varies from 4 to 30 mg. Relief of symptoms may not occur for a day or two because the drug is not very soluble and has a slow onset and long duration of action.

Methylprednisolone (Medrol). Methylprednisolone is available in 2-, 4-, 8-, 16-, 24-, and 32-mg tablets and sustained-release capsules containing 2 and 4 mg for oral administration. Dos-

age is individually determined, but in general, it is about two thirds that of either prednisone or prednisolone. Suppressive doses for severe conditions range from 20 to 60 mg daily; for less severe conditions the initial daily dosage may be from 4 to 40 mg. The daily dose is divided into four parts and is given after meals and at bedtime with food. The daily maintenance dose is frequently about half the initial dose. The drug is also available for injection (Depo-Medrol for intramuscular injection, Solu-Medrol for intramuscular or intravenous injection).

Prednisolone sodium phosphate (Hydeltrasol). This drug is more soluble than prednisolone or its acetate or tebutate. After parenteral (intravenous or intramuscular) administration it has a rapid onset and short duration of action. It is administered parenterally (20 mg/ml) and topically to the skin, eye, or external ear.

Dexamethasone (Decadron, Deronil, Gammacorten). Dexamethasone is a fluorinated synthetic glucocorticoid structurally similar to hydrocortisone. It is a particularly potent antiinflammatory agent (30 times more than hydrocortisone). In contrast to cortisone and hydrocortisone, it may exhibit diuretic effects in patients made edematous by the administration of other adrenocortical hormones. Dexamethasone lacks mineralocorticoid activity and hence is not suited to replacement therapy for adrenal insufficiency. It is used primarily for its antiinflammatory and antiallergic effects.

Dexamethasone is administered orally or topically. As is true for other adrenal steroids, the dosage varies considerably, depending on the severity of the symptoms to be controlled and the response of the patient. Usual dose ranges from 0.5 to 10 mg daily. The drug is marketed in 0.25-, 0.5-, 0.75-, 1.5- and 4-mg tablets, as an elixir containing 0.1 mg/ml, and as an aerosol and cream.

Dexamethasone sodium phosphate. This drug is a derivative of dexamethasone, is more soluble than dexamethasone, and is suited for injection (intramuscular, intravenous, and intrasynovial).

Betamethasone (Celestone). Betamethasone is structurally similar to dexamethasone and

TABLE 28-2 Relative potency of glucocorticoids in treatment of nonendocrine disease

Corticoid	Potency (relative to cortisone)	Trade name	Equivalent dose (mg)	Approximate plasma half-life (minutes)	Range of biologic half-life (hours)
Cortisone	1	Cortogen Acetate Cortone Acetate	25	90	8 to 12
Hydrocortisone	1.2	Cortril Cortef Hydrocortone	20	90	8 to 12
Prednisone	4 to 5	Meticorten Paracort Deltasone	5	> 200	18 to 36
Prednisolone	4 to 5	Delta-Cortef Hydeltra Meticortelone Paracortol Sterane	5	> 200	18 to 36
6-Methylprednisolone	5 to 6	Medrol	4	> 200	18 to 36
Triamcinolone	4 to 8	Aristocort Kenacort	4	> 200	18 to 36
Dexamethasone	16 to 30	Decadron Deronil Dexameth Gammacorten Hexadrol	0.75	> 300	36 to 54
Betamethasone	16 to 30	Celestone	0.6	> 300	35 to 54

has an approximately equal level of potency. It is administered orally and is available in 600 mg tablets. A suspension containing betamethasone sodium phosphate and betamethasone acetate (repository) is available for intramuscular or local injection.

Triamcinolone (Aristocort, Kenacort). Triamcinolone is a potent glucocorticoid that is said to produce effects comparable to prednisolone but with lower dosage. It apparently is less likely to produce retention of sodium and water than many of the related compounds and seemingly does not affect excretion of potassium except after large doses. Prolonged use and large doses, however, bring about negative protein and calcium balance and impaired carbohydrate metabolism, as well as symptoms of hyperadrenalism. It is administered orally and is available in 1-, 2-, 4-, 8-, and 16-mg tablets. The usual initial dose varies from 8 to 60 mg daily, given in divided portions. Maintenance dosage is determined in relation to each patient.

Triamcinolone acetonide (Aristocort, Acetonide, Kenalog). This is a derivative of triamcinolone. It is available as a suspension for injection containing 10 and 40 mg/ml in 5-ml vials. It is available as a cream, a lotion, an ointment, and a spray for the treatment of acute and chronic dermatoses.

Fluprednisolone (Alphadrol). This synthetic drug differs from prednisolone by having a fluorine atom, which increases its antiinflammatory activity to 2.5 times that of prednisolone. Range of dose is 2.5 to 30 mg daily. It is available in 1.5-mg tablets. The equivalent dose to cortisone (25 mg) is 1.5 mg.

Meprednisone (Betapar). This synthetic drug differs from prednisolone by the substitution of a methyl group for a hydrogen group. Its actions are similar to those of dexamethasone. It is available in 4-mg tablets. Range of dose is 8 to 60 mg daily, depending on the underlying disease and its severity. A dose of 4 mg is equivalent to 25 mg cortisone.

Side effects and toxic effects. Although

prednisone, prednisolone, and closely related compounds may achieve their effects with lower dosage, their capacity to produce many of the same side effects as cortisone and hydrocortisone continues to pose problems. A gain in weight, abnormal growth of hair on the face (hypertrichosis), the development of supraclavicular fat pads, increase in blood pressure, euphoria, emotional instability, undue fatigability, and menstrual irregularities are symptoms of a developing hypercortisonism that are more difficult to treat than to prevent. Postmenopausal women and young children are especially susceptible to the adrenal steroids and are more likely to develop hypercortisonism than younger women or men. Many physicians recommend that the patient be kept on doses that can be tolerated even though all symptoms may not be completely relieved. The patient should also have the benefit of other therapy.

Beclomethasone dipropionate (Vanceril, Beclovent) inhaler

Beclomethasone is a synthetic corticosteroid chemically related to prednisolone that has high antiinflammatory activity. Systemic absorption occurs rapidly from respiratory and gastrointestinal tissues, with excretion in the feces and urine (less than 10%).

Uses. Beclomethasone is indicated for long-term corticosteroid treatment for symptomatic control of bronchial asthma. It should be considered after bronchodilator and/or cromolyn failure or when oral steroids are producing undesirable side effects. Use of this drug in patients not receiving systemic steroids (withheld because of concern over potential adverse reactions) and in those inadequately controlled with nonsteroidal measures has resulted in improvement in pulmonary function within 1 to 4 weeks.

"Stable" asthmatic patients receiving systemic steroids have some difficulty when switching to beclomethasone therapy because of slow recovery from impaired adrenal function (slow resumption of adrenal function). This suppression of adrenal function may last up to 1 year. Beclomethasone may be effective for such patients and may permit significant reduction in the oral corticosteroid dosage. The slow rate of withdrawal is emphasized. During withdrawal from systemic steroids some patients exhibit symptoms such as joint and/or muscle pain, lassitude, and depression.

Preparation, dosage, and administration. This metered dose oral inhaler has 200 doses per inhaler (10 mg/dose); each activation of the inhaler releases about 50 μg into the adapter. The usual adult dosage is two inhalations (100 μg) three or four times daily. Individuals with severe asthma may initially administer 12 to 16 inhalations three to four times daily and adjust dosage downward to correspond with response, but they must not exceed 20 inhalations daily. Children 6 to 12 years receive one or two inhalations three to four times daily based on response, not to exceed 10 inhalations daily. The nurse should instruct the patient who is also using a bronchodilator by inhalation (for example, isoproterenol) in addition to the beclomethasone to use the bronchodilator first to enhance penetration of the steroid into the bronchial tree. Several minutes should elapse before using the steroid inhaler to reduce the potential toxicity of the flurocarbon propellants.

Side effects and toxic effects. Patients may complain of hoarseness or dry mouth. Localized infections with *Candida albicans* or *Aspergillus* have occurred frequently in the mouth and pharynx and occasionally in the larynx. Deaths caused by adrenal insufficiency have occurred during and after transfer from systemic corticosteroids to aerosol beclomethasone. Suppression of hypothalamic-pituitary-adrenal (HPA) function (reduction of early morning plasma cortisol levels) has been reported in adults receiving 1600 μg daily for 1 month. During periods of stress (trauma, surgery, infections) or severe asthmatic attacks, a patient transferred from systemic steroids (oral tablets) will require supplementary treatment with additional systemic steroids (oral tablets) for a short course with gradual tapering as symptoms subside. The nurse should warn the patient that the steroid inhaler is not useful in aborting an acute attack but that catecholamine inhalation product is useful for this purpose. The patient should be told also that it may be weeks before the full benefit of the steroid inhaler is realized.

The steroid inhaler is contraindicated in treatment of status asthmaticus or other acute asthmatic episodes needing intensive measures.

The nurse should encourage the patient to carry a warning card indicating the need for supplementary systemic steroids during stressful periods or a severe asthma attack. After patients are withdrawn from systemic corticosteroids, they require a number of months for HPA function recovery. During this time patients exhibit signs and symptoms of adrenal insufficiency when exposed to stress (hypotension, weight loss, particularly gastroenteritis). The beclomethasone inhaler does not provide the systemic steroid necessary for coping with these emergencies. Before discharging the patient the nurse should encourage the patient to see the physician to have routine tests of adrenocortical function done to assess the risks of adrenal insufficiency in emergency situations. This can include measurement of early morning resting cortisol levels.

Patients transferred from systemic steroid therapy should be told by the nurse that they may experience unmasked allergic conditions previously suppressed (rhinitis, conjunctivitis, and eczema).

NASAL FORM

A nasal inhaler of beclomethasone dipropronate (Vancerase, Beconase) is indicated for symptomatic relief of seasonal or perennial rhinitis that is refractory to conventional treatment. Improvement appears within 1 to 5 days and is significant within 14 days. The nasal inhaler is also contraindicated in respiratory tuberculous infection and in untreated fungal, bacterial, or systemic viral infection. Rarely reported are transient nasal bloody discharges, nasal mucosa ulcerations, and localized *Candida albicans* in the nasopharynx region after intranasal administration. Irritation and burning in the nose and sneezing attacks are reported immediately following the intranasal administration. Each activation of this device delivers 42 μg beclomethasone for about 200 doses. This device is to be used at regular inter-

vals; it is not useful to prevent acute attacks. Therefore, nasal vasoconstrictors (sympathomimetics) or oral antihistamines are used until the therapeutic effects of intranasal beclomethasone are reached. Use in children under 12 years of age is not established.

Dosage and administration. Initially, one inhalation (activation) is given in both nostrils two to four times daily, then maintained up to one nasal inhalation in both nostrils three times daily. The patient may be told to use a nasal vasoconstrictor during the first week before beginning beclomethasone intranasal administration. This is done to decrease excessive nasal mucous secretion or nasal mucous edema, which impairs delivery of the drug to its site of action.

MINERALOCORTICOIDS
Aldosterone

Aldosterone, the primary mineralocorticoid in humans, is synthesized in the adrenal zona glomerulosa, which is the outer edge of the adrenocortical tissue below the adrenal capsule. Aldosterone production is maintained primarily by the renin-angiotensin system and the concentration of circulating serum potassium concentration. A drop in the circulating arterial volume stimulates volume receptors in the juxtaglomerular apparatus. As a result renin (a proteolytic enzyme) is produced and acts on angiotensinogen, which is synthesized by the liver to form angiotensin I. The renin and the angiotensinogen produce the decapeptide, angiotensin I. When the angiotensin I passes through the pulmonary circulation two amino acids are cleared from it to form an octapeptide, angiotensin II. Angiotensin II stimulates the adrenal zona glomerulosa to produce aldosterone. Aldosterone promotes sodium reabsorption in the kidney at the distal convuloted tubule to preserve extracellular fluid volume. In the normal patient aldosterone secretion is stimulated by a decrease in circulating volume (loss of blood, excessive diuresis, low salt intake, etc.) and increased potassium levels. Aldosterone secretion is suppressed by an elevation of sodium levels in the blood (for example, by excessive dietary salt intake). It restricts the loss of sodium and its accompanying anions, chloride and bicarbonate, and thereby helps maintain extracellular fluid volume. It also maintains acid-base and potassium balance.

In adrenal insufficiency, aldosterone deficit occurs, sodium reabsorption is inhibited, and potassium excretion decreases. Hyperkalemia and mild acidosis occur. In adrenalectomy, the loss of aldosterone leads to an overall reduction of sodium reabsorption and a powerful and uncontrolled loss of extracellular fluid. Plasma volume drops and a state of hypovolemic shock may ensue. This may cause death unless a mineralocorticoid, salt, and water are administered. In excessive doses, aldosterone increases potassium excretion, and unless dietary intake compensates for the loss, hypokalemia results, and acidification of the urine occurs leading to metabolic alkalosis.

Aldosterone is much more potent in its electrolyte effects than desoxycorticosterone. Aldosterone has not yet established a therapeutic status comparable to that of desoxycorticosterone. Its use has been limited because of its cost and relative unavailability and because it must be administered intramuscularly.

The amount of aldosterone secreted by the adrenal cortex is apparently affected by the concentration of sodium in body fluids rather than by the stimulation of the adrenal cortex by ACTH.

Desoxycorticosterone acetate (Doca Acetate, Percoten)

For some years desoxycorticosterone was the only potent steroid available that had selective action in favoring water and salt retention in the patient with Addison's disease. This hormone was lifesaving in the treatment of persons with low or absent adrenocortical function. Desoxycorticosterone was originally obtained by chemical synthesis and has been found in adrenal glands in only trace levels.

Desoxycorticosterone acetate is a white, crystalline powder, insoluble in water and slightly soluble in vegetable oils. In small amounts it has been isolated from the adrenal cortex and is synthesized as the acetate.

The activity of desoxycorticosterone acetate

appears to be limited to the metabolism of sodium, potassium, and water. It is particularly effective in correcting defects in the sodium-potassium balance. It promotes the retention of the sodium ions and water and the excretion of potassium. The site of action is probably the renal tubule of the kidney, where reabsorption is modified. It has no noticeable effect on carbohydrate and protein metabolism and no antiinflammatory effects.

·Patients with chronic adrenal insufficiency, such as patients with Addison's disease, may progress satisfactorily with the administration of desoxycorticosterone and sodium chloride. Some physicians prefer to use cortisone and hydrocortisone with sodium chloride along with maintenance doses of desoxycorticosterone. In acute adrenal insufficiency adrenocortical extract, cortisone, hydrocortisone, and desoxycorticosterone as well as other adrenal steroids may be used. Patients treated only with desoxycorticosterone are highly affected by states of stress or infections, and an addisonian crisis may be precipitated.

Since the advent of newer drugs, desoxycorticosterone acetate is not used as widely as in the past. Desoxycorticosterone acetate and pivalate are effective in partial replacement therapy for adrenocortical insufficiency caused by Addison's disease and for treatment of the salt-losing adrenogenital syndrome.

Preparation, dosage, and administration. The following are preparations available of desoxycorticosterone acetate.

Desoxycorticosterone acetate, DOCA (Doca Acetate, Percorten, Decortin, Decosterone); desoxycortone acetate. This is available as a solution for injection (5 mg/ml) and in 125-mg implant pellets that have an effect for 8 to 12 months. One pellet is implanted for each 0.5-mg daily maintenance dose of DOCA. The solution is given by intramuscular injection.

The oral and intramuscular maintenance dose of desoxycorticosterone acetate varies from 1 to 5 mg daily, depending on the response of the patient and the intake of sodium chloride (the higher the intake of salt, the lower the requirement of adrenal steroid). In the management of an acute crisis 5 to 15 mg once or twice a day may be needed along with cortisone or other adrenal steroids.

Sterile desoxycorticosterone pivalate suspension. This is a microcrystalline repository suspension of the drug. One injection lasts approximately 4 weeks for the patient with Addison's disease. It is administered intramuscularly. The usual dose is 50 mg.

Side effects and toxic effects. When large doses of desoxycorticosterone are given, patients may develop edema, pulmonary congestion, or congestive heart failure, and even death may result. A fair number of patients develop hypertension after several months or years of receiving this drug. The blood pressure should be taken periodically, and if hypertension develops, the dosage of the steroid and probably also the salt intake should be carefully adjusted. Excessive loss of potassium may account for electrocardiographic changes and sudden attacks of weakness.

Fludrocortisone acetate (Florinef)

Fludrocortisone acetate is a derivative of hydrocortisone acetate and is marketed as a lotion, as an ointment for topical application, and as a tablet (0.1 mg) for oral administration. It has intense sodium-retaining effects. The usual oral dose for Addison's disease is 0.1 to 0.2 mg daily. The plasma half-life is over 200 minutes and the biologic half-life ranges from 18 to 36 hours.

This synthetic adrenogenital steroid possesses very potent mineralocorticoid properties and high glucocorticoid activity. Because of its marked effect on sodium retention, the use of fludrocortisone in the treatment of conditions other than those indicated is not advised.

In Addison's disease, the combination of fludrocortisone with a glucocorticoid such as hydrocortisone or cortisone provides substitution therapy approximating normal adrenal activity with minimal risks of unwanted effects.

The dose for salt-losing adrenogenital syndrome is 0.1 to 0.2 mg daily. If transient hypertension develops the dose is reduced to 0.05 mg daily. The nurse should advise the patient to arrange periodic checking of the serum electrolyte levels (especially advisable during prolonged therapy) and to adopt dietary salt restriction. Use of a potassium supplement may be necessary.

ADRENAL STEROID SUPPRESSANT
Aminoglutethimide (Cytradren)

Action and results. By inhibiting the enzymatic conversion involved in hormone secretion, aminoglutethimide inhibits cholesterol conversion to pregnenolone, thus causing decreased secretion of endogenous cortisol and a fall in plasma estradiol and estrone. To overcome the endogenous cortisol inhibition a reflex rise in ACTH occurs. If endogenous cortisol secretion becomes to low, 20 to 30 mg hydrocortisone orally in the morning is adequate replacement. A mineralocorticoid (fludrocortisone) may be given as replacement for aldosterone suppression from adrenocortical hypofunction. Most of the parent drug is excreted in the urine within 24 hours. The half-life has not been established but is found to decrease by about half (from 13 hours to 7 hours) after 6 to 32 weeks of treatment with 1 g/day.

Uses. The approved indication is suppression of adrenal function until appropriate surgical intervention is possible in certain patients with Cushing's syndrome. There is no effect on the underlying causes of the disease state. Cushing's syndrome caused by benign adrenocortical tumor, ectopic ACTH–secreting tumors, adrenal carcinoma, bilateral adrenal hyperplasia, and excess ACTH secretion will respond to this therapy. Pituitary-dependent Cushing's syndrome does not respond because the increasing ACTH levels are responding to decreasing glucocorticoid levels. Unapproved indications for the use of this drug are prostate carcinoma and breast carcinoma (when the neoplasm contains estrogen receptors).

Dosage and administration. Therapy is initiated in a hospital (for monitoring) with one tablet (250 mg) taken every 6 hours four times daily, with morning cortisol monitoring performed. Plasma cortisol levels are reduced from one-half to two-thirds of pretreatment levels within 3 months of treatment. If adequate suppression is not achieved, the dose is increased at a rate of 250 mg daily every 1 to 2 weeks, not exceeding 2 g/day.

Side effects and toxic effects. Early in therapy hypothyroidism may be seen as a result of the thyroxine synthesis inhibition. This hypothyroidism responds to thyroid replacement. Later in therapy a reflex rise in TSH returns the depressed thyroxine levels to normal. In hypertensive patients with low renin plasma levels hypotension may occur. Two thirds of patients treated over 4 weeks experience transient side effects as drowsiness and lethargy (because of the metabolite glutethimide), allergic and hypersensitivity reactions, morbiliform skin rash, nausea, and anorexia. Because of the cortical hypofunction, precaution is needed in patients undergoing stress such as surgery, trauma, and acute illness. It is contraindicated in pregnancy since it potentially may cause fetal harm. Hypotension (weakness and dizziness) due to aldosterone suppression requires blood pressure monitoring. Other side effects reported are tachycardia, myalgia, masculinization and hirsutism in females, precocious sexual development in males, transient leukopenia, neutropenia, agranulocytosis, and pruritus. Aminoglutethimide increases the metabolism of dexamethasone but not of hydrocortisone. Elevations in SGOT and alkaline phosphatase are seen.

NURSING IMPLICATIONS

The adrenal cortex is at maximal activity between 2 AM and 8 AM and is minimal between 4 PM and midnight; therefore the corticosteroid should be given before 9 AM to minimize the adrenocortical suppression. The corticosteroid will suppress adrenocortical activity the least when given at the time of maximal activity in the morning. The nurse should encourage the patient to take the daily doses with breakfast (before 9 AM); if more than one dose is taken daily doses should be taken in evenly spaced intervals. Patients should be instructed to have identification stating they are undergoing long-term steroid therapy. The patient should notify the physician if there is an unusual gain in weight, lower extremity swelling, muscle weakness, psychic manifestations, facial puffing,

irregular menstrual cycle, prolonged sore throat, cold, fever, or infection.

The nurse should discuss with the patient and the family the consequences of taking large doses of corticosteroids for long periods. These consequences can include disturbances of fluids and electrolytes, susceptibility to infection, hyperglycemia and glycosuria, reactivation of bleeding or perforation of peptic ulcers, myopathy, psychosis, osteoporosis, and Cushing's syndrome.

Pancreas

The pancreas is a gland that lies transversely across the posterior wall of the abdomen. Its function in the body is to secrete a limpid colorless fluid that digests proteins, fats, and carbohydrates. It also produces internal secretions—insulin and glucagon—that have an effect on blood sugar levels in the body.

Insulin is a hormone secreted by the beta cells of the islets of Langerhans in the pancreas. It is a protein that, upon hydrolysis, yields a number of amino acids. In its crystalline state it appears to be chemically linked with certain metals (zinc, nickel, cadmium, or cobalt). Normal pancreatic tissue is rich in zinc, a fact that may be of significance in the natural storage of the hormone. Insulin consists of two polypeptide chains and contains 48 amino acids, the exact sequence of which is known. Insulin is stored in the beta cells as a larger protein known as *proinsulin*.

Since relatively small amounts of insulin are necessary in the body tissues, it is thought that insulin acts as a catalyst in cellular metabolism.

Carbohydrate metabolism is controlled by a finely balanced interaction of a number of endocrine factors (adrenal, anterior pituitary, thyroid, and insulin), but the particular phase of carbohydrate metabolism that is affected by insulin is not entirely known. When insulin is injected subcutaneously, however, it produces a rapid lowering of the blood sugar. This effect is produced in both diabetic and nondiabetic persons. Moderate amounts of insulin in the diabetic animal promote the storage of carbohydrate in the liver and also in the muscle cells, particularly after the feeding of carbohydrate. In the normal animal there is also an increase in the deposit of muscle glycogen but apparently no increase in the level of liver glycogen. In both diabetic and nondiabetic individuals the oxygen consumption increases and the respiratory quotient rises.

Glucagon, like insulin, is a pancreatic extract and is thought to oppose the action of insulin. Glucagon is a product of the alpha cells of the islets of Langerhans. Glucagon acts primarily by mobilizing hepatic glycogen and converting it to glucose, which produces an elevation of the concentration of glucose in the blood.

DIABETES MELLITUS

Diabetes mellitus is a heterogeneous metabolic disease characterized particularly by an inability to utilize carbohydrate. It is a state in which there is an ineffective insulin action because of decreases effectiveness of insulin at the tissue site or a decreased insulin availability. Obesity, certain drugs, viruses, autoimmune phenomena, genetic predisposition, and age may have a role in its development. The blood sugar becomes elevated, and when it exceeds a certain amount, the excess is secreted by the kidney (glycosuria). Symptoms include increased appetite (polydipsia), thirst (polyphagia), weight loss, increased urine output (polyuria), weakness (fatigue), and itching such as pruritus vulvae.

In diabetes mellitus there is a failure to store glycogen in the liver, although the conversion of glycogen back to glucose or the formation of glucose from other substances (gluconeogenesis) is not necessarily impaired. As a result, the level of blood sugar rapidly rises. This derangement of carbohydrate metabolism results in an abnormally high metabolism of proteins and fats. The ketone bodies, which result from oxidation of fatty acids, accumulate faster than the muscle cells can oxidize them, resulting in the development of ketosis and acidosis. The course of untreated diabetes mellitus is progressive. The symptoms of diabetic coma and acidosis are directly or indirectly the result of the accumulation of acetone, beta-hydroxybutyric acid, and diacetic acid. Respirations become rapid and deep, the breath has an odor of acetone, the blood sugar is elevated, the patient becomes dehydrated, and stupor and coma develop unless treatment is promptly started.

The American Diabetes Association and the International Diabetes Federation have approved new classifications of diabetes. The traditional terms "juvenile-onset diabetes" and "maturity-onset diabetes" have been replaced by the designations Type I (or IDDM—insulin-dependent diabetes mellitus) and Type II (or NIDDM—non-insulin-dependent diabetes mellitus) respectively.

The International Classification of Diabetes Mellitus and Other Categories of Glucose Intolerance is logically arranged in order from clinical disease down to nonclinical statistical risk.

Type I: Insulin-dependent diabetes mellitus (IDDM)—This clinical category was formerly named by the following: juvenile diabetes (JD), Juvenile-onset diabetes (JOD), Ketesis-prone diabetes and brittle diabetes. The clinical characteristics are as follows:
1 Little or no endogenous insulin is produced.
2 Exogenous insulin is required to sustain and maintain life.
3 Patients usually are young but are not exclusively young.
4 Often islet-cell antibodies are present.
5 Causes are believed to be genetic, environmental, or acquired.
6 Abnormal immune responses are found.

Type II: Non-insulin-dependent diabetes mellitus (NIDDM)—This clinical category was formerly named by the following: adult-onset diabetes (AOD), maturity-onset diabetes (MOD), ketosis-resistant diabetes, stable diabetes, and maturity-onset diabetes of youth (MODY). The clinical characteristics are as follows:
1 Variable amounts of endogenous insulin are produced.
2 Patients may need exogenous insulin to avoid hyperglycemia.
3 Ketosis is usually restricted to periods of infection or other stress.
4 Patients are of any age but usually over 40 years.
5 Most affected persons are obese. Cause is believed to be involved with genetic and environmental factors. This type of diabetes is

divided into subtypes of obese (Type II A) or nonobese (Type II B).

Diabetes mellitus associated with other conditions or syndromes—This clinical category was formerly named secondary diabetes. The clinical characteristic is that Diabetes is accompanied by conditions known or suspected to be causative, including as pancreatic or hormonal disease, drug or chemical toxicity, insulin receptor abnormalities, and certain genetic syndromes.

Impaired glucose tolerance (IGT), Type A (nonobese) or Type B (obese)—This clinical category was formerly named by the following terms: asymptomatic diabetes, chemical diabetes, subclinical diabetes, borderline diabetes, and latent diabetes. The clinical characteristics are as follows:
1 Glucose levels are between those of normal persons and diabetic persons.
2 Patient has above-normal susceptibility to atherosclerotic disease.
3 Renal and retinal complications occur but generally do not become clinically significant.

Gestational diabetes (GDM)—This clinical category has had no change in names. The clinical characteristics are as follows:
1 This condition begins or is recognized during pregnancy.
2 Glucose intolerance is possibly transitory but recurs frequently.
3 An above-normal risk of perinatal complications exists.

Previous abnormality of glucose tolerance (PrevAGT)—This nonclinical statistical risk category was formerly named latent diabetes and prediabetes. The clinical characteristics include a normal glucose tolerance test despite a previous history of hyperglycemia. This category includes formerly obese diabetic persons who eliminated glucose intolerance by weight loss.

Potential abnormality of glucose tolerance (PotAGT)—This second nonclinical statistical risk category was formerly named potential diabetes and prediabetes. The clinical characteristics are that the individual has no previous or existing glucose intolerance but is likely to become diabetic. Included are persons who are closely related to diabetic patients, those who have evidence of islet-cell antibodies, mothers of babies who weighed over 9 pounds at birth, some American Indian tribes (for example, the Pima), and obese patients.

Diabetes mellitus is usually treated with exogenous insulin, diet, and exercise. Glucose and insulin promote the formation and retention of glycogen in the liver, and the oxidation of fat in the liver is arrested. Therefore, the rate of formation of acetone bodies is slowed and the acidosis is checked. Other supportive measures such as the restoration of the fluid and electrolyte balance of the body are exceedingly important in its treatment.

Insulin has its principal use in the control of symptoms of diabetes mellitus when this disease cannot be satisfactorily controlled by diet and exercise alone. Certain mild cases of the disease can be treated by diet alone, but many patients require insulin in order to live active and useful lives. The dosage must be determined for each individual patient and can best be done when the patient is under the direct observation of the physician for a period of time. A number of factors determine the amount of insulin needed by the patient, and a patient's needs are not always constant. Adjustments in dosage may be necessary if infection is present, if the patient has an anesthetic, if emotional strain and stress are prominent, or if his activity is increased or decreased.

It is important that the symptoms of diabetes be adequately controlled. The more nearly the blood chemistry of the diabetic patient is restored to normal, the more normal his metabolism and nutrition will be, and the less degenerative damage will occur in organs such as the eye and heart. It is also very important not to induce hypoglycemic reactions.

Insulin has been used also in some hospitals for the purpose of producing hypoglycemic shock for its effect on the patient with schizophrenia. It is a dangerous treatment with a relatively high mortality rate and should be used only by those who are well equipped, qualified, and familiar with the procedure. It has been replaced, to a great extent, by electroshock therapy and other drugs.

Low-dose regular insulin therapy is used in treating diabetic ketoacidosis, a medical emergency. Diabetic ketoacidosis is the result of an insulin-deficient metabolism that alters the utilization of fat, carbohydrate, and protein and leads to hyperglycemia, glycosuria, electrolyte deficits (sodium, potassium, nitrogen, magnesium chloride, phosphate), dehydration, hypovolemia, hyperosmolarity, ketonemia and ketonuria, metabolic acidosis, and impairment of cardiovascular and respiratory systems when arterial pH is less than 7. Treatment is centered around administration of regular insulin and intravenous fluid therapy. Low-dose continuous insulin infusion (8 to 10 units/hour) or frequent, small intravenous regular insulin injections at the same dosage are employed along with careful monitoring and the use of an IV infusion pump to control the infusion rate.

To prevent episodic recurrences of ketoacidosis the nurse should discuss with the patient and family the observance of the following precautions: use a regimented pattern of diabetic control; never omit antidiabetic drugs, particularly when a secondary illness is manifested; consume clear liquids and eat smaller meals when illness occurs; when ill, frequently test urine for ketones and sugar; and notify the family physician of secondary illness. The family and patient should know that the following factors may lead to diabetic ketoacedosis: insulin-dependent diabetes mellitus, omission of insulin, infections, cerebrovascular accidents/stroke, myocardial infarction, pregnancy, trauma, surgery, and stress (especially emotional).

Recently substantial progress has been achieved in the treatment of diabetes mellitus by diet control, the use of newer insulins, and the concepts of management of diabetes using the sulfonylurea agents. New information has surfaced relating the role of insulin receptors to certain disease states affected particularly in diabetes.

The future of diabetic therapy may include (1) the synthesis of human insulin by bacteria genetically altered by recombinant DNA technology (Eli Lilly & Co.), (2) islet-cell and/or pancreas transplantation, and (3) external and implanted continuous insulin infusion pumps.

HYPOGLYCEMIC AGENTS
Insulin preparations

A number of different types of insulin preparations are used in medicine. All preparations have the same fundamental pharmacologic action. Differences are those related to the time and duration of absorption of the injected insulin into the circulation, providing faster or slower, shorter or more prolonged effects. Table 28-3 presents some of these commercially available insulins.

All insulin preparations are stable as long as the vials are protected from extreme heat or cold. Vials of insoluble preparations (all except regular insulin) should be rotated between the hands and inverted end to end several times before a dose is withdrawn. A vial should not be shaken vigorously or the suspension made to foam.

Insulin is given subcutaneously into the loose connective tissues of the body, usually into the arms or thighs. It cannot be given by mouth because it is destroyed by digestive enzymes. Regular insulin is usually given about 15 to 30 minutes before meals. It is somewhat irritating, and since the tissues of the diabetic patient are likely to be less resistant to the invasion of pathogenic organisms than normal tissue, the technique used in administration of insulin should be flawless. The same site of injection should not be used repeatedly, but a plan of rotation should be followed so that the same site is not used more often than once a month.

There is evidence that indicates that altering the insulin injection sites from the leg to the abdomen or arm has the effect of accelerating the absorption of insulin and diminishes the postprandial rise in plasma glucose. Varying the insulin injection sites within the same anatomic region rather than between different regions may diminish daily fluctuation or variations in insulin absorption and in metabolic control in insulin-dependent diabetic patients.

There is no average dose of insulin for the diabetic person; each patient's needs must be determined individually. These needs are frequently determined by testing for glycosuria and ketonuria. Unless complications are present, insulin is not used if the patient's glucose tolerance is sufficiently high to permit him to have a diet sufficient for light work.

Dosage of insulin is expressed in units rather than in milliliters or minims. Insulin injection is standardized that each milliliter contains 40 or 100 USP units. One insulin unit will, on the average, promote the metabolism of approximately 1.5 g dextrose. To estimate the necessary insulin dosage for the patient the physician must know how much dextrose will be obtained from the diet and what the patient's glucose tolerance is—how much insulin the

TABLE 28-3   Tabulation of some commercially available insulins

Type of insulin	Time and route of administration	Time of onset (hours after administration)	Peak action (hours after administration)	Duration of action (hours)	Time when glycosuria most likely to occur	Time when hypoglycemia most likely to occur	Species source
Insulin injection (regular, crystalline zinc*) (pH 7.2; Zn 0.01-0.04 mg/100 units), clear	Intravenously (emergency); 15 to 20 minutes before meals; subcutaneously	Short acting (rapid) within 1 hour	2 to 4	5 to 7	During night	10 AM to lunch	Beef, pork, beef-pork
Semilente* (amorphous zinc) (pH 7.2; Zn 0.140-0.25 mg/100 units), turbid or cloudy	30 to 45 minutes before breakfast; deep subcutaneously; never intravenously	Short acting (rapid)—within 1 to 3 hours	2 to 8	12 to 16	During night	Before lunch	Beef-pork
Lente* (combination of 30% semilente and 70% ultralente) (pH 7.2; Zn 0.14-0.25 mg/100 units), turbid or cloudy	1 hour before breakfast; deep subcutaneously; never intravenously	Intermediate-acting (slow)—within 2 to 4 hours	6 to 12	24 to 28	Before lunch	3 PM to dinner	Beef, pork, beef-pork
NPH (neutral-protamine-Hagedorn) or Isophane (pH 7.2; Zn 0.016-0.04 mg/100 units), turbid or cloudy	1 hour before breakfast; subcutaneously	Intermediate-acting (slow)—within 3 to 4 hours	6 to 12	24 to 28	Before lunch	3 PM to dinner	Beef, pork, beef-pork
Protamine zinc (PZI) (pH 7.2; Zn 0.15-0.25 mg/100 units), turbid or cloudy	1 hour before breakfast; subcutaneously	Slow-acting (very prolonged)—within 4 to 6 hours	14-24	24 to 36+	Before lunch and at bedtime	2 AM to breakfast	Beef, pork, beef-pork
Ultralente* (pH 7.2; Zn 0.14-0.25 mg/100 units), turbid or cloudy	1 hour before breakfast; deep subcutaneously; never intravenously	Prolonged very slow-acting—8 hours	18 to 24	36+		During night; early morning	Beef-pork

*Contains no modifying protein (protamine or globin).

patient is able to make for himself. Insulin must be regularly administered and must be accompanied by carefully estimated diets of known composition.

On March 24, 1980, the U.S. Food and Drug Administration discontinued certification of all 80-unit insulin products. This was done in an attempt to standardize insulin usage and reduce the risks for potential error arising from the availability of two high-concentration insulin preparations (U-80 with 80 units/ml and U-100 with 100 units/ml). The nurse will receive a significant number of questions regarding insulin conversions by many patients previously maintained on U-80 insulin. The concentrations of U-40, U-100, and U-500 insulin will be available. The labels on the insulin will continue to have the same colors (U-40 is red, U-100 is black) and the color of insulin syringe packages will remain the same (U-40 red and U-100 orange).

In the near future U-40 insulin may also be replaced by U-100 insulin. The following advantages are expected to result from the conversion to U-100 insulin:

1 It will standardize the concentration of all insulin available to all diabetic persons.
2 It will eliminate serious dosage errors occurring when using U-40 insulin with U-80 syringes and vice versa.
3 It will provide compatibility with the metric system.

Symptoms of overdosage. The symptoms of hypoglycemia develop in the patient who is given an overdose of insulin or in the patient with hyperinsulinism as a result of certain changes in the pancreas. When caused by an overdose of insulin, the fall in blood sugar is in proportion to the amount of insulin given. In humans, toxic symptoms occur when the blood sugar falls below 79 mg/100 ml. The point at which the symptoms become noticeable varies greatly, however. For each person there is a level at which severe symptoms or the convulsive stage of hypoglycemia is reached. The symptoms of hypoglycemia depend on the speed with which it develops. Symptoms resulting from protamine zinc insulin are especially insidious.

Early symptoms include a feeling of weakness, sweating, nervousness and anxiety, pallor

or flushing, and a vague feeling of apprehension. If the patient does not receive treatment, the symptoms may be intensified with the development of aphasia, convulsive seizures, coma, and even death. When the first mild symptoms are noted, the patient should receive treatment at once. Prolonged hypoglycemia is associated with diminished oxygen consumption and irreparable injury of the nervous system. Symptoms of hypoglycemia are quickly relieved by the administration of a soluble carbohydrate in the form of orange juice or two or three lumps of sugar by mouth or a soluble carbohydrate intravenously if the patient is comatose.

Ambulatory patients learn to recognize sudden hunger, sweating, and nervousness as subjective signs of insulin overdosage and carry a few lumps of sugar or sugar candy with them. A night nurse may find a diabetic patient asleep but in a pool of perspiration, which would indicate that he was having an insulin reaction and he should be awakened and given a soluble carbohydrate.

Other untoward effects. Repeated injections of insulin at the same site may cause local reactions of the subcutaneous tissues. These can be avoided by changing the exact site of injection.

Some patients experience a disturbance of vision thought to result from a change in the crystalline lens of the eye. This disappears after a few weeks. Edema of the face and sometimes of the extremities is observed occasionally, especially in young women. This, too, tends to disappear, but if troublesome it may necessitate restriction of sodium chloride and the use of a mild diuretic.

A few patients exhibit allergic reactions in the form of urticaria, redness, and itching in the region where the insulin has been injected. These symptoms can usually be controlled by changing to a different species/source of insulin.

Zinc may be involved significantly in some patients presenting with an insulin allergy. Improved purification processes for insulin have decreased the incidence of insulin allergy. The allergic reactions are of the local, delayed hypersensitivity type, are self limiting, and resolve with further insulin administration. In more stubborn cases the mixing of antihistamines or corticosteroids with the insulin has provided some relief, and substitution of pork, beef, or lente insulin for NPH insulin has been useful. Screening for this potentially remediable allergic response to the zinc may be accomplished by intradermal skin testing using sterilized zinc sulfate solution with patients presenting with stubborn insulin allergic reactions.

Insulin resistance. An occasional diabetic patient fails to respond to an ordinary therapeutic dose of insulin. In these cases, there has developed what is known as insulin resistance. Enormous doses (200 units or more daily) may be required to lower the blood-sugar level and to prevent acidosis. The cause of this condition is not entirely understood. In some instances it appears to be caused by the formation of antibodies, and in other cases it is thought to result from disturbance of the pituitary, adrenal, or thyroid glands. Most patients respond to large doses of insulin.

In vivo insulin resistance is a manifest feature of obesity. A major cause of insulin resistance in obese patients is the reduction of insulin receptors in the cells of a wide variety of tissues. An important regulatory function is the plasma insulin level. In obesity hyperinsulinemia is a paramount feature and a low receptor situation may occur concurrently with it. (The opposite may occur in anorexia nervosa, where there may be hypoinsulinemia without obesity. In anorexia nervosa there is a large number of insulin receptors.) The simple therapy of weight reduction corrects both the metabolic abnormalities of hyperinsulinemia and the decreased insulin receptors in the obese diabetic patient. The resultant increase in receptor numbers yields an increase in sensitivity to insulin. There is a direct relationship between the amount of weight loss and the degree of increase in insulin receptors. High-carbohydrate diets in nonobese patients with reduced insulin receptors leads to a marked improvement in glucose transport activity in cells and in vivo sensitivity.

Drug interactions

Insulin and sulfonylurea. There is no evidence to date that routine addition of a sulfonylurea to insulin therapy for a patient will result in enhanced control, though there is a recognized increase in receptor numbers and other evidences of the extrapancreatic action of sulfonylureas. There are some unusual situations where utilization of a sulfonylurea for a patient who requires insulin may enhance therapy, such as the severely insulin-resistant state where the patient requires massive amounts of insulin yet possesses adequate endogenous insulin secretion (C peptide function). The sulfonylurea may break the insulin resistance.

The increase in the activity of insulin receptors with weight reduction may overcome the antagonism to insulin activity that is imposed by reduced insulin-receptor activity. Where hyperglycemia continues to prevail, the sulfonylurea therapy is capable of intensifying the insulin receptor interaction.

Insulin and cardiotonic glycosides. Caution must be exercised when insulin is administered to patients concurrently receiving cardiotonic glycosides, because insulin affects serum potassium levels. For example, digitalis effects are enhanced by low serum potassium levels and are decreased by high serum potassium levels.

Preparation, dosage, and administration

Regular insulin injection. This is an aqueous solution of the active principle of the pancreas that affects the metabolism of glucose. This preparation is marketed in 10-ml vials in strengths of 40, 100, and 500 USP units/ml of the injection. The maximum degree of lowering of the blood sugar occurs in 2 or 3 hours. The onset of its activity is 1 hour, and the duration of activity is 6 to 8 hours.

Protamine zinc insulin suspension; protamine zinc insulin injection. This is a preparation of insulin to which has been added an appropriate amount of protamine and a zinc salt, in a suspension of minute particles which has the effect of slowing absorption. The effects produced by protamine zinc insulin are the same as those of insulin, except that the blood sugar–lowering action is much more prolonged. It may be used in those cases where the unmodified insulin does not provide control of symptoms unless it is given in several daily doses or in cases where lack of control is evidenced by frequent hypoglycemic reaction, ketosis, or pronounced fluctuations in levels of blood sugar. Usually protamine zinc insulin is administered either in the morning, 30 minutes to 1½ hours before breakfast, or in the evening, 1 hour before supper or before retiring. Its maximum blood sugar–lowering action is about 14 to 24 hours after administration. Its onset of action is 4 to 6 hours, and its duration of action is 24 to 36 hours or longer.

Isophane insulin suspension (NPH insulin). This drug is a modified protamine zinc insulin. N indicates that it is a neutral solution; P stands for protamine zinc insulin; and H means that it originated in Hagedorn's laboratory. It is marketed in concentrations of 40 or 100 USP units/ml suspension. Its action places it between globin insulin and protamine zinc insulin. Its onset of action is within 2 hours, while peak effect is reached in 6 to 12 hours, and the duration of its action is 24 to 28 hours. Isophane insulin may be mixed with regular insulin. It is an intermediate-acting insulin preparation and should not be used when a quick-acting insulin is needed. It is given only by subcutaneous injection.

Insulin zinc suspension (lente insulins). Lente insulins consist of insulin precipitated with zinc and resuspended in an acetate buffer rather than a phosphate buffer, which is used in other insulin preparations. By varying the way the insulin is prepared it is possible to obtain suspensions that contain particles of different size and form. It has been found that the larger crystals produce a longer but less intense effect, and this preparation is known as ultralente insulin; its action resembles that of protamine zinc insulin. Semilente insulin contains smaller particles, and its action falls between that of NPH and crystalline insulin. It is officially known as prompt insulin zinc suspension. Insulin zinc suspension (lente insulin) contains a mixture of ultralente and semilente insulins. Lente insulins are available in quantities of 40 or 100 units/ml suspension. The duration of lente insulin is much like that of NPH insulin, and the two can be used interchangeably. Its characteristics of action place it between regular insulin and protamine zinc insulin.

The principal advantage of the lente insulins

is their lack of sensitizing substances such as protamine or globin. They are useful for the treatment of diabetic patients who are allergic to other types of insulin or for those whose disease is difficult to control.

Insulin zinc suspension, extended, includes the ultralente insulins, which are made of larger particles of zinc insulin. The injection should be made deep into subcutaneous tissue but not into muscle, and it should never be given intravenously. The usual time of administration is in the morning before breakfast. The dosage must be individualized for each patient. It is not used in the treatment of acidosis or for conditions that demand a rapid-acting insulin.

Pork insulins. A new purified pork insulin is available known as Iletin II, Pork Insulin U-100. Pork insulin is available in the various types— regular, NPH, protamine zinc, and lente. The pork insulin products differ from previous pork insulin preparations in that they have undergone additional steps of chromatographic purification. The regular (concentrated or U-500) Iletin is also available in the Iletin II pork purified insulin. This new chromatographic purification procedure reduces minor protein components in crystalline insulin preparations and reduces the levels of noninsulin substances. Patients who should be considered for use of Iletin II include those who are taking the monospecies pork insulin, those who are taking mixed beef-pork or beef insulin and have persistent local or systemic allergy, or patients taking mixed beef-pork or beef insulin who develop insulin lipodystrophy.

The improvement of gel-filtration chromatrography elution profiles with the ion-exchange chromatography elution profile produced an improved single peak assessment of the purification assay process. The term "single peak" does not refer to the time or action of insulin but only the assessment profile of purification assay.

Since the introduction of the single-peak insulin, the incidences of lipodystrophy and insulin allergy have substantially declined.

The terms "monocomponent" and "single component" refer to further purification of insulin. These are contaminated to a lesser degree by insulin fragments (somatostatin, glu-

TABLE 28-4 Currently available oral sulfonylurea hypoglycemic agents

Generic name	Trade name and tablet strengths	Metabolism and excretion	Dose range (smallest effective dose to maximum dose)	Serum half-life (hours)	Usual duration of hypoglycemic effects (hours)	Daily dose frequency
Tolbutamide	Orinase; 250 and 500 mg	Carboxylated in liver to inactive metabolites; excreted in urine	0.5 to 3 g	4 to 6	6 to 12 (short)	Usually divided
Acetohexamide	Dymelor; 250 and 500 mg	Reduced in liver to active metabolite (2½ times greater in hypoglycomic activity than parent); excreted in urine	0.25 to 1.5 g	1.6 parent 5.3 metabolite	12 to 24 (medium-long)	Single or divided
Tolazamide	Tolinase; 100, 250, and 500 mg	Several (six) metabolites (less active than parent); excreted in urine	0.1 to 1 g	7	Up to 20 hours, (average 10 to 14) (short to medium)	Single or divided
Chlorpropamide	Diabinese; 100 and 250 mg	Metabolized (less than 80%) in liver; 20% excreted in urine unchanged	0.1 to 0.75 g	30 to 36	Up to 60 (prolonged)	Single
Second generation sulfonylurea agents						
Glyburide (glibenclamide)	Daonil (Europe), Micronase (Europe), Diabeta (Canada); 1.25, 2.5, 5, 10 mg	Metabolized in liver to inactive metabolites; excreted in urine, bile, and feces	2.5 to 30 mg	Biphasic 3.2 and 10	Up to 24 (average 10 to 16) Medium-long	Single or divided
Glipizide	Minidiab (Europe); 5 and 10 mg	Metabolized in liver; excreted in urine	2.5 to 40 mg	3 to 4	Up to 24 (6 to 12 average) Medium-long	Single or divided

cagon, pancreatic polypeptide, proinsulin, intermediates, arginine insulin, insulin ethyl esters, desamido insulins, unidentified proteins) and may give less insulin resistance for IgG increments (decreasing immunogenicity).

It is possible that a small number of patients using the new purified insulin formulations may require a slight modification in dosage. Patients should seek medical supervision about their dosages with new purified insulin before using the purified insulin formulations (improved single-peak or purified single or mono-component). The dose may be slightly reduced initially to avoid the risk of hypoglycemia and the patient carefully monitored.

Biosynthetic human insulin. The fusion of genetic materials from different species of living organisms has produced biosynthetic human insulin, or production of human insulin by cloning. Recombinant DNA (genetic engineering or gene splicing to recombine DNA) provides techniques for the separation and insertion of single genes from one organism (for example humans) into a host bacteria (such as *E. coli*). The recombined genes are then reproduced within the host bacteria and coded for the desired bacterial protein production. The viable laboratory-made organism becomes a "living factory" because this functional host cell is capable of producing human insulin. The gene responsible for producing human insulin is now transferred to the genes of *E. coli* bacteria by cloning.

The biosynthetic human insulin is identical to human endogenous insulin and will be available for commercial distribution. The recombinant DNA insulin will decrease the occurrence of allergic and other reactions experienced among some diabetic persons currently using available animal pancreatic gland sources. Long-range predictions (20 years) indicate a possible diminished supply of animal source insulin, and the biosynthetic human insulin provides a vehicle to meet future demands for insulin.

Oral hypoglycemic agents

In the early days of insulin therapy many attempts were made to obtain a preparation or modification of insulin active after oral administration. None was successful, and it is unlikely that any can be, since polypeptides and proteins are both susceptible to destruction in the gastrointestinal tract and are poorly absorbed in an intact state.

In recent years certain drugs have been found that do have blood sugar–lowering or "insulin-like" action when given by mouth. They are principally the group of sulfonylureas. These compounds were originally discovered after observing that some of the antibacterial sulfonamides had hypoglycemic effects. These drugs are sometimes called "oral insulins," although this definitely is incorrect, since, chemically, they are completely different from insulin. They also differ from insulin in origin and mode of action. Table 28-4 presents these agents that are available for clinical practice.

Traditionally sulfonylureas were thought to operate by stimulating insulin secretion. Research has indicated that these drugs may also alter cell-receptor sensitivity to insulin. Sulfonylureas may increase the ability of insulin to bind to various cells and increase the number of insulin receptors. Changes in insulin receptors may be an important factor in the insulin resistance that exists among some persons with maturity-onset diabetes. It is possible that sulfonylurea agents not only affect the availability but also the action of insulin, and it is this effect on insulin action that may be mediated through alterations in insulin receptors. Additionally, the sulfonylureas may affect the responsiveness of the liver to insulin, independent of changes in the receptors.

Prolonged administration of sulfonylureas produces blood glucose lowering but plasma insulin levels remain unaltered. The subsequent effects of blood glucose appear to be improved sensitivity of beta cells or extrapancreatic effects occurring in the liver and on insulin sensitivity of peripheral tissues. The precise mechanism of long-term sulfonylureas is uncertain.

Sulfonylureas appear to increase insulin sensitivity of the peripheral tissues, and they enhance the insulin sensitivity of the pancreas. Ambient insulin concentration is therefore not the sole factor influencing insulin receptors.

The mechanism of action for the sulfonylurea agents is that of stimulation of insulin secretion in the acute situation, but in long-term therapy there is a hypoglycemic effect of sulfonylurea that is unrelated to any acute insulin secretion.

The sulfonylureas are metabolized in the liver to both active (acetohexamide, tolazamide) and inactive (chlorpropamide, tolbutamide) metabolites and excreted in the urine. They are most effective, therefore, in relatively mild diabetes when there is still some reserve islet capacity, such as the adult patient in whom the diabetes is recognized after the age of 30 years and who can be controlled with less than 40 units of insulin per day. They are less effective or ineffective in (severe diabetes or juvenile diabetes) in which it is presumed that no functional islet tissue is left to respond.

Although much interest and enthusiasm have greeted the sulfonylureas and although these drugs have considerable scientific importance, they cannot be said to have fully replaced insulin in the treatment of diabetes. Nurses should recognize that the need for instruction that stresses dietary restrictions is even greater for patients receiving oral hypoglycemic agents than for those taking insulin, and it must be remembered that these patients, too, must be taught how and when to test for glycosuria and ketonuria, to maintain diet and personal hygiene, and to recognize dangerous symptoms. Since insulin is indispensable for management of complications, the patient must also be instructed in the use of insulin.

It must be noted that sulfonylurea drugs depress radioactive iodide uptake and may cause misleading results in diagnostic tests.

Controversy has developed about these drugs since findings from studies indicate that diet and oral hypoglycemic therapy was no more effective than diet alone, and perhaps even less effective, for the prevention of complications and reduction of cardiovascular mortality. The University Group Diabetes Program, concluded in 1970 that maturity-onset diabetic patients treated with diet plus tolbutamide had a higher rate of cardiovascular deaths than patients treated with diet alone or diet plus insulin. A later publication confirmed these results in relation to phenformin (no longer marketed in the United States). An FDA audit found that although certain errors and discrepancies marred this study, none appeared to invalidate the conclusions on tolbutamide and phenformin.[1]

Side effects and toxic effects. The most commonly seen secondary effects of oral hypoglycemics are as follows:

hypoglycemia (this may persist for several days)—headache, nervousness, weakness, fatigue, dizziness, malaise, tingling sensations
gastrointestinal—anorexia, nausea, vomiting, diarrhea, abdominal pain, gastrointestinal bleeding
skin rashes—exfoliative dermatitis, erythema, urticaria (hives), photosensitivity
blood dyscrasias—leukopenia, thrombocytopenia, agranulocytosis, anemias
diuretic effects—with acetohexamide, tolazamide, glyburide
antidiuretic effects—dilutional hyponatremia from chlorpropamide
others—cholestatic jaundice, adverse reactions with alcohol (disulfiram-like reaction—vasomotor effect), possible relationship with cardiovascular disease death

Patients taking the oral sulfonylurea antidiabetic drugs tolbutamide and chlorpropamide experience alcohol intolerance similar in effect but milder (abdominal pain, etc.) than that associated with disulfiram and metronidazole. Tolbutamide and alcohol interact by multiple mechanisms and cause unpredictable fluctuations in serum glucose levels. The most serious side effects are symptoms of severe hypoglycemia. Because of the unpredictability of these reactions the nurse must caution patients about excessive alcoholic intake (and medications containing alcohol) when the patient is begun on therapy with the oral sulfonylureas. Alcohol also has the ability to increase the rate of metabolism of tolbutamide and other sulfonylureas when there is long-term consumption of excessive quantities of alcohol. Tolbutamide is one of the drugs for which there are distinct differences in effects among occasional drinkers as opposed to chronic alcoholics. Whereas short-term consumption of large amounts of alcohol increases tolbutamide's half-life, the chronic alcoholic's consumption causes a significant decrease in tolbutamide's half-life. The half-life of tolbutamide is about 50% shorter in abstaining alcoholics than in nondrinkers.

Oral hypoglycemic agents may also interfere with some enzymatic reactions in the liver, and therefore their use for patients with hepatic damage is not recommended. The incidence of toxicity seems to be low. It is important that the diabetic patient observe dietary restrictions as carefully as when taking insulin.

Some patients develop allergic reactions that may require that administration of the hypoglycemic agent be stopped and that therapy with insulin be resumed. Patients should be carefully instructed concerning the limitations of tolbutamide and other sulfonylureas. Overdosage produces characteristic hypoglycemic reactions.

Drug interactions. Diabetic control changes when a second drug is added to or deleted from a course of therapy of a diabetic patient controlled with an antidiabetic agent. This necessitates a change in the antidiabetic drug dose or careful monitoring. Some drugs reported to have a hyperglycemic effect are beta blocking drugs, corticosteroids, diazoxide, diuretics, epinephrine, phenytoin, and thyroid preparations. Some drugs reported to cause an increased hypoglycemic effect are beta blocking drugs, chloramphenicol, coumarin anticoagulants, guanethidine, monoamine oxidase inhibitors, oxyphenbutazone, phenylbutazone, probenecid, salicylates, steroids (anabolic), and sulfonamides. The beta blocking drugs prevent the appearance of premonitory signs and symptoms (pulse rate and blood pressure changes) of acute hypoglycemia. Labile diabetic patients who are maintained on these drugs should be cautioned since the hypoglycemic attacks may be accompanied by a precipitous elevation in blood pressure. Sulfonylureas may decrease the effect of thyroid preparations and enhance the activity of barbiturates. The nurse should strongly discourage the frequent consumption of alcohol, as described earlier.

Preparations, dosage, and administration

Tolbutamide (Orinase). Tolbutamide is effective for the treatment of diabetes mellitus of the stable type without acute complications such as acidosis or ketosis. This drug, a sulfonylurea derivative, is marketed in 250- and 500-mg tablets for oral administration. Therapeutic trial with this drug is initiated with 3 g on the first

day and 2 g on the second day; then dosage is gradually reduced until the minimum dose for satisfactory control of blood sugar has been determined. Maintenance dosage may vary from 0.5 to 2 g/day. The drug is preferably given in 2 or 3 divided doses and after meals. Traces of the drug have been found in plasma 1 hour after administration, the drug has a serum half-life of about 4 to 6 hours, and the duration of action is 6 to 12 hours. Diabetic patients require close medical supervision, especially when the drug is first tried.

When tolbutamide therapy is begun, it will frequently be effected with a concurrent, gradual reduction of insulin dosage. During this conversion period, the nurse must be alert to the occurrence of hypoglycemic reactions that might indicate a need for modification of the dosage schedules.

Sodium tolbutamide. Orinase Diagnostic Sodium tolbutamide is used as a diagnostic aid for pancreatic islet cell adenoma and is available in 1-g vials with diluent.

Carbutamide. This drug causes allergic reactions in human beings and has not been released for use in the United States.

Tolazamide (Tolinase). Tolazamide is a sulfonylurea compound pharmacologically related to tolbutamide, but it is absorbed more slowly. The average serum half-life of tolazamide is 7 hours, with a duration of action of about 12 to 24 hours. Tolazamide is administered orally in doses ranging from 100 mg to 1 g daily. It is available in 100-, 250-, and 500-mg tablets. Dosage in excess of 1 g is not recommended. Side effects are similar to those of other sulfonylurea drugs. The diuretic effect of tolazamide, acetohexamide, and glyburide may be caused by inhibition of activity of the antidiuretic hormone at the renal tubule.

Chlorpropamide (Diabinese). Chlorpropamide belongs to the sulfonylurea group and has a serum half-life of 30 to 36 hours, and a duration of action up to 60 hours. It may be given in a single daily dose. The drug is available in 100- and 250-mg scored tablets (D shaped tablets) for oral administration. A dosage in excess of 750 mg daily is not recommended. Side effects are similar to those of other sulfonylurea drugs but may be more severe. The patient must be observed closely during the first 6 weeks of therapy. Hypersensitivity reactions may occur and are an indication for discontinuation of the drug. The drug may also prolong the action of sedatives and hypnotics. It is contraindicated in pregnancy, severe hepatic or renal dysfunction, other endocrine dysfunction, and Raynaud's disease. Water retention and dilutional hyponatremia (inappropriate antidiuretic hormone syndrome) are reported in edema-prone patients (like those with congestive heart failure or hepatic cirrhosis). Alcohol intolerance occurs more often than with other sulfonylureas.

Acetohexamide (Dymelor). Acetohexamide is a sulfonylurea compound closely related to tolbutamide but about twice as potent. It is available in 250- and 500-mg scored tablets, and its usual dosage range is from 250 mg to 1.5 g. Side effects resemble those of other sulfonylureas.

The uricosuric property of acetohexamide with therapeutic doses may have application in the diabetic patient with gout; the combined serum half-life of parent and metabolite is 6 to 8 hours (the parent compound has a serum half-life of about 1.6 hours and that of the metabolite is 5.6 hours). The duration of action is 12 to 24 hours.

Phenformin hydrochloride. This is not a sulfonylurea compound but a biguanide derivative. Phenformin is only available in the United States from the FDA (Division of Metabolism and Endocrine Drug Products) under an investigational new drug (IND) application because of the high risk of lactic acidosis observed with this biguanide hypoglycemic agent. The indications for phenformin to be applied in the IND are as follows: noninsulin dependent diabetes, nonketotic elevated blood glucose, symptoms such as polydipsia, symptoms uncontrolled by diet and sulfonylureas, intolerance or allergy to sulfonylureas; threatened loss of patient's occupation due to the hypoglycemia from insulin, hazard of hypoglycemia to patient or others, or inability of patient to have insulin administered due to disability, no practical alternative or no access to assistance.

Lactic acidosis is described as elevated lactate levels, increased lactate-to-pyruvate ratio, lowered blood pH, and azotemia. The incidence of lactic acidosis in patients treated with phenformin ranges from 0.25 to 4 cases per 1000 treatment years. The onset of lactic acidosis is signaled with nausea, vomiting, hyperventilation, malaise, or abdominal pain. The nurse should alert the patient to discontinue the drug if any of these symptoms develop and immediately notify the attending physician. Alcohol and phenformin potentiate the mutual tendencies to elevate blood lactate levels; therefore, the nurse should caution the patient receiving phenformin to avoid the consumption of alcohol (including alcohol-containing drugs such as over-the-counter drugs).

Its exact mode of action has not been clearly defined, but phenformin seems to act by supplementing insulin effects in peripheral utilization of glucose. Its effectiveness requires the presence of some insulin, either exogenous or endogenous. It has been used in combination therapy with sulfonylureas when either drug alone does not produce maximal results. Side effects may include an unpleasant, metallic or bitter taste, anorexia, cramps, nausea, and sometimes vomiting and diarrhea.

HYPERGLYCEMIC AGENTS
Glucagon

Glucagon is effective in the treatment of severe functional hypoglycemic reactions in patients who are receiving insulin therapy for diabetes or during insulin shock therapy in psychiatric patients. A patient in hypoglycemic coma will usually respond 5 to 20 minutes after being given an injection of glucagon. However, in most patients, after the initial rise in the concentration of glucose in the blood, it will fall to normal or hypoglycemic levels within 1½ hours. In order to prevent the patient from relapsing into coma after he has been aroused by glucagon, dextrose or another readily absorbable sugar is administered. Because patients who receive glucagon require close medical supervision, the drug is only recommended for emergency home use by self-administration. Glucagon requires available liver glycogen and is therefore of no value in states of adrenal insufficiency, chronic hypoglycemia, or starvation.

When diluted for intravenous administration, 5% dextrose injection is the solution of choice, because in combination with chloride salts (sodium chloride, potassium chloride, calcium chloride, etc.) a precipitate will develop. The nurse must remember this caution when injecting the glucagon into an intravenous infusion drip being administered. A solution of glucagon and dextrose will be stable for a period of 24 hours if stored at room temperature. The patient with insulin-dependent diabetes mellitus (juvenile-type diabetes) will not have as great a response in blood glucose levels to glucagon administration as will the non-insulin-dependent diabetes mellitus patient (mature or adult-type stable diabetic). Supplementary carbohydrate (to restore liver glycogen and prevent secondary hypoglycemia) products should also be given as soon as possible to the patient. The nurse must consider the possible use of parenteral glucose-dextrose 50% (if the patient fails to respond to the glucagon) because of the deleterious effect of sustained cerebral hypoglycemia and potential for cortical damage.

Glucagon is a potent inhibitor of smooth muscle action and is useful as a diagnostic aid in gastrointestinal x-rays. It is suggested for use in acute diverticulitis to reduce pain and restoration of bowel function. Its ability to relax smooth muscle has found additional usefulness to relax the esophageal smooth muscle in patients with esophageal rings or a small hiatal hernia presenting with acute aphagia to permit passage of a food bolus obstruction.

Glucagon acts on adenylcyclase but not on beta receptors. Thus it is effective in patients receiving beta blockers.

Preparation, dosage, and administration. Glucagon is available in vials containing powder suitable for injection. One milliliter of diluent is used for each milligram of glucagon. The usual dosage for the diabetic patient is 0.5 to 1 mg. If the patient does not respond in 20 minutes, an additional one to two doses may be given. The drug may be given by intravenous, intramuscular, or subcutaneous injection.

Side effects and toxic effects. Nausea and vomiting are the most frequent side effects observed in patients who have received glucagon, but these effects may be caused by hypoglycemia rather than the drug. Hypotensive reactions immediately after the administration of glucagon have also been reported. Because glucagon is an agent of protein derivation with

unknown potential toxicity, nurses need to be alert to detect early signs of hypersensitivity. Glucagon has a positive inotropic effect (ventricular tachycardia and fibrillation) on the heart similar to that caused by the catecholamine, but it is not blocked by the beta blockers. As a vasoactive drug it can increase hepatic blood flow to increase elimination as various drugs (propranolol, lidocaine, etc.).

Diazoxide (Proglycem)

Diazoxide administered orally produces a prompt dose-related increase in blood glucose level primarily by inhibition of insulin release from the pancreas and an extrapancreatic effect. The hyperglycemic effect begins within an hour and lasts up tp 8 hours with normal renal function. Other pharmacologic actions include increases in pulse rate, serum uric acid levels (due to decreased excretion), and serum free fatty acid levels and a decrease in chloride excretion. In the presence of hypokalemia the hyperglycemic effects are potentiated. The resultant hyperglycemia is reversed by insulin or tolbutamide. The inhibition of insulin release by diazoxide is antagonized by alpha adrenergic blocking agents.

Diazoxide is 90% serum protein bound, is excreted by the kidneys, and has a plasma half-life by the intravenous route of about 30 hours. Limited data have shown an oral route serum half-life for adults ranging from 24 to 36 hours and in children 9.5 to 24 hours; impaired renal function and overdosage prolongs the half-life.

Oral diazoxide is used in the management of organic (nonfunctional) hypoglycemia caused by hyperinsulinism associated with an inoperable islet cell adenoma, carcinoma, or extrapancreatic malignancy in adults and in children. It is also used in leucine sensitivity, islet cell hyperplasia, and nesidioblastoses. A confirmed diagnosis of these conditions is required for its use, since it is contraindicated in functional hypoglycemia. Safety in pregnancy has not been established.

Preparation, dosage, and administration. Diazoxide is available in 50- and 100-mg capsules and chocolate-mint suspension containing 50 mg/ml (available with a calibrated dropper). The usual *child-adult* daily dosage is 3 to 8 mg/kg, divided into two or three equal doses every 8 to 12 hours; for infants and newborns the dose is 8 to 15 mg/kg.

Side effects and toxic effects. Overdosage causing marked hyperglycemia associated with ketoacidosis will respond to prompt insulin administration and restoration of fluid and electrolytes. The nurse must keep in mind the long half-life (30 hours) of this drug when treating the symptoms of overdosage; a period of a week is required for observation to monitor the blood sugar levels for stabilization within normal limits. Sodium and fluid retention, resulting from the antidiuretic property, is the most common serious adverse reaction in young infants and adults and may lead to congestive heart failure in patients with compromised cardiac reserve. Serious but infrequent adverse reactions include diabetic ketoacidosis and hyperglycemic hyperosmolar nonketotic coma that will respond to insulin administration and fluid and electrolyte restoration and balance. Hirsutism of the lanugo type occurs in children and women. Hyperglycemia or glycosuria requires a dose reduction. Gastrointestinal intolerance, tachycardia, palpitations, elevation of serum uric acid, thrombocytopenia, and neutropenia are also among the adverse reactions.

The occurrence of ketoacidosis and hyperglycemic hyperosmolar nonketotic coma may be reduced by careful patient education directed at monitoring urine for sugar and ketones (especially under stressful conditions) and prompt notification to the physician of abnormal findings or unusual symptoms.

Drug interactions. The following drug interactions have been observed when a patient is taking diazoxide:

1 Enhancement of oral anticoagulants
2 Decreased antidiabetic effects of oral antidiabetic agents and insulin
3 Enhanced hyperglycemic, hyperuricemic, and antihypertensive effects of thiazide diuretics and thiazide-like drugs

NURSING IMPLICATIONS

A newly diagnosed diabetic individual has much to learn about his disease and its therapy. Without a good understanding the progression of the disease will proceed much more rapidly, with complications such as gangrene, infections, and hypoglycemic shock or coma occurring more frequently. The nurse plays a large part in counseling and in the education of diabetic patients. Many nursing staffs of hospitals have established regular diabetic classes for the diabetic patient, but they do not replace the one-to-one contact that a nurse has with a diabetic patient during hospitalization.

The box below is a guideline that a nurse can use in interacting with a diabetic patient. The information communicated should enhance the patient's understanding of the dis-

---

Patient education and counseling guidelines

1. Patient information, injection techniques, rotation of sites, aseptic technique, effects of stress, diet, hyperglycemic drug control, urine testing
2. Patients' individual knowledge and acceptance of altered life-style
   a. Definition of diabetes (hereditary implication)
   b. Action and function of insulin and oral hypoglycemic agents
   c. Mechanisms and causes of diabetes
   d. Three hallmarks of diabetes management
      (1) Diet
      (2) Exercise
      (3) Insulin/oral sulfonylurea
   e. Hypoglycemic plans (glucagon use), signs, prevention, treatment
   f. Hyperglycemic plans, signs, prevention, treatment
   g. Chronic complications (awareness)
3. Expression of the patients' reactions or inner feelings of this state
   a. Anticipated compliance or noncompliance
   b Individualized plan to enhance compliance
   c. Compliance with this life-style
   d. Family involvement (supportive)
4. Alcoholic beverages
5. Drug interactions
6. Major complications of diabetes mellitus
   a. Three major complications
      (1) Diabetic ketoacidosis
      (2) Hyperglycemic hyperosmolar nonketoic coma
      (3) Minor small and large vessel disease of eye, kidney, heart, brain
   b. Diabetic peripheral neuropathy
   c. Peripheral vascular disease
7. Family and individual acceptance as key to success in management, learning, and techniques
8. Referral to community resources

ease and of the therapy in order to promote optimal care at home so that he can live a normal, productive life.

In coping with each crisis or change, diabetic patients and their family may go through five stages of adjustment: denial, anger, bargaining, depression, and finally acceptance. To emphasize, for example, the depression stage—the nurse may consider depression as secondary to this chronic illness (diabetes mellitus). In the diabetic individual, a suicide attempt may take a passive form, such as failing to take insulin or the oral agents, ignoring the warning signs of impending coma, or using poor diet control measures.

Summary of nursing considerations

Hormones are natural chemical substances that act after being secreted into the bloodstream from the ductless, or endocrine, glands. Hormones from various endocrine glands work in concert to obtain physiologic control of vital processes. Their relationship may be synergistic or antagonistic, allowing for flexibility and control. Following are the six major areas in which hormones play a crucial regulatory role: (1) control and coordination of the secretory and motor activities of the digestive tract, (2) control of energy production, (3) control of composition and volume of extracellular fluid, (4) adaptation, such as acclimatization and immunity, (5) growth and development, and (6) reproduction and lactation. The wide range of onset and duration of hormonal activiy contributes to the flexibility of the endocrine system.

Hormones may exert their effects by (1) controlling the formation or destruction of some intracellular regulator, such as cyclic AMP, (2) controlling protein synthesis, and (3) controlling membrane permeability and the movement of ions and other substances.

In common usage, hormones refer to those well-recognized and chemically specific products of the various endocrine glands that are released in small amounts and that have specific well-defined physiologic effects on metabolism. The list of major hormones includes products of the secretions of the anterior and poste-

rior pituitary, the thyroid hormone, insulin and glucagon from the pancreas, epinephrine and norepinephrine from the adrenal medulla, several potent steroids from the adrenal cortex, and the gonadal hormones of both sexes. The secretion of many of these hormones is regulated by chemical mediators released by the hypothalamus.

In medicine these substances are generally used in two ways: (1) for replacement when a patient lacks sufficient endogenous hormone, exemplified by the use of insulin in diabetes or the use of adrenal steroids in Addison's disease, and (2) for pharmacologic effects beyond those of replacement, exemplified by the use of large doses of the adrenal steroids for their antiinflammatory effects.

QUESTIONS

FOR STUDY AND REVIEW

1 Name the various tropic hormones produced by the pituitary gland and their target organs.
2 What is meant by "negative feedback"; by "positive feedback"?
3 Explain the therapeutic use and action of corticotropin.
4 What is the corticosteroid circadian rhythm for persons on a "normal" day-night schedule? How might this rhythm influence the pharmacologic response to corticosteroids when *time* of administration is taken into consideration?
5 Explain the therapeutic use for vasopressin.
6 How are thyroid hormones biosynthesized? How does this knowledge help you to understand thyroid therapy?
7 Which drugs are used to treat hypothyroidism? Discuss their pharmacologic effects. What side effects and toxic effects can result from these drugs?
8 What advantage do the synthetic thyroid preparations have over desiccated thyroid?
9 Which drugs are used to treat hyperthyroidism? Discuss their pharmacologic effects. What side effects and toxic effects can occur from these drugs?
10 What adverse effects can occur with radioactive iodine?
11 What is the therapeutic use of calcitonin?
12 Explain the therapeutic uses for cortisone.
13 What common side effects can occur from cortisone therapy?
14 When is the use of steroids contraindicated?
15 Prepare a teaching plan for the patient who must be maintained on steroid therapy.
16 Discuss methods for controlling hypoglycemic

reactions due to insulin therapy; for preventing lipodystrophy.

17 For what type of diabetic condition is the oral hypoglycemic agent indicated? Name two.

18 Discuss insulin resistance.

19 Discuss insulin allergy.

20 Prepare a teaching plan for a diabetic patient.

REFERENCE

1. Audit confirms conclusions of UGDP study on oral diabetes drugs, FDA Drug Bull. **8**(6):1979.

BIBLIOGRAPHY

GENERAL

A.M.A. drug evaluations, ed. 4, New York, 1980, John Wiley & Sons, Inc.

Avery, G.S., editor: Drug treatment, ed. 2, 1981, ADIS Press.

Goth, A.: Medical pharmacology, ed. 10, St. Louis, 1981, The C.V. Mosby Co.

Guthrie, D.W., and Guthrie, R.A., editors: Nursing management of diabetes mellitus, St. Louis, 1977, The C.V. Mosby Co.

Lewis, A.J., editor: Modern drug encyclopedia, ed. 14, New York, 1977, Dun-Donnelley Publishing Co.

Modell, W., editor: Drugs of choice, 1980-1981, St. Louis, 1980, The C.V. Mosby Co.

THYROID HORMONES AND DRUGS

Blum, A.S.: The medical management of hyperthyroidism, Ration. Drug Ther. **8**:1, 1974.

Edelman, I.S.: Thyroid thermogenesis, N. Engl. J. Med. **290**:1303, 1974.

Hallal, J.C.: Thyroid disorders, Am. J. Nurs. **77**:418, 1977.

Hershman, J.M.: Clinical application of thyrotropin-releasing hormone, N. Engl. J. Med. **290**:886, 1974

Mackin, J.F., and others: Thyroid storm and its management, N. Engl. J. Med, **291**:1396, 1974.

Menendez, C.E., and others: Thyrotoxic crisis and myxedema coma, Med. Clin. North Am. **57**:1467, 1973.

Mills, L.C.: Drug treatment in thyroid disease, Semin. Drug Treat. **3**:337, 1974.

Selenkow, H.A.: Thyroid dysfunction, diagnosis and therapy, Primary Care **1**:23, 1974.

HORMONES OF THE ADRENAL GLAND

Dluhy, R.G., and others: Pharmacology and chemistry of adrenal glucocorticoids, Med. Clin. North Am. **57**:1155, 1973.

Ganong, W.F., and others: ACTH and the regulation of adrenocortical secretion, N. Engl. J. Med. **290**:1006, 1974.

National Diabetes Data Group, Diabetes **28**:1039, 1979.

Newton, D.W., and others: You can minimize the hazards of corticosteroids, Nursing '77 **7**(6):26, 1977.

Rose, L.I., and Saccar, C.: Choosing corticosteroid preparation, Am. Fam. Phys. **17**:198, 1978.

Singer, B.: Adrenal corticosteroids—physiological considerations, Br. Med. J. **1**:36, 1972.

HORMONES FROM THE PANCREAS

Askew, G.B., and Letcher, K.I.: Oral hypoglycemic agents, Nursing '75 **5**(8):45, 1975.

Cahill, J.F.: Glucagon, N. Engl. J. Med. **288**:157, 1973.

Coleman, W.B., and others: Insulin allergy, Ann. Allergy **29**:283, 1971.

Elenbaas, R.M., and Forni, P.J.: Management of insulin allergy and resistance, Am. J. Hosp. Pharm. **33**:491, 1976.

Fajans, S.S., and others: What is diabetes? Definition, diagnosis and course, Med. Clin. North Am. **55**:793, 1971.

Feldman, J.M., and others: Tests for glucosuria. An analysis of factors that cause misleading results, Diabetes **22**:115, 1973.

Fletcher, H.P.: The oral antidiabetic drugs: pro and con, J. Am. Nurs. **76**:596, 1976.

Flier, J.S., and others: Receptors, antireceptor antibodies and mechanisms of insulin resistance, N. Engl. J. Med. **300**:413, 1979.

Free, A.H.: A test for blind diabetics to estimate urine glucose, Diabetes **22**(Suppl. 1):319, 1973.

Galloway, J.A., and others: New forms of insulin, Diabetes **21**:637, 1972.

Galloway, J.A., and others: A comparison of acid regular and neutral regular insulin, Diabetes **22**:471, 1973.

Garafano, C.: Travel tips for the peripatetic diabetic, Nursing '77 **7**(8):44, 1977.

Genuth, S.M.: Constant intravenous insulin infusion in diabetic ketoacidosis, J.A.M.A. **223**:1348, 1973.

Guthrie, D.W.: Exercise, diets and insulin for children with diabetes, Nursing '77 **7**(2):48, 1977.

Hayter, J.: Five points in diabetic care, Am. J. Nurs. **76**:594, 1976.

Kahn, C.R., and Rosenthal, A.S. Immunologic reaction to insulin, Diabetes Care **2**:2806, 1978.

Karam, J.H., and others, Antidiabetic drugs after the University Group Diabetes Program (UGDP), Annu. Rev. Pharmacol. **15**:351, 1975.

Koivisto, V.A., and Felig, P.: Alterations in insulin absorption and in blood glucose control associated with varying insulin sites in diabetic patients, Ann. Intern. Med. **92**(1):59, 1980.

Kryston, L.J., and Shaw, R.A.: The rationale for the use of drugs in the treatment of diabetes mellitus, Semin. Drug Treat. **3**:365, 1974.

Morris, H.C. Pharmacology of corticosteroids in asthma and allergy: principles and practice, St. Louis, 1978, The C.V. Mosby Co., pp. 469-480.

Owen, G.E., and others: Managing insulin dependent diabetic patients, Postgrad Med. **59**:127, 1976.

Pilkis, S.J., and Park, C.R.: Mechanism of action of insulin, Annu. Rev. Pharmacol. **14**:365, 1974.

Polefsky, J.M.: The insulin receptor: its role in insulin resistance of obesity and diabetes, Diabetes **25**:1154, 1976.

Prince, M.H., and Olefsky, J.M. Direct in vitro effect of a sulfonylurea to increase human fibroblast insulin receptor, J. Clin. Invest. **66**:608, 1980.

Prout, T.E., and others: The UGDP controversy. Clinical trials versus clinical impressions, Diabetes **21**:1035, 1972.

Schumann, D.: Coping with the complex, dangerous, elusive problem of those insulin-induced hypoglycemic agents, Nursing '74 **4**(4):56, 1974.

Seltzer, H.: A summary of criticisms of the findings and conclusions of the University Group Diabetes Program (UGDP) Diabetes **21:**976, 1972.

White, P.: Diabetes mellitus in pregnancy, Clin. Perinatol. **1:**331, 1974.

Wolfe, L.: Insulin: paving the way to a new life, Nursing '77 **7**(11):38, 1977.

ADRENAL STEROID SUPPRESSANT

Harland, J.S., and others: Aminoglutethimide: metabolism and effects on steroid synthesis in vivo, J. Endocrinol. **87**(2):31, 1980.

Murray, F.T., and others: Serum aminoglutethimide levels: studies of serum half-life, clearance, and patient compliance, J. Clin. Pharmacol. **19:**704, Nov.-Dec. 1979.

Robinson, M.G.: Aminoglutethimide: medical adrenalectomy in the management of carcinoma of the prostate: a review after 6 years, Br. J. Urol. **52:**328, 1980.

Santen, R.J., and Wells, S.A.: The use of aminoglutethimide in the treatment of patients with metastatic carcinoma of the breast. Cancer **46:**1066, 1980.

CHAPTER 29

Drugs affecting human development and sexuality

JAMES S. WOODS

Reproduction and sexual development

Among the most important attributes of all living creatures is the ability to reproduce themselves. Although the most vital functions associated with reproduction are performed within one living body, specialization in higher reproduction between two sexes, from which the contribution of both is essential if the reproductive process is to be completed. In human beings the function of the reproductive process in both sexes is highly complex, involving not only the reproductive organs but other endocrine organs and the brain as well. Many specific hormones, several of which have been isolated as chemical entities, also play a major role in the physiologic aspects of reproduction. Despite the many advances toward understanding reproduction, however, the mechanisms regulating some aspects of the reproductive process and the interrelationships of the known hormones remain undetermined.

The reproductive system of the human female consists of the ovaries, uterine (fallopian) tubes, uterus, and vagina; in the male it consists of the testes, seminal vesicles, prostate gland, bulbourethral glands, and penis. The reproductive organs of both the male and the female are largely under the control of the endocrine glands. The ovaries and testes are known as gonads and not only produce ova and sperm cells but also form endocrine secretions that initiate and maintain the secondary sexual characteristics in men and women. When gonadal function diminishes and finally ceases, the secondary sexual characteristics gradually change and reproductive function ceases. The period of change is marked in women by the cessation of menses and is known as the menopause. In men diminution of output of the sex hormone also occurs in later life, but it is less clearly definable and is sometimes called the male climacteric.

Pituitary gonadotropic hormones

The organ that exerts the chief gonadotropic influence in the body is the pituitary gland, also called the hypophysis. In the human being the pituitary gland is a reddish gray, oval structure, about 10 mm in diameter, located in the base of the brain just behind the optic chiasm as an extension of the floor of the thalamus. The pituitary is composed of different types of tissue embryologically derived from two sources: (1) a neural component originating from the thalamus and (2) a buccal component developing upward from the ectoderm of the oral cavi-

ty. The terms "adenohypophysis" and "neurohypophysis," or "anterior lobe" and "posterior lobe," are used to differentiate the buccal and neural components, respectively.

The anterior lobe is the largest and most essential part of the pituitary gland, comprising about 70% of its total weight. The most characteristic function of the anterior pituitary is the elaboration of hormones that influence the activities of other glands, particularly those of the endocrine system. Such hormones, called *tropic* hormones, are carried by the blood to other target organs and aid in maintaining those glands or in stimulating production of other hormones. When present in excess, tropic hormones induce first functional and later morphologic hypertrophy of their target organs. In contrast, atrophy and decline in function of many endocrine glands occur as a result of pituitary hypofunction or after hypophysectomy.

The pituitary hormones that are principally responsible for development and maintenance of sexual gland function are the *gonadotropins*. These substances influence the normal functions of the testes and ovaries. Follicle-stimulating hormone (FSH) stimulates the development of the ovarian (graafian) follicles up to the point of ovulation in the female; in the male FSH stimulates the development of the seminiferous tubules and promotes spermatogenesis. Luteinizing hormone (LH), or interstitial cell–stimulating hormone (ICSH), acts in the female to promote the growth of the interstitial cells in the follicle and the formation of the corpus luteum; in the male, ICSH stimulates the growth of interstitial cells in the testes and promotes the formation of the hormone androgen. A third hormone is known as the luteotropic hormone (LTH), or luteutropin; it is identical with the lactogenic hormone, or prolactin. In the female FSH initiates the cycle of events in the ovary. Under the influence of both FSH and LH the graafian follicle grows, matures, secretes estrogen, ovulates, and forms the corpus luteum. LTH promotes the secretory activity of the corpus luteum and the formation of progesterone. In the absence of LTH the corpus luteum undergoes regressive changes and fails to make progesterone.

The clinical use of the pituitary gonadotropic hormones has been handicapped by the lack of sufficiently refined preparations. Commercial preparations often contain other proteins and inert substances that make injections painful and make allergic reactions possible.

Some degree of success has accompanied the use of these gonadotropic extracts when used in the treatment of amenorrhea. Fröhlich's syndrome (adiposogenital dystrophy), sterility, undescended testicle (cryptorchidism), and hypogenitalism. Lack of success in treatment can sometimes be attributed to the fact that when a deficiency of one of the pituitary hormones exists, it is more than likely that there is a deficiency in a number of others that may not be of a direct gonadotropic nature.

There are no official gonadotropic preparations from the anterior pituitary gland.

Nonpituitary gonadotropic hormones

Chorionic gonadotropin (Follutein, Antuitrin-S, A.P.L.); human chorionic gonadotropin (Pregnyl)

Certain gonadotropic substances are formed by the placenta during pregnancy in the human female and in certain animals. One such substance, human chorionic gonadotropic hormone (HCG), differs from pituitary gonadotropins both biologically and chemically. It produces little of the follicle-stimulating effect but affects principally the growth of the interstitial cells and the secretion of luteal hormone. In women it is capable of prolonging the luteal phase of the menstrual cycle. Its normal role seems to be to enhance and prolong the secretion of the corpus luteum during early pregnancy. HCG does not initiate the formation of corpus luteum, nor does it appear to be able to restore a regressing corpus luteum.

In the male, HCG stimulates the interstitial cells of the testes, causing them to increase production of androgen, which in turn promotes the growth and development of accessory sex organs.

Chorionic gonadotropin has also been found in the blood of pregnant mares, but HCG is preferred therapeutically because it is of human origin and it does not induce the formation of antihormones in the patient. It is believed to be the substance that forms the basis of some pregnancy tests (Friedman's and Aschheim-Zondek). HCG was originally thought to come from the anterior pituitary gland, but it is now recognized as coming from the placenta.

HCG is effective for treatment of cryptorchidism not caused by anatomic obstruction and in selected cases of male hypogonadism secondary to pituitary failure. HCG is also helpful in the treatment of female infertility when used with human menopausal gonadotropin (see the following section).

Chorionic gonadotropin, a water-soluble gonadotropic substance and a glycoprotein containing about 12% galactose, is available in vials containing 5000, 10,000, and 20,000 units. One unit is equal to the gonadotropic activity of 1 mg if the international standard powder (IU) of chorionic gonadotropin.

Dosage for cryptorchidism in boys and hypogonadism in men is 4000 IU three times weekly for 3 weeks. Therapy in boys should be discontinued if there is evidence of precocious sexual maturity. Dosage for anovulation is 5000 to 18,000 IU. Chorionic gonadotropin is given intramuscularly but never intravenously.

Adverse reactions to HCG include headache, irritability, restlessness, edema, depression, tiredness, precocious puberty, gynecomastia, and pain at the injection site.

Human menopausal gonadotropin (Pergonal)

Human menopausal gonadotropin (HMG) is a purified preparation of gonadotropic hormones extracted from the urine of postmenopausal women. It contains both lutcinizing (LH) and follicle-stimulating hormones (FSH) in a 1:1 ratio, 75 IU of each hormone. HMG is used to promote follicular growth and maturation in women with secondary anovulation. To induce ovulation, therapy with HMG must be followed by the administration of HCG. The dose is 75 IU of FSH and 75 IU of LH given intramuscularly daily for 9 to 12 days, followed by 10,000 units of HCG 1 day after the last dose of HMG. If there is evidence of ovulation but no pregnancy, this dosage regimen may be repeated for two more courses before the dose is increased to 150 IU FSH and 150 IU LH daily for 9 to 12 days followed by 10,000 IU HCG 1 day later. The same dose may be repeated for two or more courses if there is evidence of ovulation but no pregnancy.

There is marked variability in individual responses to HMG. Monitoring of urinary estrogen permits the clinician to determine the dose and duration of treatment according to the patient's response. Pregnancy occurs in 20% to 45% of patients within four to six treatment cycles. Although a higher pregnancy rate is obtained with larger doses, the degree of hyperstimulation is also greater. To prevent hyperstimulation, HCG should be withheld when the urinary estrogen level is higher than 150 µg in 24 hours. Abortions occur in about 25% of the patients.

Adverse effects associated with HMG treatment include nausea and vomiting, diarrhea, and fever. Mild hyperstimulation is evidenced by ovarian enlargement, flatulence, and abdominal discomfort, which usually last 1 to 3 weeks and require no treatment. Severe hyperstimulation, which usually occurs within 2 weeks after therapy, is evidenced by weight gain, ascites, pleural effusion, oliguria, hypotension, and hypercoagulability, for which hospitalization is required. These patients should have daily determinations of fluid intake and output, body weight, hematocrit, serum and urinary electrolytes, and urinary specific gravity. Patients with significant ovarian enlargement following ovulation should refrain from sexual intercourse because of the danger of hemoperitoneum from ruptured ovarian cysts. Ovarian rupture with intraperitoneal hemorrhage may require surgery.

The patient and her partner should be informed about complications from HMG and about the frequency and potential hazards of multiple births. Reports place the incidence of multiple births in patients treated with HMG at 17% to 53%.

HMG treatment is contraindicated in patients with overt thyroid and adrenal dysfunction, infertility other than secondary ovarian failure, abnormal vaginal bleeding of undetermined cause, ovarian cysts, and pregnancy.

Female sex hormones (ovarian hormones)

The ovaries, in addition to their function of providing ova, manufacture and secrete steroid hormones that control secondary sex characteristics, the reproductive cycle, and the growth and development of the accessory reproductive organs in the female. Two main types of hormones are secreted by the ovary: (1) the *follicular*, or *estrogenic*, hormones (estrogens) produced by the cells of the developing graafian follicle; and (2) the *luteal* or *progestational* hormones (progestogens) derived from the corpus luteum that is formed in the ovary from the ruptured follicle. Normal development and activity of the reproductive organs depend in part on the proper balance between these hormones, which are secreted in sequence under the influence of the gonadotropins of the anterior pituitary gland.

ESTROGENS

The follicular hormone is responsible for the development of the sex organs at puberty and for the secondary sex characteristics—growth and distribution of hair, texture of skin, distribution of body fat, growth of breasts, and character of voice and maintenance of these characteristics throughout adult life. The follicular hormone apparently exists not as an entity but as a number of related polymorphic forms that differ in their activity. These substances, which exhibit similar estrogenic activity, are called estrogens. The group includes both the natural estrogens and the synthetic substances that have similar effects in the body.

Chemistry. The naturally occurring estrogens are steroids in which ring "A" is a benzene (aromatic ring) in place of the saturated ring of the other major steroids. The primary natural estrogen believed to be secreted by the follicle is estradiol (estrin), so named for the two hydroxyl groups.

Both estrone (Theelin) and estradiol are naturally occurring estrogens. In the body estrone can be converted into estradiol and vice versa. There are a number of other naturally occurring estrogens.

The synthetic estrogens include both *steroid* and *nonsteroid* forms. The steroid forms include modifications of the naturally occurring steroid estrogens so as to increase potency (ethinyl estrogens). The more important group, however, consists of the nonsteroid synthetic estrogen compounds that do not closely resemble the natural estrogens chemically yet have remarkably similar pharmacologic action. A typical member of this group is diethylstilbestrol.

Natural estrogenic substances are found in a variety of places in both plants and animals. They are found in the blood of both sexes, testicular fluid, feces, bile, and the urine of pregnant women and pregnant mares. Estrogens have also been found and isolated from the adrenal gland. These substances vary somewhat chemically in accordance with the source.

Pharmacologic action and result. When estrogenic substances (natural or synthetic) are injected into immature animals such as rats, they are capable of hastening sexual maturity and producing estrus. In these animals the vaginal epithelium changes after the administration of estrogens and appears as it does in mature animals. This is the basis of bioassay and standardization of preparations of these substances.

When estrogens are administered in doses that compare favorably with the amount normally secreted by the ovaries, the effect is like that produced by the natural secretion of these glands. When estrogens are administered in larger amounts than these, however, other effects may be produced.

One effect is that of inhibiting hyperactivity of the pituitary gland. Increased activity of the pituitary gland is believed to occur at menopause or after surgical removal of the ovaries. This may cause symptoms such as flushing, sweating, and hot flashes. The administration of estrogen prevents hyperactivity of the pituitary gland at least temporarily or while the estrogen continues to be given.

When estrogens are administered, the same changes occur in the myometrium and endometrium as occur naturally; the myometrium and endometrium proliferate (cells reproduce rapidly). When the estrogen is withdrawn, uterine bleeding frequently occurs. It sometimes occurs even with continued administration of the estrogen.

Estrogens naturally stimulate the development of the breasts, that is, the development of the ducts in the gland and possibly both the ducts and the alveoli. Whether this occurs as a direct action on the mammary gland or because of indirect effect on the pituitary gland is not clear. Estrogens are known to inhibit the secretion of milk.

Estrogens exhibit effects in other parts of the body, such as the skeletal system. Large doses inhibit the development of the long bones by causing premature closure of the epiphyses and by preventing the formation of bone from cartilage (endochondral bone formation). On the other hand, some aspects of the bone formation are augmented by the presence of estrogens, and when these substances are lacking, osteoporosis may develop, such as is seen in women after menopause.

Estrogens resemble the hormones made in the adrenal cortex in that large doses affect water and electrolyte balance and are prone to cause retention of sodium and development of edema. Their ability to do this is much less significant than that of the adrenal steroid hormones, however. It is known that the estrogen level in the blood is high just prior to menstruation, and at this time retention of water and electrolytes is recognized as a cause of gain in weight.

Some of the responses to estrogens in the body can be antagonized by the administration of androgens (male hormones), and the reverse is also true.

Uses. Estrogens are used for a variety of conditions in which there is a deficiency of these substances, such as to relieve certain symptoms associated with menopause. At menopause the normal endocrine balance is disturbed by the gradual cessation of ovarian function. The pituitary gland apparently attempts to compensate for the lack of ovarian activity by temporary hyperfunction. Symptoms caused by this compensatory reaction respond well to estrogenic therapy because large doses of ovarian hormones depress the secretion of the gonadotropic hormones of the anterior pituitary. Vasomotor disturbances and headache can often be relieved. Symptoms that are of psychic origin do not respond to this type of therapy as a rule. The estrogenic substances may be administered orally, intravaginally, or parenterally. Both the dosage and the method of administration must be decided in relation to the individual patient. Postmenopausal osteoporosis has also been treated with estrogens with symptomatic but not roentgeno-graphically visible benefit.

Senile vaginitis and kraurosis vulvae respond well to estrogen therapy. Some lower urinary tract infections that are part of post-menopausal atrophy have also been successfully treated with estrogens.

A major use of estrogens is in contraceptive therapy. (See the section on oral contraceptives in this chapter.)

Functional uterine bleeding, failure of ovarian development, and acne have been known to exhibit positive responses to estrogen therapy.

Estrogenic material may also serve as a substitute for castration for the relief of discomfort associated with prostatic carcinoma and its metastasis. Limited palliative effect has also been noted in postmenopausal women who have inoperable breast cancer with metastasis to the soft tissues.

Preparation, dosage, and administration
NATURAL ESTROGENS

Estrone (Theelin). Estrone is a crystalline estrogenic substance that is marketed in 1- and 5-ml ampules or 10- and 15-ml vials containing estrone in oil or aqueous suspension. The concentration varies from 1 mg/ml for the preparation in oil and from 1 to 5 mg/ml for the aqueous suspension. Estrone is also available in vaginal suppositories containing 0.2 mg of the drug; dose is one suppository daily. For menopausal symptoms the drug is usually administered intramuscularly, 0.1 to 1.5 mg/weekly in single or divided doses. For dysfunctional uterine bleeding 2 to 5 mg is administered daily until bleeding is controlled.

Piperazine estrone sulfate (Ogen). This prepa-

ration has the same actions and uses as estrone. It is administered orally. Tablets containing 0.75, 1.5, and 3 mg are available. For the control of menopausal symptoms the dosage is usually 1.5 to 3 mg daily; for the treatment of senile vaginitis and pruritus vulvae, 1.5 to 4.5 mg; for breast engorgement, 4.5 mg at intervals of 4 hours for five doses; and for dysfunctional uterine bleeding, 3.75 to 7.5 mg daily until flow ceases.

Estradiol (Aquadiol, Progynon). This drug is derived from estrone and marketed as an aqueous suspension and in pellets, tablets, and suppositories. Preparations for injection contain 0.25 to 1 mg/ml. Estradiol is 10 times more potent than estrone except when administered intravaginally; by this route both are effective at the same dosage level. For replacement therapy dose is 0.5 to 1.5 mg two or three times weekly.

Estradiol benzoate (Progynon Benzoate, Ovocylin Benzoate), oestradiol benzoate. This form is less subject to destruction in the tissues than the parent substance and hence is suitable for parenteral administration (intramuscularly). Dosage varies from 0.5 to 1.5 mg two or three times weekly, depending on the condition and the severity of symptoms.

Estradiol dipropionate (Ovocylin Dipropionate). Estradiol depropionate is absorbed more slowly than estradiol, but in other respects its effects are similar to other estradiol compounds. It is administered intramuscularly as a solution in oil and is available in 10- and 30-ml vials containing 1 mg of drug/ml. Dosage ranges from 1 to 5 mg given every 1 or 2 weeks.

Estradiol cypionate (Depo-Estradiol Cypionate.) This preparation may produce more prolonged effects than the estradiol compounds mentioned previously, and injection of 5 mg may cause effects to persist for 3 to 4 weeks. It is available as an oil solution, 1 or 5 mg/ml. It is administered by intramuscular injection. For maintenance effects 1 to 5 mg may be administered weekly for 2 to 3 weeks and then every 3 or 4 weeks.

Ethinyl estradiol (Estinyl, Feminone), ethinyloestradiol. Ethinyl estradiol is a potent estrogen made suitable for oral administration. It is available in tablets, 0.02, 0.05, or 0.5 mg. Dosage varies greatly with the condition treated. For control of menopausal symptoms 0.02 to 0.05 mg is given daily.

CONJUGATED ESTROGENS

Conjugated estrogens (Premarin). This preparation contains water-soluble, conjugated forms of mixed estrogens from the urine of pregnant mares. The principal estrogen present is sodium estrone sulfate. These preparations are available in tablets for oral administration. They are also available as topical creams and lotions and as a powder for injection (intramuscular or intravenous). The action and uses of conjugated estrogens are similar to those of other estrogens. Dosage of 0.3 to 1.25 mg daily and cyclically is usually sufficient to control menopausal symptoms. Senile vaginitis and pruritus vulvae are usually relieved with doses of 1.25 to 3.75 mg. For palliation of breast cancer a daily oral dose of 30 mg is recommended. For dyfunctional uterine bleeding 3.75 to 7.5 mg is given daily for 3 to 5 days or until bleeding stops.

SYNTHETIC ESTROGENS

Diethylstilbestrol (DES), stilboestrol. Diethylstilbestrol is a relatively inexpensive synthetic estrogenic substance that duplicates practically all known actions of the natural estrogens. It is relatively active when given orally or parenterally. Diethylstilbestrol is effective for treatment of menopausal syndrome, female hypogonadism, amenorrhea, female castration, and primary ovarian failure. It is available in plain tablets, enteric-coated tablets, and capsules for oral administration, in solution for injection, and in the form of vaginal suppositories. These dosage forms are available in wide range of concentrations. The average oral dose for treatment of menopausal symptoms is 0.2 to 0.5 mg daily. The dosage is reduced if discomfort results. For the suppression of lactation, 5 mg once or twice daily 2 to 4 days is considered sufficient; for prostatic cancer, 3 mg daily (intramuscularly) reduced to 1 mg daily or 0.5 mg three times a day (orally); and for the palliation of mammary cancer, the daily oral dose recommended for initial treatment is 15 mg, which is

increased according to the tolerance of the patient. Dosage of all preparations should be kept at the minimum necessary for the relief of symptoms.

Side effects are relatively common after oral administration and include nausea, vomiting, and headache. Vaginal carcinoma has been associated with diethylstilbestrol given to pregnant women. This malignancy appears many years later in the daughters of such women. Thus its use is contraindicated during pregnancy.

Diethylstilbestrol dipropionate. This form is prescribed for the same conditions for which other estrogenic substances are used. It is given intramuscularly in oil and has a rather prolonged effect; hence, reactions such as nausea, vomiting, headache, and dizziness occur less frequently than with free diethylstilbestrol. It is also administered orally as tablets. Dosage for the relief of menopausal symptoms is 0.5 to 2 mg two or three times a week; larger doses are required for suppression of lactation and for the treatment of prostatic cancer.

Dienestrol (Synestrol). This is a nonsteroid estrogen that can be administered orally. It is said to cause fewer side effects than diethylstilbestrol and is less potent. Dosage for the relief of menopausal symptoms is 0.1 to 1.5 mg daily. Larger doses, up to 15 mg daily, may be ordered for the patient with mammary cancer. Dose for postpartum breast engorgement is 1.5 mg daily for 7 days. Dienestrol also can be given subcutaneously and intramuscularly. It is available in 0.1-, 0.5-, and 10-mg tablets for oral administration; in a suspension for injection, 50 mg/10 ml; and as a vaginal cream containing 0.1 mg/g.

Chlorotrianisene (TACE). This drug in general shares the actions and uses of other estrogenic substances, although it exhibits some points of difference The compound is stored in body fat, from which it is slowly released. Therefore, its action extends beyond the time when administration of the drug has been discontinued. It is effective in the relief of mammary engorgement, but its use in large amounts is not recommended for cancer of the breast of patients beyond the age of menopause because it may induce uterine bleeding. Average oral dose for relief of menopausal symptoms is 12 to 25 mg daily; in cases of prostatic cancer, 12 to 25 mg daily; and for relief of mammary engorgement, 50 mg daily (to be continued only for 1 week). To suppress lactation, 72 mg is given twice daily for 2 days; the first dose should be given within 8 hours after delivery. It is available in 12-, 25-, and 72-mg capsules.

Hexestrol. This is a compound that is less potent and less toxic than diethylstilbestrol. It is used for many of the same conditions for which the latter estrogen is used. It is available in 1- and 3-mg tablets for oral administration. The dosage recommended for the control of menopausal symptoms is 2 to 3 mg, which is reduced as the symptoms are brought under control.

Methallenestril (Vallestril); benzestrol (Benzestrol); promethestrol dipropionate (Meprane Dipropionate). These are additional synthetic estrogens that produce effects similar to those produced by diethylstilbestrol.

The synthetic estrogens offer the advantage of ease of administration, since they can be given orally, and they are also relatively inexpensive.

Side effects and toxic effects. Side effects seen in connection with estrogen therapy frequently include nausea and vomiting, diarrhea, and skin rash. The symptoms are usually mild and related to dosage, potency of the compound, and route of administration. Other symptoms include edema and an increased amount of calcium in the blood of patients who have been given prolonged therapy. Adjustment of dosage, substitutions of another estrogen, and perhaps parenteral rather than oral administration may relieve the gastrointestinal symptoms. Periodic tests of the blood and of renal function are recommended. Tenderness of nipples and breast engorgement may occur in young women, and males may manifest gynecomastia.

Estrogens are carcinogenic when administered experimentally in animals that have an inherited sensitivity to certain types of carcinoma. Many clinicians believe that estrogens are therefore contraindicated for women who have a personal or family history of malignancy of the reproductive system. Estrogens are used, however, for patients having inoperable breast cancer.

Drug interactions. Estrogens can influence blood coagulation, and there is evidence that they increase incidence of thrombophlebitis and thromboembolism. Thus, when given concurrently with oral anticoagulants, dosage of anticoagulants must be adjusted.

Estrogens enhance the antiinflammatory effect of corticosteroids, and dose of the latter drugs should be adjusted.

PROGESTERONE AND PROGESTOGENS

The secretion of progesterone by the corpus luteum is under the influence of one of the pituitary hormones, LTH. The chemical structure of progesterone resembles that of the estrogens and also the androgens. The chemistry of progesterone and related compounds differs from that of the estrogens in that ring "A" is not aromatic and there is also a two-carbon side chain at the 17 position. Chemically, this group is closely related to the adrenal steroids.

Progesterone functions in the preparation and maintenance of the lining of the uterus for the implantation and nourishment of the embryo. It supplements the action of estrogen in the effects on the uterus and also in the mammary glands. It suppresses ovulation during pregnancy and keeps the uterus in a quiescent state by decreasing the irritability of the uterine muscle. Progesterone also decreases the sensitivity of the uterus to oxytocin and ergonovine. After the third month of pregnancy its production takes place in the placenta.

Progesterone injections cause the uterine endometrium to convert the proliferative phase to the secretory, or progestational, phase. It also induces proliferation of the secretory elements of the breast, and it causes an increase in the cornified vaginal epithelium.

Progesterone was formerly obtained from the corpus luteum, but it is now prepared synthetically because the naturally occurring hormone is inactivated or extremely weak in its effect when taken orally.

Progesterone is effective for use in amenorrhea and abnormal uterine bleeding from hormonal imbalance. In the treatment of amenorrhea, responsiveness to progesterone depends on the priming of the endometrium with estrogen.

Some progestogens are components of oral contraceptives, which suppress ovulation. Norethindrone and norethynodrel are more effective in this respect than are other progestogens.

Preparation, dosage, and administration

Progesterone (Gesterol, Lutocylin, Lipo-Lutin, Progestin, Proluton). This preparation is available in an oil solution or aqueous suspension for injection. It is ineffective when given orally. The solution in oil is administered intramuscularly and the suspension may be administered subcutaneously. It is given in doses up to 25 mg or more daily. Intramuscular dose for amenorrhea is 25 mg three times weekly during the last 2 weeks of the calculated menstrual cycle after estrogen therapy during the first 2 weeks of the cycle. Dose for functional uterine bleeding is 5 to 10 mg daily for 3 to 5 days, repeated every 4 weeks for 3 to 4 months. For threatened abortion a dose of 5 to 50 mg daily may be given; for dysmenorrhea, 10 to 25 mg is given daily for the week prior to menstruation. Progestasert is an intrauterine device that releases 65 µg progesterone daily for 1 year.

Norethindrone (Norlutin). Norethindrone is a semisynthetic compound chemically related to ethisterone and testosterone. It produces effects similar to those produced by progesterone but is about twice as potent and it has some androgenic qualities. It is effective for the treatment of amenorrhea and abnormal uterine bleeding caused by hormonal imbalance and endometriosis. When administered at certain times during the menstrual cycle, the drug apparently inhibits ovulation, and continuous administration causes delay of menstruation for prolonged periods of time. Norethindrone has been used successfully in suppressing ovulation when given with estrogen. On the other hand, when given to women who are amenorrheic but who have received estrogen therapy, the drug will usually produce bleeding within 24 to 72 hours after administration has been stopped. It is being used chiefly for the treatment of patients who have amenorrhea, menstrual irregularity, endometriosis, and infertility. It is available in

5-mg tablets and is administered orally in doses of 5 to 20 mg daily. For endometriosis up to 30 mg daily may be given.

Norethynodrel. This drug is a synthetic progestogen similar to norethindrone but with fewer androgenic qualities. It is available for clinical use in combination with mestranol, an estrogen, and is marketed under the name of Enovid. As such, it is used to provide cyclic control, to prevent breakthrough bleeding, and to suppress ovulation. It is available in 2.5-, 5-, and 10-mg tablets with varying amounts of mestranol.

Medroxyprogesterone acetate (Provera). This synthetic substance differs from progesterone mainly in that it is active after oral administration. It can be used for all conditions for which progesterone is indicated and is more potent than ethisterone. It is available in 2.5- and 10-mg tablets or as a suspension for injection. It has no inherent estrogenic activity, and priming with estrogen is necessary. Drowsiness has been reported as a side effect.

Hydroxyprogesterone caproate (Delalutin). A synthetic derivative of progesterone, hydroxyprogesterone caproate is a great deal like progesterone except that it has a longer duration of action after parenteral administration. Duration of action is 7 to 17 days. It is available in oil solution, 250 mg/2 ml, for intramuscular injection. The usual single dose is 125 to 250 mg, and one dose every 4 weeks may be sufficient in treatment of menstrual disorders and ovarian and uterine dynfunction. It is also effective as a presumptive test for pregnancy and as a test for endogenous estrogen. It is ineffective for treatment of postpartum pains, ovarian deficiency, and senile vaginitis. Priming with estrogen is necessary.

Side effects and toxic effects. Preparations of progesterone or related compounds appear to have a low order of toxicity. Patients occasionally have gastrointestinal symptoms, headache, dizziness, and allergic manifestations. Cases have been reported in which masculinization of female infants occurred in connection with the administration of progesterone to the mothers during pregnancy.

Prolonged high dosages of progestogens may

cause gastrointestinal disturbances, edema and weight gain, headache and vertigo, oligomenorrhea, and breast congestion.

Male sex hormones (androgens)

Normal development and maintenance of male sex characteristics depend on adequate amounts of the male sex hormones, the androgens. All androgenic compounds have a steroid nucleus. In fact, natural estrogens, androgens, and some of the hormones of the adrenal cortex all exhibit an interesting similarity in their structural formulas.

There are at least five steroidal hormones that manifest androgenic activity, and all are derivatives of androsterone. The most potent is testosterone, which is chemically similar to progesterone. Androgens chemically similar to testosterone are excreted in the urine and are usually referred to as 17-ketosteroids because there is a ketone group attached to carbon 17 of the steroid structure. It should be remembered, however, that the urinary 17-ketosteroids are products of the adrenal cortex in both men and women.

Action and clinical effects. The androgens function in the development and maintenance of the male sex organs. Administration to immature males causes growth of the genitals and the appearance of secondary sex characteristics. Androgen replacement is indicated in the amelioration of androgen deficiency. When a high concentration of androgenic substances is maintained in the circulation, anterior pituitary secretion is inhibited and spermatogenesis is retarded.

In mammals both sexes form male and female hormones, although they are antagonistic to each other. The administration of testosterone to women can suppress menstruation and cause atrophy of the endometrium.

Androgens are also potent anabolic agents, since they stimulate the formation and the maintenance of muscular and skeletal protein. They bring about retention of nitrogen (essential to the formation of protein in the body) and enhance storage of inorganic phosphorus, sulfate, sodium, and potassium.

The anabolic effects of androgens are of particular significance in the treatment of patients who are paraplegic as a result of trauma to the spinal cord and in whom the maintenance of adequate nutrition, prevention of atrophy in muscles and bones, and prevention as well as treatment of decubitus ulcers constitute serious problems. Similar problems are encountered in the care of patients who are chronically ill or malnourished or who have a wasting disease such as cancer.

Uses. Androgens have been used in replacement therapy for patients with hypogonadism and eunuchoidism. They produce marked changes in sex organs, body contour, and voice, provided the deficiency state has not been present for a prolonged period. In contrast, androgens have little effect on senile men or on patients with psychogenic impotence. They may increase libido in women.

Androgens have been employed in the treatment of cryptorchidism either alone or in combination with gonadotropic substances.

Androgens have also been used in the treatment of dysmenorrhea and menopausal states and for the suppression of lactation and breast engorgement. Favorable results are sometimes obtained from their use to relieve subjective symptoms associated with the male climacteric, just as estrogens are of value in relieving symptoms of the menopause in women.

Androgens have been employed for palliative relief of advanced inoperable cancer of the breast, although the mechanism of action is not clear. Subjective improvement (improved appetite, gain in weight, relief of pain) seems to be a major part of this effect. Improvement is temporary and seldom exceeds 1 year. Androgens are preferred for patients with breast cancer prior to or during menopause, since estrogens may promote the development of the cancer at this time.

Preparation, dosage, and administration

Testosterone. Testosterone produces effects similar to those of testosterone propionate. It is available in 75-mg pellets, as an aqueous injectable suspension of 25, 50, and 100 mg/ml, and as tablets for oral and sublingual administration. The usual dose is 10 mg daily by the buccal route, or 25 mg intramuscularly twice a week to once daily. The rate of absorption by the buccal route is unpredictable.

For male hypogonadism three 75-mg testosterone pellets are implanted subcutaneously into the medial aspect of each thigh using a pellet injector. These pellets are effective for the treatment of eunuchism, eunuchoidism, and the male climacteric.

Testosterone propionate (Oreton). Testosterone propionate is *effective* for male hypogonadism, eunuchism, eunuchoidism, male climacteric androgen deficiency, prevention of postpartum pain and breast engorgement, and palliation of breast cancer. This preparation is available in 10-mg buccal tablets (these are held in the space between the teeth and cheek) and as a solution for intramuscular injection containing 50 and 100 mg/ml. The usual dose is 25 mg two to four times a week, with a usual range of dose of 25 to 150 mg weekly, depending on the response obtained and the effect desired. From 5 to 10 mg daily may be sufficient as maintenance doses for therapy in men. For relief of symptoms of breast cancer, 150 to 300 mg weekly in several doses may be administered. Since there is marked variation in sensitivity to testosterone, virilism may occur in females even with small doses of the drug. This preparation is synthesized from cholesterol or extracted from bull testes.

Testosterone enanthate (Delatestryl). Testosterone enanthate has a therapeutic use similar to that of testosterone propionate. This preparation is administered as a solution in oil and provides a prolonged effect of 3 weeks or more. The usual intramuscular dose is 100 to 400 mg every 2 to 4 weeks.

Methyltestosterone (Oreton-M, Metandren). The therapeutic use of this drug is similar to that of testosterone propionate. Methyltestosterone is available in 10- and 25-mg tablets for oral administration, in 5- and 10-mg buccal tablets, and in 5- and 10-mg tablets for sublingual administration. Absorption from the buccal membranes is more effective than from the gastrointestinal tract. The indications and actions of this compound are essentially the same as those for testosterone propionate. The usual oral dose is 10 mg three times a day. Range of dose is 10 to 50 mg daily. Doses for the suppression of lactation are larger. Dosage for breast cancer is 50 to 200 mg daily. Dosage is adjusted according to the needs and response of the patient.

Testosterone cypionate (Andronate). Although similar to testosterone propionate, this drug has the advantage of more prolonged androgenic effects. It is available in solution at 50, 100, and 200 mg/ml for intramuscular injection. Treatment is normally given at intervals of 1 or 2 weeks for androgen deficiency.

Norethandrolone (Nilevar). This compound is a synthetic androgen that is chemically and pharmacologically related to testosterone. Its androgenic properties are less significant than its anabolic effects. Patients receiving anabolic hormones such as norethandrolone should be on high-calorie, high-protein diets, if possible. The drug is administered orally or intramuscularly in amounts that range from 30 to 50 mg daily in divided doses. Preparations are available in solution at 25 mg/ml and in 10-mg tablets for oral administration.

Fluoxymesterone (Halotestin, Ultandren). Fluoxymesterone is a synthetic halogenated derivative of methyltestosterone. It is available in 2-, 5-, and 10-mg tablets for oral administration. It is several times more potent than methyltestosterone from the standpoint of both androgenic and anabolic activity. The dosage for androgen deficiency varies from 2 to 10 mg daily. The dosage for anabolic effects ranges from 4 to 10 mg, and 10 to 30 mg daily has been used for palliation of breast cancer.

Nandrolone phenpropionate (Durabolin); phenylpropionate. This drug is a synthetic steroid hormone related to norethandrolone. Similarly, its anabolic effects are prominent while androgenicity is low. This drug is administered intramuscularly, and the usual adult dosage ranges from 25 to 50 mg once weekly.

Side effects. Effects that are regarded as untoward in the female include deepening of the voice, hirsutism (excessive growth of hair), flushing, acne, regression of the breasts, enlargement of the clitoris, and general masculinization. In prepuberal boys androgen treatment may produce pubic hair development, phallic enlargement, and increased frequency of erections. Premature epiphyseal closure may occur in children who are given anabolic steroids to stimulate growth. Less prominent but probably more serious effects include retention of sodium, potassium, water, and chloride, which can contribute to heart failure. Jaundice has occasionally been observed after the administration of methyltestosterone and norethandrolone. Nausea and gastrointestinal upsets occur occasionally. Patients receiving androgens should be observed carefully for hypercalcemia and the appearance of edema. The latter can sometimes be controlled with the use of diuretics and a diet low in salt.

Contraindications. Androgens are contraindicated for patients with prostatic cancer and serious cardiorenal dysfunction. They are also contraindicated in pregnant women because of possible masculinization of the female fetus.

Oral contraceptives
OVULATORY SUPPRESSANTS

Contraception is as old as history and has been practiced in many forms, including the use of mechanical devices and ingestion of various herbs. Not until recently, however, has there been any consistent measure of reliability in these practices. The introduction of Enovid in 1960 dramatically demonstrated the unfailing suppression of ovulation by a combination of progesterones and estrogens. This event was preceded by a decade of research, the elucidation of which was largely the responsibility of Rock, Pincus, and Garcia. Evidence of the contraceptive effect of norethynodrel was published by this group in 1956 and followed by a number of controlled studies, most notably in Puerto Rico. By 1965 refined forms of this drug multiplied, and more than 5 million American women were using oral contraceptives.

Few drugs have been studied as ambitiously and intensively as have the oral contraceptives because of (1) the interest aroused concerning the effects these drugs might have on the human body when hormone levels and relationships are altered for the sole purpose of prevent-

ing conception, (2) the need for a simple method of population control in densely populated countries, and (3) the desire by many couples for planned parenthood.

Pharmacologic action and result. The development of the oral contraceptives was based on the knowledge that ovulation did not occur during pregnancy and that large amounts of estrogen and progesterone were produced by the extended function of the corpus luteum and by placental secretion.

In addition, a review of physiology of the menstrual cycle reveals the following.

1 Ovulation is dependent on the anterior pituitary gland to secrete two hormones: FSH (for maturation of the ovum) and LH (for release of the mature ovum from the ovary).
2 The hypothalamus regulates the secretion of these hormones by the anterior pituitary by secreting hormones known as releasing factors.
3 Large amounts of estrogen (secreted by the maturing follicle and, following ovulation, by the corpus luteum) inhibit the hypothalamic releasing factors, which inhibits FSH and LH release and blocks ovulation.
4 Progesterone (secreted by the corpus luteum) inhibits the hypothalamic releasing factor for LH, which also interferes with ovulation.
5 Estrogen and progesterone are responsible for endometrial buildup; decreased production of estrogen and progesterone results in endometrial sloughing and menstrual bleeding.

From this information it can be readily understood why the administration of progesterone derivatives and estrogenic substances prevents ovulation without preventing menstruation and why these substances are the ingredients of oral contraceptives.

It is generally accepted that oral contraceptives act, at least in part, by inhibiting the secretion of gonadotropins from the pituitary gland. Other possible actions may include a direct inhibitory effect on the ovary, changes in tubal motility, or changes in the endometrium that would result in failure of implantation of fertilized ova.

The combination of drugs rapidly transforms the early secretory stage of the endometrium to one resembling secretory exhaustion. The drug is therefore judged effective because the estrogen encourages proliferative change

TABLE 29-1 Composition and doses of some oral contraceptives

Mg—estrogen	Mg—progestin	Trade name
Combinations*		
0.02 Ethinyl estradiol	0.3 Norgestrel	Lo/Ovral
0.02 Ethinyl estradiol	1 Norethindrone	Loestrin 1/20; Zorane 1/20
0.03 Ethinyl estradiol	1.5 Norethindrone	Loestrin 1.5/30; Zorane 1.5/30
0.035 Ethinyl estradiol	0.4 Norethindrone	Ovcon-35
0.035 Ethinyl estradiol	0.5 Norethindrone	Brevicon; Modicon
0.05 Mestranol	1 Norethindrone	Norinyl 1 + 50; Ortho-Novum 1/50
0.05 Ethinyl estradiol	0.5 Norgestrel	Ovral
0.05 Ethinyl estradiol	1 Ethynodiol diacetate	Demulen
0.05 Ethinyl estradiol	1 Norethindrone	Ovcon-50; Zorane 1/50
0.05 Ethinyl estradiol	1 Norethindrone acetate	Norlestrin, 1
0.05 Ethinyl estradiol	2.5 Norethindrone acetate	Norlestrin, 2.5
0.06 Mestranol	10 Norethindrone	Ortho-Novum, 10 mg
0.035 Ethinyl estradiol	1 Norethindrone	Ortho-Novum, 1/35
0.075 Mestranol	5 Norethynodrel	Enovid 5 mg
0.08 Mestranol	1 Norethindrone	Norinyl 1 + 80; Ortho-Novum 1/80
0.035 Ethinyl estradiol	1 Norethindrone	Norinyl 1 + 35
0.10 Mestranol	1 Ethynodiol diacetate	Ovulen
0.10 Mestranol	2 Norethindrone	Norinyl, 2 mg; Ortho-Novum, 2 mg
0.10 Mestranol	2.5 Norethynodrel	Enovid-E
0.15 Mestranol	9.85 Norethynodrel	Enovid, 10 mg
Minipills†		
—	0.35 Norethindrone	Micronor; Nor-QD
—	0.075 Norgestrel	Ovrette
Postcoital‡ (Not generally recommended)		
25 Diethylstilbestrol	—	—

Adapted from Goodman, L., and Gilman, A., editors: The pharmacological basis for therapeutics, ed. 6, New York, 1980, Macmillan Inc., p. 1440.

*Combination tablets are taken for 20 or 21 days and off for 7 or 8 days. These preparations are listed in order of increasing content of estrogen.

†Minipills are taken daily continually.

‡25 mg twice daily for 5 days within 72 hours after sexual intercourse; *see* text for limited indications.

that inhibits ovulation, while progesterone ensures that withdrawal bleeding will be physiologic, prompt, and brief.

Preparation, dosage, and administration. Although the use of exogenous estrogenic substances alone will inhibit ovulation, undesirable bleeding frequently occurs during the latter phase of the cycle. If estrogen levels are increased to prevent this, severe nausea and breast tenderness occur. It is for these reasons that estrogens are combined with progesterones in oral contraceptives.

Since naturally occurring progesterone is inactivated or extremely weak in its effect when taken orally and must be given by injection to be effective, the progestogens (steroidal compounds related to progesterone) have been developed. The majority of the oral contraceptives contain a synthetic progestogen, either norethynodrel or norethindrone.

Norethynodrel is a basic progestin, while norethindrone is a more androgenic progestin.

The latter is sometimes recommended for patients experiencing excess side effects from estrogen, such as greater weight gain and amenorrhea. Norethynodrel, on the other hand, is good for patients with oily skin, acne, hirsutism, and breakthrough bleeding.

Three methods of oral contraception are available: one is termed combination therapy, a second method is called low dosage progestogens (minipill), and a third method is postcoital contraception. Table 29-1 lists composition and doses of oral contraceptives used in these three methods. Sequential oral contraceptives have been withdrawn from the market as a result of increased incidence of endometrial pathology.

Combination therapy consists of taking tablets containing a progestogen and an estrogen.

In this therapy, 20 tablets are taken during each menstrual cycle. The first day of menstruation is day 1; on day 5 the first tablet is taken regardless of whether menstruation has ceased. One tablet is then taken each day for the next 20 days. Menstruation will occur within 2 to 7 days after the last tablet has been taken. The fifth day after the start of menstruation, the cycle begins again. The combination method of therapy is very effective. Most authorities claim it to be 100% effective; failures are the result of missed dosage.

It is important that women who are considering use of oral contraceptives should be instructed with respect to the following information.

1 The woman should take one tablet every day for the 20-day period without fail. Eliminating one tablet may lead to ovulation or breakthrough acyclic bleeding.
2 If breakthrough bleeding occurs, administration of the drug should be continued and the physician should be consulted. What may be required is a different balance of estrogen or a different progestogen. Breakthrough bleeding may occur only in the first cycles of treatment until the woman adjusts to the hormones. Spotting or slight brownish discharge is not breakthrough bleeding, and it eventually disappears. If bleeding is similar to that of menses, the woman is usually advised to stop taking the drug and begin the medication again 5 days later, beginning a new cycle.
3 Even if menses does not occur following completion of a medication cycle, the woman should be cautioned to begin another medication cycle on the seventh day and not to wait for menstruation to begin, since ovulation may occur within 9 or 10 days after stopping the medication. Ovulation can occur in the presence of a delayed or missed menstruation.
4 Women who ovulate early or have a shortened menstrual cycle (21 days or less) should be cautioned to use another method of birth control during the first medication cycle. Under steroid therapy, these women wil usually convert to a 28-day cycle.
5 The woman should be instructed to establish a definite pattern for taking the tablet at the same time each day; however, anytime within a 24-hour period is adequate.
6 The woman should be examined and reevaluated for oral contraceptive therapy at least once yearly and should report any untoward symptoms to her physician.

Side effects. Analysis of the side effects of oral contraceptives is difficult because of the different drugs and drug combinations used, the different dosages, and individual differences. Since ovarian hormones influence all body systems either directly or by their influence on other endocrine glands and metabolism, a variety of side effects can be expected to occur. Known adverse effects on the body systems resulting from estrogen-progestogen combinations include the following. More experience with norethindrone-only preparations is needed to determine its adverse effects.

Gastrointestinal. Nausea is a common effect, particularly during the first 2 or 3 months. Vomiting, an increase or decrease in appetite, abdominal pain, diarrhea, and constipation also occur. The absorption of folate, a water-soluble vitamin, is decreased, causing anemia in some women.

Alterations in liver function have been reported. Jaundice, cholestasis, and some liver cell degeneration have been noted. Patients with a history of liver disease, such as hepatitis, may be more likely to develop these effects.

Cardiovascular. There is general, but not universal, agreement that there is a cause-effect relationship between oral contraceptives and thromboembolic phenomena. In the United States a study of the morbidity of thrombophlebitis indicated a fourfold increase with use of oral contraceptives; in Great Britain studies show a three- to tenfold increase. The British study also showed a higher death rate for users of oral contraceptives than for nonusers, and a higher death rate for older users (35 to 44) than younger users (20 to 34). Another study in Great Britain showed a three- to fourfold increase in postoperative thromboembolic disease for patients taking oral contraceptives.

There is some indication that thromboembolism is related to estrogen dosage, and it is recommended that the lowest effective dose be used.

Oral contraceptives increase the number of platelets and may increase their tendency to clump; other blood clotting factors are also increased. In addition, intimal thickening of arteries and veins has been reported, as well as abnormal vein dilation, which may cause venous stasis. All of these factors may explain the increased risk of thromboembolism in users of oral contraceptives.

Migraine headache has been intensified in

some women with a previous history of migraine, and in some women onset of migraine occurred with use of oral contraceptives. Therapy for these patients should be discontinued.

Hypertension has occurred. Estrogen-progestogen combinations increase the amount of renin produced by the kidney, which in turn increases the production of angiotensin, a potent pressor substance. Blood pressure determinations should be made before therapy and regularly during therapy.

A cooperative study in the United States, Sweden, and Great Britain showed that incidence of thromboembolic disease was lower in women with type O blood. The reason for this is unknown.

Endocrine. Estrogens decrease the rate of corticosteroid metabolism, but there is no evidence that they cause adrenal dysfunction. Thyroid function tests are altered but thyroid function does not seem to be affected.

Menses usually occurs 6 to 10 weeks after discontinuance of oral contraceptive therapy. In some women inhibition of ovarian function may require the use of clomiphene or gonadotropins.

Reproductive. The cervix may undergo hyperplasia and hypersecretion of the cervical glands and increased vascularity. Regression of the myometrium has been noted, and tenderness and fullness of the breasts may occur. Estrogens and progestogens have been detected in human milk, but its long-range effect on the offspring is not known. There are no definitive data to prove or disprove an association between oral contraceptives and breast or uterine cancer.

Central nervous system. Mood changes are common with the use of oral contraceptives; some women experience a sense of well-being and a release of tension; for others there is increased tension, irritability, and depression. Both increase and decrease in libido have been reported.

A few rare cases of severe ophthalmic disorders have been reported. Users of oral contraceptives experience more difficulty with contact lenses than nonusers.

Cutaneous. A variety of skin reactions may occur, including chloasma, acne, and pruritus.

Contraindications. Contraindications include a history of thromboembolic disease, hepatic disease, mammary or genital carcinoma, large uterine fibroids, migraine headache, asthma, epilepsy, and blood dyscrasias. Oral contraceptives should not be taken if pregnancy is suspected because of the danger of possible masculinization of the fetus.

MINIPILL

Contraceptive tablets containing only the progestogen, norethindrone, at a very low dose level of 0.35 mg is known as the minipill. Trade names for the minipill include Micronor and Nor-QD. Dosage is one tablet daily without interruption. These preparations probably exert their contraceptive action by reducing the penetrability of the sperm in the cervical mucus, by interfering with luteal function by suppressing the secretion of gonadotropins, and by interfering with the implantation of the ovum. The minipill does not prevent ovulation. The minipill is believed to be slightly less effective as a contraceptive than the contraceptives containing both estrogen and progestogen. The dropout rate appears to be higher for the minipill than for the combination tablets, which is believed to be a result of a significant incidence of unpredictable bleeding patterns.

POSTCOITAL CONTRACEPTIVES

Work is in progress on the development of effective "morning after" postcoital drugs. Such preparations involve the utilization of high doses of estrogens and are thought to act by preventing implantation of the fertilized ovum. Their effectiveness is directly related to the amount given. The most commonly used postcoital preparations are diethylstilbestrol (DES), conjugated estrogens, and ethinyl estradiol.

DES has been used in the past on a large number of patients; it shortens transit time for the fertilized ovum into the uterine cavity. DES is contraindicated for patients with blood clotting disorders, impaired liver function, a history of thrombophlebitis, cancer of the breast or uterus, or undiagnosed abnormal uterine bleeding.

DES must not be given to pregnant women; every effort should be made to be certain the patient is not pregnant before treatment is started. If at all possible, a pregnancy test should be performed before instituting postcoital contraceptive therapy. If it should be determined that a patient received DES while pregnant, the patient should be informed about the risk of vaginal or cervical cancer occurring in her female offspring, and she should be given the option of deciding whether or not the pregnancy should be terminated.

DES is available in 25-mg tablets for use as a postcoital contraceptive. It is administered orally in a dosage of 25 mg twice a day for 5 days beginning not later than 72 hours (but preferably 24 hours) after sexual intercourse. This dosage can prevent pregnancy but it cannot terminate pregnancy. Patients must be warned that to be effective the full course of treatment must be taken regardless of the nausea that commonly occurs.

DES should be used only as an emergency measure and not as a routine means of birth control; repeated use should be avoided.

CONTINUOUS ACTION DRUGS

Several attempts have been made toward developing continuous action drugs that are effective in providing contraceptive protection for women for a prolonged time. Among those that have received the greatest attention are medroxyprogesterone acetate and quinestrol.

Medroxyprogesterone acetate (Depo-Provera)

Medroxyprogesterone acetate has proved to be an exceedingly effective contraceptive drug when administered at 3- to 6-month intervals at doses of 150 to 300 mg. Higher doses can provide even longer prevention against pregnancy. Medroxyprogesterone is thought to act through several mechanisms, which include interference with gonadotropin release at the hypothalamic level with suppression of ovulation, thinning of the endometrium, and thickening of the cervical mucous lining. Advantages are the minimal reliance required of the patient and relatively simple administration. The risk of failure is very low.

Prolonged or irregular bleeding has been reported in 10% to 40% of women taking medroxyprogesterone. The incidence of this effect decreases with the number of injections received. Amenorrhea is present in about 20% of the patients after 1 month of therapy and increases to 80% after 3 years. The most serious potential side effect observed has been prolonged, or possibly permanent, infertility following cessation of medroxyprogesterone use. Of those attempting to conceive following cessation of treatment, 66% do so by 9 months and 75% by 1 year; average time to conception from last injection is about 11 months. This drug should not be used by lactating women, since the effects of this drug on the neonate are not known.

Quinestrol (Estrovis)

Quinestrol is a synthetic estrogen that has been formulated in a "pill-a-month" preparation. Quinestrol is a highly potent, orally active derivative of ethinyl estradiol. Its extended action is attributed to its storage in and slow release from adipose tissues in the body—one dose of 5 mg is sufficient to cause an estrogenic response for 6 to 14 weeks. A monthly dose of 5 mg inhibits ovulation. The major problem now experienced with quinestrol is the erratic and unpredictable rate of release of the drug from fat stores, which can predispose to difficulty in establishing a cyclic pattern and lead to contraceptive failure.

ALTERNATIVES TO ORAL CONTRACEPTION

The woman who is reluctant to expose herself to the possibility of hormonal secondary effects should seek effective alternative modes of contraception.

Intrauterine devices (IUDs) have a very high effectiveness that may rely on the mild inflammation created in the uterine lining. Adverse effects can include cramping, heavier menstrual flow, occasional expelling of the IUD, allergy to copper (Copper-T, Cu-7, Tatum-T), pelvic inflammatory disease and sterility, uterine or cervical perforation, septic abortion, or ectopic pregnancy (located outside the uterus). Progestasert (progesterone-containing IUD) is associated with as high an incidence of ectopic pregnancy in women as in those not using any contraception.

Diaphragms, if used with a spermicide, are fairly effective. There are no serious side effects, but they should not be used if cystitis is frequent. They must be inserted before intercourse and left in place for 6 to 8 hours.

Intravaginal foams, creams, jellies, and tablets (Semicid, Encare) that are spermicidal are somewhat less effective, with a 15% first-year failure rate. They must be inserted 10 to 15 minutes before intercourse and give protection for 2 hours afterward. Burning and irritation of the vagina or penis are common.

Condoms are rubber sheaths that must be fitted over the erect penis. They are somewhat effective and have no serious side effects; they provide some protection against sexually transmitted diseases.

Female sterilization (tubal ligation or "tying the tubes") and male sterilization (vasectomy) are each 100% effective and should be considered permanent and irreversible. Minor, treatable surgical complications may ensue.

Literature comparing the contraceptive options is available from the Food and Drug Administration, Department of Health and Human Services, Rockville, Md. 20857.

MALE ORAL CONTRACEPTIVES

Although the chemical contraceptives available today are for utilization only by women, there has been some research into the development of oral contraceptive agents for men. Unfortunately, this area is plagued with problems, most of which bear either on male sexuality or on male reproductive physiology. Foremost is the presumption that men will not use chemical contraceptives because of fear of psychologic and clinical effects on libido and masculinity. These fears are not completely unfounded, since adverse effects on sexual physiology have been observed with spermatogenic agents. Thus the pharmaceutical industry has been slow to institute research programs in this

area. Another problem lies in the complexity of the male reproductive system. Experimental drugs that block spermatogenesis, such as the nitrofurans, thiophenes, hydrazines, and sex steroids, require approximately 2 months between drug action and contraceptive effectiveness. In addition, the Antabuse-like effect of some of these agents, which produce acute toxic effects in persons taking them in combination with alcohol, limits their use in contemporary society, where alcohol consumption is often associated with sexual activity.

A more effective approach to controlling fertility in the male has been proposed to lie in the use of agents that will interfere with the fertilizing capacity of spermatozoa in the epididymis. Such drugs as cyproterone acetate and the alpha chlorohydrins may someday be suitable for this purpose.

Ovulatory stimulants and drugs used for infertility

Anovulation is physiologic in patients who are pregnant, breast feeding, and postmenopausal. It becomes a suspected pathologic condition in women with abnormal bleeding or infertility. The incidence of anovulation is unknown and cannot be ascertained, but diagnostic tests may determine its presence.

Methods of ovulation induction include use of gonadotropins, thyroid preparations, cortisone preparations, estrogens, and synthetic agents.

GONADOTROPINS

Both HCG and HMG have been used as ovulatory stimulants in the treatment of female infertility; the dosages and regimens have been described earlier in this chapter. HCG is sometimes given along with clomiphene citrate (see the following section on synthetic agents) as an intramuscular injection just before ovulation, and it is always given in conjunction with the more potent drug, HMG. In cases of male infertility caused by poor sperm quality, HCG has been used to stimulate the interstitial cells of the testes to produce testosterone, which may in turn improve sperm motility. Tests of the ability of HMG to improve sperm levels have proved inconclusive.

THYROID PREPARATIONS

Thyroid preparations are used in hypothyroid or hyperthyroid conditions, which are often associated with anovulation.

CORTISONE PREPARATIONS

Cortisone preparations suppress adrenal activity, thereby decreasing androgen and estrogen secretions and encouraging release of human pituitary gonadotropins. This treatment is appropriate when adrenal gland dysfunction is etiologic in anovulation, as in adrenogenital syndrome.

ESTROGENS

These hormones act to induce ovulation in two ways: (1) by stimulating the release of pituitary gonadotropin and increasing secretion of FSH and LH and (2) by making the ovary more responsive to the influence of gonadotropin. Short-term therapy may stimulate the ovary, but long-term estrogen therapy depresses gonadotropin, which results in anovulation.

SYNTHETIC AGENTS

Several synthetic agents have recently become available. The mode of action of these drugs in inducing ovulation is not yet well established, but they may act either directly on the enzyme systems, suppressing estrogen production and secondary stimulation of gonadotropin, or directly on the hypothalamus, pituitary gland, or both, stimulating secretion of gonadotropin.

Side effects with any of these therapies are common, including gastrointestinal disturbances similar to those in pregnancy, breakthrough bleeding, abdominal pain, and weight gain.

Clomiphene citrate (Clomid)

This drug bears a close structural relationship to the potent synthetic estrogen chlorotrianisene (Tace). Its mechanism of action is not definitely known but it may compete with estrogen at the hypothalamic level, causing an increase in secretion of the hypothalamic

releasing factor and a resultant increase in the pituitary gonadotropins LH and FSH and, consequently, ovarian stimulation. It is generally suitable for patients with amenorrhea of pituitary origin, the Stein-Leventhal syndrome, and the Chiari-Frommel syndrome. Dosage is 50 to 100 mg daily for 5 to 7 days. Short-term therapies have been found more effective than long-term ones. Side effects include hot flashes and the presence of ovarian enlargement with or without cyst formation. Clomiphene is teratogenic in some animals, and it should not be given to pregnant women. Visual abnormalities such as blurred vision have been reported. If these occur, the drug should be stopped. Other adverse effects include nausea, cyclic ovarian pain (mittelschmerz), breast engorgement, and abnormal uterine bleeding. These effects disappear when the drug is stopped. Incidence of ovulation has been ascertained as 76% in one study, although further research is needed. Pregnancy occurs in 25% to 30% of patients treated. Multiple pregnancies may occur in 10% of patients.

Drugs affecting the uterus

The uterus is a highly muscular organ that exhibits a number of characteristic properties and activities. The smooth muscle fibers extend longitudinally, circularly, and obliquely in the organ. The uterus has a rich blood supply, but when the uterine muscle contracts, blood flow is diminished. Profound changes occur in the uterus during pregnancy. The human uterus increases in weight during pregnancy from about 50 g to approximately 1000 g. Its capacity increases tenfold in length, and new muscle fibers may be formed. These changes are accompanied by changes in response to drugs. Since the uterine smooth muscle responds sensitively to many drugs, the uterus of virgin guinea pigs or rabbits is used in standardizing a number of drugs that have a stimulating action on smooth muscle.

The uterus, both in situ and when excised, contracts rhythmically. Both pendular and peristaltic movements may be seen. In non-gravid animals, peristaltic movements are relatively slight and, just as in the intestine, pauses occur between peristaltic contractions. These peristaltic movements vary greatly with the condition of sexual activity. Movements are depressed early in pregnancy but increase later. Parturition is accomplished by powerful peristaltic waves, which cause labor pains.

Drugs that act on the uterus include (1) those that increase the motility of the uterus and (2) those that decrease uterine motility.

Drugs that increase uterine motility
OXYTOCICS

In the human being, stimulation of either the sympathetic or the parasympathetic division of the autonomic nervous system may bring about increased uterine contractions. However, autonomic agonist drugs are not useful for affecting the motility of the uterus because they lack the desired selectivity. Hence drugs that exert a selective action on the smooth muscle of the uterus, such as oxytocics, are used for this purpose.

The most commonly used oxytocics are alkaloids of synthetic oxytocin and ergot, although many other drugs may exhibit some effect on uterine motility.

Oxytocin is one of two hormones secreted by the posterior pituitary; the other hormone is vasopressin (antidiuretic hormone, ADH). Both are peptides containing eight amino acids. Because of the similarity in their structures, oxytocin has some vasopressor activity and vasopressin some oxytocic activity.

Oxytocin means "rapid birth," derived from its ability to contract the pregnant uterus. It also facilitates milk ejection during lactation.

The nonpregnant uterus is relatively insensitive to oxytocin, but during pregnancy uterine sensitivity to oxytocin gradually increases, with the uterus being most sensitive at the termination of pregnancy. Oxytocin secretion may precede and possibly trigger delivery of the fetus. Large amounts of oxytocin have been detected in the blood during the expulsive phase of delivery. It is believed that oxytocin is released in response to stretching of the uterine cervix and vagina. A positive feedback mechanism may be operant; that is, more forceful contractions of uterine muscle and greater stretching of the cervix and vagina result in more oxytocin release. Oxytocin acts directly on the myometrium, having a stronger effect on the fundus than on the cervix.

Suckling and auditory or visual stimuli related to suckling, such as the mother seeing her baby or hearing the child cry, causes release of oxytocin, which in turn causes contraction of the smooth muscle of the mammary gland and milk ejection (a conditioned reflex).

Preparation, dosage, and administration
Oxytocin injection, synthetic (Pitocin, Syntocinon, Uteracon). Oxytocin is used to induce active labor or to increase the force and rate of existing contractions during delivery. It is also used to contract uterine muscle and decrease hemorrhage after delivery of the placenta. Occasionally it is used to promote milk ejection when ineffective ejection is believed to be caused by inadequacy of breast feeding.

Oxytocin can be given by intravenous, intramuscular, subcutaneous, intranasal, or buccal routes. The intravenous infusion dose is 1 ml of oxytocin added to 500 or 1000 ml of 5% dextrose or normal saline and infused at an initial rate of 0.5 to 0.75 ml/minute. The rate is carefully increased until an optimal uterine response is obtained (three or four contractions in 10 minutes). The infusion should be stopped or the rate of flow decreased if a change in fetal heart tones occurs, contractions become excessive, or the uterus fails to relax following contractions.

For emergency treatment of postpartum bleeding 0.6 to 1.8 units oxytocin is diluted with 3 to 5 ml of sodium chloride and slowly injected. Effects occur within 15 to 60 seconds.

For control of postpartum bleeding the desired dose is 3 to 10 units given by intramuscular injection. Effects by this route appear in 3 to 7 minutes and persist for 30 to 60 minutes.

Buccal administration consists of placing one or more tablets in the buccal space (inner cheek) every 30 minutes until the desired uterine response is obtained or a total of 15 tablets (3000 units) has been given. This method of administration is less precise and less reliable than intravenous administration, since rate of absorption is unpredictable. Thus, continuous, careful supervision is vital.

The nasal spray is used to promote milk ejection for breast feeding. The usual dose is one spray into one or both nostrils 2 to 3 minutes before nursing.

Contraindications. Oxytocin is usually contraindicated during the first stage of labor. If used when the cervix is undilated and rigid, severe laceration and excessive trauma are likely to occur. It is contraindicated in malpresentation of the fetus, severe toxemia, fetal distress, severe medical conditions such as cardiovascular disease, and predisposition to uterine rupture (multiparas, previous cesarean section, or uterine surgery).

Side effects. Synthetic oxytocin produces fewer side effects and is less toxic than the older (now obsolete) preparation from the posterior pituitary of domesticated animals. The synthetic preparation lacks the vasopressin and protein components.

Water intoxication may occur when large doses of oxytocin have been infused for long periods. Allergic reactions may also occur. When used injudiciously, oxytocin can cause maternal death because of uterine rupture, hypertensive crisis, and cerebral hemorrhage. Pelvic hematomas, bradycardia, and arrhythmias also occur. Arrhythmias may also occur in the fetus, and fetal deaths have been reported.

Oxytocin and related drugs should be used only in the hospital and only with continuous medical supervision. Special emphasis should be placed on monitoring maternal blood pressure, fetal heart tones, and the strength and duration of uterine contractions. Prolonged contractions of the uterus may result in diminished blood flow and decreased oxygen to the fetus.

ERGOT ALKALOIDS

Ergot is the dried sclerotium (mycelium) of the parasitic fungus *Claviceps purpurea*, which grows on many species of grain, especially rye, where it forms long black bodies on the ears of the rye. The parasite is especially prevalent when the weather is moist and warm and grows predominantly in the grain fields of North America and Europe. Ergot was known as an obstetric herb to midwives long before it was recognized by the medical profession. Today ergot growth is carried out in fermentation vats in factories.

Active constituents. Both levorotatory and dextrorotatory alkaloids have been isolated from ergot, but only the levorotatory compounds are pharmacologically significant. All ergot alkaloids are derivatives of lysergic acid in which substitutions have been made at the carboxyl group.

The entire large group of ergot alkaloids can be divided into three groups: ergotamine, ergotoxine, and ergonovine. Members of each group have certain common chemical features and pharmacologic actions. The first two have a polypeptide chain substituted at the carboxyl group of lysergic acid, whereas alkaloids of the ergonovine group are chemically simpler and contain a relatively small isopropyl side chain.

Pharmacologic actions. Ergot alkaloids have three major actions in the body: smooth muscle stimulation (particularly of blood vessels and the uterus), adrenergic blockade, and central nervous system effects.

1 *Smooth muscle stimulation.* All smooth muscle is stimulated by the ergot alkaloids. The action is a direct one. This action is pronounced in the natural alkaloids but reduced in the hydrogenated derivatives.

   a. *Oxytocic effect.* Like oxytocin, the ergot alkaloids stimulate contractions of the uterine muscle in the pregnant uterus. In early stages of pregnancy the uterus is not very sensitive to the alkaloids; therefore, they cannot be used as abortifacients. During the third trimester uterine sensitivity increases. Oxytocin is used for induction and stimulation of labor. Ergonovine and methylergonovine are drugs of choice for the prevention of postpartum bleeding. Reduction of bleeding results from contraction of the uterine wall around the bleeding vessels at the placental site. Very high doses cause sustained uterine contracture.

   b. *Vasoconstriction.* All blood vessels are constricted by ergot alkaloids, with the larger arteries being the most sensitive. Arteries may show localized narrowings and even occlusions, which may lead to thrombosis and gangrene. Ergotamine is useful in the treatment of migraine headache for its vasoconstricting effect on cerebral vessels, but decreased flow in peripheral, mesenteric, and coronary arteries can result in ischemia of the respective tissues.

In large doses, ergot alkaloids cause a definite rise in blood pressure. This effect is more likely to be evoked in hypertensive subjects than in those with normal blood pressure.

2 *Adrenergic blockade.* In high doses some of the ergot alkaloids block the vasoconstricting action of the catecholamines (norepinephrine) in laboratory animals. However, this effect does not occur with therapeutic doses in humans.

3 *Central nervous system effects.* The dehydrogenated alkaloids inhibit sympathetic activity and produce a slight fall in blood pressure and bradycardia.

Preparation, dosage, and administration

Ergonovine maleate (Ergotrate); Ergometrine maleate, methylergonovine maleate (Methergine); methylergometrine maleate. These preparations are used primarily after delivery of the placenta to produce firm uterine contractions and to decrease uterine bleeding. They are also used for postabortal hemorrhage and during the puerperium to hasten involution of the uterus. They can be given orally since they are readily absorbed from the gastrointestinal tract. Effects occur 2 to 5 minutes after intramuscular injection and 3 to 5 minutes after oral administration.

Preparations are available in 1-ml ampules containing 0.2 mg/ml and as tablets containing 0.2 mg. The usual intramuscular dose is 0.2 mg, which may be repeated in 2 to 4 hours. The usual oral dose is 0.2 mg three or four times a day usually for 2 days (maximum, 1 week). Intravenous injections may be used in emergency situations, but this route of administration carries a high risk and the patient should be monitored.

Side effects. Side effects may include nausea and vomiting, dizziness, headache, cramps, dyspnea, and chest pain. Allergic reactions have been reported. Elevated blood pressure and bradycardia may occur; these effects are less frequent and less pronounced with methylergonovine than with ergonovine. Increased sensitivity to ergot alkaloids is seen in hepatic disease (the liver probably metabolizes the drug), and in febrile and septic states.

Contraindications. Ergot alkaloids are contraindicated in obliterative vascular disease, liver disease, and kidney disease. They are also contraindicated for induction of labor and threatened spontaneous abortion.

Prolonged use is not recommended since ergotism may develop, although authenticated reports of its occurrence have not been published.

PROSTAGLANDINS

Prostaglandins are an important class of natural substances that are synthesized in most mammalian tissues. As derivatives of prostanoic acid, the prostaglandins comprise a family of more than a dozen closely related substances with many varied biologic actions. Among these are smooth muscle stimulation or depression, vasoconstriction or dilation, inhibition of platelet aggregation, inhibition of gastric secretion, depression of the corpus luteum, and induction of sodium excretion. The best studied prostaglandins are those of the E and F series. E series prostaglandins (PGE_1, PGE_2) tend to be vasodilators and smooth muscle depressants. Those of the F series tend to be pressors in some species (dogs, rats) and depressors in others (cats, rabbits). The 1 and 2 series have 1 and 2 double bonds, respectively, in the side chains. The primary action tends to be on cell membranes. Although the precise mechanisms of action of the prostaglandins are not yet understood, they are currently thought to modify or inhibit the action of adenyl cyclase, which alters the formation of cyclic AMP, the mediator of most hormone actions in the cell.

Clinical studies indicate that prostaglandins are important in the physiology of labor. In some animals, such as sheep, prostaglandins appear prior to the onset of labor and not as a consequence of it. Karim in 1968 successfully induced term labor with prostaglandins using PGF_2 or PGE_2. Additional studies have shown conflicting results, which may have resulted from study design. More refined studies using an inducibility score indicate PGF_2 is just as effective as synthetic oxytocin for inducing term labor in woman with similar degrees of inducibility.

Prostaglandins are also being investigated

as abortifacients in the second trimester of pregnancy. A major drawback with this approach is the occurrence of undesirable side effects.

Dinoprost tromethamine (PGF$_2\alpha$-THAM, Prostaglandin F$_2$ Alpha Tromethamine, Prostin F2 Alpha)

Dinoprost is the tromethamine salt of the naturally occurring compound, prostaglandin F$_2$ alpha (PGF$_2\alpha$). It produces contraction of the gravid uterus similar to that of the term uterus during labor. Contractions are usually adequate for delivery; however, dinoprost-induced abortion may be incomplete. It is believed that the drug acts directly on the myometrium. Dinoprost also stimulates gastrointestinal smooth muscle; large doses cause bronchoconstriction, hypertension, and alteration in heartbeat.

After administration dinoprost is widely distributed in the maternal and fetal bodies. It is rapidly metabolized in the maternal lungs and liver. Metabolites of the drug are excreted within 24 hours, primarily via the urine.

Dinoprost has been administered intravenously and orally for induction of term labor; for evacuation of the uterus in missed abortion, fetal death in late pregnancy, and hydatidiform mole; and as a contraceptive agent.

Preparation, dosage, and administration. Dinoprost is available for injection in 4- and 8-ml ampules containing 5 mg drug/ml. Dinoprost is approved by the FDA for intraamniotic instillation to terminate pregnancy during the second trimester. Before injecting the drug, 1 ml of amniotic fluid should be withdrawn by transabdominal tap. If the amniotic fluid contains blood, dinoprost should not be administered.

After intraamniotic instillation of 40 mg dinoprost, maximum plasma level of the drug occurs in about 2 hours. The half-life of the drug in amniotic fluid is 3 to 6 hours, while the plasma half-life is reported to be less than 1 minute. Abortion usually occurs in about 20 hours in 50% of patients, with most patients aborting within 48 hours following an initial dose of 40 mg dinoprost, with 10 to 40 mg given 24 hours later.

Side effects. Vomiting occurs in more than 50% of patients and nausea, abdominal cramps, or uterine pain occurs in about 25%. Diarrhea and lactation, which may last several days, may also occur. Bronchoconstriction, tachycardia, and hypertension can occur if the drug is inadvertently administered into the maternal circulation.

The following reactions have been reported after prostaglandin treatment: pain, which may be epigastric, substernal, or located in the leg or shoulder; headache; flushing; diaphoresis; coughing and wheezing; convulsions; paresthesias; breast tenderness; hyperventilation; and a burning sensation in the eyes or breasts. Other reactions that have been reported include uterine rupture, urinary retention, bronchospasm, hematuria, polydipsia, and second-degree heart block.

Precautions. Dinoprost must be used cautiously in patients with a history of asthma, glaucoma, hypertension, epilepsy, or cardiovascular disease.

If used before the cervix is adequately dilated, cervical perforation or cervicovaginal fistulas may result. Since cervical trauma can occur without symptoms, patients should be carefully examined following uterine evacuation.

Dinoprost is contraindicated in patients with acute pelvic inflammatory disease. Animal studies indicate that dinoprost may be potentially teratogenic.

Drug interactions. Aspirin appears to increase the time interval between administration of dinoprost and abortion, and it may therefore be advisable to avoid use of aspirin when dinoprost has been given.

Drugs that decrease uterine motility

There are times when inhibition of uterine contractions is indicated, as when a patient begins premature labor or when uterine tone is high and contractions are unusually frequent and uncoordinated. Drugs that combat these conditions include certain depressants of the central nervous system as well as several that act directly on uterine smooth muscle.

Ethyl alcohol given intravenously and the

beta receptor stimulants metaproterenol (Alupent), ritodrine (Premar), and isoxsuprine (Vasodilan) have been used as uterine relaxants with varying degrees of success. Ritodrine appears to be a powerful uterine relaxant. Until drugs are clinically available that specifically relax the uterus with minimal side effects, bed rest and sedation remain the most acceptable means for arresting premature labor.

Drugs used in toxemia of pregnancy

Toxemia of pregnancy (preeclampsia and eclampsia) is a syndrome characterized by sodium and water retention and severe generalized vasoconstriction. These complications of pregnancy develop in the order mentioned but do not seem to have a cause-and-effect relationship. Drugs used in the treatment of toxemia of pregnancy include thiazide diuretics, magnesium sulfate preparations, and various antihypertensive drugs.

THIAZIDE DIURETICS

Therapy with thiazide diuretics such as diazoxide (Hyperstat I.V. Injection), which are started prior to the onset of the vasoconstrictor component of the toxemia syndrome, decreases the likelihood of progression of the illness and may have a general prophylactic value in high-risk patients. However, it is not clear whether both the renal and the vascular actions of the drug contribute to this effect. After severe hypertension has developed, a much more rapidly effective drug is required. At this stage the blood pressure appears to respond to the drugs commonly used for the emergency control of blood pressure in much the same manner as do pressure elevations of other etiology. Intravenous diazoxide consistently, effectively, and safely lowers the blood pressure in toxemia and has been reported to produce very favorable results in this condition.

MAGNESIUM SULFATE PREPARATIONS

Magnesium sulfate, when administered parenterally, produces depression of both the central nervous system and all muscular tissue (smooth, skeletal, cardiac). Because of its depressant effects on uterine smooth muscle, magnesium sulfate is one of the most important drugs in the treatment of toxemia of pregnancy. It is also effective in counteracting uterine tetany that may occur after large doses of oxytocin.

Magnesium sulfate is available for intramuscular or intravenous injection in 10%, 25%, and 50% concentrations. Various dosage schedules have been used for preeclampsia or eclampsia. An initial dose of 4 g magnesium sulfate in 250 ml 5% dextrose may be given intravenously; this dose may be followed by 4 to 5 g intramuscularly into each buttock. Intramuscular doses of 4 to 5 g may then be given at 4-hour intervals as needed, depending on the patient's response. Usual range of dose is 1 to 10 g daily. Determinations should be made of the patient's serum magnesium levels and urinary excretion of magnesium. Effective anticonvulsant serum level ranges from 2.5 to 7.5 mEq/liter.

When magnesium sulfate is given intravenously, the effect is immediate and duration of action is about 30 minutes. When magnesium sulfate is given intramuscularly, onset of action occurs in about 1 hour and duration of action is 3 to 4 hours. For uterine tetany, 1 to 2 g is usually given intravenously. Intravenous injections should be given slowly and the patient should be observed carefully for signs of magnesium toxicity. An injectable form of calcium, usually 10 to 20 ml 10% calcium gluconate, should be readily available for use in case severe central nervous system depression occurs. Calcium is a specific antidote for magnesium toxicity.

Adverse reactions and precautions. Premonitory symptoms of magnesium toxicity include "feeling hot all over" and extreme thirst. Disappearance of the patellar reflex is a useful clinical sign to detect the onset of magnesium toxicity. Patellar reflex loss usually occurs when the serum magnesium level exceeds 4 mEq/liter.

Adverse effects include flushing, sweating, hypotension, depression of reflexes, flaccid paralysis, hypothermia, circulatory collapse, and depression of cardiac and central nervous system function. The most immediate danger to life is respiratory paralysis; mechanical respiratory assistance may be necessary to support life. Abrupt injection of large doses of magnesium sulfate can cause cardiac arrest. A patient receiving magnesium sulfate parenterally *should never be left alone.* If repeated doses are given, knee jerk reflexes should be tested before each dose and if absent, no further magnesium should be given until reflexes return to normal. Respiration rate should be counted before each dose; a rate of 16 per minute should be present before each dose. In addition, urine output should be 100 ml or more during the 4 hours before each dose.

Intravenous magnesium should not be given during the 2 hours preceding delivery since magnesium may cause neuromuscular or respiratory depression in the infant. Intramuscular magnesium usually does not adversely affect the newborn.

Drug interactions. Additive central nervous system effects occur when narcotics, barbiturates, general anesthetics, or other central nervous system depressants are given concomitantly with magnesium sulfate; thus dosages of these drugs must be carefully adjusted. Excessive neuromuscular blockade can occur if a neuromuscular blocking agent (such as tubocurarine) is given to a patient receiving parenteral magnesium sulfate. In digitalized patients, if calcium is used to treat magnesium toxicity, heart block may occur and extreme caution is required.

ANTIHYPERTENSIVE DRUGS

Veratrum alkaloids, reserpine, and hydralazine are antihypertensive agents that have been used most frequently in the past to control blood pressure in cases of toxemia. However, in comparison with diazoxide, *Veratrum* alkaloids are much more difficult to control; reserpine is usually less effective, acts more slowly, and produces nasal congestion that can cause serious respiratory difficulties in the newborn; and hydralazine produces even more disturbing and unpleasant side effects. Hence the use of alternative drugs, such as those already described in the treatment of toxemia, is indicated when possible.

Drugs affecting the fetus and neonate
Role of the placenta in drug transfer to the fetus

There have been numerous scientific advances in recent years that have brought about heightened interest in and attention to the effects of maternal medications on the fetus and the newborn infant. Paramount among these is the recognition that virtually all substances ingested by the mother, whether intentionally or otherwise, are likely to reach the fetus through the maternal circulation or the neonate through the milk. Drugs taken by the mother during pregnancy are of particular concern in this respect because of the potentially harmful effects these drugs or their metabolites may have on the developing conceptus. The extent to which substances in the maternal blood reach the fetus depends primarily on the functioning of the placenta, the organ that provides the only communication between the fetus and the outside world through the mother.

An important aspect of placental function is the ability of the organ to transfer materials to the fetus against a concentration gradient and therefore ensure that adequate amounts of substances essential for fetal growth and development are present. The recognition that the placenta plays an active and selective role in transfer mechanisms is relatively recent. For years the use of the term "placental barrier" typified the concept of the placenta as an organ whose prime function was to protect the fetus against injury and infection and to provide a physical barrier to the passage of noxious substances from mother to fetus. It is now recognized, however, that essentially all substances ingested by the pregnant woman may reach the fetus in either original or metabolized form by active or passive transplacental transport processes.

In the case of substances required for fetal development, the majority of essential nutrients, including vitamins, amino acids, and ions such as calcium, are actively transported from mother to fetus against a concentration gradient. An adequate level of these essential nutrients is maintained on the fetal side of the placenta through the continued selective activity of the placental cells. On the other hand, drugs and many exogenous compounds are considered to cross the placenta by a simple diffusion process. An exception to this rule is the rare case when drugs have a structural similarity to endogenous substances that are normally transported by active processes. The rate at which placental transfer occurs by simple diffusion is governed by standard physiochemical considerations and depends on the concentration of the substance on the maternal side of the barrier, the thickness of the membrane and the surface area available for transfer, and a diffusion constant unique to the substance being transferred. The value of the diffusion constant depends on the molecular size and spatial conformation, ionic dissociation, and lipid solubility of the chemical in question. The last property is of particular importance for drug transfer to the fetus in that the passage of lipid-soluble substances across the placenta, as with other membranes, is accelerated in comparison with substances that are less fat soluble. As a rule, therefore, one would expect poor fetal penetration of highly ionized drugs with low lipid solubility, such as tubocurarine, and more rapid transfer of drugs with high lipid solubility and low degrees of dissociation, such as thiopental. Overall, this rule is a useful and valid concept, but its application is limited to individual cases when genetic and environmental circumstances may affect drug transport processes. It should also be recognized that any substance, regardless of physiochemical properties, will eventually reach the fetus if present in sufficient concentration in the maternal circulation.

Chemical teratogenesis

Embryogenesis represents a finely balanced interplay of cell proliferation, differentiation, migration, and organogenesis. It is a precisely programmed sequence of events, repeating itself in detail for every zygote of a species. Teratogenesis refers to the process by which chemical agents alter the embryogenic process in such a way that defects of one or another organ

system are produced. Because each step in embryogenesis may depend on a previous one, and because numerous tissues and organs develop at precise stages of gestation, the timing of chemical exposure is critical with respect to its teratogenic potential.

During the early phase of cell proliferation no malformations can be induced. At this time all teratogens have nonspecific all-or-none effects; the embryo may be killed, but if it survives it becomes a normal individual. All cells at this stage may be so much alike that no selectively toxic action is possible on those that will eventually form particular organ systems. Alternatively, damaged cells that have undergone partial differentiation may still be replaced by others that escaped injury. Very late in fetal development it is also difficult to produce abnormalities, since the processes of organogenesis have been largely completed. In each species there is, therefore, a relatively short period of sensitivity to teratogens, when early organogenesis is in progress. In the human being the timetable of embryologic development suggests a period extending roughly from the third week through the third month of pregnancy. At 20 days after fertilization the cephalocaudal segmentation of the embryo into somites is just beginning. These segments are the precursors of the axial skeleton and musculature. At about 30 days the limb buds make their appearance, and by 60 days organ differentiation in the fetus (now about 30 mm long) is well underway. Accordingly, rubella-induced malformations of the eye, ear, and heart occur principally between the fourth and eighth weeks. Thalidomide interference with limb formation is chiefly a hazard of the same period—the second month of pregnancy.

It was, in fact, the thalidomide catastrophe, 1960 to 1961, that brought to public attention the fact that ingestion during pregnancy of drugs having no apparent toxic effect on the mother could produce serious fetotoxic effects resulting in congenital malformations in the newborn. Thalidomide was introduced in the late 1950s in West Germany, England, and other European countries as a tranquilizing drug. It was effective and seemed remarkably free of toxic side effects. Although the typical therapeutic dose was about 100 mg, patients recovered from ingestion of as much as 14 g taken with suicidal intent. Shortly after the introduction of thalidomide into therapy, there was an increase in the number of infants born with phocomelia, a shortening or complete absence of the limbs. These were interesting observations, since at the University Pediatric Clinic in Hamburg, for example, not a single case of phocomelia had been seen in the decade 1949 to 1959. In 1959 there was a single case; in 1960, 30 cases; and 1961, 154 cases. Comparable increases in the frequency of this anomaly, previously almost unknown, occurred simultaneously in many parts of the world where thalidomide was in use. Finally, in November 1961, a study suggested an association between phocomelia and the ingestion of thalidomide by pregnant women. Subsequent investigations in several countries indicated that in practically every case of phocomelia the mother had taken thalidomide between the third and eighth weeks of pregnancy. Sometimes only a few doses during the critical period sufficed.

The critical period for each kind of malformation produced in the human fetus has been established by careful retrospective analysis. When thalidomide was taken 35 to 36 days after the last menstrual period (approximately 21 to 22 days gestation), absence of the external ears and paralysis of the cranial nerves resulted. Three to 5 days later (about 24 to 27 days of gestation), the phocomelia effect was at its maximum; 1 or 2 days later, similar defects of the legs occurred. The sensitive period terminated 48 to 50 days after the last period (34 to 36 days of gestation), with the production of hypoplastic thumbs and anorectal stenosis.

Thalidomide was withdrawn from the market at the end of 1961, and the outbreak of phocomelia subsided promptly. In the United States the drug had not been approved by the FDA and was therefore never in general use. The total number of infants throughout the world who were deformed by thalidomide is estimated to be approximately 10,000. Although phocomelia is the most obvious and directly disabling abnormality, congenital malformations of the internal organs are also common in the affected children.

The thalidomide disaster represents the worst that can happen with respect to effects of a drug ingested by the mother of the fetus. However, the experience served to bring drug-induced teratogenesis out of the realm of laboratory curiosity and into the public arena. It focused attention on the requirement for more exhaustive drug testing, as well as on the need for a more effective system for disseminating information on possible adverse gestational drug effects, both to pregnant women and to the general public. A listing of drugs in current or potential use and an indication of their possible effects on the fetus or newborn is given in Table 29-2. It should be particularly noted that the estrogens or progestins, if taken during the first 3 to 4 months of pregnancy, can increase risk of birth defects, especially limb and heart defects. A higher incidence of birth defects can be found when conception immediately follows discontinuance of oral contraceptives. Those who discontinue taking oral contraceptives should therefore use another form of contraception for at least 3 months before attempting to conceive. Other drugs suspected of causing serious adverse effects in the fetus include tetracyclines (discolors teeth), barbiturates (addiction), tranquilizers, phenytoin, or antineoplastic drugs (cleft palate or lip), vaccines, alcohol (a component of many over-the-counter cold remedies), nicotine, and some obstetric analgesics. The FDA has established five categories (A, B, C, D, X) for labeling prescription drugs according to their potential for being teratogens. Category A applies to drugs for which well-controlled studies have failed to demonstrate risk to the fetus.

Effects of maternal drug ingestion on the nursing infant

The nursing infant may be the unintended recipient of drugs administered to the mother. Foreign compounds are known to be excreted into the milk of nursing mothers, and these compounds may then be ingested by the infant while nursing.

Studies of drug effects on the breast-fed infant are primarily available through retrospective studies or anecdotal reports. In these

T A B L E   2 9 - 2   **Effects of maternal medication on the fetus and newborn**

Agent	Effect
Anesthesia (inhalation)	
Halothane (Fluothane)	No significant depression if given for short duration
Enflurane (Enflane)	No significant depression if given for short duration
Nitrous oxide	No significant depression if oxygen concentration administered to mother is adequate (20% or more)
Anesthesia (local)	
Lidocaine (Xylocaine)	Crosses placenta readily; adverse effects on the fetus not established
Mepivacaine (Carbocaine)	May depress infant by direct drug effect or indirectly via maternal hypotension when used for regional anesthesia (spinal or epidural procedures)
Procaine (Novocaine)	
Tetracaine (Pontocaine)	
Antibacterials	
Ampicillin (Amcill)	No untoward effect; safe use in pregnancy not established
Cephalexin (Keflex)	Crosses placenta; only 50% of infants will have bacteriostatic levels in cord blood or amniotic fluid when mother has adequate serum levels
Cephalothin (Keflin)	No untoward effect; safe use during pregnancy and in infants under 1 month of age not established
Chloramphenicol	"Gray syndrome" (gastrointestinal irritability, circulatory collapse, death) in newborn treated with this drug; never proved to occur in newborn if drug given only to mother
Erythromycin	No untoward effects demonstrated; safe use during pregnancy not established
Isoniazid (INH)	Unconfirmed, retrospective, and circumstantial evidence of psychomotor retardation
Kanamycin	Ototoxicity suspected but not proved in infants born to mothers treated for extended periods
Lincomycin (Lincocin)	Crosses placenta rapidly, fetal blood levels equal ¼ maternal blood levels; no untoward effects recorded
Metronidazole (Flagyl)	No untoward effect known; crosses placental barrier readily; not recommended during first trimester
Nitrofurantoin (Furadantin)	Megaloblastic anemia in fetus with glucose-6-phosphate dehydrogenase deficiency
Novobiocin	Increase in hyperbilirubinemia if newborn treated; not proved to occur via maternal treatment
Penicillin	No untoward effect
Sulfonamides	Sulfonamides displace protein-bound bilirubin and can cause kernicterus in fetus and in newborn infants
Sulfadiazine (Microsulfon)	
Sulfamethoxypyridazine (Midicel)	
Sulfisoxazole (Gantrisin)	
Streptomycin	Hearing loss (rare) in infants of mothers having prolonged treatment in early pregnancy due to eighth cranial nerve damage
Tetracycline (Achromycin)	Staining of deciduous teeth and hypoplasia of enamel, inconclusive association with congenital cataracts, potential for bone growth retardation but not proved to occur in utero
Chlortetracycline (Aureomycin)	
Oxytetracycline (Terramycin)	
Demeclocycline (Declomycin)	
Anticoagulants	
Dicumarol	Risk of fetal hemorrhage, particularly if mother overtreated
Heparin (Heprinar)	No untoward effect; does not cross placenta
Warfarin (Coumadin)	Risk of fetal hemorrhage, particularly if mother overtreated; reports of malformed infants with hypoplastic nasal structures
Anticonvulsants	
Phenytoin (Dilantin)	Increased incidence of midline clefts, congenital heart disease, eye defects, and coagulation defect
Trimethadione (Tridione)	Abortion; malformations, mental retardation
Antidiabetic agents	
Chlorpropamide (Diabinese)	Respiratory distress and neonatal hypoglycemia, teratogenic effects suspected but not proved, neonatal thrombocytopenia
Insulins	No proved untoward effect
Tolbutamide (Orinase)	Effects suspected but not proved; not recommended for use in diabetic women who may become pregnant; some reports of diverse multiple congenital abnormalities

T A B L E 2 9 - 2 Effects of maternal medication on the fetus and newborn—cont'd

Agent	Effect
Antihistamines and antiemetics Cyclizine (Marezine) Meclizine (Bonine)	No evidence of adverse effects in the newborn; not generally recommended for use during pregnancy
Antimalarial agents Chloroquine (Aralen)	Abnormal retinal pigmentation reported after maternal treatment for lupus erythematosis; congenital deafness has been reported when mother treated with high doses
Quinine (Coco-Quinine)	Early reports of ototoxicity and congenital malformations unsubstantiated by other clinicians, danger of fetal damage probably minimal
Antineoplastic agents Methotrexate (Amethopterin)	Congenital anomalies; hypertelorism
Cytarabine (ARA-C)	Reports of intrauterine growth retardation and fetal death
Mercaptopurine (Purinethol)	Hemolytic anemia of the newborn
Antithyroid agents Methimazole (Tapazole)	All antithyroid drugs cross placenta and can result in fetal goiters and hypothyroidism
Sodium iodide, ^{131}I Propylthiouracil (PTU)	Permanent fetal thyroid suppression (^{131}I)
Barbiturates Amobarbital (Amytal) Pentobarbital (Nembutal) Phenobarbital Secobarbital (Seconal) Thiamylal (Surital) Thiopental (Pentothal)	All barbiturates and thiobarbiturates cross placenta; in usual clinical doses they cause minimal fetal depression, decreased neonatal responsiveness and inhibited ability to suck; phenobarbital induces microsomal enzymes to increase conjugation of bilirubin in the newborn
Beta blocking agents Propranolol (Inderal)	Crosses placenta, results in beta adrenergic blocking effects in fetus, depressing circulatory responses of the newborn
Keratolytics Podophyllum Resin (Podoben)	Maternal absorption resulted in peripheral neuropathy and fetal death in utero (drug is antimitotic used for venereal warts and granuloma inguinale)
Digitoxin	When administered during eighth month of pregnancy may cause digitalis intoxication of fetus
Diuretics Chlorothiazide (Diuril) Hydrochlorothiazide (HydroDIURIL)	Thrombocytopenia Thrombocytopenia
Fungistatic agents Griseofulvin (Fulvicin-U/F)	No untoward effect
Intravenous fluids	Electrolyte imbalance possible, usually hyponatremia (lethargy, poor muscle tone, poor color)
Hallucinogens Lysergic acid diethylamide (LSD)	Fetal neural tube defects have been reported to be more common in infants born to users of LSD, but these patients were also taking other drugs such as marijuana and amphetamines. (Extensive review of literature suggests no untoward chromosomal or teratogenic effects of LSD itself.)
Narcotics Alphaprodine (Nisentil) Codeine Heroin Levophanol (Levo-Dromoran) Meperidine (Demerol) Methadone (Dolophine) Morphine	Depression of fetal respiration; decreased responsiveness of newborn. Depresses neonatal psychophysiologic function. Infants born to narcotic addicts develop withdrawal symptoms of hyperirritability, shrill cry, and vomiting. Can be fatal. Intrauterine growth retardation and prematurity more common. No reports of fetal or infant death resulting from methadone treatment of mother, but infant shows typical withdrawal symptoms, which can be more difficult to treat and more prolonged than with heroin
Narcotic antagonists Levallorphine (Lorfan) Naloxone (Narcan)	Decreases neonatal depression caused by narcotic
Nicotine (smoking)	Reports of intrauterine growth retardation, conflicting reports about long-term developmental effects of maternal smoking, no definite deleterious effect demonstrated

Continued.

T A B L E 2 9 - 2 Effects of maternal medication on the fetus and newborn—cont'd

Agent	Effect
Salicylates	
Aspirin	Congenital defects more common in women taking salicylates in first trimester, no cause-and-effect relationship proved; inhibits platelet aggregation and causes hemorrhagic tendency in newborn, may predispose to prolong pregnancy by inhibiting prostaglandin biosynthesis, salicylate poisoning can occur in fetus with maternal overdose
Sedatives	
Alcohol (heavy consumption during pregnancy)	Growth deficiency; fetal alcohol syndrome
Chloral hydrate (Noctec)	No significant effect; crosses placenta; withdrawal symptoms in newborn similar to those seen with opiates; not recommended in pregnancy
Ethchlorvynol (Placidyl)	
Skeletal muscle relaxants	
Decamethonium bromide (Syncurine)	In usual clinical doses, drugs do not cross placenta and do not cause any noticeable effect on fetus or newborn
Gallamine triethiodide (Flaxedil)	
Succinylcholine chloride (Anectine)	
Steroids	
Betamethasone (Decadron)	Accelerates pulmonary maturation, salutary effects on fetus (or newborn) not entirely substantiated
Cortisone acetate (Cortistan)	Possible relationship to cleft palate and fetal death; not definitely proved in humans
Dexamethasone (Decadron)	Some reports of placental insufficiency syndrome, fetal distress during labor, and fetal death
Prednisolone (Cordrol)	
Prednisone (Fernisone)	
Progesterone (Progestin)	Masculinization of female fetus, implicated in development of multisystem anomalies and development of congenital heart defects
Diethylstilbestrol (DES)	Delayed development of adenosis and adenocarcinoma of vagina in female infant, vaginal cancer in teenage girls born to mothers on DES during pregnancy
Testosterone	Masculinization of female fetus
Thyroid compounds	
Desiccated thyroid extract (Dathroid)	Crosses the placenta but no known untoward effect on fetus or newborn
Liothyronine (Cytomel)	
Tranquilizers	
Chloridiazepoxide (Librium)	Crosses placenta; no untoward effects demonstrated to date
Chlorpromazine (Thorazine)	No definite effect on fetus substantiated; extrapyramidal effects may appear in newborn if drug is given during last trimester; jaundice also reported; possibility of permanent neurologic damage cannot be excluded
Diazepam (Valium)	Crosses placenta; neonatal respiratory depression, hypotonia, and hypercapnia; lower newborn body temperature
Meprobamate (Equanil, Miltown)	No untoward effect on human fetus substantiated; crosses placental barrier; safe use in pregnancy not established
Prochlorperazine (Compazine)	Same as for chlorpromazine
Tricyclic antidepressants	
Imipramine (Tofranil)	Anecdotal reports of craniofacial and CNS lesions; several large studies have refuted these findings
Vitamins	
Vitamin D (Calciferol)	Anecdotal reports of hypercalcemia and cardiovascular lesions resembling vitamin D intoxication; maternal intake should not be excessive
Vitamin K and analogs	Administration to mother results in hyperbilirubinemia of newborn
Menadione sodium bisulfite (Kappadione)	
Phytonadione (AquaMephyton)	

instances the population as well as the data may be limited. It is obviously not feasible to conduct in vivo research where the well-being of the subjects would be seriously compromised. Thus current information concerning pharmacologic effects is drawn largely from what has already occurred or from animal studies in which the findings are questionable in terms of their applicability to human beings.

This portion of the chapter is directed to what has already been documented or is strongly suspected about drug effects on infants of nursing mothers. From it, some practical application may be drawn for therapy and for patient counseling and teaching.

SYNTHESIS AND COMPOSITION OF MILK

The mammary tissue, where milk is synthesized, is a compound, tubule-alveolar gland. The secretory, or alveolar, cells are surrounded by myoepithelial cells having contractile properties, which permits the transfer of milk from alveoli into the duct system. Proteins, carbohydrates, and fats are the most important natural components of milk.

The initiation of synthesis and secretion of milk is a highly complex hormonal interaction achieved by the combined effects of estrogens and progesterones interacting with FSH and LH. Milk production begins slowly; just prior to parturition the levels of estrogen and progesterone fall, and progesterone's inhibitory effect on prolactin release by the pituitary is withdrawn. Under the influence of prolactin, the alveolar cells become highly secretory. As the infant begins to stimulate the breast by sucking, a release of oxytocin from the posterior pituitary occurs, which affects the contractility of the myoepithelial cells, and a flow of milk is established. This is called the "milk ejection reflex."

Lactation may be inhibited by the administration of androgens and estrogens, either separately or in combined form. The timing and the dosage are the most important factors in eliciting response. Low dosages of progesterone or estrogen preparations, used in contraceptive therapy to suppress ovulation, may diminish lactation. If contraceptive therapy is begun after adequate milk production is established, lactation is not affected but the composition of the milk may be. For example, ethinyl estradiol augments milk protein content.

THE PRESENCE OF DRUGS IN MILK

In the maternal circulation drugs differ in their binding to plasma proteins. It is the unbound fraction that exerts the pharmacologic action and can be metabolized and excreted. Any endogenous or exogenous substance may compete with the drug and its binding to albumin, which may result in its displacement and augment its passage into the mammary duct system. In this instance the amount available for infant ingestion is increased. It is important to note that an isolated measurement of the concentration of a drug in milk is misleading unless it can be correlated with the total quantity ingested and absorbed by the infant.

The mammary gland is a relatively unimportant route for total drug excretion. However, this must not detract from the fact that foreign substances may appear in the milk and be ingested by the infant.

Small, water-soluble molecules (urea, antipyrine, alcohol) pass through biologic membranes by simple diffusion. Other drugs, such as sulfonamides, are bound to milk proteins. The passage of larger molecules depends on their lipid solubility and state of ionization; they pass through in a lipid-soluble, nonionized form. Drugs with low lipid solubility will diffuse rather slowly. Milk is an emulsion of fat in water, and the relative concentration of each component varies with and within each feeding. There is less fat concentration in the first milk the infant receives as compared to the last at any given feeding. Also, the time of day will determine the composition of milk, primarily in terms of fat content. Usually the fat content is higher in the morning. This consideration becomes important when dealing with drugs like pentobarbital and secobarbital. Since they are more lipid soluble, these drugs tend to transfer into milk as its fat content rises.

Types of effects. There is a lack of adverse reaction by infants to most drugs ingested with breast milk. However, this should not obscure the possibility of minimal or nondemonstrable effects, which may produce individual homeostatic complications.

Cumulative effect. An additive factor is seen with repeated administration of drugs that bind to fat tissue or to tissue proteins. These materials remain in the body for long periods. As an example, free chlorpromazine has been detected in tissues 18 months after discontinuation of the drug. It is not known at this time what impact this may have on the infant.

Effect on activity of drug-metabolizing enzymes. Some foreign compounds are known to increase the activity of drug-metabolizing enzymes located in the liver microsomes. Higher activity of these enzyme systems results in faster termination of drug action and also accelerates the hydroxylation of endogenous substances such as steroids. The long-term consequences of these phenomena are not known. In humans, phenobarbital and phenytoin are known inducers of drug metabolism by the liver, and they are excreted in breast milk. It is also known that the hepatic drug-metabolizing enzyme system in infants is immature with respect to that of the adult, which could predispose the infant to toxicity from drugs excreted unmetabolized in the milk.

Genetic defect. Persons with certain hereditary metabolic defects may adversely react to drug doses which are too small to produce pharmacologic action in normal subjects. For example, the presence of sulfamethoxypyridazine in the breast milk has been known to cause hemolytic anemia in an infant lacking the enzyme glucose-6-phosphate dehydrogenase.

Alteration of homeostatic functions. Such alteration will facilitate effects by other agents. For example, a hypocoagulability state is likely to follow anticoagulant therapy of the mother. However, this effect may go unrecognized unless mechanical or surgical trauma to the infant occurs.

Interference with normal physiologic functions. Modification of infant thyroid function may result from maternal ingestion of iodides or thyroid preparations. This action would render the neonate vulnerable to the development of goiter and hyperthyroidism.

Hypersensitivity. It is possible for the infant to develop hypersensitivity reactions following exposure to medication via breast milk. This is most likely to occur when doses are administered to both infant and mother, as in congenital syphilis, so that excessive amounts reach the infant.

Table 29-3 lists various drugs excreted in human milk and their possible effects on the nursing infant. Should a condition exist or occur that necessitates the use of one or more drugs with known or suspected effects on the nursing infant, lactation should be suppressed.

Discontinuance of breast-feeding. It is rarely necessary for the mother to discontinue nursing because of drug content in breast milk. A mother who has elected to breast-feed her infant usually wants to succeed and persevere in this psychologic and physiologic relationship. Often she is convinced that the advantages exceed any possible disadvantages or inconvenience. Breast-feeding has many positive features, such as assisting uterine involution, providing optimal nutrition (which includes a degree of antibody protection to the newborn), giving opportunity for consistent rest, and offering the close physical contact needed for mother/infant interaction.

Breast-feeding should be discontinued on a medical basis:

1 When the drug is so potent that minute amounts may have profound effect on the infant (radioactive products, steroids, anticoagulants, antineoplastics)
2 When the substance has significant antigenic properties (penicillin and its congeners)
3 When the mother exhibits evidence of decreased renal unction and is taking medication that might involve the breast as a secondary means of excretion.
4 When the mother has ingested a toxic substance such as a heavy metal (mercury) or benzene products
5 When the mother has a serious illness, is in recognizable negative calcium or nitrogen balance, or has a notable vitamin deficiency

Drugs affecting sexual behavior

An important part of human development is the attainment of a sexual identity and the ability to live as a sexual being. The realization of these objectives has become increasingly complicated in recent years in light of changing definitions of societal sex roles for both men and women, as well as the widespread availability, utilization, and even abuse of drugs that can modify sexual behavior. Unfortunately, much of current drug practice is shrouded in ignorance or misconception about the effects of drugs on sexual function. It is therefore important from a health care perspective to acquire and provide as much insight as possible regard-

Text continued on p. 911.

TABLE 29-3 **Drugs excreted in human milk and the possible significance for nursing infants**

Drug	Excreted	Quantity excreted	Significance
Antihistamine drugs			
Diphenhydramine (Benadryl)	Yes		Not significant in therapeutic doses to affect child
Trimeprazine tartrate (Temaril)	Yes		Not significant in therapeutic doses to affect child
Tripelennamine (Pyribenzamine)	Yes		Only bovine studies reported to date; apparently not enough is excreted to be significant in therapeutic doses
Antiinfective agents			
Amantadine (Symmetrel)	Possible		Not to be administered; personal correspondence with the manufacturer suggests it will be found in maternal milk; may cause vomiting, urinary retention, skin rash
Ampicillin (Polycillin, Amcill, Omnipen, Penbritin, Principen, others)	Yes	0.7 µg/ml	Not significant in therapeutic doses to affect child
Carbenicillin disodium (Pyopen, Geopen)	Yes	0.265 µg/ml 1 hour after administration of 1 g	Not significant in therapeutic doses to affect child
Cephalexin (Keflex)	No		
Cephalothin (Keflin)	No		
Chloramphenicol (Chloromycetin)	Yes	Half blood level 2.5 mg/100 ml	Infants have underdeveloped enzyme system, immature liver and renal function, may not have glycuronide system adequately developed to conjugate chloramphenicol; caution advised
Chloroquine (Aralen)	No	After daily dose of 0.6 g no traces could be found in milk of 105 subjects	Not significant in therapeutic doses to affect child
Demeclocycline (Declomycin)	Yes	0.2-0.3 mg/500 ml	Not significant in therapeutic doses to affect child
Erythromycin (Ilosone, E-mycin, Erythrocin)	Yes	0.05-0.1 mg/100 ml. 3.6-6.2 µg/ml	Higher concentrations have been reported in milk than in plasma
Isoniazid (Nydrazid)	Yes	0.6-1.2 mg/100 ml; same concentration in milk as in maternal serum	Infant should be monitored for possible signs of isoniazid toxicity
Kanamycin (Kantrex)	Yes	1 g given intramuscularly gave a concentration of 18.4 µg/ml	Infant should be monitored for possible signs of kanamycin toxicity
Lincomycin (Lincocin)	Yes	0.5-2.4 µg/ml	Not significant in therapeutic doses to affect child
Mandelic acid	Yes	0.3 g/24 hr following maternal dose of 12 g/day	Not significant in therapeutic doses to affect child
Methacycline (Rondomycin)	Yes		Same precautions as with tetracyclines
Methenamine (Hexamine)	Yes		Not significant in therapeutic doses to affect child
Metronidazole (Flagyl)	Yes	Level comparable to serum	Apparently not significant in therapeutic doses; caution should be exercised due to its high milk concentration
Nalidixic acid (NegGram)	Yes	3.9 µmg/liter	Not significant in therapeutic doses; however one case of hemolytic anemia in an infant was attributed to nalidixic acid

From O'Brien, T.E.: Excretion of drugs in human milk, Nurs. Dig. **3**(4): 25, 1975.

Continued.

T A B L E 29-3 Drugs excreted in human milk and the possible significance for nursing infants—cont'd

Drug	Excreted	Quantity excreted	Significance
Antiinfective agents—cont'd			
Nitrofurantoin (Furadantin)	Yes		Not significant in therapeutic doses to affect child
Novobiocin (Albamycin, Cardelmycin)	Yes	0.36-0.54 mg/100 ml	This antibiotic has been used to treat infections among infants with no untoward effects reported
Oxacillin (Prostaphlin)	No		
Paraamino salicylic acid	No		
Penethamate (Leocillin)	No	24-74 µg/100 ml	Animal study suggests it be avoided
Penicillin G potassium	Yes	Up to 6 units/100 ml	Controversy exists among clinicians; some feel that the risk of sensitivity symptoms must be looked for, others feel the small amount is insignificant; parent should be told to inform physician that infant has been exposed to penicillin
Penicillin, benzathine (Bicillin)	Yes	10-12 units/100 ml	Clinical need should supersede possible allergic responses
Pyrimethamine (Daraprim)	Yes		Detected in human milk but no conclusions drawn; apparently not significant in therapeutic doses
Quinine sulfate	Yes	0-0.1 mg/100 ml after maternal dose of 300-600 mg	Not significant in therapeutic doses to affect child
Sodium fusidate	Yes	0.2 µg/ml	Not significant in therapeutic doses to affect child
Streptomycin	Yes	Present for long periods in slight amounts given as dihydrostreptomycin	Risk should outweigh benefit of nursing; to be avoided
Sulfanilamide	Yes	After maternal dose of 2-4 g daily 9 mg/100 ml in milk	Not significant in therapeutic doses; may cause a rash
Sulfapyridine	Yes	3-13 mg/100 ml after maternal dose of 3 g daily	To be avoided; has caused skin rash
Sulfathiazole	Yes	0.5 mg/100 ml after dose of 3 g/day	Not significant in therapeutic doses to affect child
Sulfisoxazole (Gantrisin)	Yes	Concentration similar to plasma level	To be avoided, during first 2 postpartum weeks; may cause kernicterus
Tetracycline HCl (Achromycin, Steclin, Sumycin, others)	Yes	0.5-2.6 µg/ml after maternal dose of 500 mg qid	Not enough to treat an infection in an infant; however, it has been hypothesized that there may be a sufficient amount to cause discoloration of the teeth in the infant; the antibiotic, however, may be largely bound to the milk calcium
Antineoplastics			
Cyclophosphamide (Cytoxan)	Yes		To be avoided, as are other antineoplastic drugs; nursing should be discontinued
Autonomic drugs			
Atropine sulfate (ingredient in many products, both prescription and nonprescription)	Yes	Less than 0.1 mg/100 ml	Should not be administered for two main reasons: (1) it inhibits lactation, and (2) it may cause atropine intoxication in the infant

T A B L E 2 9 - 3 **Drugs excreted in human milk and the possible significance for nursing infants—cont'd**

Drug	Excreted	Quantity excreted	Significance
Carisoprodol (Soma, Rela)	Yes	May be present in breast milk at concentrations four times maternal plasma	Not to be administered, based upon manufacturer's recommendation; infant may be exposed to a series of adverse reactions ranging from CNS depression to gastrointestinal upset
Ergot (Cafergot)	Yes		Avoid whre possible; may cause symptoms in infants ranging from vomiting and diarrhea to weak pulse and unstable blood pressure
Hyoscine	Yes	Trace amounts	Not significant in therapeutic doses to affect child
Mepenzolate bromide (Cantil)	No		
Methocarbamol (Robaxin)	Yes	Small amounts	Not significant in therapeutic doses to affect child
Propantheline bromide (Pro-Banthine)	No		
Scopolamine	Yes		Not significant in therapeutic doses to affect child
Blood formation and coagulation			
Dicumarol	Yes		Therapeutic doses can be administered without deleterious effect on infant; infant should be monitored with mother
Ethyl biscoumacetate (Tromexan)	Yes	0-0.17 mg/100 ml; no correlation with dosage	Not significant in therapeutic doses; infant should be monitored with mother
Iron	Yes		Not significant in therapeutic doses to affect child
Ferrous sulfate Iron-dextran (Feosol, Imferon)			
Phenindione (Hedulin, Dindevan)	Yes		To be avoided; may produce a prothrombin deficiency in infant; one case of massive hematoma reported in an infant receiving drug in maternal milk
Warfarin sodium (Coumadin)	Yes		Infant should be monitored with mother; benefit should outweigh possible risk
Cardiovascular drugs			
Dextrothyroxine (Choloxin)	Yes		Not significant in therapeutic doses to affect child
Guanethidine (Ismelin)	Yes		Not significant in therapeutic doses to affect child
Methyclothiazide, deserpidine (Enduronyl)	Yes		Same precautions as with reserpine and thiazide diuretics
Methyldopa (Aldomet)	Yes		Studies performed on bovines; nothing reported in humans
Propranolol (Inderal)	No		
Reserpine (Serpasil, others)	Yes		May produce galactorrhea
Central nervous system drugs			
Alcohol	Yes	Small amounts	It appears that moderate amounts of alcohol have little, if any, effect on the nursing infant

Continued.

T A B L E 2 9 - 3 **Drugs excreted in human milk and the possible significance for nursing infants—cont'd**

Drug	Excreted	Quantity excreted	Significance
Central nervous system drugs—cont'd			
Amitriptyline (Elavil)	No		
Aspirin	Yes	Moderate amounts	It could cause a bleeding tendency by interfering with the function of the infant's platelets or by decreasing the amount of prothrombin in the blood. Risk is minimal if mother takes aspirin just after nursing and if the infant has an adequate store of vitamin K
Barbital (Veronal)	Yes	4-5 mg of diethylbarbituric acid/500 ml of milk detected after a single dose of 500 mg	Significant quantities, avoid administration; produced marked sedation in infant
Barbiturates	Yes		It appears that in therapeutic doses the barbiturates have little or no effect on the infant; one case was reported where high doses had a hypnotic effect on one infant; it is best to avoid administering, since barbiturates serve as inducing agents for hepatic drug metabolizing enzymes
Bromides (Bromo-Seltzer; many nonprescription sleeping aids)	Yes	0-6.6 mg/100 ml	Not to be administered; reactions range from rash to drowsiness
Caffeine	Yes	1% of that ingested	Not significant in usual amounts to affect child
Chloral hydrate (Noctec, Somnos)	Yes	0-1.5 mg/100 ml	Not significant in therapeutic doses
Chlorazepate (Tranxene)	Yes		Not to be administered based upon manufacturer's recommendation; may cause drowsiness
Chlordiazepoxide (Librium)	Yes		Not significant in therapeutic doses to affect child
Chloroform	Yes		One study performed in 1908 reported that a nursing infant slept for 8 hours; not significant in therapeutic doses
Chlorpromazine (Thorazine)	Yes	4.15 mg/ml after daily dose of 200 mg in dogs	Not significant; may cause galactorrhea
Codeine	Yes		Not significant in therapeutic doses to affect child
Cycloheptenyl ethyl barbituric acid (Medomin)	Yes		Not significant in therapeutic doses to affect child
Desipramine (Norpramin)	No		
Dextroamphetamine (Dexedrine)	No		
Diacetylmorphine (heroin)	Yes		Not enough to prevent withdrawal in addicted infants
Diazepam (Valium)	Yes	51 mg/ml after 4 days of diazepam; 28 mg/ml of N-demethyldiazepam	Recent studies recommend that this drug be avoided during nursing; infant reported as lethargic and experienced weight loss; may cause hyperbilirubinemia
Diphenhydramine (Benadryl)	Yes		Not significant in therapeutic doses to affect child
Flutenamic acid (Arlef)	Yes		Excreted in small amounts; no recommendations

T A B L E 29-3 **Drugs excreted in human milk and the possible significance for nursing infants—cont'd**

Drug	Excreted	Quantity excreted	Significance
Hydroxyphenbutazone (Tandearil)	Yes	0 in 53 of 55 mothers	Conflicting reports; both conclude that it would have no significant effect in therapeutic doses
Imipramine (Tofranil)	No		
Indomethacin (Indocin)	Yes		Not significant in therapeutic doses to affect child
Lithium carbonate (Eskalith, Lithane, Lithonate)	Yes	Same in child's serum as in mother's milk, 0.3 mEq/liter	Infant should be monitored for possible signs of lithium toxicity
Mefenamic acid (Ponstel)	Yes		Not significant in therapeutic doses to affect child
Meperidine (Demerol)	Yes		Not significant in therapeutic doses to affect child
Meprobamate (Miltown, Equanil)	Yes	Present in milk two to four times maternal plasma level	Infant should be monitored for possible signs of meprobamate toxication if therapy is to be continued
Mesoridazine besylate (Serentil)	Yes		Not significant in therapeutic doses to affect child
Morphine	Yes	Small amounts	Not significant in therapeutic doses to affect child
Pentazocine (Talwin)	No		
Phenobarbital (Luminal, others)	Yes		To be avoided where possible; serves as an inducing agent for hepatic drug metabolizing enzymes
Phenylbutazone (Butazolidin)	No	0.63 mg/100 ml 1½ hours after mother injected (IM) with 750 mg	No side effects noted among group studied, but because of possible lethal reactions infant should be closely monitored
Phenytoin (Dilantin)	Yes		Not significant in therapeutic doses although one case of methemoglobinemia was associated with phenytoin
Piperacetazine (Quide)	Yes		Manufacturer suggests it may have a great potential for excretion in milk
Primidone (Mysoline)	Yes		To be avoided, may cause undue somnolence and drowsiness
Prochlorperazine (Compazine)	Yes	0.4-1.5 mg/100 ml in dogs after daily dose of 200 mg	Not significant in therapeutic doses to affect child
Propoxyphene HCl (Darvon)	Yes	0.4% of dose to mother found in stomach of nursing rat	Not significant in therapeutic doses to affect child
Salicylates	Yes	1.0-3.0 mg/100 ml of sodium salicylate detected 4 hours after maternal dose of 4 g	Not significant in therapeutic doses; high doses (5 g/day) have been reported to cause a rash in infant
Thiopental sodium (Pentothal)	Yes		Not significant in therapeutic doses to affect child
Thioridazine (Mellaril)	Yes		Not significant in therapeutic doses to affect child
Tranylcypromine (Parnate)	Yes		Not significant in therapeutic doses to affect child
Trifluoperazine (Stelazine)	Yes	0.4-1.5 mg/100 ml in dogs after daily dose of 200 mg	Not significant in therapeutic doses to affect child

Continued.

TABLE 29-3 Drugs excreted in human milk and the possible significance for nursing infants—cont'd

Drug	Excreted	Quantity excreted	Significance
Diagnostic agents			
Carotene (natural product found in carrots)	Yes		One incident reported where infant turned yellow; mother ate 2-3 lb of carrots per week; not significant in average quantities
Iopanoic acid (Telepaque)	Yes		Not significant in therapeutic doses to affect child
Electrolytic, caloric, and water balance			
Cyclamate (Sucaryl)	Yes		Not significant in therapeutic doses to affect child
Cyclopenthiazide (Navidrix)	No		
Furosemide (Lasix)	No		
Hydrochlorothiazide (Hydro-Diuril, Esidrix, others)	Yes		To be avoided, based on manufacturer's recommendation; no specific adverse effects reported in infants to date
Spironolactone (Aldactone)	No		
Thiazides	Yes		To be avoided based on manufacturer's recommendation; no specific adverse reactions reported in infants to date
Expectorants and cough preparations			
Potassium iodide	Yes	3 mg/100 ml	To be avoided, may affect infant's thyroid
Gastrointestinal drugs			
Aloe	Yes		Controversial, one author claims it may give rise to catharsis in some infants; others feel its presence is insignificant
Anthraquinone (Dorbane, Dorbantyl, Danthron, Peri-Colace, Doxidan, Dialose-Plus)	Yes		One animal study found it present in milk and in "significant" amounts; another human study did not detect it; a third human study detected it and felt it best not to administer it to nursing mothers, as it may cause catharsis in the infant
Cascara	Yes		Avoid where possible; reported to have increased gastric motility in infant
Emodin (found in cascara sagrada)	Yes		Avoid where possible; reported to have increased gastric motility in infant
Phenolphthalein (found in many nonprescription laxative products)	Yes		Not significant in therapeutic doses to affect child
Rhubarb	Yes		Not significant in therapeutic doses to affect child
Senna	Yes		Not significant in therapeutic doses; high doses may cause diarrhea in nursing infant
Hormones and synthetic substitutes			
Carbimazole (Neo-Mercazole)	Yes		Not to be administered; antithyroid may cause goiter in nursing infant
Chlormadione (Estalor-21)	Yes		Possible effects must be weighed against risk of pregnancy

T A B L E 2 9 - 3 Drugs excreted in human milk and the possible significance
for nursing infants—cont'd

Drug	Excreted	quantity excreted	Significance
Chlorotrianisene (TACE)	Yes		Avoid where possible estrogenic substances may be in breast secretions
Contraceptives (oral)	Yes		Possible effects must be weighed against risk of pregnancy; may inhibit lactation if administered during first prenatal weeks; possible gynecomastia in male infant
Corticotropin	Yes		Destroyed during passage through gastrointestinal tract; its presence in milk is unimportant
Cortisone	Yes		No human study; among animals a 50% lower weight than control, retarded sexual development, exophthalmos
Dihydrotachysterol (Hytakerol)	Yes		May cause hypercalcemia
Estrogen (oral contraceptives)	Yes	0.17 µg/100 mg	Possible effects must be weighed against risk of pregnancy
Ethisterone (Pranone)	Yes		To be avoided; may cause significant skeletal advancement
Fluoxymesterone (Halotestin, Ora-testryl, Ultandren)			Used to suppress lactation
Iodides (nonradioactive)	Yes	After a dose of 0.6 g (as potassium salt) 68 mg was recovered	To be avoided, chronic use may affect infant's thyroid gland
Liothyronine sodium (Cytomel)	No		
Lyndiol	Yes		To be avoided; caused a diminution in milk protein and milk fat
Lynestrenol (oral contraceptive under investigation)	Yes		Possible effects must be weighed against risk of pregnancy
Medroxyprogesterone actates (Provera)	No		
Mestranol (estrogenic compound found in several oral contraceptives)	Yes		Possible effects must be weighed against risk of pregnancy
Norethindrone (Norlutin)	Yes		Possible effect must be weighed against risk of pregnancy
Norethisterone ethanate (progesterone contraceptives)	Yes		Possible effects must be weighed against risk of pregnancy
Norethynodrel (Enovid)	Yes	1.1% of dose	Possible effects must be weighed against risk of pregnancy
Phenformin HCl (DBI)	Yes		Not significant; does not exert hypoglycemic effect on normal subject
Pregnane-3 (α), 20 (β)-diol	Yes		Although it may cause unconjugated hyperbilirubinemia in breastfed infants it was regarded as not being significant enough to stop nursing
Thiouracil	Yes	Higher in milk than in blood 9-12 mg/100 ml	To be avoided; may cause goiter in nursing infatn or agranulocytosis
Thyroid	Yes		Not significant in therapeutic doses to affect child
Tolbutamide (Orinase)	Yes		Not significant in therapeutic doses to affect child

Continued.

TABLE 29-3 Drugs excreted in human milk and the possible significance for nursing infants—cont'd

Drug	Excreted	Quantity excreted	Significance
Radioactive agents			
Gallium 67 (gallium citrate)	Yes		Avoid where possible; radionuclides are generally contraindicated during nursing, or nursing should be temporarily stopped
Iodine, radioactive (^{131}I)	Yes	Total in 48 hours of milk; 1.3 µCi after maternal dose of 29.5 µCi	To be avoided; affects infant's thyroid gland
Sodium, radioactive, as sodium chloride	Yes	0.5%-1.3% of dose per liter of milk	Not significant in therapeutic dose, although it is best to avoid the radionuclides if possible
Serums, toxoids, and vaccines			
Diphtheria antibodies	Yes	Less than 0.30% of dose administered	Of no value in conferring passive immunity to infant
Skin and mucous membrane preparations			
DDT	Yes	5 mg/100 ml	The concentration is higher in human milk than in bovine milk; DDT poisoning
Vitamins			
Calciferol (vitamine D)	Yes		Caution advised; may cause hypercalcemia
Cyanocobalamin (vitamin B_{12})	Yes	0.1-0.4 µg/liter	Not significant in therapeutic doses to affect child
Folic acid	Yes	0.7 µg/liter	Not significant in therapeutic doses to affect child
Phytonadione (vitamin K_1, AquaMEPHYTON)	Yes		Not significant in therapeutic doses to affect child
Thiamine (vitamine B_1) deficiency	Yes	10-13 µ/liter	A lack of this B vitamn in the nursing mother (beriberi) causes the excretion of a toxic substance, methylglyoxal, which has caused infant death
Miscellaneous agents			
Allergens (eggs, wheat flax seed, peanuts, cottonseed, etc.)	Yes		May cause allergic response in sensitive child
Colchicine	Yes		A 1929 study indicated that this drug may pass into milk; no adverse effect reported
Fluorides (found in many toothpastes)	Yes		Not significant in quantities ingested; excess could affect tooth enamel
Hexachlorobenzene	No		Avoid use as an insecticide; has caused infant mortality
Mercury	Yes		Environmental contaminant; signs of mercury intoxication and CNS effects
Nicotine	Yes	0.4-0.5 mg/liter; 11 to 20 cigarettes/day	In moderation, no effect; not more than 20 cigarettes/day
Ribonucleic acid (RNA)	Yes		Particles from human milk contain a reverse transcriptase and high molecular weight RNA that serves as a template; these particles have two features diagnostic of known RNA tumor viruses

ing such effects. The purpose of this section is to consider recent developments from biomedical and clinical research regarding the effects of drugs in common usage on sexual behavior in humans.

Drugs that may impair libido and sexual function

Drugs that have an adverse effect on sexual function and activity may do so through an overall depressive effect on the central nervous system, through a more specific action on a portion of the autonomic nervous system that affects sexual function, or through a combination of both. Male potency in particular seems to be susceptible to the effects of drugs that interact with the autonomic nervous system. This section describes some of these drugs, which comprise a surprisingly large variety of clinically administered and prescribed agents in use today.

The autonomic nervous system consists of nerves, ganglia, and plexuses that are distributed throughout the body to provide innervation for the automatic function of various body organs. Included under the control of this system are the sex organs and associated glands and blood vessels. The two main anatomic divisions of the autonomic nervous system, the sympathetic (adrenergic) outflow and the parasympathetic (cholinergic) outflow, are viewed as physiologic antagonists. Often, however, these systems function cooperatively, as in their synergistic effect on sexual function.

In the male adrenergic impulses produce ejaculation by causing contraction of the prostate and seminal vesicles in association with an effect on the bulbocavernous and ischiocavernous muscles. Drugs that block adrenergic impulses may affect ejaculatory function as a result of sympathetic blockade.

On the other hand, parasympathetic stimulation controls penile erection. This response is secondary to congestion of the vascular sinuses in the corpora resulting from parasympathetic nerve action in the venous channels. Drugs that interfere with parasympathetic nerve transmission will block this function.

Ganglionic blocking agents, which may simultaneously block both sympathetic and parasympathetic nerve function, may result in complete impotence and therefore sexual dysfunction.

ANTIHYPERTENSIVE DRUGS

Some drugs have been successfully used in the treatment of high blood pressure because of the vasodilation they produce by means of blockade of the sympathetic nervous system. Such adrenergic inhibition, however, occasionally results in impotence and concomitant decrease in sexual function. Guanethidine (Ismelin) and reserpine (Serpasil), which act partially by depleting the adrenergic nerve transmitter norepinephrine, (originating from nerve endings) or by blocking release of the transmitter from the nerve terminal, may produce impotence by inactivation of the nervous mechanisms responsible for sexual function. Experiments with guanethidine have shown that erectile potency, ability to ejaculate, and intensity of climax were all reduced significantly during use of this drug. Similar observations have been made with reserpine, which additionally has central effects that lead to a decrease in libido and to male impotence. In women reserpine has been shown to block ovulation, cause infertility and pseudopregnancy, and induce lactation. All these actions may have a profound effect on sexual function and behavior.

Anticholinergic drugs and especially those with ganglionic blocking activity may also produce impotence and other untoward effects on sexual function. In addition to guanethidine, which falls into this category, mecamylamine (Inversine) and trimethaphan (Arfonad) are used as antihypertensive agents and are included in this group. Since these drugs may block both sympathetic and parasympathetic innervation of the sex organs, both erectile capability and ejaculatory function may be affected during their use.

Another drug used in the treatment of hypertension is spironolactone (Aldactone), a diuretic. This drug acts by displacement of aldosterone in the kidneys, thus interfering with the normal resorption of sodium ions. Sexual dysfunction in both men and women has been reported in association with the use of this drug. Amenorrhea was observed in six women who took spironolactone for 9 months, with normal menses returning within 2 months after drug therapy was discontinued. Gynecomastia and impotence in men have also been observed during spironolactone therapy.

ANTIDEPRESSANTS

Depression includes emotional disorders ranging from mild despondence without somatic manifestations to severely retarded states and suicidal risks. In contemporary society, characterized by increased demands on both time and ability as a way of life, depression and its manifestations are becoming more and more common. Depression is usually accompanied by decreased sexual drive, interest, and activity.

Treatment of depression by either psychologic support or relief from stressful conditions often results in a return of normal sexual interest and behavior. Often, however, the use of antidepressant drug therapy is recommended. Some such agents, unfortunately, have the inherent capacity to promote the development of impotence and to adversely affect other aspects of sexual behavior. Thus the positive aspects of these drugs resulting from mood elevation may be counterbalanced by the negative effects of these drugs on sexual function.

Two categories of antidepressant drugs are currently in use. The first group consists of chemicals known as tricyclic compounds and includes imipramine (Tofranil), desipramine (Norpramin, Pertofrane), amitriptyline (Elavil), nortriptyline (Aventyl), and protriptyline (Vivactil). Although the antidepressant effects of these drugs is not clearly understood, their peripheral anticholinergic effects are similar to those produced by the antihypertensive agents. The untoward effects on sexual function are attributed primarily to the anticholinergic actions of these drugs. Thus the tricyclic compounds are most often associated with the development of male impotence.

The second group of drugs used as antidepressants are the monoamine oxidase (MAO) inhibitors. These drugs are also used as antihypertensive agents. Their primary mechanism of action is blockade of the enzyme monoamine oxidase in the brain and in adrenergic nerve terminals. Substances normally oxidized by MAO, especially serotonin and norepinephrine, therefore accumulate and in some way produce stimulation of mood.

Two types of MAO inhibitors are currently available for clinical or therapeutic use: the hydrazine derivatives, which include phenelzine sulfate (Nardil) and pargyline (Eutonyl). Impotence may result from the use of these drugs because of their tendency to block peripheral ganglionic nerve transmission.

ANTIHISTAMINES

Histamine is a naturally occurring substance that possesses a variety of physiologic properties, including smooth muscle stimulation, mediation of the inflammatory response, and cardiovascular effects. Antihistaminic drugs act as competitive inhibitors of histamine at physiologic receptor sites and prevent its action. Well-known examples of such drugs include diphenhydramine (Benadryl), promethazine (Phenergan), and chlorpheniramine (Chlor-Trimeton). These drugs are annually consumed by millions for use as antiemetics, as mild sedatives, and for the control of allergy and cold symptoms. Most antihistamines display anticholinergic effects such as dryness of the mouth, urinary retention, and constipation. Continuous use of these drugs may result in interference with sexual activity. This effect is presumably mediated by means of the blockade of parasympathetic nerve impulses to the sex glands and organs.

ANTISPASMODICS

For the most part, antispasmodic drugs are quaternary ammonium compounds. Their primary effect is relaxation of the smooth muscle of the gastrointestinal tract, bilary tract, ureter, and uterus. Because these drugs may act as ganglionic blocking agents, postural hypotension and impotence may result from their use. Drugs in this category include methantheline (Banthine), glycopyrrolate (Robinul), hexocyclium (Tral), and poldine (Nacton).

SEDATIVES AND TRANQUILIZERS

A wide variety of sedatives and tranquilizers has become available in recent years. Many of these drugs have both direct and indirect effects on sexual interest and capability. Two of the most frequently used classes of tranquilizers include the phenothiazines and the benzodiazepine compounds. Several minor categories of sedative drugs may also affect sexual function.

Phenothiazines comprise one of the most widely used classes of drugs in medical practice today. More than 30 phenothiazines with a broad spectrum of action are currently available. Known as the major tranquilizers, phenothiazines are primarly used in the treatment of psychosis, but they have additional use as antiemetics and analgesics. Chlorpromazine (Thorazine, Megaphen) is the bestknown example; others include prochlorperazine (Compazine), thioridazine (Mellaril), and mesoridazine (Serentil). Although the details of the mechanism of the sedative effect of the phenothiazines are not fully understood, these drugs are thought to act by modifying sensory input into the reticular formation of the brainstem. The sedative effect may partially account for a decrease in interest in sexual activity of persons undergoing phenothiazine therapy.

In addition to their central effects, these drugs exert a variety of peripheral actions that may also contribute to inhibition of sexual function. Phenothiazines decrease skeletal muscle tone and block cholinergic synapses at both muscarinic and nicotinic receptors. Inhibition of various adrenergic impulses may occur as well. Impotence, decreased libido, and ejaculation disorders have been reported in cases of patients taking phenothiazines. Failure to ejaculate has been reported in men treated with thioridazine, although erection and orgasm do not appear to be affected. Ejaculation problems have also been reported in association with the use of chlorprothixene (Taractan) and mesoridazine (Serentil).

Chlorpromazine may also influence sexual function by affecting the endocrine glands, possibly through acting on the hypothalamus. In animal studies phenothiazine derivatives have been shown to cause a suppression of hypothalamic and pituitary function, resulting in decreased secretion of hormones affecting the function of sex organs in both males and females. Chlorpromazine has been shown to be spermicidal in dogs and to reduce the copula-

tion rate of male rats. Regressive and atrophic changes in the testes of experimental animals receiving phenothiazines have also been reported. Chlorpromazine has been shown to reduce urinary levels of gonadotropins as well as estrogens and progestins. As with reserpine, chlorpromazine blocks ovulation, suppresses estrous cycles in animals, induces lactation, and maintains a decidual reaction. The release of pituitary gonadotropins by relatively small doses of chlorpromazine has been shown to delay ovulation and menstruation in female patients. Prolonged amenorrhea has been reported to accompany treatment with certain phenothiazine derivatives.

Benzodiazepine compounds comprise the second widely used class of tranquilizing drugs. The two best known are chlordiazepoxide (Librium) and diazepam (Valium). As mild tranquilizers, both drugs are used in the treatment of anxiety, as skeletal muscle relaxants, and in the treatment of alcoholism. Impairment of sexual function has been associated with the effects of chlordiazepoxide and diazepam on the activity of both cholinergic and adrenergic facets of the autonomic nervous system. As with the phenothiazine derivatives, ejaculation problems have been reported for patients using chlordiazepoxide. Aspermia, the absence of ejaculation during coitus or masturbation, has also been reported in association with the use of chlordiazepoxide. The definitive sedative and relaxing activity of these drugs may also account for the decreased interest in sexual activity observed in patients using them. Alternatively, the efficacious use of these tranquilizers has been considered of value in the treatment of sexual impotence and other problems involving sexual performance.

Several other types of drugs used in the treatment of psychologic problems have been shown to depress sexual activity in human beings. Benperidol, a sedative and mild tranquilizer, has been shown to have antilibidinous effects in men. In a study of sex offenders, benperidol was effective in abolishing sexual desire and the ability to maintain an erection. Failure to ejaculate without concomitant alteration of erection or orgasm has been reported in patients treated with phenoxybenzamine (Dibenzyline), an alpha adrenergic blocking agent once used as an adjunct to psychiatric therapy. The potent sympatholytic effects of this drug have been advanced to account for the adverse effects on sexual function. Lithium carbonate has also been associated with disturbed sexual function in patients treated with this drug for mania.

ETHYL ALCOHOL

Ethyl alcohol deserves to be considered for its effects on human sexual function and behavior as a drug of individual and unique notoriety. Revered for centuries as a sexual stimulant and cure of all ills, alcohol is in fact a depressant and is recognized today to have far greater social than therapeutic value. Although a sedative, alcohol in moderate amounts may help to enhance sexual activity by relieving anxieties and loosening the inhibition that often shroud sexual behavior. Beyond a certain limit, however, neither desire nor virility will overcome the depression of physical capability that occurs under its influence.

Studies on the pharmacologic action of alcohol have shown that the central nervous system is more affected by alcohol than any other system of the body. Electrophysiologic studies suggest that alcohol exerts its first depressant effect on the reticular activating system, a part of the brain responsible for the integration of activity in various parts of the nervous system. The cortex is thus released from integrating control, with the result that various processes related to thought and motor activities become disrupted. The first mental processes to be affected are those related to sobriety and self-restraint. The result is a less inhibited and less restrained approach to sexual behavior and other activities normally inhibited by previous training or experience. Subsequent to the continued consumption of alcohol, however, the brain becomes narcotized, reflexes become retarded, blood vessels are dilated, and the capacity for sexual function is diminished. In addition, alcohol produces a severe diuretic effect, which also interferes with sexual function.

Alcohol may also precipitate a negative social orientation with regard to sexual behavior. Alcohol overindulgence by males has been shown to be a frequent cause of forcible sexual assault on females. In a study in which various types of sexual offenders were assessed for frequency of offense, drunk persons constituted 12% to 16% of reported incidents. In these cases alcoholic consumption had not ensued to the point of physical incapacitation but rather to a stage characterized by confusion, belligerence, and misinterpretation, resulting in violent antisocial acts. Thus, although initially permitting a less inhibited approach to sexual behavior, alcohol eventually decreases the capability and enjoyment of sexual activities through both physical incapacitation and depression of a rational approach to sexual behavior.

BARBITURATES

Barbiturates, such as amobarbital (Amytal), pentobarbital (Nembutal), secobarbital (Seconal), and thiopental (Pentothal), are sedative-hypnotic drugs that produce a wide range of general depressant effects on all nervous tissues. As with alcohol, these drugs, when taken in prescribed dosage, produce relaxation, hypnosis, and sleep with concomitant depression of a wide range of body functions, including sexual performance and ability. With prolonged use or overdose barbiturates can cause respiratory failure and death. Withdrawal following continued heavy consumption of barbiturates may precipitate convulsions. There is no rationale for their usege in altering sexual behavior in human beings.

SEX HORMONE PREPARATIONS

In recent years it has been observed that sex hormones may act on parts of the central nervous system and other organs of the body to influence sexual and aggressive behavior, as well as mood and emotional outlook. Thus variations in female hormones may produce anxiety, irritability, and depression, whereas male hormones are associated with aggression and increased sexual interest. Currently, there is growing evidence that the sexual drives of both men and women may be influenced by treatment with sex hormones. In one study male hormones prescribed to women were shown to increase sexual interest and enjoyment, whereas male patients with the female hormone estrogen almost always experienced a decrease or cessation of libido.

These observations have now been extended to the production of synthetic sex hormone preparations, many of which have been shown to influence sexual behavior. The antiandrogen steroid, cyproterone acetate, decreases libido and potency and has been successfully used in the treatment of hypersexuality in adult males. Synthetic estrogens and progesterones have, of course, found wide acceptance as oral contraceptive agents. Another class of synthetic sex hormones are the anabolic steroids, which are derivatives of the male sex hormone, testosterone. These drugs, which include methandrostenolne (Dianabol), nandrolone phenpropionate (Durabolin), and norethandrolone (Nilevar), are used clinically to promote nitrogen retention and weight gain in elderly or undernourished patients. In recent years considerable controversy has arisen over the use and misuse of these drugs by athletes and other postpubertal persons to promote muscle growth and endurance. When used by normally developed, well-nourished individuals, the anabolic effects of these drugs on strength and development are questionable. These is even considerable evidence that sexual activity may be adversely affected by these drugs because of their antigonadotropic effects on sexual function. These effects have been dramatically demonstrated in men treated with norethandrolone for 8 to 25 weeks who showed loss of libido, decreased potency, diminished testicular size, and azoospermia. Although recovery from most of these effects occurred in most patients within 6 months after treatment was stopped, testicular morphology remained abnormal, and it was questionable whether normal sexual function would ever be regained.

METHADONE

Methadone, a drug widely used in heroin withdrawal and narcotics maintenance programs, has been found to produce both serious fertility problems and impaired sexual performance in male users of the drug. Fertility changes are associated with a pronounced reduction in the size and secretory activity of the secondary sex organs, resulting in extremely low ejaculate volume and low sperm motility. Whether this condition is reversible after withdrawal from the drug is not yet known, although animal studies suggest that normal secondary sex organ function will return after discontinuance of methadone treatment.

Drugs that may enhance libido and sexual function

The search for substances that increase sexual potency or drive has existed almost as long as civilization itself. Inscriptions found in the ruins of ancient cultures have described the preparation of "erotic potions," and an endless number of "aphrodisiacs" have been described since then to modern times. In contemporary society the continuous proliferation of drugs and chemicals that modify mood and behavior has enhanced the claim that many such drugs have aphrodisiac properties, and more and more agents are considered by some to fulfill this purpose.

In reality there are no known drugs that specifically increase libido or sexual performance, and every chemical taken for this purpose, without medical advice and especially in combination with other drugs, poses the danger of drug interaction or overdose. However, a number of pharmacologically active agents are capable of temporarily modifying both physiologic responsiveness and subjective perception in such a manner as to enhance the enjoyment, if not the fulfillment, of the sex act. Some of these agents are considered in this section.

Cantharis

Cantharis (cantharidin, Spanish fly), a legendary sexual stimulant, is in reality a powerful irritant and potent systemic poison. A powder made from dried beetles (*Cantharis vesicatoria*) found in southern Europe, cantharis is capable of producing severe illness characterized by vomiting, diarrhea, abdominal pain, and shock. When taken internally, it causes irritation and inflammation of the genitourinary tract and dilation of the blood vessels of the penis and clitoris, producing in some instances prolonged erections or engorgement, usually without an increase in sexual desire. Deaths have been reported from the promiscuous use of cantharis as an aphrodisiac. It is currently recognized that cantharis is not an effective sexual stimulant, and it is seldom used in modern medical practice.

Yohimbine

Another natural substance with supposed aphrodisiac properties is yohimbine, an alkaloid derived from the west African tree *Corynanthe yohimbe.* Yohimbine produces a competitive alpha adrenergic blockage of limited duration and antidiuresis, probably from the release of an antidiuretic hormone. Although yohimbine stimulates the lower spinal nerve centers controlling erection, there is no convincing evidence that it acts as a sexual stimulant. It currently has no therapeutic uses.

Narcotics and psychoactive agents

The use of drugs such as morphine, heroin, cocaine, marijuana, LSD, and amphetamines as aphrodisiacs has become somewhat prevalent in contemporary society, and there is little doubt that these agents can under certain circumstances enhance the enjoyment of the sexual experience for some. More commonly, however, there is a decrease in sexual behavior for those who try them. The reason for such variation in responsiveness is that these agents have no particular properties that specifically increase sexual potency but rather they tend to affect the user according to the particular circumstances under which they are used. Thus the state of mind of the individual user and the amount consumed contribute considerably to the effect achieved. As with alcohol, these drugs act on the central nervous system to release inhibitions, which are often the cause of problems involving sexual behavior; taken in excess or too often, however, these drugs will have the opposite response and will inhibit sexual drive and function.

Recent studies have shown that both morphine and heroin in sufficient doses produce marked reduction in sexual activity in men and women users. In men nonemissive erections and impotence can result. The reduction in sexual potency is complicated in narcotics users who are concomitantly taking other types of

drug therapy, especially considering the potent addicting powers of the narcotic agents.

Marijuana (cannabis), an extract of the *Cannabis sativa* plant, is considered by many to be a sexual stimulant. However, as with alcohol, its effect results indirectly from relaxation and release of inhibitions surrounding sexual activity. The active ingredient in marijuana is tetrahydrocannabinol; the pharmacologic effects resulting from smoking marijuana depend on the personality of the user, the dose, and the prevailing circumstances. Most commonly, the effects of marijuana are a distortion of time and an enhanced suggestibility, producing the illusion that sexual climax is somewhat prolonged. Thus the subjective consideration of the user of marijuana as an aphrodisiac may enhance enjoyment of the sex act. Studies on the properties of marijuana for a specific effect on sexual behavior, however, have shown that it has no such properties. On the contrary, there is evidence that marijuana smokers have a higher incidence of decreased libido and impaired potency than nonusers. In addition, chronic intensive use of marijuana has been shown to depress plasma testosterone levels in healthy males and has produced gynecomastia in some users.

Lysergic acid diethylamide (LSD) is another drug that, although considered an aphrodisiac by some, has potentially untoward effects on sexual function and behavior. As with marijuana, any alteration of sexual performance produced by LSD is principally subjective; the effects of this drug are almost entirely on the central nervous system. Little response, if any, has been seen in other organ systems that can be attributed to a direct effect of LSD, and there is no biochemical or pharmacologic evidence to support the contention that LSD or similar drugs contain any sex-stimulating properties. On the other hand, the repeated use of LSD may produce serious psychologic problems, which could have an overall adverse effect on sexual interest or activity. The use of LSD during pregnancy may cause a higher rate of malformed babies or stillbirths than in nonusers.

Amphetamines (Benzedrine, Dexedrine, Methedrine) have also been utilized for the purpose of stimulating sexual function. These drugs have a powerful central stimulant action, in addition to peripheral alpha and beta sympathomimetic effects. The main results of an oral dose of 10 to 30 mg are wakefulness and alertness, mood elevation, increased motor and speech activity, and often elation and euphoria. Physical performance is usually improved, and fatigue can be prevented or reversed. The effects of amphetamines on sexual performance, however, are quite inconsistent. At moderate dosage levels there is seldom any effect on sexual behavior, aside from the accompanying elevation of mood or reversal of fatigue. Doses in the range of 20 to 50 mg have been reported to alter sensations so as to enhance the orgasmic feeling. However, higher doses, such as 1 g taken intravenously, will produce loss of interest and withdrawal from sexual activity.

Amphetamines, along with other psychoactive agents, will do little to promote the enjoyment of sexual activity and may produce in the long run adverse psychologic and physical effects that may reduce sexual interest and capability.

OTHER DRUGS THAT MAY STIMULATE SEXUAL BEHAVIOR

A number of clinically used or experimental drugs have been shown to enhance sexual interest or potency in both patients and laboratory animals. This effect seems to occur independent of their prescribed intention or use.

L-Dopa

Levodihydroxyphenylalanine (L-dopa) is a natural intermediate in the biosynthesis of catecholamines in the brain and peripheral adrenergic nerve terminals. In the biologic sequence of events it is converted to dopamine, which in turn serves as a substrate of the neurotransmitter norepinephrine. L-Dopa has been used with gratifying success in the treatment of Parkinson's syndrome, a disease of the basal ganglia characterized by dopamine deficiency. When L-dopa is administered to a parkinsonian patient, amelioration of the symptoms is observed, presumably because of the conversion of the drug to dopamine. Recently it has been observed that patients, especially elderly men, who are

being treated with L-dopa experience a sexual rejuvenation. It was to this effect that the sexual stimulating powers of L-dopa have been attributed. Consequently, studies with younger men complaining of decreased erectile ability have similary shown that L-dopa increases libido and incidence of penile erections. Overall, however, these effects were short-lived and did not promote satisfactory sexual function and potency. Thus it is conceded that L-dopa is not a true aphrodisiac but that increased sexual activity experienced by parkinsonian patients treated with L-dopa reflects an improvement of well-being, along with partial recovery of normal sexual functions that were impaired by Parkinson's disease.

p-Chlorophenylalanine (PCPA)

PCPA, a drug chemically related to L-dopa, has been claimed to have potent aphrodisiac properties in laboratory animals. Currently, considerable controversy characterizes the potential sex-stimulating powers of this drug, which is used experimentally as a selective blocker of serotonin biosynthesis in the brain. In one report, PCPA, when used with the monoamine oxidase inhibitor phenelzine, significantly increased the sexual deficiency. The sexual improvement paralleled the amelioration of headaches and mood. Since PCPA has not yet come into clinical usage, it is not known what direct effects it may have on human libido or sexual ability.

Amyl nitrite

Amyl nitrite, a drug used in the treatment of angina pectoris, is alleged to enhance sexual activity in humans. As a vasodilator and smooth muscle stimulant, amyl nitrite has been reported to intensify the orgasmic experience if inhaled at the moment of orgasm. This effect is probably the result of relaxation of smooth muscles and consequent vasodilation of the genitourinary tract. No effects of amyl nitrite on libido or sexual function have been reported.

Vitamin E

Much has been said in recent years about the positive effects of vitamin E (alpha-tocopherol)

TABLE 29-4 Drug effects on human sexual behavior

Drug or drug category	Principal effect	Probable mechanism of action

Antihypertensives
  Guanethidine (Ismelin)
  Mecamylamine (Inversine)
  Reserpine (Serpasil)
  Spironolactone (Aldactone)
  Trimethaphan (Arfonad)
	Negative	Peripheral blockade of nervous innervation of sex glands

Antidepressants
  Amitriptyline (Elavil)
  Desipramine (Norpramin, Pertofrane)
  Imipramine (Tofranil)
  Nortriptyline (Aventyl)
  Pargyline (Eutonyl)
  Phenelzine sulfate (Nardil)
  Protriptyline (Vivactil)
  Tranylcypromine sulfate (Parnate)
	Negative	Central depression; peripheral blockade of nervous innervation of sex glands

Antihistamines
  Chlorpheniramine (Chlor-Trimeton)
  Diphenhydramine (Benadryl)
  Promethazine (Phenergan)
	Negative	Blockade of parasympathetic nervous innervation of sex glands

Antispasmodics
  Glycopyrrolate (Robinul)
  Hexocyclium (Tral)
  Methantheline (Banthine)
  Poldine (Nacton)
	Negative	Ganglionic blockage of nervous innervation of sex glands

Sedatives and tranquilizers
  Benperidol
  Chlordiazepoxide (Librium)
  Chlorpromazine (Thorazine, Megaphen)
  Chlorprothixene (Taractan)
  Diazepam (Valium)
  Mesoridazine (Serentil)
  Phenoxybenzamine (Dibenzyline)
  Prochlorperazine (Compazine)
  Thioridazine (Mellaril)
	Negative
	
	Transiently positive
		Central sedation; blockade of autonomic innervation of sex glands; suppression of hypothalamic and pituitary function
		Tranquilization and relaxation

Ethyl alcohol	Negative Transiently positive	Central depression; suppression of motor activity; diuresis Release of inhibitions; relaxation
Barbiturates	Negative	Central depression; suppression of motor activity; hypnosis

Sex hormone preparations
  Cyproterone acetate
  Methandrostenolone (Dianabol)
  Nandrolane phenpropionate (Durabolin)
  Norethandrolone (Nilevar)
	Negative	Antiandrogenic effects on sexual function; loss of libido; decreased potency

Methadone	Negative	Suppresses secondary sex organ function in male
Cantharis (Spanish fly)	Negative	Irritation and inflammation of genitourinary tract, systemic poisoning
Yohimbine	Questionable	Stimulation of lower spinal nerve centers

Narcotics and psychoactive drugs
  Amphetamines
  Cocaine
  Heroin
  LSD
  Marijuana
  Morphine
	Negative
	
	Transiently positive
		Central depression; decreased libido and impaired potency
		Release of inhibitions; increased suggestibility; relaxation

L-Dopa and p-chlorophenylalanine (PCPA)	Questionable	Improvement of well-being
Amyl nitrite	Questionable	Vasodilation of genitourinary tract; smooth muscle relaxation
Vitamin E	Questionable	Supports fertility in laboratory animals

Adapted from Woods, J.S.: Drug effects on human sexual behavior. In Woods, N.F.: Human sexuality in health and illness, ed. 2, St Louis, 1979, The C.V. Mosby Co.

on sexual performance and ability in human beings. Unfortunately, there is little scientific rationale to substantiate such claims. The primary reasons for attributing a positive role in sexual performance to vitamin E come mainly from experiments on vitamin E deficiency in laboratory animals. In such experiments the principal manifestation of this deficiency is infertility, although the reasons for this condition differ in males and females. In female rats there is no loss in ability to produce apparently healthy ova, nor is there a defect in the placenta or uterus. However, fetal death occurs shortly after the first week of embryonic life, and fetuses are reabsorbed. This situation can be prevented if vitamin E is administered any time up to the fifth or sixth day of embryonic life. In the male rat the earliest observable effect of vitamin E deficiency is immobility of spermatozoa, with subsequent degeneration of the germinal epithelium. However, there is no alteration in the secondary sex organs or diminution of sexual vigor, although the latter may occur with continued vitamin E deficiency. Because of experimental results such as these, it has been thought that vitamin E could restore or preserve virility, fertility, sexual interest, potency, and endurance in humans. There is no evidence to support any of these contentions, but since sexual performance is often influenced by mental attitude, a person who believes vitamin E may improve sexual prowess may actually find such improvement.

A listing of drugs that may affect libido and sexual functioning is given in Table 29-4.

Drugs used to treat sexually transmitted and related diseases

Sexually transmitted diseases (STDs) have reached epidemic proportions in America. They are increasingly frequent among teenagers, who show an incredible lack of knowledge about these conditions. For example, one study showed that 40% of 200 adolescent girls thought that taking birth control pills would prevent venereal disease.

STDs are spreading mainly because sexual activity is increasing, especially among young people, because symptoms may be minimal and spread easily, because sexual partners are not always informed by the one afflicted, and because barrier methods of contraception such as the condom have lost favor. Dilemmas associated with STDs include embarrassment, inconvenience, pain, itch, alienation, sterility, and death.

Table 29-5 lists common sexually transmitted diseases and conditions and their usual treatment. Note that the FDA has announced that there is no evidence that vaginal sulfonamides can be considered effective for infections caused by *Candida*, *Trichomonas*, or *Haemophilus* (*Gardnerella* [new classification under study]).

Though most STDs are often more symptomatic in women, both partners should usually be treated to prevent recurrence. Patients should be forewarned that topical self-treatment of mucous membranes for discomfort by benzocaine or cortisone compounds occasionally results in incapacitating local allergic reactions. Measures effective in preventing STDs include selectivity in coital partners, prompt hygiene, avoidance of actions that promote vaginal pH changes (oral contraception, broad-spectrum antibiotic therapy, untreated diabetes mellitus, alkaline soaps and bubble baths), mild douching after menses, and substitution of the condom as a mechanical barrier to organism transmission. Topical application of cultured yogurt is thought to facilitate healthful pH in the vagina.

TOXIC SHOCK SYNDROME

Toxic shock syndrome is a severe illness characterized by sudden onset of high fever with vomiting, diarrhea, and myalgia, followed by the development of hypotension and possibly shock. A sunburnlike rash is present during the acute phase, and 10 days after onset there is a desquamation (peeling) of the skin of the palms and soles of the feet. Trauma resulting from tampon use during menses and the bacterium *Staphylococcus aureus* have been implicated. Beta-lactamase-resistant antistaphylococcal antibiotics are recommended as particularly effective in preventing recurrences.

TABLE 29-5 Common sexually transmitted diseases or conditions*

Condition	Cause	Symptoms	Treatments
Gonorrhea (the second most commonly reported communicable disease, following upper respiratory infection)	*Neisseria gonorrhoeae*	May be variable At first, creamy yellow discharge and burning sensation on urination Often unnoticed by women	Procaine penicillin G, 4.8 million units in one dose IM (half in each buttock) Tetracycline, 1.5 g in one dose, then 0.5 g every 6 hours for 4 days† Ampicillin, 3.5 g† Spectinomycin, 2 g. IM Doxycycline hyclate, orally (Children's dosages vary)
Herpes	Herpes simplex virus (HSV), type 2 and occasionally type 1 (usually orally transmitted)	Painful, itching vesicles on genitals up to 20 days after contact and lasting 2 to 3 weeks Fever with flu-type symptoms and burning sensation during urination	Strict cleanliness 0.19% 2-deoxy-D-glucose gel may be used experimentally although efficacy has not been completely established
Syphilis	*Treponema pallidum*	Stage 1: small, reddish, painless papule on genitals lasting up to 5 weeks Stage 2: body rash, enlarged nodes, fever, sore throat, malaise Stage 3: internal and external ulcers, arthritis, hypoesthesias, impaired function of major organ systems and nervous system	Procaine penicillin G, 600,000 units IM for 8 days Benzathine penicillin G (Bicillin), 2.4 million units IM Tetracycline 0.5 g qid for 20 days Erythromycin, same as tetracycline Other dosage schedules for congenital or progressive disease
Nongonococcal urethritis (NGU)	Many possible organisms; almost half caused by a chlamydia bacterium	Discharge Burning sensation during urination Often unnoticed by the female	Tetracycline orally (investigational)
Candidiasis (formerly moniliasis)	*Candida* (formerly *Monilia*) *albicans*—yeastlike organism	Vaginitis with vulvar pruritus Thick, white discharge Male can be a carrier only	Mild acid (vinegar) douches Vaginal tablets, cream, or gel forms of either: Nystatin for 14 days‡ Clotrimazole for 7 days‡ Miconazole for 7 days‡ Others: chlordantoin, proprionic acid and salts, candicidin

*Several conditions may be concurrent.
†Probenecid, 1 g orally, is also administered.
‡Preferred therapy.

T A B L E 2 9 - 5 **Common sexually transmitted diseases or conditions—cont'd**

Condition	Cause	Symptoms	Treatments
Trichomoniasis	*Trichomonas*—protozoa	Vaginitis with vulvar pruritus Yellow-green discharge and burning sensation Male can be a carrier only	Metronidazole (Flagyl), 250 mg orally bid for 10 days or tid for 5 days, or 2 g in 1 day
Nonspecific vaginitis (prior to 1955)	Bacteria: *Haemophilus vaginalis; Corynebacterium vaginalis; Gardnerella vaginalis* (classification now under consideration)	Gray, homogenous, odorous vaginal discharge No vulvitis or vaginitis Male asymptomatic	Oral therapy for 5 days: metronidazole (Flagyl), 250 mg tid or 500 mg bid Cephradine (Anspor), 250 mg qid Cephalexin (Keflex), 500 mg qid Ampicillin, 500 mg qid‡ Tetracycline, 500 mg qid
Pediculosis	*Phthirus pubis*—crab lice	Intense pruritus over pubic/genital area; Lice ova seen on pubic hair Occasionally small blood spots on underwear	Gamma benzene hexachloride (Kwell) lotion, cream, or shampoo, applied thinly on hair and skin of pubic area and surrounding skin
Scabies	*Sarcoptes scabiei*—mites	Intense itch in genital area, areas between fingers, and on forearms 4 to 6 weeks after contact, especially at night	Gamma benzene hexachloride (Kwell) lotion or cream, total body application Crotamiton (Eurax) cream or lotion, total body application twice within 24 hours

BENIGN BREAST DISEASE

These are conditions such as adenosis and fibrocystic breast changes that are characterized by pain and swellings of the breasts at various times, frequently premenstrually, from the ages of about 25 to 40. Elimination from the diet of methylxanthines (in coffee, tea, colas, chocolate) theophylline, and theobromine has been shown to cause some breast nodules of fibrocystic disease to regress and disappear until the substance is resumed.

Summary of nursing considerations

Human reproduction is a highly complex process involving the coordinated activities of the reproductive organs, various endocrine glands, and the brain. Many specific hormones play a major role in the physiologic regulation of reproduction. The reproductive organs are largely under the control of the pituitary gland. The ovaries and the testes are known as gonads and produce not only ova and sperm, respectively, but also form secretions that initiate and maintain the secondary sexual characteristics. When gonadal function diminishes, the secondary sexual characteristics gradually change and reproductive function ceases. The period of change is marked in women by cessation of menses and is known as the menopause. In men diminution of sex hormone output is called the male climacteric.

The hormones concerned with ovarian function include the anterior pituitary hormones, which are required for the normal development and function of the gonads, the gonadotropic hormones of placental origin, and the ovarian hormones themselves. The ovarian hormones include the naturally occurring steroids, the synthetic and partly synthetic steroids, and the nonsteroid compounds such as stilbestrol, which have an ovarian, hormonelike function.

The development of oral contraceptives was based on the knowledge that ovulation did not occur during pregnancy and that large amounts of estrogen and progesterone were produced by the extended function of the corpus luteum and by placental secretion. The administration of progesterone derivatives and estrogenic substances prevents ovulation without preventing menstruation, thus these substances are the ingredients of oral contraceptives. It is generally accepted that oral contraceptives act, at least in part, by inhibiting the secretion of gonadotropins from the pituitary gland. Such oral contraceptives are called ovulatory suppressants. Other possible actions may include a direct inhibitory effect on the ovary, changes in the tubal motility, or changes in the endometrium that would result in failure of implantation of fertilized ova. This described the postcoital contraceptive method. The combination of drugs (ovulatory stimulants) rapidly transforms the early secretory stage of the endometrium to one resembling secretory exhaustion. Oral contraceptive drugs are therefore judged effective because the estrogen encourages proliferative change that inhibits ovulation, while progesterone ensures that withdrawal bleeding will be physiologic, prompt, and brief.

The uterus is a highly muscular organ that exhibits a number of characteristic properties and activities. Drugs that act on the uterus include those that increase motility (oxytocin, ergot, prostaglandins), those that decrease motility (central nervous system depressants and sedatives) and those used for toxemia of pregnancy (diuretics, magnesium sulfate, antihypertensives).

Maternal medications affecting the fetus and nursing infant are receiving increased attention. The importance of the nurse's role as teacher and fetal advocate should be emphasized. Since the thalidomide tragedy of 1961, the placenta has not been considered an effective barrier against untoward drug influences on the developing fetus. The number of medications administered to pregnant women has multiplied; the fetus may be potentially more threatened from these agents than from delivery and the agents used during delivery. The basic problem occurs when drugs are given without justification or without thorough knowledge of contraindications, proper dosage, adverse reactions, and possible interaction effects with other therapy.

The attainment of sexual identity and the ability to live as a sexual being are an important part of human development. Many drugs that are ingested for medical or social purposes may act to alter libido and sexual capabilities. Drugs that have an adverse effect on sexual functioning may do so either through a depressive effect on the central nervous system or through a more specific effect on the portion of the autonomic nervous system that controls sexual function. Drugs used to enhance libido and sexual activity seem to act primarily through a central effect, producing increased suggestibility, release of inhibitions, and relaxation. However, there are no known drugs that specifically increase libido and sexual performance. Every chemical taken without medical advice, especially in combination with other drugs, poses the danger of compounding the adverse effects on sexual function in the user. In view of the widespread use of drugs in contemporary society, the health practitioner has an increasing responsibility to be informed of the possible effects of drug usage on sexual function and to provide informative counseling to patients regarding the possible consequences of specific drug actions on sexual capability.

QUESTIONS

FOR STUDY AND REVIEW

1 When is oxytocin used? What precautions should be taken with this drug? Compare its use with that of ergonovine.
2 Discuss the use of prostaglandins in obstetrics.
3 Discuss the use of magnesium sulfate in the treatment of toxemia of pregnancy.
4 Through library research explain the pros and cons of estrogen therapy in the prevention and treatment of osteoporosis in postmenopausal women.
5 Through library research prepare and give a

report on the relationship between stilbestrol and cancer.

6 Explain the therapeutic action of the estrogen-progestogen oral contraceptives.

7 Identify some common side effects and some contraindications of oral contraceptive therapy.

8 Explain the therapeutic use and pharmacologic action of clomiphene (Clomid).

9 Describe the objectives of androgen therapy.

10 How can drug effects on the fetus be determined?

11 What effect does alcohol have on libido and sexual response?

12 What effect on sexual response can be expected with the administration of:
a an adrenergic blocking drug?
b a parasympathetic blocking drug?

13 Interview a nurse working in a prenatal clinic, a family nurse practitioner, or an obstetrician to determine what instructions are provided to their pregnant patients concerning the use of medicines during pregnancy.

14 Interview a pregnant patient to determine what instructions she has received concerning over-the-counter drugs, alcohol, smoking, and prescribed drugs.

15 What effect do the following drugs have on the nursing infant when ingested by the mother?
a aspirin   f thyroid
b phenobarbital   g nicotine
c diazepam (Valium)   h penicillin
d cascara   i anticonvulsants
e oral contraceptives   j alcohol

16 Through library research obtain a recent article on drugs affecting sexuality, the fetus, or the nursing infant and prepare and give a report on the information to your class.

BIBLIOGRAPHY

Adlercreutz, H.: Hepatic metabolism of estrogens in health and disease, N. Engl. J. Med. **290**:1081, 1974.

Ammann, A.J., and Steihm, E.R.: Immune globulin levels in calcium and breast milk from formula and breastfed infants, Proc. Soc. Exp. Biol. Med. **122**:1098, 1966.

Apt, L., and Gaffney, W.: Congenital eye abnormalities from drugs during pregnancy. In Leopold, I.H., editor: Symposium on ocular therapy, vol. 7, St. Louis, 1974, The C.V. Mosby Co.

Ayd, F.J.: Excretion of psychotropic drugs in human breast milk, Internat. Drug Therapy Newsletter **3**:9, 1973.

Banner, E.A.: Vaginitis, Med. Clin. North Am. **58**:763, 1974.

Barnardo, D., Strothers, I., and Sharrett, M.: Breast milk, jaundice and the pill, Br. Med. J. **2**:348, 1972.

Beacham, D.W., and Beacham, W.D.: Synopsis of gynecology, St. Louis, 1977, The C.V. Mosby Co.

Beeson, P.B., and McDermott, W., editors: Textbook of medicine, ed. 15, Philadelphia, 1980, W.B. Saunders Co.

Benton, B.: Stilbestrol and vaginal cancer, Am. J. Nurs. **74**:900, 1974.

Blough, H.A., and Giuntoli, R.L.: Successful treatment of human genital herpes infections with 2-Deoxy-D-glucose, J.A.M.A. **241**(26): 2798, 1979.

Boreus, L.O.: Fetal pharmacology, New York, 1973, Raven Press.

Bowes, W.A.: Obstetrical medication and infant outcome: a review of the literature. Monog. Soc. Child Dev. **35**:3, 1970.

Burt, R.A.P.: The fetal and maternal pharmacology of some of the drugs used for relief of pain in labour, Br. J. Anaesth. **43**:824, 1971.

Butts, P.: Magnesium sulfate in the treatment of toxemia, Am. J. Nurs. **77**:1294, 1977.

Catz, C.S., and Giacoia, G.P.: Drugs and metabolites in human milk. In Galli, C., Jacini, G., and Pecile, A., editors: Dietary lipids and postnatal development, New York, 1973, Raven Press.

Check, W.: Benign breast lumps may regress with change in diet, J.A.M.A. **241**(12):122, 1979.

Chinn, P.L.: Child health maintenance: concepts in family centered care, St. Louis, 1974, The C.V. Mosby Co.

Chung, H.J.: Arresting premature labor, Am. J. Nurs. **76**:810, 1976.

Cicero, T.J., and others: Function of the male sex organs in heroin and methadone users, N. Engl. J. Med. **292**:882, 1975.

Colbrinik, R., Hood, T., and Chusid, E.: The effects of narcotic addiction on the newborn infant, Pediatrics **9**:288, 1952.

Cooke, I.D.: The menopause, Br. J. Hosp. Med. **7**:581, 1972.

Cowart, M., and Newton, D.: Oral contraceptives: how best to explain their effects to patients, Nursing '76 **6**(6):44, 1976.

Cushman, P., Jr.: Sexual behavior in heroin addiction and methadone maintenance, N.Y. State J. Med. **72**:1261, 1972.

Cutting, W.C.: Handbook of pharmacology: the actions and uses of drugs, ed. 5, New York, 1972, Appleton-Century-Crofts.

Dennerstein, G.J.: Vaginitis: diagnosis and treatment, Drugs **4**:419, 1972.

Desmond, M.M.: Obstetric medication and infant behaviour, Anesthesiology **40**:111, 1974.

Drill, V.A.: Oral contraceptives: relation to mammary cancer, benign breast lesions, and cervical cancer, Annu. Rev. Pharmacol. **15**:367, 1975.

Eckstein, H., and Jack, B.: Breastfeeding and anticoagulant therapy, Lancet **1**:672, 1970.

Erkkola, R., and Kanto, J.: Diazepam and breastfeeding, Lancet **1**:1235, 1972.

Fairley, K.F., and others: Sterility and testicular atrophy related to cyclophosphamide therapy, Lancet **1**:568, 1972.

Forfar, J.O., and Nelson, M.M.: Epidemiology of drugs taken by pregnant women: drugs that may affect the fetus adversely, Clin. Pharmacol. Ther. **14**:632, 1973.

Ganong, W.F.: Review of medical physiology, ed. 2, Los Altos, Calif., 1965, Lange Medical Publications.

Garcia, C.-R., and Rosenfeld, D.L.: Contraceptive methods. In Human fertility: the regulations of reproduction, Philadelphia, 1977, F.A. Davis Co.

Gardner, H.L.: *Haemophilus vaginalis* vaginitis after twenty-five years, Am. J. Obstet. Gynecol. **137**(3):385, 1980.

Gay, G.R., and Sheppard, C.W.: Sex in the drug culture, Med. Asp. Human Sex. **6:**28, 1972.

Ginsburg, J.: Placental drug transfer, Annu. Rev. Pharmacol. **11:**387, 1971.

Gladstone, G.R., and others: Propranolol administration during pregnancy: effects on the fetus, J. Pediatr. **86:**962, 1975.

Gochfeld, M.: Pesticides and the nursing mother, Pediatrics **50:**169, 1972.

Goldstein, A., Aronow, L., and Kalman, S.M.: Chemical teratogenesis, In Goldstein, A., Aronow, L., and Kalman, S.M.: Principles of drug action, New York, 1968, Harper & Row, Publishers, Inc.

Goodman, L.S., and Gilman, A., editors: The pharmacological basis of therapeutics, ed. 6, New York, 1980, Macmillan Inc.

Graber, E.A., and Barber, H.R.K.: The case for and against estrogen therapy, Am. J. Nurs. **75:**1766, 1975.

Graedon, J.: The people's pharmacy—2, New York, 1980, Avon Books.

Greaves, G.: Sexual disturbances among chronic amphetamine users, J. Nerv. Ment. Dis. **155:**363, 1972.

Greenwald, P., and others: Prenatal stilbestrol experience of mothers of young cancer patients, Cancer **31:**568, 1973.

Herbst, A.L., and others: Effects of maternal DES ingestion on the female genital tract, Hosp. Pract. **10:**51, 1975.

Hill, R.M.: Drugs ingested by pregnant women, Clin. Pharmacol. Ther. **14:**654, 1973.

Hoover, R., and others: Menopausal estrogens and breast cancer, N. Engl. J. Med. **295:**401, 1976.

Individual differences in composition of milk, Br. Med. J. **1:**253, 1954.

Isler, V., and others: Cycle pattern and pregnancy rate following combined clomiphene-estrogen therapy, Obstet. Gynecol. **41:**602, 1973.

Janerich, D.T., and others: Oral contraceptives and congenital limb reduction defects, N. Engl. J. Med. **29:**697, 1974.

Jensen, E.V., and DeSombre, E.R.: Estrogen-receptor interactions, Science **182:**126, 1973.

Juchau, M.R., and Dyer, D.C.: Pharmacology of the placenta, Pediatr. Clin. North Am. **19:**65, 1972.

Kantor, H.I., and others: Estrogen for older women. A three year study, Am. J. Obstet. Gynecol. **116:**115, 1973.

Kaplan, H.S.: The new sex therapy, New York, 1974, Brunner/Mazel, Inc.

Karim, S.M.M., and Hillier, K.: Prostaglandins: pharmacology and clinical application, Drugs **8:**176, 1974.

Kastrup, E.K., editor: Facts and comparisons, St. Louis, 1980, Facts and Comparisons, Inc.

Kaufman, R.H.: The origin and diagnosis of nonspecific vaginitis, N. Engl. J. Med. **303**(11):637, 1980.

Kistner, R.W.: The use of clomiphene citrate in the treatment of anovulation, Semin. Drug Treat. **3:**159, 1973.

Knowles, J.A.: Breast milk: a source of more than nutrition for the neonate, Clin. Toxicol. **7:**69, 1974.

Knowles, J.C.: Effects on the infant of drug therapy in nursing mothers, Drug Ther. Bull. **3:**May, 1973.

Lanier, A.P., and others: Cancer and stilbestrol: a follow-up of 1,719 persons exposed to estrogens in utero and born 1943-1959, Mayo Clin. Proc. **48:**793, 1973.

Lawrence, R.A.: Breast-feeding, a guide for the medical profession, St. Louis, 1980, The C.V. Mosby Co.

Lerch, C., and Bliss, V.J.: Maternity nursing, ed. 3, St. Louis, 1978, The C.V. Mosby Co.

Lin, T.J., and others: Clinical and cytologic responses of post-menopausal women to estrogen, Obstet. Gynecol. **41:**97, 1973.

Lindsey, R., and others: Long-term prevention of post-menopausal osteoporosis by oestrogen, Lancet **1:**1038, 1976.

Mack, T.M., and others: Estrogens and endometrial cancer in a retirement community, N. Engl. J. Med. **294:**1262, 1976.

Mann, J.I., and Inman, W.H.W.: Oral contraception and death from myocardial infarction, Br. Med. J. **2:**245, 1975.

Mandelli, M., and others: Placental transfer of diazepam and its disposition in the newborn, Clin. Pharmacol. Ther. **17:**564, 1975.

Marx, J.L.: Estrogen drugs: do they increase the risk of cancer? Science **191:**838,1976.

Mellin, G.W.: Drugs in the first trimester of pregnancy and the fetal life of homo sapiens, Am. J. Obstet. Gynecol. **90:**1168, 1963.

Menning, B.: Infertility: a guide for the childless couple, Englewood Cliffs, N.J., 1977, Prentice-Hall, Inc.

Millar, J.H.D., and Nevin, N.C.: Congenital malformations and anticonvulsant drugs, Lancet **1:**328, 1973.

Mirkin, B.L.: Perinatal pharmacology and therapeutics, New York, 1976, Academic Press, Inc.

Money, J., and Anke, E.: Man and woman, boy and girl, Baltimore, 1972, The Johns Hopkins University Press.

Morrison, J.C., and others: Metabolites of meperidine related to fetal depression, Am. J. Obstet. Gynecol. **115:**1132, 1973.

Nelson, M.M., and Forfar, J.: Association between drugs administered during pregnancy and congenital abnormalities of the fetus, Br. Med. J. **1:**523, 1971.

Noble, I.M.: Prescribing in pregnancy, Practitioner **212:**657, 1974.

Novak, E.R., and Woodruff, J.D., editors: Gynecologic and obstetric pathology, ed. 8, Philadelphia, 1979, W.B. Saunders Co.

Odell, W.D., and Molitch, M.E.: The pharmacology of contraceptive agents, Annu. Rev. Pharmacol. **14:**413, 1974.

Odell, W.D., and Swerdloff, R.S.: Male hypogonadism, West. J. Med. **124:**446, 1976.

O'Brien, T.E.: Excretion of drugs in human milk, Am. J. Hosp. Pharm. **31:**844, 1974.

Physicians' desk reference, ed. 34, Oradell, N.J., 1980, Medical Economics Co.

Progestasert IUD and ectopic pregnancy, FDA Drug Bull. **8**(6):37, Dec. 1978-Jan. 1979.

Rane, A., and Sjoqvist, F.: Drug metabolism in the human fetus and newborn infant, Pediatr. Clin. North Am. **119:**37, 1972.

Rothballer, A.A.: Aggression, defense, and neurohumors, Brain Function **5:**135, 1972.

Sartwell, P.E., and others: Epidemiology of benign breast lesions: lack of association with oral contraceptive use, N. Engl. J. Med. **288:**551, 1973.

Schnider, S.: A review: fetal and neonatal effects of drugs in obstetrics, Anesth. Analg. **45:**372, 1966.

Schultz, H.W.: Drugs and pregnancy, review article reprint from Pharmindex, January, 1974.

Shapiro, S., and others: Anticonvulsants and parental epilepsy in the development of birth defects, Lancet 1:272, 1976.

Smithells, R.W., and Morgan, D.M.: The transmission of drugs by the placenta and breasts, Practitioner 204:14, 1970.

Soika, C.: Combatting osteoporosis, Am. J. Nurs. 73:1001, 1973.

Speidel, B.D., and Meadow, S.R.: Epilepsy, anticonvulsants and congenital malformations, Drugs 8:354, 1974.

Stevenson, R.E.: The fetus and the newly born infant: influences of the prenatal environment, ed. 2, St. Louis, 1977, The C.V. Mosby Co.

Stock, R.J., and others: Vaginal douching. Current concepts and practices, Obstet. Gynecol. 42:141, 1973.

Swerdloff, R.S., and others: Complications of oral contraceptive agents—a symposium, West. J. Med. 122:20, 1975.

Symposium on drugs and the unborn child. Clin. Pharmacol. Ther. 14(4, Part 2):619, 1973.

Thompson, D.L., and Frame, B.: Involutional osteopenia: current concepts, Ann. Intern. Med. 85:789, 1976.

Timby, B.: Ovulation method of birth control, Am. J. Nurs. 76:928, 1976.

Turksoy, R.N.: Induction of ovulation with the use of human menopausal gonadotropins in anovulatory infertile women, Semin. Drug Treat. 3:177, 1973.

Vessey, M.P., and others: Oral contraceptives, and breast cancer. Progress report of an epidemiological study, Lancet 1:941, 1975.

Wilson, J.D.: Recent studies on the mechanism of action of testosterone, N. Engl. J. Med. 287:1284, 1972.

Wilson, J.T.: Developmental pharmacology: a review of its application to clinical and basic science, Annu. Rev. Pharmacol. 12:423, 1972.

Woods, J.S.: Drug effects on human sexual behavior. In Woods, N.F.: Human sexuality in health and illness, ed. 2, St. Louis, 1979, The C.V. Mosby Co.

UNIT TEN

DERMATOLOGIC PREPARATIONS

CHAPTER 30

Dermatologic agents

The skin

The skin is the largest organ of the body, but absorption from the skin is unpredictable, poor, and uncertain. The flat cells of the outermost layer of the skin contain keratin, a substance that serves to waterproof the skin and to prevent absorption of water and other substances. Absorption is affected, however, by the presence of sweat glands and of sebaceous glands, which are epidermal appendages that penetrate the dermis. Hair follicles, pigment cells, nerve endings, nerve networks, and blood vessels as well as collagenous and elastic fibers all contribute to the functions of the skin. Although the skin is not known for its powers of absorption, drugs that cannot penetrate the horny first layer are sometimes absorbed by way of the sebaceous or sweat glands. Absorption is increased if the skin is macerated either by water or perspiration. It is more likely to occur if the epidermis is thin, as it is in the axilla, eyelids, or skin of a child. Absorption will take place rapidly from raw or denuded surfaces.

Methyl salicylate rubbed on the skin can be found in the urine in 30 minutes. Alcohol and volatile solvents promote absorption. The nature of the vehicle (see Table 30-1) affects absorption—drugs that are fat soluble can be absorbed more rapidly than water-soluble drugs, and natural fats make a better vehicle to carry the drug into the skin than do substances such as petrolatum.

Drugs may be concentrated in the skin in small amounts. Silver, copper, arsenic, mercury, bromides, borates, phenol, salicylates, antipyrine, methylene blue, and phenolphthalein may be deposited in the skin and sweat glands, and this may explain the skin eruption sometimes noticed after their use. Many other drugs can be the cause of skin eruption.

A wide range of drugs are used in dermatology, some for systemic and others for local effects as listed below:

Specific
    Acne products
    Antipsoriatics
    Antiseborrheics
    Burn preparations
    Diaper rash products
    Poison ivy products
    Sunscreens
General
    Antibiotics
    Antifungal agents
    Antihistamines
    Antiseptics/germicides
    Bath products
    Cauterizing products
    Corticosteriods and combinations
    Corticosteroid/antibiotic combinations
    Emollients

T A B L E 3 0 - 1 **Dermatologic vehicles**

Surface, disease	Base	Effect	Examples/notes
Dry and scaly (e.g., psoriasis, dry eczema, ichthyosis)	Ointment	Occlusive emollient	Soft white or soft yellow paraffin Emulsifying ointment Synthetic bases Lanolin (may sensitize)
Moist or dry (e.g., eczema in various stages)	Cream	Cooling, emollient and moisturizing	Oily cream Aqueous cream Cetomacrogol cream Synthetic bases (preservatives may sensitize)
Acutely inflamed; wet and oozing (e.g., weeping eczema and other bullous diseases)	Lotions	Drying, soothing and cooling	Saline solution Calamine lotion Aluminium accetate solution Potassium permanganate solution
Lichenified (e.g., eczema); oozing (e.g., eczema)	Pastes	Protective, prevents spreading of active ingredient Dries wet areas	Zinc compound paste Lassar's paste Coal tar paste–impregnated bandages protect eczema from scratching Paste used as vehicle for dithranol in psoriasis
Flexures, especially if sore and moist (e.g., intertrigo, flexural eczema and psoriasis, candidiasis)	Dusting powders	Lessen friction and are drying	Talc dusting powder; zinc starch and talc can be used as a vehicle for other antifungal drugs
Flexures (e.g., intertrigo, candidiasis, ulcers)	Paints	Drying	Castellani's magenta paint Better than powders for very moist areas

Adapted from Hunter, 1973; From Avery, G.S.: Drug treatment, ed 2, Brooklyn, 1980, Adis Press USA Inc., p. 418.

Irrigating sterile solutions
Keratolytics
Local anesthetics
Ointment and lotion bases
Rubs and liniments
Scabicides and/or pediculicides
Skin protectants
Tar-containing products
Wet dressings

It is impossible in a textbook of this kind to present more than a superficial discussion of dermatologic agents. The student, therefore, should refer to specialty texts devoted to dermatology and dermatologic therapy.

Skin disorders

Reactions or disorders of the skin are manifested by symptoms such as itching, pain, or tingling and by signs such as swelling, redness, papules, pustules, blisters, and hives. Some common dermatologic disorders in the United States are listed below:

Acne vulgaris (cystic acne and acne scars)
Atopic dermatitis
Dyshidrotic eczema
Folliculitis
Fungus infections (tinea pedis, tinea unguium, tinea versicolor, tinea cruris)
Hand eczema
Herpes simplex
Lichen simplex chronicus
Psoriasis
Seborrheic dermatitis
Verruca vulgaris
Vitiligo

A reaction of the skin that makes the patient uncomfortable or unsightly may be attributable to or related to sensitivity to drugs, allergy, infection, emotional conflict, hormonal imbalance, or degenerative disease. Sometimes the cause of the skin disorder is unknown and the treatment may be empiric in the hope that the right remedy will be found.

Dermatologic diagnosis includes physical inspection, personal and family medical history, and laboratory tests including blood and urine tests, cytodiagnosis, and biopsy. The physical examination of the skin sometimes includes the use of Wood's light. This instrument provides long-wave ultraviolet light, which is helpful in detecting hair and skin infected with fungi that fluorescence and in aiding in differentiation of hypopigmented areas and depigmented areas of the skin. The potassium hydroxide 10% (KOH) test aids in diagnosis of mycotic infection. The solution will disintegrate keratin, disclosing, under microscopic examination, mycelia (vegetative part as filaments), fungal elements, and hyphae (which acquire food). Other tests include the Tzanck test for epidermal giant cells (seen in herpes zoster viral infections, usually with inclusion bodies, and in pemphigus vulgaris without bodies), biopsy, and patch tests. The dermatophyte test medium is a fast-acting medium that creates a marked color change when a dermatophyte is grown in it. The box on p. 932 lists the nature of different types of lesions and some of the conditions associated with them.

When the nature of the lesion has been established, its characteristics should be defined according to size, shape, surface, and color.

The next step is to discover the distribution of the rash. In some diseases the diagnosis can be made from the distribution, and in others, it is of much assistance. The inference should not be drawn, however, that because a disease is not found in its common pattern of distribution that it can be excluded. For example, psoriasis is commonly found on the extensors, but occasionally it will be seen as a solitary lesion in the external ear. A basal cell carcinoma is most common on the face, but occasionally it occurs on the trunk. On the other hand, rosacea only attacks those areas of the face that flush.

The regional distribution of common conditions is shown in the box on p. 933 (several diseases may overlap or occur simultaneously but in different areas).

Table 30-2 is a summary of the vast number of dermatologic reactions from drugs and their characteristic lesions and sequelae. The nurse always needs to be cognizant of a patient's drug history and current therapy to relate such lesions and sequelae to the appropriate cause; this often saves the patient many unnecessary and uncomfortable diagnostic examinations and lessens the anxiety of the medical team. Simply discontinuing a particular drug often resolves a complicated dermatologic problem or sequelae of unknown origin.

Text continued on p. 940.

Different types of lesions and some of the conditions associated with them

Atrophy
Senile skin
Lupus erythematosus

Bullae
Contact dermatitis (poison ivy)
Dermatitis herpetiformis
Drug eruptions (sulfonamides, bar-
    biturates)
Erythema multiforme
Herpes zoster
Impetigo
Insect bites
Pemphigoid
Pemphigus

Crusts
Any ulcerating disease
Any vesicular or bullous dermatitis

Depigmentation
Albinism
Vitiligo

Hyperkeratosis
Corns
Ichthyosis

Hyperpigmentation
Addison's disease
Chloasma
Cushing's disease
Freckles
Hemochromatosis
Neurofibromatosis
Pregnancy

Macules
Addison's disease
Drug eruptions
Freckles
Measles
Nevus flammeus
Neurofibromatosis (café-au-lait
    spots)
Vitiligo

Nodules
Basal cell carcinoma
Chilblains
Erythema induratum
Erythema nodosum
Hemangiomas
Keratoacanthoma
Lipomas
Molluscum contagiosum
Neurofibromas
Syphilis
Warts

Papules
Acne
Basal cell carcinoma (rodent ulcer)
Granuloma pyogenicum
Melanoma
Molluscum contagiosum
Pigmented nevi
Tuberculids
Warts
Xanthomas

Plaques
Atopic dermatitis
Lichen planus
Lupus erythematosus
Paget's disease of the nipple
Psoriasis
Seborrheic dermatitis

Pustules
Acne
Chickenpox
Folliculitis
Herpes simplex
Herpes zoster
Rosacea
Smallpox

Scaly macules
Pityriasis rosea
Pityriasis versicolor
Seborrheic dermatitis
Tinea corporis

Scaly papules
Atopic dermatitis
Contact dermatitis
Lichen planus
Localized neurodermatitis
Psoriasis
Syphilis

Scars
Any ulcerating disease

Ulcers
Basal cell carcinoma
Bedsores
Self-inflicted conditions, e.g.,
    dermatitis artefacta
Squamous cell carcinoma
Syphilitic gummas
Trauma
Tuberculosis
Venous stasis

Vegetative
Condylomas
Squamous cell carcinoma
Warts

Vesicles
Atopic dermatitis
Burns
Chickenpox
Contact dermatitis
Dermatitis herpetiformis
Herpes simplex
Herpes zoster
Insect bites
Scabies

Wheals
Insect bites
Urticaria

·om Solomons, B.: Lecture notes on dermatology, ed. 4, Oxford, London, 1977, Blackwell Scientific Publications, Ltd., pp. 17-21.

Regional distribution of common dermatological conditions

Abdomen
Candidiasis
Drug eruptions
Pityriasis rosea
Psoriasis
Scabies
Seborrheic warts
Urticaria

Anogenital area
Candidiasis
Contact dermatitis
Herpes simplex
Intertrigo
Lichen planus
Pediculosis pubis
Pruritus
Psoriasis
Scabies
Seborrheic dermatitis
Syphilis
Tinea cruris (in males)
Warts

Arms
Contact dermatitis
Lichen planus
Psoriasis

Axillae
Boils
Candidiasis
Contact dermatitis
Pediculosis
Seborrheic dermatitis
Tinea

Back
Acne
Pityriasis rosea
Psoriasis
Seborrheic dermatitis
Seborrheic warts

Chest
Acne
Pityriasis rosea
Pityriasis versicolor
Psoriasis
Seborrheic dermatitis
Seborrheic warts

Ears
Contact dermatitis
Lupus cerythematosus
Neoplasm
Otitis externa
Psoriasis
Seborrheic dermatitis

Eyelids
Contact dermatitis
Neoplasms
Warts
Xanthelasma

Face
Acne
Contact dermatitis
Impetigo
Infantile eczema
Lupus erythematosus
Neoplasms
Rosacea
Sebaceous cysts
Seborrheic dermatitis
Seborrheic warts

Feet
Atopic dermatitis
Contact dermatitis
Corns
Dyshidrosis
Psoriasis
Tinea
Warts

Hands
Atopic dermatitis
Contact dermatitis
Dyshidrosis
Hyperhidrosis
Scabies
Warts

Legs
Contact dermatitis
Erythema nodosum
Insect bites
Lichen planus
Neurodermatitis
Psoriasis
Purpura
Varicose dermatitis

Lips
Cheilitis
Contact dermatitis
Herpes simplex
Leukoplakia
Neoplasms

Mouth
Aphthous stomatitis
Leukoplakia
Lichen planus
Neoplasms
Pemphigus

Scalp
Alopecia
Pediculosis
Psoriasis
Sebaceous cysts
Seborrheic dermatitis
Tinea

Apart from these visible signs, there are other aids to diagnosis in some conditions.

From Solomons, B.: Lecture notes on dermatology, ed. 4, Oxford, London, 1977, Blackwell Scientific Publications, Ltd., pp. 17-21.

TABLE 30-2   Life-threatening drug-induced skin eruptions

Drug eruptions	Drugs involved	Reported sequelae
Exofollative dermatitis	Aminosalicylic acid (PAS)	Hepatitis, hemolytic anemia
	Antidiabetics, oral	
	Arsenicals	
	Barbiturates	
	Carbamazepine (Tegretol)	
	Demeclocycline (Declomyein)	
	Diphtheria and tetanus toxoids and pertussis vaccine, absorbed and Salk poliomyelitis vaccine	Death; probably caused by penicillin in the poliovirus vaccine
	Furosemide (Lasix)	
	Gold	
	Griseofulvin (Grifulvin)	Lymphadenopathy
	Hydroflumethiazide (Saluron)	
	Isorbide (Isordil)	
	Measles virus vaccine	
	Mercury	
	Methotrimeprazine (Levoprome)	
	Nitrofurans	
	Nitroglycerin	
	Oral antidiabetics	
	Oxyphenbutazone (Tandearil)	
	Penicillin	
	Phenindione (Hedulin)	Hepatitis, nephritis
	Phenothiazines	
	Phenylbutazone (Butazolidin)	
	Phenytoin (Dilantin)	Atypical lymphocytes, hypoproteinemia, hepatosplenomegaly
	Streptomycin	
	Sulfamethoxypyridazine (Midicel)	Death
	Sulfasalazine (Azulfidine)	
	Sulfisomide (Elkosin)	
	Sulfonamides	
	Tetracyclines	
Stevens-Johnson syndrome (erythema multiforme)	Aminophenazone	
	Ampicillin	
	Antipyrine	
	Arsenicals	
	Barbiturates	
	Carbamazepine (Tegretol)	
	Chloramphenicol	
	Chlorpropamide (Diabinese)	
	Clindamycin	
	Codeine	
	Cold preparation 666	
	Mephenytoin (Mesantoin)	
	Novobiocin	
	Oxyphenbutazone (Tandearil)	
	Paramethadione	
	Penicillin	
	Phenolphthalein	

From Martin, E.W.; Hazards of medication, ed. 2, Philadelphia, 1978, J.B. Lippincott Co.

T A B L E 3 0 - 2 Life-threatening drug-induced skin eruptions—cont'd

Drug eruptions	Drugs involved	Reported sequelae
	Phenylbutazone (Butazolidin)	
	Phenytoin (Dilantin)	Death
	Phenytoin and trimethadione	Lupus erythematosus occurred simultaneously
	Rifampin (Rifadin, Rimactane, etc.)	
	Salicylates	
	Salizopyrine	
	Sulfadimethoxine (Madribon)	
	Sulfamethoxypyridazine (Kynex, Midicel)	Death; 2 out of 14 cases
	Sulfasalazine (Azulfidine)	
	Sulfisomidine (Elkosin)	
	Thiacotazone (Amithiozone)	Death
	Thiazides	
	Thiouracil	
	Trimethadione (Tridione) and phenobarbital	Lupus erythematosus with subsequent medication
	Triple sulfas (Sulphatriad)	
	Tetracycline	
Toxic epidermal necrolysis (Lyell's syndrome)	Acelaziamide (Diamox)	
	Antihistamines	
	Antipyrine	
	Barbiturates	
	Chenopodium oii	Death
	Dapsone	
	Diallylbarbituric acid	
	Diphtheria	
	Ethylmorphine HCl (Didial)	
	Gold salts	
	Ipecac	
	Methyl salicylate	
	Neomycin sulfate	
	Nitrofurantoin (Furadantin)	Death; cause questionable
	Opium powder	
	Oxyphenbutazone (Tandearil)	
	Penicillin	
	Pentazocine (Talwin)	
	Phenobarbital	
	Phenolphthalein	
	Phenylbutazone (Butazolidin)	Death; 1 out of 4 cases
	Phenytoin (Dilantin)	Death
	Procaine penicillin, aqueous injection and oral mixed sulfonamide preparation	
	Sulfadimethoxine (Madribon)	Death; leukopenia
	Sulfamethoxypyridazine (Kynex, Midicel)	
	Sulfasalazine (Azulfidine)	
	Sulfathiazole	Death
	Sulfisomidine (Elkosin)	
	Sulfonamides	
	Tetracycline	

Continued.

TABLE 30-2 **Life-threatening drug-induced skin eruptions—cont'd**

Drug eruptions	Drugs involved	Reported sequelae
Lupus erythematosus	Aminosalicylic acid	
	Chlorpromazine (Thorazine)	
	Chlortetracycline (Aureomycin)	
	Corticosteroid withdrawal	
	Digitalis (long term)	
	Ethosuximide (Zarontin)	
	Gold compounds (long term)	
	Griseofulvin	
	Guanoxan	
	Hydantoin anticonvulsants	
	Hydralazine (Apresoline)	
	Isoniazid (Nydrazid)	
	Isoquinazepon	
	Mephenytoin (Mesantoin)	
	Methyldopa (Aldomet)	
	Methysergide	
	Methyithiouracil	
	Oral contraceptives (mestranol?)	
	Oxyphenbutazone (Tandearil)	
	Para-aminosalicylic acid (PAS)	
	Penicillamine	
	Penicillin	
	Phenobarbital (long term)	
	Phenylbutazone (Butazolidin	
	Phenytoin (Dilantin)	
	Practolol	
	Primidone (Mysoline)	
	Procainamide (Pronestyl)	
	Propylthiouracil	
	Reserpine (long term)	
	Rifampin (Rifadin, Rimactane, rifampicin)	
	Streptomycin	
	Sulfadiazine	
	Sulfadimethoxine	
	Sulfamethoxypyridazine (Kynex)	
	Sulfasalazine (Azulfidine)	
	Sulfonamides (long acting)	
	Tetracycline	
	Thiazides (long term)	
	Trimethadione (Tridione, Troxidone)	

From Martin, E.W.; Hazards of medication, ed. 2, Philadelphia, 1978, J.B. Lippincott Co.

Photosensitizers

Acetohexamide (Dymelor)
Acridine preparations (slight)
Agave lechuguilla (amaryllis)
Agrimony
9-Aminoacridine
Aminobenzoic acid
Amitriptyline (Elavil, etc.)
Anesthetics (procaine group)
Angelica
Anthracene
Antimalarials
Arsenicals

Barbiturates
Bavachi (corylifolia)
Benzene
Benzopyrine
Bergamot (perfume)
Bithionol (Actamer, Lorothi-dol)
Blankophores (sulfa deriva-tives)
Bulosemide (Jadit)
Bromchlorsalicylanilid
4-Butyl-4-chlorosalicylanilide

Carbamazepine (Tegretol)
Carbinoxamine d-form (Twis-ton R-A)
Carbutamide (Nadisan)
Carrots, wild
Cedar oil
Celery
Chlorophyll
Chlorothiazide (Diuril)
Chlorpromazine (Thorazine)
Chlorpropamide (Diabinese)
Chlortetracycline (Aureomy-cin)
Citron oil
Citrus fruits
clover
Coal tar
Contraceptives, oral

Demeclocycline (Declomycin, demethylchlortetracycline)
Desipramine (Norpramin, Per-tofrane)
Dibenzopyran derivatives
Dicyanine-A
Diethylstilbestrol
Digalloyl trioleate (sunscreen)
Dill
Diphenhydramine hydrochlo-ride (Benadryl)

Eosin (slight)
Estrone

Fennel
Fluorescein dyes
5-Fluorouracil

Furocoumarins (bergamot oil)
Glyceryl p-aminobenzoate (sunscreen)
Gold salts
Grass (meadow)
Griseofulvin (Fulvicin)

Hematoporphyrin
Hexachlorophene (rare)
Hydrochlorothiazide (Esidrix, HydroDiuril)

Imipramine HCl (Tofranil)
Isothipencyl (Theruhistin)
Isothipendyl (Theruhistin)

Lady's thumb (tea)
Lantinin
Lavender oil
Lime oil

Meclothiazide (Enduron)
Mepazine (Pacatal)
9-Mercaptopurine
Methotrimeprazine (Levo-prome)
Methoxsalen (Meloxine, Oxso-ralen)
5-Methoxypsoralen
8-Methoxypsoralen
Monoglycerol para-aminoben-zoate
Mustards

Nalidixic acid (NegGram)
Naphthalene
Nortriptyline (Aventyl)

Oxytetracycline (Terramycin)

Para-dimethylaminoazoben-zene
Paraphenylenediamine
Parsley
Parsnips
Penicillin derivates (Griseoful-vin)
Perloline
Perphenazine (Trilafon)
Phenanthrene
Phenazine dyes
Phenolic compounds
Phenothiazines (dyes [methy-lene blue, toluidine blue], etc.)
Phenoxazines
Phenylbutazone (Butazolidin)
Phenytoin (Dilantin)
Pitch and pitch fumes
Porphyrins
Prochlorperazine (Compazine)
Promazine hydrochloride (Sparine)

Profriptyline (Vivactil)
Promethazine hydrochloride (Phenergan)
Psoralens (perfume)
Pyrathiazine hydrochloride (Pyrrolazote)
Pyridine

Quinethazone (Hydromox)
Quinine

Rose Bengal perfume (slight)
Rue

Salicylanilides
Salicylates
Sandalwood oil (perfume)
Silver salts
Smartweed (tea)
Stilbamidine isethionate
Sulfacetamide
Sulfadiazine
Sulfadimethoxine
Sulfaguanidine
Sulfanilamide (slight)
Sulfamerazine
Sulfamethazine
Sulfapyridine
Sulfathiazole
Sulfonamides
Sulfisomidine (Elkosin)
Sulfonylureas (antidiabetics)

Tetrachlorsalicylanilide (TCSA)
Tetracyclines
Thiazides (Diuril, HydroDiu-ril, etc.)
Thiophene
Thiopropazate dihydrochlo-ride (Dartal)
Tolbutamide (Orinase)
Toluene
Tribromosalicylanilide (TBS), (deodorant soaps)
Trichlormethiazide (Metahy-drin)
Tridione
Triethylene melamine (TEM)
Triflupromazine hydrochlo-ride (Vesprin)
Trimeprazine tartrate (Temar-il)
Trimethadione (Tridione)
Tripyrathiazine
Trypaflavine
Trypan blue

Vanillin oils

Water ash

Xylene

Yarrow

From Martin, E.W.: Hazards of medication, ed. 2, Philadelphia, 1978, J. B. Lippincott Co.

Drugs causing an acneform reaction

ACTH
Androgenic hormones
Bromides
Corticosteroids
Cyanocobalamin
Hydantoins
Iodides
Methandrostenolone (Dianabol)
Methyltestosterone (Metandren, etc.)
Oral contraceptives

Drugs causing purpura

ACTH
Allopurinol (Zyloprim)
Amitriptyline (Elavil, Endep, etc.)
Anticoagulants
Barbiturates
Carbamides
Chloral hydrate
Chlorothiazide (Diuril)
Chlorpropamide (Diabinese)
Chlorpromazine (Thorazine)
Corticosteroids
Digitalis
Fluoxymesterone
Gold salts
Griseofulvin (Grifulvin)
Iodides
Mepesulfate
Meprobamate
Oxyphenbutazone (Tandearil)
Penicillin
Phenylbutazone (Butazolidin)
Quinidine
Rifampin (Rifadin, Rimactame, rifampicin)
Sulfonamides
Thiazides
Trifluoperazine

Drugs causing urticaria

ACTH
Amitriptyline
Barbiturates
Bromides
Chloramphenicol (Chloromycetin)
Dextran
Enzymes
Erythromycin (Erythrocin, Ilotycin)
Griseofulvin (Grifulvin)
Hydantoins (Dilantin, etc.)
Insulin
Iodides
Iodopyracet (Diodrast)
Meprobamate (Equanil, Miltown)
Meperidine (Demerol)
Meprobamate
Mercurials
Nitrofurantoin (Furadantin)
Novobiocin
Opiates
Penicillin
Penicillinase
Pentazocine (Talwin)
Phenolphthalein
Phenothiazines
Propoxyphene (Darvon)
Rifamoin (Rifadin, Rimactane, rifampicin)
Salicylates
Serums
Streptomycin
Sulfonamides
Tetracyclines
Thiouracil

Drugs causing alopecia

Alkylating agents
Anticoagulants
Antimetabolites
Bleomycin (Blenoxane)
Mepesulfate
Mephenytoin (Mesantoin)
Methimazole
Methotrexate
Norethindrone acetate (Norinyl, Noriestrine, Ortho-Novum)
Quinacrine
Oral contraceptives
Sodium warfarin (Coumadin)
Trimethadione (Tridione)
Triparanol (Mer-29)

Drugs causing morbilliform reactions

p-Aminosalicylic acid (PAS)
Anticonvulsants
Anticholinergics
Antihistamines
Barbiturates
Chloral hydrate
Chlordiazepoxide (Librium)
Chlorothiazide (Diuril)
Chlorpromazine (Thorazine)
Gold salts
Griseofulvin (Grifulvin)
Hydantoins (Dilantin, etc.)
Insulin
Meprobamate
Mercurials
Methaminodiazepoxide
Novobiocin
Organic extracts
Para-aminosalicylic acid
Penicillin
Phenothiazines
Phenylbutazone (Butazolidin)
Quinacrine (Atabrine)
Salicylates
Serums
Streptomycin
Sulfonamides
Sulfones
Tetracyclines
Thiouracil

Drugs causing lichenoid reactions

Amiphenazole (Daptazole)
Chloroquine
Gold salts compounds
Organic arsenicals
Para-aminosalicylic acid
Quinacrine (Atabrine, mepacrine)
Quinidine
Thiazides

From Martin, E.W.: Hazards of medication, ed. 2, Philadelphia, 1978, J.B. Lippincott Co.

Drugs causing fixed eruptions

Acetanilid
Acetarsone
Acetophenetidin
Acetylsalicylic acid
Aconite
Acriflavine
Aminopyrine
Amobarbital
Amodiaquine
Amphetamine sulfate
Anthralin
Antimony potassium tartrate
Antipyrine
Arsphenamine
Barbital
Barbiturates
Belladonna
Bismuth salts
Bromides
Chloral hydrate
Chlorguanide
Chloroquine
Chlorothiazide and sun
Chlorpromazine
Chlortetracycline
Cinchophen
Copaiba
Dextroamphetamine
Diacetyldiphenotisatin
Diallybarbituric acid
Diethylstilbestrol
Digilanid
Digitalis
Dimenhydrinate (Dramamine)
Dimethylamine acetarsone
Diphenhydramine (Benadryl)

Disulfiram and alcohol
Eosin
Ephedrine
Epinephrine
Ergot alkaloids
Erythrosin
Eucalyptus oil
Formalin
Frangula
Gold compounds
Griseofulvin (Grifulvin)
Iodine
Ipecac
Ipomea
2-Isopropyl-4-pentenoyl urea
   (Sedormid)
Karaya gum
Magnesium hydroxide
Meprobamate
Mercury salts
Methenamine
Neoarsphenamine
Opium alkaloids
Oxophenarsine
Oxytetracycline (Terramycin)
Para-aminosalicylic acid
Penicillin
Phenacetin
Phenazone
Phenobarbital
Phenolphthalein
Phenylbutazone (Butazoiidin)
5-Phenylethylhydantoin
Phenylhydantoin
Phenytoin (Dilantin)
Phosphorus

Potassium chlorate
Pyrimidine derivatives
Quinacrine
Quinidine
Quinine
Reserpine
Salicylates
Santonin
Saccharin
Scopolamine
Sodium salicylate
Sterculia gum
Stramonium
Streptomycin
Strychnine
Sulfadiazine
Sulfaguanidine
Sulfamerazine
Sulfamethazine
Sulfamethoxypyridazine (Kynex)
Sulfapyridine
Sulfarsphenamine
Sulfathiazole
Sulfisoxazole (Gantrisin)
Sulfobromophthalein sodium
Sulfonamides
Tetracyclines
Thiambutosine
Thiram and alcohol
Thonzylamine HCl (Neohetramine)
Tripelennamine (Pyribenzamine)
Trisodium arsphenamine sulfate
Tryparsamide
Urease
Urginin
Vaccines and immunizing agents

Drugs causing contact dermatitis

Acriflavine
Amethocaine
Antazoline
Antazoline and phenocide
Antazoline and pyribenzamine
Antihistamine
Arsphenamine
Atabrine

Bacitracin (occupational)
Benzocaine
Benzoyl peroxide and
   chlorhydroxyquinoline
Bleomycin (Blenoxane)

Cetrimide
Chloramphenicol

Chlorcyclizine
Chlorhexidine
Chlorhydroxyquinaline and
   benzoyl peroxide
Chlorxylenol
Chlorphenesin
Chlorpromazine
Colophony
Crotamiton
Cyclomethycaine

Diphenhydramine
Domiphen

Ephedrine

Formaldehyde

Halogenated phenolic
   compounds
Hedaquinium chloride

Iodine
Iodochlorhydroxyquinoline
Isoniazid (occupational)

Lanolin
Meprobamate
Mepyramine (Pyrilamine)
Mercurials
Mercury

Neomycin
Nitrofurazone
Novobiocin

om Martin, E.W.: Hazards of medication, ed. 2, Philadelphia, 1978, J.B. Lippincott Co.

Continued.

Drugs causing contact dermatitis—cont'd

Para-aminosalicylic acid	Procaine and other anesthetics	Spiramycin (occupational)
Parabens	Promethazine	Streptomycin
Penicillin	Propamidine	Sulfonamides
Peru balsam	Pyribenzamine and antazoline	Sulfur and salicylic acid ointment
Phenindamine		
Phenocide and antazoline	Quinacrine (Atabrine)	Tetracyclines
Phenol	Quinine	Thiamine
Potassium hydroxyquinoline sulfate		Thimerosal (Merthiolate)
	Resorcin	

Dermatologic preparations

As previously stated, dermatologic products are so vast in number it would be difficult to cover them all in this chapter. However, to serve as a guide to the major groups of products, Table 30-3 has been included to give an idea of the types of products and their ingredients used for various dermatologic indications.

For the sake of simplicity, this section will be divided into three major groups of dermatologic products: vehicles, prophylactic agents, and therapeutic agents. Some dermatologic vehicles include those listed in Table 30-1; others include solutions, baths, soaps, wet dressings, and soaks. Prophylactic agents include sunscreens, protectives, and antiseptics and disinfectants. Therapeutic agents include the antiinfectives, and antiinflammatory corticosteroids, keratolytic agents, acne products, stimulants and irritants, topical anesthetics, and burn products for second- and third-degree burns. Although the treatment of scabies and pediculosis is often included in dermatologic discussions, this topic is covered in Chapter 25. The antiseptics and disinfectants that are classified as dermatologic agents will also not be included, since they were presented in Chapter 23.

Vehicles
EMOLLIENTS

Emollients are fatty or oily substances that may be used to soften or soothe irritated skin and mucous membrane. An emollient may also serve as a vehicle for application of other medicinal substances. Olive oil and liquid petrolatum are frequently used to cleanse dry areas that would be irritated by water.

Fixed oils. Fixed oils are used as emollients and include olive oil, flaxseed oil, and cottonseed oil.

Glycerin (Glycerol). In pure form glycerin tends to have a drying effect, but when diluted with water or rose water, it is useful for application to irritated lips and skin.

Lanolin; hydrous wool fat. Lanolin is made by combining the purified fat of sheepswool with 25% to 30% water. It is used as an ointment base. It does not become rancid, and as much as twice its weight of water can be incorporated with it. It has a somewhat unpleasant odor. It requires dilution for use in ointments, and from 20% to 100% of petrolatum may be added for this purpose.

Hydrophilic ointment, aqueous cream. Hydrophilic ointment is an ointment in which the oil is dispersed in the continuous water phase. It is an oil-in-water emulsion, and when medicaments are incorporated, the wetting agent in the emulsion enables the drugs to come in more direct contact with the skin and sebaceous glands. It is less greasy and more easily washed off than other ointments. Inflamed or irritated skin is often intolerant of this kind of ointment.

Petrolatum; soft paraffin (petroleum jelly). Petrolatum is a purified, semisolid mixture of hydrocarbons derived from petroleum and used as a vehicle for medicinal agents for local application. It is an important ointment base.

Plastibase. Plastibase is a type of ointment base that contains 95% liquid petrolatum and

TABLE 30-3   Topical dermatologic products and their ingredients

Product	Ingredients
Acne products	Benzoyl peroxide alone and in combination; sulfur products; tetracycline topical solution; erythromycin topical solution; clindamycin topical solution; combination products containing antiseptics, antimicrobials, astringents, corticosteroids, keratolytics, and solvents; medicated bars containing detergents, keratolytics, and surfactants; liquid cleansers containing keratolytics and organic solvents; abrasive cleansers containing granules of polyethylene, aluminum oxide feldspar and keratolytics, surfactants, and antiseptics; tretinoin, retinoic acid, or vitamin A acid
Antipsoriatic products	Coal tar derivatives alone and in combination with corticosteroids, salicylic acid, phenol, and cresol; anthralin; ammoniated mercury
Antiseborrheic products	Selenium sulfide; tar derivatives; povidone-iodine; pyrithione zinc; chlorosene; parachlorometaxylenol; sulfacetamide; antiseborrheic combinations with keratolytics, antipruritics, antibacterials, antimicrobials, antiseptics, local irritants, antifungals, antiinfectives, and steroids (for antiinflammatory and vasoconstrictor activity)
Burn products	Nitrofurazone; mafenide; silver nitrate; tannic acid; silver sulfadiazine
Topical diaper rash products	Antimicrobials; astringents; lubricants; protectives; anticandidal agents
Poison ivy products	Adsorbents; anesthetics; antihistamines; antiseptics; astringents; counterirritants; demulcents; inactivator of ivy toxin urushiol; protectants; clindamycin
Sunscreens	Chemical barriers: benzophenones, PABA and PABA esters, cinnamates, others such as menthyl anthranilate, digalloyl trioleate; physical barriers: red petrolatum, titanium dioxide, zinc oxide
Antibiotic products	Bacitracin; chloramphenicol; chlortetracycline; erythromycin; neomycin; tetracycline; combinations including polymyxin B, oxytetracycline, gramicidin
Antiseptic/germicidal products	Iodine compounds: iodine, providone-iodine, poloxamer-iodine; mercury compounds: thimerosal, merbromin, phenylmercuric nitrate, mercocresols; hexachlorophene; chlorhexidine gluconate; benzalkonium chloride; oxychlorosene sodium; silver compounds such as mild silver protein; miscellaneous antiseptics: hexylresorcinol, bismuth-formic-iodide
Antifungal products	Undecylenic acid; triacetin (glyceryl triacetate); iodochlorhydroxyquin (clioquinol); miconazole; acrisorcin; haloprogin; tolnaftate; clotrimazole; nystatin; amphotericin; combinations including caprylate, propionic acid and salts, benzoic acid, sodium thiosulfate, keratolytics as salicylic acid, astringents as tannic acid, boric acid as astringent/antiseptic
Antihistamine products	Antihistamines: phenyltoloxamine, pyrilamine maleate, methapyrilene, chlorpheniramine maleate, diphenhydramine, tripelennamine; antihistamines in combination with anesthetics, antipruritics, and astringents
Bath products	Colloidal materials and emollient oils: lanolin, fatty acid esters, mineral, polyoxyethylene fatty esters, soybean oil, colloidal oatmeal, colloidal sulfur, balsam peru, soya protein
Cauterizing products	Dichloracetic acid; silver nitrate
Corticosteroids and combinations	Amcinonide; betamethasone salts (dipropionate, valerate, benzoate); clocortolone pivulate; desonide; dexamethasone and salts; flumethasone; fluocinolone and salts; fluocinonide; desoximethasone; diflorasone diacetate; flurandrenolide; fluorometholone; halcinonide; hydrocortisone (as Cortaid sold without a prescription); methylprednisolone; prednisolone; triamcinolone acetonide; combinations with antifungals, keratolytics, antipruritics, local anesthetics, astringents, antihistamines, vasoconstrictors, peeling and drying agents, antibiotics
Emollients	Dexpanthenol; vitamin E; urea (carbamide); vitamin A and D as cod liver oil
Irrigating sterile solutions	Physiologic solutions of sodium salts (chloride, acetate, gluconate), dextrose, potassium salts (chloride, monobasic phosphate), dibasic sodium phosphate heptahydrate, magnesium salts (sulfate, chloride)
Keratolytics	Salicylic acid, cantharidin
Local anesthetics	For skin: benzocaine (ethyl aminobenzoate), butamben picrate, cyclomethycaine sulfate, dibucaine, dimethisoquin hydrochloride, diperodon, lidocaine, pramoxine, tetracaine; for mucous membrane: benzocaine, cocaine, cyclomethycaine sulfate, dyclonine, hexylcaine, lidocaine, tetracaine; combinations are found with various products of almost all classes of topical agents
Rubs and liniments	Analgesics (salicylates, triethanolamine), counterirritants (methyl salicylate, camphor, menthol, eugenol, eucalyptol, thymol); local anesthetics; vasodilators (methacholine chloride)

Continued.

TABLE 30-3 Topical dermatologic products and their ingredients—cont'd

Product	Ingredients
Scabicides and/or pediculicides	Gamma benzene hexachloride (Lindane); crotamiton; pyrethrins; piperonyl butoxide; petroleum distillate; tetrahydronaphthalene; isobronyl thiocyanoacetate, precipitated sulfur 6% in petrolatum
Skin protectants	Silicone, lanolin, starch
Tar-containing topical combinations	Coal tar and derivatives; antipruritics; mild local anesthetics; counterirritants such as menthol; astringents; antiseptic protective such as zinc oxide; keratolytics and precipitated sulfur; salicylic acid; topical antiseptic such as ammoniated mercury
Wet dressings and soaks	Burow's solution (aluminum acetate solution) or modified Burow's solution (aluminum chloride hexahydrate); Dalibour solution (zinc and copper sulfate camphor); lime sulfur solution

5% polyethylene; it is a hydrophobic base.

Polysorb anhydrous, aquaphor. There are absorbent ointment bases that will combine with water or aqueous solutions of drugs.

Rose water ointment. Rose water ointment is a plesant smelling water-in-oil emulsion of the cold cream type. It contains spermaceti and white wax as emulsifying agents in addition to expressed almond oil, sodium borate, rose water, oil of rose, and distilled water. Nonallergic cold creams do not contain perfume, to which some patients are intolerant.

Cold cream. Cold cream is like rose water ointment except that mineral oil is substituted for almond oil or persic oil.

Theobroma oil (cacao or cocoa butter). Theobroma oil is a fixed oil that is expressed from the roasted seeds of *Theobromo cacao.* It is a yellowish white solid having a faint, agreeable odor and a bland taste resembling chocolate. It is used chiefly for making suppositories and, to some extent, as a lubricant for massage and for application to sore nipples.

White ointment. White ointment is a mixture of white wax and white petrolatum. It is mostly petrolatum with a little white wax added to give it stiffness. It is used as an ointment base.

Yellow ointment. Yellow ointment contains yellow wax and petrolatum.

Zinc oxide ointment. Zinc oxide ointment contains 20% zinc oxide in a base of liquid Petrolatum and white ointment.

Zinc ointment. Zinc ointment contains 15% zinc oxide in a base of simple ointment.

Vitamin A and D ointment. Vitamin A and D ointment contains vitamin A and vitamin D in a lanolin-petrolatum base or vanishing cream base (for example, Clocream).

Vitamin E. Vitamin E may aid in controlling dry or chapped skin and is used as a deodorant with questionable effectiveness.

Urea or carbamide (Aquacare, Nutraplus, Carmol). Urea or carbamide promotes hydration and softens keratin in dry skin and hyperkeratotic conditions. The available forms are cream and lotions in range of 2% to 40% urea.

Combination products. Combination products to lubricate and moisturize the skin contain various emollients and other ingredients. Some examples of combination products are Allercreme skin lotion; Lubriderm; Keri Lotion; Dermassage; Nivea oil, cream, and lotion; Neutrogena lotion and oil; Purpose Dry Skin Cream; LactiCare Lotion; and Nutraplus lotion and cream.

Bath preparations. Emollient preparations used as bath dermatologic preparations often contain colloidal material, such as oatmeal and sulfur, and various oils, such as mineral oil, lanolin oil, and soybean oil, which aid in humectant, emollient, and soothing action. Examples of these products are Aveeno Colloidal Oatmeal, Alpha-Keri therapeutic bath oil, and lubriderm Bath Oil.

SOLUTIONS AND LOTIONS

Soothing preparations may also be liquids that carry an insoluble powder or suspension, or they may be mild acid or alkaline solutions, such as boric acid solution, limewater, or aluminum subacetate used as wet dressings and soaks. The bismuth salts (the subcarbonate or the subnitrate) and starch are also commonly used for their soothing effect.

Aluminum acetate solution (Burow's solution). This mild protein precipitant coagulates bacterial and serum protein and contains 545 ml aluminum subacetate solution and 15 ml glacial acetic acid in 1000 ml aqueous medium. It is diluted with 10 to 40 parts of water before application. This may be prepared from Domeboro or Bluboro products.

Aluminum subacetate solution. This preparation contains 145 g aluminum sulfate, 160 ml acetic acid, and 70 g precipitated calcium carbonate in 1000 ml aqueous medium. It is applied topically after dilution with 20 to 40 parts of water as a wet dressing.

Calamine lotion. Prepared calamine, zinc oxide, bentonite magma, glycerin, and calcium hydroxide solutions are included in this lotion. It is a soothing lotion used for the dermatitis caused by poison ivy, insect bites, prickly heat, and so on. It is patted on the involved skin area and is available with an antihistamine, diphenhydramine, as Caladryl lotion.

Zinc stearate. Zinc stearate is a compound of zinc and variable proportions of stearic and palmitic acids. It contains about 14% zinc oxide and is similar to zinc oxide. It is used as a dusting powder, but caution should be observed with its use, particularly around infants, to prevent inhalation of the powder.

BATHS

Baths may be employed to cleanse the skin, to medicate it, or to reduce temperature. The usual method of cleansing the skin is by the use of soap and water, but this may not be tolerated in skin diseases. In some cases even water is not tolerated and inert oils must be substituted. Persons with dry skin should bathe less frequently than those with oily skin. It is possible to keep the skin clean without a daily bath. Nurses are sometimes accused of overbathing hospital patients, causing the patient's skin to become dry and itchy. An oily lotion is preferable to alcohol (isoprophyl or ethyl) for dry skin.

To render baths soothing in irritative conditions, bran, starch, or gelatin may be added in the proportion of about 1 to 2 ounces per gallon of water. Oils such as Alpha-Keri, Lubath, and oilated oatmeal in a proportion of 1 ounce to the tub of water decrease the drying effect of water and thus help to relieve the itching of a sensitive, xerotic skin.

SOAPS

Ordinary soap is the sodium salt of palmitic, oleic, or stearic acids or mixtures of these. Soaps are prepared by saponifying fats or oils with the alkalies. The fats or oils used vary considerably. The oil used for castile soap is supposed to be olive oil. Some soaps are made with coconut oil to which the skin of some persons is sensitive. Soaps contain glycerin unless it has been removed from the preparation. The consistency of the soap depends on the predominating acid and alkali used.

Although all soaps are relatively alkaline, the presence of an excess of free alkali or acid will constitute a potential source of skin irritation.

Medicated soaps contain antiseptics and other added substances, such as cresol, thymol, and sulfur, but soaps per se are antiseptic only insofar as they favor the mechanical cleansing of the skin.

The belief that soap and water are bad for the complexion is erroneous for the most part. A clean skin helps to promote a healthy skin. The soap used in maintaining a clean skin should be mild and contain a minimum of irritating materials.

Soaps are irritating to mucous membranes, and they are used in enemas mainly because of this action. They are also used in the manufacture of liniments and tooth powders. One of the mildest soaps is shaving soap.

Prophylactic agents
PROTECTIVES

Protectives are soothing, cooling preparations that form a film on the skin. Protectives, to be useful, must not macerate the skin, must prevent drying of the tissues, and must keep out light, air, and dust. Nonabsorbable powders are usually listed as protectives, but they are not particularly useful because they stick to wet surfaces and have to be scraped off and do not stick to dry surfaces at all.

Collodion. Collodion is a 5% solution of pyroxylin, or guncotton, in a mixture of ether and alcohol. When collodion is applied to the skin, the ether and alcohol evaporate, leaving a transparent film that adheres to the skin and protects it.

Flexible collodion. Flexible collodion is a mixture of collodion with 2% camphor and 3% castor oil. The addition of the latter makes the resulting film elastic and more tenacious. Styptic collodion contains 20% tannic acid and is, therefore, astringent as well protective.

Nonabsorbable powders. Nonabsorbable powders include zinc stearate, zinc oxide, certain bismuth preparations, talcum powder, and aluminum silicate. The disadvantages associated with their use have been mentioned previously.

Although it is safe to say that no substances known at present can stimulate healing at a more rapid rate than is normal under optimal conditions, preparations that act as bland protectives may help by preventing crusting and trauma. In some instances they may reduce offensive odors.

SUNBURN PREPARATIONS

Sunburn is an acute erythema caused by too long an exposure to the rays of the sun. In some cases, especially if a large area is involved, it may be serious, and the skin surface should be treated as in any serious burn. Exposure to the sun should be done gradually, a few minutes each day, when a general tan is desired. As would be true for any minor partial-thickness burn, when the epithelium is intact and remains so, ordinary protective demulcents or emollients are sufficient to allay irritation.

The use of sunscreens such as para-aminobenzoic acid and its esters, benzophenones and cinnamates can minimize the absorption of ultraviolet rays by the skin, which causes sunburn. These preparations, however, are only of value in preventing sunburn if they are applied before intense sun exposure.

Physical sunscreens such as zinc oxide, red petrolatum, or titanium dioxide are the most effective in preventing a sunburn, but cosmetically they are not appealing to most people.

Therapeutic agents
ANTIINFECTIVES

Antiinfectives include topical antibiotics and antifungal agents in this section. They will be discussed throughout under other headings as well.

ANTIBIOTICS

The most frequent causative organisms of skin infections are *Streptococcus pyogenes* and *Staphylococcus aureus.* Folliculitis, impetigo, furuncles, carbuncles, and cellulitis often result from these organisms. These common skin disorders are infections for which topical antibiotics would be applied. Only some of the agents follow; other topical antibiotics will be discussed under other headings such as acne products and antifungals.

Bacitracin. Bacitracin is very useful in the local treatment of infectious lesions. Bacitracin is most often used in an ointment (Bacguent), although it can be used to moisten wet dressings or as a dusting powder. It is odorless and nonstaining and its use seldom results in sensitization; however, allergic contact dermatitis has occurred.

Neomycin. Neomycin has been used successfully in the treatment of a number of infections of skin and mucous membrane. It is applied topically, but occasionally it irritates the skin; allergic contact dermatitis is reported especially when used on stasis ulcers. An ointment (Mycitracin) combining *neomycin, bacitracin, and polymyxin B* may be more efficacious in mixed infections than when these agents are used singly.

In conditions where absorption of neomycin may occur (burns, trophic ulceration, and so forth), there is the potential of nephrotoxicity, ototoxicity, and neomycin hypersensitivity reactions. This risk is seen more frequently in patients with compromised renal function, patients with extensive burns (over 20% of area), and patients using other aminoglycoside antibiotics. Sensitization may occur to any of the antibiotic ingredients, and prolonged use may produce overgrowth of fungi. Photosensitivity is reported with topical gentamicin.

The possibility of hypersensitivity occurs with chloramphenicol when used topically and the additional risk of bone marrow hypoplasia, blood dyscrasias, itching, burning angioneurotic edema, urticaria, and vesicular and maculopapular dermatitis.

ANTIFUNGAL AGENTS

There are few fungi that produce keratinolytic enzymes to provide for their existence on skin. There are three infectious fungi that can cause local fungal infections without systemic effects: *Microsporum, Trichophyton,* and *Epidermophyton.* The possibility of a mixed infection with these fungi must never be overlooked.

Fungi exist in a moist, warm environment, preferably in dark areas (such as in shoes and socks). Tinea pedis (athlete's foot, ringworm of the foot) is most commonly encountered. Immunologic mechanisms may have an important role in fungal control. The triad for suspicion for fungal infections is an immunologic deficit, a specific fungi involvement, and the skin condition.

The stratum corneum is a layer of dead desquamated cells that are shed normally or are dissolved in sebum. The fungi invade this layer and cause inflammation and induce sensitivity when they penetrate the epidermis and dermis. Since the stratum corneum is shed daily, the ability to spread or transmit the fungi is by contact.

Miconazole nitrate (MicaTin). Miconazole nitrate is an antifungal that inhibits growth of common dermatophytes. It is commonly used for tinea pedis (athlete's foot), tinea cruris (ringworm of the groin), and tinea capitis (ringworm of the scalp) caused by *Trichophyton (rubrum* and *mentagrophytes)* and *Epidermophyton floccosum,* cutaneous candidiasis (moniliasis), and tinea versicolor *(Pityrosporon orbiculare).* The last two are nondermatophytic fungi. The product Monistat-7 is indicated for the local treatment of vulvovaginal candidiasis (moniliasis). Miconazole should be discontinued if sensitivity or chemical irritation develops. Contact with the eyes should be avoided; burning, irritation, and maceration may occur.

Miconazole is available in a cream and lotion, both 2%, and in a water-miscible base. The cream should be applied sparingly and smoothly over the affected area twice daily (morning and evening), avoiding maceration, and once daily for tinea versicolor; for intertriginous (skin chafe on opposing surfaces) areas the lotion should be used. Patients with tinea versicolor exhibit clearing after 2 weeks of treatment. Common dermatophyte infections are relieved within 1 month. Pruritus is relieved within 1 week, and early clinical improvement is seen within 2 weeks; *Candida* is treated for 2 weeks to reduce recurrence.

Haloprogin (Halotex). Haloprogin is an antifungal agent for treatment of superficial fungal skin infections. It is used for topical treatment of tinea (pedis, cruris, corporis, manuum [hands]) caused by *Trichophyton (rubrum, tonsurans, mentagrophytes), microsporum canis,* and *Epidermophtyon floccosum* and tinea versicolor caused by *Pityrosporon orbiculare,* which appear in scales as hyphal elements and spores. A cream and a solution (1%) are available.

Side effects reported include local irritation, burning sensation, scaling, vesicle formation, maceration, and pruritus. If these reactions occur, haloprogin should be discontinued. If no improvement from treatment occurs after 4 weeks, reevaluation of diagnosis and treatment is in order. Halaprigin should be applied to affected areas liberally twice daily for 2 to 3 weeks; interdigital lesions require at least 4 weeks of therapy.

Clotrimazole (Lotrimin, Mycelex). Clotrimazole is a broad-spectrum antifungal agent that inhibits the growth of yeasts and pathogenic dermatophytes. It is used for topical treatment in the inhibition of growth of pathogenic dermatophytes and *Malassezia furfur.* There is an additional indication for vulvovaginal candidiasis (moniliasis) in vaginal tablets and creams (Gyne-Lotrimin, Mycelex-G). Its systemic use is in the treatment of generalized candidiasis. Clotrimazole's use in pregnancy (first trimester) is only recommended when the benefit is essential to the welfare of the childbearing patient.

The side effects are not common but can include erythema, stinging, blistering, peeling, edema, pruritus, urticaria, and general skin irritation.

The drug is available in cream and solution (both 1%). It is gently massaged into the affected and surrounding areas twice daily (morning and evening). Clinical improvement (relief of pruritus) is seen within 1 week of therapy. As with other antifungal agents, if no improvement is seen within 4 weeks, the patient is to be reevaluated.

Tolnaftate (Tinactin, Aftate). Tolnaftate is a nonsensitizing synthetic fungicidal agent; it generally does not sting or irritate intact or broken skin. The mode of action is unknown. It is used for treatment of fungal infections, caused by *Trichophyton, Microsporum,* and *Epidermophyton,* and tinea versicolor, caused by *Malassezia furfur.* The scalp should be treated with the cream or solution, and an oral antifungal agent (griseofulvin) is needed to treat onychomycosis or chronic infections of scalp, palms, and soles in conjunction with tolnaftate. Tolnaftate is not effective against *Candida albicans.* As with other antifungals, a 4-week period is needed for treatment.

This product does not require a prescription. The available forms are cream, gel, powder, and aerosol (for powder and liquid), all having 1% strength. Because of their drying effect, powders are recommended for use in intertriginous areas and naturally moist skin areas. Daily hygiene to prevent reinfection includes the use of powder forms. All dosage forms relieve burning, itching, and soreness within 24 hours and eliminate symptoms within 6 weeks. The powder must be kept from contact with the eyes. The infected areas should be washed and dried morning and evening and a ½-inch ribbon of cream should be applied, rubbing gently on the infected area while spreading the cream evenly. The solution application is generally 2 to 3 drops massaged gently over the infected area after washing and drying. The powder is sprinkled on all areas of infection and inside shoes and socks. The treatment is continued to prevent remission in those susceptible to tinea.

Potassium permanganate solution (1:100 to 1:10,000). This antimicrobial solution is sometimes prescribed for foot soaks for epidermophytosis of the feet (athlete's foot). It is inexpensive and odorless but leaves brown stains on fabrics, skin, and nails.

Benzoic and salicylic acid ointment (Whitfield's Ointment). This ointment contains salicylic ointment. It is used for epidermophytosis of the feet.

Nystatin (Mycostatin). Nystatin is an antibi-otic substance used to treat infections of the skin and mucous membranes caused by *Candida albicans.* Vaginal infections are treated with suppositories or tablets, each containing 100,000 units, once or twice daily. An ointment and cream are available (100,000 units) for moniliasis of the skin and should be applied to the affected area once to several times a day.

Griseofulvin (Fulvicin, Grifulvin). Griseofulvin is an important addition to the treatment of superficial fungous infections, particularly those caused by the trichophyton and microsporon organisms. It is given orally in a dosage of 1 g/day (in children the dosage is decreased by half). It has a fungistatic action by combining with the keratin of skin, hair, and nails. Topical therapy should be continued while the griseofulvin is ingested. It is available in 250-mg tablets for oral administration.

Nursing implications for fungal disorders. The nurse may encourage the patient with a superficial fungal infection to practice adequate hygienic principles to discourage growth. Some of the principles are: (1) the affected area should be dry and aerated, and clothing that is warm or that causes an occlusive environment of moisture should be avoided; (2) the body areas may be kept dry by using powders (with or without antifungal ingredients) to prevent maceration; (3) before applying the antifungal medication, the patient should wash the area with mild soap and water and dry; (4) friction or trauma of the area may be avoided by not wearing tight-fitting clothing, which causes friction; clothing should be laundered daily.

ANTIINFLAMMATORY CORTICOSTEROIDS

Topical corticosteroids are generally indicated for relief of inflammatory dermatoses. They also offer the benefit of lessening systemic corticosteroid side effects and allowing direct contact with the localized lesion. Table 30-4 lists some of the most commonly used corticosteroids in practice currently.

The effectiveness of the topical corticosteroids is due to their antiinflammatory, antipruritic, and vasoconstrictor actions. Topical corticosteroids may also stabilize epidermal lysosomes in the skin. A correlation exists between

TABLE 30-4   Glucocorticoids for topical use

Generic name	Trade name(s)	Generic name	Trade name(s)
Amcinonide	Cyclocort cream (0.1%)	Fluorometholone	Oxylone cream (0.025%)
Betamethasone-17-ben-zoate	Benisone Uticort gel (0.025%) Cream (0.025%)	Flurandrenolide	Cordran Cream (0.05%, 0.025%) Ointment (0.05%, 0.025%) Lotion (0.05%) Tape (4 µg/cm²)
Betamethasone dipro-pionate	Diprosone Aerosol (0.7%) Cream (0.64%) Lotion Ointment	Halcinonide	Halciderm Halog Cream (0.1%, 0.025%) Solution (0.1%) Ointment (0.1%, 0.025%)
Betamethasone-17-val-erate	Valisone Cream (0.12%, 0.012%) Ointment (0.12%) Lotion (0.12%) Aerosol (0.18%)	Hydrocortisone	Cort-Dome Cream (0.5%, 1.0%) Lotion (0.5%, 1.0%)
Clocortolone pivalate	Cloderm (0.1%)	Hydrocortisone acetate	Cortaid (0.025%, 0.05%) Cream Ointment Lotion Cortef ointment (1.0%, 2.5%) Carmol-HC (urea 10%) cream (1.0%) Neo-Cortef (neomycin) cream (1.0%, 2.5%)
Desonide	Tridesilon Cream (0.05%) Ointment (0.03%)		
Dexamethasone	Aeroseb-Dex Decadermin estergel (0.01%) Decaspray Aerosol (0.01%)		
Desoximetasone	Topicort emollient cream (0.24, 0.05%)	Hydrocortisone-17-val-erate	Westcort cream (0.2%)
Diflorasone diacetate	Florone Cream (0.05% propylene glycol solvent emulsified hydrophil Ointment (0.05%) emollient base Arlamol-E solvent	Methylprednisolone ac-etate	Medrol acetate topical cream (0.25%, 1.0%)
		Prednisolone	Meti-Derm Cream (0.5%) Aerosol (50 mg/150-g container)
Flumethasone pivalate	Locorten cream (0.03%)	Triamcinolone aceton-ide	Kenalog Cream (0.0%, 0.025%, 0.5%) Ointment (0.1%, 0.025%, 0.5%) Lotion (0.1%, 0.025%) Spray Mycolog (nystatin, neomycin, gramicidin) Ointment Cream Aristocort Cream (0.5%, 0.1%, 0.025%) Ointment (0.1%, 0.025%) Gel (0.1%)
Fluocinolone acetonide	Synalar Cream (0.025, 0.01%) Ointment (0.025%) Solution (0.01%) Synalar-HP cream (0.2%) NeoSynalar (neomycin combination) cream (0.025%) Fluonid Cream (0.025%, 0.01%) Ointment (0.025%) Solution (0.01%)		
Flucocinonide	Lidex Cream (0.05%) Ointment (0.05%) Lidex-E (0.05%) water-washable emollient base Topsyn gel (0.05%)		

the potency and the therapeutic efficacy (box on p. 948). The vehicle (aerosol, cream gel, lotion, ointment, solution, and tape) in which the corticosteroid is placed also alters the vaso-constrictor property and the therapeutic efficacy. Ointment bases and propylene glycol both enhance the penetration of the corticosteroid and its vasoconstrictor effects. The lotion form is well suited for hairy areas or a lesion that is oozing and wet whereas creams and ointments are well suited for dry, scaling, thickened, and pruritic areas. Sprays are suited for the scalp. All vehicles used influence absorption and therapeutic effect.

The percutaneous penetration rate after application also influences therapeutic effica-

Corticosteroids in order of potency*
(Vasoconstrictor assay comparisons)

I. Cyclocort Cream (0.1%)
Diprosone ointment (0.05%)
Florone cream (0.05%)
Florone ointment (0.05%)
Halog cream (0.1%)
Lidex cream (0.05%)
Lidex ointment (0.05%)
Topicort cream (0.25%)
Topsyn gel (0.05%)

II. Aristocort cream (0.5%)
Diprosone cream (0.05%)
Benisone gel, Unicort gel (0.025%)
Valisone ointment (0.1%)

III. Aristocort ointment (0.1%)
Cordran ointment (0.05%)
Kenalog ointment (0.1%)
Synalar HP cream (0.2%)
Synalar ointment (0.025%)
Valisone lotion (0.1%)

IV. Cloderm cream (0.1%)
Cordran cream (0.05%)
Kenalog cream (0.1%)
Kenalog lotion (0.025%)
Synalar cream (0.025%)
Valisone cream (0.1%)
Westcort cream (0.2%)

V. Desonide cream (0.05%)
Locorten cream (0.03%)

VI. Topicals with hydrocortisone (Cortaid), dexamethasone, flumethasone (Locorten), prednisolone (Meti-Derm), and methylprednisolone (Medrol)

Modified from Stoughton, 1972.
*I is the most potent Group, and potency decreases with each group to Group VI, which is least potent. No significant differences in agents exist within a group so they are in alphabetical sequence. The vasoconstrictor assay may not correlate with clinical efficacy.

cy. It is limited by three factors: Rate of dissolution, rate of diffusion, and drug penetration rate (the skin itself as a barrier). The skin is selectively permeable by having regional variations in absorptive capacity. Since most topical corticosteroids are in suspensions (ointments, creams, lotions), the addition of a solvent to the product can enhance drug dissolution, which may improve absorption. The sebum, enzymes, and perspiration of the skin convert topical suspensions to solutions only partially, needing the inclusion of a solvent in the vehicle to increase the rate of dissolution and to overcome the barrier to penetration) the dissolution barrier).

If extensive areas are covered or if the occlusive technique (to be discussed later) is employed, an increased systemic absorption of the corticosteroid is also seen, specifically in children and infants and where there are large areas of altered skin.

Administration. For moist lesions a small amount of cream or lotion should be gently rubbed into the affected region two to four times daily until it disappears. For dry, scaly lesions an ointment is applied in a thin film to the affected area two to three times daily. A hairy application site requires the parting of the hair to permit a more direct contact with the lesion.

Regional differences of the skin offer differences in penetration of the topical corticosteroids. The existence of the stratum corneum acts as an essential barrier to penetration, and its thickness is related to the degree of penetration it permits. The mucous membranes are devoid of this layer, thus permiting rapid penetration. The vulvar and scrotal regions have a thin stratum corneum offering little barrier to steroid penetration; the eyelids also have a thin stratum corneum. Side effects (including adrenal suppression) resulting from systemic absorption may occur from corticosteroid topical application in these areas.

Since side effects may also be attributed to excessive use by the patient, the overcompliance may be compensated for by the use of an adjunctive topical lubricating cream without steroids applied three times daily. If overcompliance is not a problem, the use of the potent penetrating product, diflorasone diacetate ointment, Florone, requiring a once daily dosage would be a choice not to be overlooked. This once daily application has the potential for minimizing certain side effects (for example, systemic absorption or atrophy). This ointment has good hydration, moisturizing, and lubricating (through the serum corneum to the epidermis) properties because of the petrolatum, and the steroid solvent Arlamol E can be applied at night. The need for occlusion necessitates that the steroid be kept in place for about 5 to 6 hours, applying a cream in the morning and the ointment at night. This will be cosmetically acceptable to the patient and may further patient acceptance and compliance.

To avoid systemic steroid complications from topical use the adult dosage of corticosteroids in the first category (boxed material on p. 948) should be maintained below 100/week. In children under 5 years of age, hydrocortisone (as hydrocortisone acetate) should be the drug of first selection for topical corticosteroid therapy, since it is much less potent than the fluorinated corticosteroids. Hydrocortisone valerate (Westcort, 0.2% cream) has a better potential for sequelae than the flourinated steroids.

Side effects and toxic effects. Side effects reported with corticosteroid topical products are acneiform eruptions (with high-potency steroids on sebaceous gland areas or under occlusive dressings); allergic contact dermatitis, burning sensations; dryness; irritation; itching; hypopigmentation; purpura (bruising—diffuse atrophy leads to vulnerable capillaries); hirsutism (with high-potency steroids, on face and scalp); overgrowth of bacteria, fungus, and virus; hypertrichosis; and folliculitis.

The following are seen more frequently with occlusive dressings: Cushing's syndrome, striae (stretch marks), skin atrophy, maceration of the skin, secondary infection, and ocular effects (glaucoma, cataracts).

A shiny erythema with telangiectasia (a skin spot from a dilated blood vessel) occurs in skin treated with long-term topical steroid therapy, and an acnelike eruption may develop on perioral skin if a fluorinated steroid is applied to the face. As little as 0.25 μg of a fluorinated topical product may cause intermittent suppression of the pituitary-adrenal axis if the steroid is absorbed continuously through the skin. When the skin is broken, absorption is enhanced by an occlusive dressing, which can increase the effects of a potent topical fluorinated steroid.

Contraindications. Contraindications are previous histories of allergy to corticosteroids, presence of infections (for example, fungal and tuberculosis of the skin), and presence of sequelae as a result of previous corticosteroid reaction for example, telangiectasia, dermal atrophy, and striae.

Topical corticosteroids should *not* be used extensively in large amounts or for prolonged periods of time on pregnant patients because of the potential risk of fetal abnormalities (established in laboratory animals).

Occlusive dressing technique. The technique of applying an occlusive dressing (as for management of psoriasis and persistent inflammatory dermatoses) is generally done in the following manner.

1 Remove the superficial scaling before the topical application. Soak the affected area in a bath to soften scales and provide ease in removal by brushing, picking, or gentle rubbing. Remove the crusts, scales, and dried exudates during this cleansing procedure. Shave or clip the hair in the treatment area to permit direct contact of the topical steroid with the skin and to permit easy removal. This will prevent the development of odor under the occlusive dressing.
2 Rub the topical steroid into the affected area thoroughly.
3 An occlusive dressing of pliable plastic nonporous film such as polyethylene, Saran-Wrap, or a plastic bag (cleaning bag or Handi Wrap) is used to cover the affected area. To provide more moisture, a slightly dampened cloth or gauze may be placed over the area before applying the plastic film. The use of polyethylene gloves is convenient for treatment of the hands and fingers; a plastic garment bag (not for children) can be used for treatment of lesions of the trunk and buttocks; for the scalp the use of a shower cap is convenient.
4 Seal the edges of the dressing to adjacent normal unaffected skin with tape or suitable wrapping (at least 7 to 8 hours, preferably 12 to 24 hours).
5 The dressing may be removed during the day and reapplied nightly for patient convenience. During the day when the dressing is removed, the patient may use a steroid cream or lotion applied sparingly. More resistant cases may necessitate the dressing to be in place for 3 to 4 days to achieve a better response.
6 Continue the therapy for a few days after the lesions have cleared so that relapse does not occur prematurely as a result of a too abrupt cessation of therapy.

Some precautions observed in occlusive therapy are described as follows:

1 In the hospital environment there is an increased potential of secondary infection from resistant strains of staphylococci, so the use of occlusive dressings is cautioned.
2 Generally an occlusive dressing is not used on areas where the stratum corneum penetration barrier is removed such as weeping, exudative lesions, since there is a potential for systemic absorption. Systemic absorption is seen when large amounts of steroids are used topically over large areas, when steroids are used for a long time in an airtight occlusive dressing to enhance absorp-

tion, and when the epidermal layer is broken.

3 If miliaria or folliculitis occurs, the occlusive dressing should be discontinued and the use of cool water compresses without occlusion may be instituted.

4 The occlusive dressing may cause thermal homeostasis impairment leading to body temperature elevation, which necessitates discontinuance of the occlusive dressing.

Nursing implications. To enhance patient compliance the reasons for the occlusive dressing procedure should be described to the patient. This technique intensifies percutaneous penetration of the topical steroid and concentrates the medication in the area where it is most needed.

The nurse should be aware that the patient may purchase over-the-counter (OTC) hydrocortisone in 0.25% or 0.5% dosage strengths in ointments, creams, lotions, and aerosol sprays. This topical corticosteroid does not require a prescription.

The age of the skin affects absorption of the potent fluorinated corticosteroids; the very young and the very old have skin that is more permeable.

Other factors that influence the rate and extent of percutaneous absorption are the partition coefficient (degree of division between the vehicle and the skin) of the drug, hydration of the skin, drug concentration, pH effect, skin temperature elevations, and skin condition (inflamed or abraded).

If prolonged treatment is required, the clinical monitoring of plasma cortisol levels monthly by the physician until the steroid is discontinued would be prudent. Most side effects are temporary and resolve when the topical steroid is discontinued.

ACNE PRODUCTS

Acne vulgaris involves an intrafollicular hyperkeratinization that leads to the formation of a keratin plug at the base of the pilosebaceous follicle; it afflicts 30% to 85% of adolescents. The reduction and removal of sebum and bacteria, specifically *Propionibacterium acnes,* are the target of therapy. Being anaerobic, *P. acnes* lives deep within the follicle, producing lipase, protease, hyaluronidase, and lecithinase. It is thought that the *P. acnes* tranforms the sebum glycerides into free fatty acids that irritate the follicle wall, which ruptures and releases the fatty acids producing inflammatory reactions. Treatment in acne therapy may include (1) removal of keratin plugs, (2) decreasing the amount of *P. acnes,* (3) lowering the amounts of free fatty acid formation, (4) decreasing the sebum production, and (5) effectively improving the appearance of the patient for psychosocial benefit.

Of the many forms of treatment modalities in acne therapy only the topical forms of benzoyl peroxide, tetracycline, erythromycin, clindamycin, and tretinoin will be discussed here.

Tretinoin (retinoic acid, vitamin A acid, Retin-A)

Tretinoin is an irritant that stimulates epidermal cell turnover, which causes skin peeling; this reduces the free fatty acids and horny cell adherence within the comedone.

Its use is in the treatment of acne vulgaris in which comedones, pustules, and papules predominate. Tretinoin is available in cream (0.05% and 0.1%), gel (0.025% and 0.01%), liquid (0.05%), and saturated swab (0.05%) dosage forms. It is applied before retiring each night by covering the area lightly. Some patients may require less frequent applications or use a lower percentage strength, and others may respond to the higher percentage dosage forms. Results may be seen after 2 or 3 weeks; it may take up to 6 weeks for optimal effects, after which a lower strength may be used to maintain therapy.

Side effects and toxic effects. Excessive red, edematous, blistered, or crusted skin may be seen in patients with sensitive skin; temporary alterations in pigmentation are sometimes seen; and susceptibility to ultraviolet light is seen. These reactions are all reversible on discontinuation of therapy. The patient should be warned to keep this drug away from the mucous membranes, eyes, mouth, and nose. Its use may cause a feeling of warmth and stinging with peeling.

Patients with sunburned skin, skin sensitive to ultraviolet light, or skin exposed to weather extremes (wind and cold) must exercise caution and not use tretinoin until the skin has recovered. Severe local erythema and peeling at the application site is reported.

The patient must avoid medicated or abrasive cleansers, soaps, and cosmetics that have a drying effect and those with high alcohol concentrations, since they will interact with the tretinoin. Redness, peeling, and discomfort are seen with excessive or overzealous use.

Drug interactions. The possible interactions with concomitant topical use are seen with peeling agents such as benzoyl peroxide, resorcinol, salicylic acid, and sulfur, which result in excessive keratolytic and peeling effects. However, these products may be applied on alternating days.

Benzoyl peroxide

Benzoyl peroxide slowly and continuously liberates active oxygen, producing antiseptic, drying, and keratolytic actions. The release of oxygen into the pilosebaceous area creates unfavorable growth conditions for *P. acnes* and reduces the release of the fatty acids from sebum. Additionally, the drying vehicle (a gel or lotion) aids in shrinking the papules or pustules but does not have an effect on comedones or cysts.

Benzoyl peroxide has been approved for the clinical use and treatment of acne. This agent is available in the following dosage forms: creams, gels, and lotions in 5% and 10% strengths. It will bleach fabric and possibly hair if contact is made over prolonged periods. Its application will produce warmth, stinging, redness, drying, and peeling. The beneficial signs of peeling and drying should not alarm the patient; they occur within 4 days of therapy. Benzoyl peroxide is applied once daily for the first few days and increased or decreased as therapeutic results indicate.

An adverse reaction is painful irritation, which necessitates cessation of this agent. It should be kept away from the nose, eyes, mouth, and mucous membranes. Hypersensitivity is reported. Use on inflamed denuded or thin skin is to be avoided.

TOPICAL ANTIBIOTICS

Topical antibiotics used in the treatment of acne (clindamycin, erythromycin, tetracycline, meclocycline) have unknown mechanisms of action. Therefore the postulated mechanisms of action of these antibiotics are antiinflammatory or inhibitory or suppressive of acne-causing bacteria and the reduction of short-chain free fatty acids of the surface lipids.

Clindamycin phosphate (Cleocin T topical solution)

Topical clindamycin efficacy in the treatment of acne is reported to be equal to or better than oral tetracycline therapy and superior to topical erythromycin or topical tetracycline therapy. The solution concentration is an equivalent of 10 mg/ml of clindamycin in 50% isopropyl alcohol with propylene glycol and water. This is one of the most widely used topical antibiotic indicated in the treatment of acne vulgaris. Skin phosphatases, by hydrolysis, convert the clindamycin phosphate to the antibacterial active clindamycin base.

The affected skin is first washed and dried before a thin layer is sparingly applied in a dabbing motion. When the applicator tip becomes dry, the bottle should be inverted and the automatic spring-loaded valve tip should be depressed several times until it is moist.

A thin film is applied twice daily directly from the applicator bottle (30 or 60 ml). The fingers and hands do not directly apply this product. The unique applicator system allows efficient and economic delivery and stability for 24 months.

Approximately 10% of a dose penetrates and is absorbed in the stratum corneum layer. Clindamycin has appeared in the urine without detectable activity in the plasma and with detectable activity in comedonal extracts. After topical application, there is an inhibition of acne-causing bacteria and reduction of free fatty acids on the skin surface.

Side effects and toxic effects. The alcohol base may cause transient burning and irritation to the eye, nose, mouth, abraded skin, and other mucous membranes. This irritation can be overcome with the application of cool water. Gastrointestinal reactions (diarrhea and colitis) owing to potential systemic absorption have been reported. If diarrhea occurs, a large bowel endoscopy should be considered. Irritations and staining of skin, sensitization, gram-negative folliculitis, *Staphylococcus aureus*, erythema, rashes, and contact dermatitis have been reported.

Cross-resistance exists with lincomycin and antagonism with erythromycin. Contraindications demonstrated by hypersensitivity to any form of clindamycin or lincomycin may apply to the topical preparation. During the patient interviews the nurse should inquire about any previous sensitivity not only to clindamycin but also to other antibiotics or allergens, and atopic patients should be questioned since some absorption may possibly occur through the skin.

Tetracycline topical solution (Topicycline)

Topical tetracycline, used in treating acne vulgaris, is directly applied to the pilosebaceous unit (hair follicle and sebaceous gland), which is most numerous on the face, back, chest, and upper arms. Systemic tetracycline decreases the amount of free fatty acids present in acne lesions, but the mechanism by which topical tetracycline therapy improves acne is unknown.

Topical tetracycline produces serum levels of 0.1 μg/ml, which is less than 7% of that produced by a 500 mg/day oral dose. Liver damage in patients with renal impairment using topical tetracycline is unlikely, but it should be considered. No data are available regarding the use of topical tetracyclines in pregnant women, and no established data are available concerning its use during lactation.

Tetracycline is generously applied twice daily (morning and evening) to affected areas until the skin is wet. Because of the 40% ethanol and other components, the eyes, nose, mouth, and mucous membrane areas should be avoided. Normal use of cosmetics is permitted. Transient stinging or burning may occur. The slight yellow superficial coloring of the skin of light-complected patients may be washed off. Under a source of ultraviolet light (sun, sunlamp), the treated areas will fluoresce.

Meclocycline sulfosalicylate (Meclan) cream

Meclocycline sulfosalicylate is a topical oxytetracycline derivative that is indicated in the treatment of acne vulgaris. The mode of action is not clearly understood. The percutaneous absorption resulting from prolonged use of this tetracycline derivative necessitates cautious monitoring of patients with hepatic or renal dysfunctions. No adequate well-controlled studies have been made in pregnant women or nursing mothers. Among the reported adverse reactions are a few instances of acute contact dermatitis and skin irritation. Excessive application may result in temporary follicular staining and fabric staining. Application of this nonalcoholic vanishing cream is done in the morning and evening or less often depending on patient response.

Erythromycin topical solution (A/T/S, Eryderm, Staticin)

Erythromycin topical solution is indicated for the treatment of acne vulgaris. With this product, an overgrowth of antibiotic-resistant organisms may occur.

Erythromycin topical solution is applied with the fingertips and hands each morning and evening to the affected areas. These areas are to be washed and rinsed and patted dry; after application, the hands and fingers should be washed.

Frequently described adverse reactions include erythema, desquamation, tenderness, dryness, pruritus, oiliness, and acne. A generalized urticarial reaction requiring systemic steroid therapy has been reported with the use of this agent.

Hypersensitivity to erythromycin or the other components of the solution (alcohol, propylene glycol) is a contraindication to its use. Its safe use in pregnancy and lactation has not been established. Erythromycin topical solution should not be used near the eyes, nose, mouth, and other mucous membranes. A cumulative irritant effect may occur with concomitant use of peeling, desquamating, or abrasive agents.

KERATOLYTICS

Keratolytics (keratin dissolvers) are drugs that soften scales and loosen the outer horny layer of the skin. Salicylic acid and resorcinol are drugs of choice. Their action makes possible the penetration of other medicinal substances by cleaning the lesions involved. Salicylic acid is particularly important for its keratolytic effect in local treatment of scalp conditions, warts, corns, fungous infections, acne, and chronic types of dermatitis. It is used up to 20% in ointments, plasters, or collodion for this purpose.

BURN PRODUCTS

It is said that approximately 6000 or more people die each year of thermal injury in the United States alone. The chief cause of death is shock, a fact of considerable significance in any effective plan of treatment.

Burns cause lesions of the skin accompanied by pain. The burn may be caused by heat (thermal burn), chemical cauterizing agents (chemical burns), or electricity (electrical burns). Sources may be friction, lightning, or electromagnetic energy sources (ultraviolet light, x-rays, lasers, or atomic explosion). The types of burns that result from various sources are relatively specific and diagnostic.

Consideration of what takes place in the damaged tissues clarifies many points of treatment. At first there is an altered capillary permeability in the local injured area. That is, the permeability is increased and a loss of plasma and weeping of the surface tissues result. If the burn is at all extensive, considerable amounts of plasma fluid may be lost in a relatively short time. This depletes the blood volume and causes a decreased cardiac output and diminished blood flow. Unless the situation is rapidly brought under control, irreparable damage may result from the rapidly developing tissue anoxia. Lack of sufficient oxygen and the accumulation of waste products from inadequate oxidation result in loss of tone in the minute blood vessels, and the increased capillary permeability then extends to tissues remote from those suffering the initial injury. Thus a generalized edema often develops and the vicious cycle once established tends to be self-perpetuating. One of the aims in the treatment of burns is therefore, to stop the loss of plasma insofar as it is possible and replenish that which is lost as quickly as possible.

Partial- or full-thickness burns must be thought of as open wounds with the accompanying danger of infection. The infection must be prevented or treated. The treatment, however, must be such that it will not bring any further destruction of tissue or of the small islands of remaining epithelium from which growth and regeneration can take place.

When burns are divided into three degrees, they are classified by the depth of skin involved within a geographic designation. First-degree burns involve only the epidermis, causing erythema with characteristic dry painful reddening and edema without blistering or vesiculation (for example, overexposure to sun or flash burn). Second-degree burns involve the epidermis extending into the dermis and may be superficial or involve deep dermal necrosis. Epithelial regeneration may extend from the deep skin appendages such as hair follicles and sebaceous glands that penetrate the dermis. This burn is characterized by a moist, blistered, very painful surface (for example, flash or scald burns from nonviscous liquids). Third-degree burns involve destruction of the entire dermis and epidermis characterized by white, lustrous, or opaque skin; dry, leathery skin; or coagulated, charred skin without sensation as a result of the destruction of nerve endings (for example, flame burns or hot viscous liquids). Deep third-degree burns extend into subcutaneous fat, muscle, or bone; they cause scarring and may require skin grafting.

The severity of electrical burns depends on the amount of voltage received, the condition of the skin (for example, cuts, abrasions, and moisture, which lower resistance), and contraction of flexor muscles, which inhibits release from the power source. This may result in cardiac systole, ventricular fibrillation, or nervous system paralysis, which can lead to respiratory arrest. Electrical burns develop necrosis of more tissue than thermal burns. Electrical burns are of three types: In Type I, the electrical current causes effects on blood vessels such as occlusion, thrombosis, or tissue destruction. In Type II, electrical burns from high-tension currents (for example, an electrical arc) produce a crater in the skin. Type III electrical burns are similar to flame burns because the arc flame ignites the patient's wearing apparel.

Chemical burns occur after contact with acid or alkali; the initial treatment is water irrigation of the affected area followed by neutralization. Chemical burns may occur in the mouth and appear as a white slough owing to necrosis of the epithelium and underlying connective tissues.

First aid treatment of burns. An important first aid treatment for minor and major burns, regardless of cause (chemical, electric, thermal), is to immediately cool the wound to remove irritants, decrease inflammation, and constrict blood vessels; this reduces the permeability of the blood vessels and checks edema formation. Cold tap water can be used to thoroughly flush the wound and to cool hot clothing. The more quickly the wound is cooled, the less tissue damage there is likely to be, and the more rapid will be the recovery. No greasy ointments, lard, butter, or dressings should be applied, since these agents will inhibit loss of heat from the burn, which will increase both discomfort and tissue damage. The burn may be left exposed to the air or cold wet compresses may be applied until the patient can be transported to a place where he can receive medical attention.

Prevention and treatment of infection. Penicillin and streptomycin are frequently used for the early treatment of burned patients other than those with a minor partial-thickness burn and an intact skin. These agents are given parenterally during the first few days, and are then discontinued until debridement has been performed or until there is evidence of infection. Some physicians believe that in the treatment of burns that are not grossly contaminated it may be better to wait until there is evidence of infection, obtain a culture, and follow with the antibiotic of choice.

A booster dose of tetanus toxoid is given to the patient who has been previously immunized, and active immunization is started for those not previously immunized.

Mafenide acetate (Sulfamylon)

One of the most important therapeutic agents developed to combat burn infection in avascular tissue has been the discovery of mafenide acetate. Mafenide (a sulfonamide) is a water-soluble ointment that is applied topically to the burn wound with sterile gloves following wound cleansing and debridement. The exposure method of therapy is preferred, although occasionally dressings may be applied; however, this may result in tissue maceration.

The ointment (applied with a sterile gloved hand) forms a protective coating over the burn. It rapidly diffuses through partial (second-degree) and full-thickness (third-degree) burns and has proved to be one of the most effective means for preventing and retarding bacterial invasion in burn wounds. It has decreased deaths resulting from septicemia and decreased extension of the wound from infection. It has decreased the number of burn cases requiring plastic surgery or skin grafting. However, eschar separation is delayed.

Mafenide acetate is relatively nontoxic. It is rapidly broken down in the body and eliminated via the kidneys. Since this drug is a strong carbonic anhydrase inhibitor, acidosis may occur, usually compensated by hyperventilation. The patient should be carefully observed for any signs resulting in respiratory alkalosis. If rapid or labored respirations occur, the ointment should be washed off the wound. Therapy can be interrupted for 2 to 3 days without impairing the bacterial control of the wound.

Mafenide may cause some discomfort when first applied (in ¹⁄₁₆-inch layer once or twice daily)—a burning sensation may occur that lasts from a few minutes to as long as an hour.

This is a highly stable drug. It remains active for several years and does not need to be refrigerated except in tropical countries.

Silver nitrate

An aqueous solution of silver nitrate 0.5% has been used extensively in some burn centers during the past few years. As a 0.5% solution it is a relatively safe antiseptic agent for gram-negative bacteria. Dressings soaked in silver nitrate 0.5% are applied early to the burn; the dressings must be kept moist and must not be allowed to dry, which would cause precipitation of silver salts into the wound and irritation. Concentrations of silver nitrate above 1% produce tissue necrosis; concentrations below 0.5% are not antiseptic. Silver nitrate stains anything with which it comes in contact. The brown or black tissue discoloration is usually not permanent. Silver nitrate solution 0.5% is a hypotonic solution, and when it is used on extensive burns or for extensive periods of time it may cause electrolyte imbalance. Serum electrolytes should be frequently determined and patients observed for symptoms of sodium or potassium depletion (change in behavior, confusion, and so on); blood sample color (brownish) is indicative of methemoglobinemia.

Silicone fluid (dimethyl polysiloxane)

Silicone fluid has been used to treat hand burns. The hands are placed in plastic bags containing silicone fluid. This is a stable agent; it is inert, has a low specific gravity, and is not harmful to normal or burned skin. The bouyancy of the silicone fluid is a result of its low specific gravity. This permits the patient to move his fingers freely without great discomfort.

Silver sulfadiazine (Silvadene)

Silver sulfadiazine is an antiinfective agent with broad antimicrobial activity against many gram-negative and gram-positive bacteria and yeast. It is particularly effective against *Pseudomonas* organisms. It is produced by the reaction of silver nitrate with sulfadiazine. Silver sulfadiazine acts only on the cell membrane and cell wall to produce its bactericidal effect.

Silver sulfadiazine is used in second- and third-degree burns for the prevention and treatment of infection. Control of infection may prevent the conversion of infected second-degree burns resulting in necrosis. Since silver sulfadiazine is not a carbonic anhydrase inhibitor, it does not alter acid-base balance; neither does it alter electrolyte balance nor stain tissues, linen, or dressings. Silver sulfadiazine softens eschar, facilitating eschar removal and preparation of the wound for grafting.

Silver sulfadiazine is available as a 1% cream to be applied topically to cleansed, debrided burn wounds once or twice daily. It should be applied with a sterile gloved hand to a thickness of about 1/16 inch. Burn wounds should be continuously covered with the cream. If the cream is removed by patient activity, it should be reapplied. Daily bathing and debriding are important. Dressings may or may not be used.

Therapy is usually continued until satisfactory healing has occurred or the wound is ready for grafting. Since silver sulfadiazine inhibits bacterial growth, delayed eschar separation may occur, necessitating escharotomy to prevent contractures.

Pain, burning, and itching occur infrequently following application of the silver sulfadiazine cream.

Silver sulfadiazine may cause a hypersensitivity reaction; if this occurs, the drug should be discontinued. Hemolysis may occur in patients with glucose-6-phosphate dehydrogenase deficiency.

When applied to extensive areas of the body, significant amounts of the drug may be absorbed, producing adverse reactions characteristic of the sulfonamides. Renal function in these patients should be monitored and the urine examined for sulfa crystals.

Silver sulfadiazine may cause kernisterus is not recommended for pregnant women or premature or newborn infants, but is useful in pediatric burn patients.

TOPICAL ANESTHETICS

Antipruritics are drugs given to allay itching of skin and mucous membranes. There is less need for these preparations as the constitutional treatment of patients with skin disorders is better understood. Dilute solutions containing phenol as well as tars have been widely used. They may be applied as lotions, pastes, or ointments. Dressings wet with potassium permanganate 1:4000, aluminum subacetate 1:16, boric acid, or physiologic saline solution may cool and soothe and thus prevent itching. Lotions such as calamine or calamine with phenol (phenolated calamine) and cornstarch or oatmeal baths may also be used to relieve itching.

Local anesthetics such as dibucaine and benzocaine may decrease pruritus, but their use is not recommended because of their high sensitizing and irritating effects. The application of hydrocortisone in a lotion or ointment in a strength of 0.5% to 1% has proved to be one of the best methods of relieving pruritus and decreasing inflammation. It has the additional advantage of possessing a low sensitizing index.

It may be necessary to administer sedatives that have a systemic effect. Some physicians prefer not to use barbiturates because they decrease cortical control of the scratch reflex. Trimeprazine, one of the phenothiazine derivatives, is said to be effective for the relief of itching. Trimeprazine tartrate is administered orally. The usual dose for adults is 2.5 mg four times a day.

In addition to the aforementioned measures to relieve itching, preparations of ergotamine are used to relieve the generalized itching associated with jaundice, cirrhosis of the liver, Hodgkin's disease, and so on. Ergotamine tartrate is one of the preparations and there are others. One of the others is dihydroergotamine, which is said to relieve itching in a way similar to ergotamine tartrate without producing the common undesirable side effects of that preparation (nausea, vomiting, and cardiovascular reactions).

Other preparations used to relieve itching related to allergic reactions are the antihistaminic drugs. Calamine and Benadryl, marketed under the name of Caladryl, are examples of combined drugs given to relieve itching.

STIMULANTS AND IRRITANTS

Stimulants are those substances that produce a mild irritation and in that way promote healing and the disappearance of inflammatory exudates. Most of the irritant drugs exert a stimulating effect when applied in low concentrations. Examples of preparations that may have a stimulating effect are the tars obtained from the destructive distillation of wood and coal.

Tars, when diluted, act as antiseptics as well as irritants. Official preparations include juniper tar, coal tar, and prepared coal tar. The tars are sometimes prescribed in the treatment of psoriasis and chronic eczematous dermatitis. The official tars are seldom employed full strength. Coal tar is the most antiseptic but also the most irritant, and it has the most disagreeable odor. Ichthammol, derived from destructive distillation of coal, is used in the form of an ointment for eczema and seborrheic conditions of the skin.

Compound benzoin tincture is useful as a stimulant and protective for skin ulcers, bedsores, cracked nipples, and fissures of the lips, anus, and the like.

Preparations made of red blood cells also have been used to stimulate healing of indolent wounds and ulcers.

Summary of nursing considerations

A wide range of drugs are used in dermatology, some for systemic and others for local effects. Drugs may be excreted by the skin in small amounts. Silver, copper, arsenic, mercury, bromides, borates, phenol, salicylates, antipyrine, methylene blue, and phenolphthalein may be deposited in the skin and sweat glands, possibly explaining the skin eruption sometimes noticed after their use. Many other drugs can be the cause of skin eruption. Reactions or disorders of the skin are manifested by symptoms such as itching, pain, or tingling and by signs such as swelling, redness, papules, pustules, blisters, and hives.

The nurse must be cognizant of the following factors when caring for patients receiving topical drug therapy:

1 Overtreatment is often difficult to avoid.
2 Topical drugs have a sensitizing potential.
3 There is often a lack of uniform responsiveness of patients to topical therapy.
4 Fair-complexioned individuals are less tolerant of topical drugs than darker complexioned persons.
5 Infants, children, and the elderly usually react unfavorably to drying preparations such as "shake lotions" (for example, calamine lotion) and alcoholic solutions.
6 Action of topical drugs may be greatly enhanced under occlusive dressings.
7 Bland toilet soaps are preferred for patients with sensitive skin (for example, Neutrogena, Dove); medicated soaps should be avoided.

To serve as a guide to the major groups of dermatologic products, Table 30-3 has been included to give an idea of the types of compounds and their ingredients that are used for treating various kinds of dermatologic conditions. For the sake of simplicity, these compounds have been divided into three major groups: vehicles, prophylactic agents, and therapeutic agents.

The vehicles include emollients and solutions along with lotions, baths, and soaps. Protectants and sunburn preparations, on the other hand, are employed as prophylactic agents. Protectives are soothing, cooling preparations that form a film on the skin. Protectives, to be useful, must not macerate the skin, must prevent drying of the tissues, and must keep out light, air, and dust. Nonabsorbable powders are usually listed as protectives but they are not particularly useful because they stick to wet surfaces and have to be scraped off and do not stick to dry surfaces at all. Finally, the therapeutic agents that vary in number and type are used to treat specific dermatologic conditions.

QUESTIONS

FOR STUDY AND REVIEW

1 What are some of the nursing problems unique to the care of patients with disorders of the skin?
2 Define each of the following and give an example of each:
   a. Emollients
   b. Keratolytics
   c. Antipruritics
3 Which topical preparations are readily availalbe in your clinical facility for pruritus? for dry skin? for denuded or excoriated areas?
4 What preparations are used in your hospital for prevention or treatment of decubitus ulcers?
5 Select a common skin disorder (for example, acne, athlete's foot, sunburn), and determine the over-the-counter preparations available in one or more pharmacies. Note the type and amount of ingredients in each preparation. Through library research, obtain information to support or refute the safety and effectiveness claims for the various preparations.
6 What secondary reactions have been reported with the use of corticosteroid topical products?
7 Name some sunscreen compounds that are used to prevent sunburn. When should these agents be applied and why?

BIBLIOGRAPHY

A.M.A. drug evaluations, ed. 4, New York, 1980, John Wiley & Sons, Inc.

Ayers and Mihan: Acne vulgaris and lipid peroxidation: new concepts in pathogenesis and treatment, Int. J. Dermatol. **17:**305, 1978.

du Vivier, A., and Stoughton, R.B.: Acute tolerance to effects of topical glucocorticosteroids, Br. J. Dermatol. **94:**25, 1976.

Feldman, R.J., and Maibach, H.I.: Regional variation in percutaneous penetration of 14C-cortisol in man, J. Invest. Dermatol. **48:**181, 1967.

Goodman, L.S., and Gilman, A.: The pharmacological basis of therapeutics, ed. 6, New York, 1980, Macmillan, Inc.

Goth, A.: Medical pharmacology, ed. 10, St. Louis, 1981, The C.V. Mosby Co.

Hawkins, K.: Wet dressings: putting the damper on dermatitis, Nursing '78 **8**(2):64, 1978.

Hunter, J.A.A.: The structure and function of skin in relation to therapy, Br. Med. J. **4:**340, 1973.

Hunter, J.A.A.: The basis of skin therapy, Br. Med. J. **4:**411, 1973.

Kligman, A.M.: An overview of acne, J. Invest. Dermatol. **62:**268, 1974.

Maibach, H.I., and Stoughton, R.B.: Topical corticosteroids. In Azarnoff, D.L., editor: Steroid therapy, Philadelphia, 1975, W.B. Saunders Co.

Matus, N.R.: Topical therapy: choosing and using the proper vehicle, Nursing '77 **7**(11):8, 1977.

McKenzie, A.W.: Percutaneous absorption of steroids, Arch. Dermatol. **86:**611, 1962.

McKenzie, A.W., and Stoughton, R.B.: Method for comparing percutaneous absorption of steroids, Arch. Dermatol. **86:**608, 1962.

Melski, J.W., and Arndt, K.A.: Topical therapy for acne, N. Engl. J. Med. **302**(9):503, 1980.

Modell, W.: Drugs of choice, St. Louis, 1980-1981, The C.V. Mosby Co.

Ninman, C., and Shoemaker, P.: Human amniotic membrane for burns, Am. J. Nurs. **75:**1468, 1975.

North, C., and Weinstein, G.: Treatment of psoriasis, Am. J. Nurs. **76:**410, 1976.

Proceedings of Workshop on Dermatology, Clin. Pharmacol. Ther. **16:**861, 1974.

Rook, A., and others: et al.: Textbook of dermatology, ed. 2, Oxford, 1974, Blackwell Scientific Publications, Ltd.

Scoggins, R.B., and Kliman, R.: Relative potency of percutaneously absorbed corticosteroids in the suppression of pituitary-adrenal function, J. Invest. Dermatol. **45:**347, 1965.

Solomons, B.: Lecture notes on dermatology, ed. 4, Oxford, 1977, Blackwell Scientific Publications, Ltd.

Soter, N.A., and others: Clinical dermatology, N. Engl. J. Med. **289:**189, 1973.

Stoughton, R.B.: Bioassay system for formulations of topically applied glucocorticosteroids, Arch. Dermatol. **106:**825, 1972.

Stoughton, R.B.: Topical antibiotics for acne vulgaris, current usage, Arch. Dermatol. **115:**486, 1979.

White, M.G., and Asch, M.J.: Acid-base effects of topical mafenide acetate in the burned patient, N. Engl. J. Med. **284:**1281, 1971.

Debriding agents

The decubitus ulcer (bedsore or pressure sore) is a break in the skin and underlying tissue that is caused by abnormal and sustained pressure or friction being exerted over the bony prominences of the body by the object upon which the body part rests. It results in ischemic necrosis.

There are many contributing causes to this condition that must be treated, among which are the following: obesity or malnutrition; debilitation; a shearing force on the lower body if the head of the bed is raised more than 30 inches; a loss of sensation of pressure or pain; muscle atrophy and motor paralysis, as a result of a reduction in the amount of adipose tissue between skin and underlying bone; poor nutrition because of anemia, hypoproteinemia, and deficiencies in vitamins, minerals, and trace elements (such as zinc); trauma; incontinence; edema; infection; heat and moisture (maceration); and local circulatory interference.

Prevention and treatment of decubitus ulcers are centered around treatment of underlying causes, providing a well-balanced nutritional state, and minimizing or eliminating the pressure or friction causing vascular stasis and tissue damage. The following are some preventive and treatment measures that the nurse may employ to reduce the occurrence of decubitus ulcers.

1 Change the patient's position frequently (every 2 hours day and night).
2 Maintain a clean, dry, and wrinkle-free bed. Bed-

clothes should be smooth rather than coarse and should be changed frequently.
3 Provide active and passive exercise to increase muscle and skin tone and to improve vascularity, or use a whirlpool.
4 Position the patient with pillows and pads, not exceeding a 30-inch elevation of the head.
5 Use sheepskin, polystyrene, and foam rubber pads and heel protectors to relieve pressure. Place them on a mattress in direct contact with the patient's skin. The mattress should be free of surface bulges and indentations, having a uniform flat surface, to prevent friction or wrinkles.
6 Use an alternating pressure mattress pad covered with one layer of sheet, to promote circulation and reduce the occurrence of tissue ischemia.
7 Massage the patient's back with nonalcoholic skin lotion, covering the bony prominences of the ankles, coccyx, elbows, heels, hips, knees, shoulders, and other areas having thin layers of subcutaneous tissue.
8 Provide meticulous skin hygiene, with frequent inspections for abnormal alterations. Wash gently with warm water and mild nondetergent soap, rinse, and blot dry with a soft towel. An emollient lubricating lotion may be used following washing to keep the skin soft.
9 Keep the skin of incontinent patients dry and clear of urine and fecal contamination, since maceration from moisture promotes tissue breakdown and predisposes patients to infection. Trimmed nails prevent self-inflicted injury caused by scratching of the skin.
10 Maintain nutritional support and adequate fluid intake with a diet high in protein, vitamins, minerals, and trace elements. The patient's hemoglobin level should be 12 g/100 ml or more.)
11 Necrotic decubitus ulcers often require debride-

ment by surgical or adjunctive topical intervention methods.

12 Treatment regimens are based on the extent of skin involvement.

Enzymes

Enzymes are proteins that act as catalysts for chemical reactions in living systems. The characteristics attributed to catalysts are *speed*, *efficiency*, and *specificity*. Catalysts accelerate chemical reactions, increasing the rapidity of the reaction by as much as a thousandfold, a millionfold, or more. Catalysts consistently produce a particular response without being changed themselves in the process. Furthermore, enzymes act only on a certain substance (absolute specificity) or closely related substances (group specificity) and no other substance.

Enzymes are usually soluble in cellular fluid or can be adsorbed; some enzymes adhere to membranous structures within the cell. Enzymes can split organic substances with which they come in contact into small, highly diffusible substances.

Most enzymes contain the suffix "ase" in their name plus the name of the substrate on which they act. For example, collagenase acts on and degrades collagen; hyaluronidase acts on hyaluronic acid, a ground substance of connective tissue. Enzymes are also grouped according to the reactions they catalyze. For example, proteolytic enzymes hasten the hydrolysis of proteins.

Since enzymes are proteins, they may be antigenic and cause toxic reactions of an immunologic type. Enzymes are biologically active in the presence of certain cofactors such as ions (Ca^{++}, Mg^{--}, and so on) or a nonprotein organic compound such as a vitamin. A cofactor involved during catalysis is termed a *coenzyme*.

The enzymes discussed in this chapter are used topically for *chemical debridement*—that is, the removal, by enzymatic digestion, of necrotic and injured tissue, clotted blood, purulent exudates, or fibrinous accumulations in wounds. This action cleans the wounds and facilitates healing. System is antibiotic therapy and topical antibiotic or antiseptic therapy may be used in conjunction with enzymatic debridement to control or inhibit infection.

Hyaluronidase; hyaluronidase for injection (Wydase)

Hyaluronic acid is a polysaccharide that is an essential component of intercellular ground substance. It is present in the form of a gel in many parts of body tissues, where it serves as intercellular cement and acts as a barrier to the diffusion of invading substances.

Hyaluronidase is a mucolytic enzyme prepared from bovine testes. It is capable of hydrolyzing and depolymerizing hyaluronic acid. It acts as a spreading factor to facilitate absorption and distribution of injected fluids and to facilitate hypodermoclysis. The drug is used as an adjunct in subcutaneous urography, since it improves resorption of radiopaque agents. Hyaluronidase is also used to increase diffusion and absorption of local accumulations of transudates and edema and to resolve hematomas.

Hyaluronidase is especially useful in facilitating administration of fluids by hypodermoclysis, particularly in infants and young children. The resulting increased rate of dispersion and absorption of the injected fluid reduces tissue tension and pain. The rate of absorption, however, should not be greater than that of an intravenous infusion. Special care must be exercised when the drug is administered to children—the speed and total volume administered must be controlled to avoid overhydration. If the drug is injected directly into an infected area, the infection will spread.

If an intravenous solution containing a drug with marked vasoconstrictor action (for example, noradrenalin) infiltrates surrounding tissue, hyaluronidase along with phentolamine may be injected subcutaneously into the infiltrated area. Phentolamine helps relieve the vasoconstrictor action of noradrenalin, and hyaluronidase enhances resorption of the infiltrated fluid. These actions will help prevent tissue necrosis if the drugs are administered early during the infusion infiltration.

In ophthalmic surgery, hyaluronidase is injected with an anesthetic to enhance anesthesia and akinesia (that is, to decrease muscle movement).

Preparation, dosage, and administration. Hyaluronidase is available in a stable dried form in vials containing 150 and 1500 N.F. units and in a solution for injection, 150 units in 1-ml or 10-ml vials. A dose of 150 units is dissolved in 1 ml isotonic sodium chloride solution and is then added to 1000 ml of fluid for hypodermoclysis, or it is injected into the proposed site of the clysis. For children, 15 units is added to each 100 ml solution. The drip rate should not exceed 2 ml/minute.

Side effects and toxic effects. Hyaluronidase has a low level of toxicity, but caution is recommended when it is administered to patients with infections. It should not be injected into or around infected areas, since it will spread the infection by the same mechanism of action that causes spread of injected solutions. Hypersensitivity to this substance sometimes occurs, especially in patients with a history of allergy. Skin testing before administration is recommended.

Sutilains (Travase)

Sutilains is a sterile preparation of proteolytic enzymes isolated from culture filtrates of *Bacillus subtilis*. It is five to sixteen times greater in its action than chymotrypsin. It dissolves and aids in the removal of only nonviable or undenatured protein in necrotic tissue and purulent exudate from open wounds and ulcers resulting from second- and third-degree burns, decubiti, peripheral vascular disease, and trauma. If dissolution does not occur in 24 to 48 hours, the drug should be discontinued.

Preparation. Sutilains is prepared as an ointment containing 82,000 casein units/g ointment base (15-g tubes). It must be refrigerated at a temperature between 2° and 10° C.

A wound should be thoroughly cleansed with water or isotonic sodium chloride solution and left wet before a thin layer of sutilains ointment is applied. The area should then be covered with loose wet dressings. This procedure should be repeated three or four times daily. A moist environment is necessary for this agent's enzymatic activity. The enzymatic activity of sutilains is unaffected by neomycin, mafenide, streptomycin, or penicillin. The optimal pH range of activity is 6 to 6.8.

Side effects and precautions. Side effects are mild; they include transient pain, paresthesia, bleeding, and transient dermatitis. If bleeding or dermatitis occurs, the drug should be discontinued. Although systemic allergic reactions have not been reported, the drug is capable of causing an antibody response. This drug must be kept away from the eyes; if contact occurs, the eyes should be rinsed with copious amounts of sterile water.

Contraindications. Sutilains should not be applied to wounds communicating with major body cavities, wounds with exposed major nerves or nerve tissue, neoplastic ulcers, or wounds in women of childbearing age.

Drug interactions. The use of detergents and antiseptics (benzalkonium chloride, hexachlorophene, iodine, nitrofurazone) concomitantly should be avoided because of possible substrate denaturation of sutilains. Compounds containing metallic ions, such as thimerosal, interfere with the action of the enzyme.

Papain (Panafil)

Panafil Ointment contains papain and 10% urea. Since at physiologic pH values papain does not digest collagen significantly, the denaturing agent urea is added to act on collagen. Chlorophyll derivatives are also added to this product for deodorization. Panafil White Ointment has no chlorophyll.

Papain is used for enzymatic debridement and promotion of healing of surface lesions where healing is retarded by local infection, necrotic tissue, fibrinous or purulent debris, or eschar. It is applied once or twice daily and covered with gauze. Hydrogen peroxide must not be used to irrigate the lesion with each redressing, because it inactivates the papain. All accumulated liquefied necrotic material must be removed before redressing. Side effects of occasional itching and a burning or stinging sensation are associated with the first application to necrotic tissue in dermal wounds.

Trypsin (Granulex)

Granulex aerosol spray contains trypsin, balsam of Peru, and castor oil with an emulsifier. It is indicated for treatment of decubitus ulcers, varicose ulcers, debridement of eschar, dehiscent wounds, and sunburn. The trypsin acts to debride eschar and necrotic tissue. The balsam of Peru improves circulation in the capillary bed. The castor oil acts as a protective and lessens premature epithelial desiccation and cornification. The aerosol form allows treatment without the extraneous pain caused by physical wound contact.

The can should be shaken well, and the wound should be coated rapidly and moderately (not in excess). Granulex should not be sprayed on fresh arterial clots, and the eyes should be covered (or patient's head turned away from the direction of spray) to avoid eye contact. The spray is used at least twice daily or as often as necessary.

Fibrinolysin and desoxyribonuclease ointment (Elase)

The proteolytic enzymes fibrinolysin and desoxyribonuclease are derived from bovine plasma and pancreas, respectively. Purulent exudates consist of fibrinous material and nucleoprotein. Desoxyribonuclease attacks desoxyribonucleic acid, and fibrinolysin (plasmin) acts on fibrin of blood clots and fibrinous exudates. The mechanism of action is fibrinolytic activity on denatured proteins (devitalized tissue); protein elements of living cells are unaffected.

A product that contains the two enzymes in combination with chloromycetin is also available. The added bacteriostatic properties inhibit bacterial protein synthesis by interfering with transfer of activated amino acids from soluble ribonucleic acid to ribosomes in infected lesions. Systemic antibiotics are also indicated.

Elase is used to debride inflamed and infected lesions, including surgical wounds, ulcerative lesions (trophic, decubitus, stasis, arteriosclerotic), second- and third-degree burns, and wounds resulting from circumcision or episiotomy. Other indications include cervicitis and irrigation of infected wounds and superficial hematomas near fatty tissue.

Allergic reactions have been observed in persons who are sensitive to bovine source materials, mercury compounds (thimerosal, a mercury derivative, is used as a preservative in

the ointment base of Elase), or chloromycetin.

Application techniques are those listed in the discussion of nursing implications at the end of this chapter. Changing the dressing at least once daily—preferably two or three times daily—is recommended. Local hyperemia has been reported.

The topical solution may be used in a spray or a wet dressing. Elase is also available as a dry powder in vials.

Collagenase (Santyl, Biozyme-C)

Collagenase is an enzymatic debriding agent derived from *Clostridium histolyticum*. It is capable of degrading both denatured and undenatured collagen. Other proteolytic enzymes act only on denatured collagen. Thus it is claimed that collagenase produces more effective debridement by acting on collagen at the wound edges, where necrotic slough is anchored. These actions promote the formation of granulation tissue and the epithelization of dermal ulcers and burned tissue.

The optimal pH range for collagenase is 6 to 8; a local pH alteration outside this range will decrease the enzymes' activity. In addition, the activity is adversely affected by detergents, soaps, cleansing agents, hexachlorophene, heavy metal ions (as found in antiseptics, iodine, thimerosal, mercury compounds, and silver nitrate), boric acid, and soaks such as Burow's solution (which has a low pH and contains a metal ion). If any of these heavy metal ion or acidic solutions are thought to have been used prior to application of collagenase, a thorough cleansing irrigation of the area with normal saline should be performed to remove the agents. Hydrogen peroxide, Dakin's solution, and sterile normal saline are compatible with collagenase. This ointment should be applied only within the area of the lesion, since a transient erythema has been reported as a cutaneous reaction on the wound surface or the area adjacent to the lesion. This reaction may be prevented by applying a protectant (for example, zinc oxide paste) around the lesion.

Collagenase can be inactivated by irrigating the lesion with an acidic solution such as Burow's solution (pH 3.6 to 4.4). Collagenase should be applied once daily. If the wound is deep, collagenase should be applied directly with a wooden tongue depressor or spatula. The application should be repeated if the dressing area is soiled (for example, because of incontinence). Before collagenase is applied, the area is cleansed of debris by gentle rubbing with a gauze pad saturated with hydrogen peroxide, Dakin's solution, or sterile normal saline. The ulcer should be patted dry with a clean gauze pad. If infection is present, a topical antibacterial agent (for example, neomycin-bacitracin-polymyxin B solution or powder) is applied directly to the ulcer surface.

The average time for complete debridement of dermal ulcers and decubiti with collagenase is about 11 days. This time permits debridement of necrotic tissue and establishment of granulation tissue. Topical enzymes used for debriding may increase the risk of bacteremia in the debilitated patient; this may necessitate monitoring of these patients for systemic bacterial infections. The ointment does not have to be refrigerated; it is stored at room temperature. Collagenase is available in 25-g jars, with 250 units/g in white petrolatum.

NURSING IMPLICATIONS

The following are aspects of care for patients being treated with topically applied enzymatic drugs (not the nonenzymatic agents).

1 Before topical application of enzymes, the wound should be thoroughly cleansed with a solution that does not inactivate the enzyme (for example, physiologic saline or sterile distilled water). Solutions containing metal or acidic ions should be avoided, to prevent inactivation of the enzymes. As much necrotic tissue should be removed with forceps and scissors as can be readily removed. All previously applied ointment should be removed before new ointment is applied to the substrate.
2 Delibilitated patients should be carefully monitored, since debriding enzymes increase the risk of bacterial infection.
3 Thick eschar should be crosshatched with a No. 11 blade for adequate contact of enzyme to the substrate.
4 Ointment should be applied directly to the wound with a tongue depressor or spatula and then covered with sterile gauze, or it can be applied with a sterile gauze pad that is then placed over the wound. A bandage and/or tape should then be used to hold the dressing in place.

5 Ointment or jelly preparations should be confined to the wound. The surrounding healthy tissue (or skin) should be protected from the enzyme. (For example, zinc oxide paste can be used.)
6 The treated lesion should be kept moist and protected from drying.
7 The enzyme must be in direct contact with the wound for a sufficient length of time.
8 Patients should be observed for allergic or sensitivity reactions—for example, determatitis and febrile reactions.
9 To avoid delayed healing, the enzyme should be discontinued when the wound is clean and debrided.

Nonenzymatic agent

Dextranomer (Debrisan)

Dextranomer is a hydrophilic dextran polymer in the form of small beads (0.1 to 0.3 mm in diameter); it is used for cleansing only a secreting wound. Each gram of beads absorbs about 4 ml of fluid from a secreting lesion or wounds. This rapid action continues until all the beads are saturated. The assumption of a grayish yellow color by the beads indicates that they are saturated and ready for removal. The spaces between the beads produce a powerful dehydrating suction force—up to 200 mm Hg. Low-molecular-weight substances in the secretions of wound exudates (for example, toxins, peptides) are drawn up (absorbed) within the beads. The higher molecular weight substances (plasma, protein, fibrinogen, split products) are absorbed in the spaces between adjacent swollen beads. Thus application of dextranomer to the surface of a secreting wound removes exudates and particles that impede tissue repair and increase wound healing time.

Secreting or exudative wounds for which dextranomer can be used include venous stasis ulcers, decubitus ulcers, infected traumatic and surgical wounds, and infected burns.

The contents of each container should be used for only one patient, to limit cross-contamination. If the wound is a cratered decubitus ulcer, the nurse should allow for expansion of the beads by not packing the wound tightly. During the first few days, as the edema is reduced, the wound itself may appear larger in size than it did before treatment.

Preparation, dosage, and administration. Dextranomer is available in 4-g packages and 60- and 120-g containers. To initially prepare the wound, it should be irrigated with sterile water or saline and the area should be left moist. The beads should cover the wound surface to a depth of 3 mm (⅛ to ¼ inch) (for example 4 g of beads covers a wound or ulcer 1½ × 1½). The wound should be lightly bandaged to hold the beads in place. The degree of wound secretion determines the number of dressing changes (usually one or two daily; profuse secretion may necessitate three or four dressing changes). Changes are done before full saturation of the beads (grayish yellow color), to prevent drying and to facilitate bead removal by irrigation (for example, sterile water, saline). A patient occasionally may experience some minor pain during dressing changes. The nurse should be aware that if the beads are spilled on the floor, the floor becomes slippery, creating a work hazard.

Summary of nursing considerations

Enzymes are proteins that act as catalysts for chemical reactions in living systems. Characteristics attributed to catalysts are speed, efficiency, and specificity. Enzymes are usually soluble in cellular fluid or can be adsorbed or adhere to membranous structures within the cell. The enzymes discussed in this chapter are used topically for chemical debridement of wounds to facilitate healing. Antibiotic therapy may be used in conjunction with enzymatic debridement to control or inhibit infection.

QUESTIONS

FOR STUDY AND REVIEW

1 Explain what is meant by the term "chemical debridement."
2 Discuss the uses of and differences between the following drugs:
Dextranomer
Collagenase
Sutilains
3 How should enzymes be stored?
4 Discuss the nursing care important to patients receiving topical enzymatic preparations.
5 Discuss the drug interactions of collagenase.
6 Discuss the effectiveness and mechanisms of action of dextranomer.

BIBLIOGRAPHY

A.M.A. drug evaluations, ed. 4, New York, 1980, John Wiley & Sons, Inc.

Bell, W.R., and others: The urokinase-streptokinase pulmonary embolism trial (phase II) results, Circulation **50:**1070, 1974.

Douglas, A.S.: Blood coagulation and fibrinolysis in clinical practice, Clin. Haematol. **2:**1, 1973.

Heel, R.C., and others: Dextranomer: a review of its general properties and therapeutic efficacy, Drugs **18:**89, 1979.

Modell W., editor: Drugs of choice 1980-1981, St. Louis, 1980, The C.V. Mosby Co.

Morgan, J.E.: Topical therapy for pressure ulcers, Surg. Gynecol. Obstet. **141**(6):945, 1975.

National Cooperative Study: The urokinase pulmonary embolism trial, Circulation **47**(Suppl. II), April, 1973.

Nierman, M.M.: Treatment of dermal and decubitus ulcers, Drugs **15:**226, 1978.

Parish, L.C., and Collins, E.: Decubitus ulcers: comparative study, Cutis **23:**106, 1979.

Shapira, E., Gilade, A., and Newman, Z.: Use of water-insoluble papain (WIP) for debridement of burn eschar and necrotic tissue, preliminary report, Plast. Reconstr. Surg. **52**(3):279, 1973.

Streptokinase and urokinase, Med. Lett. Drugs Ther. **20**(8):37, 1978.

Tibbutt, D.A., and others: Comparison of streptokinase and heparin in life-threatening pulmonary embolism, Br. Med. J. **1:**343, 1974.

Vasconex, L.O., Schneider, W.J., and Jurkiewics, M.J.: Pressure sores, Curr. Probl. Surg. **14**(4):62, 1977.

UNIT ELEVEN

TOXICOLOGY

CHAPTER 32

Poisons and antidotes

Poisoning

Poisonings are common in the United States; only a percentage are actually reported. About 2 million cases occur each year, with about 5000 fatalities. Most poisonings are *accidental* and caused by drug intoxication. Some poisonings are *suicide* attempts. *Criminal* poisonings are rare, since modern scientific methods permit highly accurate detection of poisons and most large cities maintain toxicologic laboratories in conjunction with law enforcement agencies. *Industrial* poisonings are prevalent, since modern technology exposes humans to numerous toxic agents in exhaust gases, radioactive substances, insecticides, and the like.

Two thirds of the accidental poisonings occur in children under age 5. According to the National Clearinghouse for Poison Control, ingestions of toxic substances by children younger than 5 years old are generally deemed to be accidental; ingestions by older children are more likely to be true suicide attempts, a "cry for help." Occurrences in children under 1 year of age are usually accidental medication overdoses by parents; from 1 to 5 years, the curious, experimenting, or hungry child is usually the initiator.

Morbidity and mortality from accidental poisonings in children under 5 years old have dropped, in part, it is thought, because of public awareness of the potential hazards in children's environment and because of the proliferation of childproof containers. Unfortunately, this encouraging trend is not reproduced in other age categories—a cause for continuing concern.

Currently the most frequent substance involved in adult poisoning is a medication, most often a tranquilizer or sedative. Children most often ingest plants, household cleansers, antihistamines or medications for colds, perfumes, or vitamins and minerals. However, they suffer the most toxic effects from the nonprescription medications they ingest. Though aspirin poisonings in children are dropping in frequency, the increased trade in acetaminophen products has been accompanied by increasing numbers of reports of poisonings with them. This is a trend that warrants close attention because acute overdose by acetaminophen can produce centrilobular hepatic necrosis.

DETECTION OF POISONS

Toxicology is the study of poisons, their action and effects, methods for their detection, and diagnosis and treatment of poisoning. A poison can be defined as any substance that in relatively small amounts can cause death or serious bodily harm by chemical action. All drugs are potential poisons when used improperly or in excess dosage. Poisoning may be *acute* or *chronic*. In acute poisoning the effects are immediate. In chronic poisoning the effects are insiduous as a result of cumulative effects of small amounts of poison absorbed over a prolonged period of time. Chronic poisoning causes chronic illness that may or may not be reversible.

Nurses may be confronted by a suspected poisoning in many ways. A mother or neighbor may call, upset that her small child has taken one of her contraceptive pills, or a patient may accidentally drink the glass of peroxide mixture that had been intended as a mouthwash, or a teenager may be brought into the emergency room unarousable. Often the nurse is alone in the situation, yet speedy detection and treatment are essential.

Cues that typically point to poisoning are the occurrence of sudden, violent symptoms such as severe nausea, vomiting, diarrhea, collapse, or convulsions. It is important to find out (if possible) what poison has been taken and how much. Additional information that might prove helpful to the physician in making a diagnosis includes answers to questions or reports of observed phenomena, as follows:

1 Any reports of poison contacted by the victim should be noted.
2 Occurrence in the "at-risk" age group of children 1 to 5 years old may be significant.
3 Report of a history of previous poisonings or ingestion of foreign substances should be noted.
4 Diverse symptoms or signs referrable to multiple organ system involvement that defy diagnosis are important.
5 Is there a history of suicidal intent or thought?
6 Did the symptoms appear suddenly in an otherwise healthy individual? Did a number of persons become ill about the same time (as might happen in food poisoning)?
7 Is there anything unusual about the person, his clothing, or his surroundings? Is there evidence of burns about his lips and mouth? Are the gums discolored? Are there needle (hypodermic) pricks, pustules, or scars on the exposed and accessible surfaces of the body? Does the individual have dilated or constricted pupils? (These may be seen in examination of drug addicts.) Is there any skin rash or discoloration?
8 The odor of the breath, the rate of respiration, any difficulty in respiration, and cyanosis should be noted.
9 The quality and rate of the pulse should be noted.
10 If vomitus is seen, what is its appearance and its odor? Is or was vomiting accompanied by diarrhea or abdominal pain?
11 Any abnormalities of stool and urine should be noted; change in color or the presence of blood may be significant.
12 For signs of involvement of the nervous system, the presence of excitement, muscular twitching, delirium, difficulty in speech, stupor, coma, constriction or dilation of the pupils, and elevated or subnormal temperature should be looked for.

Coma caused by drug overdose is characterized by the following categories:

Grade I—patient asleep but easily aroused, reacts to painful stimuli, deep tendon reflexes present, pupils normal and reactive, ocular movements present, and vital signs stable
Grade II—pain response absent, deep tendon reflexes depressed, pupils slightly dilated but reactive, and vital signs stable
Grade III—deep tendon and pupillary reflexes absent, and vital signs stable
Grade IV—respiration and circulation depressed

Table 32-1 will further assist in differentiating the signs of coma of toxic origin from those of coma resulting from structural neurologic damage. The nurse should refrigerate in a covered container all specimens of vomitus, urine, or stool in case the physician wishes to examine them and perhaps turn them over to the proper authority for analysis. This is of particular importance not only in making or confirming a diagnosis but also in the event that the case has medicolegal significance.

Any of the signs listed earlier should be noted carefully for report to the Poison Control Center or physician in charge. However, full

TABLE 32-1 Signs of coma of toxic origin differentiated from signs of coma resulting from structural neurologic damage (to be used as corroborating guide only)

Signs	Structural neurologic damage	Toxic neurologic effects
Motor activity	Spasticity	Flaccidity
Pupillary reactions	Absent or variable	Present
Toe-to-head progression of signs	Yes	No
Blood pressure	May increase early; may decrease later	Usually decreases

Adapted with permission from Howard C. Mofenson: Poison control manual, 1979, unpublished data.

reliance on signs and symptoms for clear-cut diagnosis and poison identification is fraught with danger, since these incidents may occur concurrently with an episode of acute disease, especially in children (for example, aspirin intoxication), and symptoms may be similar or otherwise confusing. Likewise, more than one substance may be responsible for the signs of poisoning observed. Onset may also vary, depending on the amount of substance taken, when it was taken (in relation to meals), and in what form it was taken (solutions ingested will act faster than toxins in solid form).

A loose working definition of toxic dose of the average medication has been determined to be a dose that is five times the amount of the usual therapeutic dose. Unknown but crucial information about the volume of a liquid seen to be ingested can be estimated by the following rule of thumb: the volume of one swallow of a liquid by a child under 5 years old is about 5 ml; in the adult it is about 15 ml.

Another clue in determining whether a toxic amount of any substance could have been ingested can be found in the type of packaging. Spray aerosol containers, pump containers,

and squeeze tubes rarely are the cause of poisoning. The label wording will also provide clues. The contents can be assumed to be extremely toxic if the label states "Call physician immediately," if it states "Danger—Poison," or if it gives any antidote information. If the label notes "Danger—Poison," "Warning," or "Caution," it is automatically assumed to have toxic potential. The label "Keep Out of Reach of Children," however, if unaccompanied by any of the other warnings, usually infers only minimal toxicity except under unusual conditions.

Not all substances commonly ingested accidentally are toxic if small amounts are taken on only one occasion. The Poison Control Center must be consulted and careful observations made, or course, but it is helpful for householders to know this so as to be selective in stocking supplies and in making certain other judgments. A list of some frequently ingested products that are *usually nontoxic* in small amounts is given as follows:

Abrasives, bleaches (sodium hypochlorite, less than 5%)
Cigarettes, cigars

T A B L E 3 2 - 2 Toxidromes that may suggest certain drug poisonings or overdoses

Signs	Inference	Signs	Inference
Agitation, panic, depression Beet-red skin color Dilated pupils Dry skin with fever Hallucinations	Atropine Scopolamine	Pulmonary congestion Salivation	
		Ataxia ⎫ Drowsiness ⎬ No alcohol odor to breath Slurred ⎭ speech	Barbiturates Sedative-hypnotics Tranquilizers
Argumentativeness Arrhythmias Diarrhea Dilated pupils Dry mouth with fetid odor Headache Hyperactivity Sweating Tachycardia Tremors	Amphetamines	Arrhythmias Coma Convulsions	Tricyclic antidepressants: imipramine (Tofranil), amitriptyline (Elavil)
		Fever Hyperpnea Vomiting	Salicylates
Euphoria or coma Pinpoint pupils Slow respirations	Opiates	Ataxia Oculogyric crisis (coordinated deviation of eyes, usually upward) Torsion head and neck syndrome	Phenothiazines
Involuntary defecation Involuntary urination Lacrimation Miosis	Organophosphates Mushrooms (particularly genus *Amanita* or *Galerina*)		

Adapted with permission from Howard C. Mofenson: Poison control manual, 1979, unpublished data.

Cosmetics, perfume, cologne
Glues, rubber cement
Hydrogen peroxide (medicinal, 3%)
Indelible pen or Magic Markers
Matches
Paint (latex)
Pencil (graphite or coloring)
Play-Doh
Soaps, shampoos, detergents (except dishwasher detergents)
Toothpaste (with or without fluoride)

In assisting with poisoning diagnosis and toxic substance identification, nurses (especially in the emergency room) and nurse practitioners should familiarize themselves with certain clusters of signs associated with common drug poisonings or overdoses. These have been called "toxidromes" and are listed in Table 32-2. Other common single signs and their associated causative toxins are listed in Table 32-3.

Certain presumptive laboratory screening tests may be performed to help establish a more definitive diagnosis or for medicolegal reasons, but treatment should not be based solely on these tests, nor should treatment be delayed awaiting test results. Specimens of urine, blood, stool, or emesis; the results of the first lavage; and/or the suspect substance may need to be tested. Therefore all such products should be saved under refrigeration for analysis. X-ray films of the abdomen may identify the presence of radiopaque substances such as certain medications, lead in paint chips, or other heavy metals such as arsenic, bismuth, iron, or thallium. Challenge doses of specific antidotes may be given to test for reversal of symptoms. However, the typical nursing situation in poisoning incidents calls for immediately contacting the nearest Poison Control Center.

POISON CONTROL CENTERS*

There are over 600 poison control centers in the continental United States, Hawaii, Alaska, the Virgin Islands, Guam, Puerto Rico, the Canal Zone, and the District of Columbia. Most are located near hospitals or in emergency rooms of large community hospitals. Their telephone numbers are listed in the local telephone book. Many are open 24 hours every day and are

*The address of the coordinating agency for all poison control centers is the National Clearinghouse for Poison Control Centers, U.S. Department of Health and Human Services, Food and Drug Administration—Division of Poison Control, 5660 Fishers Lane, Room 1345, Rockville, Maryland 20857.

T A B L E   3 2 - 3   **Single signs that suggest the presence of certain toxins**

Sign	Inference	Sign	Inference
Abdominal colic	Black widow spider bite Heavy metals Withdrawal from narcotic depressant	Convulsions or muscle twitching	Alcohol Amphetamines Antihistamines Boric acid Camphor Chlorinated hydrocarbon insecticides (DDT) Cyanide Lead Organophosphate insecticides Plants: azalea, iris, lily-of-the-valley, water hemlock Salicylates Strychnine Withdrawal from drugs: barbiturates, benzodiazepines (Valium, Librium), meprobamate
Ataxia	Alcohol Barbiturates Bromides Carbon monoxide Hallucinogens Heavy Metals Organic solvents Phenytoin (Dilantin) Tranquilizers		
Coma and drowsiness	Alcohol (ethyl) Antihistamines Barbiturates, other hypnotics Carbon monoxide Opiates Salicylates Tranquilizers	Paralysis	Botulism Heavy metals

Adapted with permission from Howard C. Mofenson: Poison control manual, 1979, unpublished data.

T A B L E 3 2 - 3   Single signs that suggest the presence of certain toxins—cont'd

Sign	Inference	Sign	Inference
	Plants (poison hemlock, etc.)		Methanol
	Triorthocresyl phosphate (plasticizer)		Withdrawal from narcotic depressants
Oliguria/anuria	Carbon tetrachloride	Nystagmus on lateral gaze	Barbiturates
	Ethylene glycol (antifreeze)		Minor tranquilizers (meprobamate, benzodiazepines), phenytoin (Dilantin)
	Heavy metals		
	Hemolysis due to naphthalene, plants, etc.	Pinpoint	Mushrooms (muscarinic)
	Methanol		Opiates
	Mushrooms		Organophosphate insecticides
	Oxylates		
	Petroleum distillates	Respiratory alterations	
	Solvents	Increased	Amphetamines
Oral signs			Barbiturates (early sign)
Breath odors			Carbon monoxide
Acetone	Acetone		Methanol
	Alcohol (methyl or isopropyl)		Petroleum distillates
	Phenol		Salicylates
	Salicylates	Paralysis	Botulism
Alcohol	Ethyl alcohol		Organophosphate insecticides
Bitter almonds	Cyanide		
Coal gas	Carbon monoxide	Slowed or depressed	Alcohol
Garlic	Arsenic		Barbiturates (late sign)
	Dimethyl sulfoxide (DMSO)		Opiates
	Phosphorus		Tranquilizers
	Organophosphate insecticides	Wheezing/pulmonary edema	Mushrooms (muscarinic)
	Thallium		Opiates
Oil of wintergreen	Methyl salicylate		Organophosphate insecticides
Petroleum	Petroleum distillates		Petroleum distillates
Violets	Turpentine	Skin color changes	
Dryness	Amphetamines	Jaundice	Aniline dyes/coal tar colors
	Antihistamines		Arsenic
	Atropine		Carbon tetrachloride
	Narcotic depressants		Castor bean
Salivation	Arsenic		Fava bean
	Corrosive substances		Mushroom
	Mercury		Naphthalene (moth repellent/insecticide)
	Mushrooms		Yellow phosphorus
	Organophosphate insecticides	Red flush	Alcohol
	Thallium		Antihistamines
Pulse rate changes			Atropine
Increased	Alcohol		Boric acid
	Amphetamines		Carbon monoxide
	Atropine		Nitrites
	Ephedrine		Tricyclic antidepressants
Slowed	Digitalis	Cyanosis	Aniline dyes
	Lily-of-the-valley		Carbon monoxide
	Narcotic depressants		Cyanide
			Nitrites
Pupillary changes			Strychnine
Dilated	Amphetamines	Violent emesis (with or without hematemesis)	Aminophylline
	Antihistamines		Bacterial food poisoning
	Atropine		Boric acid
	Barbiturates (when combined with coma)		Corrosives
	Cocaine		Fluoride
	Ephedrine		Heavy metals
	LSD		Phenol
			Salicylates

staffed to (1) answer specific questions from the public or from professionals about identification of ingredients in trade named products, (2) estimate their toxicity, and (3) suggest specific treatment for poisonings. They also handle calls about drug abuse, suicide, food poisoning, dog bites, insect bites, snake bites, drugs and breast-feeding, and teratogenic drugs.

Poison control centers can be highly instrumental in reducing the number of poisonings (aside from treatment). They provide annual nationwide statistical analyses of poisonings by category, which help clarify the magnitude of the problem. Poison control centers also make available a wide selection of pamphlets, resources, and presentations to educate the public and professionals alike to the ubiquity of poisons in the environment and procedures to follow in dealing with poisons.

CLASSIFICATION AND MECHANISMS OF ACTION OF POISONS

The classification of poisons is as broad as the classification of drugs, since any drug is a potential poison when used in excess.

Poisons may be classified in various ways. They may be grouped according to chemical classifications as organic and inorganic poisons; as alkaloids, glycosides, and resins; or as acids, alkalies, heavy metals, oxidizing agents, halogenated hydrocarbons, and so on.

Another way in which they may be grouped is by locale of exposure—poisons found in the home, poisons encountered in industry, poisons encountered while camping, and so on.

Still another way in which poisons may be classified is according to the organ or tissue of the body in which the most damaging effects are produced. Some poisons injure all cells they contact. Such chemical substances are sometimes called protoplasmic poisons or cytotoxins. Others have more effect on the kidney (nephrotoxins), the liver (hepatotoxins), or the blood or blood-forming organs.

Poisons that affect chiefly the nervous system are called neurotoxins or neurotropic poisons. They must be studied separately, because different symptoms characterize each one. Symptoms of toxicity have been mentioned in connection with each of these drugs as they were presented in previous chapters. Although

symptoms of this group of poisons are to some extent specific, it is also true that certain symptoms are encountered repeatedly and are associated with a large number of poisons. Drowsiness, dizziness, headache, delirium, coma, and convulsive seizures always indicate central nervous system involvement. On the other hand, dry mouth, dilated pupils, and difficult swallowing are associated with overdosage of atropine or one of the atropine-like drugs; ringing in the ears, excessive perspiration, and gastric upset are associated with salicylate overdosage.

Many of the central nervous system depressants cause death by producing excessive depression or respiration and respiratory failure. The general anesthetics, barbiturates, chloral hydrate, and paraldehyde are examples of such drugs.

Many times the precise mechanism of action is not known; death may be caused by respiratory failure but exactly what happens to cause depression of the respiratory center may not be known.

Central nervous system stimulants such as pentylenetetrazol and strychnine in toxic amounts cause convulsive seizures, exhaustion, and depression of vital centers.

It is apparent that the human body depends on a constant supply of oxygen if various physiologic functions are to proceed satisfactorily. Anything that interferes with the use of oxygen by the cells or with the transportation of oxygen will produce damaging effects in cells and in some cells faster than in others. Carbon monoxide from automobile engines and unvented gas heaters is one of the most widely distributed toxic agents. It poisons by producing hypoxia and finally asphyxia. Carbon monoxide has a great affinity for hemoglobin and forms carboxyhemoglobin. Thus the production of oxyhemoglobin and the free transport of oxygen is interfered with, and oxygen deficiency soon develops in the cells. Unless exposure to the carbon monoxide is terminated quickly and before 40% of hemoglobin has been changed to carboxyhemoglobin, the anoxia may produce serious brain damage; death occurs when 60% of the hemoglobin has been changed to carboxyhemoglobin.

The cyanides act somewhat similarly in that

they bring about cellular anoxia, but they do so in a different manner. They inactivate certain tissue enzymes so that cells are unable to utilize oxygen. Death may occur very rapidly.

Curare and the curariform drugs in toxic amounts bring about paralysis of the diaphragm, and again the victim dies from lack of oxygen.

Certain drugs have a direct effect on muscle tissue from the body such as that of the myocardium or the smooth muscle of the blood vessels. Death results from the failure of circulation or cardiac arrest. The nitrites, potassium salts, and digitalis drugs may exert toxic effects of this type.

Arsenic is an example of a protoplasmic poison or cytotoxin. Compounds of arsenic inhibit many enzyme systems of cells, especially those that depend on the activity of their free sulfhydryl (SH) groups. The arsenic combines with these SH groups and makes them ineffective. Hence extensive tissue damage in the body occurs.

Methyl alcohol owes its toxic effect to an intermediate product of metabolism—formic acid. This produces a severe acidosis, lowered pH of the blood, reduced cerebral blood flow, and decreased consumption of oxygen by the brain. There is also a selective action on the retinal cells of the eye, but the exact cause of this injury is unknown.

Benzene is an example of a poison that acts by inhibiting the formation of all types of blood cells. In some instances the precursor of one type of blood cell is injured more than another. Depression of the formation of any of the blood cells can cause death.

The strong acids and alkalies denature and destroy cellular proteins. Examples of corrosive acids are hydrochloric, nitric, and sulfuric acids. Sodium, potassium, and ammonium hydroxides are examples of strong or caustic alkalies. Locally these substances cause destruction of tissue, and death may result from hemorrhage, perforation, or shock. Corrosive poisons may also cause death by altering the pH of the blood or other body fluids, or they may produce marked degenerative changes in vital organs such as the liver or the kidney.

TREATMENT OF POISONED VICTIMS

Since the emphasis is on *prompt* treatment, health care may often in these emergencies be best served by quick action by informed bystanders at the scene who apply first aid measures while help is sought from the poison control center and transportation to a hospital, clinic, or physician's office is arranged. A first aid chart that offers instruction for poisoning emergencies is included here as an example (p. 974) to delineate specific actions for different types of poisonings:

The caller to the Poison Control Center should bring to the telephone the following information (if available):

1 Physical appearance of the substance
2 Odor, color, and texture; distinguishing characteristics of the substance
3 Trade name or chemical name if known
4 Purpose or what the substance was meant to be used for
5 Label statements relating to "poison" content or flammability

After the events of the suspected poisoning have been thoroughly assessed and problems analyzed, including the identification of the substance if possible, prompt nursing actions must be instituted. Nursing management will be guided by four major goals:

1 Vital functions (respirations, circulation, etc.) will be maintained, supported, or restored.
2 The toxic substance will be removed or eliminated from the system as soon as possible.
3 The action of certain specific poisons may be counteracted, reversed, or antagonized by specific antidotes.
4 Recurrences will be reduced or prevented.

Based on the priority of nursing problems in each poisoning episode, these goals may best be implemented simultaneously or in order of need. Prompt removal of the poison or supportive care may be all the treatment needed.

Support of vital functions. Basic to the treatment of poisoning is intensive supportive therapy, good nursing care, and a minimum of dangerous invasive interventions. The nursing care of the poisoned patient should focus on restoration, support, and maintenance of such vital functions as ventilation, circulation, and acid-base and fluid-electrolyte balance. Emotional support for the patient and others involved in this crisis is crucial.

POISON CONTROL CENTERS

First aid for possible poisoning

Remember: Any non-food substance may be poisonous!

1. Keep all potential poisons—household products and medicines—out of the reach of small children.
2. Use "safety caps" (child-resistant containers) as intended to avoid accidents.
3. Have 1 oz. Syrup of Ipecac in your home and in your first aid kit for camping, travel, etc.
4. Keep your Poison Center's and your physician's phone number handy.

If you think an accidental ingestion has occurred:

1. Keep calm—do not wait for symptoms—call for help promptly!
2. Find out if the substance is toxic—Your Poison Control Center or your physician can tell you if a risk exists and what you should do.
3. Have the product's container or label with you at the phone.
   a. If a poison is on the skin:
   Immediately remove affected clothing.
   Flood involved parts of body with water, wash with soap or detergent and rinse thoroughly.
   b. If a poison is in the eye:
   Immediately flush the eye with water for 10 to 15 minutes.
   c. If a poison is inhaled:
   Immediately get the person to fresh air. Give mouth to mouth resuscitation if necessary.
   d. If vomiting has been recommended:
   Give one tablespoon of Ipecac syrup followed by a glass (8 oz.) of clear liquid (water, juices, or carbonated beverage). If the patient doesn't vomit within 15 to 20 minutes, give another tablespoon of Ipecac and more water. Do *not* use salt water. It can be dangerous.

Never induce vomiting if:

1. The victim is in *coma* (unconscious).
2. The victim is *convulsing* (having a fit or a seizure).
3. The victim has swallowed a *caustic* or *corrosive* (e.g. lye).

For reemphasis:

1. Always call to be certain of possible toxicity before undertaking treatment.
2. Never induce vomiting until you are instructed to do so.
3. Do not rely on the label's antidote information—it may be out of date—call instead!
4. If you have to go to an Emergency Room, take the tablets, capsules, container, and/or label with you.
5. Don't hesitate to call your Poison Center or your doctor a second time if the victim seems to be getting worse.

Adapted from American Association of Poison Control Centers, William O. Robertson, M.D., Secretary. From Physician's desk reference for nonprescription drugs, ed. 2, Oradell, NJ, 1981, Medical Economics Co. Reprinted by permission.

A general overall assessment and history should be performed quickly and competently to determine the extent of any impairments of body systems or particular susceptibilities. Expert nursing care is essential to observe the following for information indicating impending complications:

1 Level of consciousness
2 Vital signs—Temperature may elevate with certain CNS stimulants and salicylates. Transient cardiac arrhythmias may occur; anticipate obtaining an electrocardiogram. Pulmonary congestion, airway obstruction, or apnea is common; aspiration of vomitus can occur; turning, deep breathing, coughing, and suctioning may be crucial. Ausculation may demonstrate a need for chest x-ray examination, suctioning, tracheostomy, endotracheal intubation, blood gas determinations, supplemental oxygen and a respirator/ventilator, etc. Initiation of intravenous infusion may be anticipated.

It is also essential that positioning to prevent aspiration of vomitus be done and that mouth care be attended to promptly after emesis. Moderate amounts of plain water by mouth (if a gag or swallow reflex is present) may be all that is needed to dilute or effectively inactivate many ingested poisons.

Close attention to developing problems and responsive intervention can often fend off the need for more aggressive medical therapies, which tax the already tenuous condition of the poisoned patient.

Removal or elimination of poison. Careful evaluation of the patient who has been affected by a toxic substance is essential to determine which of the foregoing steps take priority and by which route the poison should be removed or eliminated, if necessary. The route is largely determined by the manner of the poisoning. Ingested substances can be removed from the gastrointestinal tract directly from the stomach; transit time through the colon may be speeded up to decrease the potential for absorption of the substance; or if the substance has probably already been assimilated into the system or was injected, attempts may be made to remove or filter it from the bloodstream. Contact poisons may be flushed from the skin, eyes, and other external areas by copious volumes of plain flowing water from a pitcher or other container. Soapy warm water is needed to remove organic solvents and tenacious oils. Inhaled toxins are treated by removing the patient to fresh air and administering artificial respiration or oxygen and other supportive measures as necessary.

Various methods exist for the removal or elimination of poisons from the gastrointestinal tract or systemic circulation: emesis, gastric lavage, cathartics, diuretics, dialysis, or, occasionally, blood exchange transfusions or hemoperfusion through charcoal or exchange resins. There are numerous approaches to treatment of the poisoning emergency; each must be tailored by clinical judgment to individual patient needs.

The most generally effective method is the most natural one—emesis, the sooner the better—*unless emesis is contraindicated.* (See contraindications in box above.) If vomiting does

---

Contraindications for induced emesis in poisonings

No emetic should be given if:

1. Presence of protective airway reflexes (gag and cough) is questionable or is not demonstrable.
2. Convulsions are present or impending.
3. Corrosive substances (for example, lye) or convulsion-inducing substances have been taken.
4. Substance is a petroleum distillate (for example, kerosene, gasoline) and less than 1 to 2 ml/kg body weight has been ingested.
5. Victim is pregnant (depending on clinical judgment, however).

The decision may be made to induce emesis despite prior administration of an emetic, since the attempt may well be worth a try. If activated charcoal has been administered, lavage may be recommended.

Adapted with permission from Howard C. Mofenson: Poison control manual, 1979, unpublished data.

not or cannot occur naturally, use of one of the common emetics is the preferred treatment. Commonly used is syrup of ipecac (*never* fluid extract of ipecac, which is 14 times more concentrated and has been responsible for a number of deaths), or apomorphine, a narcotic emetic that causes a reflex action of the vomiting center in the brainstem. Apomorphine can cause severe, protracted emesis and should be used with extreme caution and with naloxone hydrochloride (Narcan) on hand. Naloxone is a narcotic antagonist used to counteract any respiratory depression resulting from the use of apomorphine.

Syrup of ipecac probably acts both centrally and locally; it directly stimulates the vomiting center, and it has an irritant effect on gastric mucosa. The usual dose for adults is 15 to 30 ml, followed by 200 to 300 ml of water, milk, or fruit juice, or as much fluid as the patient can drink. For children under 1 year of age a 7.5-ml dose is given; children from 1 to 5 years old receive a 15-ml dose; and those over 5 years, a 30-ml dose.

Vomiting usually occurs in 15 to 30 minutes. The dose may be repeated once after 20 minutes if the first dose is not effective.

If vomiting does not occur within 30 minutes, gastric lavage should be performed, since ipecac is a cardiotoxic if absorbed and may cause conduction disturbances, atrial fibrillation, or myocarditis.

Syrup of ipecac is available without a prescription in 1-ounce (30-ml) bottles bearing the following instructions:
1 For emergency use to cause vomiting in poisoning. Before using, call physician, poison control center, or hospital emergency room immediately for advice.
2 Warning—Keep out of reach of children. Do not use if strychnine, corrosives such as alkalies (lye) and strong acids, or petroleum distillates such as kerosene, gasoline, fuel oil, coal oil, paint thinner, or cleaning fluid have been ingested.

It is recommended that syrup of ipecac be kept in every home, particularly where there are children.

If the patient is conscious, drug-induced vomiting is usually preferable to gastric lavage, particularly in children, since aspiration of vomitus is less likely to occur. Nurses should employ the necessary measures to reduce the likelihood of aspiration of vomitus (proper positioning of patient). Occasionally, induction of vomiting may be facilitated by stimulating the pharynx but time should not be wasted in repeated futile attempts.

Apomorphine, although more dangerous to use, may be used to induce vomiting when more rapid emesis is necessary; it is effective within 1 to 15 minutes after administration. The single dose (which may *not be repeated)* is 0.1 ml/kg body weight, resulting in a dose range of 2 to 10 mg. Adults are usually given 5 to 6 mg; children between 1 and 2 years of age are usually given 1 to 2 mg. The fact that apomorphine comes in a 6-mg tablet that requires crushing and diluting with 3 ml of sterile water for subcutaneous injection make for some awkwardness, delay, and questionable accuracy or potency of the produced solution (the crushed powder will account for some of the resultant volume, so that it cannot be said with certainty that 1 ml of solution contains an evenly distributed 2 mg of this potent CNS depressant).

If emesis cannot be induced, gastric lavage should be begun *except* under most of the same contraindicating conditions (that is, untreated convulsions, absent reflexes, corrosives, etc.). Lavage *may* be preferred treatment for pregnant women and for patients who have ingested more than 2 ml/kg body weight of a petroleum distillate (the latter should have endotracheal intubation to protect the airway). Lavage may be contraindicated in the presence of cardiac arrhythmias.

An Ewald or Jacques orogastric tube No. 28 or No. 30 for children and No. 34 or No. 36 French for adults and several liters of half-strength saline solution are used for lavage. A nasogastric tube is too narrow to be effective. Stomach contents should be aspirated first and saved for toxicologic analysis if necessary. Then repeat lavage should be done in amounts of about 50 ml for children and 100 ml for adults until returns are clear. (Remember that dead space in the tube itself accounts for 20 to 25 ml of fluid.) Neither emesis nor lavage is guaranteed to empty the stomach completely, however.

When emesis or lavage is complete, activated charcoal may be instilled or swallowed to act as an adsorbent. Activated charcoal adsorbs a large variety of substances, both simple and complex. It is used as an adjunct in the treatment of oral poisonings with heavy metals, mercuric chloride, strychnine, phenol, atropine, phenolphthalein, oxalic acid, poison mushrooms, aspirin, and most drugs. It is not effective for poisoning with cyanide, DDT, ethanol, methanol, caustic alkalies, ferrous sulfate, boric acid, organophosphates, or carbonate.

For emergency treatment of adults or children, 5 to 50 g of the powder is mixed with tap water to form a slurry with the consistency of thick soup; this is taken orally by the patient or passed through a lavage tube. A dose of 50 g is used routinely by some emergency centers; the dose may be as high as 120 g. In general, the dose should be 10 times the estimated weight of the ingested substance. To improve palatability a small amount of a flavoring agent (for example, cherry), concentrated fruit juice, or chocolate powder may be added to the slurry; ice cream or sherbet should not be used, since these substances decrease the adsorptive capacity of the charcoal. Tablets or capsules of charcoal should not be used for treatment of poisoning, since they are less effective than the powder.

If ipecac syrup is to be used to induce vomiting, it is given before administering activated charcoal, since the charcoal will adsorb the syrup. Activated charcoal should be given as soon after poison ingestion as feasible.

The charcoal mixture need not be removed from the stomach afterward because there are no known adverse effects. If left in, it can serve as a marker to indicate the point at which there is a probable end to further gastrointestinal absorption of the ingested poison.

Administration of activated charcoal and ion exchange resins such as cholestyramine and colestipol, if given within 1 hour, may prevent intestinal reabsorption of some drugs that normally undergo recycling through the liver and thereby facilitate intestinal elimination. Digitoxin and phenprocoumon toxicity has been effectively treated this way. Paraquat, which is a lethal weed killer used on some marijuana plants and which is extremely rapidly absorbed from the gastrointestinal tract, is known to bind strongly to Fuller's earth and bentonite, but these adsorbents must be given too early to be practical. Cholestyramine binds to acidic drugs such as acetaminophen, but again, it must be given almost immediately.

Other ways used to block or eliminate toxins from the system include forced diuresis, cathartics and enemas, dialysis, hemoperfusion, and exchange transfusions. These methods should be reserved as treatment under certain conditions and for specific poisons; they are not universally effective and are much less commonly used than emesis or lavage.

Diuresis may be effective if the poison is one in which the total body clearance of active substance depends largely on renal clearance. For example, if only 1% of a drug dose is normally excreted in the urine, even a twenty-fold increase in renal clearance will not be clinically significant. When performed, diuresis may be forced by infusing 1 to 2 liters of fluid per hour or by administration of mannitol, an osmotic diuretic. Hazards related to fluid overload, especially in conditions of heart failure, organ edema, renal failure, or acid-base imbalances, are obvious.

In addition, changing the pH of the urine may enhance excretion of certain drugs. Alkalinization by administering sodium bicarbonate or other bases is particularly effective in salicylate overdoses, and probably in phenobarbital and 2,4-dichlorophenoxyacetic acid (weed killer, 2,4-D). It is reported to be questionably effective for some barbiturates and amitriptyline. Forced acid diuresis is probably more potentially hazardous, but is often recommended for poisoning with amphetamines, quinine, and fenfluramine (Pondimin), despite lack of full documentation of efficacy.

Cathartics and enemas are sometimes used to enhance toxin elimination and to cut down potential for absorption via the gastrointestinal tract. However, this is unlikely, since absorption is usually rapid and occurs in the upper small intestine. Castor oil or cathartics such as sodium sulfate or magnesium sulfate (Epsom Salt) are used in overdoses of glutethimide (Doriden), a nonbarbiturate hypnotic, or short-acting barbiturates, among others. Efficacy has not been established.

Clearance of poisons directly from the blood stream by peritoneal dialysis or hemodialysis, hemoperfusion, or transfusion is occasionally done to augment other measures previously discussed. These more complex methods may be ineffective, overly taxing to the poisoned patient, unnecessary, or even harmful in some instances. There are not enough well-controlled studies to prove efficacy yet. The degree to which they may be useful depends in part on the properties of the substance (that is, whether it freely circulates or whether it is bound to plasma proteins or to tissues). Various lists of substances amenable to dialysis exist; some substances for which dialysis has *not* proved useful are as follows*:

Amitriptyline (Elavil)
Anticholinergics
Antidepressants
Antihistamines
Atropine
Chlordiazepoxide (Librium)
Desipramine hydrochloride (Pertofrane)
Diazepam (Valium)
Digitalis

*Adapted from Krupp, M.A., and Chatton, M.J.: Current medical diagnosis and treatment 1979, Los Altos, Calif. 1979, Lange Medical Publications, p. 981.

Diphenoxylate hydrochloride (Lomotil)
Glutethimide (Doriden)
Hallucinogens
Imipramine (Tofranil)
Methaqualone (Quaalude)
Methyprylon (Noludar)
Narcotic opiate depressants (for example, heroin)
Nortriptyline (Aventyl)
Oxazepam (Serak)
Phenelzine sulfate (Nardil)
Propoxyphene (Darvon)

The following are some common criteria for considering dialysis:

1 Presence of potentially lethal levels of a dialyzable substance
2 Presence of high levels of a substance that breaks down into dialyzable poisons
3 When usual supportive or corrective measures will not suffice to prevent further damage (for example, coma, apnea, shock, or hyperthermia)
4 When major degradation or excretion routes are damaged, blocked, or otherwise dysfunctional (for example, renal or liver failure)
5 Often when the patient is pregnant (hemodialysis)

Though hemodialysis is more efficient for short-term dialysis, peritoneal dialysis may be less hazardous and may be continued over a longer period of time. Hemoperfusion is a more promising technique. Studies seem to show that there is more efficient removal of drugs when heparinized blood can be passed through a column packed with adsorbents such as activated charcoal or, better yet, newer exchange resins such as polacrilin (Amberlite). Possible complications include embolism; loss of white cells, platelets, and fibrinogen; and hemorrhage.

Table 32-4 lists some specific poisons with associated symptoms and the appropriate emergency treatment.

Text continued on p. 983.

TABLE 32-4 **Some specific poisons, symptoms, and emergency treatment***

Poison	Symptoms†	Treatment‡
Acetaminophen (paracetamol in Great Britain)—Datril, Tempra, Tenlap, Tylenol, Valadol	First, anorexia, nausea, vomiting. Liver function tests are elevated. Then jaundice, hypoglycemia, encephalopathy, renal failure, myocardiopathy, thrombocytopenia.	See antidote protocol for *N*-acetylcysteine (Mucomyst) as investigational drug. Emesis/lavage and activated charcoal. Otherwise purely symptomatic treatment. (See text.)
	Hepatic toxicity can be caused by a single dose of 200 to 250 mg/kg body weight. A 25-g dose is potentially fatal.	Hepatic lesions are reversible over a few weeks or months.
Alcohol (ethanol)	*Acute:* Central nervous system depression with decreased inhibitions and higher mental processes, gastric irritation with nausea and vomiting, hypoglycemia with seizures, hypothermia, jaw spasms, extensor rigidity, positive Babinski sign, ketoacidosis, convulsions, fever, cerebral edema with severe headache, coma.	Gastric lavage with tap water, or emesis. Give 4 g sodium bicarbonate. Maintain airway; support respirations; get blood gas, alcohol, and glucose levels. Oral or intravenous glucose is given as needed for hypoglycemia/ketoacidosis. Diazepam is given as needed for hyperexcitability or vomiting.
	Chronic: Vitamin and mineral deficiencies, polyneuropathy, myopathy, chronic gastritis, cirrhosis, pancreatitis, anemias, thrombocyte and granulocyte deficiencies.	
Amphetamines, psychedelic drugs—Cocaine, LSD, mescaline, etc.§	Central nervous system stimulation, paranoia, visual hallucinations, but oriented to time and space.	Provide secure environment, presence of familiar persons; "talking down" the patient. Sedative barbiturates and diazepam may be helpful.
	Mydriasis, increased blood pressure and pulse, hyperreflexia, tremor, piloerection, muscular weakness, fever, and occasionally drowsiness, nausea, and decreased urine output.	Give follow-up for symptoms, depression. Provide conservative, supportive measures.

*Treatment may vary with the individual situation and clinical judgment.
†Symptoms will vary with the concentration of poison in the body.
‡See text for specific antidote therapies.
§Toxicity usually involves more than a single substance.
‖Most common examples.
¶Highly addicting with narrow margin of safety, especially in combination with ethanol.

TABLE 32-4 Some specific poisons, symptoms, and emergency treatment—cont'd

Poison	Symptoms	Treatment
Arsenic (found in weed killers, insecticides, sheepdip, rodenticides, and so on)	Rapidity of onset of symptoms related to whether or not poison is taken with food. Odor of garlic on breath and stools. Faintness, nausea, difficulty in swallowing, extreme thirst, severe vomiting, gastric and mouth pain, "rice water" stools, oliguria, hematuria, albuminuria, cold clammy skin, skeletal muscle cramps. Collapse and death.	Induce emesis with ipecac syrup. Give 0.5 to 10 g of activated charcoal in a glass of water followed by repeated lavage with warm water or weak sodium bicarbonate solution or by an emetic (warm water) repeated until vomiting occurs. Give intravenous fluids. Allow sedation, analgesics. Dimercaprol (BAL) is the antidote of choice; penicillamine is an alternate. Keep patient warm. Relieve pain and diarrhea.
Barbiturates (sleep inducers, anticonvulsants, sedatives)—amobarbital (Amytal), pentobarbital (Nembutal), phenobarbital (Luminal), secobarbital (Seconal), thiopental (Pentothal), and others	Similar to alcohol intoxication. Deep sleep or stupor occasionally preceded by confusion, excitement. Later, coma, with sluggish or absent reflexes. Extremes in respiratory rate. Shock with decreased blood pressure, pinpoint pupils, weak and thready pulse. Death from respiratory failure, hypostatic pneumonia, or pulmonary edema. Very early there will be sluggishness in actions, thinking, and speech; poor memory; faulty judgment; narrow attention; emotional lability; untidy grooming; suicidal tendencies. Also, nystagmus, strabismus, diplopia, vertigo, positive Romberg sign, superficial reflexes, skin rashes. Concurrent use of amphetamines is also common.	Gradual withdrawal for the chronic user. General supportive care for all: Keep warm; turn; see to hydration, nutrition, etc. For acute poisoning, emesis or lavage after passing endotracheal tube if less than 2 hours since ingestion; hemodialysis may be effective. Pressor agents and use of ventilators may be necessary.
Carbon monoxide (present in coal gas; exhaust gases from inadequately vented combustion engines, especially cars)	Tissue anoxia. Symptoms vary with concentration of carbon monoxide in blood. Headache, dizziness, impaired hearing and vision, vomiting, yawning, drowsiness, confusion, loss of consciousness. Slow respiration, rapid pulse. Coma, cherry-red or dusky lips and nail beds.	Remove patient to fresh air; provide artificial respiration; give high concentration of oxygen, preferably under positive pressure. Intravenous glucose and prednisone as needed for cerebral edema. Bed rest for 48 hours. Keep patient warm.

Caustics/corrosives
  Acids
    Contact or ingested—carbolic or crude creosol (disinfectants), hydrochloric‖ (metal cleaners, soldering), nitric‖ and oxalic (cleaning solutions), sulfuric (auto batteries) acids
	Parts in contact with acid are first white, later brown or yellow.
	Coagulation necrosis with somewhat superficial tissue damage.
	Pain; thirst, difficulty breathing, speaking, swallowing; circulatory collapse; death from asphyxia.
		Avoid stomach tube, emesis (danger of perforation), or sodium bicarbonate (danger of gaseous distention/rupture).
		Give copious amounts of water.
		Relieve pain and treat shock.
		Corticosteroid therapy possibly effective.
		Keep patient warm and quiet.

Inhaled, volatile—Bromine, chlorine, fluorine, iodine	Cough, dyspnea, pulmonary edema.	Remove from area. Inspect skin and clothing. Treat pulmonary edema.
Alkalis (identifiable by "soapy" or slippery texture)	Deep penetrating tissue destruction (for example, esophageal perforation) with possibly severe scarring and stricture formation. Symptoms similar to acid ingestion; additionally, bloody vomitus and stools. Mucous membranes white and swollen; mouth, throat, and lips swell.	If liquid agent, prepare for possible esophagoscopy and/or surgery. Avoid stomach tube and emesis. Give large amounts of water. Corticosteroid therapy possibly effective in presence of burns. Relieve pain and treat shock.

Continued.

TABLE 32-4 Some specific poisons, symptoms, and emergency treatment—cont'd

Poison	Symptoms	Treatment
Caustics/corrosives—cont'd Alkalis—cont'd Contact or ingested—ammonia, automatic dishwasher detergent, caustic soda (soapmaking), Clinitest tablets, lime (building construction), potash (lye, drain chemicals[1]), potassium hydroxide, sodium hydroxide	Skin cold and clammy, hypotension, rapid pulse, violent vomiting, great anxiety.	
Cyanides—rodent and rat killers, metal polishes, commercial fumigants	An odor of oil of bitter almonds on the breath. Headache, rapid breathing, dyspnea, asphyxia, palpitation of heart, feeling of tightness in chest, cyanosis, convulsions, hypotension, sweating. Death may come within a few minutes.	Prompt treatment sometimes successful. Immediately remove poison by an emetic (ipecac syrup or apomorphine) or lavage. Remove to fresh air if poison taken by inhalation. Give amyl nitrite (several pearls broken into gauze and given by inhalation), followed by 1% sodium nitrite intravenously slowly, in 10-ml doses, to a total of 50 ml in an hour; follow this by slow intravenous administration of sodium thiosulfate (50 ml of a 25% solution). Oxygen, artificial ventilation, and blood transfusion may be necessary in presence of deepening cyanosis despite apparent recovery (methemoglobinemia). Antidote dosages based on hemoglobin level; assess blood pressure frequently.
Hydrocarbons or petroleum distillates (present in kerosene, gasoline, naphtha, cleaning fluids, paint thinner, charcoal lighter fluid, benzene—most dangerous effect in blood-forming tissue)	*Ingestion* (more hazardous because of potential for aspiration to occur during ingestion and treatment): Symptoms of intoxication similar to those of alcohol; burning sensation in mouth, esophagus, and stomach. Vomiting, dizziness, tremor, muscle cramps, confusion, fever, dullness. Cold, clammy skin; weak, irregular pulse; thirst; convulsions; unconsciousness; coma. Pulmonary symptoms include cough, cyanosis, bloody sputum, rales, edema, pneumonia. Death from respiratory failure. *Inhalation:* Visual difficulties, transient euphoria, headache, nausea. Death from respiratory failure.	Avoid emetics and lavage usually unless large amounts have been swallowed. Use emesis if more than 2 ml/kg body weight ingested or if there are dangerous additives involved; lavage after endotracheal intubation if more than 2 ml/kg ingested *and* there is loss of gag reflex, convulsions, or dyspnea. Emesis is precluded in ingestion of (1) high viscosity, low volatility products such as oils in home fuel, lubrication, machine oil (unless it contains triorthoresyl phosphate); (2) tar, asphalt, glues, greases, petroleum jelly, mineral oil.
MAO inhibitors—phenelzine (Nardil), tranylcypromine (Parnate)	*Acute:* Agitation, hallucinations, hyperreflexia, fever, and convulsions may appear late. *Chronic:* Mostly excess central nervous system stimulation, convulsions, and orthostatic hypotension.	Measures supportive to the maintenance of normal temperature, respirations, blood pressure, and fluid-electrolyte balance.

TABLE 32-4 Some specific poisons, symptoms, and emergency treatment—cont'd

Poison	Symptoms	Treatment
Nonbarbiturate sedatives—chloral hydrate, ethchlorvynol (Placidyl),¶ glutethimide (Doriden—toxic near 2.5 to 4 mg/day),¶ methaqualone (Quaalude),¶ methyprylon (Noludar),¶ paraldehyde. Benzodiazepines in large doses: Chlordiazepoxide (Librium), Diazepam (Valium—toxicity increased in intramuscular or intravenous doses or in combination with other drugs/ethanol), flurazepam (Dalmane), oxazepam (Serax), etc.	*As a group:* Extinction of inhibitions, ataxia, clumsiness, nystagmus, excess sedation, possible coma and death. Drug dependency and withdrawal symptoms. *Glutethimide:* Occasionally sudden apnea on being touched, hypotension, dilated pupils, no gag or corneal reflexes, coma. *Diazepam:* Respiratory or circulatory insufficiency.	*Glutethimide:* Intubate first, then lavage and give intravenous fluids. Recommended medications are intramuscular ephedrine, neosynephrine, intravenous benzedrine, intramuscular sodium benzoate. Provide respiratory system support and urinary catheterization as needed. Hemodialysis may be considered. Admit for close surveillance. *Diazepam:* lavage may be too late to prevent absorption. Supportive care may be sufficient even with large doses (300 to 400 mg).
Opiates, opioids (having morphine-like pharmacologic actions)—codeine, heroin, hydromorphone hydrochloride (Dilaudid), meperidine hydrochloride (Demerol), methadone (Methadon, Dolophine), morphine sulfate and hydrochloride, oxycodone (Percodan), pentazocine (Talwin), powdered opium (Pantopon), propoxyphene (Darvon), etc.	Depending on the drug, dosage, and duration of use, varied symptoms may be seen. The typical triad may be present: (1) depressed respirations, (2) pinpoint pupils (dilated if severely hypoxic), (3) coma. Respiratory rate may be 2 to 4 min and irregular; cyanosis. Hypotension directly related to decreased respiratory exchange. Urine output and body temperature are decreased. Pulmonary edema, shock can occur. Frank convulsions and death usually attributable to respiratory failure.	Gradually reduce dosage if chronic user, or substitute methadone, etc., for opiates. Maintain vital functions, especially airway, and provide ventilation. Give naloxone as antagonist (see Table 32-6). Position to prevent pneumonia and complications of shock, coma.
Organophosphorous insecticides—HEPT, Malathion, Parathion, TEPP, etc.	Headache, dizziness, anorexia, nausea, vomiting, diarrhea, blurred vision, abdominal pain, dyspnea, wheezing, chest pain, sweating, salivation, tearing, confusion. Cyanosis, respiratory failure, muscular twitching. Collapse.	Remove secretions, maintain patent airway. Decontaminate skin with soapy water or tincture of green soap. Induce vomiting, give milk by mouth. Give oxygen, artificial respiration to combat shock; intubate as needed. Atropinization is mandatory as soon as cyanosis has been relieved. *Adults:* give 2 to 4 mg atropine intravenously; repeat at 5- to 10-minute intervals until signs of atropine toxicity appear (dry flushed skin, tachycardia, mydriasis). *Children:* give 0.5 to 1 mg intravenously or intramuscularly every 10 to 15 minutes. Mild degree of atropinization should be maintained for 48 hours. Pralidoxime (Protopam) also given if poisoning is severe (see text). Perform gastric lavage if poison ingested. Maintain close supervision for 72 hours.

Continued.

TABLE 32-4 Some specific poisons, symptoms, and emergency treatment—cont'd

Poison	Symptoms	Treatment
Plants		
House and garden, various plant parts (seeds often contain a compound that releases cyanide when eaten)	Varied, including irritation and swelling of the mouth, tongue, throat; nausea, vomiting, diarrhea; irregular pulse; hypotension; convulsions; occasionally kidney damage.	Varied, depending on plant and part ingested: emesis or lavage, then supportive and symptomatic care as needed. For example, give atropine, 2 mg subcutaneously for decreased blood pressure; phentolamine for increased blood pressure; alkalinize urine with sodium bicarbonate, 5 to 15 g, every 4 hours to prevent precipitation of hemoglobin in the kidneys, as needed. Control convulsions as needed. Treatment may vary with species involved.
Mushrooms (genus *Amanita*, causal agent most frequently fatal)	Confusion, excitement, thirst, nausea, vomiting, diarrhea, wheezing, salivation, bradycardia, small pupils (muscarinic effects) or dilated pupils, tremors, collapse or death.	Induction of emesis or lavage; possible catharsis. For muscarinic symptoms give atropine sulfate, 1 to 2 mg subcutaneously, every 30 minutes as needed. Give sedatives for excitement. Increase oral and intravenous fluids. Treat shock.
Psychopharmacologic agents (antipsychotics, mood stabilizers, antidepressants, sedatives—make up the single most frequently encountered group of toxins treated by Poison Control Centers according to the latest accounting)—butyrophenones (haloperidol [Haldol]—also used in Tourette's syndrome); phenothiazines: chlorpromazine (Thorazine), thioridazine (Mellaril), trifluoperazine (Stelazine), triflupromazine (Vesprin)	Excess sedation, hypotension. Extrapyramidal effects: parkinsonian syndrome, akathisia (constant walking, no agitation) acute dystonic reactions (facial grimacing, seen at start of therapy), tardive dyskinesia (involuntary mouth movements and choreiform movements of extremities). Symptoms pronounced in elderly clients.	Phenothiazines: gastric lavage; admit to intensive care unit for at least 3 days; monitor vital signs, cardiac signs. Give diazepam for seizures. Treat hypertension very cautiously. Give sponge baths for fever. Give lidocaine for arrhythmias. Physostigmine intramuscularly or intravenously slowly has been effective in reversing anticholinergic central nervous system effects.
Salicylates—acetylsalicylic acid: aspirin	Respiratory alkalosis first appears, then metabolic acidosis—hyperpnea, flushed face, tinnitus, hyperthermia, abdominal pain, vomiting, dehydration, bleeding, tremor/convulsions, pulmonary edema, coma.	Induce emesis or aspirate stomach without fluids, then lavage with 2 to 4 L warm tap water and activated charcoal. Draw blood for pH, sodium, chloride, and potassium levels. Titrate intravenous fluids with serum electrolyte levels. Give phytonadione, 0.1 mg/kg body weight, once intramuscularly to correct prothrombin levels. Transfusion may be given for low platelet counts. Dialysis may be considered. Give sponge baths for fever.
Tricyclic antidepressants—amitriptyline (Elavil), imipramine (Tofranil)	*Acute:* fever, hypertension, seizures, coma. In children cardiac arrhythmias may occasionally be seen.	Induce emesis or perform a gastric lavage. Control convulsions with diazepam 0.2 mg/kg IV. Give physostigmine salicylate 2 mg IM or IV. See text. Maintain respirations.

PREVENTION OF POISONING

The renewed focus in nursing on primary care and its corollary, prevention, applies readily to poisonings. Prevention has always been the bailiwick of nursing, and other disciplines are beginning to take part. Combined efforts with drug information centers and other health professionals and creative approaches have already had an impact on the frequency of certain categories of drug poisoning, notably aspirin poisoning.

Various creative graphic symbols are now appearing on labels of poisonous substances to alert the adult and/or nonreading child to the potential hazard contained therein. "Mr. Yuk," an ugly, green-faced, scowling image, is one of these.

Tricky-to-open caps appear to delay if not totally prevent childrens' indiscriminate use of medicines. Others who have no need for these caps can request medication in the familiar easy-to-open caps.

There is much to learn about toxins in our environment, both apparent and potential, and therefore much to do in the way of poison prevention, but concerted, thoughtful efforts have already had a positive effect on statistics.

Antidotes

The number of antidotes for specific toxins is minimal (Table 32-5); there is no widely accepted "universal antidote." Delaying nursing care while specific substance identification is made and the antidote sought may be more injurious in the long run. Antidotes can be as toxic as the original poison if not used appropriately.

Antidotes are more effective after the stomach is empty. The correct dose to reverse toxicity depends on the specific drug involved, its half-life, and severity of toxicity shown. Antidotes work by any of the following mechanisms: (1) antagonizing or stimulating receptor sites that have been rendered hyperfunctional or dysfunctional by the poison; (2) interfering with enzyme inhibition; (3) administering the product of metabolism that has been interfered with; (4) inhibiting the biotransformation of a substance to a poisonous metabolite; (5) giving an agent that inactivates the toxic product; (6)

TABLE 32-5 Antidotes for specific drugs and poisons

Poison	Specific antidote
Acetaminophen (Tylenol, Datril, over-the-counter cold preparations)	N-acetylcysteine (Mucomyst),* 2-aminoethanethiol (Cysteamine)*
Alcohol (methanol) and ethylene glycol	Alcohol (ethanol)
Anticholinergics (atropine)	Physostigmine salicylate
Carbon monoxide	Oxygen administered under high pressure
Coumarin anticoagulants	Vitamin K, clotting factors
Cyanide	Amyl nitrite, sodium nitrite, sodium thiosulfate
Ethylene glycol (antifreeze)	Alcohol (ethanol)
Heavy metals:	
Arsenic	Dimercaprol (BAL)
Copper	Penicillamine (Cuprimine)
Iron	Deferoxamine (Desferal)
Lead	Dimercaprol, penicillamine, calcium disodium edetate (CaEDTA)
Mercury	Dimercaprol, deferoxamine
Nitrates and nitrites	Methylene blue
Opiates	Naloxone (Narcan)
Organophosphates (insecticides)	Atropine sulfate, pralidoxime (2-PAM)
Phenacetin (over-the-counter preparations)	Methylene blue
Tricyclic antidepressants	Physostigmine salicylate

*Not yet FDA approved (see text).

chelation (forming highly stable complexes, tying up the substance—usually a heavy metal such as iron); (7) producing immunotherapy—the use of antidrug antibodies to bind and inactivate drugs (for example, there is a report of severe digoxin poisoning reversed with sheep digoxin–specific antibodies); and (8) reducing compounds that have bound tightly to oxygen in the bloodstream.

N-Acetylcysteine (Mucomyst)

Though now used effectively as an antidote for acetaminophen poisoning, N-Acetylcysteine has not been officially approved by the FDA for this purpose except as an investigational drug, under supervision. Such approval is anticipated soon. However, it has been fully accepted in clinical practice as a mucolytic agent for some time. The protocol for its supervised use as an antidote can be obtained by writing or calling the Rocky Mountain Poison Control Center at 1-800-525-6115. Individual trials of both cysteamine and L-methionine as antidotes for acetaminophen have also been run, but neither has FDA approval at present, although one institution does give cysteamine with success.

Criteria for use of this protocol in treatment of acetaminophen poisoning are as follows:

1 Awareness of the legal ramifications in using an investigational drug
2 History of ingestion of 7.5 g or more of acetaminophen
3 Time of ingestion must be known to within 2 hours and ingestion must have been within the preceding 24 hours
4 Serum level of acetaminophen must be above 150 μg/ml within 4 hours after ingestion

Informed consent must be obtained since this is still experimental and an investigational drug.

Dosage. *N*-Acetylcysteine is given after lavage either by mouth or by Miller-Abbott tube. The protocol specifies a loading dose of 140 mg/kg body weight of a 20% solution with follow-up doses of 70 mg/kg every 4 hours for 17 doses. The drug should only be diluted in cola, orange juice, or grapefruit juice. Other important detailed instructions are included in the official protocol.

Ethyl alcohol (ethanol)

Useful as an antidote in poisoning involving methanol (found in Sterno, wood alcohol, and ethylene glycol "permanent" antifreeze), ethyl alcohol interferes with metabolism and the formation of toxic metabolites. It is given as a 100-proof (50%) solution by intravenous infusion at 1 ml/kg body weight (diluted to not more than a 5% solution), followed by 0.5 to 1 ml/kg every 2 hours orally or intravenously for 4 days, with blood levels carefully monitored. Sodium bicarbonate or sodium lactate may also be given. Delirium, if present, may be controlled by pentobarbital sodium, 100 mg, every 6 to 12 hours.

Physostigmine salicylate (Antilirium)

Physostigmine salicylate is used in anticholinergic poisonings, for belladonna alkaloid poisoning, and overdosage of some antihistamines. Physostigmine inhibits the action of cholinesterase and thereby prolongs and exaggerates the effect of acetylcholine. Its actions are therefore similar to those of parasympathetic stimulation.

Dosage. Physostigmine comes in 2 mg/2 ml ampules. Usual range of dose is 0.5 to 4 mg intramuscularly or intravenously for two to three doses for adults. The lowest effective dose possible should be used. The initial dose in adults is 2 mg intramuscularly or intravenously. It is given slowly over 2 to 3 minutes (1 mg/minute) intravenously and may be repeated every 5 minutes if anticholinergic effects persist, to a maximum total of 6 mg. Intramuscularly it may be repeated every 20 minutes, to a maximum of 6 mg.

The initial dose for children is 0.5 mg intramuscularly or intravenously; this may be repeated every 5 minutes, to a total of 2 mg intravenously, or given every 20 minutes, to 2 mg intramuscularly.

Contraindications and side effects. Contraindications are many, including the presence of asthma, diabetes, gangrene, cardiovascular disease, and mechanical obstruction of the gastrointestinal or urinary tracts. It is a drug definitely not for routine use in mild cases of poisoning. It should be discontinued if excessive parasympathetic signs are noted: for example, increased salivation, emesis, or involuntary urination or defecation.

Amyl nitrite
Sodium nitrite
Sodium thiosulfate

The sequential administration of these drugs provides effective antidotal therapy for cyanide poisoning if the drug has been mostly removed from the stomach. They act by producing methemoglobin, which binds with the cyanide and renders it impotent. Methemoglobin can be produced by an inhalation of a fresh ampule of amyl nitrite for 30 seconds every 2 minutes (a fresh ampule must be crushed for use every 3 minutes). Intravenous administration of sodium nitrite should follow as soon as possible. A dose of 10 mg/kg (0.33 ml/kg of 3% sodium nitrite) is infused intravenously at a rate of 2.5 to 5 ml/minute. The adult dose is 10 to 15 ml, repeated once if necessary.

An intravenous dose of sodium thiosulfate is given 15 minutes after the nitrite infusion is finished. A dose of 1.65 ml/kg of 25% sodium thiosulfate is run at 2.5 to 5 ml/minute. The adult dose is 20 to 50 ml, repeated once if necessary.

Methemoglobin and hemoglobin levels must be monitored during this therapy. Possible hypotension must be assessed, and epinephrine should be available.

Dimercaprol (BAL in oil)

Dimercaprol (BAL in oil) is a highly effective antidote for use in arsenic, gold and mercury, and somewhat effective in copper and lead poisoning (ethylenediamine tetraacetate [EDTA] is given in combination with BAL for the latter); it is not effective in poisoning involving Freon or cadmium. Other antidotes are very useful for the treatment of some other intoxications caused by heavy metals. Most important are calcium disodium edetate and penicillamine.

Dimercaprol was developed during World War II as an antidote for the arsenic-containing blister gas lewisite, hence, the name "BAL" for "British anti-lewisite." It was used to decontaminate the skin and eyes of persons who had been in contact with the gas, but later it was found to be of value in the treatment of various forms of arsenic poisoning.

Dimercaprol is a colorless liquid with a rather offensive odor. It is dispensed in a 10% solution in peanut oil for intramuscular injection. One milliliter contains 100 mg dimercaprol.

Arsenic compounds produce their toxic effects by combining with the sulfhydryl groups of enzymes, which are necessary for normal metabolism. As a result, the processes of oxidation and reduction in the tissues are seriously hindered. Dimercaprol interferes with this combination, forms a stable combination with the arsenic, neutralizes its toxic effects, and hastens its excretion.

Dimercaprol is also indicated in the treatment of gold and mercury poisoning. Treatment should begin as soon as possible after poisoning has occurred. In mercury poisoning, if treatment does not occur within 2 hours, irreversible, extensive renal damage may occur.

Results in the treatment of poisoning from other heavy metals are disappointing or inconclusive, but dimercaprol may be used as an adjunct in treating lead and copper toxicity.

Dosage. In the treatment of mild arsenic or gold poisoning, the dose is 2.5 to 5 mg/kg body weight, given by deep intramuscular injection four times daily the first 2 days, reduced to two injections on the third day, and then daily for the next 10 days. In severe arsenic or gold poisoning 3 mg/kg body weight is given intramuscularly every 4 hours for the first 2 days, then four times on the third day, and then twice daily for 10 days. In mercury poisoning the dosage is 5 mg/kg body weight initially, then 2.5 mg/kg one or two times daily for 10 days. In lead poisoning, the intramuscular dose is 4 mg/kg body weight every 4 hours for 5 days, given along with EDTA.

After intramuscular injection, maximum plasma concentrations occur in 30 to 60 minutes. The drug is excreted or metabolized in 4 hours.

Side effects. Adverse effects from dimercaprol are usually mild and transitory. Frequent side effects are a rise in blood pressure, tachycardia, and pain and sterile abscesses at the injection site. This drug gives the patient's breath an unpleasant odor. It may cause nausea and vomiting, headache, a burning sensation of the mouth, throat, and eyes, a constricting sensation in the chest, muscular aching, tingling in the extremities, anxiety, restlessness, lacrimation, and salivation.

Fever occurs commonly in children. High doses may cause capillary damage, coma, and convulsions.

Precautions. Dimercaprol is potentially nephrotoxic. Since the dimercaprol-metal complex breaks down easily in an acid medium, the urine should be kept alkaline to protect the kidneys.

Its use is contraindicated in hepatic insufficiency except for postarsenical jaundice.

Penicillamine

Penicillamine is used to treat copper poisoning and to remove copper from the body in hepatolenticular degeneration (Wilson's disease). It may also be used as a chelator of lead, arsenic, iron, and mercury. It is derived from the degradation of penicillin, but it has no antibacterial activity.

Dosage. Pencillamine should be given in the acute phase at 100 mg/kg/day divided into four oral doses for 5 days. For the chronic phase, 30 to 50 mg/kg/day is divided into four doses. Pyridoxine, 10 to 25 mg, should be given once a day.

The recommended oral dose of penicillamine is 250 to 300 mg every 6 to 8 hours. The maximum dosage for adults is 1 g daily. The drug should be given on an empty stomach between meals and at bedtime to avoid interference with dietary metals. For young children and infants over 6 months of age, the daily dose is 250 mg dissolved in fruit juice. Onset of action of penicillamine is 30 minutes; peak effect occurs in 2 to 3 hours. Dosage must be individualized by determining the urinary excretion of copper. Patients receiving penicillamine for copper chelation should be on a low-copper diet; food such as chocolate, nuts, shellfish, liver, mushrooms, and broccoli should be avoided. In addition, patients should take 25 mg pyridoxine daily, since the drug increases the body's requirement for this vitamin. It should be noted that penicillamine may inhibit wound healing. Cross-sensitivity to penicillin may exist. Penicillamine may also be give for cystinuria.

Side effects. Rashes, blood dyscrasias, and renal damage may occur following the use of penicillamine. The drug is relatively safe, however, and adverse effects do not occur frequently. Patients should be carefully observed for hypersensitivity reactions. Urinalysis and blood examinations should be performed every 3 days for the first 2 weeks of therapy, every 10 days for the next 3 or 4 months, and then monthly until therapy is terminated. If hematuria, leukopenia, thrombocytopenia, or increased proteinuria occurs, the drug should be discontinued until normal values are obtained. If therapy is reinstituted, the dose should be small and increments made cautiously.

Deferoxamine (Desferal)

Deferoxamine binds iron, converts it to a less toxic form, and promotes its excretion. Consequently, it is useful in the treatment of iron poisoning and in diseases such as hemochromatosis in which there is a chronic accumulation of iron in the body. The complex formed when deferoxamine is combined with

iron is a reddish color. Since the complex is excreted through the urinary tract, the urine of patients with this drug will be reddish brown. The drug seems to have little effect on hemoglobin levels.

Preparation, dosage, and administration. Deferoxamine is available in vials of 500 mg of lyophilized powder. The powder is readily dissolved by adding 2 ml sterile water for injection. Intramuscular injection is the preferred route of administration. The intramuscular dosage in moderate cases of iron poisoning is 50 mg every 6 to 12 hours up to a maximum of 2 g and not to exceed 6 g in 24 hours. The adult intramuscular dosage is 1 to 2 g every 6 to 8 hours, to a maxium dose of 6 g in 24 hours. In severe cases of shock deferoxamine is given intravenously as a 5% solution at a rate not to exceed 15 mg/kg/hour. Assessment for the development of hypotension or apnea is essential. The subcutaneous route should be avoided, since it may cause severe tissue irritation and damage. Likewise, the oral route should not be used as it increases iron absorption.

Side effects. Deferoxamine is well tolerated, and adverse effects are infrequent. Mild rash or pruritus may occur. Rapid intravenous injection may cause hypotension, apnea, tachycardia, erythema, and urticaria. Pain and tissue irritation may occur at the injection site. Patients receiving long-term therapy have reported allergic reactions, blurred vision, fever, diarrhea, and leg cramps. Cataracts have been reported after prolonged deferoxamine therapy but not after short-term therapy. Deferoxamine can lower blood sugar and serum calcium levels and increase blood coagulability; thus these parameters should be monitored. Its use is contraindicated in patients with severe renal impairment.

Calcium disodium edetate (Calcium Disodium Versenate, CaEDTA)

Calcium disodium edetate is most useful in the treatment of lead poisoning. It combines with heavy metal in the body to form nonionized, water-soluble complexes that are readily excreted by the kidneys; it is given along with BAL.

CaEDTA is also used diagnostically in cases of suspected lead poisoning. If the 24-hour urinary excretion of lead is 500 μg or more per liter following administration of the drug, a diagnosis of poisoning may be made before clinical symptoms and irreversible damage occur.

It is effective for reduction of blood and depot lead in acute and chronic lead poisoning and lead encephalopathy; it is probably effective for the treatment of other heavy metal poisonings and in the removal of radioactive and nuclear fission products such as plutonium.

Given intravenously, it has a half-life of 20 to 60 minutes; about 50% is excreted in the urine in 1 hour and 95% in about 24 hours. Thus adequate kidney function is vital during therapy. Intravenous infusions may be given prior to the first drug dose to establish urine flow; however, fluids should be carefully titrated so that sudden increases in intracranial pressure do not occur (a potential danger if there is lead encephaopathy), yet adequate urine volume is maintained. Urine volume should be assessed continuously and daily urinalysis performed to determine if there is increased proteinuria, red blood cells, or large renal epithelial cells; if these occur, the drug should be discontinued immediately, since this indicates increased renal damage. It must be used cautiously in patients with tuberculosis or renal disease.

CaEDTA interferes with the action of zinc insulin by forming a chelate with zinc. Thus these two drugs should not be given concurrently. CaEDTA may deplete trace element metals (for example, copper, magnesium) from the body. Its safe use during pregnancy has not been established.

Preparation, dosage, and administration. CaEDTA is available for injection in 5-ml ampules (1 g each, or 200 mg/ml), and in 500-mg tablets, but it should not be given orally as it is a gastrointestional tract irritant and may enhance lead absorption. Dosage depends on severity of intoxication, patient's size, results of treatment, and patient's tolerance. CaEDTA may be administered by subcutaneous, intramuscular (children), or intravenous injection (adults).

Lead encephalopathy is quite common among children (rare in adults) and has an alarmingly high mortality. A single preliminary dose of dimercaprol prior to CaEDTA administration has been found by some investigators to be highly effective in reducing the death rate. The stomach should be emptied of lead prior to treatment with CaEDTA.

Intramuscular administration is preferred for children. Dosage should not exceed 50 mg/kg/day for mild cases of lead poisoning and may be evenly divided into three doses a day for 3 to 5 days for young children, twice a day for older children. Four days without therapy should intervene before a second course is given, if it is necessary. Procaine hydrochloride should be added to CaEDTA to minimize pain at the injection site (1 ml of 1% procaine solution to each milliliter of CaEDTA, or crystalline procaine should be used to decrease intramuscular injection volume).

For intravenous administration, an ampule of 1 g/5 ml should be diluted with 250 to 500 ml normal saline solution or D_5W and administered over no less than a 1-hour period. This may be done twice a day for up to 5 days. If another course is necessary, a 2-day interruption of therapy should intervene. Maximum dosage is 50 mg/kg/day.

Side effects. If more than the recommended dosage is used, renal damage may occur, particularly in children. Symptoms of acute lead poisoning, particularly cerebral symptoms, may be aggravated at the beginning of therapy. If this happens, dosage should be reduced.

Malaise, excessive thirst, paresthesias, sudden fever and shaking chills, headache, nausea and vomiting, and lacrimation may occur 4 to 8 hours after infusion of the drug.

Precautions. Since CaEDTA may produce eletrocardiographic changes, the patient's heart should be monitored for irregularities. CaEDTA may be toxic if used alone in lead encephalopathy. Patients should be hydrated first and urine flow established.

Contraindications. CaEDTA should not be given to patients with anuria or severe renal disease.

Methylene blue

Methylene blue is used to counteract methemoglobinemia when the methemoglobin level is 40 mg/100 ml or if dyspnea is present after intoxication by aniline dyes or nitrites (occasionally as a result of excesses in cured foods, especially in children), and in certain enzyme-deficient states challenged by the administration of acetanilid or the sulfonamides. Methylene blue apparently acts as a catalyst to reduce methemoglobin to hemoglobin. It also has mild bacteriostatic properties. It is inferior to other antidotes for cyanide poisoning.

Dosage. Methylene blue is given intravenously in a 1% solution at a dose of 1 to 2 mg/kg body weight over a 5 to 10-minute period, and may be repeated once in 4 hours (common adult dose is 6 to 12 ml). The dosage must be carefully controlled, since excessive doses of methylene blue have caused methemoglobinemia, hemolysis, and depression of the central nervous system. Very large doses (500 mg) have caused nausea, abdominal and precordial pain, dizziness, headache, sweating, and confusion.

Naloxone injection (Narcan)

Naloxone is extremely useful to reverse the respiratory depression of opiate overdose. It is the only commercially available antagonist used for pentazocine overdose. One milligram of naloxone blocks the effects of 25 mg heroin. A dose of 5 mg/kg has been given without ill effects to neonates whose respirations are depressed by maternal therapeutic doses of morphine or meperidine. Artificial ventilation may suffice, however, and may be the preferred treatment of addicts to avoid the precipitation of hazardous withdrawal syndromes.

Naloxone has replaced nalorphine (Nalline) and similar substances that can cause central nervous system depression; naloxone has no similar depressant properties. It competes with opiates for receptor sites.

Naltrexone is another drug very similar to naloxone in action and effects.

Precautions. The nurse should anticipate possible vomiting and act to prevent aspiration by proper position of the patient and preparation of equipment for intubation if necessary.

Preparation, dosage, and administration. Naloxone is available in 1-ml ampules and 10-ml multidose vials (0.4 mg/ml). The initial dose for children is 0.01 mg/kg body weight given intramuscularly or intravenously; if respirations do not improve markedly in 2 minutes, a second, larger dose may be given. According to Moore and others, repeated doses of naloxone may be necessary until the narcotic is metabolized and excreted. The usual adult dose is 0.4 mg, but higher doses, up to 1.2 to 2 mg, may be necessary and should be titrated with respiratory rate and depth. Increases toward a normal respiratory rate may be noted within 1 to 2 minutes, and there may be a transient "overshoot" response. The effects of naloxone may last for 2 to 3 hours.

Atropine sulfate

Atropine in large doses is valuable in the treatment of poisoning by anticholinesterase organophosphorous insecticides (for example, parathion, dimpylate, and malathion—in descending order of toxicity. It is also used to antagonize cholinergic effects of neostigmine or other anticholinesterase agents given in the treatment of myasthenia gravis and similar disorders. It is a specific antidote when used cautiously for the "rapid type" of mushroom poisoning (*Amanita muscaria* and some other fungi), but not for the "delayed type." It is used as a significant priming supplement to stimulate respirations before pralidoxime is given as combination therapy. It is also commonly given preoperatively to decrease oral and respiratory secretions, to prevent laryngospasm, and on other occasions to increase heart rate.

Dosage. Treatment by atropine in poisoning is usually aggressive. Following an initial intravenous injection of 2 to 4 mg, a 2-mg dose (1/30 grain) should be repeated every 3 to 10 minutes until muscarinic symptoms disappear (postganglionic nerve-ending stimulation in cardiac and smooth muscle and glands, producing depressed cardiovascular action, increased gastrointestinal activity, increased sweating and salivation, and pupillary constriction) or if they reappear. Mild atropinization should be maintained by the oral administration of 1 to 2 mg at intervals of several hours as long as there are symptoms.

Side effects and toxic effects. Atropine has a wide margin of safety; the lethal dose of atropine has been stated to be 10 to 15 mg for children and 100 mg for adults, but victims of organophosphate poisoning can tolerate larger doses. Signs of toxicity include depressed respirations, central nervous system excitation, restlessness, irritability, delirium, and hallucinations, extending to respiratory and circulatory failure, coma, and paralysis. Ataxia, restlessness, delirium, fright, and aggressive behavior are *early* signs of toxicity. People living in tropical or subtropical climates are particularly sensitive to atropine effects.

Contraindication. The main contraindication to administration of atropine is glaucoma.

Pralidoxime chloride (2-PAM, Protopam)

Pralidoxime is a cholinesterase reactivator used as an antidote for poisoning by organophosphate insecticides, which inactivate cholinesterase in the body. Pralidoxime breaks down the binding between the organophosphate compound and cholinesterase, liberating the cholinesterase, which can then destroy accumulated acetylcholine.

The reactivation of cholinesterase occurs primarily at the neuromuscular junction of skeletal muscles; little reactivation occurs at autonomic effector sites, and even less in the central nervous system. Pralidoxime is used to reverse respiratory muscle paralysis. However, it is relatively ineffective on the respiratory center, and atropine sulfate, 1 to 4 mg intravenously must be given initially as soon as cyanosis is overcome by mechanical ventilation to relieve respiratory depression from accumulated acetylcholine at this site. In mild poisonings atropine therapy alone may suffice. Pralidoxime is most effective if given immediately after poisoning. Blood should be drawn to measure cholinesterase levels before giving pralidoxime.

Preparation, dosage, and administration. Pralidoxime is available in 20-ml vials containing 1 g powder and in 500-mg tablets. It is administered intravenously (or intramuscularly or subcutaneously if the intravenous route is not feasible) in a dosage of 1 to 2 g in 100 ml saline for adults at a rate of no more than 500 mg/minute (preferably over 15 to 30 minutes). This may be repeated cautiously after 1 to 2 hours. The children's infusion uses 25-40 mg/kg body weight of a 5% to 10% solution given slowly. Dosage should be reduced for patients with renal insufficiency.

Side effects. Pralidoxime may cause dizziness, diplopia, blurred vision, nausea, tachycardia, increased blood pressure, hyperventilation, laryngospasm, and muscular weakness/

rigidity, especially with rapid injection rates.

Contraindications. Pralidoxime is contraindicated in poisoning with insecticides carbaril (Sevin) or dimpylate (Diazinon) because it may potentiate the existing toxicity.

Summary of nursing considerations

Toxicology is the study of poisons, their action and effects, methods for their detection, and diagnosis and treatment of poisoning. A poison can be defined as any substance that in relatively small amounts can cause death or serious body harm by chemical action. All drugs are potential poisons when used improperly or in excess dosage. Poisoning may be acute, when the effects are immediate, or chronic, when the effects are insidious as a result of cumulative effects of small amounts of poison absorbed over a prolonged period of time.

A nurse's immediate attention is imperative when poisoning is suspected. The nurse should send for a physician and apply suitable first-aid measures. There is reason to suspect that a poison has been taken when sudden, violent symptoms occur, such as severe nausea, vomiting, diarrhea, collapse, or convulsions. It is important to find out (if possible) what poison has been taken and how much. Tables 32-3 and 32-4 list common poisoning agents, signs and symptoms, and emergency treatment. Attempts are being made to educate the public by means of the establishment of poison centers, dissemination of information, and adoption of a universal poison symbol recognizable by children.

Treatment of poisoning involves support of vital functions and removal of the poison or administration of a suitable antidote. First-aid measures for poisoning are outlined on p. 974.

QUESTIONS

FOR STUDY AND REVIEW

Circle the answer of your choice.
  1 Which of the following conditions would lead you to suspect acute poisoning?
   a. gradual loss of weight
   b. anorexia, undue lassitude
   c. onset of sudden violent symptoms
   d. weakness, anemia, headache

2 Which of the following factors is likely to be the crucial one in the successful treatment of early and acute poisoning?
   a. amount of supportive treatment
   b. immediate removal of poison from the body
   c. control of shock
   d. administration of the right antidote
3 Which of the following kinds of antidotes are represented when sodium chloride solution is used in the treatment of silver nitrate poisoning?
   a. chemical
   b. physical
   c. universal
   d. physiologic
4 If you were working in the chemistry laboratory and splashed some hydrochloric acid in your eye, what is the first thing you would do?
   a. rush to the emergency room or health center
   b. search for a weak base and instill some in your eye
   c. neutralize the acid with solution of sodium hydroxide
   d. wash eye with copious amounts of plain water
5 BAL (British anti-lewisite) is a recommended antidote for poisoning from:
   a. hydrocarbons
   b. strong acids
   c. phenolic compounds
   d. certain heavy metals
6 Death from carbon monoxide is likely to be caused by:
   a. changes in bone marrow
   b. damage to liver and kidney
   c. depression of heart
   d. anoxia
7 Death from a poison like methyl alcohol is likely to result from:
   a. destruction in the kidney
   b. perforation, hemorrhage, or both
   c. acidosis
   d. depression of the respiratory center
8 Which of the following statements best explains why children are often poisoned by medicines left around the house?
   a. children are naturally curious about things
   b. children mistake sweet-tasting tablets or pills for candy
   c. children like to explore new things with their mouths
   d. children like to imitate other members of the household
9 Which of the following would you do if present at the scene of a poisoning and the patient had been vomiting?
   a. note odor and color of the vomitus before flushing down the toilet
   b. save a specimen of vomitus and add a preservative if possible
   c. save a specimen of vomitus (an early one if possible) for the physician
   d. discard emesis as fast as possible to avoid offense to the patient
10 For what type of emergency situation is naloxone given? For what type of poisoning is atropine employed?

BIBLIOGRAPHY

Arena, J.M.: Treatment of some common household poisonings, Pharmacol. Phys. 3(9):1, 1969.
Arena, J.M.: The clinical diagnosis of poisoning, Pediatr. Clin. North Am. 17:477, 1970.
Arena, J.M.: Poisoning: toxicology, symptoms and treatment, ed. 3., Springfield, Ill., 1974, Charles C Thomas, Publisher.
Arena, J.M.: Poisoning: treatment and prevention, J.A.M.A. 232:1272, 1975.
Aronow, R., and others: Phencycliding overdose: an emerging concept of management, Am. Coll. Emergency Physicians 7(2):56, 1978.
Avery, G.S.: Drug treatment, Sydney, 1980, ADIS, Bulletin, National Clearinghouse for Poison Control Centers, U.S. Department of Health, Education and Welfare, Rockville, Md., April 1980.
Bailey, B.O.: Acetaminophen hepatotoxicity and overdose. Am. Fam. Physician 22:83, July 1980.
Barer, J., and others: Fatal salt poisoning from salt used as an emetic, Am. J. Dis. Child 125:889, 1973.
Bean, J.: Use of bethanechol to treat anticholinergic side effects of tricyclic antidepressants and phenothiazines, Hosp. Pharmacy 15(6):317, 1980.
Bourne, P.G., editor: A treatment manual for acute drug abuse emergencies, Rockville, Md., 1974, National Clearinghouse for Drug Abuse Information, National Institute on Drug Abuse.
Calesnick, B.: Tricyclic antidepressant toxicity, Am. Fam. Physician 21(6):104, 1980.
Cashman, T.M., and Shirley, H.C.: Emergency management of poisoning, Pediatr. Clin. North Am. 17:525, 1970.
Caranasos, G.J., and others: Drug-induced illness leading to hospitalization, J.A.M.A. 228:713, 1974.
D'Anrea, V.: Psychoactive drugs, Menlo Park, 1977, Benjamin Cummings Co.
Deichmann, W.B., and Gerarde, H.W.: Toxicology of drugs and chemicals, New York, 1969, Academic Press, Inc.
Dimijian, G.G., and Radclat, F.A.: Evaluation and treatment of the suspected drug user in the emergency room, Arch. Intern. Med. 125:162, 1970.
Dove, A.K.: Pharmacologic principles in the treatment of poisoning, Pharmacol. Phys. 3(7):1, 1969.
Dove, A.K.: Poisoning from common household products, Pediatr. Clin. North Am. 17:569, 1970.
Driesbach, R.H.: Handbook of poisoning: diagnosis and treatment, ed. 8, Los Altos, Calif., 1980, Lange Medical Publications.
Duffy, T.P., editor: Poisoning. In Harvey, A.M., and other editors: The principles and practice of medicine, New York, 1976, Appleton-Century-Crofts.
Editorial: Childhood poisoning: prevention and first aid management, Br. Med. J. 4:483, 1975.
Evans, L.E.J., and others: Treatment of drug overdosage with naloxone, a specific narcotic antagonist, Lancet 1:452, 1973.

Gellis, S.S., and Kagan, B.M., editors: Accident and emergencies. In Current pediatric therapy, vol. 6, Philadelphia, 1980, W.B. Saunders Co.

Goodman, L.S., and Gilman, A.: The pharmacological basis of therapeutics, ed. 6, New York, 1980, Macmillan, Inc.

Greensher, J., and others: Activated charcoal updated, J. Am. Coll. Emergency Physicians **8**:7, July 1979.

Hill, J.B.: Salicylate intoxication, N. Engl. J. Med. **288**:1110, 1973.

Joselow, M.M., Louria, D.B., and Brawder, A.A.: Mercurialism: environmental and occupational aspects, Ann. Intern. Med. **76**:119, 1972.

Kempshield, J.H., and others: Dialysis of poisons and drugs, annual review, Trans. Am. Soc. Artif. Intern. Organs **19**:590, 1973.

Keyvan-Larijarni, H., and Tannenberg, A.: Methanol intoxication, Arch. Intern. Med. **134**:293, 1974.

Krogh, C.: Toxicities in perspective—Acetylsalicylic acid and acetaminophen, Can. Pharmaceutical J. **113**:169, 1980

Laurence, F.H., and others: Activated charcoal: a forgotten antidote, Maine Med. Assoc. **63**:311, 1975.

Lawrence, R.A., and Haggerty, R.J.: Household agents and their potential toxicity, Mod. Treat. **8**:511, 1971.

Leape, L.L., and others: Hazards, to health—liquid lye, N. Engl. J. Med. **284**:578, 1971.

Loomis, T.A.: Essentials of toxicology, Philadelphia, 1978, Lea & Febiger.

Lovejoy, F.: Priorities in poisoning, Emergency Med., p. 265, Feb. 15, 1979.

Maher, J.F.: Nephrotoxicity of drugs and chemicals, Pharmacol. Phys. **4**:1, 1970.

Mann, J.B., and Sandberg, D.H.: Therapy of sedative overdosage, Pediatr. Clin. North Am. **17**:617, 1970.

Matthew, H.: Gastric aspiration and lavage, Clin. Toxicol. **3**:179, 1970.

Matthew, H.: Acute poisoning: some myths and misconceptions, Br. Med. J. **1**:519, 1971.

Matthew, H., and Lawson, A.A.H.: Treatment of common acute poisonings, ed. 2, Edinburgh, 1972, Churchill Livingstone.

Mennear, J.H.: The poisoning emergency, Am. J. Nurs. **77**:842, 1977.

Mofenson, H.C.: Poison control manual, East Meadow, N.Y., 1979, Nassau County Medical Center Poison Control Center, unpublished.

Mofenson, H.C., and Greensher, J.: Poisoning—an update, Clin. Pediatr. **18**(3):, 1979.

Moore, R.A., and others: Nalaxone, J. Dis. Child. **134**(2):156, 1980.

Morgan, J.P., and Joel, L.S.: Phencyclidine, N.Y. State J. Med.: 2035, 1978.

Murphy, J.V.: Intoxication following the ingestion of elemental zinc, J.A.M.A. **212**:2119, 1970.

Page, L.B.: Mushroom poisoning, editorial; West. J. Med. **132**(1):66, 1980.

Parcel, G.S.: First aid in emergency care, St. Louis, 1977, The C.V. Mosby Co.

Parkhouse, J., Pleuvry, B.J., and Rees, J.M.H.: Analgesic drugs, Oxford, 1979, Blackwell Scientific Publications.

Parry, M., and Wallach, R.: Ethylene glycol poisoning, Am. J. Med. **57**:143, 1974.

Pascoe, D.J.: Poisoning. In Pascoe, D.J., and Grossman, M., editors: Quick reference to pediatric emergencies, Philadelphia, 1973, J.B. Lippincott Co.

Peper, K.W., and Griner, P.F.: Suicide attempts with drug overdose. Outcomes of intensive vs. conventional floor care, Arch. Intern. Med. **134**:703, 1974.

Rodman, M.J.: Poisoning treatment and prevention, R.N. **35**:51, 1972.

Ross, J.F.: The management of the presuicidal, suicidal, and postsuicidal patient, Ann. Intern. Med. **75**:441, 1971.

Rumack, B.H., and Temple, A.R.: Management of the poisoned patient, Princeton, 1977, Science Press.

Schreiner, G.E.: Dialysis of poisons and drugs—annual review, Trans. Am. Soc. Artif. Intern. Organs **16**:544, 1970.

Silver, H.K., Kempe, C.H., and Bruya, H.B.: Handbook of pediatrics, ed. 11, Los Altos, Calif., 1975, Lange Medical Publications.

Sjogvist, F., and Alvan, G.: Pharmacological principles in the management of accidental poisoning, Pediatr. Clin. North Am. **17**:495, 1970.

Stracener, C.E., and Scherz, R.G.: Experiences with safety containers for prevention of accidental childhood poisoning, Northwest Med. **63**:334, 1970.

Tennant, F.S.: Complications of propoxyphene abuse, Arch. Intern. Med. **132**:191, 1973.

Tong, T.G.: Poisoning and its treatment, Part 1. Incidence and clinical signs of poisoning and toxic overdose, Nurse Pract. **2**(2):35, 1976.

Tong, T.G.: Poisoning and its treatment, Part 2. Treatment of poisoning and toxic overdose, Nurse Pract. **2**(3):29, 1977.

APPENDIX

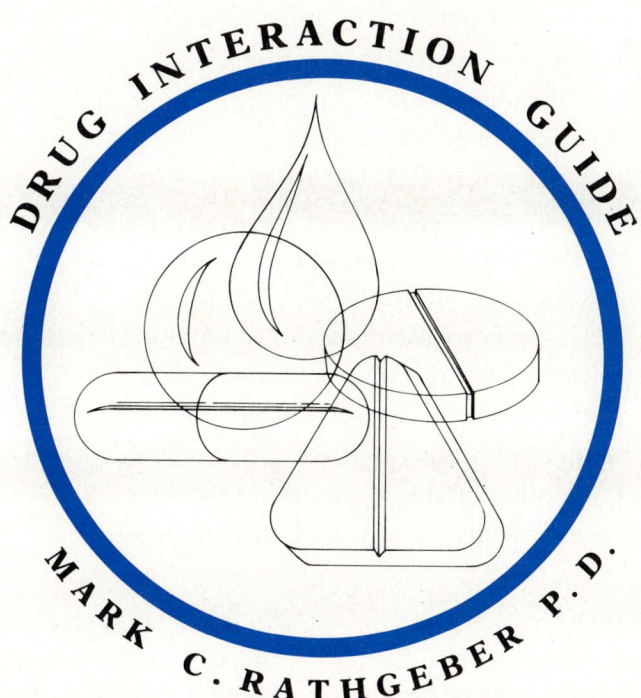

DRUG INTERACTION GUIDE

MARK C. RATHGEBER P.D.

DRUG INTERACTION GUIDE

Table of contents

HOW TO USE THE APPENDIX

When the interaction of two or more prescription or over-the-counter (OTC) products is in question, look up each individual product in the index following Chart 18. All prescription drugs are listed by both trade name and corresponding generic name. The trade name refers the reader to the generic name and indicates the charts containing the interaction in question.

Column 4 of each chart lists OTC/food items that may interact with the prescription drugs listed in column 1 to produce side effects noted in the introduction to that chart. Most OTC and household remedies are listed in the charts and may not be listed individually in the index. Chart 1 deals primarily with OTC drugs, household remedies, and their interactions.

Prescription medications primarily used in the injectable form and some anesthetics are listed in Chart 18 and may not be listed individually in the index.

Dedication and acknowledgements

The Drug Interaction Guide is dedicated to all members of the health care profession devoted to furthering the best of health. I would like to acknowledge all those associated with making the guide possible, along with Susan Mantia of Washington University Medical Center, Ben Hesselberg, R.Ph., and The C.V. Mosby Company for making this information available in this text.

Logo is by Sharon Powers.

CHART 1 Over-the-counter drug interactions

	Any of these OTC drugs may interact with	➡ any of these OTC/food items as described in introductory material.	
This chart deals strictly with products that can be bought over the counter and points out the potentially hazardous reactions that may occur. As described in the chart, the combination of alcohol-containing products can increase the damage to the stomach lining and possibly cause blood loss. Also described in this chart is the combination of alcohol-containing OTC products that, when combined with other OTC antihistamine-containing products, may cause drowsiness. Although some cough and cold remedies cause drowsiness when taken alone, combination compounds the decrease in alertness. When selecting a product in the OTC category it is always advisable to evaluate the ingredients to avoid any further complications with other OTC products or prescription medications, as pointed out in this and following charts. The OTC products that interact with other prescription medications are described in the following charts.	Alcoholic beverages Beer Cheracol, Cheracol D Cosanyl-DM Creo-Terpin, Creo-Terpin Plus Demazin Syrup Dristan Cough Formula Histadyl E.C. Neo-Synephrine Tablets Novahistine-DH and Novahistine Expectorant Nyquil Pertussin Robitussin, Robitussin-AC, Robitussin DM Triaminic Expectorant Valadol Liquid Vicks Formula 44 Cough Mixture	A.P.C. and A.P.C. Compound A.S.A., A.S.A. Compound Alka-Seltzer Alka-2 Allerest Anacin products Arthritis Strength Bufferin Ascriptin Aspergum Aspirin Bayer products Bufferin Cama Chlorpheniramine products Chlor-Trimeton Compoz Conar Contac Coricidin products Coryban-D Capsules Demazin Dormin Ecotrin Empirin compound Excedrin 4-Way Cold Tablets Histadyl E.C. Measurin Midol Neo-Synephrine Tablets Novahistine products Nyquil Nytol	PAC Pamprin Phensal Pyrilamine Robitussin-AC Sinutab Sleep-Eze Sodium salicylate Sominex Sudafed Plus Triaminic liquids Triaminicin Triaminicol Vanquish Vicks Formula 44 Cough Mixture

CHART 2 Antihistamine interactions

	Any of these prescription drugs may interact with	any of these prescription drug groups	and result in this interaction.	OTC/food items
The drugs listed in Chart 2, column 1, are antihistamines, and antihistamine combinations. The combinations listed usually contain a decongestant such as pseudoephedrine or phenylpropanolamine. Indications, depending on the type of antihistamine, include allergies, nasal congestion and drainage, and watery eyes. Antihistamines are commonly employed to aid in the treatment of nausea, vomiting, dizziness, vertigo, and insomnia. Hydroxyzine (Atarax, Vistaril) is an antihistamine but is also indicated to be useful in the management of pruritus resulting from allergic conditions and contact dermatoses. Antihistamines can potentiate other central nervous system–acting drugs, so special precautions should be exercised when these are used in conjunction, especially with narcotics, barbiturates, and alcohol. Antihistamines may cause anticholinergic effects, such as dry mouth, which could be relieved by chewing gum. Smoking tends to cause further irritation and should be avoided. If nausea or upset stomach is a problem, the medication should be taken with food or milk. The interactions denoted here between antihistamines and OTC drugs should be avoided since an increased potential for severe drowsiness or decrease in mental alertness may occur.	Azatadine (Optimine) Brompheniramine (Dimetane) Chlorpheniramine (Chlor-Trimeton, Teldrin) Clemastine (Tavist) Cyproheptadine (Periactin) Dexchlorpheniramine (Polaramine) Dimetapp Diphenhydramine (Benadryl) Disophrol Drixoral Naldecon Nolamine Novafed-A Ornade Promethazine (Phenergan) Pyribenzamine Tripelennamine (PBZ) Triprolidine (Actidil)	Acenocoumarol (Sintrom) Anisindione (Miradon) Bishydroxycoumarin (Dicumarol) Griseofulvin (Fulvicin, Grifulvin) Oral contraceptives Oxyphenbutazone (Tandearil) Phenindione (Hedulin) Phenprocoumon (Liquamar) Phenylbutazone (Azolid, Butazolidin) Phenytoin (Dilantin) Warfarin (Coumadin)	This interaction can cause a decrease in the effectiveness of the prescription drugs listed in column 2.	A.R.M. Alcoholic products Allerest Bayer Decongestant Cold Tablets Beer Cheracol, Cheracol D Coldene Compoz Conar Contac Coricidin Coryban-D Cosanyl-DM Creo-Terpin Demazin Dormin Dristan Dristan Cough Formula Histadyl E.C. Neo-Synephrine Novahistine Nyquil Nytol Pertussin Pyrilamine Robitussin-AC & Robitussin DM Sinutab Sleep-Eze Sominex Super Anahist Tea Plus Triaminicin Triaminicol Vicks Formula 44 products Vicks Sinex products
		Atropine products Belladonna products (Donnatal) Dicyclomine (Bentyl) Furazolidone (Furoxone) Glycopyrrolate (Robinul) Isocarboxazid (Marplan) Pargyline (Eutonyl) Phenelzine (Nardil) Procarbazine (Matulane) Propantheline (Pro-Banthine) Tranylcypromine (Parnate) Trihexphenidyl (Artane)	The combination of these medications may cause constipation, dry mouth, blurred vision, urine retention, and possible increased heart rate. Also a possibility of decreased mental alertness may occur. See below for additional prescription drug–prescription drug interactions involving antihistamines listed in column 1.	

CHART 2 Antihistamine interactions—cont'd

Any of these prescription drugs may interact with	any of these prescription drug groups ▶	and result in this interaction. ▶	OTC/food items
Azatadine (Optimine) Brompheniramine (Dimetane) Chlorpheniramine (Chlor-Trimeton, Teldrin) Clemastine (Tavist) Cyproheptadine (Periactin) Dexchlor- pheniramine (Polaramine) Dimetapp Diphenhydramine (Benadryl) Disophrol Drixoral Naldecon Nolamine Novafed-A Ornade Promethazine (Phenergan) Pyribenzamine Tripelennamine (PBZ) Triprolidine (Actidil)	Amobarbital (Amytal) Chloral hydrate (Noctec) Chlordiazepoxide (Librium) Chlorpromazine (Thorazine) Clonazepam (Clonopin) Clorazepate (Tranxene, Azene) Codeine-containing products Cyclobenzaprine (Flexeril) Diazepam (Valium) Esgic Ethchlorvynol (Placidyl) Fiorinal Fluphenazine (Prolixin) Flurazepam (Dalmane) Glutethimide (Doriden) Hydroxyzine (Atarax, Vistaril) Librax Limbitrol Lorazepam (Ativan) Meprobamate (Equanil, Miltown) Oxazepam (Serax) Oxybutynin (Ditropan) Pentobarbital (Nembutal) Perphenazine (Trilafon) Phenobarbital (Luminal) Prazepam (Centrax) Prochlorperazine (Compazine) Promazine (Sparine) Propoxyphene (Darvon, Darvocet) Secobarbital (Seconal) Thioridazine (Mellaril) Thiothixene (Navane) Triclofos (Triclos) Trifluoperazine (Stelazine) Tuinal	The combination of the medications listed in column 2 with the drugs in column 1 could cause an increase in the likelihood of central nervous system depression. Such a combination could result in drowsiness, dizziness, blurred vision, loss of appetite, and a decrease in mental alertness. Caution must be exercised if operating any type of machinery or driving. It is not advisable to drink alcoholic beverages while taking any of these medications as this may compound the problem of adverse side effects.	

CHART 3 Antidiabetic drug interactions

	Any of these prescription drugs may interact with	any of these prescription drug groups ➤	and result in this interaction. ➤	OTC/ food items
The hypoglycemic agents listed in Chart 3, column 1, aside from insulin, are sulfonamide derivatives devoid of antibacterial effects. These oral agents aid in the stimulation of synthesis of endogenous insulin in the patient with functional pancreatic beta cells. Contraindications include fever, infections, surgery for severe trauma, ketosis, acidosis, coma, and pregnancy. Transient side effects may include loss of appetite, nausea, and stomach upset. Prolonged discomfort, sore throat, low fever, diarrhea, or dark urine may warrant a change in dosage or discontinuation of the medication. The OTC interactions denoted here involve the cough and cold preparations that could alter the dosage or increase the potential for nausea or stomach upset. Alcoholic beverages should always be avoided, and aspirin or salicylate products could also lower one's blood glucose level when used in combination with these medications.	Acetohexamide (Dymelor) Chlorpropamide (Diabinese) Insulin Tolazamide (Tolinase) Tolbutamide (Orinase)	Acetazolamide (Diamox) Bendroflumethiazide (Naturetin) Benzthiazide (Exna) Chlorothiazide (Diuril) Chlorthalidone (Hygroton) Dichlorphenamide (Daranide) Ethacrynic acid (Edecrin) Ethoxyzolamide (Cardrase, Ethamide) Furosemide (Lasix) Hydrochlorothiazide (Esidrix, HydroDiuril) Methazolamide (Neptazane) Methyclothiazide (Enduron) Metolazone (Diulo, Zaroxolyn) Polythiazide (Renese) Quinethazone (Hydromox) Steroids (Prednisone) Trichlormethiazide (Metahydrin, Naqua)	Reaction may cause an increase in blood glucose level, which could result in excessive thirst and urination (hyperglycemic effect). Drugs in column 2 may work against diabetic medication in column 1. Notify physician if loss of appetite, nausea, or vomiting is noticed. See Chart 7 for additional listing of steroids that can cause this same effect.	Alcoholic beverages Beer Cheracol and Cheracol D Coldene Coryban-D Cosanyl-DM Creo-Terpin Demazin Syrup Dristan Cough Formula Histadyl E.C. Neo-Synephrine Elixir Novahistine-DH and Novahistine Expectorant Nyquil Pertussin Robitussin, Robitussin-AC, and Robitussin DM Triaminic Expectorant Valadol Liquid Vicks Formula 44 Cough Mixture
		Alcoholic products Clofibrate (Atromids) Furazolidone (Furoxone) Guanethidine (Ismelin Sulfate) Isocarboxazid (Marplan) Metoprolol (Lopressor) Nadolol (Corgard) Oxyphenbutazone (Tandearil) Pargyline (Eutonyl) Phenelzine (Nardil) Phenylbutazone (Azolid, Butazolidin) Procarbazine (Matulane) Propranolol (Inderal) Tranylcypromine (Parnate)	Reaction may cause a decrease in blood glucose level leading to hunger (excessive), numbness, fatigue, headache, drowsiness, or sweating (hypoglycemic effect). If this occurs use candy or lump sugar to offset this adverse reaction.	

CHART 4 Anticoagulant interactions

	Any of these prescription drugs may interact with	any of these prescription drug groups ➤	and result in this interaction. ➤	OTC/ food items
The medications listed in Chart 4, column 1, are probably the most critical group to monitor in terms of interactions. Since these agents are highly but weakly bound to plasma protein (albumin), a significant potential for displacing these drugs by other drugs exists. Even though a particular drug is known to interact with an anticoagulant, it is often difficult to predict a certain patient's response, and thus close monitoring of the patient is mandatory. The in vivo effect of depressing factors VII, IX, X, and II (prothrombin) depends on the dosage of the drug administered. Oral anticoagulants have no effect on established thrombosis and do not reverse any tissue damage. The aim of treatment is to prevent further complications. Adverse reactions range from prolonged or excessive bleeding from nose, gums, and cuts to black stools, vomiting, unusual menstrual flow, prolonged diarrhea, headaches, fever, and loss of appetite. The description of the OTC interactions listed here are described in column 3.	Acenocoumarol (Sintrom) Anisindione (Miradon) Bishydroxy-coumarin (Dicumarol) Phenindione (Hedulin) Phenprocoumon (Liquamar) Warfarin (Coumadin)	Acetohexamide (Dymelor) Allopurinol (Zyloprim) Chloral hydrate (Noctec) Chlorpropamide (Diabinese) Cimetidine (Tagamet) Clofibrate (Atromid-S) Methandrostenolone (Dianabol) Naldixic acid (NegGram) Oxymetholone (Anadrol) Oxyphenbutazone (Oxalid, Tandearil) Phenylbutazone (Azolid, Butazolidin) Sulfinpyrazone (Anturane) Thyroid preparations Tolazamide (Tolinase) Tolbutamide (Orinase)	Drug interaction may result in an increased likelihood of increasing the activity of the anticoagulant drugs listed in column 1. See Chart 16 for analgesics that may cause this same effect.	The OTC drugs listed could increase the activity of therapeutic medication and lead to excessive bleeding. The foods listed are high in vitamin K and could reduce the effectiveness of an anticoagulant drug. A.S.A. and A.S.A. Compound Aspirin Alka-Seltzer and Alka-Seltzer Plus. Alka-2 A.P.C. Arthritis Strength Bufferin Ascriptin & Ascriptin A/D Aspergum Bayer products Bufferin Cama Coricidin products Dristan Tablets Ecotrin Empirin compound Excedrin and Excedrin PM 4-Way Cold Tablets Measurin Midol PAC Pamprin Phensal Sodium salicylate Sominex Super Anahist Triaminicin Tablets Vanquish Leafy green vegetables, for example, cabbage, spinach, kale, cauliflower, alfalfa
		Amobarbital (Amytal) Butabarbital (Butisol) Carbamazepine (Tegretol) Ethchlorvynol (Placidyl) Glutethimide (Doriden) Pentobarbital (Nembutal) Phenobarbital (Luminal) Rifampin (Rifadin, Rimactane) Secobarbital (Seconal) Tuinal Vitamin K (Synkayvite) Other prescription drugs including antihistamines (Chart 2), steroids (Chart 7), and alcoholic beverages could produce unpredictable responses to medication, and a physician should be consulted before using these drugs.	Drug interaction may result in an increased likelihood of decreasing the activity of the anticoagulant drugs listed in column 1. See the diuretics (Chart 10) and oral contraceptives (Chart 6), which may cause this same result.	

CHART 5 Antiparkinsonism drug interactions

	Any of these prescription drugs may interact with ➡	any of these prescription drug groups ➡	and result in this interaction. ➡	OTC/ food items
The medications listed in Chart 5, column 1, are referred to as "antiparkinsonism agents." Since the depletion of dopamine in the brain can cause the involuntary movements, levodopa products are used to cross the blood-brain barrier and then are converted to dopamine. Dopamine itself does not cross the barrier. In the combination product (Sinemet), carbidopa aids in preventing the systemic decomposition of levodopa, thus allowing more medication to reach the brain. These medications should be used with caution or not at all in patients with a history of peptic ulcers or those who are pregnant or nursing. The OTC interactions here involve reducing or reversing the beneficial effects of levodopa products when combined with foods or drugs containing pyridoxine (vitamin B_6). If a vitamin supplement is necessary, Larobec is one product formulated not to contain any pyridoxine.	Levodopa products Bendopa Bio/DOPA Dopar Larodopa L-Dopa Parda Sinemet	Furazolidone (Furoxone) Isocarboxazid (Marplan) Pargyline (Eutonyl) Phenelzine (Nardil) Procarbazine (Matulane) Tranylcypromine (Parnate) Chlorpromazine (Thorazine) Fluphenazine (Prolixin) Haloperidol (Haldol) Mesoridazine (Serentil) Perphenazine (Trilafon) Piperacetazine (Quide) Prochlorperazine (Compazine) Promazine (Sparine) Thioridazine (Mellaril) Trifluoperazine (Stelazine) Triflupromazine (Vesprin)	The mixing of antidepressant or antianxiety agents with the medications listed in column 1 may cause a severe increase in blood pressure, flushing, and palpitations. Various phenothiazine tranquilizers may block or diminish the effectiveness of the prescription medications in column 1. Other tranquilizers should be used with caution. Methyldopa (Aldomet) may increase dopa products' effect, while phenytoin (Dilantin) and papaverine (Pavabid) may diminish the effects. See Chart 13 for additional antianxiety agents that could also cause decreased effects of prescription drugs in column 1.	Allbee-T Beminal-500 Corn Cynal Hexa-Betalin Liver Orexin Pyridoxine tablets Stresstabs 600 Trophite Vio-Bec Vitamin B complex Vitamin B_6 tablets Yeast

CHART 6   Oral contraceptive interactions

	Any of these prescription drugs may interact with	any of these prescription drug groups	and result in this interaction.	OTC/ food items

The oral contraceptives suppress ovulation by increasing the level of estrogen and progestin, which inhibit the follicle-stimulating hormone and luteinizing hormone. Oral contraceptives are also employed for their supplemental effect in other conditions.
 	
These medications should not be used if any of the following conditions are present or suspected: breast cancer, history of cerebrovascular accidents, neoplasms, pregnancy, nursing, or abnormal vaginal bleeding. The individual package insert should be consulted for additional warnings and precautions.
 	
Cigarette smoking increases the risk of serious cardiovascular side effects with estrogens and should be avoided. These risks also increase with age and amount of smoking.
 	
The first group of OTC interactions denoted here involves those vitamins that may be depleted when taking contraceptives and should be corrected by supplementing diet with an OTC product containing these vitamins.
 	
The second group, vitamin A products, if taken in excess, could lead to an accumulation of vitamin A within the system.
	Brevicon
	Demulen
	Enovid
	Loestrin
	ModiCon
	Norinyl
	Norlestrin
	Ortho-Novum
	Ovcon
	Ovral
	Ovulen
		Ampicillin (Polycillin, Principen)
		Antihistamines (see Chapter 2)
		Oxyphenbutazone (Tandearil)
		Phenylbutazone (Azolid, Butazolidin)
		Phenytoin (Dilantin)
		Rifampin (Rifadin, Rimactane)
			An increased possibility of breakthrough bleeding or spotting and decrease in the effectiveness of the pill may occur. Another form of contraception may be advisable in these instances. When combining these interacting drugs see Chart 2, column 1, for detailed list of antihistamines that may cause the same effect.	Cyanocobalamin (vitamin B_{12})
				Folic acid
				Pyridoxine (vitamin B_6)
				Vitamin E
				Vitamin A products:
				  Adabee
				  Cod liver oil concentrate
				  Dayalets
				  Mi-Cebrin
				  Myadec
				  Optilets-500
				  Super-D products
				  Theragran
				  Vitamin A

		Acenocoumarol (Sintrom) Anisindione (Miradon) Bishydroxycoumarin (Dicumarol) Phenindione (Hedulin) Phenprocoumon (Liquamar) Warfarin (Coumadin)	The blood-thinning drugs listed in column 2 may be decreased in their effectiveness. Onset and cessation of bleeding should be closely monitored.	

CHART 7 Steroid interactions

	Any of these prescription drugs may interact with ▶	any of these prescription drug groups ▶	and result in this interaction. ▶	OTC/food items
The medications listed in Chart 7, column 1, are referred to as "steroids," or more specifically, adrenocortical steroids. With the exception of fludrocortisone they are all glucocorticoids. Indications include endocrine, rheumatic, allergic, dermatologic, ophthalmic, respiratory, hematologic, and neoplastic conditions. Individual drug monographs should be consulted. Stressful situations, vaccinations, and surgery should be avoided while receiving steroid therapy. Patients predisposed to ulcers or who are pregnant or nursing require special monitoring or discontinuance of steroid medication, which is primarily completed by a gradual decrease in the dosage. Adverse reactions that may require immediate medical attention involve, but are not limited to, sodium and fluid retention, muscle weakness, nausea, persistent thirst, frequent urination, increased intraocular pressure, and blurred vision. The salicylate- or alcohol-containing OTCs listed here can complicate and increase the potential for nausea, ulceration, or decrease in the steroid effectiveness.	Betamethasone (Celestone) Cortisone (Cortone) Dexamethasone (Decadron, Hexadrol) Fludrocortisone (Florinef) Hydrocortisone (Cortef, Hydrocortone) Methylprednisolone (Medrol) Prednisolone (Delta-Cortef) Prednisone (Deltasone, Meticorten) Triamcinolone (Aristocort, Kenacort)	Acetazolamide (Diamox) Bendroflu-methiazide (Naturetin) Benzthiazide (Exna) Chlorothiazide (Diuril) Chlorthalidone (Hygroton) Dichlorphenamide (Daranide) Digifortis (Pil-Digis) Digitoxin (Crystodigin, Purodigin) Digoxin (Lanoxin) Ethacrynic acid (Edecrin) Ethoxzolamide (Cardrase, Ethamide) Furosemide (Lasix) Gitalin (Gitaligin) Hydrochloro-thiazide (Esidrix, HydroDiuril) Methazolamide (Neptazane) Methyclothiazide (Enduron) Metolazone (Diulo, Zaroxolyn) Polythiazide (Renese) Quinethazone (Hydromox) Trichlormethiazide (Metahydrin, Naqua)	This combination may cause an increase in the effect of the heart medications in column 2. Too much potassium may be lost, and a physician should be notified if shortness of breath, fatigue, prolonged nausea, abdominal pain, cramps, and blurred vision are noticed. The diuretics listed in column 2 may also increase loss of potassium, so it is imperative to have frequent checkups. See Charts 3 and 9 for additional steroid reactions.	A.P.C. and A.P.C. Compound A.S.A. and A.S.A. Compound Alcoholic products Alka-Seltzer Alka-2 Allerest Anacin products Arthritis Strength Bufferin Ascriptin Aspergum Aspirin Bayer products Bufferin Cama Chlorpheniramine products Chlor-Trimeton Compoz Conar Contac Coricidin products Coryban-D Capsules Demazin Dormin Ecotrin Empirin compound Excedrin 4-Way Cold Tablets Histadyl E.C. Measurin Midol Neo-Synephrine Tablets Novahistine products Nyquil Nytol PAC Pamprin Phensal Pyrilamine Robitussin-AC Sinutab Sleep-Eze Sodium salicylate Sominex Sudafed Plus Triaminic liquids Triaminicin Triaminicol Vanquish Vicks Formula 44 Cough Mixture
		Amobarbital (Amytal) Chloral hydrate (Noctec, Somnos) Flurazepam (Dalmane) Glutethimide (Doriden) Pentobarbital (Nembutal) Secobarbital (Seconal) Tuinal	The sedatives or hypnotics (sleeping medications) listed in column 2 may reduce a steroid's effectiveness.	

C H A R T 8 Antispasmodic interactions

	Any of these prescription drugs may interact with	any of these prescription drug ➤ groups	and result in this ➤ interaction.	OTC/food items
The prescription drugs listed in Chart 8, column 1, are referred to as "antispas-modics." Most of these products are used in gastrointestinal disorders, yet some are used primarily in urinary, kidney, and allergic disorders. Since these products may cause some drowsiness, dizziness, or blurred vision, the CNS depressants should be avoided. If dryness of the mouth occurs, relief could be accomplished by chewing gum. If this persists or if a skin rash, flushing, or eye pain develops, further medical attention is necessary. Some of these drugs can decrease perspiration, which could lead to fever or heat stroke, so it is advisable to remain, when possible, in a cool environment. Antacids, if used along with any of these products, should not be taken at the same time. An hour or two should be allowed between them. The OTC interactions noted here can compound the problem of dry mouth, blurred vision, or drowsiness, and these product combinations should be avoided if possible.	Atropine products Belladonna products Benztropin mesylate (Cogentin) Dicyclomine (Bentyl) Glycopyrrolate (Robinul) Librax Propantheline (Pro-Banthine) Trihexyphenidyl (Artane)	Amitriptyline (Elavil, Endep) Chlorpromazine (Thorazine) Cyclobenzaprine (Flexeril) Desipramine (Norpramin, Pertofrane) Disopyramide (Norpace) Haloperidol (Haldol) Imipramine (Tofranil) Meperidine (Demerol) Nortriptyline (Aventyl) Oxybutynin (Ditropan) Prochlorperazine (Compazine) Quinidine (Cin-Quin)	The combination of these medications may cause constipation, dryness of mouth, blurred vision, urine retention, and possible increased heart rate. If to combine the drugs must be used in combination, physician may need to reduce the dose of one or both drugs. Refer to Chart 2 for additional interactions of antispasmodics and antihistamines.	Allerest A.R.M. Bayer Decongestant Cold Tablets Chlorpheniramine Chlor-Trimeton Compoz Conar Contac Coricidin Coryban-D Capsules Demazin Dormin Dristan Histadyl E.C. Neo-Synephrine Tablets Novahistine products Nyquil Nytol Pyrilamine Robitussin-AC Sinutab Sleep-Eze Sominex Super Anahist Tea Plus Triaminic liquids Triaminicin Triaminicol Vicks Formula 44 Cough Mixture Vicks Sinex products

CHART 9 Heart medication interactions

	Any of these prescription drugs may interact with →	any of these prescription drug groups →	and result in this interaction. →	OTC/food items
The medications listed in Chart 9, column 1, are referred to as "cardiac glycosides." They increase the force of myocardial contraction and the refractory period of the atrioventricular (A-V) node. Indications include congestive heart failure, atrial fibrillation, flutter, and tachycardia, but these medications are contraindicated in ventricular fibrillation. Lowered potassium levels sensitize the myocardium to the glycosides, and toxic levels may be reached even with usual dosages. Many arrhythmias for which digitalis is advised closely resemble those reflecting toxic digitalis levels. Nausea and vomiting may also be associated with toxic levels, along with a loss of appetite, weakness, diarrhea, blurred vision, and yellow or green halos around objects. The first group of OTC interactions involves antacids, which, if taken *at the same time*, could decrease the effectiveness of the glycoside. The second group of antiasthmatic products could cause or complicate arrhythmias while a patient is undergoing digitalis therapy.	Digifortis (Pil-Digis) Digitoxin (Crystodigin, Purodigin) Digoxin (Lanoxin) Gitalin (Gitaligin)	Acetazolamide (Diamox) Bendroflu-methiazide (Naturetin) Benthiazide (Exna) Chlorothiazide (Diuril) Chlorthalidone (Hygroton) Dichlorphenamide (Daranide) Ethacrynic acid (Edecrin) Ethoxzolamide (Cardrase, Ethamide) Furosemide (Lasix) Hydrochlorthiazide (Esidrix, HydroDiuril) Methazolamide (Neptazane) Methyclothiazide (Enduron) Metolazone (Diulo, Zaroxolyn) Polythiazide (Renese) Quinethazone (Hydromox) Trichlormethiazide (Metahydrin, Naqua)	Although these drugs are sometimes used together, there is a possibility of a decreasing potassium level, which could lead to toxic levels of a heart pill. A physician should be notified if any of the signs explained in the introduction to Chart 9 or leg cramps are noticed. Steroids (Chart 7) and licorice may also cause a loss in potassium. See Chart 10 for more information on the diuretics listed in column 2. If any potassium supplements (KCl, Kato, K-Lyte, Kaon, Kaochlor, and so on) must be taken, checkups should be frequent to ensure that levels are not too high.	Aludrox Aluminum hydroxide Amphojel Anacin Arthritis Formula Antacids Ascriptin Camalox Dristan Gelusil Kaolin/pectin (Kaopectate) Maalox Magnesium hydroxide Magnesium trisilicate Milk of Magnesia Mylanta Adrenalin Asthmanefrin Breatheasy Bronkaid Mist Epinephrine Histadyl E.C. Medihaler-EPI Primatene Mist Solution A Vaponefrin Va-Tro-Nol
		Metoprolol (Lopressor) Nadolol (Corgard) Propranolol (Inderal) Phenytoin (Dilantin) Reserpine (Serpasil) Reserpine combination (see Chart 11)	The drugs in column 2 are sometimes used together with heart medications, yet could result in irregular heartbeat. Pulse should be taken regularly and any changes in pulse or persistent dizziness should be reported to a physician. See Chart 3 for additional reactions on some of the prescription drugs in column 2.	

CHART 10 Diuretic interactions

	Any of these prescription drugs may interact with	any of these prescription drug ➤ groups	and result in this ➤ interaction.	OTC/food items
The medications listed in Chart 10, column 1, are referred to as "diuretics." The range of indication includes, but is not limited to, hypertension, edema, cardiac conditions, and renal dysfunction. The carbonic anhydrase inhibitors listed are also sometimes employed in the treatment of glaucoma. The thiazide diuretics tend to cause a depletion of potassium and sodium; thus, close monitoring of potassium levels is necessary, especially in cardiac conditions requiring digitalis therapy. Lowered potassium levels may be indicated by weakness, leg cramping, and joint or foot pain. Spironolactone (Aldactone Aldactazide) and triamterene (Dyazide, Dyrenium) are used to help conserve the loss of potassium, and additional potassium ion supplements may not be necessary or even harmful. The OTC alcoholic interactions denoted here involve products that could increase the potential for severe hypotension and drowsiness. The decongestant products listed could negate the antihypertensive effect or cause an increase in blood pressure.	Acetazolamide (Diamox) Bendroflu-methiazide (Naturetin) Benthiazide (Exna) Chlorothiazide (Diuril) Chlorthalidone (Hygroton) Dichlorphenamide (Daranide) Ethacrynic acid (Edecrin) Ethoxzolamide (Cardrase, Ethamide) Furosemide (Lasix) Hydrochlorthiazide (Esidrix, HydroDiuril) Methazolamide (Neptazane) Methyclothiazide (Enduraon) Metolazone (Diulo, Zaroxolyn) Polythiazide (Renese) Quinethazone (Hydromox) Trichlormethiazide (Metahydrin, Naqua)	Digifortis (Pil-Digis) Digitoxin (Crystodigin, Purodigin) Digoxin (Lanoxin) Gitalin (Gitaligin)	Although this combination of a heart tablet (column 2 drugs) with a diuretic is often used to treat various illnesses, the diuretic could decrease the potassium level, which could lead to toxic levels of the heart pill. Frequent checkups are recommended, and a physician should be notified if any weakness, leg cramps, shortness of breath, abdominal pain, or blurred or yellow vision is noticed. See Chart 9 for other heart medication interactions. See Charts 3, 4, and 7 for diuretic interactions.	Adrenalin Alcoholic products Alconefrin Allerest capsules and spray A.R.M. Asthmanefrin Bayer Decongestant Breatheasy Bromo-Quinine Bronkaid Caffeine Coffee Coldene Contac Coricidin Cough Syrup and Nasal Mist Coricidin-D Coryban-D Cosanyl-DM Demazine Repetabs & Syrup Dimacol Dristan tablets, capsules, and liquid Epinephrine Fedrazil 4-Way Cold Tablets and Nasal Spray Histadyl E.C. Medihaler-EPI Neo-Synephrine products No Doz Novahistine products Nyquil Ornacol Ornex Orthoxicol Phenylephrine Phenylpropanol-amine Primatene Privine Romilar Cough Syrup Sinutab Cold Tablets and Sinutab II Solution A Sudafed Super Anahist Tea Tea Plus Triaminic products Triaminicol Trind Ursinus Va-Tro-Nol Vicks Inhaler
		Acenocoumarol (Sintrom) Anisindione (Miradon) Bishydroxy-coumarin (Dicumarol) Phenindione (Hedulin) Phenprocoumon (Liquamar) Warfarin (Coumadin) See Chart 11 for additional prescription drugs used for high blood pressure (antihypertensives).	Drug interactions could result in an increased likelihood of decreasing the activity of the anticoagulant drugs in column 2. See Chart 4 for more anticoagulant interactions. Lithium (Eskalith) should be used with caution when combined with diuretics.	

CHART 11 Antihypertensive interactions

	Any of these prescription drugs may interact with ➤	any of these prescription drug groups ➤	and result in this interaction.	OTC/ food items
The medications listed in Chart 11, column 1, are referred to as "antihypertensives." The diuretic antihypertensives are discussed in Chart 10.

When initiating therapy, transient drowsiness or dizziness may occur, and thus the patient should avoid sudden changes in posture and balance. If medications are changed or discontinued, it is advisable to gradually reduce the dosage over a period of days.

Adverse reactions that may require further medical attention might include persistent hypotension, fever, fatigue, chills, sore throat, diarrhea, or swelling.

The following antihypertensives are listed in other charts: clonidine (Catapres, Combipres) (see Chart 14), metoprolol (Lopressor), nadolol (Corgard), and propranolol (Inderal) (see Charts 3 and 9).

The OTC interactions denoted here involve products that could cause or complicate severe drowsiness and dizziness. OTC cold remedies that contain a decongestant should be avoided since an unpredictable response may occur. This should be explained to any patient taking reserpine products, since these naturally tend to cause nasal congestion. A saline nasal spray may be the only product necessary to control this problem without further complications. | Guanethidine (Esimil, Ismelin) Hydralazine (Apresazide, Apresoline) Methyldopa (Aldomet, Aldoril) Reserpine (Serpasil, Reserpoid) Reserpine combinations: Demi-Regroton Diupres Diutensin-R Exna-R Hydropres Hydroserpine Metatensin Naquival Regroton Salutensin Ser-Ap-Es | Furazolidone (Furoxone) Isocarboxazid (Marplan) Pargyline (Eutonyl) Phenelzine (Nardil) Procarbazine (Matulane) Tranylcypromine (Parnate) | This combination may result in a severe increase in blood pressure, fever, convulsion, or dizziness. A physician should be notified if persistent headache, sore throat, diarrhea, or any irregular heartbeat is noticed. See also Chart 15 for other antidepressants that could cause a change in blood pressure when used in combination.

Although combinations of different antihypertensive drugs are used together to aid in the control of blood pressure, certain combinations should be avoided or monitored very closely. Propranolol, metoprolol, and nadolol may interact with prazosin (Minipress) or reserpine and reserpine combinations. Hydralazine may interact with minoxidil (Loniten). These reactions could produce severe low blood pressure with resultant dizziness or produce irregular heartbeat. | Alcoholic beverages Beer Cheracol Coryban-D Cosanyl-DM Creo-Terpin Demazin Dristan Cough Formula Histadyl E.C. Neo-Synephrine tablets Novahistine products Nyquil Pertussin Robitussin Triaminic Expectorant Vicks Formula 44 Cough Mixture |

CHART 12   Antibiotic interactions

The medications listed in Chart 12, column 1, are referred to as "tetracycline" or "tetracycline-combination antibiotics." The combination products contain an antifungal agent to help decrease or eliminate the severity of a diarrhea side effect in those susceptible. Skin sensitivity to the burning rays of the sun is a common occurrence when taking these medications; it is therefore advisable to use a sunscreen agent for protection. Avoidance of these medications is advisable if one is pregnant or nursing. They should also be avoided in infants and young children to prevent any damage to tooth enamel or discoloration of the teeth. Dosage should be taken on an empty stomach, 1 hour before a meal or 2 hours after, unless otherwise directed. A change in medication or dosage may be indicated if severe diarrhea or skin rash occurs. The OTC interactions denoted here involve products that may comply with the tetracycline product and thus result in a decrease in absorption with resultant lower therapeutic levels of the antibiotic.	Any of these prescription drugs may interact with	any of these prescription drug groups	and result in this interaction.	OTC/ food items
	Achromycin V Achrostatin V Bristacycline Cyclopar Kesso-Tetra Mysteclin-F Panmycin QID Tet Robitet SK-Tetracycline Sumycin Tetrachel Tetracycline Tetracyn Tetrex V-Tet	Ampicillin (Polycillin, Principen) Bactocill Cloxacillin (Tegopen) Dicloxacillin (Dycill, Dynapen) Oxacillin (Prostaphlin) Penicillin Penicillin G potassium (Pentids) Penicillin V potassium (Ledercillin, Pen·Vee K, V-Cillin K, Veetids)	A decrease in the effectiveness of the drugs in either column 1 or 2 may occur. The mixing of these drugs should be avoided unless otherwise directed.	Iron preparations Fer-In-Sol Ferrous sulfate Milk & dairy products Antacids & products containing calcium, aluminum, or magnesium Alka-Seltzer Plus Alka-2 Aludrox Aluminum hydroxide Amphojel Anacin Arthritis Formula Ascriptin Bufferin Calcium Calcium carbonate Cama Camalox Creamalin Dicarbosil Antacid Tablets Di-Gel Dristan Tablets Gelusil Maalox & Maalox Plus Magnesium hydroxide Magnesium trisilicate Milk of Magnesia Mylanta and Mylanta III Rolax Titralac Triaminicin Tums Vanquish
		Acenocoumarol (Sintrom) Anisindione (Miradon) Bishydroxy-coumarin (Dicumarol) Phenindione (Hedulin) Phenprocoumon (Liquamar) Warfarin (Coumadin)	An increase in the effect of the blood-thinning drugs in column 2 may occur, which could result in hemorrhage or unusual bleeding.	

CHART 13 Antianxiety medication and sedative interactions

	Any of these prescription drugs may interact with ▶	any of these prescription drug groups ▶	and result in this interaction. ▶	OTC/ food items
Although the medications listed in Chart 13, column 1, include antianxiety drugs, sedatives, hypnotics, antipsychotics, and tranquilizers, they are grouped this way since they have similar or common interactions. The therapeutic indications of these groups involve, but are not limited to, allergic disorders, nausea, tension, insomnia, muscular disorders, and epilepsy. Other anticonvulsants may also interact in a similar manner as these agents; therefore a full package insert should be consulted. An adjustment in dosage or medication may be warranted if excessive drowsiness, fatigue, difficulty in concentrating, dizziness, nightmares, irritability, muscle spasm, or dependence develops or if the patient becomes pregnant. Combination of any of the column 1 drugs may increase central nervous system depression and should be avoided if possible. The OTC interactions involved here increase the potential for severe central nervous system depression and may still cause this effect a day or two after the prescription medication has been discontinued. Caution should be exercised when in any activity requiring mental alertness.	Amobarbital (Amytal) Chloral hydrate (Noctec) Chlordiazepoxide (Limbitrol, Librium) Chlorpromazine (Thorazine) Clonazepam (Clonopin) Clorazepate (Azene, Tranzene) Diazepam (Valium) Ethchlorvynol (Placidyl) Fluphenazine (Prolixin) Flurazepam (Dalmane) Glutethimide (Doriden) Hydroxyzine (Atarax, Vistaril) Lorazepam (Ativan) Meprobamate (Equanil, Miltown) Oxazepam (Serax) Pentobarbital (Nembutal) Perphenazine (Trilafon) Phenobarbital (Luminal) Prazepam (Centrax) Prochlorperazine (Compazine) Promazine (Sparine) Secobarbital (Seconal, Tuinal) Triclofos (Triclos) Trifluoperazine (Stelazine) Thioridazine (Mellaril) Thiothixene (Navane)	Amitriptyline (Elavil, Endep) Amoxapine (Asendin) Cyclobenzaprine (Flexeril) Desipramine (Norpramin, Pertofrane) Doxepin (Adapin, Sinequan) Etrafon Imipramine (Tofranil) Limbitrol Maprotiline (Ludiomil) Nortriptyline (Aventyl, Pamelor) Triavil Trimipramine (Surmontil)	The combination of the drugs in column 1 with any of the medications in column 2 may increase the likelihood of central nervous system depression. This may cause confusion, depression, drowsiness, unusual weakness, slurred speech, headache, or lack of mental alertness. A person taking these medications, whether a drug in column 1, a drug in column 2, or a combination of drugs in both columns, should be familiar with his or her reaction to the medication before driving or undertaking a job requiring mental alertness. See Chart 2, column 1, drugs, the antihistamines, which could also cause severe nervous system depression and drowsiness if combined with the medications in column 1.	Alcoholic products Allerest A.R.M. Bayer Decongestant Cold Tablets Beer Cheracol & Cheracol D Coldene Compoz Conar Contac Coridin Coryban-D Cosanyl-DM Creo-Terpin Demazin Dormin Dristan & Dristan Cough Formula Histadyl E.C. Neo-Synephrine Novahistine Nyquil Nytol Pertussin Pyrilamine Robitussin-AC & Robitussin-DM Sinutab Sleep-Eze Sominex Super Anahist Synephricol Tea Plus Triaminicin Triaminicol Vicks Formula 44 Cough Mixture Vicks Sinex

CHART 14 Antidepressants-I interactions

	Any of these prescription drugs may interact with	➤ any of these prescription drug groups	➤ and result in this interaction.	OTC/food items
The medications listed in Chart 14, column 1, are referred to as "antidepressants." Some of these medications also have antianxiety effects. Others may be used in enuresis, and one is primarily a muscle relaxant but interacts like a tricyclic.	Amitriptyline (Elavil, Endep) Amoxapine (Asendin) Cyclobenzaprine (Flexeril) Desipramine (Norpramin, Pertofrane)	Clonidine (Catapres, Combipres) Guanethidine (Esimil, Ismelin)	The drug reaction here can block the blood-pressure-lowering effect of the drugs listed in column 2. A physician may need to adjust the dosage required.	Alcoholic products Allerest A.R.M. Bayer Decongestant Cold Tablets Beer Cheracol and Cheracol D
Often these medications may require up to 4 weeks of therapy before noticeable improvement may be seen. Discontinuance of therapy should be gradual to avoid headache or nausea.	Doxepin (Adapin, Sinequan) Etrafon Imipramine (Tofranil) Limbitrol Maprotiline (Ludiomil) Nortriptyline (Aventyl, Pamelor) Triavil Trimipramine (Surmontil)	Furazolidone (Furoxone) Isocarboxazid (Marplan) Pargyline (Eutonyl) Phenelzine (Nardil) Procarbazine (Matulane) Tranylcypromine (Parnate)	This reaction could cause a severe increase in blood pressure and lead to fever, excitement, convulsions, coma, and possible circulatory collapse. This combination of drugs should be avoided.	Coldene Compoz Conar Contac Coricidin Coryban-D Cosadein Cosanyl-DM Creo-Terpin Demazin Dormin Dristan & Dristan Cough Formula
Transient drowsiness or dryness of the mouth may be experienced when first beginning these medications. If a sore throat develops, further medical attention may be required to adjust or discontinue medication. Drowsiness or blurred vision may occur, which may be transient. Persons predisposed to glaucoma should be monitored closely. The OTC interactions involving alcohol-containing products may result in an increased potential for severe drowsiness and decreased mental alertness. An unpredictable response to the sympathomimetics may occur when combined with the prescription drugs in column 1.		Amphetamine (Benzedrine) Benzphetamine (Didrex) Chlorphentermine (Pre-Sate) Dextroamphetamine (Dexedrine) Diethylpropion (Tenuate, Tepanil) Ephedrine products Epinephrine products Methamphetamine (Desoxyn) Phendimetrazine (Bontril, Plegine) Phenmetrazine (Preludin) Phenteramine (Fastin, lonamin)	This combination may increase or decrease the effects of the drugs in column 2. This could lead to such varied side effects as increased blood pressure and severe headache. Caution should be exercised if these groups are combined. See Charts 13 and 15 for additional antidepressant interactions.	Histadyl E.C. Neo-Synephrine Novahistine Nyquil Nytol Penetro Pertussin Pyrilamine Robitussin-AC & Robitussin-DM Sinutab Sleep-Eze Sominex Super Anahist Synephricol Tea Plus Triaminicin Triaminicol 2/G DM Vicks Formula 44 Cough Mixture Vicks Sinex products

CHART 15 Antidepressants-II interactions

	Any of these prescription drugs may interact with	any of these prescription drug groups	and result in this interaction.	OTC/food items

The drugs listed in Chart 15, column 1, are referred to as "monoamine oxidase (MAO) inhibitors." Although the major effects are antidepressant, some are used for anxiety or in chemotherapy procedures.
 	
Because of the potency of these drugs they require special precautions and considerations when used. Transient drowsiness, dizziness, weakness, or blurred vision may occur. If these symptoms persist or severe headaches, rash, dark urine, jaundice, sore throat, or diarrhea occurs, the dosage or drug may need to be changed.
 	
Since the effects of MAO inhibitors may last for up to 2 weeks after discontinuing use, no interacting drug should be started within this period of time.
 	
The interacting OTC and food products listed here could cause severe hypertension, fever, excitement, and convulsions if combined. Therefore it is of the utmost importance to avoid these products high in tyramine and sympathomimetics. Alcohol-containing products should also be avoided if possible.
	Furazolidone (Furoxone)
	Isocarboxazid (Marplan)
	Pargyline (Eutonyl)
	Phenelzine (Nardil)
	Procarbazine (Matulane)
	Tranylcypromine (Parnate)
		Antidepressants (see Chart 14)
		Ephedrine products
		Guanethidine (Esimil, Ismelin)
		Levodopa (Dopar, Larodopa)
		Meperidine (Demerol)
		Methyldopa (Aldomet, Aldoril)
		Methylphenidate (Ritalin)
		OTC diet aids (see Chart 14)
		Phenylephrine (Neo-Synephrine)
		Phenylpropanol-amine (Propadrine)
		Pseudoephedrine (Sudafed)
		Reserpine (Serpasil)
		Reserpine-containing drugs (see Chart 11)
		Tyramine
			A combination of this type could result in a lethal reaction. Concurrent use of any of the drugs in column 2 with any of the medication in column 1 may cause sudden and severe high blood pressure, fever, excitement, and convulsions.
			
			The MAO inhibitors in column 1 should not be combined with any of these drugs, nor should they be used for 14 days after discontinuing an MAO inhibitor.
			
			See Charts 2, 3, 4, 11, and 14 for additional MAO inhibitor interactions.
				Cheeses:
				  Cheddar
				  Emmenthaler
				  Gruyere
				  Stilton
				  Brie
				  Camembert
				Coffee
				Chocolate
				Cola (excessive)
				Fermented sausages, for example, fermented bolognas, salamis, summer sausage, pepperoni
				A.R.M.
				Adrenalin
				Alconefrin
				Allerest capsules and spray
				Asthmanefrin
				Bayer Decongestant Cold Tablets
				Breatheasy
				Bromoquinine
				Bronkaid
				Cheracol Cold Capsules
				Coldene
				Contac
				Coricidin-D
				Cosanyl-DM
				Demazin
				Dimacol
				Dristan
				Epinephrine

C H A R T 1 5 Antidepressants-II interactions—cont'd

Any of these prescription drugs may interact with ➤	any of these prescription drug groups ➤	and result in this interaction.	OTC/food items
Furazolidone (Furoxone)			Fedrazil
Isocarboxazid (Marplan)			Histadyl E.C.
Pargyline (Eutonyl)			Medihaler-EPI
Phenelzine (Nardil)			Beer
Procarbazine (Matulane)			Red wines, for example, Chianti, Sherry
Tranylcypromine (Parnate)			Bananas
			Figs (canned)
			Avocados
			Fava or yeast extract
			Chicken liver
			Beef liver
			Neo-Synephrine
			No-Doz
			Nyquil
			Ornacol
			Ornex
			Orthoxicol
			OTC diet aids
			Phenylephrine
			Phenylpropanol-amine
			Primatene
			Privine
			Romilar Cough Syrup
			Sinutab
			Solution A
			Sudafed
			Super Anahist
			Tea
			Tea Plus
			Triaminic products
			Triaminicol
			Trind
			Ursinus
			Va-Tro-Nol
			Vicks Sinex
			4-Way cold products

CHART 16 Analgesic interactions

	Any of these prescription drugs may interact with	any of these prescription drug ▶ groups	and result in this ▶ interaction.	OTC/food items
The medications listed in Chart 16, column 1, are referred to as "analgesics." The majority are more specifically referred to as "nonsteroidal antiinflammatory agents"; these help control pain and inflammation by a reduction in prostaglandin synthesis. These medications should be taken with food or milk to minimize the potential for stomach distress or bleeding of the intestinal mucosa. Patients with a history of allergies to aspirin, bleeding problems, or ulcers may not tolerate these medications. Skin rash, tinnitus, blurred vision, swelling, or unusual weight gian may require a change in dosage or drug. Dizziness may be transient with these medications. The OTC interactions denoted here involve products containing aspirin, salicylates, or alcohol, which in combination can increase the severity of stomach distress and/or bleeding. Propoxyphenc (Darvon, Darvocet) and products containing codeine may react similarly with these OTC products. Aspirin and salicylate products can decrease the effectiveness of the other prescription analgesics.	Aspirin/salicylate products Fenoprofen (Nalfon Ibuprofen (Motrin) Indomethacin (Indocin) Meclofenamate (Meclomin) Naproxen (Anaprox, Naprosyn) Oxyphenbutazone (Oxalid, Tandearil) Phenylbutazone (Azolid, Butazolidin) Sulindac (Clinoril) Zomepirac (Zomax)	Acenocoumarol (Sintrom) Anisindione (Miradon) Bishydroxy-coumarin (Dicumarol) Phenindione (Hedulin) Phenprocoumon (Liquamar) Warfarin (Coumadin)	When used in combination there is an increase in the likelihood and severity of increasing the effectiveness of the prescription drugs in column 2. This could result in bruising, increased bleeding, or hemorrhage. Some of the prescription drugs in column 1 may not have as much of an effect (for example, Zomax) but still could affect bleeding time. Probenecid (Benemid) and sulfinpyrazone (Anturane) should normally not be combined with the column 1 drugs (especially with Indocin).	Alcoholic beverages Alka-Seltzer Alka-2 Anacin A.P.C. Bufferin A.S.A. and A.S.A. compound Ascriptin Aspergum Aspirin Bayer products Beer Cama Cheracol Coricidin Coryban-D Cosanyl-DM Creo-Terpin Demazin Syrup Dristan Cough Formula and Dristan Decongestant Tablets Ecotrin Empirin Excedrin 4-Way Cold Tablets Histadyl E.C. Measurin Midol Neo-Synephrine Novahistine Nyquil PAC and PAC Compound Pamprin Pepto-Bismol Pertussin Phensal Robitussin Sodium salicylate Sominex Super Anahist Triaminic Expectorant Triaminicin Vanquish Vicks Formula 44 Cough Mixture

CHART 17 Chemotherapeutic drug interactions

	Any of these prescription drugs may interact with ➤	any of these OTC/food items as described in column 1.	Any of these prescription drugs may interact with ➤	any of these prescription drug groups ➤	and result in this interaction. ➤
The antineoplastic drugs listed in Chart 17 are primarily used in various neoplastic disorders, although methotrexate is sometimes used in psoriatic conditions. The full product description should be consulted when questioning these medications. Persistent diarrhea, fever, chills, sore throat, unusual bleeding, bruising, or jaundice may warrant a change in dosage or drug. Nursing or pregnancy should be avoided for at least 8 weeks following therapy. The patient should avoid stressful situations and maintain a well-balanced diet. The OTC reactions noted here show that if fluorouracil is used orally, acidic foods taken at the same time could significantly decrease the effectiveness of fluorouracil. The OTC interactions regarding methotrexate point out that salicylates can increase the toxic side effects of methotrexate if the two are combined. Methotrexate can also decrease the effects of fluorouracil.	Fluorouracil (5-Fu) Methotrexate	Acidic foods, for example, orange juice Alka-2 Alka-Seltzer Anacin Products A.P.C. Arthritis Strength Bufferin A.S.A. and A.S.A. Compound Ascriptin Aspergum Aspirin Bayer products Bufferin Cama Coricidin products Dristan Ecotrin Empirin Excedrin 4-Way Cold Tablets Measurin Midol PAC and PAC Compound Pamprin Pepto-Bismol Phensal Sodium salicylate Sominex Super Anahist Triaminicin Vanquish	Azathioprine (Imuran) Cyclophosphamide (Cytoxan) Mercaptopurine (Purinethol) Procarbazine (Matulane; see Chart 15)	Allopurinol (Zyloprim)	Even though this combination of two interacting drugs may often be prescribed by the physician, it is usually with a decrease in the dosage or strength of the drugs in column 1. This is done to avoid any toxic or adverse side effects.

CHART 18 Injectable drug and anesthetic interactions

Any of these prescription drugs may interact with ➡	any of these prescription drug groups ➡	and result in this interaction.
Heparin sodium	A.S.A. and salicylates Anticoagulants (oral) (Chart 4)	An increase in the anticoagulant effect may occur; patients should be monitored protime. Guaifenesin (Robitussin) and dipyridamole (Persantine) may react with heparin and lead to increased chance of bleeding.
Methotrimeprazine (Levoprome)	Antihypertensives (Chart 11)	An increase in antihypertensive effect resulting in severe hypotension may occur.
	CNS depressants MAO inhibitors (Chart 15)	There is an increase in central nervous system depression and severe and toxic reactions. Avoid MAO inhibitor combination.
	Anticholinergics Succinylcholine chloride (Anectine)	This combination results in decreased blood pressure and effects on the central nervous system from stimulation to delirium. Extrapyramidal symptoms or tachycardia may occur.

Muscle relaxants
  Depolarizing:
    Decamethonium (Syncurine)
    Succinylcholine (Anectine)
  Nondepolarizing:
    Gallamine (Flaxadil)
    Pancuronium (Pavulon)
    (Metubine)
    Tubocurarine
	Anesthetics
	Lithium (Lithane, Eskalith)
	Lidocaine (Mylocaine)
	Clindamycin (Cleocin)
	Lincomycin (Lincocin)
	Quinidine (CinQuin)
	Procainamide (Pronestyl, Procan)
	colymycin-M
	Polymixin B (Aerosporin)
		These combinations result in prolongation in neuromuscular blockade. Respiratory depression or apnea may occur.
		
		Amphotericin B (Fungizone) and aminoglycosides react with muscle relaxants (see below).

Diazoxide (Hyperstat I.V.)	Thiazide diuretics Antidiabetic agents (Chart 3)	Enhanced hyperglycemic effect and hypertension occur. Hyperglycemic effects occur.
	Anticoagulants (Chart 4)	These combinations cause increased anticoagulant effect and possible hemorrhage.
Amphotericin B (Fungizone)	Muscle relaxants (see above) Aminoglycoside (see below) Digitalis (Chart 9)	Increased skeletal muscle effect due to potassium loss occurs. There is an increased possibility of nephrotoxicity. Hypokalemia and increased digitalis toxicity are possible.
	Steroids (Chart 7)	These combinations result in increased potassium loss and possible decrease in infectious resistance, sometimes used together to control drug reaction.

CHART 18 Injectable drug and anesthetic interactions—cont'd

Any of these prescription drugs may interact with	➤ any of these prescription drug groups ➤	and result in this interaction.
Methoxyflurane (Penthrane)	Tetracyclines (Chart 12)	These combinations may cause nephrotoxicity and should be avoided.
Mercaptomerin (Thiomerin)	Digitalis (Chart 9)	These may result in hypokalemia with resultant digitalis toxicity.
Doxorubicin (Adriamycin) Dannorubiecin (Cerubidine)	Cyclophosphamide (Cytoxan)	An increase in cardiotoxicity may occur.
Aminoglycosides Amikacin (Amikin) Gentamicin (Garamycin) ˻Neomycin Kanamycin (Kantrex) Streptomycin Tobramycin (Nebcin)	Anesthetics (see below) Muscle relaxants (see above) Ether Sodium citrate	These combinations result in a possible increase in skeletal muscle response and severe possibility of respiratory paralysis.
	Diuretics Ethacrynic acid (Edecrin) Furosemide (Lasix)	These result in ototoxicity and should be avoided if possible.
	Colistimethate (Coly-Mycin M) Polymixin B (Aerosporin) Viomycin (Viocin) Cephaloridine (Loridine)	There is an increased potential of nephroxicity/neurotoxicity and neuromuscular block with polypeptides. Concurrent use should be avoided if possible. Cephaloridine could increase toxicity when used with diuretics above.
Anesthetics	Metaraminol (Aramine) Epinephrine preparations Dopamine (Intropin)	Ventricular arrhythmias may occur.
	Antihistamines (Chart 2) MAO inhibitors (Chart 15) Methyldopa (Aldomet, Aldoril) *Rauwolfia* alkaloids and reserpine combinations (Chart 11)	Severe increase in hypotension/hypertension and/or central nervous system depression could occur. Physicians should allow 10 to 14 days after discontinuing MAO inhibitors and *Rauwolfia* products before administering anesthetics.
Anesthetics with vasoconstrictor, for example, lidocaine (Xylocaine) with epinephrine	MAO inhibitors (Chart 15) Tricyclic antidepressants (Chart 14) Phenothiazines	Severe hypotension and/or hypertension may occur. Sufficient time should be allowed after discontinuing drugs in column 2 before administering.

DRUG INTERACTION GUIDE

INDEX

A

Acenocoumarol, Charts 2,4,6,10,12
Acetazolamide, Charts 3,7,9,10
Acetohexamide, Charts 3,4
Achromycin V; *see* Tetracycline
Achrostatin V; *see* Tetracycline
Actidil; *see* Triprolidine
Adapin; *see* Doxepin
Adrenalin, Charts 9,10,15; *see also* Epinephrine
Aldactazide; *see* Spironolactone
Aldactone; *see* Spironolactone
Aldomet; *see* Methylopda
Aldoril; *see* Hydrochlorothiazide and Methyldopa
Allopurinol, Charts 4,7
Amitriptyline, Charts 8,13,14,15
Amobarbital, Charts 2,4,7,13
Amoxapine, Charts 8,13,14,15
Amphetamine, Chart 14
Ampicillin, Charts 6,12
Amytal; *see* Amobarbital
Anadrol; *see* Oxymetholone
Analgesics, Chart 16
Anaprox; *see* Naproxyn
Anesthetics, Chart 18
Anisindione, Charts 2,4,6,10,12,16
Antacids, Charts 9,12
Antianxiety medications, Charts 2,13
Antibiotics, Chart 12
Anticoagulants, Chart 4
Anticonvulsants, Charts 2,13
Antidepressants-I, Chart 14
Antidepressants-II, Chart 15
Antidiabetic medications, Charts 3,4
Antihistamines, Charts 2,4,8,13,15
Antihypertensives, Chart 11
Antiparkinson drugs, Chart 5
Antispasmodics, Charts 2,8
Anturane; *see* Sulfinpyrazone
Apresazide; *see* Hydralazine
Apresoline; *see* Hydralazine
Aristocort; *see* Triamcinolone
Artane; *see* Trihexphenidyl
Asendin; *see* Amoxapine
Atarax; *see* Hydroxyzine
Ativan; *see* Lorazepam
Atromid-S; *see* Clofibrate
Atropine products, Charts 2,8
Aventyl; *see* Nortriptyline
Azathioprine, Chart 17

Azatidine, Chart 2
Azene; *see* Clorazepate
Azolid; *see* Phenylbutazone

B

Bactocill, Chart 12
Bananas, Chart 15
Belladonna products, Charts 2,8
Benadryl; *see* Diphenhydramine
Bendopa; *see* Levodopa
Bendroflumethiazide, Charts 3,7,9,10
Benemid; *see* Probenecid
Bentyl; *see* Dicyclomine
Benzedrine; *see* Amphetamine
Benzphetamine, Chart 14
Benzthiazide, Charts 3,7,9,10
Benztropin Mesylate, Charts 2,8
Betamethasone, Chart 7
Bio/DOPA; *see* Levadopa
Bishydroxycoumarin, Charts 2,4
Bontril; *see* Phendimetrazine
Brevicon, Chart 6
Bristacycline; *see* Tetracycline
Brompheniramine, Chart 2
Butabarbital, Charts 4,13
Butazolidin; *see* Phenylbutazone
Butisol; *see* Butabarbital

C

Carbamazepine, Chart 4
Cardrase; *see* Ethoxzolamide
Catapres; *see* Clonidine
Celestone; *see* Betamethasone
Centrax; *see* Prazepam
Cheeses, Chart 15
Chemotherapy, Chart 17
Chlor-Trimeton; *see* Chlorpheniramine
Chloral hydrate, Charts 2,4,7,13
Chlordiazepoxide, Charts 2,13
Chlorpheniramine, Chart 14
Chlorpromazine, Charts 2,5,13
Chlorpropamide, Charts 3,4
Chlorthalidone, Charts 3,7,9,10
Chlorothiazide, Charts 3,7,9,10
Cimetidine, Chart 4
Cin-Quin; *see* Quinidine
Clemastine, Chart 2
Clinoril; *see* Sulindac

O

Optimine; *see* Azatidine
Oral contraceptives, Chart 6
Orinase; *see* Tolbutamide
Ornade, Chart 2
Ortho-Novum, Chart 6
Ovcon, Chart 6
Ovral, Chart 6
Ovulen, Chart 6
Oxacillin, Chart 12
Oxalid; *see* Oxyphenbutazone
Oxazepam, Charts 2,13
Oxybutynin, Charts 2,8
Oxymetholone, Chart 4
Oxyphenbutazone, Charts 2,3,4,6,16

P

Pamelor; *see* Nortriptyline
Panmycin; *see* Tetracycline
Parda; *see* Levodopa
Pargyline, Charts 2,3,5,11,14,15
Parnate; *see* Tranylcypromine
PBZ; *see* Tripelennamine
Pen·Vee K; *see* Penicillin V potassium
Penicillin, Chart 12
Penicillin G potassium, Chart 12
Penicillin V potassium, Chart 12
Pentids; *see* Penicillin G potassium
Pentobarbital, Charts 2,4,7,13
Peritactin; *see* Cyproheptadine
Perphenazine, Charts 2,5,13
Pertofrane; *see* Desipramine
Phendimetrazine, Chart 14
Phenelzine, Charts 2,3,5,11,14,15
Phenergan; *see* Promethazine
Phenindione, Charts 2,4,6,10,12,16
Phenmetrazine, Chart 14
Phenobarbital, Charts 2,4,13
Phenprocoumon, Charts 2,4,6,10,12
Phenteramine, Chart 14
Phenylbutazone, Chart 2,3,4,6,16
Phenylephrine, Chart 15
Phenylpropanolamine, Chart 15
Phenytoin, Charts 2,6,9
Pil-Digis; *see* Digitalis
Piperacetazine, Chart 5
Placidyl; *see* Ethchlorvynol
Plegine; *see* Phendimetrazine
Polaramine; *see* Dexchlorpheniramine
Polycillin; *see* Ampicillin
Polythiazide, Charts 3,7,9,10
Potassium chloride, Chart 9
Prazepam, Charts 2,13
Prazosin, Chart 11
Pre-Sate; *see* Chlorphenteramine
Prednisolone, Chart 7
Prednisone, Chart 7
Preludin; *see* Phenmetrazine
Principen; *see* Ampicillin
ProBanthine; *see* Propantheline
Probenecid, Chart 16
Procarbazine, Charts 2,3,5,11,14,15

Prochlorperazine, Charts 2,5,8,13
Prolixin; *see* Fluphenazine
Promazine, Charts 2,5,13
Promethazine, Chart 2
Propadrine; *see* Phenylpropanolamine
Propantheline, Charts 2,8
Propoxyphene, Chart 2
Propranolol, Charts 3,9,11
Prostaphlin; *see* Oxacillin
Pseudoephedrine, Charts 2,15
Purinethol; *see* Mercaptopurine
Purodigin; *see* Digitoxin
Pyribenzamine, Chart 2
Pyridoxine, Chart 5

Q

QID Tet; *see* Tetracycline
Quide; *see* Piperacetazine
Quinethanzone, Charts 3,7,9,10
Quinidine, Chart 8

R

Regroton; *see* Reserpine
Renese; *see* Polythiazide
Reserpine, Charts 9,11,15
Reserpine combinations, Charts 9,11,15
Rifadin; *see* Rifampin
Rifampin, Charts 4,6
Rimactane; *see* Rifampin
Ritalin; *see* Methylphenidate
Robinul; *see* Glycopyrrolate
Robitet; *see* Tetracycline

S

Salutensin; *see* Reserpine
Sausages, Chart 15
Secobarbital, Charts 2,4,7,13
Seconal; *see* Secobarbital
Sedatives, Charts 2,13
Ser-Ap-Es; *see* Hydrochlorothiazide, Hydralazine, and Reserpine
Serentil; *see* Mesoridazine
Sinemet; *see* Levodopa
Sinequan; *see* Doxepin
Sintrom; *see* Acenocoumarol
6-MP; *see* Mercaptopurine
SK-Tetracycline; *see* Tetracycline
Solution A, Chart 9
Sparine; *see* Promazine
Spironolactone, Chart 10
Stelazine; *see* Trifluoperazine
Steroids, Charts 3,7
Stresstabs 600, Chart 5
Sudafed; *see* Pseudoephedrine
Sulfinpyrazone, Charts 4,16
Sulindac, Chart 16
Sumycin; *see* Tetracycline
Surmontil; *see* Trimipramine
Synkavite; *see* Vitamin K

INDEX

Page numbers in *italics* indicate illustrations.
Page numbers followed by *n* indicate footnotes.
Page numbers followed by *t* indicate tables.

Aliphatic compounds as neuroleptics, 329-330

Aliphatic dimethylamine subgroup of phenothiazine derivatives, side effects and dose equivalents of, 322*t*

Alka-2, dosage of, 500*t*

Alkaline sclerosing of veins from barbiturate abuse, 375

Alkaloids
belladonna, for diarrhea, 523-524
description of, 29-30
ergot, as adrenergic blocking drug, 441-442
opium, causing opiate-like dependence, 367
plant, in cancer chemotherapy, 809

Alkalosis
metabolic, in hypokalemia, 688
respiratory, from salicylates, 187
systemic, from bicarbonate antacids, 501*t*

Alkylating agents in cancer chemotherapy, 808-809

Allergenic extracts, purpose, preparation, storage, and alerts of, 784*t*

Allergens, excretion of, in breast milk, 910*t*

Allergic conditions, agents used in, 487-489

Allergic contact dermatitis; *see* Dermatitis, contact, allergic

Allergic reactions
to antimicrobial agents, 716-717
prevention and treatment of, 746
to calcitonin, 829
common manifestations of, in human, 485*t*
to deferoxamine, 986
to drugs, assessment for, 71
to ergot alkaloids, 892
to eye, steroids for, 551-552
to heparin, 647
to isoniazid, 739
to local anesthetics, 263
to mumps virus vaccine, 776*t*
to nicotinyl tartrate, 628
to opiates, 148
to oxytocin, 891
to PAS, 740
to penicillins, 720-721
to phenothiazines, 325-326
to progesterone, 880
to tetanus immune globulin, human, 782*t*
to tetracyclines, 731
to thiazide-type diuretics, 667
to tricyclic antidepressants, 341
to vaccine protein from, rabies vaccine, duck embryo vaccine, 783*t*
to vitamin B₁₂, 641

Allergic skin reactions to influenza virus vaccine, 778*t*

Allergy(ies)
associated with histamine, 484
drug, 56

Allopurinol
for gout, 205-206
interaction of
with azathioprine with, 204
probenecid, 207

Almonds, bitter, toxins causing, 971*t*

Aloe, excretion of, in breast milk, 908*t*

Alopecia
abused drugs causing, 367
from azathioprine, 203
from chloroquine phosphate, 202
from cimetidine, 504
from clofibrate, 598
drugs causing, 938
from heparin, 647
from tricyclic antidepressants, 341
from valproic acid, 220

Alpha blocking agents, 440-442

Alpha Chymar; *see* Alpha-chymotrypsin

Alpha-chymotrypsin in cataract extraction, 554

Alphadrol; *see* Fluprednisolone

Alseroxylon for hypertension, 612

AlternaGEL
acid-neutralizing capacity of, 498*t*
dosage of, 500*t*

Alu-Cap, dosage of, 500*t*

Aludrox, acid-neutralizing capacity of, 498*t*

Aludrox suspension, sodium content of, 501*t*

Aludrox tablets, sodium content of, 501*t*

Aluminum acetate solution in dermatologic preparations, 943

Aluminum carbonate gel, basic, as antacid, dosage of, 500*t*

Aluminum hydroxide for diarrhea, 522

Aluminum hydroxide gel as antacid, dosage of, 500*t*

Aluminum phosphate gel as antacid, dosage of, 500*t*

Aluminum subacetate solution in dermatologic preparations, 943

Alupent; *see* Metaproterenol sulfate

Alurate; *see* Aprobarbital

Alu-Tab, dosage of, 500*t*

Alu-Tabs, sodium content of, 501*t*

A.M.A. Drug Evaluations, 77

Amantadine hydrochloride
excretion of, in breast milk, 903*t*
for parkinsonism, 290-291
for viral infections, 744

Ambilhar; *see* Niridazole

Amblyopia
in chronic alcoholism, 182
toxic
from ethchlorvynol abuse, 376
from ibuprofen, 194

Amcill; *see* Ampicillin

Amcill-S; *see* Ampicillin sodium

Amebiasis
chemotherapy of, 793
drugs for, 788*t*
general treatment of, 795*t*

Amebic meningoencephalitis, primary, drugs for, 788*t*

Amebicides
chemotherapy of, 793-795
classification of, 794

Amenorrhea from tricyclic antidepressants, 138

Americaine; *see* Benzocaine

American cutaneous leishmaniasis; *see* *Leishmania mexicana*

American Hospital Formulary Service, 77

American Journal of Nursing, 77

American mucocutaneous leishmaniasis; *see* *Leishmania braziliensis*

Amethocaine hydrochloride for local anesthesia, 260

Amethopterin; *see* Methotrexate

Amicar; *see* Aminocaproic acid

Amides for local anesthesia, 256

Amigen; *see* Protein hydrolysate injection

Amikacin, 729

Amikacin sulfate, routes of administration of, 727*t*

Amikin; *see* Amikacin

Amiloride as distal tubule diuretic, 671

Amino acid solution for parenteral nutrition, 684-685

Amino acids in parenteral nutrition, 682

Aminocaproic acid as antifibrinolytic drug, 652

Aminoglutethimide, 853-854

Aminoglycosides, 727-730
actions of, 727
drug interactions with, 746*t*
interactions of, with nondepolarizing neuromuscular blocking drugs, 278*t*
nursing implications of, 729-730
pharmacokinetics of, 727
results of, 727
routes of administration of, 727*t*
side effects and toxic effects of, 727-728

Aminophylline
for angina, 596
as bronchodilator, 465

Aminopyrine, interaction of phenylbutazone with, 200

Aminosalicylic acid for tuberculosis, 740
route of administration of, 739*t*

Aminosyn; *see* Amino acid solution

Amitone, dosage of, 500*t*

Amitriptyline hydrochloride
as antidepressant, 344
comparison of, with other tricyclic antidepressants, 340*t*
effect of, on sexual behavior, 919*t*
excretion of, in breast milk, 906*t*
interaction of, with pargyline, 620
poisoning from, symptoms and treatment of, 981*t*
toxidromes suggesting, 969*t*

Ammonia as reflex respiratory stimulant, 474

Ammoniated mercury ointment for infectious diseases, 757

Ammoniated mercury ophthalmic ointment for infectious diseases, 756

Ammonium carbonate as bronchomucotropic drug, 458

Ammonium chloride, 672-673
as bronchomucotropic drug, 458

Ammonium chloride injection for replacement therapy, 678-679

Amnesia
in hypercalcemia, 692
obstetric
barbiturates for, 170
meperidine for, 151
retrograde, from ethchlorvynol withdrawal, 376

Amobarbital
as anticonvulsant, parenteral use of, 211*t*
dosage, administration, and length of action of, 170
plasma half-life values for, 168*t*
poisoning from, symptoms and treatment of, 979*t*

Amodiaquine hydrochloride as antimalarial drug, 791-792

Amoxapine
as antidepressant, 346
comparison of, with other tricyclic antidepressants, 340*t*

Amoxicillin, 722

Amoxicillin trihydrate, route of administration of, 720*t*

Amoxil; *see* Amoxicillin trihydrate

Amphetamine phosphate for severe alcoholic intoxication, 181

Amphetamine sulfate, 225

Amphetamines
abuse of, 361, 382-384
acute intoxication of, signs and symptoms of, 365
as anorexigenic, 225
as central nervous system stimulants, 224-226
effect of, on sexual behavior, 919*t*
illicit drug adulterants of, 365
interaction of, with bicarbonate antacids, 501*t*
poisoning from, symptoms and treatment of, 978*t*
as psychostimulants, 336-337
street names for, 382
toxidromes suggesting, 969*t*
types of, 382

Amphojel
acid-neutralizing capacity of, 498*t*
dosage of, 500*t*

Amphojel suspension, sodium content of, 501*t*

Amphotericin B
drug interactions with, 747*t*

Cefadyl; *see* Cephapirin
Cefamandole, 724
Cefazolin, 724
Cefotaxime sodium, 724
Cefoxitin, 724
Celbenin; *see* Methicillin sodium
Celestone; *see* Betamethasone
Cells, goblet, 450
Cellulitis
    from diazoxide, 617
    in opiate toxicity, 368
Celontin; *see* Methsuximide
Celospor; *see* Cephacetrile
Central and peripheral sympathetic inhibitor
        drugs for hypertension, 611-613
Central nervous sympathomimetics, abuse of,
        382-384
Central nervous system (CNS)
    components of, 135, 136-139
    depressants of, 142-185
        alcohols as, 178-185; *see also* Alcohol(s)
        analgesics as, 142-162; *see also* Analge-
            sic(s)
        contraindications to, 166
        hypnotics as, 162-185; *see also* Hypnot-
            ics
        interaction of
            with barbiturates, 167*t*
            with benzodiazepines, 313
            with diphenhydramine, 289
            with diphenoxylate, 525
            with droperidol, 249
            with fentanyl, 249
            with opiates, 524
            with valproic acid, 221
        sedatives as, 162-185; *see also* Sedatives
    depression of
        from cocaine, 261
        from fenfluramine, 228
        from local anesthetics, 263
        from loperamide overdose, 526
        from phenytoin, 214
    drug actions on, 135-142
    drugs affecting, 135-230
        excretion of, in breast milk, 905*t*
    effects of dantrolene on, 276
    effects of lidocaine on, 587
    effects of monoamine oxidase inhibitors on,
        348
    effects of oral contraceptives on, 886
    effects of propranolol on, 590
    effects of thyroid hormones on, 832
    emotions and, 302-304
    excitation of, from penicillins, 720
    functions of, 135-136, 405
    in hypercalcemia, 692
    stimulants of, 222-228
        amphetamines as, 224-226
        analeptics as, 222-227
        anorexiants as, 227-228
        nonamphetamine, 226-227
        for nonpsychotic mental disorders, 354-
            355
        xanthines as, 222-224
    stimulation of, from acetaminophen over-
        dose, 162
    synaptic transmission in, 139-142
    toxic effects of lithium on, 353*t*
    toxic effects of local anesthetics on, 263
Central sympathetic inhibitor drugs for hy-
        pertension, 608-611
Centrax; *see* Prazepam
Cēpacol mouthwash, 496
Cephacetrile, 724
Cephalexin, 724
    excretion of, in breast milk, 903*t*
Cephaloglycin, 724
Cephaloridine, 724
Cephalosporins, 723-725
    drug interactions with, 747*t*
    interactions of probenecid with, 207
    nursing implications of, 725

Cephalosporins—cont'd
    oral, 724-725
    parenteral, 723-724
        and oral, 725
    side effects and toxic effects of, 723
Cephalothin sodium, 723-724
    excretion of, in breast milk, 903*t*
Cephapirin, 724
Cephradine, 725
Cerebellum
    anatomy and physiology of, 138
    functions of, behavioral-emotional, 302
Cerebral arterial disease, atherosclerosis and,
        597
Cerebral cortex; *see* Cortex, cerebral
Cerebral excitement from trihexyphenidyl
        overdose, 288
Cerebral hemorrhage from oxytocin, 891
Cerebral medulla, effects of caffeine on, 223
Cerebral palsy, spasticity of
    benzodiazepines for, 311
    dantrolene for, 275
Cerebral spasticity, 269
Cerebrospinal nervous system; *see* Central
        nervous system (CNS)
Cerebrovascular accident, spasticity follow-
        ing, benzodiazepines for, 311
Cerebrovascular disease, antiinflammatory
        agents for, 185
Cerebrum
    effects of morphine and opium on, 144-
        145
    functions of, behavioral-emotional, 302
Cestode infections, drugs for, 801
Cetylpyridinium chloride for infectious dis-
        eases, 762
Chagas' disease; *see* Trypanosoma cruzi
Chalazion, definition of, 547
Chancroid, sulfonamides for, 735
Chancroid infection, tetracyclines for, 730
Charcoal, activated, for diarrhea, 522, 523
Charcocaps; *see* Charcoal, activated
Cheilosis in riboflavin deficiency, 702
Chel-Iron; *see* Ferrocholinate
Chemical assay, definition of, 9, 24
Chemical name of drug, 28, 41
Chemical teratogenesis, 896-897
Chemotherapy
    antineoplastic; *see also* Antineoplastic
        agents
        combination, 815
        drug administration in, double-syringe
            technique for, 817
        nursing implications in, 815-817
    definition of, 3
    of parasitic diseases, 787-803
Chenodeoxycholic acid as digestant, 506
Chest
    constricting sensation in
        from benzonatate, 475
        from dextran 40, 658
        from dimercaprol, 985
    dermatologic conditions of, 933
    pain in
        from alcohol abuse, 380
        constricting, from monoamine oxidase
            inhibitors, 348
        from ergot alkaloids, 892
        from mannitol, 672
        from metolazone, 668
Children
    administration of drugs to, 108-115
        intramuscular, 111-112
        intravenous, 113-114
        oral, 110-111
        rectal, 112
    drug actions in, 54
    drug dosage for, conditions influencing,
        114
    eardrop instillation in, 113
    eyedrop instillation in, 113
Chilling from benzonatate, 475

Chills
    from acetaminophen overdose, 162
    from amphotericin B, 742
    from anxiolytics, 309
    from dantrolene, 276
    from droperidol, 248
    from glutethimide abuse, 376
    in heroin withdrawal, 369
    from hespan, 658
    from hydralazine hydrochloride, 616
    from mannitol, 672
    from metolazone, 668
    in pyrogenic reaction to intravenous infu-
        sion, 687
    shaking, from calcium disodium edetate,
        987
Chlophedianol hydrochloride as cough sup-
        pressant, 476
Chlor-Trimeton; *see* Chlorpheniramine
Chloral hydrate
    abuse of, 373
    excretion of, in breast milk, 906*t*
    interaction of, with coumarin drugs, 167
    poisons from, symptoms and treatment of,
        981*t*
    as sedative-hypnotic, 175-176
Chloramine-T for infectious diseases, 759
Chloramines for infectious diseases, 758-759
Chloramphenicol, 732
    drug interactions with, 747*t*
    excretion of, in breast milk, 903*t*
    interaction of
        with barbiturates, 167*t*
        with oral hypoglycemics, 865
    for ocular infections, 547-548
Chloraseptic mouthwash, 496
Chlorcyclizine hydrochloride for allergic con-
        dition, 488
Chlordiazepoxide hydrochloride
    abuse of, 381
    for alcohol withdrawal, 311-312
    as anxiolytic, 314-315
        side effects of, 309*t*
    effect of, on sexual behavior, 919*t*
    excretion of, in breast milk, 906*t*
    interaction of disulfiram with, 184
    for labor and delivery, 312
    poisoning from, symptoms and treatment
        of, 981*t*
Chlorhexidine gluconate for infectious dis-
        eases, 761
Chloride, interaction of, with sutilains, 960
Chlorine for infectious diseases, 758
Chlormadione, excretion of, in breast milk,
        908*t*
Chloroform
    excretion of, in breast milk, 906*t*
    for general anesthesia
        history of, 235
        properties of, 239*t*
    interactions of, with catecholamines, 428
Chloromycetin; *see* Chloramphenicol
P-Chlorophenylalanine (PCPA), effect of, on
        sexual behavior, 917, 919*t*
Chlorophyll complex perles for hemostasis,
        654
Chloroprocaine hydrochloride for local anes-
        thesia, 258
Chloroptic; *see* Chloramphenicol
Chloroquine, excretion of, in breast milk,
        903*t*
Chloroquine hydrochloride as antimalarial
        drug, 791
Chloroquine phosphate
    as anthelmintic drug, 801
    as antimalarial drug, 791
    for rheumatoid arthritis, 201-202
Chlorosis as iron-deficiency condition, 638
Chlorothiazide for hypertension, 621-622
Chlorotrianisense
    excretion of, in breast milk, 909*t*
    as synthetic estrogen, 878-879

Desyrl - antidepressant for elderly w cardiov & dvasc mean
(Trazodone)

Diethyl ether; *see* Ether
Diethylcarbamazine citrate for nematode infections, 800
Diethylpropion hydrochloride
  as anorexiant, 227-228
  for obesity management, 382
Diethylstilbestrol (DES) as synthetic estrogen, 878
Diethylstilbestrol dipropionate as synthetic estrogen, 878
Diffusion in passive transport, 45
Di-Gel, acid-neutralizing capacity of, 498t
Digestants, 505-506
Digilanid, 573
Digitaline Nativelle; *see* Digitoxin
Digitalis, 567-576
  actions of, 568-569
  administration of, 571
    intravenous, digitalis toxicity due to, 575
  for atrial fibrillation, 570
  chemical composition of, 567-568
  for congestive heart failure, 567, 570
  contraindications to, 575
  dosages of, 571-572, 574t
  increased sensitivity to, in hypokalemia, 688
  interaction of
    with antacids, 502
    with bretylium, 591
    with bulk-forming laxatives, 517
    with calcium antacids, 501t
    with catecholamines, 428
    with dobutamine, 433
    with heparin, 647
  intoxication from, treatment of, 575
  introduction of, in eighteenth century, 4
  in myocardial contraction, 562
  pharmacokinetics of, 569-570
  powdered, 572
    administration and dosage of, 574t
  precautions with, 575
  preparations of, 571-573
    choice of, 571-572
    nursing implications for, 575-576
    purple foxglove, 572-573
    standardization of, 571
    white foxglove, 573
  results of, 568-569
  side effects and toxic effects of, 574-575
  toxicity of
    lidocaine for, 586
    predisposing factors to, 574-575
  uses of, 570-571
    prophylactic, 570-571
  ventricular dysrhythmias from, phenytoin for, 588
Digitalis glycoside, interaction of, with adrenal corticosteroids, 842
Digitalis tincture, 572
  administration and dosage of, 574t
Digitalization
  and choice of preparations, 571-572
  rapid, digitalis toxicity due to, 575
Digitoxin
  administration and dosage of, 574t
  effects of, on fetus and newborn, 899t
  interaction of barbiturates with, 167t
  preparation, dosage, and administration of, 572-573
Digoxin, 573
  administration and dosage of, 574t
  interaction of adsorbents with, 522
Dihydrocodeinone bitartrate, 149-150
  as cough suppressant, 475
Dihydroergocornine dihydroergocristine dihydroergokryptine mesylate as adrenergic blocking drug, 442
Dihydroindolone, derivatives of, as neuroleptic, 335
Dihydromorphinone as cough suppressant, 475

Dihydrotachysterol, 828
  excretion of, in breast milk, 909t
  for hypocalcemia, 691
Dihydroxyaluminum aminoacetate as antacid, 500t
1,25-Dihydroxycholecalciferol; *see* Calcitriol
Diiodohydroxyquin for amebicides, 794
Diisopropyl fluorophosphate; *see* Isofluorophate
Dilantin; *see* Phenytoin
Dilator muscle of eye, anatomy and physiology of, 533-534
Dilaudid; *see* Hydromorphone hydrochloride
Diloxanide-furoate for amebicides, 794
Diluents of respiratory secretions, 456
Diluted sodium hypochlorite solution for infectious diseases, 758
Diluting segment diuretics, 666-668
Dimenhydrinate
  as antiemetic, 506
  for motion sickness, 490
Dimercaprol for specific drugs and poisons, 985
Dimetane; *see* Brompheniramine maleate
Dimethisoquin hydrochloride for topical anesthesia, 262
Dimethyl polysiloxane; *see* Silicone fluid
Dindevan; *see* Phenindione
Dinoprost tromethamine to increase uterine motility, 893
Dioctyl calcium sulfosuccinate; *see* Calcium docusate
Dioctyl sodium sulfosuccinate; *see* Sodium docusate
Diothane; *see* Diperodon
Di-Paralene; *see* Chlorcyclizine hydrochloride
Dipaxin; *see* Diphenadione
Diperodon for topical anesthesia, 262
Diphenadione as anticoagulant drug, 650
Diphenhydramine hydrochloride
  for allergic conditions, 488
  for colds, 477
  effect of, on sexual behavior, 919t
  excretion of, in breast milk, 903t, 906t
  for parkinsonism, 289
Diphenidol hydrochloride as antiemetic, 506-507
Diphenoxylate hydrochloride for diarrhea, 525-526
Diphenylhydantoin; *see* Phenytoin sodium
Diphtheria, erythromycin for, 726
Diphtheria and tetanus toxoids, and pertussis vaccine, adsorbed, purpose, preparation, storage, and alerts of, 781t
Diptheria antibodies, excretion of, in breast milk, 910t
Diphyllobothrium latum, drugs for, 799t
Dipivefrin hydrochloride for glaucoma, 539-540
Diplopia
  from carisoprodol, 271
  from ethchlorvynol abuse, 376
  in hypocalcemia, 690
  from pralidoxime, 989
  from sulindac, 199
Dipyridamole
  for angina, administration, dosage, and action of, 595t
  as antiplatelet drug, 651
  for arterial thrombi, 643
Dipyrone, interaction of phenylbutazone with, 200
Direct-acting cholinergic drugs, 416-417
Direct respiratory stimulants, 473-474
  functions of, 478-479
Disalcid; *see* Salsalate
Disc, slipped, diazepam for, 311
Discoloration of skin, abused drugs causing, 367
Disinfectant(s), 751-753
  mechanisms of action of, 752

Disinfectant(s)—cont'd
  oral, sodium perborate solution as, 496-497
  organism sensitivity to, 752
Disinhibition
  from barbiturate abuse, 374
  from ethyl alcohol abuse, 374
  from phenobarbital abuse, 375
Disintegration of drugs, drug actions and, 44
Disipal; *see* Orphenadrine hydrochloride
Disodium cromglycate; *see* Cromolyn sodium
Disodium edetate for hypercalcemia, 692
Disopyramide phosphate for cardiac dysrhythmias, 584-585
Disorientation
  from diphenidol, 507
  from flurazepam, 317
  in hypercalcemia, 692
  in hypomagnesemia, 693
  from lidocaine, 587
  from mannitol, 542
  from marijuana abuse, 387
  from tricyclic antidepressants, 339
Disseminated BCG infection from Bacillus Calmette-Guérin vaccine, 779t
Dissociative anesthesia, 247
Distal convoluted tubule, effect of diuretics on, 664
Distal tubule diuretics, 670-671
Distention
  from chlorothiazide, 622
  from cyclopropane, 242
Distortions, perceptual, from ethchlorvynol withdrawal, 376
Disulfiram for chronic alcoholism, 182, 184-185, 380
Diuresis
  from bromocriptine, 294
  from carbonic anhydrase inhibitors, 541
  from desmopressin acetate, 827
  hypomagnesemia due to, 693
  in poison treatment, 977
  from urea, 543
Diuretic effects of oral hypoglycemics, 864
Diuretics, 662-674
  classification of, 664-671
  diluting segment, 666-668
  distal tubule, 670-671
  effects of
    on fetus and newborn, 899t
    on tubular function in nephron, 663-664
  hypercalcemia from, 692
  for hypertension, 621-622
  interactions of, with catecholamines, 428
  loop, 668-670
  mercurial, 669-670
  osmotic 671-672
  proximal tubule, 665-666
  thiazide; *see* Thiazide diuretics
  use of, 662
  water as, 672
  xanthine, 672
Diuril; *see* Chlorothiazide
Dizziness
  from albuterol, 464
  from anticholinergics, 287, 524
  from anxiolytics, 309
  from baclofen, 270
  from bretylium, 591
  from bromocriptine, 294
  from carbamazepine, 221
  from central skeletal muscle relaxants, 269-270
  from chlorphenesin carbamate, 271
  from cimetidine, 492, 504
  from cyclandelate, 628
  from cyclobenzaprine hydrochloride, 273
  from dantrolene, 276
  from diphenidol, 507
  from diphenoxylate, 526

Drug(s)—cont'd
cardiovascular, excretion of, in breast milk, 905t
causing acneform reaction, 938
causing alopecia, 938
causing contact dermatitis, 939-940
causing fixed eruptions, 939
causing lichenoid reactions, 938
causing morbilliform reactions, 938
causing urticaria, 938
for cestode infections, 801
characterization of, 28-42
cholinergic; see Cholinergic drugs
cholinergic blocking; see Cholinergic blocking drugs
classification of, 30-31
clinical experience with, value of, 6
coloring substances for, 37
concentrations of
effect of, on drug absorption, 47-48
minimum effective, 53
contraindications to, assessment for, 71
control of, international, 20
controlled, regulation of, by Canadian Food and Drugs Act, 17
corticosteroid; see Corticosteroids
craving for, in heroin withdrawal, 369
cumulation of, 57
data on
in assessment, 67-70
exploring, 77-78
definition of, 3
delivery systems for, 37, 40t, 42
dependence on, 57
for dermatology, 929
designated, regulation of, by Canadian Food and Drugs Act, 17-18
development of, 11-13, 24-25
dispensing systems for, 83-86
floor stock, 83
individual order, 83
unit dose, 83-85
distribution of, 48-49
barriers to, 48-49
in pediatric patients, 114-115
dosage of; see Dosage of drugs
dosage forms of, 33-36
effectiveness ratings for, 14-15
effects of
evaluation of, 117-119
on mind, 124
primary, 70-71
on respiratory center, 468-473
toxic, 70-71; see also Toxicity
evaluation of, 11-13, 24-25
excretion of, 50-51
fantasies about, 122-123
flavoring agents for, 496
half-life of, biologic, 51
for helminthiasis, 799t
hematologic, 633-660
idiosyncratic reactions to, 56-57
incompatibilities of, 75-76t, 76-77
infertility, 888-889
information references on, 77-78
interactions of, 57, 71-77; see also specific drug
with alcohol, 73-74
with cigarette smoking, 74
enzyme alterations and, 73-74
with foods, 72-73
with other drugs, 72
intramuscularly injectable, compatibility of, 75-76t
intravenous infusion of, 107
legend, definition and control of, 14
legislation on, 13-20
in Canada, 16-20, 25-26
in United States, 13-16, 25t
liability for, 16
malabsorption of, food-induced, 72-73
measurement systems for, 90-92

Drug(s)—cont'd
metabolism of, 49-50
drug interactions and, 72
misuse of, definition of, 359
for motion sickness, 489-490
mucosal constrictor, 476-477
for myasthenia gravis, 417-418
names of, 28-29, 41
for nematode infection, 798-800
nursing responsibilities related to, 5-6
orders for; see Orders for drugs
parasympatholytic; see Cholinergic blocking drugs
parasympathomimetic, 415-416
use of, 414-415
peripheral vascular, 605-630
antihypertensives as, 606-627; see also Antihypertensive drugs
antihypotensives as, 627-628
peripheral vasodilators as, 628-629
pharmaceutical preparations of, 31-37, 38-40t, 41-42
pharmacologic types of, causing opiate-like dependence, 367
physical dependence on, definition of, 362
plant, active constituents of, 29-30
plasma binding of, drug distribution and, 48
prescribing of, by nurses, legislation on, 21
presence of, in milk, 901-902
proprietary, control of, 129-130
psychic dependence on, definition of, 362
psychoactive, effect of, on sexual behavior, 919t
receptor sites for, actions at, drug interactions and, 72
regimens for, common, 816t
restricted, regulation of, by Canadian Food and Drugs Act, 18
self-administration of, 124-130; see also Self-medication
for sexually transmitted diseases, 918, 921
solubility of, effect of, on drug absorption, 46
solutions of, 31-33, 38t, 41
sources of, 29-30, 41
stability of, 37, 40-41
standards for, 9-11, 24-25
storage of, 37, 40-41, 85-86
storage reservoirs for, drug distribution and, 48
summation of effects of, 57
surface-active, for respiratory system, 456
suspensions of, 31-32, 38t, 41
symbolic meaning of, 122-124
sympatholytic, use of, 415
sympathomimetic; see Adrenergic drugs
synergism of, 57
tachyphylaxis from, 57
teaching patients about, 117
teratogenic effects of, 49
therapy with; see Pharmacotherapeutics
thrombolytic; see Thrombolytic drugs
tolerance to, 57
for toxemia of pregnancy, 894-895
toxic effects of, 70-71
transport of
active, 45
passive, 45
for trematode infections, 800
uses of, 5
Drug Efficacy Study Implementation (DESI), 14-15
Drug enzyme interaction theory of drug action, 52
Drug fever
from gold compounds, 201
from propylthiouracil, 840
Drug information centers as information sources, 78

Drugs of Choice, 78
Dryvax; *see* Smallpox vaccine
Duct, collecting, effect of diuretics on, 664
Durabolin; *see* Nandrolone phenpropionate
Duranest; *see* Etidocaine
Durham-Humphrey Amendment to Food and Drug Act, 14, 25t
Duricef; *see* Cefadroxil
Dyclone; *see* Dyclonine hydrochloride
Dyclonine hydrochloride for topical anesthesia, 262
Dyes for infectious diseases, 755
Dymelor; *see* Acetohexamide
Dynapen; *see* Dicloxacillin sodium
Dynorphin in central nervous system, 142
Dyrenium; *see* Triamterene
Dysarthria from benzodiazepines, 313
Dyscrasias, blood; *see* Blood, dyscrasias of
Dyskinesia
from levodopa-carbidopa combination, 293
from phenothiazines, 326-327
tardive, persistent, from phenothiazines, 327-328
Dysmenorrhea
acetaminophen for, 161
antiinflammatory agents for, 185
naproxen sodium for, 195-196
Dyspepsia from zomepirac, 192
Dysphagia
abused drugs causing, 366
from allergenic extracts, 784t
from dantrolene, 276
from glutethimide abuse, 376
from metoclopramide, 528
from molindone, 335
Dyspnea
in congestive heart failure from quinidine overdose, 582
in disulfiram reaction, 184
from dobutamine hydrochloride, 433, 628
from doxapram, 473
from epinephrine, 459
from ergot alkaloids, 892
from histamine, 486
in hypocalcemia, 690
in methyl alcohol poisoning, 183
in thiamine deficiency, 700
from thyroid overdose, 834
Dysrhythmias, cardiac
abused drugs causing, 366
automaticity disturbance causing, 576
conductivity disturbance causing, 576-579
from cyclopropane, 242
from digitalis toxicity, 574
from dipivefrin, 540
from dobutamide, 628
from doxapram, 473
drugs for, 576-592
classification of, 577-579
group I-A, 579-585
group I-B, 585-588
group II, 588-590
group III, 590-591
group IV, 591-592
from edrophonium, 286
heart block causing, 577
in hypervitaminosis D, 699
from levodopa, 292
from lithium, 353t
from local anesthetics, 263
from methylphenidate, 227, 354, 355
in opiate toxicity, 368
from oxytocin, 891
from phenylbutazone, 200
from propoxyphene overdose, 160, 373
reentry phenomenon causing, 577, 578t
from succinylcholine, 283
from thyroid overdose, 834
from tricyclic antidepressants, 339, 342
Dystonia(s)
from metoclopramide, 528, 529

Neo-calglucon = CA⁺⁺ Supplement *(handwritten annotation)*